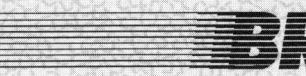

ESSENTIALS OF
Paramedic Care

Workbook
SECOND EDITION

Robert S. Porter

BRYAN E. BLEDSOE, DO, FACEP, EMT-P
Adjunct Associate Professor of Emergency Medicine
The George Washington University Medical Center
Washington, DC
and
Emergency Physician
Midlothian, Texas

ROBERT S. PORTER, MA, NREMT-P
Senior Advanced Life Support Educator
Madison County Emergency Medical Services
Canastota, New York
and
Flight Paramedic
AirOne, Onondaga County Sheriff's Department
Syracuse, New York

RICHARD A. CHERRY, MS, NREMT-P
Clinical Assistant Professor of Emergency Medicine
Technical Director for Medical Simulation
Upstate Medical University
Syracuse, New York

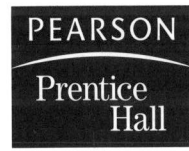

Upper Saddle River, New Jersey 07458

Publisher: Julie Levin Alexander
Publisher's Assistant: Regina Bruno
Executive Editor: Marlene McHugh Pratt
Senior Managing Editor for Development: Lois Berlowitz
Project Development: Triple SSS Press Media Development
Assistant Editor: Matthew Sirinides
Director of Marketing: Karen Allman
Executive Marketing Manager: Katrin Beacom
Marketing Coordinator: Michael Sirinides
Director of Production and Manufacturing: Bruce Johnson
Managing Editor for Production: Patrick Walsh
Production Liaison: Faye Gemmellaro
Production Editor: Heather Willison/Carlisle Publishing Services
Manufacturing Manager: Ilene Sanford
Manufacturing Buyer: Pat Brown
Senior Design Coordinator: Cheryl Asherman
Cover Design: Blair Brown
Cover Photography: Eddie Sperling
Composition: Carlisle Publishing Services
Printing and Binding: Banta Harrisonburg
Cover Printer: Phoenix Color

Studentaid.ed.gov, the U.S. Department of Education's Website on college planning assistance, is a valuable tool for anyone intending to pursue higher education. Designed to help students at all stages of schooling, including international students, returning students, and parents, it is a guide to the financial aid process. This Website presents information on applying to and attending college, as well as on funding your education and repaying loans. It also provides links to useful resources, such as state education agency contact information, assistance in filling out financial aid forms, and in introduction to various forms of student aid.

NOTICE ON CARE PROCEDURES

It is the intent of the authors and publisher that this Workbook be used as part of a formal EMT-Paramedic program taught by qualified instructors and supervised by a licensed physician. The procedures described in the Workbook are based upon consultation with EMT and medical authorities. The authors and publisher have taken care to make certain that these procedures reflect currently accepted clinical practice; however, they cannot be considered absolute recommendations.

The material in this Workbook contains the most current information available at the time of publication. However, federal, state, and local guidelines concerning clinical practices, including, without limitation, those governing infection control and universal precautions, change rapidly. The reader should note, therefore, that the new regulations may require changes in some procedures.

It is the responsibility of the reader to familiarize himself or herself with the policies and procedures set by federal, state, and local agencies as well as the institution or agency where the reader is employed. The authors and the publisher of this Workbook disclaim any liability, loss, or risk resulting directly or indirectly from the suggested procedures and theory, from any undetected errors, or from the reader's misunderstanding of the text. It is the reader's responsibility to stay informed of any new changes or recommendations made by any federal, state, and local agency as well as by his or her employing institution or agency.

NOTICE ON CPR AND ECC

The national standards for Cardiopulmonary Resuscitation (CPR) and Emergency Cardiovascular Care (ECC) are reviewed and revised on a regular basis and may change slightly after this manual is printed. It is important that you know the most current procedures for CPR and ECC, both for the classroom and your patients. The most current information may be obtained from the appropriate credentialing agency.

Copyright © 2007 by Pearson Education, Inc., Upper Saddle River, New Jersey 07458. Pearson Prentice Hall. All rights reserved. Printed in the United States of America. The publication is protected and Copyright and permission should be obtained from the publisher prior to any prohibited reproduction, storage in a retrieval system, or transmission in any form or by any means, electronic, mechanical, photocopying, recording, or likewise. For information regarding permission(s), write to: Rights and Permissions Department.

Pearson Prentice Hall™ is a trademark of Pearson Education, Inc.
Pearson® is a registered trademark of Pearson plc.
Prentice Hall® is a registered trademark of Pearson Education, Inc.

Pearson Education Ltd.
Pearson Education Singapore, Pte. Ltd.
Pearson Education Canada, Ltd.
Pearson Education—Japan
Pearson Education Australia PTY, Limited

Pearson Education North Asia Ltd.
Pearson Educación de Mexico, S.A. de C.V.
Pearson Education Malaysia, Pte. Ltd.
Pearson Education, Upper Saddle River. NJ

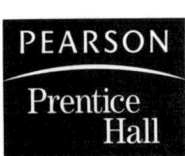

10 9 8 7 6 5 4
ISBN 0-13-171164-4

Dedication

To Kris and sailing: Pleasant distractions from writing about and practicing prehospital emergency medicine.

CONTENTS
Self-Instructional Workbook
Essentials of Paramedic Care
SECOND EDITION

Introduction to the Self-Instructional Workbook ix
How to Use the Self-Instructional Workbook xi
Guidelines to Better Test-Taking xiii

DIVISION 1: Introduction to Advanced Prehospital Care 1

CHAPTER 1 Introduction to Advanced Prehospital Care 3
Part 1: Introduction to Advanced Prehospital Care 3
Part 2: EMS Systems 5
Part 3: Roles and Responsibilities of the Paramedic 13
Part 4: The Well-Being of the Paramedic 18
Part 5: Illness and Injury Prevention 28
Part 6: Ethics in Advanced Prehospital Care 31

CHAPTER 2 Medical/Legal Aspects of Advanced Prehospital Care 35

CHAPTER 3 Anatomy and Physiology 45
Part 1: The Cell and the Cellular Environment 45
Part 2: Body Systems 50

CHAPTER 4 General Principles of Pathophysiology 77
Part 1: How Normal Body Processes Are Altered by Disease and Injury 77
Part 2: The Body's Defenses against Disease and Injury 84

CHAPTER 5 Life-Span Development 93

CHAPTER 6 General Principles of Pharmacology 99
Part 1: Basic Pharmacology 99
Part 2: Drug Classifications 109

CHAPTER 7 Intravenous Access and Medication Administration 127
Part 1: Principles and Routes of Medication Administration 127
Part 2: Intravenous Access, Blood Sampling, and Intraosseous Infusion 137
Part 3: Medical Mathematics 144

CHAPTER 8 Airway Management and Ventilation 147

CHAPTER 9 Therapeutic Communications 161

v

DIVISION 2: Patient Assessment	**167**
CHAPTER 10 History Taking	169
CHAPTER 11 Physical Exam Techniques	175
CHAPTER 12 Patient Assessment in the Field	195
CHAPTER 13 Clinical Decision Making	211
CHAPTER 14 Communications	217
CHAPTER 15 Documentation	225

DIVISION 3: Trauma Emergencies	**233**
CHAPTER 16 Trauma and Trauma Systems	235
CHAPTER 17 Blunt Trauma	239
CHAPTER 18 Penetrating Trauma	247
CHAPTER 19 Hemorrhage and Shock	253
CHAPTER 20 Soft-Tissue Trauma	263
CHAPTER 21 Burns	277
CHAPTER 22 Musculoskeletal Trauma	289
CHAPTER 23 Head, Facial, and Neck Trauma	301
CHAPTER 24 Spinal Trauma	315
CHAPTER 25 Thoracic Trauma	323
CHAPTER 26 Abdominal Trauma	333

DIVISION 4: Medical Emergencies	**341**
CHAPTER 27 Pulmonology	343
CHAPTER 28 Cardiology	355
Part 1: Cardiovascular Anatomy and Physiology, ECG Monitoring, and Dysrhythmia Analysis	355
Part 2: Assessment and Management of the Cardiovascular Patient	391
CHAPTER 29 Neurology	419
CHAPTER 30 Endocrinology	437
CHAPTER 31 Allergies and Anaphylaxis	447
CHAPTER 32 Gastroenterology	453

CHAPTER 33 Urology and Nephrology 463

CHAPTER 34 Toxicology and Substance Abuse 475

CHAPTER 35 Hematology 495

CHAPTER 36 Environmental Emergencies 505

CHAPTER 37 Infectious Disease 521

CHAPTER 38 Psychiatric and Behavioral Disorders 535

CHAPTER 39 Gynecology 541

CHAPTER 40 Obstetrics 547

DIVISION 5: Special Considerations/Operations **555**

CHAPTER 41 Neonatology 557

CHAPTER 42 Pediatrics 569

CHAPTER 43 Geriatric Emergencies 589

CHAPTER 44 Abuse and Assault 613

CHAPTER 45 The Challenged Patient 619

CHAPTER 46 Acute Interventions for the Chronic-Care Patient 631

CHAPTER 47 Assessment-Based Management 643

CHAPTER 48 Operations 651
  Part 1: Ambulance Operations 651
  Part 2: Medical Incident Management 657
  Part 3: Rescue Awareness and Operations 667
  Part 4: Hazardous Materials Incidents 678
  Part 5: Crime Scene Awareness 691

CHAPTER 49 Responding to Terrorist Acts 701

Workbook Answer Key 707

National Registry of Emergency Medical Technicians Practical Evaluation Forms 719

Emergency Drug Cards 735

INTRODUCTION
To the Self-Instructional Workbook
Essentials of Paramedic Care
SECOND EDITION

Welcome to the self-instructional workbook for *Essentials of Paramedic Care*. This workbook is designed to help guide you through an educational program for initial or refresher training that follows the guidelines of the 1998 U.S. Department of Transportation EMT-Paramedic National Standard Curriculum. The workbook is designed to be used either in conjunction with your instructor or as a self-study guide you use on your own.

This workbook features many different ways to help you learn the material necessary to become a paramedic, including those listed below.

Features

Review of Chapter Objectives
Each chapter of *Essentials of Paramedic Care* begins with objectives that identify the important information and principles addressed in the chapter reading. To help you identify and learn this material, each workbook chapter reviews the important content elements addressed by these objectives as presented in the text.

Content Self-Evaluation
Each chapter of *Essentials of Paramedic Care* presents an extensive narrative explanation of the principles of paramedic practice. The workbook chapter (or chapter part) contains between 10 and 90 multiple-choice questions to test your reading comprehension of the textbook material and to give you experience taking typical emergency medical service examinations.

Chapter Parts
Several chapters in *Essentials of Paramedic Care* are long and contain a great deal of subject matter. To help you grasp this material more efficiently, the workbook breaks these chapters into parts with their own objectives and content review.

National Registry Practical Evaluation Forms
Supplemental materials found at the back of the workbook include the National Registry Practical Evaluation Forms. These or similar forms will be used to test your practical skills throughout your training and, usually, for state certification exams. By reviewing them, you have a clearer picture of what is expected of you during your practical exam and a better understanding of the type of evaluation tool that is used to measure your performance.

Emergency Drug Cards
This workbook contains alphabetized three-by-five-inch cards that present the names/classes, descriptions, indications, contraindications, precautions, and routes and dosages of drugs the paramedic is most likely to encounter in prehospital care. Detach the cards and use them in flash card fashion. Practice until you can give the correct route, dosage, indications, and contraindications for each drug.

Acknowledgments

Contributors

We wish to acknowledge the extraordinary talents and efforts of the following people who contributed chapters to this workbook. In developing study guides, questions, and activities, they have upheld the highest standards of EMS instruction.

Division 4
Beth Lothrop Adams, MA, RN, NREMT-P
EMS Quality Manager
Fairfax County Fire Department
Fairfax County, Virginia

Elizabeth Coolidge-Stolz, MD
Medical Writer, Health Educator
North Reading, Massachusetts

Division 5
Bob Elling, MPA, REMT-P
Professor of Management
American College of Prehospital Medicine
Faculty Member
Hudson Valley Community College of Prehospital Emergency Medicine
Schenectady, New York

Reviewers

The reviewers listed below provided many excellent suggestions for improving this workbook. Their assistance is greatly appreciated.

Blaine Griffiths, BSAS, RN, NREMT-P
Youngstown State University
Youngstown, Ohio

David M. Habben, NREMT-P
EMS Consultant
Boise, Idaho

Edward B. Kuvlesky, NREMT-P
Battalion Chief
Indian River County EMS
Indian River County, Florida

Matthew R. Streger, MPA, NREMT-P
Deputy Commissioner
Cleveland Emergency Medical Services
Cleveland, Ohio

Scott Vahradian, EMT-P
Santa Cruz, California

K. Lee Watson, NREMT-P
Martinsville-Henry County Rescue Squad
Martinsville, Virginia

The author and the publisher gratefully acknowledge the contributions of the following in the preparation of this workbook. We thank him for his skill, conscientiousness, and dedication to excellence:

Tony Crystal, Sc.D., EMT-P, RPhT
Director, Emergency Medical Services
Lake Land College
Mattoon, Illinois

How to Use
The Self-Instructional Workbook
Essentials of Paramedic Care
SECOND EDITION

The self-instructional workbook accompanying *Essentials of Paramedic Care* may be used as directed by your instructor or independently by you during your course of instruction. The recommendations listed below are intended to guide you in using the workbook independently.

- Examine your course schedule and identify the appropriate text chapter or other assigned reading.

- Read the assigned chapter in *Essentials of Paramedic Care* carefully. Do this in a relaxed environment, free of distractions, and give yourself adequate time to read and digest the material. The information presented in *Essentials of Paramedic Care* is often technically complex and demanding, but it is very important that you comprehend it. Be sure that you read the chapter carefully enough to understand and remember what you have read.

- Carefully read the Review of Chapter Objectives at the beginning of each workbook chapter (or part). This material includes both the objectives listed in *Essentials of Paramedic Care* and narrative descriptions of their content. If you do not understand or remember what is discussed from your reading, refer to the referenced pages and reread them carefully. If you still do not feel comfortable with your understanding of any objective, consider asking your instructor about it.

- Take the Content Self-Evaluation at the end of each workbook chapter (or part), answering each question carefully. Do this in a quiet environment, free from distractions, and allow yourself adequate time to complete the exercise. Correct your self-evaluation by consulting the answers at the back of the workbook, and determine the percentage you have answered correctly (the number you got right divided by the total number of questions). If you have answered most of the questions correctly (85 to 90 percent), review those that you missed by rereading the material on the pages listed in the answer key and be sure you understand which answer is correct and why. If you have more than a few questions wrong (less than 85 percent correct), look for incorrect answers that are grouped together. This suggests that you did not understand a particular topic in the reading. Reread the text dealing with that topic carefully, and then retest yourself on the questions you got wrong. If incorrect answers are spread throughout the chapter content, reread the chapter and retake the Content Self-Evaluation to assure that you understand the material. If you don't understand why your answer to a question is incorrect after reviewing the text, consult with your instructor.

- When you have completed *Essentials of Paramedic Care* and its accompanying workbook, prepare for a course test by reviewing both the text in its entirety and your class notes.

If, during your completion of the workbook exercises, you have any questions that either the textbook or workbook doesn't answer, write them down and ask your instructor about them. Prehospital emergency medicine is a complex and complicated subject, and answers are not always black and white. It is also common for different EMS systems to use differing methods of care. The questions you bring up in class, and your instructor's answers to them, will help you expand and complete your knowledge of prehospital emergency medical care.

The authors and Brady Publishing continuously seek to assure the creation of the best materials to support your educational experience. We are interested in your comments. If, during your reading and study of material in *Essentials of Paramedic Care*, you notice any error or have any suggestions to improve either the textbook or workbook, please direct your comments via the Internet at the following address:

harrier@localnet.com

You can also visit the Brady website at:
www.bradybooks.com/paramedic

GUIDELINES TO BETTER TEST-TAKING

The knowledge you will gain from reading the textbook, completing the exercises in the workbook, listening in your paramedic class, and participating in your clinical and field experience will prepare you to care for patients who are seriously ill or injured. However, before you can practice these skills, you will have to pass several classroom written exams and your state's certification exam successfully. Your performance on these exams will depend not only on your knowledge but also on your ability to answer test questions correctly. The following guidelines are designed to help your performance on tests and to better demonstrate your knowledge of prehospital emergency care.

1. Relax and be calm during the test.

A test is designed to measure what you have learned and to tell you and your instructor how well you are doing. An exam is not designed to intimidate or punish you. Consider it a challenge, and just try to do your best. Get plenty of sleep prior to the examination. Avoid coffee or other stimulants for a few hours before the exam, and be prepared.

Reread the text chapters, review the objectives in the workbook, and review your class notes. It might be helpful to work with one or two other students and ask each other questions. This type of practice helps everyone better understand the knowledge presented in your course of study.

2. Read the questions carefully.

Read each word of the question and all the answers slowly. Words such as "except" or "not" may change the entire meaning of the question. If you miss such words, you may answer the question incorrectly even though you know the right answer.

EXAMPLE:
The art and science of Emergency Medical Services involves all of the following EXCEPT:

- A. sincerity and compassion.
- B. respect for human dignity.
- C. placing patient care before personal safety.
- D. delivery of sophisticated emergency medical care.
- E. none of the above

The correct answer is C, unless you miss the "EXCEPT."

3. Read each answer carefully.

Read each and every answer carefully. While the first answer may be absolutely correct, so may the rest, and thus the best answer might be "all of the above."

EXAMPLE:
Indirect medical control is considered to be:

- A. treatment protocols.
- B. training and education.
- C. quality assurance.
- D. chart review.
- E. all of the above

While answers A, B, C, and D are correct, the best and only acceptable answer is "all of the above," E.

4. Delay answering questions you don't understand and look for clues.

When a question seems confusing or you don't know the answer, note it on your answer sheet and come back to it later. This will ensure that you have time to complete the test. You will also find that other questions in the test may give you hints to answer the one you've skipped over. It will also prevent you from being frustrated with an early question and letting it affect your performance.

EXAMPLE:

Upon successful completion of a course of training as an EMT-P, most states will:

    A. certify you. (correct)
    B. license you.
    C. register you.
    D. recognize you as a paramedic.
    E. issue you a permit.

Another question, later in the exam, may suggest the right answer:

The action of one state in recognizing the certification of another is called:

    A. reciprocity. (correct)
    B. national registration.
    C. licensure.
    D. registration.
    E. extended practice.

5. Answer all questions.

Even if you do not know the right answer, do not leave a question blank. A blank question is always wrong, while a guess might be correct. If you can eliminate some of the answers as wrong, do so. It will increase the chances of a correct guess.

EXAMPLE:

When a paramedic is called by the patient (through the dispatcher) to the scene of a medical emergency, the medical control physician has established a physician/patient relationship.

    A. True
    B. False

A true/false question gives you a 50 percent chance of a correct guess.

The hospital health professional responsible for sorting patients as they arrive at the emergency department is usually the:

    A. emergency physician.
    B. ward clerk.
    C. emergency nurse.
    D. trauma surgeon.
    E. both A and C (correct)

A multiple-choice question with five answers gives a 20 percent chance of a correct guess. If you can eliminate one or more incorrect answers, you increase your odds of a correct guess to 25 percent, 33 percent, and so on. An unanswered question has a 0 percent chance of being correct.

Just before turning in your answer sheet, check to be sure that you have not left any items blank.

Don't Make the Test Your First Emergency! Get Your Test Prep Materials from Brady.

Brady has everything you need to help you succeed in your paramedic course, as well as important tools for success on your national/state exams and your career beyond. Here are a few of our related titles.

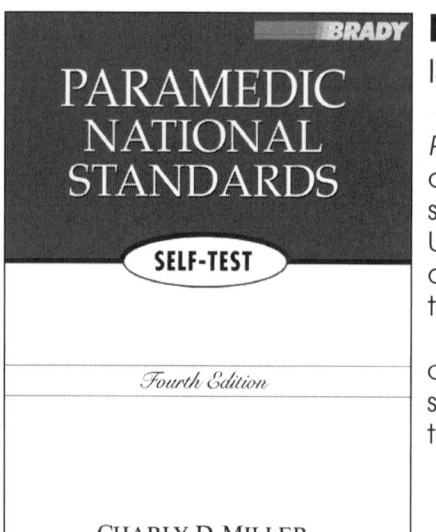

Paramedic National Standards Self-Test, 4th ed.
ISBN: 0-13-110500-0   Charly D. Miller

Paramedic National Standards Self-Test is the most thorough text available to assist paramedics in preparation for national and state paramedic certification examinations. Every EMT-Paramedic U.S. Department of Transportation (DOT) objective is addressed by at least one question. This self-test text covers all possible topics that paramedics may find on their exams.

The 4th edition includes newly developed scenario-based questions along with multiple-choice questions. You will demonstrate better knowledge of the material and learn valuable test-taking skills.

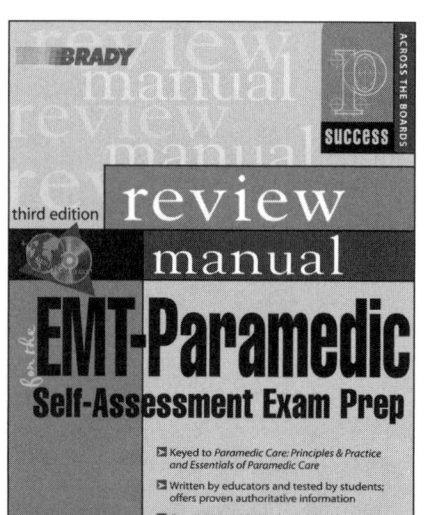

Review Manual for the EMT-Paramedic: Self-Assessment Exam Prep, 3rd ed.
ISBN: 0-13-112869-8   Cherry & Mistovich

This preparatory text blends a comprehensive collection of practice exam questions with helpful test-taking tips. With rich content review, this test preparation is a blueprint for success across the boards. A CD-ROM is bound with the book, containing additional practice exams.

Test Prep Online—Go to www.prenhall.com/emtachieve to register and start preparing today.

To see the wide variety of titles we publish for all levels of EMS and Fire, check out our online catalog at www.bradybooks.com.

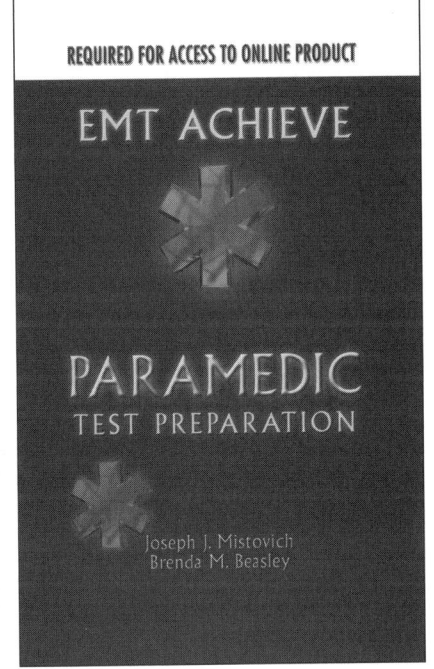

EMT-Achieve: Paramedic Test Preparation
ISBN: 0-13-221737-6   Mistovich & Beasley

EMT-Achieve: Paramedic Test Preparation is an Internet-based online test preparation product. Four 180-question tests contain questions across the major content areas—airway and breathing, cardiology, medical emergencies, pediatrics, operations, and trauma—found in national and state examinations. In addition, each of the six content areas has one 25-question test.

Once you take a test, you can immediately see your results, which makes it easy to target areas of improvement. All test questions have rationales, and many are reinforced with text, photos, and illustrations.

Go to www.prenhall.com/emtachieve to register.

To order:
Ask your local bookstore for these review titles or log onto www.bradybooks.com

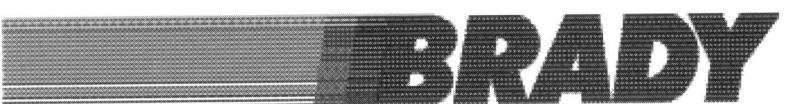

Essentials of Paramedic Care

Division 1

Introduction to Advanced Prehospital Care

Chapter 1

Introduction to Advanced Prehospital Care

Part 1: Introduction to Advanced Prehospital Care

Review of Chapter Objectives

With each chapter of the Workbook, we identify the objectives and important elements of the textbook content. Because Chapter 1 is lengthy, it has been divided into parts. You should review items in these parts and refer to the text pages listed if any points are not clear.

After reading Part 1 of this chapter, you should be able to:

1. **Describe the relationship between the paramedic and other members of the allied health professions.** pp. 6–7

   The paramedic is the highest-level prehospital care provider and leader of the prehospital care team. He or she is a member of the allied health care professions and specifically a member of the ancillary health care professions, which include health care professionals other than physicians and nurses. Paramedics are credentialed or licensed by an appropriate state or provincial agency and approved by their system's medical directors.

2. **Identify the attributes and characteristics of the paramedic.** p. 7

   Paramedics must possess the knowledge, skills, and attitudes consistent with the expectations of the public and the profession. This includes recognizing that you are an essential component in the continuum of care and an advocate for the patient. As a paramedic, you must be flexible enough to work within the various types of EMS systems and adjust to the ever-changing emergency environment. You must be a confident leader, accept the challenges of your profession, have excellent judgment, communicate effectively, develop a rapport with a great diversity of patients, and function independently in a very unstructured environment.

3. **Explain the elements of paramedic education and practice that support its stature as a profession.** p. 7

   The 1998 U.S. Department of Transportation's EMT-Paramedic: National Standard Curriculum describes an intensive course of education with a great emphasis on anatomy, physiology, and pathophysiology. This material provides a broad foundation for your understanding of the human body and its injury and illness. Once you complete initial training, you are expected to continue your education, both to expand your knowledge of prehospital care and to ensure that you remain practiced and ready to employ those skills used less frequently. Further, you and other members of the profession must commit to supporting research both to define and improve skills and care procedures that benefit patients and to identify those that do not. Only through research can the paramedic profession continue to grow and earn respect for the work of its members. Despite its relative youth, the field of emergency medical services enjoys growing public recognition as an important segment of the health care professions. However, this status must not be taken for granted.

4. **Define and give examples of the expanded scope of practice for the paramedic.** p. 8

Currently there are four areas in which the scope of practice for EMT-Paramedics has been expanded. They include critical care transport, primary care, industrial medicine, and sports medicine. Critical care transport is a specialization directed at the needs of critically ill or injured patients as they are moved from one care facility to another. During this transport, paramedics often use equipment far more advanced and complex than that found on standard ambulances. With the changing nature of the health care market and increasing specialization of health care facilities, this realm of expanded scope is growing. Primary care is the movement of the paramedic into more traditional health care roles in such places as emergency departments, outpatient clinics, physicians' offices, urgent care centers, and patients' homes. Industrial medicine is the field in which specially trained paramedics provide on-site services including emergency care, safety inspection, accident prevention, medical screening, and vaccinations in the work place. Sports medicine sets the paramedic as a partner with the athletic trainer while providing emergency care and advising whether an injured player should return to the game or continue competition.

Content Self-Evaluation

Each of the chapters in this Workbook includes a short content review. The questions are designed to test your ability to remember what you read. At the end of this Workbook, you can find the answers to the questions as well as the pages where the topic of each question was discussed in the text. If you answered a question incorrectly or are unsure of the answer, review the pages listed.

MULTIPLE CHOICE

_____ 1. The modern ambulance is best described as a(n):
   A. rapid patient transport vehicle.
   B. vehicle for horizontal transport.
   C. mobile emergency room.
   D. mobile intensive care unit.
   E. automated care delivery center.

_____ 2. While required to be licensed, registered, or credentialed, paramedics still may only function as approved by and under the direct supervision of the system's medical director.
   A. True
   B. False

_____ 3. The expanding role of the paramedic may place him in the role of:
   A. public educator.
   B. health promoter.
   C. injury and illness prevention advocate.
   D. facilitator of access to care.
   E. all of the above

_____ 4. The paramedic is held accountable to which of the following?
   A. the public
   B. the system medical director
   C. the employer
   D. his or her peers
   E. all of the above

4 ESSENTIALS OF PARAMEDIC CARE

_____ 5. The best way to ensure that you meet the expectations of the public, peers, and the system medical director is to:
   A. know your protocols.
   B. attend all ongoing education sessions.
   C. record everything well on the prehospital care report.
   D. always act in the best interest of the patient.
   E. act confident and in control while you provide care.

_____ 6. Which of the following is NOT a characteristic of a professional paramedic?
   A. confident leadership
   B. excellent judgment
   C. strong opinions about ethnic groups
   D. ability to develop a rapport with a wide variety of patients
   E. ability to function independently

_____ 7. Which characteristic best describes the changes made in the profession by the 1998 DOT National Standard Curriculum?
   A. It provided algorithms for most situations paramedics face.
   B. It raised the standards of education for the paramedic.
   C. It allowed the paramedic to prescribe more drugs.
   D. It required stronger math, English, and communication skills.
   E. all of the above

_____ 8. For years, paramedic practice was based on anecdotal data and tradition.
   A. True
   B. False

_____ 9. Which of the following is an example of the expanded scope of practice for paramedics?
   A. critical care transport   D. sports medicine
   B. primary care   E. all of the above
   C. industrial medicine

_____ 10. A tactical paramedic is likely to provide support to which of the services listed below?
   A. fire service   D. law enforcement
   B. utility company   E. all of the above
   C. search and rescue

Part 2: EMS Systems

Review of Chapter Objectives

After reading Part 2 of this chapter, you should be able to:

1. **Describe key historical events that influenced the national development of Emergency Medical Services (EMS) systems.** pp. 9–12

   There is a long history of individuals providing care in the out-of-hospital setting, beginning in ancient times. The cardinal events in the history of EMS include the first organized use of patient transport (and the ambulance) by Jean Larrey, chief surgeon for Napoleon. While simply a horse-drawn cart called an ambulance volante (flying ambulance), it represented the first recognized attempt to bring the injured from the field to medical care. Wars continued to be the impetus to improve out-of-hospital care. The American Civil War, World Wars I and II, and the Korean and Vietnamese conflicts all brought substantial changes to field care and transport. The war in Vietnam saw a greater reduction in mortality associated with immediate care in the field and rapid access to surgery than was the case in any previous conflict. However, the single greatest event in the development of modern-day EMS was the National Highway Safety Act of 1966. This act, for the first time and on a national level, recognized emergency medical services and financially supported their development. Under that act, and its establishment of the Department of Transportation (DOT) as overseeing agency, the nation soon had the first national EMS training curriculum, new criteria for ambulance design (the KKK specifications), and the creation of state-led agencies to coordinate EMS development. Later federal legislation created EMS systems through the guidance of the Department of Health, Education, and Welfare, and since then several federal initiatives have continued to improve the nation's EMS system, mostly under the leadership of the DOT.

2. Define the following terms:

Certification p. 16
Certification is a process by which an agency or association grants recognition to an individual who meets its qualifications.

EMS systems p. 8
An emergency medical services system is a comprehensive network of personnel, equipment, and resources established to deliver aid and emergency medical care to the community.

Ethics p. 53
Ethics are rules or standards for conduct of a particular group or profession.

Health care professional p. 17
Health care professionals are properly trained and licensed or certified providers of health care.

Licensure p. 16
Licensure is a process by which a governmental agency grants permission to engage in an occupation based on an applicant's attaining a required competency sufficient to ensure the public's protection.

Medical direction pp. 13–14
Medical direction is the guidance of the actions of prehospital care providers by a physician associated with the emergency medical services system. Medical direction may be on-line or off-line medical direction and includes the physician's involvement in and supervision of personnel education, personnel and equipment selection, protocol development, quality improvement, and advocacy for the EMS system and the patient.

Peer review p. 21
Peer review is a process of evaluation of the quality of conduct or actions performed by members of a group or profession that is undertaken by other members of that group or profession.

Profession p. 16
A profession is a vocation requiring advanced education or training in a specialized body of knowledge and/or skills.

Professionalism p. 21
Professionalism is the conduct or qualities that characterize a practitioner in a particular field or profession.

Protocols p. 14
Protocols are policies and procedures addressing primarily triage, treatment, transport, and transfer of patients as well as special circumstances and events within the EMS system.

Registration p. 16
Registration is the listing of your name and essential information within a particular record of a certifying organization.

3. **Identify national groups important to the development, education, and implementation of EMS as well as the role of national associations, the National Registry of EMTs, and the roles of various EMS standard-setting agencies.** pp. 17–18

The National Association of EMTs, the National Registry of EMTs, the National Association of State EMS Directors, the National Association of Emergency Physicians, the National Council of State EMS Training Coordinators, and other like associations provide leadership, advise national regulatory bodies, and establish standards for performance related to the provision of emergency medical care. These organizations serve to guide the continuing development, initial and ongoing EMS education, and implementation and coordination of EMS systems nationally.

National associations identify standards for performance in EMS and advocate for patient care and the professional stature of their members. The National Registry of EMTs maintains a national standard, through testing, at the Basic, Intermediate, and Paramedic levels of EMT training. Other standard-setting agencies establish the criteria and standards for system performance. For example, the Joint Committee on Educational Programs for the EMT-Paramedic sets standards for institutions educating paramedics. The American Heart Association sets standards for basic and advanced cardiac life support. The American College of Emergency Physicians recommends a list of ALS equipment for ambulances. The American College of Surgeons establishes a listing of essential BLS ambulance equipment.

4. **Identify the standards (components) of an EMS system as defined by the National Highway Traffic Safety Administration.** p. 11

NHTSA has defined the following components for EMS systems:

- **Regulation and policy.** Each state must have laws, regulations, policies, and procedures that govern its EMS system.
- **Resources management.** Each state must have central control of health care resources to ensure that all patients have equal access to emergency care.
- **Human resources and training.** Each state must require that all EMS providers are taught by qualified instructors using a standardized curriculum.
- **Transportation.** Each state must ensure that patients are safely and reliably transported by ground or air ambulance.
- **Facilities.** Each state must ensure that every seriously ill or injured patient is delivered to an appropriate medical facility in a timely manner.
- **Communications.** Each state must have a system for public access to EMS along with communications among dispatchers, ambulance crews, and hospital personnel.
- **Trauma systems.** Each state should develop a system of specialized care for trauma patients including the designation of trauma centers and systems to ensure that patients arrive at the appropriate facility in a timely manner.
- **Public information and education.** EMS personnel should participate in programs designed to educate the public in injury prevention, emergency recognition, system access, and first aid.
- **Medical direction.** Each EMS system must have a physician medical director responsible for delegating medical practice to prehospital care providers and overseeing patient care.
- **Evaluation.** Each state must have a quality improvement system for continuing evaluation and upgrading of the EMS system.

5. **Differentiate among EMS provider levels: First Responder, Emergency Medical Technician-Basic, Emergency Medical Technician-Intermediate, and Emergency Medical Technician-Paramedic.** p. 17

- **First Responder.** The first responder is usually the first EMS-trained provider on the scene and is prepared to initially care for and stabilize the patient until personnel with higher levels of training arrive.
- **EMT-Basic.** The EMT-Basic is an EMS responder who meets the criteria of the U.S. DOT National Standard Curriculum for EMT-Basics and is prepared to assess, care for, and transport the patient at the basic life support level.

- **EMT-Intermediate.** The EMT-Intermediate is an EMS responder who meets the criteria of the U.S. DOT National Standard Curriculum for EMT-Intermediates and is prepared to assess, care for, and transport the patient using all EMT-Basic skills plus some advanced life support level skills such as advanced airway management, IV therapy, and administration of certain medications.
- **EMT-Paramedic.** The EMT-Paramedic is an EMS responder who meets the criteria of the U.S. DOT National Standard Curriculum for EMT-Paramedics and is prepared to assess, care for, and transport the patient using advanced patient assessment, trauma management, pharmacology, cardiology, and other medical skills. The paramedic should complete advanced cardiac life support and pediatric life support courses.

6. **Describe what is meant by "citizen involvement in the EMS system."**   **p. 14**

   Citizen involvement in the EMS system means that average members of the public can recognize a medical or trauma emergency, know how to access the EMS system, and know how to provide basic life support assistance such as hemorrhage control, CPR, and, possibly, early defibrillation prior to the arrival of EMS personnel.

7. **Discuss the role of the EMS physician in providing medical direction, prehospital and out-of-hospital care as an extension of the physician, the benefits of on-line and off-line medical direction, and the process for the development of local policies and protocols.**   **pp. 13–14**

   A paramedic functions only under the supervision and direction of a medical direction physician. That oversight is provided as either on-line medical direction or off-line medical direction. Off-line medical direction involves the physician's participation in personnel and equipment selection, training, protocol development, quality improvement, and acting as an EMS and patient advocate within the health profession. On-line medical direction consists of direct radio or phone consultation and oversight of paramedics and other prehospital care providers while they are caring for a patient. The ultimate responsibility for all care offered by the paramedic rests with the medical direction physician.

   The medical director is a physician who is legally responsible for all clinical and patient care aspects of an EMS system. Prehospital care provided by the paramedic or other EMS personnel is provided under the license of the medical director, regardless of who his or her employer is.

   The benefits of both on-line and off-line medical direction include the medical supervision of the EMS system and prehospital and out-of-hospital patient care. Among these benefits are the opportunity to practice "prehospital medicine" under the license and supervision of the medical director including use of protocols, standing orders, and algorithms developed by the medical director. Additionally, on-line medical direction provides access to direct medical consultation for EMS personnel during the care of the emergency patient.

   Protocols are developed by the medical director (in cooperation with expert EMS personnel) to address the assessment and care offered during triage, treatment, transport, and transfer of the patient. The protocols and other system policies are developed to address not only commonly encountered circumstances but also special situations such as intervener physicians, child, spouse, or elderly abuse, DNR orders, patient refusals, and the like. The protocols and policies set the standards for accountability of EMS personnel and ensure uniform, medically approved care for each and every patient.

8. **Describe the relationship between a physician on the scene, the paramedic on the scene, and the EMS physician providing on-line medical direction.**   **p. 13**

   At the scene of a medical or trauma emergency, the health care professional with the highest training specific to emergency care should be responsible for patient care. When a nonsystem-affiliated physician is at the scene (an intervener physician), the on-line medical direction physician is ultimately responsible for the patient. When on-line medical direction is not available, the paramedic may relinquish patient care responsibility to the intervener physician as long as that individual identifies him- or herself, demonstrates a willingness to assume patient care responsibilities, and agrees to provide the documentation required by the system. If treatment differs from system protocols, the intervener physician must agree to ride with the patient to the hospital.

9. **Describe the components of continuous quality improvement and analyze its contribution to system improvement, continuing medical education, and research.** pp. 20–21

Continuous quality improvement (CQI) is an ongoing effort to refine and improve the system to ensure the highest level of service possible. It involves six basic components: identifying system-wide problems, elaborating on the probable causes, listing solutions, outlining a plan of corrective action, providing resources and support to ensure success, and reevaluating the results and system performance continuously. CQI system review uses positive reinforcement and support to identify and improve patient care. It can identify areas for improvement and ways to allocate resources to make those improvements, frequently through continuing medical education. When questions arise about the benefits of care offered by a system, a CQI program can suggest research projects to investigate the real value of procedures, equipment, and protocols. The real key to effective CQI is the positive and reinforcing nature of its approach to system improvement.

10. **Describe the importance, basic principles, process of evaluating and interpreting, and benefits of research.** pp. 21–23

Research is essential to ensuring that the equipment and procedures used in the out-of-hospital setting are safe, benefit the patient, and are worth any potential risks of employing them. Research attempts to objectively evaluate the performance of interventions in an unbiased way. Research begins by asking a question (stating a hypothesis), investigating any existing research, designing a study that is unbiased and fairly measures performance, collects and analyzes data, assesses and evaluates results against the hypothesis, and reports the findings. Evidence-based medicine (EBM) evaluates research to determine which procedures in emergency medicine have a positive impact on patient outcome and which do not. This process may cause us to reevaluate the tools and procedures that were once considered standard in prehospital care.

Content Self-Evaluation

MULTIPLE CHOICE

_____ 1. An Emergency Medical Services system is a network of personnel, equipment, and resources established to deliver aid and emergency care to the community.
   A. True
   B. False

_____ 2. The date of the earliest recorded medical care procedures is:
   A. about 5,000 years ago.
   B. about 2,000 years ago.
   C. 1497.
   D. 1562.
   E. 1666.

_____ 3. In a well-developed EMS system, trained First Responders are likely to be:
   A. police officers.
   B. firefighters.
   C. life guards.
   D. teachers.
   E. all of the above

_____ 4. Which of the following was NOT a component of the Emergency Medical Services Systems Act of 1973?
   A. communications
   B. system financing
   C. training
   D. access to care
   E. system evaluation

_____ 5. The medical director is a physician who is legally responsible for all patient care offered by the system he oversees.
   A. True
   B. False

_____ 6. The intervener physician is a physician who is:
   A. not affiliated with the system of medical direction.
   B. at the scene of an emergency.
   C. a trained emergency physician.
   D. both A and B
   E. none of the above

_____ 7. When on-line medical control does not exist and an intervener physician is present, is willing to accept patient care responsibility, performs interventions consistent with the system protocols, and agrees to document the interventions as required by the system, the paramedic should:
   A. relinquish patient care responsibilities.
   B. retain patient care authority.
   C. relinquish patient care responsibilities only if the physician agrees to ride to the hospital.
   D. retain patient care responsibilities in cases of physician disagreement.
   E. none of the above

_____ 8. Off-line medical direction includes which of the following?
   A. protocols   D. quality assurance
   B. training guidelines   E. all of the above
   C. personnel selection policies

_____ 9. Which of the following is NOT one of the four "Ts" of emergency care?
   A. triage   D. transport
   B. transfer   E. treatment
   C. termination of care

_____ 10. Which of the following statements is NOT true?
   A. The ability to recognize cardiac emergencies can save lives.
   B. Over 300,000 cardiac arrests per year occur before the patient reaches the hospital.
   C. Most cardiac arrests happen immediately upon onset of symptoms.
   D. If bystanders or the patient call in time, many cardiac arrests can be prevented.
   E. all of the above

_____ 11. There are great disadvantages to dispatching EMS, fire, and police from a single control center.
   A. True
   B. False

_____ 12. The dispatch system that provides caller interrogation, predetermined response configurations, and pre-arrival instructions is:
   A. system status management.   D. caller interrogation.
   B. enhanced 911.   E. none of the above
   C. priority dispatch.

_____ 13. There may be some increased liability for a system providing prearrival instructions.
   A. True
   B. False

_____ 14. The goal of dispatch and response in an effective EMS is to have:
   A. BLS units on the scene within 4 minutes.
   B. ALS units on the scene within 8 minutes.
   C. at least 90 percent of all responses within system time limits.
   D. all of the above
   E. none of the above

_____ 15. The learning domain associated with skills is:
   A. cognitive.
   B. psychomotor.
   C. affective.
   D. didactic.
   E. dexterous.

_____ 16. The process by which a state or other governmental agency grants permission to engage in a given occupation is:
   A. licensure.
   B. certification.
   C. registration.
   D. reciprocity.
   E. tenure.

_____ 17. Granting someone recognition for meeting the qualifications of another agency is called:
   A. licensure.
   B. certification.
   C. registration.
   D. reciprocity.
   E. tenure.

_____ 18. The U.S. DOT has developed curricula for how many levels of EMS providers?
   A. 1
   B. 2
   C. 3
   D. 4
   E. 5

_____ 19. The EMS provider responsible for general patient assessment, CPR, hemorrhage control, and spinal immobilization is the:
   A. First Responder.
   B. EMT-Basic.
   C. EMT-Intermediate.
   D. EMT-Paramedic.
   E. all of the above

_____ 20. It is desirable for the EMT-Paramedic to complete which of the following courses?
   A. BTLS
   B. PHTLS
   C. PALS
   D. ACLS
   E. all of the above

_____ 21. The organization that administers practical and written exams and establishes qualifications for registration of EMT-Basics, EMT-Intermediates, and EMT-Paramedics on a national level is the:
   A. National Association of EMTs.
   B. National Registry of EMTs.
   C. National Council of State EMS Training Coordinators.
   D. Joint Review Committee on Educational Programs for the EMT-Paramedic.
   E. American College of Emergency Physicians.

_____ 22. The body that sets standards for paramedic education programs is the:
   A. Joint Review Committee on Educational Programs for the EMT-Paramedic.
   B. National Association of EMTs.
   C. National Registry of EMTs.
   D. National Council of State EMS Training Coordinators.
   E. American College of Emergency Physicians.

_____ 23. Fixed-wing aircraft are usually used for patient transports exceeding:
   A. 25 miles.
   B. 50 miles.
   C. 150 miles.
   D. 200 miles.
   E. none of the above

_____ 24. The agency responsible for establishing criteria for the design of ambulances is the:
   A. American College of Surgeons.
   B. American College of Emergency Physicians.
   C. U.S. General Services Administration.
   D. U.S. Military Assistance to Traffic and Safety Group.
   E. National Association of EMTs.

_____ 25. A standard van with a raised roof that is configured as an ambulance is categorized as which type of ambulance?
   A. Type I
   B. Type II
   C. Type III
   D. Type A
   E. Type B

_____ 26. A resource hospital is one that:
   A. accepts most patients for care.
   B. fulfills the role of the major trauma center.
   C. coordinates specialty services and ensures appropriate patient distribution.
   D. has the largest emergency department.
   E. provides restocking services for the system's ambulances.

_____ 27. A hospital designated as a receiving facility for the EMS system should have which of the following?
   A. an emergency department
   B. 24-hour emergency physician coverage
   C. surgical facilities and coverage
   D. critical and intensive care units
   E. all of the above

_____ 28. Which of the following is NOT a part of a well-designed disaster plan?
   A. mutual aid agreements among neighboring municipalities, services, and systems
   B. a rigid communications system
   C. frequent disaster plan tests and drills
   D. integration of all system components
   E. a coordinated central management agency

_____ 29. A major complaint regarding quality assurance programs is that they tend to:
   A. be one-time efforts.
   B. address only procedural issues.
   C. be punitive in nature.
   D. not examine protocol issues.
   E. create divisions among care workers on staff.

_____ 30. Continuous quality improvement differs from quality assurance in that it:
   A. emphasizes customer satisfaction.
   B. rewards or reinforces good behavior.
   C. examines billing practices.
   D. evaluates maintenance activities.
   E. all the above

_____ 31. Which of the following is NOT one of the standard rules of evidence used to evaluate a proposed change in the EMS system?
   A. There must be a basis for change.
   B. The old procedure must be deemed no longer medically acceptable.
   C. The change must be clinically important.
   D. The change must be affordable, practical, and teachable.
   E. None of the above are standard rules of evidence.

_____ 32. Ethics are best defined as:
   A. protocols and policies for conduct.
   B. rules or standards governing the performance of a profession.
   C. legal principles governing potential law suits.
   D. the four elements needed to determine negligence.
   E. justifications for actions.

_____ 33. To the patient, it may be more important to receive care from a provider who seems to be interested in him or her and empathetic than to receive the most technically correct care.
   A. True
   B. False

_____ 34. The most common source of EMS funding is:
   A. voluntary donations.
   B. direct patient payments.
   C. third-party payers.
   D. tax subsidies.
   E. residual payments.

_____ 35. The model for EMS operations that is becoming more and more popular for municipalities is the:
   A. public utility model.
   B. third service model.
   C. fire service model.
   D. volunteer model.
   E. proprietary model.

LISTING

Identify the agency or association most closely linked with the following guidelines for EMS:

36. National standard curricula for EMS providers

37. Criteria for ambulance design

38. Listing of standard equipment for Basic Life Support ambulances

39. Listing of equipment and supplies for Advanced Life Support ambulances

40. Criteria for paramedic education programs

Part 3: Roles and Responsibilities of the Paramedic

Review of Chapter Objectives

After reading Part 3 of this chapter, you should be able to:

1. Describe the attributes of a paramedic as a health care professional. pp. 27–30

The attributes of a paramedic are related to his or her stature as a health care professional and include leadership, integrity, empathy, self-motivation, appearance and personal hygiene, self-confidence, communication, time management, teamwork and diplomacy, respect, and patient advocacy.

As a paramedic, you must demonstrate leadership in order to coordinate and direct other care providers in attending to the patient. You must know the abilities of your team and ask its members to do only what they are able to do. You must demonstrate integrity to earn the respect of your peers and the medical community. You must appreciate the plight of the patient and demonstrate an understanding of his or her situation. You must be both self-confident and self-motivated to employ lifesaving procedures in the worst of conditions. You must strive for excellence in knowledge and skills and have and display confidence as you employ patient care skills. Your appearance must demonstrate a respect for both yourself and your patient. Remember that good grooming and personal hygiene both are important in presenting a professional image. You must be able to communicate effectively both orally and in writing to patients, other care providers, and physicians. You must be able to coordinate your efforts and those of others to quickly address the needs of the patient and to fulfill your responsibilities as a paramedic. You must respect others and, through demonstrating that respect, earn respect for yourself. One way of demonstrating that respect is showing a heightened sensitivity to your patient's rights as a person, including the right to confidentiality. You must become a patient advocate, promoting and ensuring that patients receive the care and attention their illness or injury requires. And finally, you must ensure that you maintain the attributes of a professional through careful delivery of your service, including mastering and refreshing skills; following protocols, policies, and procedures; checking your equipment before its use; and operating the ambulance and equipment safely.

2. **Describe the benefits of paramedic continuing education and the importance of maintaining one's paramedic license/certification.** pp. 30–31

   Continuing education helps you maintain the knowledge you acquired through your initial paramedic education and expands your own personal knowledge and skills. It helps you keep up with changes in prehospital care and is essential to maintaining your certification and ability to practice.

3. **List the primary and additional responsibilities of paramedics.** pp. 23–27

   The primary responsibilities of the paramedic include:

   - **Preparation.** You must be mentally, physically, and emotionally ready to respond to the call; know your protocols, geography, and equipment; and ensure that your vehicle and equipment are all in proper working order.
   - **Response.** You must drive responsibly, ensuring a timely, yet safe, response.
   - **Scene size-up.** You must assess the scene to determine: the safety of the scene (including identification of any hazards and the need for BSI); the number of ill or injured; the need for any additional resources; and the mechanism of injury or the nature of the illness.
   - **Patient assessment.** Once at the patient's side, you must determine whether or not the patient needs cervical immobilization as well as his or her level of consciousness (or responsiveness) and the stability of the airway, breathing, and circulation. You will then assess for specific injury or illness signs through a focused or rapid trauma assessment. You will also evaluate the patient's medical history and perform ongoing assessments.
   - **Recognition of injury or illness.** As a result of the scene size-up and patient assessment, you will identify the illness or injury and the patient's priority for care and transport.
   - **Patient management.** You will employ appropriate care procedures, guided by protocols, with your patient and, at times, consult with medical direction to further guide your care.
   - **Appropriate disposition.** Based upon the results of your assessment, the effects of the care measures you have employed, and your system's protocols, you will determine the disposition of your patient. That disposition may be transport to a level I, II, or III trauma center or to another specialized hospital, the closest hospital, or an alternative care facility. An additional possible disposition is to treat and release the patient with instructions to seek the advice of a personal physician.
   - **Patient transfer.** As the health care system becomes more complex and facilities become more specialized, you may be charged with the safe and efficient transfer of patients from one facility to another.
   - **Documentation.** At the conclusion of your patient care, you will be required to document the results of your assessment and care to ensure the continuity of patient care.
   - **Return to service.** At the end of your response, you must ensure that you, your crew, and your ambulance are ready to return to service. This includes cleaning and refueling the vehicle, maintaining equipment, and replacing supplies used during the call.

   Additional responsibilities include:

   - **Community involvement.** You should promote and participate in programs to help the community recognize when EMS is needed, how to access the system, and what to do until the ambulance arrives. Community involvement also includes participation in the development and presentation of programs to improve health—stressing a healthy diet, for example—and to reduce injury—such as promoting seat belt use.
   - **Support for primary care.** Modern health care is evolving in ways aimed at ensuring that costly resources are best directed to serve the patient. In support of this aim, you may be responsible for transporting or directing patients with minor injury or illness to alternate facilities like urgent care centers or physicians' offices.
   - **Citizen involvement in EMS.** Ordinary citizens can be highly important evaluators of the EMS system, as they are its consumers and can best say what elements of it are important to them.

Pay attention to the comments, suggestions, and criticisms of the patients/citizens you contact and pass what you learn along to the appropriate personnel in your system.
- **Personal and professional development.** To maintain and improve your ability to provide prehospital (and out-of-hospital) care, you must participate in professional development. This may include taking refresher and continuing education courses, engaging in skill maintenance exercises, and other activities.

4. **Define the role of the paramedic relative to the safety of the crew, the patient, and the bystanders.** p. 25

You must evaluate information obtained from the dispatcher and gathered during your scene size-up to identify any potential scene hazards. Then you must take action to ensure your safety and the safety of the patient, other crew members and rescue personnel, and bystanders. You must also monitor the scene during your care to ensure that no hazards develop to threaten you, your patient, fellow rescuers, or bystanders.

5. **Describe the role of the paramedic in health education activities related to illness and injury prevention.** p. 26

As EMS matures, its members will be expected to become more involved in both injury and illness prevention programs for the public. Such programs provide the most effective ways of increasing overall public health and reducing both death and disability from accidents and injuries.

6. **Describe examples of professional behaviors in the following areas:** pp. 28–30
- **Integrity.** Be honest and trustworthy in your contacts with patients, crew members, and other health care professionals. Doing this is essential to maintaining personal integrity.
- **Empathy.** You can convey empathy by attempting to understand and appreciate a patient's situation.
- **Self-motivation.** Doing your job well without direct supervision represents self-motivation.
- **Appearance and personal hygiene.** A clean, pressed shirt and trousers and well-kept hair demonstrate a good appearance and appropriate personal hygiene.
- **Self-confidence.** Displaying comfort with the application of emergency skills demonstrates self-confidence.
- **Communications.** In emergency medical services, it is essential to communicate quickly, concisely, accurately, and effectively.
- **Time management.** An emergency scene is often a chaotic place. It is imperative that you be able to organize and direct your actions and those of others quickly and efficiently to ensure that your patient receives appropriate emergency care and transport to definitive care as rapidly as possible.
- **Teamwork and diplomacy.** The emergency response is a team event, and the paramedic, as team leader, must direct many individuals to work together in the patient's best interest.
- **Respect.** Respect is demonstrated by showing regard and consideration for patients, care providers, and others. Listening to these people and indicating that you really hear what they say shows your respect for them and earns you their respect.
- **Patient advocacy.** Ensuring that the needs of your patient remain the first priority of your prehospital emergency care will help you meet your responsibility as a patient advocate.
- **Careful delivery of service.** Demonstrate professional behavior by performing your job to the highest level of excellence, by mastering and maintaining your skills and knowledge, and by conscientiously carrying out equipment checks, driving safely, and following protocols, policies, and procedures.

7. **Identify the benefits of paramedics teaching in their community.** p. 26

Teaching in your community places you in front of your "consumers" before they call for help. This gives you an opportunity to develop a positive public image and explain the workings of the system. It will also help you integrate with the other members of the health care system.

8. **Analyze how the paramedic can benefit the health care system by supporting primary care for patients in the out-of-hospital setting.** p. 25

With the increasing costs of health care, it has become necessary to ensure that the patient's needs are best matched to the available resources. This may mean that the paramedic, through assessment and consultation with the medical direction physician, may direct patients to facilities other than the emergency department.

9. **Describe how professionalism applies to the paramedic while on and off duty.** p. 28

It is essential that the paramedic displays a professional attitude toward his or her patient and the profession as a whole. This applies while both on and off duty since the public often judges a profession by the actions of its members.

Content Self-Evaluation

MULTIPLE CHOICE

_____ 1. In the past 10 years, the health care and EMS systems have seen dramatic changes in care delivery.
   A. True
   B. False

_____ 2. Prior to responding to a call, you must be:
   A. emotionally able to meet the demands of patient care.
   B. physically able to meet the demands of patient care.
   C. mentally able to meet the demands of patient care.
   D. sure the ambulance and equipment are ready for the response.
   E. all of the above

_____ 3. Prior to responding to a call, you must be familiar with:
   A. local EMS protocols.   D. neighboring EMS agencies.
   B. the local communications system.   E. all of the above
   C. local geography.

_____ 4. A call involving which of the following is least likely to require additional assistance?
   A. a single ill patient   D. hazardous materials
   B. reported use of a weapon   E. a rescue situation
   C. knowledge of previous violence

_____ 5. When a patient receives a minor injury and is transported to an alternate care facility like an outpatient clinic, this care is best described as:
   A. basic care.   D. diversion of care.
   B. primary care.   E. health maintenance.
   C. treat and release.

_____ 6. Which of the following items is NOT an essential part of the transfer of a patient between health care facilities?
   A. a verbal patient report from the transferring primary care provider
   B. a copy of the essential parts of the patient's chart
   C. the results of all diagnostic tests
   D. a summary of the patient's past medical history
   E. a summary of the patient's present medical history

_____ 7. The patient care report should normally be completed:
   A. before arrival at the emergency department.
   B. upon arrival at the emergency department.
   C. as soon as care is completed.
   D. upon arrival at your base station.
   E. either C or D

_____ 8. Which of the following is a component of returning to service after a call?
   A. refueling the ambulance
   B. restocking supplies
   C. stowing equipment
   D. reviewing the call with the crew
   E. all of the above

_____ 9. Which of the following is NOT a part of community involvement for the paramedic?
   A. teaching CPR
   B. transporting patients to alternate care facilities
   C. conducting EMS demonstrations
   D. providing prevention programs
   E. sponsoring programs that help the public recognize when to access EMS

_____ 10. What is the unique benefit of having citizen consumers involved in the development, evaluation, and regulation of the EMS system?
   A. They can help seek out alternative funding.
   B. They provide an outside objective view of the EMS system.
   C. They do not have the prejudices of most EMS providers.
   D. They can provide insight into new care procedures.
   E. all of the above

_____ 11. Which of the following is NOT an attribute of a professional?
   A. leadership
   B. excited demeanor
   C. empathy
   D. self-motivation
   E. diplomacy

_____ 12. When presented with a complex situation, a self-confident paramedic will ask for assistance.
   A. True
   B. False

_____ 13. Which of the following is NOT a method of displaying empathy?
   A. being supportive and reassuring
   B. demonstrating respect for others
   C. having a calm and helpful demeanor
   D. accepting constructive feedback
   E. understanding a patient's feelings

_____ 14. In general, the more patches you wear, the more respect you gain from patients.
   A. True
   B. False

_____ 15. Placing the patient's needs above your own represents which professional attribute?
   A. empathy
   B. diplomacy
   C. patient advocacy
   D. initiative
   E. self-confidence

MATCHING

Write the letter of the paramedic responsibility in the space provided next to the action to which it applies.

Responsibility

A. Preparation

B. Response

C. Patient assessment and management
D. Appropriate disposition
E. Patient transfer
F. Documentation
G. Return to service

Action

_____ 16. Refuel the vehicle.
_____ 17. Follow patient care protocols.
_____ 18. Transport a patient to an outpatient center.
_____ 19. Determine the mechanism of injury.
_____ 20. Record the care you provided.
_____ 21. Be familiar with local protocols.
_____ 22. Determine the patient's medical history.
_____ 23. Categorize the patient's priority for transport.
_____ 24. Take a report from the sending facility.
_____ 25. Drive responsibly and safely.
_____ 26. Deliver a patient to a level II trauma center.
_____ 27. Be mentally fit to respond to a call.
_____ 28. Check crew members for signs of stress.
_____ 29. Identify the nature of the illness.
_____ 30. Determine the seriousness of the injury.

Part 4: The Well-Being of the Paramedic

Review of Chapter Objectives

After reading Part 4 of this chapter, you should be able to:

1. **Discuss the concept of wellness and its benefits, components of wellness, and role of the paramedic in promoting wellness.** p. 31

   Wellness, or personal physical, mental, and emotional well-being, is the result of proper nutrition, basic physical fitness, safe practices to protect you from disease and injury, and the development of effective mechanisms to deal with the stress of the profession. The results of observing practices that promote wellness in your own life are a reduced incidence of work-related injury and illness, a good attitude toward the profession, and a long fruitful career in emergency medical services.

   Basic physical fitness is the muscular strength, cardiovascular endurance (aerobic capacity), and flexibility that permit you to perform the tasks associated with prehospital emergency care without risk to the musculoskeletal system.

   Good nutrition is the controlled and balanced consumption of carbohydrates, fats, proteins, vitamins, and minerals that meet the body's needs yet is not consumption in excess.

Personal protection from disease includes application of body substance isolation procedures and acquisition of proper immunizations for protection from contagious disease.

Stress and stress management involve the recognition that prehospital emergency care is a stressful profession and that stress management techniques are essential to a long career in EMS.

General safety considerations include such principles as safe lifting, ensuring a safe environment for EMS operations, safe driving practices, appropriate interpersonal relationships, and the proper dealing with habits and addictions.

The paramedic should, by example, promote basic physical fitness, proper nutrition, the following of safe practices, and the use of appropriate mechanisms to deal with job-related stress. He or she can be a model to peers, patients, and the community in general.

2. **Discuss how cardiovascular endurance, weight control, muscle strength, and flexibility contribute to physical fitness.** pp. 31–34

Cardiovascular endurance, weight control, muscular strength, and flexibility are all essential to the physical fitness required of the paramedic. Cardiovascular endurance is the measure of the heart's and blood vessels' ability to support physical exercise. Increased cardiovascular endurance improves the body's ability to accommodate the physical stress associated with patient lifting and movement and the carrying of equipment. Weight control is essential to limit cardiovascular and musculoskeletal stresses on the body. Muscular strength is achieved by regular exercise and helps keep the body ready for the stresses of lifting and moving the patient and EMS equipment. Flexibility is the strength and ease of motion through the normal range of motion of the body's major joints. Good flexibility will reduce back pain and the potential for joint and muscle injury during your EMS career.

3. **Describe the impact of shift work on circadian rhythms.** pp. 42–43

Shift work disturbs the normal biorhythms of the body, called circadian rhythms. Dramatic changes in a person's daily time schedule disturb the normal sleep/awake, appetite, hormonal, and temperature fluctuation cycles of the body and may result in drowsiness and fatigue. To diminish the negative effects of shift work, it is best to maintain a regular 24-hour sleep/awake cycle (sleeping at about the same time), even on days when you do not work.

4. **Discuss the contributions that periodic risk assessments and warning sign recognition make to cancer and cardiovascular disease prevention.** pp. 32–33

Periodic assessment of your risk for disease is important. Have frequent physical exams and examine your family history to determine the risk for cancer and cardiovascular disease. Know your cholesterol and triglyceride levels and keep them in check. Women past menopause should consider both the risks and benefits of hormonal therapy and should have periodic mammograms and pap smears with advancing age. Males should have periodic prostate exams with advancing age. Also watch for blood in the stool, changes in moles, unexplained weight loss, unexplained chronic fatigue, and unusual lumps.

5. **Differentiate proper from improper body mechanics for lifting and moving patients in emergency and nonemergency situations.** pp. 33–34

Proper lifting and moving techniques, especially when coupled with good physical fitness and good nutrition, help protect the musculoskeletal system from the high risks for injury associated with prehospital emergency care. Good posture, lifting with the leg muscles, and keeping the back straight, the palms up, and the body close to the object being lifted will reduce the potential for injury. Exhale during a lift, keep your feet apart with one foot ahead of the other, take your time, and ask for help when you think you will need it. These principles will make lifting easier and help keep you from back injury during your years of service.

6. **Describe the problems that a paramedic might encounter in a hostile situation and the techniques used to manage the situation.** pp. 45–50

Emergency responses occasionally put the caregiver into contact with hostile patients, family members, and bystanders. These individuals may affect your ability to provide care and, at the extreme, threaten you or your patient with physical harm. If there is a significant threat, remove yourself from the scene immediately. Often, however, the hostility of people at the scene can be overcome by appreciating the cultural diversity of those you treat and helping them understand that your reason for being there is to offer help. Treating everyone you attend with dignity and respect will go a long way toward establishing trust in you and in EMS providers in general.

7. **Describe the considerations that should be given to using escorts, dealing with adverse environmental conditions, using lights and siren, proceeding through intersections, and parking at an emergency scene.** pp. 46–47

Driving an emergency vehicle provides you with some privileges, but with them come some very important added responsibilities. In general, you must remain especially aware of others on the roadway and remember that they may react unexpectedly to your approach and passage. Also consider the following steps when dealing with these specific situations:

- When following an escort, be aware that some drivers may not realize that you are following from behind and may pull out in front of you.
- Adverse driving conditions (rain, snow, ice, fog) reduce visibility and traction. Give other drivers more time to see you and stop, and respect the increased stopping time and reduced maneuverability of your ambulance in these conditions.
- Lights and sirens are used to alert others of your approach and ask them to yield the right of way. However, some drivers may neither see nor hear them or may react in an unexpected manner. Be alert while using lights and sirens and anticipate the actions of others.
- Intersections pose special problems for emergency vehicles. Driving through a red light or a stop sign is dangerous because other drivers may presume they have the right of way. The situation becomes more complicated and dangerous when multiple emergency vehicles are responding. When proceeding through an intersection, and especially when passing through a red light, slow to almost a stop and keep a good lookout for other vehicles not yielding the right of way.
- Once at the scene, park so as to protect you and your crew, the patient, and other drivers. Place your emergency vehicle between traffic and the crash/care scene and be sure the lights can be seen by all oncoming traffic.

8. **Discuss the concept of "due regard for the safety of all others" while operating an emergency vehicle.** p. 47

The concept of exercising due regard for the safety of others recognizes that different drivers will react differently to the approach of emergency vehicles. This means that you must maintain an intense lookout for hazards while driving the emergency vehicle. You must anticipate the actions of other drivers on the highway, including those that are unexpected and not in keeping with the right of way given you under the law. Otherwise you may find yourself responsible for injury when your intent was to provide care or, worse, injure yourself.

9. **Describe the equipment available in a variety of adverse situations for self-protection, including body substance isolation steps for protection from airborne and bloodborne pathogens.** pp. 35–38, 45, 46–47

Equipment available to help protect you from the more common hazards of emergency medical service include helmets, footwear with toe and ankle support, body armor, reflective tape for night visibility, seatbelts, and personal protective equipment used for body substance isolation (gloves, masks, eyewear, respirators, gowns, resuscitation equipment).

Body substance isolation (BSI) practices include the use of personal protective equipment (PPE) to isolate the body from contaminants found in the air and body fluids while caring for a patient. These practices involve using protective latex or plastic gloves to protect yourself when touching a patient if there is reasonable expectation of contact with body fluids, including tears, vomit, saliva, blood, urine, fecal material, cerebrospinal fluid, or any other body fluid or substance. Masks and protective eyewear should be used whenever there is a reasonable expectation that fluid or droplets will be splattered, as is the case with arterial hemorrhage, endotracheal intubation, intensive airway care, childbirth, and the cleaning of contaminated equipment. When a patient has or is suspected of having tuberculosis or another highly contagious airborne disease, use of a special type of mask, either the high-efficiency particulate air (HEPA) or N-95 respirator, offers protection by removing small infectious particles from the air. Gowns are worn to protect clothing and the body from contamination by splashing of body fluids in extreme circumstances (like childbirth). A gown impervious to fluid movement is recommended. When possible, use disposable equipment for patient ventilation and other invasive procedures.

10. **Given a scenario where equipment and supplies have been exposed to body substances, plan for the proper cleaning, disinfection, and disposal of the items.** p. 37

When EMS equipment becomes contaminated (or possibly contaminated), it should be disposed of or properly cleaned and disinfected. Single-use devices, bandaging materials, and other disposable EMS equipment and materials should be placed in a sealed biohazard waste container and disposed of properly. Needles and other sharp contaminated items should be placed in a puncture-proof "sharps" container and disposed of properly. Equipment that has been in contact with a patient or otherwise becomes contaminated should be cleaned with soap and water, disinfected with an appropriate agent (commercial or a bleach solution), or sterilized (by heat, steam, or radiation) as per your service's policies and procedures. Any contaminated cleaning or disinfecting supplies should be disposed of properly.

11. **Describe the benefits and methods of smoking cessation.** p. 33

Smoking and the effects of nicotine are well known to be detrimental to respiratory and cardiovascular health and well linked to lung cancer. Smoking cessation programs using replacement therapy (nicotine patches), behavior modification, aversion therapy, hypnotism, and "cold turkey" approaches represent structured programs of controlled withdrawal from sociocultural, psychological, and physiological dependency on the drug. The result of a successful smoking cessation program is better respiratory and cardiovascular health and a reduced risk of respiratory infection and cancer.

12. **Identify and describe the three phases of the stress response, factors that trigger the stress response, and causes of stress in EMS.** pp. 41–43

There are three stages to the human response to stress: alarm, resistance, and exhaustion. Alarm is the initial response, more commonly known as the "fight-or-flight" response. The autonomic nervous system prepares the body to deal with a threat to its well-being by releasing hormones that increase cardiac output (increase heart rate, the strength of contraction, and preload) and blood pressure, induce pupil dilation, increase blood sugar, and relax the respiratory tree. Resistance begins as the body starts to adjust and cope with the stress. During this phase, the blood pressure and pulse rate may return to normal. The final stress response phase is exhaustion. If the exposure to stress is prolonged, the body may become exhausted and lose its ability to resist and adapt to the stressors. The individual becomes more susceptible to physical and psychological ailments.

Stress is a stimulus from the environment that affects the body. Stress can have positive effects (eustress), or it can generate negative effects (distress). Factors that induce the stress response are anything that threatens (or is perceived to threaten) the well-being of the individual. These factors include physical ones, like the threat of violence; emotional ones, like the loss of a loved one; and physiological ones, like physical fatigue or extreme hunger. Each person reacts differently to stressors, bringing his or her previous experiences into the equation.

13. **Differentiate between normal/healthy and detrimental physiological and psychological reactions to anxiety and stress.** pp. 43–44

The human stress response is the body's way of dealing with stress, and the outcome is either healthy or unhealthy. Healthy responses result in the individual's quickly adjusting to the stressor and physiologically and psychologically returning to normal. Unhealthy responses result in behavioral and physiologic manifestations like gastrointestinal disturbances, sleep disturbances, headaches, vision problems, fatigue, chest pains, confusion, a reduced attention span, poor concentration, disorientation, memory problems, inappropriate fear, panic, grief, depression, anxiety, and feelings of being overwhelmed, abandoned, or numb to emotion. A person with an unhealthy response may also experience withdrawal from normal social activities, increased use of drugs or alcohol, or inappropriate humor, silence, crying, suspiciousness, or activity levels.

EMS provides an abundant amount of stressors because of the nature of the profession. These stressors include shift work; loud pagers and sounds; poor pay; long hours; periods of boredom followed by short periods of extreme excitement; scene violence; abusive patients; vomit; blood; gory scenes; chaotic scenes; personal fears; frustration; exhaustion; demands of family members, friends, or bystanders; inclement weather; conflicts with co-workers or supervisors; hunger and thirst; and physical demands on the body, like heavy lifting. The personality traits commonly found in EMS members, a strong need to be liked and often unrealistically high self-expectations, also leave these individuals more likely to develop adverse responses to stress.

14. Describe behavior that is a manifestation of stress in patients and those close to them, and describe how that behavior relates to paramedic stress. pp. 44–45

Stress may become evident through almost any unusual behavior exhibited by the patient, family, or bystanders. It may manifest with hyper- or hypoactivity, withdrawal, suspiciousness, increased smoking, increased alcohol or drug intake, excessive humor or silence, crying spells, or any changes in behavior, communications, interactions with others, or eating habits. These behaviors can confound the assessment of the patient's mental status and place additional stress on the paramedic.

15. Identify and describe the defense mechanisms and management techniques commonly used to deal with stress, discuss research about possible problems in the use of critical incident stress management (CISM), and identify the appropriate mental health services that should be available to EMS personnel. pp. 44–45

Constructive mechanisms and management techniques used to deal with stress can be divided into two categories—immediate and long term. Immediate coping mechanisms include controlling breathing to reduce adrenaline levels and reduce heart rate, reframing thoughts to encourage or support any needed behavior on your behalf (e.g., saying to yourself "I can do this!"), and focusing your concentration on the responsibilities at hand (i.e., the needs of the patient), not the stressful problem. For long-term well-being, ensure your physical, mental, and emotional health. Exercise, watch your diet, and ensure supportive and pleasant distractions from the stress such as a non-EMS circle of friends or a vacation away from the job.

In the past, Critical Incident Stress Management (CISM) was recommended for use in emergency medical services. However, current research suggests that CISM and critical incident stress debriefing (CISD) do not appear to mitigate the effects of stress and may actually interfere with the normal grieving/healing process. There remains an important role for competent mental health professionals at multiple-casualty incidents. They should be on scene to provide psychological first aid, survey EMS providers and victims for stress-related symptoms, and be available during the 2 months post-incident to screen and council anyone displaying stress-related symptoms.

16. Given a scenario involving a stressful situation, formulate a strategy to help adapt to the stress. pp. 44–45

When you are called to a situation that places you under stress, make a conscious decision to deal with it in an appropriate manner. Immediately control your breathing by taking deep breaths and letting the air out slowly through your mouth. Repeat this as needed, and then focus your energy on the essential tasks at hand. Tell yourself "I can do it" or "I can make it through this" and attend to the immediate needs of your patient. Once the immediate stressor is removed, make sure that you take care of yourself physically, emotionally, and mentally. Talk with members of your team about the event, and identify what you have done well and areas in which you can improve. Exercise regularly, eat properly, and take a vacation or a few days off. Examine the situation and your options, decide how best to handle the situation in the long term, and go on with your life. If a situation is extremely stressful, take advantage of your system's mental health services.

17. **Describe the stages of the grieving process (Kübler-Ross) and the unique challenges for paramedics in dealing with themselves, adults, children, and other special populations related to their understanding or experience of death and dying.** pp. 38–41

The grieving patient is likely to progress through five stages of the grieving process as described by Elisabeth Kübler-Ross. Those stages include anger, denial, bargaining, depression, and acceptance. A grieving person usually progresses through these stages in order, though he or she may skip around or move back and forth between stages. In the anger stage, the person vents the frustration over the inability to control the situation or control the outcome. Denial represents the inability or refusal to accept the reality of the event or situation. Bargaining is an unrealistic attempt to change or put off the outcome. Depression represents despair over the inevitable and withdrawal into a private world. Acceptance is realization and acceptance of the event or the patient's fate.

Even though paramedics are exposed to death and dying, they don't necessarily handle these events better than other people. All people tend to move through the same stages of the grieving process, although age and the patient's special circumstances may alter the presentation of those stages. Children may not recognize the significance and finality of the event or may fear that death may soon happen to themselves or others. Adults react differently, usually experiencing a "paralyzing" feeling followed by intense grief for weeks. The intensity gradually subsides with later peaks of feeling associated with anniversaries, birthdays, and the like. The elderly usually are concerned about the effects of their death on others and their loss of independence.

18. **Given photos of various motor-vehicle collisions, assess scene safety and propose ways to make the scene safer.** pp. 46–47

The scene of an emergency is inherently dangerous, especially when it involves an auto crash. The roadway becomes a hazard as oncoming traffic may collide with your ambulance, personnel on the scene, and the wrecked auto(s). The crash produces broken glass, jagged metal, and spilled fluids that may be slippery, hot, caustic (battery acid), or flammable. If the patient involved in the crash is hostile, he or she may pose a threat to care providers as may the patient's friends and family members or other bystanders. The incident may also affect utility poles, breaking their wires to create electrical hazards. The paramedic must use caution when approaching the scene and carefully rule out hazards. If any exist, you must eliminate them or not approach the scene. Do not attempt to correct a scene hazard unless you are specifically and properly trained and equipped to handle it. Place your vehicle to caution oncoming traffic and create a barrier between you and that traffic. At all scenes with jagged metal and broken glass, wear protective clothing, including gloves, boots, helmet, and a protective coat (turnout gear). If need be, "blind" the occupants of a stopped vehicle with a spotlight until you are sure it is safe to enter the scene. If there is any possibility of blood or body fluid exposure, observe body substance isolation procedures.

Content Self-Evaluation

MULTIPLE CHOICE

_____ 1. All of the following are benefits of physical fitness EXCEPT:
   A. decreased resting heart rate.
   B. decreased resting blood pressure.
   C. increased anxiety levels.
   D. enhanced quality of life.
   E. increased resistance to disease.

_____ 2. The core elements of physical fitness include all of the following EXCEPT:
   A. disease resistance.
   B. muscular strength.
   C. flexibility.
   D. cardiovascular endurance.
   E. aerobic capacity.

_____ 3. Exercise performed against stable resistance, where muscles are exercised in a motionless manner, is called:
   A. isometric.
   B. polymeric.
   C. aerobic.
   D. isotonic.
   E. polytonic.

_____ 4. The target heart rate for a 50-year-old female with a resting heart rate of 65 is:
   A. 103.
   B. 139.
   C. 152.
   D. 170.
   E. 220.

_____ 5. Flexibility is obtained by:
   A. isometric exercise.
   B. isotonic exercise.
   C. stretching.
   D. bouncing at the end of a range-of-motion exercise.
   E. weight lifting.

_____ 6. Which of the following is NOT a major food group?
   A. grains and breads
   B. dairy products
   C. fruits
   D. meat and fish
   E. simple sugars

_____ 7. A proper and healthy diet minimizes intake of which of the following?
   A. fast foods
   B. vitamins
   C. salt
   D. protein
   E. grains

_____ 8. Which of the following does NOT increase your risk for cardiovascular disease and cancer?
   A. prolonged, chronic, and unprotected sun exposure
   B. consumption of charcoal-grilled foods
   C. eating broccoli
   D. being a postmenopausal woman
   E. elevated cholesterol levels

_____ 9. Which of the following can reduce the risk of back injury?
   A. doing abdominal crunches
   B. stopping smoking
   C. following good nutritional practices
   D. getting adequate rest
   E. all of the above

_____ 10. Which of the following is NOT part of proper lifting?
   A. positioning the load as close to the body as possible
   B. locking your back in a slightly extended position
   C. reaching while twisting to distribute weight
   D. bending your knees
   E. keeping your palms up

_____ 11. Because a person carrying a contagious disease may present without signs, you must consider the blood and body fluids of every patient you treat as infectious.
   A. True
   B. False

_____ 12. Which of the following infectious diseases is NOT transmitted via airborne pathogens?
   A. hepatitis C
   B. pertussis
   C. tuberculosis
   D. varicella
   E. rubella

_____ 13. Which of the following items of personal protective equipment is/are recommended when suctioning a patient?
   A. gloves
   B. eyewear and mask
   C. gown
   D. both A and B
   E. A, B, and C

_____ 14. Which of the following items of personal protective equipment is/are recommended when assisting a mother with childbirth?
   A. gloves
   B. eyewear and mask
   C. gown
   D. both A and B
   E. A, B, and C

_____ 15. HEPA and N-95 respirators are intended to protect against:
   A. HIV/AIDS.
   B. tuberculosis.
   C. hepatitis B.
   D. hepatitis C.
   E. bacterial meningitis.

_____ 16. Proper handwashing requires:
   A. removing rings.
   B. lathering hands vigorously.
   C. scrubbing vigorously for at least 15 seconds.
   D. scrubbing under fingernails and in creases of the knuckles.
   E. all of the above

_____ 17. Which of the following is a recommended immunization for the paramedic?
   A. tetanus/diphtheria
   B. polio
   C. hepatitis B
   D. rubella
   E. all of the above

_____ 18. Used needles are to be disposed by:
   A. placing them in a properly labeled puncture-proof container.
   B. recapping them and placing them in a biohazard bag.
   C. returning them to the pharmacy for disposal.
   D. driving them deeply into the ground.
   E. breaking them and taping them together with the tips covered.

_____ 19. Sterilization uses which of the following to kill pathogens?
   A. bleach
   B. radiation
   C. EPA-approved chemical agents
   D. pressurized steam
   E. all of the above except A

_____ 20. Which of the following represent the standard progression through the stages of grieving?
   A. anger, denial, bargaining, acceptance, depression
   B. denial, bargaining, anger, depression, acceptance
   C. denial, anger, bargaining, depression, acceptance
   D. anger, denial, bargaining, depression, acceptance
   E. depression, anger, denial, bargaining, acceptance

_____ 21. A grieving patient who is withdrawing from friends and family and is unwilling to communicate with others is most likely in which stage of loss?
   A. denial
   B. anger
   C. depression
   D. bargaining
   E. acceptance

_____ 22. Because paramedics experience death more often than the general population, they experience less stress and are better able to cope with it.
   A. True
   B. False

_____ 23. At which age are children most likely to feel that death is a temporary absence from which the deceased person will return?
   A. newborn to age 3
   B. ages 3 to 6
   C. ages 6 to 9
   D. ages 9 to 12
   E. ages 12 to 18

_____ 24. When informed of the death of a loved one, some family members may explode in anger, throw things, and scream.
   A. True
   B. False

_____ 25. When informing the family of the death of a member, use the words "dead" or "died" rather than less definitive ones such as "moved on" or "has gone to a better place."
   A. True
   B. False

_____ 26. The type of stress that has positive effects is:
   A. distress.
   B. halcion.
   C. stimulation.
   D. eustress.
   E. gravitas.

_____ 27. Which of the following is NOT a typical stressor for people working in emergency medical services?
   A. shift work
   B. violent people
   C. waiting for calls
   D. limited responsibilities
   E. thirst

_____ 28. The human response to stress progresses through three stages, in this order:
   A. resistance, alarm, exhaustion
   B. alarm, resistance, exhaustion
   C. alarm, exhaustion, resistance
   D. resistance, exhaustion, alarm
   E. exhaustion, alarm, resistance

_____ 29. The physiological phenomena that occur at approximately 24-hour intervals and regulate body temperature, sleepiness, and appetite are called:
   A. estrorhythms.
   B. circadian rhythms.
   C. lunar tidals.
   D. fatigue/rest cycles.
   E. solar epochs.

_____ 30. When you work a regular night shift, a technique that may help you maintain the appropriate awake/sleep cycle is:
   A. sleeping during one "anchor time" for both on- and off-duty days.
   B. eating well before going to bed.
   C. sleeping during the day after you work a night shift and at night when off duty.
   D. sleeping in a warm place during the day.
   E. taking short naps rather than long sleep.

_____ 31. Which of the following is a warning sign of stress?
   A. withdrawal
   B. feeling of being abandoned
   C. difficulty making decisions
   D. aching muscles and joints
   E. all of the above

_____ 32. Which of the following is NOT a healthy behavior for dealing with or reducing stress?
   A. controlled breathing
   B. remaining distant from co-workers
   C. reframing
   D. creating a non-EMS circle of friends
   E. taking a vacation

_____ 33. An example of an event that is likely to be stressful for an EMS provider is:
   A. serious injury to a child.
   B. the death of a co-worker.
   C. an EMS operation causing a civilian death.
   D. a disaster.
   E. all of the above

_____ 34. The provision of practical palliative care within hours or days of a critical event is:
   A. defusing.
   B. demobilization.
   C. critical incident stress debriefing.
   D. psychological first aid.
   E. arbitration.

_____ 35. The major problem with multi-vehicle responses is:
   A. they slow the response.
   B. they complicate communications.
   C. other drivers may yield to one vehicle and not the other.
   D. if the wrong vehicle arrives first, it may slow extrication.
   E. none of the above

_____ 36. Some cultures find eye contact impolite.
   A. True
   B. False

_____ 37. Interpersonal safety begins with effective and positive communications.
   A. True
   B. False

_____ 38. Which of the following are common roadway hazards?
   A. downed power lines
   B. spilled hazardous chemicals
   C. moving traffic
   D. adverse weather conditions
   E. all of the above

_____ 39. The paramedic attending the patient in the back of the ambulance is too busy and must move about too much to wear a seatbelt.
   A. True
   B. False

_____ 40. When driving an ambulance, a paramedic must:
   A. ignore highway regulations as necessary to reach the patient.
   B. practice due regard for the safety of others.
   C. never exceed speed limits.
   D. always use an escort vehicle.
   E. none of the above

MATCHING

Body Substance Isolation Procedures

Write the letter or letters of the appropriate personal protective equipment necessary for each of the following procedures in the space provided.

A. gloves

B. mask and eyewear

C. HEPA or N-95 respirator

D. gown

_____ 41. Suctioning

_____ 42. Childbirth

_____ 43. Endotracheal intubation

_____ 44. Patient with suspected TB

_____ 45. Serious arterial blood loss

Part 5: Illness and Injury Prevention

Review of Chapter Objectives

After reading Part 5 of this chapter, you should be able to:

1. **Describe the incidence; morbidity; mortality; and the human, environmental, and socioeconomic impact of unintentional and alleged unintentional injuries.** pp. 47–48

   Injuries are the third leading cause of death in the United States overall and the leading cause of death for individuals between the ages of 1 and 44. Nearly 70,000 deaths are nonintentional, and the largest part of these are the result of vehicle collisions, fires, burns, falls, drownings, and poisonings. For every death there are approximately 19 hospitalizations and 254 emergency department visits. The lifetime cost of trauma exceeds $114 billion.

2. **Identify health hazards and potential crime areas within the community.** pp. 50–51

   Health hazards are plentiful in a community. Homes are frequent sites of injuries to children from burns, falls, and firearm discharges. Geriatric patients also frequently fall in their homes. The home setting is also a place where paramedics are likely to encounter infants of low birth weight, patients discharged early from health care facilities, and patients having problems with medication noncompliance—all groups that are at greater likelihood for needing emergency care. Recreational and workplace injuries are also common in communities. Bars and areas with previous records of high crime rates should also be considered as potential crime areas.

3. **Identify local municipal and community resources available for physical, socioeconomic crises.** pp. 48–49, 52–53

   Establish a list of community resources in your locality that are available to assist patients in crisis. Such sites might include prenatal clinics, urgent care centers, and social services organizations that can offer food, shelter, clothing, and mental health counseling or services or referral to clinics or other forms of health care service.

4. **List the general and specific environmental parameters that should be inspected to assess a patient's need for preventative information and direction.** pp. 50–53

   Factors that should be considered when assessing the need for injury/illness prevention include the availability of prenatal care; level of public compliance with use of proper vehicular restraints for infants and children; awareness of proper firearm control measures; awareness of the dangers of drinking and driving; the home environments of geriatric patients (who are susceptible to falls); awareness of the need for patients to comply with directions for using medications; and local hospital/health organization policies involving the early discharge of patients with illness or injury. By surveying your community in these areas, you may identify parameters in which public education and direction may be beneficial in preventing illness and injury.

5. **Identify the role of EMS in local municipal and community prevention programs.** pp. 47, 48–53

   The EMS provider can promote prevention by becoming an advocate of injury prevention. This may include teaching CPR and first aid courses for the public, teaching and supporting prevention programs, and being a role model and example by following safe practices (including BSI and ensuring scene safety) him- or herself.

6. Identify the injury and illness prevention programs that promote safety for all age populations. pp. 50–53

Childhood and flu immunization programs; prenatal, well baby, and elder-care clinics; defensive driving programs; workplace safety courses; and health clinics sponsored by hospitals or health care organizations are just some examples of injury and illness prevention programs available to people across a range of ages in the community.

7. Identify patient situations where the paramedic can intervene in a preventive manner. pp. 50–53

The paramedic can intervene at the scene of an illness or injury and take advantage of a teachable moment. In a nonjudgmental, nonthreatening way, the paramedic may identify behaviors that would prevent illness or injury—for example, wearing protective equipment like seat belts in a car or helmets when biking—and instruct the patient in their use. The paramedic may also identify community risks like improperly enclosed swimming pools, which are common sites of children drowning, or poorly protected railway crossings, which are likely sites of train-versus auto collisions.

8. Document primary and secondary injury prevention data. pp. 50–53

Frequently, prehospital care reports contain or can be designed to collect information about the patient behavior regarding safe practices. Information on seat belt use, airbag deployment, medication compliance, and the like may be helpful in identifying areas in which programs promoting safe practices could reduce illness and injury. The patient care report may also identify mechanisms that frequently result in injury and suggest areas in which preventative practices or safety equipment may help reduce mortality and morbidity.

Content Self-Evaluation

MULTIPLE CHOICE

_____ 1. Injury represents the _____ leading cause of death in the United States.
   A. first
   B. second
   C. third
   D. fourth
   E. fifth

_____ 2. While injuries are often considered to be caused by accident, they are most likely predictable and preventable.
   A. True
   B. False

_____ 3. The calculation made by subtracting a person's age at death from 65 produces a result called the:
   A. years of productive life.
   B. injury risk factor.
   C. secondary span.
   D. epidemiological age.
   E. vital factor.

_____ 4. A systematic method to collect, analyze, and interpret information about injury data is a(n):
   A. injury risk program.
   B. injury surveillance program.
   C. epidemiological intervention.
   D. secondary prevention program.
   E. risk data analysis.

_____ 5. EMS providers are well distributed throughout the population, are often considered to be champions of the health care consumer, and are high-profile health care role models.
   A. True
   B. False

_____ 6. A paramedic should enter a hazardous scene only when the proper rescue, utility, or hazardous materials teams are not available.
   A. True
   B. False

_____ 7. What percentage of child deaths are the result of injuries?
   A. one third
   B. one quarter
   C. one fifth
   D. one sixth
   E. one tenth

_____ 8. The most serious injuries associated with pediatric bicycle collisions are to the:
   A. neck.
   B. head.
   C. abdomen.
   D. chest.
   E. extremities.

_____ 9. The most common cause of injury to children younger than six years old is:
   A. bicycle collisions.
   B. auto crashes.
   C. falls.
   D. abuse.
   E. fire.

_____ 10. The term *accident* does not accurately reflect the nature of auto collisions.
   A. True
   B. False

_____ 11. The greatest cause of preventable injuries in the geriatric population is:
   A. skeletal failure.
   B. motor vehicle accidents.
   C. falls.
   D. intentional mechanisms.
   E. burns.

_____ 12. The early release of patients from health care facilities to help control health care costs is likely to cause an increase in the number of EMS responses.
   A. True
   B. False

_____ 13. Which of the following is an action you should take as an EMS responder to implement injury prevention strategies?
   A. Preserve response team safety.
   B. Recognize scene hazards.
   C. Engage in on-scene education.
   D. Know your community resources.
   E. all of the above

_____ 14. The opportunity presented by an emergency call to provide information to patients/bystanders about the future prevention of such an emergency is:
   A. a prevention protocol.
   B. a teachable moment.
   C. EMS empowerment.
   D. patient/provider prevention.
   E. tertiary prevention.

_____ 15. Which of the following is a possible community resource for injury or illness prevention?
   A. childhood and flu immunization program
   B. elder-care clinic
   C. workplace safety course
   D. prenatal and well-baby clinic
   E. all of the above

Part 6: Ethics in Advanced Prehospital Care

Review of Chapter Objectives

After reading Part 6 of this chapter, you should be able to:

1. **Define ethics and morals and distinguish between ethical and moral decisions in emergency medical service.** pp. 53–54

   Morals are social, religious, or personal standards of right and wrong. Ethics are rules or standards that govern the conduct of a group or profession. Ethics and morals, along with common law, govern how we function in prehospital emergency care.
   Ethical decisions regarding patient care involve what the public and peers expect of the paramedic. Moral decisions involve the paramedic's own values of right and wrong.

2. **Identify the premise that should underlie the paramedic's ethical decisions in out-of-hospital care.** pp. 54–55

   Ultimately, the decisions made by the paramedic should be guided by the question: What is in the best interest of the patient?

3. **Analyze the relationship between the law and ethics in EMS.** p. 53

   In general, the law takes a narrower and more specific look at behavior and identifies what is wrong in the eyes of society. Ethics takes a more general view of what is right or good behavior. Laws or the results of following them may be unethical, and the law often does not resolve ethical dilemmas.

4. **Compare and contrast the criteria used in allocating scarce EMS resources.** pp. 59–60

   The most common situation regarding allocation of resources that a member of EMS is likely to face is a multiple-casualty incident (MCI). At an MCI, the triage process sorts casualties into priorities for care because patient needs outstrip the available resources. In the civilian environment, the person with the most need for care (excepting those with mortal injuries) receives care first. In the military domain, those with the least serious injuries receive care first to help maintain the fighting force (and win the battle).

5. **Identify issues surrounding advance directives in making a prehospital resuscitation decision and describe the criteria necessary to honor an advance directive in your state.** pp. 56–58

   Advance directives, such as living wills and Do Not Resuscitate orders, are ways that patients can indicate their desire for the type of medical care they wish to receive should they become incapacitated. Such directives often present ethical dilemmas for paramedics because they are trained and expected to do all that is necessary to preserve life. When a paramedic confronts a situation involving an advance directive, he or she must weigh the patient's right to autonomy against what he or she feels is in the patient's medical best interest. Whenever you are presented with an advance directive, ensure that it is valid, current, and conforms to requirements in your state for such documents. When in doubt, resuscitate.

Content Self-Evaluation

MULTIPLE CHOICE

_____ 1. Although ethical problems often have a legal aspect, most ethical problems are solved in the field and not in a courtroom.
   A. True
   B. False

_____ 2. Most codes of ethics provide specific guidance for performance of the professional.
   A. True
   B. False

_____ 3. When faced with an ethical challenge, the best guiding question is which of the following?
   A. How would I like to be treated?
   B. What would the patient want?
   C. Which actions will account for the greatest good?
   D. What is in the best interest of the patient?
   E. What actions can I defend?

_____ 4. The term that means "desiring to do good" is:
   A. benevolence.
   B. justice.
   C. beneficence.
   D. autonomy.
   E. euphylanthropnia.

_____ 5. The Latin phrase *primum non nocere* means:
   A. "Do the best you can."
   B. "Avoid mistakes."
   C. "Maintain the patient's best interests."
   D. "First, do no harm."
   E. "Treat all patients fairly."

_____ 6. Which question best describes the impartiality test for analyzing an ethical situation?
   A. Can you justify this action to others?
   B. Would you want this procedure if you were in the patient's place?
   C. Would you want this procedure performed on you if you were in similar circumstances?
   D. Will you likely be questioned about the need for this procedure later?
   E. none of the above

_____ 7. When in doubt about the validity of a DNR order or the patient's desire to be resuscitated, you should:
   A. begin resuscitation immediately.
   B. await arrival of the DNR to verify its validity.
   C. contact medical direction for advice before beginning resuscitation.
   D. not resuscitate.
   E. begin with CPR and delay advanced interventions.

_____ 8. There are no circumstances in which it is appropriate to breach patient confidentiality.
   A. True
   B. False

_____ 9. When presented with a patient who is enrolled in a health maintenance organization (HMO) whose policy states that the patient must be cared for at a member institution, you are responsible to act in the patient's best interest.
   A. True
   B. False

32 ESSENTIALS OF PARAMEDIC CARE

_____ 10. When presented with orders from a physician that do not comply with your protocols and that you believe are not in the patient's best interest, you should:
   A. follow the physician's order and report your concerns to the medical director.
   B. ask the physician to repeat or confirm the order.
   C. ask the physician for an explanation of the order.
   D. not follow the physician's order.
   E. do all except A.

Medical/Legal Aspects of Advanced Prehospital Care

Review of Chapter Objectives

After reading this chapter, you should be able to:

1. Differentiate among legal, ethical, and moral responsibilities.   p. 66

A paramedic's legal responsibility to the patient and others is defined by statute, regulation, and common law. Failure to meet this responsibility may result in criminal or civil liability. Ethical responsibilities are those actions expected of a paramedic by the health care profession and by the public. Moral responsibilities are personal values of right and wrong and are governed by conscience. Legal, ethical, and moral factors guide an individual in his or her actions as a paramedic.

2. Describe the basic structure of the legal system and differentiate civil and criminal law.   pp. 66–67

There are four primary sources of law in the United States: constitutional, common, legislative, and administrative. Constitutional law defines governmental authority and gives the individual certain rights. Common law is based upon past judge-decided cases (case law) and is a fundamental principle of our legal system. Legislative law consists of statutes enacted at the federal, state, or local level. Administrative law consists of the regulations and rules that a governmental agency uses to implement legislative law. These four sources of law affect the legal responsibilities of the practicing paramedic.

Civil law is noncriminal legal action between individuals for such things as matrimonial, contract, and personal injury disputes. It may also include civil wrongs such as assault, battery, medical malpractice, and negligence. Criminal law addresses actions against society (crimes) such as rape, murder, and burglary and will fine or imprison those found guilty.

3. Differentiate licensure and certification.   p. 68

Certification is the recognition of an individual who has met predetermined qualifications to participate in a certain activity. It may be given by a governmental or other agency or by a professional association. Licensure is a process whereby a governmental agency grants permission to an individual, after meeting certain qualifications, to engage in a particular profession. A particular state may choose to require certification, licensure, or both for a paramedic to practice.

4. List reportable problems or conditions and to whom the reports are to be made. p. 69

Each state, through statutes and administrative regulation, may require prehospital care providers to report such matters as suspected spousal abuse, child neglect and abuse, abuse of the elderly, violent crimes, and public health threats such as animal bites and communicable diseases. Reports are made to the department of health, police, or other agencies as defined in statute or regulation.

5. Define the following terms:

  a. Abandonment p. 78
  This is the termination of a patient-paramedic relationship while the patient still desires and needs care without the paramedic's providing for the appropriate continuation of care.

  b. Advance directives p. 80
  These are documents created to express the patient's treatment choices should he or she become incapacitated or otherwise unable to express a choice of treatment.

  c. Assault p. 78
  This is placing a person in apprehension of immediate bodily harm without his or her consent.

  d. Battery p. 78
  This is the unlawful touching of an individual without his or her consent.

  e. Breach of duty p. 70
  This is the failure to act with the skill and judgment expected of a similarly trained paramedic under similar circumstances.

  f. Confidentiality p. 73
  This is the principle of law that prohibits the release of medical or other information about a patient without his or her permission.

  g. Consent (expressed, implied, informed, involuntary) p. 75
  Consent is the granting of permission to treat. Expressed consent occurs when a patient gives verbal or written permission to treat. Implied consent occurs when you presume the patient would give expressed consent if he or she were able. Informed consent is consent granted by the patient who knows the necessity, nature, and risks of treatment. Involuntary consent is consent to treat a patient given by the authority of a police agency or court.

  h. Do Not Resuscitate orders p. 80
  These are advance directives that define the life-sustaining equipment or procedures that may be used if the patient's heart or respirations cease.

  i. Duty to act p. 70
  This is the formal or informal responsibility of the paramedic to provide care.

  j. Emancipated minor p. 76
  This is generally someone under 18 years of age who is married, pregnant, a parent, a member of the armed forces, or financially independent and living away from home. Such a person is often considered legally able to give informed consent.

  k. False imprisonment p. 78
  This is the restraint or transport of a patient without consent, proper justification, or authority.

  l. Immunity p. 69
  This is the exemption from legal liability.

  m. Liability p. 66
  This is the legal responsibility for one's actions. Any deviation from the duty to act or the standard of care exposes the care provider to liability.

  n. Libel p. 74
  This is the act of injuring a person's character, name, or reputation by false and malicious written statements.

  o. Minor p. 76
  A minor is a person under 18 years of age for whom a parent, legal guardian, or court-appointed custodian gives informed consent.

p. **Negligence** p. 70

This is the deviation from accepted standards of care recognized by the law for the protection of others against the unreasonable risk of harm.

q. **Proximate cause** p. 71

This is the action or inaction of the paramedic that caused or worsened the damage suffered by the patient.

r. **Scope of practice** p. 68

This is the range of duties and skills paramedics are allowed and expected to perform.

s. **Slander** p. 74

This is the act of injuring a person's character, name, or reputation by false and malicious spoken statements.

t. **Standard of care** p. 70

This is the degree of skill and judgment expected of an individual when caring for a patient and is defined by training, protocols, and the expected actions of care providers with similar training and experience, working under similar conditions.

u. **Tort** p. 67

This is a category of law dealing with civil wrongs against an individual such as negligence, medical malpractice, assault, battery, and slander.

6. **Discuss the legal implications of medical direction.** pp. 68, 72

Medical direction, both on-line and off-line, helps define the paramedic's scope of practice. Protocols, policies, and procedures as well as medical direction from an on-line physician define what is the acceptable standard of care. The system medical director is responsible for supervising the protocols and continuing education of the paramedic. The on-line medical direction physician is responsible for supervising and directing the paramedic's actions at the scene and during transport. The paramedic is responsible for ensuring that the medical care given to the patient is appropriate and in keeping with the protocols. Any breach of duty or deviation from the standard of care that results in patient injury may result in charges of negligence.

7. **Describe the four elements necessary to prove negligence.** pp. 70–71

Four elements must exist before negligence can be proven. They include the duty to act, breach of duty, actual damages, and proximate cause. The duty to act is the direct or indirect responsibility to provide the patient with care. Breach of duty is the failure to meet the standard of care associated with the patient's needs. Damages are the actual physical, psychological, or financial harm suffered by the patient. Proximate cause means that the paramedic's action or inaction directly caused or worsened the harm suffered by the patient.

8. **Explain liability as it applies to emergency medical services.** pp. 66, 70–73

Liability in EMS is the legal responsibility to provide appropriate assessment, care, and transport of the ill or injured patient. That liability extends to the system medical director and on-line medical direction physician as well as to the paramedic who supervises the actions of others while at the emergency scene. They must ensure that those they supervise follow the standard of care.

9. **Discuss immunity, including Good Samaritan statutes, as it applies to the paramedic.** pp. 69, 72

The Good Samaritan statute may offer some liability protection to someone who assists at the emergency scene if that person acts in good faith, is not grossly negligent, acts within his or her scope of practice, and does not receive payment for his or her services. In some states, Good Samaritan statutes have been expanded to include both paid and unpaid EMS providers.

Governmental immunity is a judicial doctrine that protects the government from liability unless it accepts that liability. However, most states have waived these rights, and courts are becoming increasingly likely to strike any remaining immunity down.

10. Explain necessity and the standards for maintaining patient confidentiality that apply to the paramedic. pp. 73–74

The paramedic, through his or her involvement in patient care, learns sensitive information about the patients he or she treats. To encourage patients to continue to divulge this information, paramedics must respect its confidential nature and only divulge it to those with a need to know. Information regarding a patient may be released to those continuing care, in accordance with the patient's consent to release information, as required by law, and as necessary for billing purposes.

11. Differentiate expressed, informed, implied, and involuntary consent and describe the process used to obtain informed or implied consent. pp. 75–76

Expressed consent is that given in writing or verbally, while implied consent is assumed consent from a patient who is unable to give expressed consent. Informed consent is the consent for treatment given by a patient when he or she understands the necessity, nature, risks, and alternatives to care. Involuntary consent is the consent given by the authority of a police agency or court to treat an individual.

When a patient summons an ambulance, that action suggests that he or she is asking for help and consenting to treatment. However, a paramedic is obligated to explain what he or she is going to do to and for the patient and why he or she is going to do it. The paramedic must also determine if the patient is alert, oriented, and rational enough to make a competent decision to accept or refuse care. If the patient is not able to make a rational decision regarding care, then the paramedic may need to invoke implied consent. If the patient is a minor and the legal parent or guardian cannot be reached, consent is assumed (implied consent).

12. Discuss appropriate patient interaction and documentation techniques regarding refusal of care. pp. 76–77

When a patient refuses care, the paramedic must assure and document the following: the patient was legally able and competent to make the decision; the need for care and potential consequences of refusing care were explained; on-line medical direction was consulted; the patient was directed to see his or her own physician; and the patient was directed to call the ambulance if the symptoms return or get worse. The refusal form should be signed by the patient and either a family member or a police officer. If the patient refuses to sign a refusal of treatment form, then have his or her refusal witnessed by a family member or police officer.

13. Identify legal issues involved in the decision not to transport a patient, or to reduce the level of care. pp. 77, 79

A decision not to continue the care of a patient or to relinquish care to a lesser level of provider may expose the paramedic to charges of abandonment or negligence if the patient suffers harm. This is especially true if the paramedic has initiated advanced life support procedures like starting an IV or administering a medication.

14. Describe the criteria and the role of the paramedic in selecting hospitals to receive patients. p. 79

The patient's request to be transported to a particular hospital should be honored unless his or her particular care needs demonstrate otherwise. The decision to transport a patient to a facility other than the one requested must be based upon the patient's care needs, the capabilities of the requested facility, protocols, and interaction with the on-line medical direction physician.

15. Differentiate assault and battery. p. 78

Assault threatens bodily harm, while battery is unauthorized touching. These civil and criminal actions can be avoided by the paramedic's making sure to obtain expressed consent for treatment and to explain what he or she is planning to do for the patient before doing it.

16. Describe the conditions under which the use of force, including restraint, is acceptable. pp. 78–79

The use of force to restrain a patient may be necessary when the patient is violent or poses a danger to him- or herself or to others. Then only such force and restraint should be used as is required. In conditions where force and restraint are necessary to care for a patient, the police should be involved.

17. Explain advance directives and how they impact patient care. pp. 80–81

Advance directives permit the patient to define what care he or she would desire should they become incapacitated. Advance directives include Do Not Resuscitate (DNR) orders, which limit care actions that can be taken should the patient go into cardiac or respiratory arrest. Living wills are legal documents that also prescribe the care a patient may receive, including his or her desire to donate organs and to die at home or elsewhere. State statutes usually define the authority of DNRs, living wills, and other advance directives.

18. Discuss the paramedic's responsibilities relative to resuscitation efforts for patients who are potential organ donors. pp. 80–81

When presented with a patient who is a possible organ donor, it is essential for the paramedic to maintain adequate perfusion of that organ to ensure its viability. Employ resuscitation procedures including fluid therapy, cardiac compressions, and ventilation and notify the medical direction physician that you are transporting a possible organ donor.

19. Describe how a paramedic may preserve evidence at a crime or accident scene. p. 81

Your responsibility at the crime scene is first to ensure your safety and that of your patient and then to ensure the health of the victim (your patient). If the patient is not obviously dead, initiate resuscitation and care directed at his or her injuries. Limit any movement of articles around the patient and at the scene and, if possible, document what you moved and from what location you moved it. Do not cut through clothing where objects entered the body; remove the clothing without cutting it, or cut around the openings.

20. Describe the importance of providing accurate documentation of an EMS response. pp. 81–82

Documentation establishes what was found and what was done at the emergency scene. It must be completed promptly, thoroughly, objectively, and accurately. At the same time, the confidentiality of the information obtained must be maintained. The documentation will become a part of the patient's medical record and help guide continuing patient care. It will also become a record of what you did at the emergency scene and during transport should your actions ever come into question. It may also become a legal document in a court of law when someone feels they have been injured (damaged) by someone else.

21. Describe what is required to make a patient care report an effective legal document. pp. 81–82

A patient care report must be completed in a timely manner, must be thorough, must be objective, must be accurate, and must ensure patient confidentiality to be an effective legal document.

Content Self-Evaluation

MULTIPLE CHOICE

_____ 1. The term *liability* best refers to:
- A. an illegal act.
- B. legal responsibility.
- C. an act of negligence.
- D. civil responsibility.
- E. responsibility for damages.

_____ 2. Ethical responsibilities are best described as:
   A. requirements of case law.
   B. requirements of statute law.
   C. standards of a profession.
   D. personal feelings of right and wrong.
   E. legal concepts of right and wrong.

_____ 3. Which type of law is also called statutory law?
   A. case law
   B. common law
   C. legislative law
   D. administrative law
   E. regulatory law

_____ 4. Criminal law is best described as dealing with:
   A. wrongs committed against society.
   B. conflicts between two or more parties.
   C. contract disputes.
   D. negligence.
   E. breaches of faith.

_____ 5. Which of the following is a component of a paramedic's scope of practice?
   A. protocols
   B. system policies and procedures
   C. on-line medical direction
   D. training and continuing education
   E. all of the above

_____ 6. Which of the following is NOT a common mandatory reporting event?
   A. rape
   B. spousal abuse
   C. child abuse
   D. a seizure episode
   E. animal bites

_____ 7. Governmental immunity is a likely protection for the paramedic working for a municipality.
   A. True
   B. False

_____ 8. The Ryan White CARE act provides what protection to the paramedic?
   A. It requires a notification system for contagious disease exposure.
   B. It compensates EMS providers who contract AIDS.
   C. It permits EMS review of any patient records.
   D. It grants immunity to civil litigation in cases of ordinary negligence.
   E. It defines the restraints permissible while treating a violent patient.

_____ 9. Which of the following is NOT one of the elements required to prove a charge of negligence against a paramedic?
   A. duty to act
   B. proximate cause
   C. actual damages suffered by the patient
   D. payment to the paramedic
   E. breach of duty

_____ 10. Which of the following is a duty expected of the paramedic?
   A. to respond to the scene of an emergency
   B. to conform to the expected standard of care
   C. to provide care in accordance with the system's protocols
   D. to drive, or ensure the emergency vehicle is driven, appropriately
   E. all of the above

_____ 11. The degree of care, skill, and judgment that would be expected under like or similar circumstances by a similarly trained, reasonable paramedic is:
   A. the duty to act.
   B. the scope of practice.
   C. the standard of care.
   D. a proximate cause.
   E. malfeasance.

_____ 12. *Res ipsa loquitur* is a legal term that refers to:
   A. contributory negligence.
   B. immunity from prosecution.
   C. a matter that is self-evident.
   D. the victim's liability.
   E. the reliability of evidence.

_____ 13. Which of the following may protect a paramedic from charges of negligence?
   A. Good Samaritan statute
   B. governmental immunity
   C. the statute of limitations
   D. contributory negligence
   E. all of the above

_____ 14. Although many employers and agencies carry insurance coverage, it is a good idea for a paramedic to obtain personal coverage because the agency's coverage may be inadequate.
   A. True
   B. False

_____ 15. In many states, a paramedic would be guilty of practicing without a license if, while off duty, he or she performed advanced life support skills outside his or her system of medical direction.
   A. True
   B. False

_____ 16. Which of the following is NOT an acceptable reason for the release of confidential patient information?
   A. Medical providers need it to care for the patient.
   B. A judge has signed a court order demanding its release.
   C. It is necessary for third-party billing.
   D. Other paramedics, not on the call, have requested it.
   E. The patient has made a written request for its release.

_____ 17. The act of injuring an individual's character, name, or reputation by false written statements and with malicious intent is:
   A. slander.
   B. breach of confidentiality.
   C. malfeasance.
   D. misfeasance.
   E. libel.

_____ 18. Before beginning to treat a patient, a paramedic must obtain expressed consent.
   A. True
   B. False

_____ 19. The type of consent that is given by the authority of a court is:
   A. expressed.
   B. implied.
   C. involuntary.
   D. informed.
   E. common.

_____ 20. For a patient's consent to be informed, the patient must be told and understand:
   A. the nature of the treatment.
   B. the necessity of the treatment.
   C. the risks of the treatment.
   D. the risks of refusing the treatment.
   E. all of the above

_____ 21. Once a patient has given consent for treatment, he or she may not withdraw that consent.
   A. True
   B. False

_____ 22. A minor is usually considered someone under the age of:
   A. 16.
   B. 18.
   C. 19.
   D. 21.
   E. 25.

_____ 23. Conditions that may define a person as an emancipated minor include being:
   A. married.
   B. pregnant.
   C. a parent.
   D. a member of the armed forces.
   E. all of the above

_____ 24. Once a patient has withdrawn his consent to care, it may be considered assault to encourage him to go to the hospital.
   A. True
   B. False

_____ 25. Which of the following is NOT an essential element in accepting a patient's refusal of care?
   A. The patient is conscious, alert, and rational.
   B. The patient is a minor.
   C. The patient is aware of the possible consequences of his or her decision.
   D. The patient has been advised that he or she may call again for help if necessary.
   E. The patient and/or a disinterested witness has signed a release-from-liability form.

_____ 26. Ideally, a police officer should respond to the scene of all problem patients and sign the patient care report as a witness or, if the patient poses a threat to the paramedic, accompany the paramedic and patient to the hospital.
   A. True
   B. False

_____ 27. Ending a patient–care giver relationship without providing the appropriate continuing care and without the patient's approval could be found to be:
   A. battery.
   B. defamation.
   C. nonfeasance.
   D. abandonment.
   E. assault.

_____ 28. The unlawful act of touching another person without permission is:
   A. assault.
   B. abandonment.
   C. battery.
   D. slander.
   E. libel.

_____ 29. An important question to ask yourself when considering the restraint of a patient is:
   A. does the patient need immediate treatment.
   B. does the patient pose a threat to himself.
   C. does the patient pose a threat to others.
   D. all of the above
   E. none of the above

_____ 30. If you need to use force to restrain a patient, it is best to involve law enforcement whenever possible.
   A. True
   B. False

_____ 31. Under what situation should a paramedic NOT begin resuscitation of a pulseless, nonbreathing patient?
   A. The patient is obviously dead.
   B. The patient has a valid DNR order.
   C. There is obvious tissue decomposition.
   D. There is extreme dependent lividity.
   E. all of the above

_____ 32. Do Not Resuscitate orders usually restrict care providers from:
   A. performing CPR in case of cardiac arrest.
   B. performing a "slow code."
   C. performing a "chemical code."
   D. leaving the scene until the coroner arrives.
   E. contacting medical direction.

_____ 33. If there is any doubt about the authenticity or applicability of a DNR order, a paramedic should initiate resuscitation immediately.
   A. True
   B. False

_____ 34. Which of the following statements is NOT true regarding a paramedic's responsibility at the crime scene?
   A. He or she should contact law enforcement officers if they are not on the scene.
   B. He or she should not enter the scene unless it is safe.
   C. His or her primary responsibility is to preserve the evidence at the scene.
   D. He or she should not disturb the scene unless it is necessary for patient care.
   E. He or she should document the movement of any item at the scene.

_____ 35. Which of the following is NOT required when documenting a patient care response?
   A. completing documentation promptly
   B. ensuring that documentation is accurate
   C. ensuring that documentation is subjective
   D. ensuring that patient confidentiality is maintained
   E. ensuring that documentation is thorough

Chapter 3

Anatomy and Physiology

Part 1: The Cell and the Cellular Environment

Review of Chapter Objectives

Because Chapter 3 is lengthy, it has been divided into parts to aid your study. Read the assigned textbook pages; then, progress through the objectives and self-evaluation materials as you would with other chapters. When you feel secure in your grasp of the content, proceed to the next part.

After reading Part 1 of this chapter, you should be able to:

1. Describe the structure and function of the normal cell. pp. 88–90

The cell is the basic unit of life and structured like a self-sustaining city. The cell is bound by a membrane that permits certain substances to pass to maintain electrolyte balance and permit the movement of nutrients and waste products. The fluid filling the cell is cytoplasm while small structures, called organelles, perform specific functions within the cell. All cells have the same basic structure but differentiate into ones that perform differing functions. Muscle cells cause movement; nervous cells transmit impulses. Cells of the digestive system permit absorption; gland cells secrete substances such as hormones, mucus, sweat, and saliva; all cells also excrete wastes; and respiration is the process by which they transform oxygen and nutrients into energy. Cells also enlarge and divide in a process called reproduction. Cells are organized into tissues, tissues into organs, organs into organ systems, and organ systems into an organism.

2. List types of tissue. pp. 90–91

Epithelial tissue lines internal and external body surfaces. It provides protection and specialized functions such as secretion, absorption, diffusion, and filtration. Major examples are the skin and the lining of the digestive tract.

Muscle tissue has the capability to contract when stimulated. It is of three types: cardiac muscle, found only in the heart; skeletal muscle, which is under voluntary control; and smooth muscle, found in the intestines and blood vessels, which is not under voluntary control.

Connective tissue is the most abundant tissue in the body and provides support, connection, and insulation. Connective tissue includes bone, cartilage, and fat. Blood may also be classified as connective tissue.

Nerve tissue is specialized tissue capable of transmitting electrical impulses throughout the body and makes up the brain, spinal cord, and peripheral nerves.

3. **Define organs, organ systems, the organism, and system integration.** pp. 91–94

Organs are groups of tissue that function together to provide a specific or many specific functions. Examples include the heart, brain, kidneys, or lungs. Groups of organs also function together, in organ systems, to provide functions for the human body. Such organ systems include the cardiovascular system, the respiratory system, the gastrointestinal system, the genitourinary system, the reproductive system, the nervous system, the endocrine system, the lymphatic system, the muscular system, and the skeletal system. The sum of all cells, tissues, organs, and organ systems is the organism. System integration is the dynamic organization of the cells, tissues, organs, and organ systems that provides and maintains the internal environment, homeostasis.

4. **Discuss the cellular environment (fluids and electrolytes), including osmosis and diffusion.** pp. 94–101

The body goes to great lengths to maintain a constant internal and cellular environment (homeostasis). Major factors of this environment include hydration, the movement of substances into and out of the cell, and acid–base balance.

- **Hydration.** Water composes about 60 percent of the total body weight and plays a very important role in the body's internal environment. Some 75 percent of the body's water is contained within the cells (intracellular fluid), while 7.5 percent is contained within the vascular system (intravascular fluid). The remaining water is found between cells (interstitial fluid) and in other spaces within the body. An abnormal decrease in body hydration (dehydration) may be caused by increased gastrointestinal losses, sweating, internal (third space) losses, plasma losses, or other types of losses. An abnormal increase in body water is called overhydration.
- **Electrolytes.** Electrolytes are molecules that dissociate into negatively and positively charged particles (called ions) when dissolved in water. The normal distribution of body water is dependent on the distribution of electrolytes among the body spaces (intravascular, interstitial, and intracellular).
- **Osmosis and diffusion.** Diffusion is the movement of molecules from an area of higher concentration to one of lower concentration. Osmosis is the movement of a solvent (like water) through a membrane to equalize the concentration of electrolytes on each side of the membrane. The body also moves electrolytes through cell membranes (against the osmotic gradient) by active transport and facilitated diffusion. These processes are responsible for maintaining a fluid electrolyte balance among the intravascular, interstitial, and intracellular spaces.

5. **Discuss acid–base balance and pH.** pp. 101–104

The concentration of free hydrogen ions in a fluid reflects its acidity and is noted as a logarithmic value called pH. A pH of 1 is extremely acidic, while a pH of 14 is without hydrogen ions and extremely basic (or alkalotic). The body maintains a slightly alkalotic environment by regulating the quantity of free hydrogen ions. Normal body pH ranges from 7.35 to 7.45. The body maintains its pH through a bicarbonate buffer system, the respiratory system, and the kidneys.

Content Self-Evaluation

MULTIPLE CHOICE

1. The fundamental unit of life is:
   - A. the cell.
   - B. tissue.
   - C. the organ.
   - D. the organism.
   - E. DNA.

2. One of the three main elements of a typical cell is the:
   - A. cell membrane.
   - B. cilia.
   - C. leukocyte.
   - D. eosinophil.
   - E. basophil.

_____ 3. The characteristic ability of a cell membrane to selectively permit material to pass through it is called:
   A. diffusiveness.
   B. imperviousness.
   C. semipermeability.
   D. cytoplasmicism.
   E. isotonicism.

_____ 4. The thick viscous fluid that fills the cell and gives it shape is called:
   A. ribosome.
   B. lysosome.
   C. cytoplasm.
   D. protoplasm.
   E. either C or D

_____ 5. The structure that contains the genetic material including the cell's DNA is the:
   A. endoplasmic reticulum.
   B. Golgi apparatus.
   C. nucleus.
   D. mitochondria.
   E. cytokine.

_____ 6. The compound that provides the cell with most of its energy is:
   A. DNA.
   B. phosgene.
   C. carbon dioxide.
   D. ATP.
   E. carbohydrate.

_____ 7. The tissue type that covers the internal and external body surfaces is:
   A. epithelial.
   B. smooth muscle.
   C. nerve.
   D. connective.
   E. skeletal muscle.

_____ 8. The tissue type that is mostly under voluntary control is:
   A. epithelial.
   B. cardiac muscle.
   C. nerve.
   D. connective.
   E. skeletal muscle.

_____ 9. The tissue type that provides support and insulation is:
   A. epithelial.
   B. cardiac muscle.
   C. nerve.
   D. connective.
   E. skeletal muscle.

_____ 10. The body organ system that produces most body heat is the:
   A. muscular system.
   B. gastrointestinal system.
   C. genitourinary system.
   D. endocrine system.
   E. lymphatic system.

_____ 11. The body organ system that is important in fighting disease and filtration is the:
   A. muscular system.
   B. gastrointestinal system.
   C. genitourinary system.
   D. endocrine system.
   E. lymphatic system.

_____ 12. The term that is applied to the building up and tearing down of biochemical substances to produce energy is:
   A. anatomy.
   B. physiology.
   C. catabolism.
   D. anabolism.
   E. metabolism.

_____ 13. Ductless or endocrine glands secrete directly into the circulatory system.
   A. True
   B. False

_____ 14. The natural tendency of the body to maintain a constant internal environment is:
   A. cellular equilibrium.
   B. homeostasis.
   C. metabolism.
   D. physiology.
   E. paracrine signaling.

_____ 15. The body's major baroreceptors are located in the:
  A. arch of the aorta.
  B. brainstem.
  C. lung tissue.
  D. inner ears.
  E. medulla oblongata.

_____ 16. Most of the input affecting body organs and homeostasis occurs via the positive feedback loop.
  A. True
  B. False

_____ 17. The feedback system that decreases stimulation as the target organ responds is the:
  A. positive feedback loop.
  B. negative feedback loop.
  C. decompensation system.
  D. beta adrenergic system.
  E. cholinergic loop.

_____ 18. Extracellular fluid accounts for what percentage of total body water?
  A. 75 percent
  B. 60 percent
  C. 25 percent
  D. 17.5 percent
  E. 7.5 percent

_____ 19. The fluid space found between the vascular and cellular compartments is the extracellular compartment.
  A. True
  B. False

_____ 20. A fluid that dissolves other substances is a(n):
  A. solute.
  B. electrolyte.
  C. hydrate.
  D. solvent.
  E. anhydrous.

_____ 21. Which of the following is a source of body fluid loss and dehydration?
  A. diarrhea
  B. hyperventilation
  C. pancreatitis
  D. poor nutritional states
  E. all of the above

_____ 22. The term *turgor* refers to:
  A. intense thirst.
  B. skin tension.
  C. highly concentrated urine.
  D. sunken fontanelles.
  E. extreme obesity.

_____ 23. Which element is most common in the human body?
  A. hydrogen
  B. oxygen
  C. carbon
  D. nitrogen
  E. sodium

_____ 24. A positively charged ion is a(n):
  A. anion.
  B. cation.
  C. electrolyte.
  D. dissociated element.
  E. reagent.

_____ 25. The most prevalent cation in the human body is:
  A. magnesium.
  B. chloride.
  C. potassium.
  D. bicarbonate.
  E. sodium.

_____ 26. Which of the following ions is responsible for buffering the acid concentrations in the body?
  A. magnesium
  B. chloride
  C. potassium
  D. bicarbonate
  E. sodium

_____ 27. A solution that contains more solute concentration on one side of a semipermeable membrane than on the other is said to be:
   A. hypertonic.
   B. isotonic.
   C. hypotonic.
   D. osmotic.
   E. diffused.

_____ 28. When an isotonic solution is placed in the human bloodstream, water moves in which direction?
   A. into the vascular space
   B. does not move
   C. out of the vascular space
   D. in both directions
   E. none of the above

_____ 29. When a hypertonic solution is placed in the human bloodstream, water moves in which direction?
   A. into the vascular space
   B. does not move
   C. out of the vascular space
   D. in both directions
   E. none of the above

_____ 30. The movement of a solvent from an area of higher concentration through a semipermeable membrane to an area of lower concentration is termed:
   A. diffusion.
   B. osmosis.
   C. active transport.
   D. facilitated transport.
   E. oncosis.

_____ 31. The movement of water out of and then back into the capillary as it travels through the capillary is regulated by the protein concentration within the blood and the pressure as the blood is pushed through the capillary.
   A. True
   B. False

_____ 32. The pressure that draws water into the blood because of the proteins there is called:
   A. osmolarity.
   B. osmotic pressure.
   C. hydrostatic pressure.
   D. oncotic force.
   E. filtration.

_____ 33. The movement of water out of the plasma across the capillary membrane into the interstitial space is:
   A. osmolarity.
   B. osmotic pressure.
   C. hydrostatic pressure.
   D. oncotic force.
   E. filtration.

_____ 34. The higher the pH value, the lower the concentration of hydrogen ions.
   A. True
   B. False

_____ 35. The normal pH range in the human body is:
   A. 6.9 to 7.35.
   B. 7.35 to 7.45.
   C. 7.45 to 7.8.
   D. 6.9 to 7.8.
   E. none of the above

_____ 36. Which of the following would be considered alkalosis in the human?
   A. 6.9 to 7.35
   B. 7.35 to 7.45
   C. 7.45 to 7.8
   D. 6.4 to 6.9
   E. none of the above

_____ 37. A decrease in pH of 1 would reflect which change in the concentration of hydrogen ions?
   A. 100 times as great
   B. 10 times as great
   C. 1/10th as great
   D. 1/100th as great
   E. a doubling

_____ 38. The cellular environment of the human body is slightly acidic.
   A. True
   B. False

_____ 39. The body system that responds most rapidly to a change in the pH is the:
   A. respiratory system.
   B. cardiovascular system.
   C. digestive system.
   D. buffer system.
   E. genitourinary system.

_____ 40. The addition of hydrogen ions to the bloodstream will result in an increase in carbon dioxide.
   A. True
   B. False

Part 2: Body Systems

Review of Chapter Objectives

After reading Part 2 of this chapter, you should be able to:

1. **Describe the anatomy and physiology of the integumentary system, including the skin, hair, and nails.** pp. 105–107

The integumentary system is the largest body organ, accounting for about 16 percent of weight. It provides the outer barrier for the body and protects it against environmental extremes, fluid loss, and pathogen invasion. The three-layer structure consists of:

- **Epidermis.** The epidermis is the most superficial layer of the skin and consists of numerous layers of dead or dying cells. The epidermis provides a flexible covering for the skin and a barrier to fluid loss, absorption, and the entrance of pathogens.
- **Dermis.** The dermis is the true skin. It is made up of connective tissue and houses the sensory nerve endings; many of the specialized skin cells that produce sweat, oil, and so on; and the upper-level capillary beds that allow for the conduction of heat to the body's surface.
- **Subcutaneous tissue.** The subcutaneous layer, although not a true part of the skin, works in concert with the skin to insulate the body from heat loss and the effects of trauma. It consists of connective and adipose (fatty) tissues.

Hair grows from follicles nourished by capillary beds and grows as either vellus hair (peach fuzz) or terminal (normal) hair. Arrector muscles attach to the follicle and with contraction cause the hairs to stand erect. With age the growth of hair decreases, it turns gray with decreased pigmentation, and some of the hair turns from terminal to vellus hair.

Nails are found on the distal ends of the fingers and toes and are mainly for protection. They grow from the nail root toward the tip of the digit and cover a highly vascular nail bed that gives the nail its pink color. As we age, growth decreases with decreased distal circulation, resulting in hard, thick, brittle, and yellowish nails.

2. **Describe the anatomy and physiology of the hematopoietic system, including the components of the blood, and discuss hemostasis, the hematocrit, and hemoglobin.** pp. 107–116

The components of the hematopoietic system include the blood, bone marrow, liver, spleen, and kidneys. The process of hematopoiesis forms the cellular components of blood. In the fetus, this first takes place outside the bone marrow in the liver, spleen, lymph nodes, and thymus. By the fourth month of gestation, the bone marrow begins to produce blood cells. After birth and across the span of life, bone marrow continues to fulfill this critical function, barring the development of some pathological process.

In hematopoiesis, the stem cell reproduces to maintain a constant population of cells. Some stem cells further differentiate into myeloid multipotent stem cells that, in turn, differentiate into unipotent progenitors, which ultimately mature into the formed elements of blood: red blood cells, white blood cells, and platelets. Pluripotent stem cells may also differentiate into common lymphoid stem cells, ultimately becoming lymphocytes. Erythropoietin, the hormone responsible for red blood cell production, is produced by the kidneys and, to a lesser extent, the liver. The liver also removes toxins from the blood and produces many of the clotting factors and proteins in plasma. The spleen plays an important role in the immune system with its cells that scavenge abnormal blood cells and bacteria.

The components of the blood include the white blood cells, platelets, red blood cells, and plasma. White blood cells originate in the bone marrow from undifferentiated stem cells. Leukopoiesis is the process by which stem cells differentiate into the various immature forms of the white blood cell (leukocyte). These immature forms known as blasts mature to become granulocytes, monocytes, or lymphocytes. While leukocytes provide protection from foreign invasion, each type of white blood cell has its own unique function. Healthy people have between 5,000 and 9,000 white blood cells per milliliter of blood, but the presence of an infection can cause that number to rise to greater than 16,000.

Granulocytic white blood cells are of three types: basophils, eosinophils, and neutrophils. The basophils' primary function is in allergic reactions as they are storage sites for all of the body's circulating histamine. When stimulated, they degranulate and release histamine. Eosinophils can inactivate the chemical mediators of acute allergic response, thus modulating the anaphylactic response. The neutrophils' primary function is to fight infection.

Monocytes, another of the specialized WBCs, serve as the body's trash collectors, moving throughout the body to engulf both foreign invaders and dead neutrophils. Some monocytes remain in circulation, while others migrate to other sites to further mature into macrophages. Monocytes and macrophages also secrete growth factors to stimulate the formation of red blood cells and granulocytes. Some macrophages become fixed within tissues of the liver, spleen, lungs, and lymphatic system, becoming part of the reticuloendothelial system and having the capability to stimulate lymphocyte production in an immune response.

Lymphocytes, the primary cells of the body's immune response, can be found in the circulating blood, as well as in the lymph fluid and nodes, bone marrow, spleen, liver, lungs, skin, and intestine. These highly specialized cells contain surface receptor sites specific to a single antigen and initiate an immune response in order to rid the body of such agents.

Platelets or thrombocytes function to form a plug at an initial bleeding site and secrete several factors important to clotting. The normal number of platelets ranges from 150,000 to 450,000 per milliliter. Derived from megakaryocytes that arise from an undifferentiated stem cell in the bone marrow, platelets survive from 7 to 10 days and are removed from circulation by the spleen.

Erythropoiesis, the process of RBC production, is stimulated by erythropoietin that is secreted by the kidneys when the renal cells sense hypoxia. In turn, this stimulates the bone marrow to increase red cell production resulting in increased RBC mass and thus effectively, albeit slowly, increasing the oxygen-carrying capacity of the blood.

The life span of a red blood cell is approximately 4 months, although hemorrhage, hemolysis (RBC destruction), or sequestration by the liver or spleen may significantly reduce its life span. The spleen and liver contain macrophages (a specialized type of scavenger white blood cell) that can remove damaged or abnormal cells from circulation.

Plasma is the fluid portion of the blood and is a thick, pale yellow fluid that is 90 to 92 percent water and 6 to 7 percent proteins. It also contains electrolytes, fats, carbohydrates, gases, and chemical messengers. It transports nutrients and waste products to and from the body's cells and maintains the blood's oncotic pressure. The proteins with the plasma also assist in the clotting mechanisms and buffering the blood's pH balance.

Hemostasis involves three mechanisms that work to prevent or control blood loss, including vascular spasms that reduce the size of a vascular tear, platelet plugs (an aggregate of platelets that adheres to collagen), and lastly the formation of stable fibrin clots (coagulation).

Damage to cells or to the tunica intima (innermost lining of the blood vessels) triggers the clotting or coagulation cascade. This sequence of events (cascade) can be activated by either an intrinsic pathway (trauma to blood cells from turbulence) or an extrinsic pathway (damage to vessels).

Following the intrinsic pathway: platelets release substances that lead to the formation of prothrombin activator, which in the presence of calcium converts prothrombin to thrombin. Thrombin converts fibrinogen to stable fibrin, again in the presence of calcium, which then traps blood cells and more platelets to form a clot.

The extrinsic pathway is triggered with the development of a tear in a blood vessel. When this occurs, the smooth muscle fibers in the tunica media (middle lining of the blood vessels) contract and the resultant vasoconstriction reduces the size of the injury. This action reduces blood flow through the area, effectively limiting blood loss and allowing platelet aggregation (formation of a platelet plug) and the subsequent conversion of prothrombin activator.

Clotting factors or proteins are primarily produced in the liver and circulate in an inactive state. Prothrombin and fibrinogen are the best known of these factors. Damaged cells send out a chemical message that activates a specific clotting factor. This activates each protein in sequence until a stable clot is formed.

An enzyme on the surface of the platelet membrane makes it sticky. It is this stickiness that allows platelet aggregation to occur.

Hematocrit is the packed cell volume of red blood cells per unit of blood. This measurement is obtained by spinning a sample of blood in a centrifuge to separate the cellular elements from the plasma. Red cells are by far the heaviest component of the blood, due to their carrying the iron-containing hemoglobin and settle to the bottom of the tube. Immediately above the RBCs are the white blood cells and on top is the plasma layer. The height of the RBCs in the column is divided by the total height of the tube's contents (cellular component + plasma) and is reported as a percentage. The normal range is from 40 to 52 percent, although women tend to have slightly lower levels.

Oxygen diffuses to the blood and is transported on the hemoglobin molecule. Hemoglobin is a very efficient transporter of oxygen, and each gram holds 1.34 mL of oxygen when fully saturated. As blood passes by well-oxygenated alveoli, between 98 and 100 percent of the hemoglobin is fully saturated and carries 97 percent of the oxygen in the blood. The remaining oxygen is dissolved in the blood plasma. As the oxygenated blood reaches the tissue capillaries, hemoglobin releases the oxygen. The oxygen then diffuses through the capillary wall, into the interstitial space, and then through the cell membrane.

3. **Describe the anatomy and physiology of the musculoskeletal system, including bones, joints, skeletal organization, and muscular tissue and structure.** pp. 117–138

The skeletal system is a living body system that protects vital organs, acts as a storehouse for body salts and other materials needed for metabolism, produces erythrocytes, permits us to have an upright stature, and permits us to move with relative ease through the environment. The skeletal system consists of the axial and appendicular skeletons.

The common long bone consists of a diaphysis, metaphysis, and epiphysis. The diaphysis is the hollow skeletal shaft of the long bone and contains the yellow bone marrow. It is covered by the periosteum, which contains sensory nerve fibers and initiates the bone repair cycle. The metaphysis is the transitional region between the diaphysis and the epiphysis. In this region, the thin layer of compact bone of the diaphysis shaft becomes the honeycomb of the weight-bearing epiphyseal region. The epiphysis is the articular end of the bone. Through the widening of the metaphysis and the cancellous bone underneath, the weight-bearing, articular surface distributes support over a large surface area.

Bones join at an area called a joint, where they move together to permit articulation. The actual surface of movement is the articular surface and is covered with cartilage, a smooth, shock-absorbing surface that allows free movement between the two ends of the adjoining bones. It is the actual joint surface. The joint is held together with ligaments, which are bands of connective tissue attaching bones to each other. These bands encapsulate the joint and allow some stretch, while holding the articulating bones firmly together.

The skeletal system is organized into the axial and appendicular skeletons. The axial skeleton consists of the skull, thorax, and pelvis and the cervical, thoracic, lumbar, sacral, and coccygeal spine. The appendicular skeleton consists of the upper extremity (the humerus, radius and ulna, carpals, metacarpals, and phalanges) and the lower extremity (femur, tibia and fibula, tarsals, metatarsals, and phalanges).

Muscles make up most of the body's mass, are the driving power behind body motion, and also provide most of the body's heat energy. They only have the ability to contract with force; hence, they are usually paired with one opposing the motion of the other. Muscles are usually attached by strong connective tissue called tendons. The point of attachment that remains stationary with muscle contraction is the origin, while the point of attachment that moves is the insertion.

4. **Describe the anatomy and physiology of the head, face, and neck and their relation to the physiology of the central nervous system.** pp. 138–151

Several layers of soft, connective, and skeletal tissues protect the brain. These include the scalp, the cranium, and the meninges. The scalp is a thick and vascular layer of tissue that is strong and flexible and able to absorb tremendous kinetic energy. Beneath it are several layers of connective and muscular fascia that further protect the skull and its contents and that are only connected to the skull on a limited basis. This permits the scalp to move with glancing blows and further protects the cranium.

The skull consists of numerous bones, fused together at fixed joints called sutures. These bones form a container for the brain called the cranium. The cranium is made up of three layers of bone, two thin layers of compact bone separated by a layer of cancellous bone. This construction makes the cranium both light and very strong. This vault for the brain is fixed in volume and does not accommodate any expansion of its contents. However, in the newborn and infant, the skull is more cartilaginous and more flexible, with two open areas, the anterior and posterior fontanelles. These spaces close by 18 months.

The meninges are three layers of tissue—the dura mater, the arachnoid, and the pia mater—that provide further protection for the brain. The dura mater is a tough, fibrous layer that lines the interior of the skull and spinal foramen and is continuous with the inner periosteum of the cranium. The pia mater is a delicate membrane covering the convolutions of the brain and spinal cord. The arachnoid is a web-like structure between the dura mater and pia mater. The cerebrospinal fluid fills the subarachnoid space and "floats" the brain and spinal cord to help absorb the energy of trauma.

The brain occupies about 80 percent of the volume of the cranium and is made up of the cerebrum, cerebellum, and brainstem. The cerebrum occupies most of the cranial vault and is the center of consciousness, personality, speech, motor control, and perception. It is separated into right and left hemispheres by the falx cerebri, extending inward from the anterior, superior, and posterior central skull. The cerebellum sits beneath the posterior half of the cerebrum and is responsible for fine-tuning muscular control and for balance and muscle tone. It is separated from the cerebrum by the tentorium cerebelli, a fibrous sheath that runs transverse to the falx cerebri along the base of the cerebrum. The brainstem runs anterior to the cerebellum and central and inferior to the cerebrum. It consists of the hypothalamus, thalamus, pons, and medulla oblongata. The brainstem controls the endocrine system and most primary body functions including respiration, cardiac activity, temperature, and blood pressure.

The face, consisting of several bones covered with soft tissue, protects the special sense organs of sight, smell, hearing, balance, and taste and forms and protects the upper airway and the beginning of the alimentary canal. The brow ridge (a portion of the frontal bone), the nasal bones, and the zygoma form the eye sockets and protect the eyes. The upper jaw (the maxilla) and the moveable lower jaw (mandible) provide the skeletal structures that form the opening of the mouth. Cavities within this region (sinuses) help to provide shape to the face without increasing the weight of the head. The nasal cavity provides an extended surface to warm, humidify, and cleanse incoming air. The oral cavity houses the tongue and teeth and accommodates the early physical and chemical breakdown of food.

The neck supports the head through the structure of the cervical spine and the massive muscles of the region. It is also an important region through which many important structures traverse.

The airway travels through this region, and its components include the larynx and trachea. Posterior to the trachea is the esophagus with the carotid artery and jugular vein pairs just lateral to this airway structure.

5. Describe the anatomy and physiology of the spine, including the cervical, thoracic, lumbar, and sacral spine and the coccyx. pp. 151–155

Cervical spine

The cervical spine is the vertebral column between the cranium and the thorax. It consists of seven irregular bones held firmly together by ligaments that both support the weight of the head and permit its motion while protecting the delicate spinal cord that runs through the central portion of these bones.

Thoracic spine

The thoracic vertebral column consists of 12 thoracic vertebrae, one corresponding to each rib pair. Like the cervical spine, it consists of irregular bones held firmly together by ligaments that support the weight of the head and neck and permit its motion, while protecting the delicate spinal cord that runs through the central portion of these bones.

Lumbar spine

The lumbar spine consists of five lumbar vertebrae with massive vertebral bodies to support the weight of the head, neck, and thorax. Here the spinal cord ends at the juncture between L-1 and L-2, and nerve roots fill the spinal foramen from L-2 into the sacral spine.

Sacral spine

The sacral spine consists of five sacral vertebrae that are fused into a single plate that forms the posterior portion of the pelvis. The upper body balances on the sacrum, which articulates with the pelvis at a fixed joint, the sacroiliac joint.

Coccyx

The coccygeal region of the spine consists of three to five fused vertebrae that form the remnant of a tail.

6. Describe the anatomy and physiology of the thorax, including its skeletal and muscular structure and the organs and vessels contained within it. pp. 155–160

The ribs, thoracic spine, sternum, and diaphragm define the structure of the thoracic cage. The skeletal components allow the cage to expand as the ribs are lifted upward and outward by contraction of the intercostal muscles, and the intrathoracic volume further expands as the diaphragm contracts and moves downward. The net action of this muscle movement is to increase the volume of the thoracic cage and to reduce its internal pressure. Air from the environment moves through the airway into the alveoli to equalize this pressure, and inspiration occurs. The intercostal muscles relax and the thorax settles, while the diaphragm rises back into the thorax, and the volume of the cavity decreases. This increases the intrathoracic pressure, and air rushes out to equalize with the environment. This is expiration. The pleura, two serous membranes, seal the lungs to the interior of the thoracic cage during this action and ensure that the lungs expand and contract with the changing volume of the thoracic cavity. The lungs have exceptional circulation, with capillary beds surrounding the alveoli to ensure a free exchange of oxygen and carbon dioxide between the alveolar air and the bloodstream.

The lungs fill all but the central portion of the chest cavity and are found on either side of the central structure, called the mediastinum. The mediastinum contains the heart, trachea, esophagus, major blood vessels, and several nerve pathways. The heart is located in the left central chest and is the major pumping element of the cardiovascular system. The inferior and superior vena cavae collect blood from the lower extremities and abdomen and the upper extremities, head, and neck, respectively, and return it to the heart. The pulmonary arteries and veins carry blood to and from the lungs respectively, and the aorta distributes the cardiac output to the systemic circulation. The trachea enters the mediastinum just beneath the manubrium and bifurcates at the carina into the left and right mainstem bronchi. The esophagus enters the mediastinum just behind the trachea and exits through the diaphragm.

7. **Describe the anatomy and physiology of the nervous system, including the neuron, the central nervous system (brain and spine), and the peripheral nervous system (somatic, autonomic, sympathetic, and parasympathetic divisions).** pp. 160–178

The nervous system is the body's chief control for virtually every major function. It is divided physically into the central nervous system (CNS) and peripheral nervous system (PNS). The CNS consists of the brain and spinal cord. If the body were visualized as a computer, the CNS would be the central processing unit. Basic functions, such as continuance of heartbeat and respiration, and complex functions, such as listening to Mozart and anticipating a musical passage you particularly like, are controlled by cells in the brain. Messages within the CNS, as well as those that connect it with the rest of the body, travel as nerve impulses. The complex network of nerves outside the CNS makes up the peripheral nervous system.

The messages that carry information regarding critical body functions such as respiration pass through a part of the PNS called the autonomic nervous system; these functions do not require any conscious effort to maintain them. In contrast, messages that involve voluntary, or conscious, actions and thoughts travel through the other part of the PNS, the somatic nervous system. Both the autonomic and somatic nervous systems have two parallel tracks: one of nerves that carry messages to the brain, and another that carries messages from the brain. In terms of the computer analogy, the PNS carries the various input and output messages that run between the brain and spinal cord and the rest of the body. The autonomic nervous system is also structurally and functionally broken into two parts: the sympathetic and parasympathetic nervous systems. These two parts work together to make sure the net balance of stimulatory and inhibitory messages from the brain keep body functions such as blood pressure within normal limits.

The basic structural and functional unit is the neuron, or nerve cell. Nerve cells have a body that contains the essential cell machinery of the nucleus, mitochondria, and so on. Nerve processes (usually there are many) that are capable of receiving impulses from other neurons or body cells are called dendrites. An impulse that is picked up by a dendrite travels toward the cell body. Another process, the axon, carries the impulse away from the cell body. Axons may have multiple tips, which means the neuron has the capacity to send the impulse onward to more than one other nerve or other cell. Dendrites associated with neurons of the major sense organs (such as the eye or ear) convert an environmental stimulus into a nerve impulse that can be forwarded via the axon to other nerves, and eventually the brain. Dendrites associated with neurons that monitor internal conditions such as PaO_2 also convert that information into an impulse and send it to the brain. Eventually all such information is analyzed by neurons in the brain, and response impulses travel back through the PNS. These impulses eventually affect a motor neuron, causing a muscle cell to contract, or affect another type of cell such as one in a gland. Messages cannot pass directly from an axon to a dendrite because there is a tiny physical gap, called a synapse, between each pair of neurons. As the wave of electrical depolarization (due to ion fluxes of potassium rapidly leaving the neuron and sodium rapidly entering) reaches the axon tip, it causes a chemical called a neurotransmitter to be released into the synapse. (There are multiple neurotransmitters within the body. Either acetylcholine or norepinephrine is found in the neurons of the PNS. Neurotransmitters within the CNS include dopamine and serotonin.) When the neurotransmitter crosses the synapse and is taken up by the dendrite on the other side, a wave of depolarization is started in that dendrite, and the nerve impulse is then carried toward the cell body.

Most of the CNS is protected by the bones of the cranium and spine. The spinal column is made up of 33 vertebrae running from the neck to the junction with the pelvis. There is also an inner shock-absorbing, cushioning protection system. The cells of the brain and spinal cord are bathed in cerebrospinal fluid, and there are three layers of protective membranes between the neural surface and the outer, protective bone. These meninges are called the dura mater, arachnoid membrane, and pia mater (in outer-to-inner sequence). As you look at a human brain, it has six obvious structural regions: the cerebrum, the diencephalon, the mesencephalon (or midbrain), the pons, the medulla oblongata, and the cerebellum. Sometimes, this is simplified into the terminology of the forebrain (cerebrum and diencephalon), the midbrain (mesencephalon), and the hindbrain (the brainstem—pons and medulla oblongata—and the cerebellum). The largest part of the brain, with its characteristic folded outer surfaces, is the cerebrum. The cerebrum has left and right sides, or hemispheres, which are connected physically and functionally by tissue called the corpus callosum. The cerebrum is responsible for intelligence, learning, memory, and language, as well as analysis and response to sensory and motor activities. The diencephalon is covered by the cerebrum, and it is made up of a number of vital structures: the thalamus, hypothalamus, and the limbic system. This primal part of the brain is responsible for many involuntary functions such as temperature regulation, sleep, water balance, stress response, and emotion. It also has an important role in regulating the autonomic nervous system. The brainstem consists of the mesencephalon, pons, and medulla oblongata. The mesencephalon is located between the diencephalon and the pons, and it plays a role in motor coordination. It is the major region controlling eye movement. The pons is a major connection point between the upper portions of the brain and the medulla and cerebellum. The medulla oblongata itself marks the division between the brain and the spinal cord. The major centers for control of respiration, cardiac activity, and vasomotor activity are located here. The cerebellum is located in the posterior fossa of the cranium, and it also has two hemispheres, which are closely coordinated to the brainstem and higher centers. The cerebellum coordinates fine motor movement, posture, equilibrium, and muscle tone.

The hemispheres of the cerebrum do not contain identical centers. Rather, the functional responsibilities of the cerebrum have been mapped as a whole. Important centers with clinical implications in cases such as stroke or trauma include the following: (1) speech, which is located in the temporal lobe; (2) vision, which is located in the occipital lobe; (3) personality, which is located in the frontal lobes; (4) sensory, which is located in the parietal lobes; and (5) motor, which is located in the frontal lobes. As noted previously, balance and coordination are located in the cerebellum. A last important center is called the reticular activating system (RAS), which operates in the lateral portion of the medulla, pons, and especially the mesencephalon. The RAS sends impulses to and receives messages from the cerebral cortex (the outer portion of the cerebrum). This diffuse system of interlaced cells is responsible for maintaining consciousness and the ability to respond to external stimuli.

The brain receives about 20 percent of the body's total blood flow per minute. Vascular supply to the brain is provided by two systems, a physical arrangement that provides secondary supply if one system is occluded or severed. The anterior system is the carotid, and the posterior system is the vertebrobasilar. They join at the circle of Willis before entering the structures of the brain itself. Venous drainage is via the venous sinuses and the internal jugular veins. As previously noted, there is also cerebrospinal fluid (CSF) bathing the tissues of the brain and spinal cord. Most of the intracranial CSF is found in the ventricles.

The spinal cord is 17 to 18 inches long on average in adults. It leaves the brain at the medulla and passes through an opening in the skull called the foramen magnum to enter the spinal canal. The spinal cord, which ends near the level of the first lumbar vertebra (the reason why spinal taps are done below that level), conducts impulses to and from the peripheral nervous system and locally for motor reflexes. Thirty-one pairs of nerves exit the spinal cord between adjacent vertebrae. The dorsal nerve roots carry afferent fibers, ones carrying impulses to the brain. The ventral roots carry efferent fibers, which carry impulses from the brain to the periphery. Each nerve root has a corresponding area of skin called a dermatome, to which it supplies sensation. In the field, you may be able to correlate sensory deficits to the level of a spinal cord problem. The reason why our protective motor reflexes are so fast and effective lies in the fact that the afferent and efferent impulses are coordinated in the spinal cord—they do not travel the whole way to the brain before coming back. However, because they are mediated in the spinal cord, they lack fine motor control.

The peripheral nervous system (PNS) contains 12 pairs of cranial nerves, which extend directly from the lower surface of the brain and exit through small holes in the skull, and the peripheral nerves, which exit from the spinal cord as noted previously. The nerves of the PNS control both voluntary and involuntary activities. The cranial nerves supply nervous control for the head, neck, and certain thoracic and abdominal organs. The peripheral nerves can be divided into four classes: (1) somatic sensory, afferent nerves that carry impulses concerned with touch, pressure, pain, temperature, and position; (2) somatic motor, efferent nerves that carry impulses to the skeletal (voluntary) muscles; (3) visceral (autonomic) sensory, afferent nerves that carry impulses of sensation from the visceral organs (examples being fullness in the bladder or distension of the rectum); and (4) visceral (autonomic) motor, efferent nerves that serve the involuntary cardiac muscle and the smooth muscle of the viscera and the glands.

The involuntary division of the PNS is called the autonomic nervous system, and it has two components: the sympathetic nervous system and the parasympathetic nervous system. The sympathetic system is associated with the primitive "fight or flight" response to sensory stimuli. Its major nerve roots are located near the thoracic and lumbar part of the spinal cord. Stimulation causes increased heart rate and blood pressure, pupillary dilation, rise in blood sugar, as well as bronchodilation, all responses that ready the body for stress. The neurotransmitters norepinephrine and epinephrine mediate the sympathetic nervous system's actions. Sympathetic activity is also closely correlated to activity in the adrenal medulla, tissue that is of nervous system origin and that also relies on norepinephrine and epinephrine. The parasympathetic nervous system is responsible for controlling vegetative functions such as normal heart rate and blood pressure. It is associated with the cranial nerves and the sacral plexus of nerves, and it is mediated by the neurotransmitter acetylcholine. When stimulated, it causes a decrease in heart rate, an increase in digestive activity, pupillary constriction, and a reduction in blood sugar.

8. **Describe the anatomy and physiology of the endocrine system, including the glands and other organs with endocrine activity.** pp. 177–188

There are eight major structures associated with the endocrine system located throughout the body: the hypothalamus, pituitary gland, thyroid gland, parathyroid glands, thymus, pancreas, adrenal glands, and gonads. The pineal gland is also part of the endocrine system.

The hypothalamus, located deep within the cerebrum of the brain, is the junction between the endocrine system and the central nervous system. About the size of a pea, the pituitary gland is located adjacent to the hypothalamus within the cerebrum. The pineal gland is also located adjacent to the hypothalamus. The double-lobed thyroid gland is located in the neck anterior to and just below the cartilage of the larynx. The parathyroid glands are very small and are found on the posterior lateral surface of the thyroid gland. The thymus is located in the mediastinum just behind the sternum. The pancreas is located in the upper abdomen behind the stomach and between the duodenum and the spleen. The adrenal glands are somewhat triangular in shape and are located on the superior surface of the kidneys. Gonads can be found in the lower pelvis in women, with each ovary resembling an almond in size and shape. In men, the gonads are located in the scrotum.

The endocrine system is closely linked to the nervous system and plays a critical role in our ability to maintain life by regulating many bodily functions through chemical substances called hormones. The endocrine system is made up of ductless glands, which manufacture and secrete hormones that act in adjacent tissues or travel via the bloodstream to target organs or other endocrine glands to produce specific or generalized effects. Hormones regulate metabolic activity, growth, and development, as well as mediate chemical reactions, maintain homeostatic balance, and initiate our adaptive response to stress.

9. **Describe the anatomy and physiology of the cardiovascular system, including the heart and the circulatory system.** pp. 188–200

The adult heart is roughly the size of a clenched fist, and it lies in the center of the mediastinum posterior to the sternum and anterior to the spine. Roughly two thirds of the heart lies to the left of midline, with roughly one third to the right. The bottom of the heart, the apex, lies just above the diaphragm, whereas the top of the heart, or base, lies at roughly the level of the second rib. The heart's connections with the great vessels are at the base. The heart is made up of three tissue layers: The innermost is the endocardium, which has the same type of cells as the endothelial lining of blood vessels and is continuous with the linings of the vessels entering and leaving the heart. The thickest layer is the middle layer of muscle cells, the myocardium. These unique muscle cells physically resemble skeletal muscle but have electrical properties similar to smooth muscle cells. The outermost layer of the heart is the pericardium, a protective sac made of connective tissue arranged in two layers, the visceral pericardium (also called the epicardium) and the parietal pericardium. Normally, about 25 mL of pericardial fluid is contained between the two layers of pericardium, and the heart moves freely within the pericardial sac.

The heart is made up of two side-by-side pumps, the left side and the right side. Each side has an upper chamber, the atrium, which receives blood, and a lower chamber, the ventricle, which pumps blood into other blood vessels. The atria are separated by an interatrial septum, and the ventricles are separated by an interventricular septum. The atrial walls are thin in contrast with the ventricular walls, and almost all of the heart's pumping force is generated by the ventricles. The left ventricle, which pumps blood into the aorta, has a much thicker wall than the right ventricle, which pumps blood into the pulmonary artery.

The heart contains two sets of valves that help to keep blood flowing properly through the chambers and into the aorta and pulmonary artery: The atrioventricular valves lie between each atrium and ventricle. The left atrioventricular valve is called the mitral valve, and it has two characteristic leaflets. The right atrioventricular valve is called the tricuspid valve, and it has three characteristic leaflets. When the papillary muscles that connect the valves to the walls of the heart relax, the leaflets open and blood flows from the atria into the ventricles. Special fibers called the chordae tendoneae connect the leaflets of a valve to the papillary muscles, and these fibers prevent the leaflets from prolapsing back into the atrium when the valve is open. The semilunar valves lie between the ventricles and the artery into which each empties. The left semilunar valve, or aortic valve, lies between the left ventricle and the aorta. The right semilunar valve, or pulmonic valve, lies between the right ventricle and the pulmonary artery. When these valves open, blood flows in a one-way path from the ventricles into the arteries, and backflow into the ventricles is prevented.

The superior and inferior vena cavae carry deoxygenated blood from the body to the right atrium. Blood flows through the right atrium and ventricle before entering the pulmonary artery, which carries it to the lungs. Oxygenated blood leaves the lungs through the pulmonary veins and enters the left atrium. The left ventricle pumps the blood into the aorta, which feeds the oxygenated blood into peripheral arteries to flow to the rest of the body. Pressure within the heart is markedly higher on the left than on the right because resistance to flow is higher in the peripheral circulation than it is in the pulmonary circulation. Consequently, the myocardium of the left ventricle thickens as an infant ages to the point that the adult left ventricle is markedly thicker than the right.

The circulatory system consists of two subsystems. In pulmonary circulation, blood enters the lungs via the pulmonary arteries and their smaller branches, the arterioles. It eventually flows through capillaries that form networks over alveoli, and gas exchange (movement of oxygen into the blood and carbon dioxide from the blood) takes place here. The oxygenated blood then flows into the pulmonary venules and larger pulmonary veins and enters the left atrium. The peripheral circulation begins with the aorta, which receives oxygenated blood from the left ventricle. The aorta has numerous branches. These arteries and the smaller arterioles ensure that oxygenated blood flows to all parts of the body. Oxygenated blood eventually enters capillary beds, and oxygen exchange between blood and tissues occurs. Deoxygenated blood enters smaller venules, which empty into the larger veins that return blood to the right atrium. Gas exchange occurs in capillaries because their walls are only one cell thick. This same cell layer, the endothelium, is the innermost layer of arteries and veins.

10. Describe the physiology of perfusion. pp. 200–205

Perfusion is the process by which oxygen, nutrients, waste products, and carbon dioxide are brought to and taken from the body cells. It is essential to life, and its breakdown is the process we call shock. To ensure adequate perfusion, the body requires a pump, fluid volume, and a container. The pump is the heart and for proper cardiac output, the heart must receive an adequate supply of blood (preload), have an adequate contractile force, and a proper rate of contractions. The system's fluid, blood, must be in adequate supply and fill the container, the vascular system. Additionally, the container must maintain an adequate pressure so it is able to direct blood to the tissues in need. It maintains this pressure by constricting or dilating the arterioles to maintain blood pressure. Baroreceptors monitor blood pressure and control it by changing the heart rate, strength of contraction, size of the vascular container, or the number and degree of arterioles in constriction or dilation.

11. Describe the anatomy of the respiratory system (upper and lower airway and pediatric airway) and the physiology of the respiratory system (respiration and ventilation and measures of respiratory function). pp. 205–217

The mouth, or oral cavity, is a single cavity that serves as an auxiliary air passage. The posterior upper surface is the soft palate, which moves upward and closes off the passages from the nose to the pharynx during swallowing. The nasal cavity is a hollow two-sided chamber lined with mucous membranes that warms, filters, and humidifies air as it enters the respiratory system. Its anterior openings are the nares, or nostrils. The nasal and oral cavities empty into the pharynx, or throat. The pharynx is a muscular tube that functions as the transitional area for food and air between the nose and mouth and between the esophagus and larynx.

The larynx is the tubular structure that begins the lower airway. It consists of the thyroid and cricoid cartilages, the vocal cords, the arytenoid folds, and the upper portion of the trachea. It is the "Adam's apple" located in the anterior neck. The epiglottis is a flap-like structure covering the opening of the trachea, the glottis. It closes during swallowing to prevent food or fluids from entering the trachea and respiratory system. The vallecula is a fold formed by the epiglottis and base of the tongue. The larynx opens into the trachea, a series of cartilaginous C-shaped structures that hold the airway open. The trachea divides into two mainstem bronchi at the carina. The bronchi subdivide, finally reaching the respiratory bronchioles, the alveolar ducts, and, finally, the alveoli. The alveoli are the primary exchange structures between the respiratory system and the pulmonary capillaries of the cardiovascular system for oxygen and carbon dioxide.

The gross anatomy of the pediatric airway is very similar to that of the adult but is smaller in size with smaller airway clearances and a greater proportion of soft tissue. The larynx is more superior and anterior than in the adult, and the smallest clearance of the airway is the cricoid cartilage rather than the glottis as it is in the adult. The child's tongue is proportionally larger and more easily obstructs the airway. Because of the smaller lumen size, the soft tissue swelling may obstruct the airway more quickly.

Respiration is the exchange of gases between a living organism and its environment. The volume of the thorax expands as the diaphragm contracts and displaces downward. The intercostal muscles contract, pulling the rib cage upward and outward. The muscles of the neck enhance this action as they lift the sternum. The lungs expand with the chest as the pleural seal secures the exterior of the lung to the interior of the thorax. The expansion of the lungs reduces the air pressure within them, and air flows into the alveoli. Gravity and the intrinsic elasticity of the lungs then cause the thorax to settle, the pressure within the lungs to increase, and air to be exhaled.

The air brought into the lungs contains 21 percent oxygen and very little carbon dioxide. Oxygen diffuses through the alveolar and capillary walls and is bound to the hemoglobin, while carbon dioxide diffuses in the opposite direction. The air exhaled contains about 14 percent oxygen and 5 percent carbon dioxide. The oxygen from inspired air diffuses from the alveolar space through the alveolar wall and the pulmonary capillary membrane, where it attaches to the hemoglobin of the blood. Carbon dioxide, mostly transported as bicarbonate, diffuses from the blood plasma across the capillary membrane and through the alveolar wall.

The measures of respiratory function include:

- Total Lung Capacity (TLC) is the volume of air in the lungs after a maximal inspiration, about 6 liters in the adult male.
- Tidal Volume (V_T) is the average volume of air inspired (or expired) with each breath, about 500 mL in the adult male.
- Dead Space Volume (V_D) is the portion of the tidal volume that does not reach the alveoli and is unavailable for gas exchange, about 150 mL.
- Alveolar Volume (V_A) is the amount of air that reaches the alveoli with each breath, about 350 mL.
- Minute Volume (V_{min}) is the amount of air moved in and out of the respiratory system in one minute (minute volume = tidal volume × respiratory rate).
- Alveolar Minute Volume ($V_{A\text{-}min}$) is the amount of gas that reaches the alveoli per minute.
- Inspiratory Reserve Volume (IRV) is the amount of air that can be inspired after a normal inspiration.

- Expiratory Reserve Volume (ERV) is the amount of air that can be exhaled after a normal exhalation.
- Residual Volume (RV) is the amount of air in the lungs after a maximal exhalation.
- Functional Residual Capacity (FRC) is the amount of air remaining in the lungs after a normal expiration.
- Forced Expiratory Volume (FV) is the amount of air a person can exhale after a maximal inhalation, about 4,500 mL in an adult male.

12. Describe the anatomy and physiology of the abdomen, including its divisions and the organs and vessels contained within it. pp. 217–220

The abdomen is one of the body's largest cavities, bounded superiorly by the diaphragm, laterally by the flank muscles, inferiorly by the pelvis, posteriorly by the spine and back muscles, and anteriorly by the abdominal muscles. Since most of its border is soft tissue, it is rather unprotected from injury. The abdomen contains the continuous, muscular tube of digestion, the alimentary canal. It enters the abdomen through the hiatus of the diaphragm as the esophagus. It joins the stomach, an organ that physically mixes the food with gastric juices and then sends it out and into the small bowel. The first portion of the bowel, the duodenum, mixes the digesting food with bile (a byproduct of the liver) and pancreatic juices and then begins the process of absorption. The remainder of the small bowel draws the nutrients from the food.

As the digesting food enters the large bowel it is mixed with bacteria, releasing water and any remaining nutrients. They are absorbed, and the material is pushed by peristalsis to the rectum, awaiting defecation. The bowel is a thin and vascular tube that drains its blood supply through the liver for detoxification, where some nutrients are stored and others are added to the circulation.

The liver is a large, solid organ found in the right upper quadrant, just below the diaphragm. The pancreas is a delicate organ found in the lower aspect of the upper left quadrant with a portion of it extending into the right upper quadrant. In addition to digestive juices, it manufactures insulin and glucagon. The kidneys are found deep within the flanks and filter blood to remove excess water and electrolytes. They are very vascular organs that excrete urine into the ureters through which the urine then travels to the bladder. The bladder (in the central pelvic space) rids the body of urine through the urethra. The spleen is an organ of the immune system and is very delicate and vascular, residing in the left upper quadrant.

The abdominal cavity is lined with a serous membrane, the peritoneum. It covers the anterior abdominal organs, and a double-layer sheath of it forms the omentum, which covers the anterior surface of the abdomen. The bowel is slung from the posterior wall of the abdomen by connective tissue called the mesentery that also provides perfusion to the bowel. The abdominal aorta and inferior vena cava run along the spinal column and branch frequently to serve the abdominal organs.

13. Describe the anatomy and physiology of the digestive system, including the digestive tract and the accessory organs of digestion, and also the spleen. pp. 220–223

The GI tract is a long tube that extends from the mouth to the anus and is divided structurally and functionally into different parts. In general, the GI system is divided into the upper and lower GI tracts. The upper GI tract includes the mouth, esophagus, stomach, and duodenum, whereas the lower GI tract includes the remainder of the small intestine and the large intestine, rectum, and anus. In the upper GI tract, food is ingested, and preliminary physical and chemical digestion is begun. In the lower GI tract, digestion of food is completed, nutrients are absorbed into the body, and remaining fiber, intestinal bacteria, and other materials are eliminated through the anus as feces. In addition, three additional organs, the liver, gallbladder, and pancreas, are intimately associated with the GI system both structurally (through connections with the duodenum) and functionally. The vermiform appendix, a blind sac found at the junction of the small and large intestines, does not have any apparent physiologic role in GI function but is important to you because of the inflammatory condition called appendicitis, which you will see in patients in the field.

The spleen is a structure within the immune system and sits in the left upper quadrant, just behind the stomach. It is the most fragile abdominal organ and stores a great amount of blood; hence, its injury can lead to significant hemorrhage.

14. Describe the anatomy and physiology of the urinary system, including the kidneys, ureters, urinary bladder, and urethra. pp. 223–228

The two major organs of the urinary system are the kidneys and the urinary bladder. Two major structures are the ureters and the urethra. The kidney is the critical organ of the urinary system. The kidneys perform the vital functions of the urinary system, which include:

- Maintenance of blood volume with proper balance of water, electrolytes, and pH
- Retention of key substances such as glucose and removal of toxic wastes such as urea
- Major role in regulation of arterial blood pressure
- Control of the development of red blood cells

The first two roles are achieved through the production of urine in the kidneys. The kidneys' role in regulation of blood pressure is achieved in part through control of the body's fluid volume. In addition, they produce an enzyme called renin, which acts to activate a hormone (chemical messenger) called angiotensin, which is part of a hormonal pathway that acts to retain water in the body (increase blood pressure).

The structural and functional unit within the kidney is the nephron, and each kidney contains about one million nephrons, establishing the functional reserve that most people take for granted. Blood is filtered into the first part of the nephron, the glomerulus, and then moves through a length of specialized tubule. As the fluid moves through the parts of the tubule, movement of water and some materials out of the tubule and into the blood occurs (reabsorption), as does movement of some materials out of the blood and into the tubule (secretion). The kidneys can maintain an exquisitely fine control over the relative activity of reabsorption and secretion for virtually every substance that is filtered into the glomerulus. The ability of the kidney to retain glucose, excrete wastes such as urea, and thus perform all of its vital roles is extraordinary, and life depends upon it. When kidney function is too low or nonexistent, an individual will die unless the function is replaced through artificial dialysis or through kidney transplantation. The final role of the kidney, control over development of red blood cells, is achieved through production and release of a hormone called erythropoietin, which stimulates red blood cell synthesis in the bone marrow.

Each ureter runs from a kidney to the bladder, and urine moves out of the kidney through them to reach the bladder. Because ureters are very small in internal diameter, they can become blocked by internal objects such as kidney stones. The bladder is a muscular sac that expands to hold urine. During urination, stored urine is eliminated from the bladder (and the body) through the tube called the urethra.

15. Describe the anatomy and physiology of the female reproductive system, the menstrual cycle, and the pregnant uterus. pp. 228–234

The most important female reproductive structures are located within the pelvic cavity. Essential to reproduction, these structures include the ovaries, which store eggs until maturation (once per month); the fallopian tubes, which direct the egg to the uterus; the uterus, which is a hollow chamber where the egg is fertilized and then is nurtured through the vascular uterine wall; and the vagina or birth canal. The external genitalia have accessory functions, in that they protect body openings and play an important role in sexual functioning.

A monthly hormonal cycle prepares the uterus to receive a fertilized egg. The first 2 weeks of the cycle (known as the proliferative phase) are dominated by estrogen, causing the uterine lining to thicken. In response to a surge of luteinizing hormone, ovulation takes place and an egg is released from the ovary. The secretory phase is the stage of the menstrual cycle immediately surrounding ovulation. If the egg is not fertilized, the woman's estrogen level drops sharply while the progesterone level dominates. Uterine vascularity increases in anticipation of implantation. If fertilization does not occur, estrogen and progesterone levels fall, triggering vascular changes that leave the endometrium ischemic. The ischemic endometrium is shed during the menstrual phase (menstruation), along with a discharge of blood, mucus, and cellular debris. Menstrual flow usually lasts 3 to 5 days, with an average blood loss of 50 mL.

The pregnant uterus undergoes rapid growth to support the developing fetus. Its growth displaces upward most of the contents of the abdomen and by the 32nd week of gestation fills the abdominal cavity to the lower rib margin. The uterus is a very muscular and vascular hollow organ that protects the fetus. Within it is the amniotic sac, filled with fluid that distributes the impact of trauma and protects the developing infant very well.

16. Describe the anatomy and physiology of the male reproductive system. pp. 234–235

The genitourinary system of men includes some specifically reproductive organs and structures: the testes (the primary male reproductive organs, which produce testosterone and sperm cells) and tubing called the epididymis and vas deferens, through which sperm cells leave the testes and move toward the urethra. Sperm leaves the vas deferens to enter the urethra as it passes through the substance of the other male reproductive organ, the prostate gland, which produces fluid that mixes with sperm to produce semen, the male reproductive fluid.

Content Self-Evaluation

MULTIPLE CHOICE

_____ 1. The outermost layer of the skin is the:
   A. epidermis.
   B. subcutaneous tissue.
   C. cutical.
   D. dermis.
   E. sebum.

_____ 2. Which of the following glands secrete sweat?
   A. sudoriferous glands
   B. sebaceous glands
   C. subcutaneous glands
   D. adrenal glands
   E. none of the above

_____ 3. Which of the following types of cells are found in the dermis?
   A. lymphocytes
   B. macrophages
   C. mast cells
   D. fibroblasts
   E. all of the above

_____ 4. The macrophages and lymphocytes begin the inflammation response by killing invading bodies and triggering a call for other, similar cells.
   A. True
   B. False

_____ 5. The type of hair that is short, fine, and lacks pigment is called:
   A. terminal.
   B. formative.
   C. scalioned.
   D. vellus.
   E. none of the above

_____ 6. All of the following are components of the adult hematopoietic system EXCEPT the:
   A. blood.
   B. bone marrow.
   C. thymus.
   D. liver.
   E. spleen.

_____ 7. The major determinants of blood volume are red cell mass and:
   A. erythropoietin levels.
   B. plasma volume.
   C. total body water.
   D. stem cell percentage.
   E. bone marrow volume.

_____ 8. The component of the red blood cell that is responsible for transporting oxygen is the:
   A. basophil.
   B. granulocyte.
   C. hemoglobin.
   D. neutrophil.
   E. lymphocyte.

_____ 9. The Bohr effect describes the relationship between pH and oxygen delivery in that the more acidic the blood, the more readily oxygen is released to the tissues.
   A. True
   B. False

_____ 10. All of the following will cause a right shift of the oxyhemoglobin dissociation curve and thus increase the rate that oxygen is released to the tissues EXCEPT:
   A. increased carbon dioxide.
   B. increased temperature.
   C. decreased pH.
   D. decreased activity.
   E. increased activity.

_____ 11. The term for the packed cell volume of red cells per unit of blood volume is:
   A. hematocrit.
   B. hemoglobin.
   C. red blood cell count.
   D. blood type.
   E. white blood count.

_____ 12. White blood cells that primarily function in allergic reactions to release histamine are called:
   A. lymphocytes.
   B. neutrophils.
   C. eosinophils.
   D. monocytes.
   E. basophils.

_____ 13. White blood cells that primarily function to fight infection are called:
   A. lymphocytes.
   B. neutrophils.
   C. eosinophils.
   D. monocytes.
   E. basophils.

_____ 14. T cells and B cells, which play critical roles in immunity, are types of white cells called:
   A. lymphocytes.
   B. neutrophils.
   C. eosinophils.
   D. monocytes.
   E. basophils.

_____ 15. The condition that occurs when the body develops antibodies against itself is called:
   A. acquired immunodeficiency.
   B. autoimmune disease.
   C. rejection.
   D. chemotaxis.
   E. inherited immunodeficiency.

_____ 16. Causes of the inflammatory process include all of the following EXCEPT:
   A. infectious agents.
   B. chemical agents.
   C. trauma.
   D. immunologic agents.
   E. genetics.

_____ 17. The formed blood cell components responsible for blood clotting are:
   A. red blood cells.
   B. white blood cells.
   C. lymphocytes.
   D. platelets.
   E. monocytes.

_____ 18. Which of the following is NOT a function performed by the musculoskeletal system?
   A. vital organ protection
   B. a portion of the immune response
   C. storage of material necessary for metabolism
   D. hemopoietic activities
   E. efficient movement against gravity

_____ 19. The bone cell responsible for maintaining bone tissue is the:
   A. osteoblast.
   B. osteoclast.
   C. osteocyte.
   D. osteocrit.
   E. none of the above

_____ 20. The bone cell responsible for dissolving bone tissue is the:
   A. osteoblast.
   B. osteoclast.
   C. osteocyte.
   D. osteocrit.
   E. none of the above

_____ 21. The central portion of a long bone is called the:
   A. diaphysis.
   B. epiphysis.
   C. metaphysis.
   D. cancellous bone.
   E. compact bone.

_____ 22. The transitional area between the end and central portion of the long bone is called the:
   A. diaphysis.
   B. epiphysis.
   C. metaphysis.
   D. cancellous bone.
   E. compact bone.

_____ 23. The type of bone tissue filling the end of the long bone is called the:
   A. diaphysis.
   B. epiphysis.
   C. metaphysis.
   D. cancellous bone.
   E. compact bone.

_____ 24. The covering of the shaft of the long bones that initiates the bone repair cycle is the:
   A. periosteum.
   B. peritoneum.
   C. perforating canal.
   D. osteocyte.
   E. epiphysis.

_____ 25. Immovable joints such as those of the skull are termed:
   A. synovial.
   B. synarthroses.
   C. amphiarthroses.
   D. diarthroses.
   E. A or D.

_____ 26. The elbow is an example of which type of joint?
   A. monaxial
   B. biaxial
   C. triaxial
   D. synarthrosis
   E. amphiarthrosis

_____ 27. Bands of strong material that stretch and hold the joint together while permitting movement are the:
   A. bursae.
   B. tendons.
   C. ligaments.
   D. cartilage.
   E. metaphyses.

_____ 28. The small sacs filled with synovial fluid that reduce friction and absorb shock are the:
   A. bursae.
   B. tendons.
   C. ligaments.
   D. cartilage.
   E. metaphyses.

_____ 29. Skeletal maturity is reached by age:
   A. 6.
   B. 10.
   C. 20.
   D. 40.
   E. 45.

_____ 30. The muscular system consists of about how many muscle groups?
   A. 100
   B. 200
   C. 300
   D. 500
   E. 600

_____ 31. The muscle attachment to the bone that moves when the muscle mass contracts is the:
   A. flexor.
   B. extensor.
   C. origin.
   D. insertion.
   E. articulation.

_____ 32. More than half the energy created by muscle motion is in the form of heat energy.
   A. True
   B. False

_____ 33. Which of the following is a layer of the scalp?
   A. the skin
   B. occipitalis muscle
   C. galea aponeurotica
   D. areolar tissue
   E. all of the above

_____ 34. Which of the following is NOT a bone of the cranium?
   A. frontal
   B. mandible
   C. parietal
   D. sphenoid
   E. ethmoid

_____ 35. The largest opening in the cranium is the:
   A. auditory canal.
   B. orbit of the eye.
   C. foramen magnum.
   D. tentorium.
   E. transverse foramen.

_____ 36. Place the following layers of the meninges as they occur from the cerebrum to the skull.
   A. dura mater, pia mater, arachnoid
   B. dura mater, arachnoid, pia mater
   C. arachnoid, pia mater, dura mater
   D. arachnoid, dura mater, pia mater
   E. pia mater, arachnoid, dura mater

_____ 37. The layer of the meninges that is strong and lines the interior of the cranium is the:
   A. pia mater.
   B. falx cerebri.
   C. arachnoid.
   D. dura mater.
   E. tentorium.

_____ 38. The structure that divides the cerebrum into left and right halves is the:
   A. pia mater.
   B. falx cerebri.
   C. arachnoid.
   D. dura mater.
   E. tentorium.

_____ 39. The cerebellum is the center of conscious thought and perception.
   A. True
   B. False

_____ 40. Which of the following is a function of the hypothalamus?
   A. body temperature control
   B. control of the ascending reticular activating system
   C. control of respiration
   D. responsibility for sleeping
   E. maintaining balance

_____ 41. Which of the following is a function of the medulla oblongata?
   A. body temperature control
   B. control of the ascending reticular activating system
   C. control of respiration
   D. responsibility for sleeping
   E. maintaining balance

_____ 42. While the brain accounts for only 2 percent of the total body weight, it requires 15 percent of the cardiac output and 20 percent of the body's oxygen supply.
   A. True
   B. False

_____ 43. The capillaries serving the brain are thicker and less permeable than those in the rest of the body.
   A. True
   B. False

_____ 44. The normal intracranial pressure is:
   A. 120 mmHg.
   B. 90 mmHg.
   C. 50 mmHg.
   D. 25 mmHg.
   E. less than 10 mmHg.

_____ 45. The reflex that increases the systemic blood pressure to maintain cerebral blood flow is called:
   A. the ascending reticular activating system.
   B. the descending reticular activating system.
   C. autoregulation.
   D. Cushing's reflex.
   E. mean arterial pressure.

_____ 46. Which of the following nerves is responsible for voluntary movement of the tongue?
   A. CN-I
   B. CN-III
   C. CN-VIII
   D. CN-X
   E. CN-XII

_____ 47. Which of the following is the lower and moveable jaw bone?
   A. maxilla
   B. mandible
   C. zygoma
   D. stapes
   E. pinna

_____ 48. Which of the following is the bone of the cheek?
   A. maxilla
   B. mandible
   C. zygoma
   D. stapes
   E. pinna

_____ 49. The structure responsible for our positional sense is the:
   A. ossicle.
   B. cochlea.
   C. semicircular canals.
   D. sinuses.
   E. vitreous humor.

_____ 50. Which of the following is the opening through which light travels to contact the light-sensing tissue in the eye?
   A. retina
   B. aqueous humor
   C. vitreous humor
   D. pupil
   E. iris

_____ 51. Which of the following is the light-sensing tissue in the eye?
   A. retina
   B. aqueous humor
   C. vitreous humor
   D. pupil
   E. iris

_____ 52. The white of the eye is the:
   A. sclera.
   B. conjunctiva.
   C. cornea.
   D. aqueous humor.
   E. vitreous humor.

_____ 53. The delicate, clear tissue covering the pupil and iris is the:
   A. sclera.
   B. conjunctiva.
   C. cornea.
   D. aqueous humor.
   E. vitreous humor.

_____ 54. The vertebral column is made up of how many vertebrae?
   A. 24
   B. 33
   C. 43
   D. 45
   E. 54

_____ 55. The major weight-bearing component of the vertebral column is the:
   A. spinous process.
   B. transverse process.
   C. vertebral body.
   D. spinal foramen.
   E. lamina.

_____ 56. The region of the vertebral column that has 12 vertebrae is the:
   A. cervical.
   B. thoracic.
   C. lumbar.
   D. sacral.
   E. coccygeal.

_____ 57. The region of the vertebral column that permits the greatest movement is the:
   A. cervical.
   B. thoracic.
   C. lumbar.
   D. sacral.
   E. coccygeal.

_____ 58. The region of the vertebral column that has five separate vertebrae is the:
   A. cervical.
   B. thoracic.
   C. lumbar.
   D. sacral.
   E. coccygeal.

_____ 59. The structure of the meninges of the spinal column is similar to the structure of the meninges of the cranium.
   A. True
   B. False

_____ 60. At its distal end, the spinal cord is attached to the:
   A. foramen magnum.
   B. peripheral nerve roots.
   C. sacral ligament.
   D. lumbar process.
   E. coccygeal ligament.

_____ 61. The region of the spine with the closest tolerance between the spinal cord and the interior of the spinal foramen is the:
   A. cervical spine.
   B. thoracic spine.
   C. lumbar spine.
   D. sacral spine.
   E. coccygeal spine.

_____ 62. Which of the following is located within the thorax?
   A. the heart
   B. both lungs
   C. the esophagus
   D. the trachea
   E. all of the above

_____ 63. How many rib pairs are floating ribs?
   A. 1
   B. 2
   C. 3
   D. 6
   E. 8

_____ 64. Which of the following lines is used to describe position on the chest wall?
   A. posterior axillary line
   B. anterior axillary line
   C. medial axillary line
   D. midclavicular line
   E. all of the above

_____ 65. How high does the diaphragm rise in the chest during a maximum inspiration?
   A. to the 2nd intercostal space posteriorly
   B. to the 4th intercostal space posteriorly
   C. to the 6th intercostal space posteriorly
   D. to the 8th intercostal space posteriorly
   E. to the manubrium anteriorly

_____ 66. The muscle(s) of respiration responsible for reducing the distance between ribs and helping lift the thorax is(are) the:
   A. intercostal muscles.
   B. diaphragm.
   C. sternocleidomastoid muscles.
   D. scalene.
   E. rectus abdominis.

_____ 67. The structure that separates the chest cavity from the abdominal cavity is the:
   A. mediastinum.
   B. peritoneum.
   C. perineum.
   D. diaphragm.
   E. vena cava.

_____ 68. At the beginning of and during most of expiration, the pressure within the thorax is:
   A. less than the atmospheric pressure.
   B. more than the atmospheric pressure.
   C. equal to the atmospheric pressure.
   D. first lower than and then higher than the atmospheric pressure.
   E. first higher than and then lower than the atmospheric pressure.

_____ 69. Which structures enter or exit the lungs at the pulmonary hilum?
   A. right mainstem bronchus
   B. thoracic duct
   C. pulmonary artery
   D. pulmonary veins
   E. all except B

_____ 70. The right lung has only two lobes because the heart's greatest mass is on the right.
   A. True
   B. False

_____ 71. The serous structure that ensures that the lungs expand with the thoracic cage wall and diaphragm is the:
   A. pleura.
   B. hilum.
   C. ligamentum arteriosum.
   D. lobular attachment.
   E. mediastinum.

_____ 72. Which of the following structures is NOT located within the mediastinum?
   A. thoracic duct
   B. phrenic nerve
   C. pulmonary hilum
   D. vagus nerve
   E. esophagus

_____ 73. The intercostal arteries and nerves run:
   A. behind the ribs.
   B. above the ribs.
   C. in front of the ribs.
   D. under the ribs.
   E. both A and D

_____ 74. The somatic nervous system primarily innervates the:
   A. cardiac muscle.
   B. glands.
   C. skeletal muscle.
   D. smooth muscle.
   E. respiratory system.

_____ 75. The space between the pia mater and the arachnoid membrane is the:
   A. epiarachnoid space.
   B. epidural space.
   C. subarachnoid space.
   D. subdural space.
   E. cerebral space.

_____ 76. This portion of the brain connects the two hemispheres of the cerebrum:
   A. cerebellum.
   B. cerebral cortex.
   C. corpus callosum.
   D. midbrain.
   E. diencephalon.

_____ 77. The area of the brain responsible for emotions, hormone production, and autonomic functions is the:
   A. hypothalamus.
   B. pituitary gland.
   C. pons.
   D. thalamus.
   E. medulla oblongata.

_____ 78. This portion of the brain regulates cardiovascular, respiratory, and digestive system activities:
   A. cerebellum.
   B. hypothalamus.
   C. pons.
   D. thalamus.
   E. medulla oblongata.

_____ 79. The _____ lobe of the brain is responsible for speech.
   A. frontal
   B. occipital
   C. parietal
   D. temporal
   E. semiparietal

_____ 80. The _____ system is responsible for consciousness and stimuli response.
   A. carotid
   B. limbic
   C. vertebrobasilar
   D. reticular activating
   E. cephalic

_____ 81. Which efferent fibers carry impulses to the skeletal muscles?
   A. somatic motor
   B. somatic sensory
   C. visceral motor
   D. visceral sensory
   E. visceral lymphatic

_____ 82. The _____ nervous system is mediated by epinephrine and norepinephrine.
   A. afferent
   B. parasympathetic
   C. somatic
   D. sympathetic
   E. central

_____ 83. Acetylcholine is the neurotransmitter of which nervous system?
   A. adrenergic
   B. afferent
   C. parasympathetic
   D. sympathetic
   E. central

_____ 84. The gland that is the connection between the endocrine system and the central nervous system is the:
   A. pituitary.
   B. hypothalamus.
   C. thymus.
   D. pineal.
   E. thyroid.

_____ 85. Antidiuretic hormone plays a role in maintaining fluid balance by increasing water reabsorption.
   A. True
   B. False

_____ 86. All of the following are hormones secreted by the anterior pituitary gland EXCEPT:
   A. growth hormone.
   B. oxytocin.
   C. prolactin.
   D. adrenocorticotropic hormone.
   E. thyroid-stimulating hormone.

_____ 87. In children, the thymus secretes a hormone that is critical to the maturation of T-lymphocytes, which play a significant role in:
   A. maintaining blood calcium levels.
   B. cell-mediated immunity.
   C. cellular metabolism.
   D. carbohydrate metabolism.
   E. gluconeogenesis.

_____ 88. All of the following are pancreatic hormones EXCEPT:
   A. polypeptide.   D. cortisol.
   B. glucagon.   E. insulin.
   C. somatostatin.

_____ 89. Homeostasis of blood glucose is controlled by insulin and:
   A. polypeptide.   D. cortisol.
   B. glucagon.   E. thymosin.
   C. somatostatin.

_____ 90. The substance that the alpha cells of the pancreas secrete when blood glucose levels fall is:
   A. polypeptide.   D. cortisol.
   B. glucagon.   E. insulin.
   C. somatostatin.

_____ 91. The substance secreted by the beta cells of the pancreas when blood glucose levels rise is:
   A. polypeptide.   D. cortisol.
   B. glucagon.   E. insulin.
   C. somatostatin.

_____ 92. Insulin's primary function is to:
   A. metabolize glucose at the cellular level.
   B. free glucose from muscle storage sites.
   C. increase the glucose uptake by cells.
   D. store glucose at the cellular level.
   E. enhance the function of glucagon.

_____ 93. The production of glucose by the processes of glycogenolysis and gluconeogenesis is triggered by:
   A. polypeptide.   D. cortisol.
   B. glucagon.   E. insulin.
   C. somatostatin.

_____ 94. All of the following are hormones secreted by the adrenal glands EXCEPT:
   A. epinephrine.   D. norepinephrine.
   B. cortisol.   E. aldosterone.
   C. somatostatin.

_____ 95. Glucocorticoids play a role in maintaining blood glucose levels by promoting gluconeogenesis and:
   A. decreasing glucose utilization.
   B. increasing glucose utilization.
   C. promoting salt and fluid retention.
   D. decreasing salt and fluid retention.
   E. potentiating the effects of catecholamines.

_____ 96. Catecholamines such as epinephrine and norepinephrine are hormones secreted by the adrenal medulla.
   A. True
   B. False

_____ 97. The primary function of aldosterone is to:
   A. regulate sodium and potassium excretion.
   B. regulate calcium and magnesium excretion.
   C. promote gluconeogenesis.
   D. inhibit gluconeogenesis.
   E. stimulate glucocorticoid production.

_____ 98. From innermost to outermost, the three tissue layers of the heart are:
   A. the endocardium, the pericardium, and the myocardium.
   B. the endocardium, the myocardium, and the syncytium.
   C. the endocardium, the myocardium, and the pericardium.
   D. the myocardium, the epicardium, and the pericardium.
   E. the epicardium, the myocardium, and the endocardium.

_____ 99. The small, specialized fibers that connect to the heart valve leaflets and prevent the valves from prolapsing are called:
   A. atrial strictures.
   B. chordae tendoneae.
   C. papillary muscles.
   D. semilunar structures.
   E. none of the above

_____ 100. The blood vessel that returns blood to the atria from the body is the:
   A. aorta.
   B. inferior vena cava.
   C. superior vena cava.
   D. pulmonary vein.
   E. both B and C

_____ 101. The blood supply to the left ventricle, interventricular septum, part of the right ventricle, and the heart's conduction system comes from the two branches of the left coronary artery, which are the:
   A. anterior descending artery and the circumflex artery.
   B. anterior descending artery and the posterior descending artery.
   C. circumflex artery and the posterior descending artery.
   D. circumflex artery and the marginal artery.
   E. marginal artery and the posterior descending artery.

_____ 102. The relaxation phase of the cardiac cycle is called dyastole.
   A. True
   B. False

_____ 103. Stimulation of the heart by the sympathetic nervous system results in:
   A. negative inotropic and chronotropic effects.
   B. negative chronotropic and dromotropic effects.
   C. positive chronotropic and dromotropic effects.
   D. positive inotropic and chronotropic effects.
   E. positive inotropic and dromotropic effects.

_____ 104. Specialized myocardial structures called intercalated discs enable the atria to act as an electrophysiologic syncytium and the ventricles to act as another one.
   A. True
   B. False

_____ 105. The difference between the charge of the inside of a myocardial cell and its exterior before contraction is termed:
   A. action potential.
   B. depolarization.
   C. sodium-potassium balance.
   D. resting potential.
   E. none of the above

_____ 106. The myocardial property that permits the heart cells to depolarize on their own is called:
   A. depolarization.
   B. conductivity.
   C. excitability.
   D. automaticity.
   E. conductivity.

_____ 107. The inner layer of the blood vessels are which of the following?
   A. lumen
   B. tunica intima
   C. tunica media
   D. tunica adventitia
   E. Purkinje

_____108. An inadequate delivery of oxygenated blood to body cells is:
   A. hypoxia.
   B. anoxia.
   C. hypoperfusion.
   D. ischemia.
   E. infarction.

_____109. The normal cardiac stroke volume is about:
   A. 50 mL
   B. 60 mL
   C. 70 mL
   D. 100 mL
   E. 120 mL

_____110. Which of the following affects the cardiac output?
   A. preload
   B. afterload
   C. cardiac contractile force
   D. cardiac rate
   E. all of the above

_____111. The arteriole has the ability to change its internal diameter by as much as:
   A. twice.
   B. three times.
   C. fourfold.
   D. fivefold.
   E. seven times.

_____112. Which of the following blood vessel(s) have (has) the greatest effect on blood pressure?
   A. aorta
   B. the major arteries
   C. the veins
   D. arterioles
   E. venules

_____113. The sinuses help trap bacteria and can become infected.
   A. True
   B. False

_____114. The nasal cavity is responsible for all of the functions listed below EXCEPT:
   A. warming the air.
   B. deoxygenating the air.
   C. humidifying the air.
   D. cleansing the air.
   E. the sense of smell.

_____115. The space located between the base of the tongue and the epiglottis is called the:
   A. vallecula.
   B. cricoid.
   C. arytenoid fold.
   D. epiglottic fossa.
   E. glottic opening.

_____116. Which of the following is the only bone in the axial skeleton that does not articulate with another bone?
   A. the mandible
   B. the maxilla
   C. the hyoid bone
   D. the thyroid
   E. the zygomatic bone

_____117. Which of the following correctly lists the order in which air passes through airway structures during inspiration?
   A. trachea, larynx, laryngopharynx, nasopharynx, nares
   B. nares, nasopharynx, trachea, laryngopharynx, larynx
   C. nares, nasopharynx, laryngopharynx, larynx, trachea
   D. laryngopharynx, nares, nasopharynx, larynx, trachea
   E. trachea, nares, laryngopharynx, larynx, nasopharynx

_____118. The point at which the trachea divides into the two mainstem bronchi is called the:
   A. hilum.
   B. parenchyma.
   C. vallecula.
   D. carina.
   E. pleura.

_____ 119. The mainstem bronchus that leaves the trachea at almost a straight angle is the right mainstem bronchus.
   A. True
   B. False

_____ 120. The tissue covering each lung and the interior of the thorax is the:
   A. hilum.
   B. parenchyma.
   C. vallecula.
   D. carina.
   E. pleura.

_____ 121. Which of the following is NOT one of the differences in respiration between pediatric patients and adults?
   A. The pediatric airway is smaller in all aspects.
   B. Pediatric ribs are softer and contribute less to respiration than those of adults.
   C. Children rely more on their diaphragms for breathing than adults do.
   D. The glottis is the narrowest point of the pediatric airway, while the cricoid cartilage is the narrowest point in adults.
   E. Children's teeth are softer and more prone to damage than those of adults.

_____ 122. Internal respiration occurs in the:
   A. peripheral capillaries.
   B. airway.
   C. alveoli.
   D. pulmonary capillaries.
   E. both C and D

_____ 123. Which aspect of the respiratory cycle is passive?
   A. inspiration
   B. expiration
   C. neither A nor B
   D. both A and B
   E. both A and B, but only during stress

_____ 124. The oxygenated circulation that provides perfusion for the lung tissue itself flows through the:
   A. pulmonary arteries.
   B. pulmonary veins.
   C. bronchial arteries.
   D. bronchial veins.
   E. none of the above

_____ 125. The amount of nitrogen in the air is approximately:
   A. 79 percent.
   B. 4 percent.
   C. 0.4 percent.
   D. 0.04 percent.
   E. 0.10 percent.

_____ 126. The normal oxygen saturation of hemoglobin in blood as it leaves the lungs is about:
   A. 75 percent.
   B. 85 percent.
   C. 90 percent.
   D. 95 percent.
   E. 97 percent.

_____ 127. The majority of the carbon dioxide carried by the blood is:
   A. carried by the hemoglobin.
   B. dissolved in the plasma.
   C. transported as bicarbonate.
   D. found as free gas in the blood.
   E. carried as free radicals.

_____ 128. Which of the following will reduce the carbon dioxide levels in the blood?
   A. administration of bicarbonate
   B. administration of antacids
   C. hyperventilation
   D. high-flow oxygen
   E. hypoventilation

_____ 129. Which of the following would NOT increase the production of carbon dioxide?
   A. fever
   B. airway obstruction
   C. shivering
   D. metabolic acids
   E. exercise

_____ 130. The primary center controlling respiration is located in the:
   A. medulla.   D. cerebrum.
   B. pons.   E. cerebellum.
   C. spinal cord.

_____ 131. Which of the following is the secondary or backup stimulus that causes respiration to occur?
   A. an increase in pH of the blood
   B. a decrease in pH of the blood
   C. an increase in pH of the cerebrospinal fluid
   D. a decrease in pH of the cerebrospinal fluid
   E. reduced oxygen levels in the blood

_____ 132. The amount of air moved with one normal respiratory cycle is called:
   A. minute volume.   D. dead air space.
   B. alveolar air.   E. total lung capacity.
   C. tidal volume.

_____ 133. The volume of air contained in a normal inspiration is about:
   A. 150 mL.   D. 6,000 mL.
   B. 350 mL.   E. none of the above
   C. 500 mL.

_____ 134. Which of the following abdominal organs is found in the left upper quadrant?
   A. spleen   D. sigmoid colon
   B. gallbladder   E. liver
   C. appendix

_____ 135. Which of the following abdominal organs is found in the right lower quadrant?
   A. spleen   D. sigmoid colon
   B. gallbladder   E. liver
   C. appendix

_____ 136. Which of the following abdominal organs is found in all of the abdominal quadrants?
   A. pancreas   D. sigmoid colon
   B. gallbladder   E. small bowel
   C. appendix

_____ 137. Which of the following statements is TRUE regarding the digestive tract?
   A. It is a 25-foot-long hollow tube.   D. It moves food via peristalsis.
   B. It churns food.   E. all of the above
   C. It introduces digestive juices.

_____ 138. In what order does digesting food pass through the digestive tract?
   A. duodenum, ileum, jejunum, colon   D. ileum, jejunum, colon, duodenum
   B. duodenum, jejunum, ileum, colon   E. colon, jejunum, ileum, duodenum
   C. jejunum, ileum, colon, duodenum

_____ 139. The movement of digesting material through the digestive system occurs through a process called:
   A. peristalsis.   D. emulsification.
   B. chyme.   E. evisceration.
   C. peritonitis.

_____ 140. The largest solid organ of the abdomen is the:
   A. spleen.   D. gallbladder.
   B. small bowel.   E. liver.
   C. pancreas.

_____ 141. The delicate vascular organ that performs some immune functions is the:
   A. spleen.   D. gallbladder.
   B. small bowel.   E. liver.
   C. pancreas.

_____142. The major functions of the urinary system include all EXCEPT:
   A. maintenance of blood volume.
   B. control of development of white blood cells.
   C. regulation of arterial blood pressure.
   D. maintenance of the balance of electrolytes and blood pH.
   E. removal of many toxic wastes from the blood.

_____143. BUN, or blood urea nitrogen, and creatinine are both measured in blood as part of assessment of kidney function.
   A. True
   B. False

_____144. The enzyme that is produced by the kidney and is part of the physiologic response to low blood pressure is called:
   A. aldosterone.   D. renin.
   B. angiotensin.   E. progesterone.
   C. erythropoietin.

_____145. The urethra in men is much shorter than it is in women, and this is one reason why there is a gender difference in the incidence of lower urinary tract infections.
   A. True
   B. False

_____146. Which of the following structures is part of the external female genitalia?
   A. ovary   D. vagina
   B. perineum   E. fallopian tube
   C. uterus

_____147. An elastic canal that connects the internal and external female genitalia is the:
   A. ureter.   D. vulva.
   B. urethra.   E. fallopian tube.
   C. vagina.

_____148. The layer of the uterine wall where the fertilized egg implants is the:
   A. dermametrium.   D. perimetrium.
   B. cyclometrium.   E. endometrium.
   C. myometrium.

_____149. Which of the following hormones is released by the ovaries?
   A. estrogen   D. luteinizing hormone
   B. follicle-stimulating hormone   E. thymosin
   C. gonadotropin

_____150. The menstrual cycle generally lasts:
   A. 2 weeks.   D. 9 months.
   B. 28 days.   E. 3 weeks.
   C. 7 days.

_____151. The onset of ovulation that establishes female sexual maturity is known as:
   A. menarche.   D. menstruation.
   B. menopause.   E. menacme.
   C. menses.

_____152. The _____ phase of the menstrual cycle terminates with ovulation.
   A. ischemic   D. secretory
   B. menstrual   E. fallow
   C. proliferative

_____ 153. Which process occurs during the proliferative phase of the menstrual cycle?
   A. drop in estrogen level
   B. rupture of small endometrial blood vessels
   C. shedding of the endometrium
   D. thickening of the endometrium
   E. the endometrium becomes pale

_____ 154. The age range in which menopause generally occurs is:
   A. 35 to 40 years.
   B. 40 to 55 years.
   C. 45 to 55 years.
   D. 50 to 60 years.
   E. 60 to 65 years.

_____ 155. Sperm cells are eliminated from a man's body after they move out of the testicles and pass through the following structures in first-to-last sequence:
   A. vas deferens, epididymis, urethra.
   B. ureter, epididymis, vas deferens, urethra.
   C. epididymis, vas deferens, urethra.
   D. epididymis, vas deferens, prostate gland, urethra.
   E. vas deferens, epididymis, prostate gland, urethra.

Chapter 4

General Principles of Pathophysiology

Part 1: How Normal Body Processes Are Altered by Disease and Injury

Review of Chapter Objectives

Because Chapter 4 is lengthy, it has been divided into parts to aid your study. Read the assigned textbook pages; then, progress through the objectives and self-evaluation materials as you would with other chapters. When you feel secure in your grasp of the content, proceed to the next part.

After reading Part 1 of this chapter, you should be able to:

1. **Discuss cellular adaptation, injury, and death.** pp. 241–246

    Cellular adaptation involves the ability of the body cell to change and adapt based upon normal and abnormal stresses. Cellular adaptation includes atrophy, hypertrophy, hyperplasia, metaplasia, and dysplasia.

    - Atrophy is the process of decreasing cell size due to a decrease in cell workload.
    - Hypertrophy is an increase in cell size resulting from an increase in workload.
    - Hyperplasia is an increase in the number of cells in response to an increase in workload.
    - Metaplasia is a replacement of one type of cell with another type of cell not normal for that tissue.
    - Dysplasia is an abnormal change in cell size, shape, and appearance due to an external stressor.

    Cellular injury is most commonly due to hypoxia, chemicals, infectious agents, inflammatory reactions, physical agents, nutritional factors, or genetic factors.

    - Hypoxic injury results when a cell is deprived of oxygen due to a respiratory or cardiovascular problem. Ultimately, the cell cannot efficiently produce its energy source, ATP, and acids and fluids accumulate.
    - Chemical injury results when agents such as ethanol, lead, carbon monoxide, drugs, or insecticides enter the body and injure the cell.
    - Infectious injury causes cell damage when disease-causing agents (pathogens) enter the body. These agents damage and destroy cells, create toxins, or instigate an allergic reaction.
    - Immunologic/inflammatory injury results as the body attempts to ward off invading foreign substances. Although the response is intended to attack the foreign substance, it also damages body cells.

- Physical injury results from exposure to temperature extremes, electrical current, pressure, radiation, noise, and mechanical stresses.
- Injuries due to nutritional imbalance include atherosclerosis, exacerbation of diabetes, insufficient intake of proteins, carbohydrates, lipids, vitamins, and minerals, or malnutrition and starvation.
- Genetic injury results from defective DNA that creates a predisposition toward (like diabetes) or directly causes (like sickle cell disease) a disease.

Cellular death occurs through one of two processes. They are apoptosis and necrosis.

- Apoptosis is a natural elimination of damaged, destroyed, or nonfunctioning cells. This response involves scattered individual cells and allows tissue to repair itself.
- Necrosis is the result of a pathological process and generally involves a grouping or region of cells. In necrosis, cells swell and rupture and take on a different appearance. The process disrupts the normal physiological activity of the tissue.

2. Discuss factors that precipitate disease in the human body. pp. 246–251

The body goes to great lengths to maintain a constant internal and cellular environment (homeostasis). Major factors of this environment include hydration, the movement of substances into and out of the cell, and acid–base balance.

- **Hydration.** Water composes about 60 percent of the total body weight and plays a very important role in the body's internal environment. Some 75 percent of the body's water is contained within the cells (intracellular fluid), while 7.5 percent is contained within the vascular system (intravascular fluid). The remaining water is found between cells (interstitial fluid) and in other spaces within the body. An abnormal decrease in body hydration (dehydration) may be caused by increased gastrointestinal losses, sweating, internal (third space) losses, plasma losses, or other types of losses. An abnormal increase in body water is called overhydration.
- **Electrolytes.** Electrolytes are molecules that dissociate into negatively and positively charged particles (called ions) when dissolved in water. The normal distribution of body water is dependent on the distribution of electrolytes among the body spaces (intravascular, interstitial, and intracellular).
- **Osmosis and diffusion.** Diffusion is the movement of molecules from an area of higher concentration to one of lower concentration. Osmosis is the movement of a solvent (like water) through a membrane to equalize the concentration of electrolytes on each side of the membrane. The body also moves electrolytes through cell membranes (against the osmotic gradient) by active transport and facilitated diffusion. These processes are responsible for maintaining a fluid electrolyte balance among the intravascular, interstitial, and intracellular spaces.
- **Acid–base balance.** The concentration of free hydrogen ions in a fluid reflects its acidity and is noted as a logarithmic value called pH. A pH of 1 is extremely acidic, while a pH of 14 is without hydrogen ions and extremely basic (or alkalotic). The body maintains a slightly alkalotic environment by regulating the quantity of free hydrogen ions. Normal body pH ranges from 7.35 to 7.45. The body maintains its pH through a bicarbonate buffer system, the respiratory system, and the kidneys.

3. Analyze disease risk. pp. 252–257

Disease risk arises from several sources including genetic, environmental, lifestyle, age, and gender factors. Genetic factors are transferred from parents to offspring through genes and may cause frank disease or predispose an individual to disease. Environmental factors include violence, toxins, climate, socioeconomic conditions, exposure to bacteria, and other factors. Lifestyle factors include diet, exercise, smoking, and drug use. Age results in a progressive diminution of body functions and the increasing presence of progressive diseases. Gender risk is associated with hormonal protection or predisposition to disease. Often disease risk is associated with a combination of genetic, environmental, lifestyle, age, and gender factors.

4. Describe environmental risk factors and combined effects and interaction among risk factors. pp. 252–257

Environmental risk factors include violence that may induce trauma, toxins that may cause chemical trauma, poisoning, or cancers, and adverse climates that may cause UV skin and eye damage as well as hyper- and hypothermia, frostbite, and freezing injuries. Poor water supplies, poor nutrition, inadequate housing, and poor medical care may also increase the risk for disease. Frequently, environmental and other disease risk factors combine to induce disease. Type II diabetes, for example, is associated with a familial history but is also associated with a high-fat and high-carbohydrate diet, lack of exercise, and obesity. Heart disease is associated with a familial history, diet, gender, and age factors.

5. Discuss familial diseases and associated risk factors. pp. 254–257

Diseases such as allergies, asthma, rheumatic fever, some cancers, diabetes, cardiovascular disease, cystic fibrosis, sickle cell disease, and some neuromuscular diseases are caused directly by defective genes or related to a genetic predisposition to the disease. Often these predispositions are then triggered by environmental or lifestyle factors that lead to the disease. For example, a familial history of heart disease is exacerbated with smoking, obesity, poor diet, and a sedentary lifestyle.

6. Discuss hypoperfusion. pp. 257–261

Hypoperfusion is inadequate blood flow to and past the body cells. This means that blood flow is insufficient to provide oxygen and necessary nutrients and to remove carbon dioxide and other metabolic wastes. If permitted to continue, hypoperfusion progresses and leads to failure of compensatory mechanisms, decompensation, irreversible shock, and death. Hypoperfusion (or shock) may be caused by trauma, fluid loss, myocardial infarction, infection, allergic reaction, spinal cord or brain injury, and other causes.

7. Define cardiogenic, hypovolemic, neurogenic, anaphylactic, and septic shock. pp. 261–265

Cardiogenic shock is due to the inability of the heart to pump enough blood to meet the body's needs. It is commonly caused by severe left ventricular failure secondary to a myocardial infarction or congestive heart failure. Cardiac output decreases and workload increases, while coronary artery flow decreases and myocardial oxygen demand increases. These factors begin a vicious cycle that often ends in complete heart failure.

Hypovolemic shock is due to the loss of blood volume through internal or external hemorrhage, dehydration, plasma losses from burns, excessive sweating, or third space losses. As the vascular volume decreases, the body compensates by releasing catecholamines, increasing heart rate and inducing vasoconstriction. This produces the classical signs and symptoms of shock—a rapid weak pulse, cool, clammy, ashen skin, dyspnea, anxiety, combativeness—and, ultimately, hypotension.

Neurogenic shock results from injury to the brain or spinal cord that interrupts the body's control over the vascular system. The vessels lose tone and dilate, increasing the size of the vascular container and producing a relative hypovolemia. The body's normal response is muted because the adrenal glands do not secrete catecholamines and the central nervous system cannot induce vasoconstriction. The injury may also affect the heart and respiratory system.

Anaphylactic shock is an exaggerated and severe allergic reaction to a foreign substance that enters the body. It usually occurs rapidly and may be triggered by many substances. The most severe of anaphylactic reactions are triggered when substances are injected directly into the bloodstream, as with bee and wasp stings and injected medications.

Septic shock is caused by an infection that progresses and enters the bloodstream. The toxins produced by the overwhelming infection increase capillary permeability and overcome the compensatory mechanisms, and shock results.

8. Describe multiple organ dysfunction syndrome. pp. 265–267

Multiple organ dysfunction syndrome (MODS) is a progressive impairment of two or more body organs, usually after an initial insult and apparently successful resuscitation. It is caused by an uncontrolled inflammatory response and occurs most commonly after septic shock. The syndrome is caused by an exaggerated immune response in which hormones are released, causing vasodilation, increased capillary permeability, and increased metabolic demands. The syndrome usually begins within 24 hours of the initial insult and progresses over several weeks.

Content Self-Evaluation

MULTIPLE CHOICE

_____ 1. A cell size that increases due to an increase in workload is an example of the process known as:
   A. atrophy.
   B. hypertrophy.
   C. hyperplasia.
   D. metaplasia.
   E. dysplasia.

_____ 2. An abnormal change in cell size or shape due to some external stressor is an example of the process known as:
   A. atrophy.
   B. hypertrophy.
   C. hyperplasia.
   D. metaplasia.
   E. dysplasia.

_____ 3. A blockage or reduction in the delivery of oxygenated blood to body cells is:
   A. hypoxia.
   B. anoxia.
   C. hypoperfusion.
   D. ischemia.
   E. infarction.

_____ 4. Which of the following types of cellular injuries is caused by pathogens?
   A. hypoxic
   B. chemical
   C. inflammatory
   D. immunologic
   E. infectious

_____ 5. A pathogen's virulence is described as its ability to:
   A. invade cells.
   B. destroy cells.
   C. produce toxins.
   D. produce hypersensitivity reactions.
   E. all of the above

_____ 6. A change in cellular structure due to an alteration in the permeability of the cell's membrane is:
   A. fatty alteration.
   B. anabolism.
   C. catabolism.
   D. cellular swelling.
   E. apoptosis.

_____ 7. Cellular destruction caused by an internal release of enzymes is:
   A. apoptosis.
   B. fatty change.
   C. necrosis.
   D. gangrene.
   E. hemoptysis.

_____ 8. Which of the following is NOT a type of necrosis?
   A. fatty
   B. liquefactive
   C. bilateral
   D. coagulative
   E. caseous

_____ 9. The blood component that contains proteins, electrolytes, and clotting factors is:
   A. plasma.
   B. platelets.
   C. erythrocytes.
   D. leukocytes.
   E. none of the above

_____ 10. Which of the blood components below is/are responsible for a portion of the clotting process?
   A. plasma
   B. platelets
   C. erythrocytes
   D. leukocytes
   E. A and B

_____ 11. The most desirable fluid for blood loss replacement is normal saline.
   A. True
   B. False

_____ 12. The percentage of blood accounted for by red blood cells is termed the:
   A. component count.
   B. hematocrit.
   C. hemoglobin level.
   D. oncotic pressure.
   E. leukocyte level.

_____ 13. Common signs of a transfusion reaction include:
   A. fever.
   B. chills.
   C. hives.
   D. nausea.
   E. all of the above

_____ 14. A small volume of colloid solution can be administered to a patient with a greater than expected increase in the intravascular volume.
   A. True
   B. False

_____ 15. Which of the following is NOT a colloid solution?
   A. plasmanate
   B. hetastarch
   C. dextran
   D. Ringer's solution
   E. salt-poor albumin

_____ 16. Which of the following solutions will cause a net movement of water into erythrocytes?
   A. a colloid solution
   B. a hypertonic solution
   C. a hypotonic solution
   D. an isotonic solution
   E. both A and B

_____ 17. In addition to treating the underlying cause, the care of metabolic acidosis includes ensuring adequate ventilation.
   A. True
   B. False

_____ 18. A common cause of metabolic alkalosis is the administration of:
   A. sedatives.
   B. analgesics.
   C. bronchodilators.
   D. diuretics.
   E. antibiotics.

_____ 19. Which of the following is a factor that can influence disease risk?
   A. family history
   B. environment
   C. gender
   D. lifestyle
   E. all of the above

_____ 20. Most disease processes are simply caused by either an environmental or genetic factor, rarely both.
   A. True
   B. False

_____ 21. The death rate from disease is reported as its:
   A. prevalence.
   B. morbidity.
   C. mortality.
   D. incidence.
   E. none of the above

_____ 22. People with genetic predispositions to certain diseases can frequently take actions that modify the risk factors associated with acquiring the disease.
   A. True
   B. False

_____ 23. The risk of acquiring heart disease for a person with a familial history of coronary artery disease is how many times greater than for someone without such a family history?
   A. two
   B. three
   C. four
   D. five
   E. eight

_____ 24. Hypertension is a risk factor for which of the following?
   A. stroke
   B. kidney disease
   C. cancer
   D. cardiovascular disease
   E. all except C

_____ 25. What percentage of lung cancers in women are associated with smoking?
   A. 40 percent
   B. 60 percent
   C. 70 percent
   D. 80 percent
   E. 90 percent

_____ 26. Obesity is defined as having a body weight that is over ideal body weight by:
   A. 20 percent.
   B. 25 percent.
   C. 30 percent.
   D. 35 percent.
   E. 40 percent.

_____ 27. For which of the following diseases is obesity NOT a risk factor?
   A. hypertension
   B. heart disease
   C. breast cancer
   D. vascular disease
   E. diabetes

_____ 28. Perfusion involves the exchange of which of the following between the bloodstream and body cells?
   A. carbon dioxide
   B. oxygen
   C. nutrients
   D. waste products
   E. all of the above

_____ 29. Hypoperfusion may occur with all of the following EXCEPT:
   A. low heart rate.
   B. dilated vascular container.
   C. excessive vascular constriction.
   D. reduced blood volume.
   E. excessive afterload.

_____ 30. The second stage of cellular metabolism that breaks glucose down into energy that can be used by the body requires the presence of:
   A. sodium bicarbonate.
   B. glucagon.
   C. oxygen.
   D. pyruvic acid.
   E. sodium chloride.

_____ 31. The Krebs cycle produces a chemical energy form used by the body that is called:
   A. adenosine triphosphate.
   B. lactic acid.
   C. pyruvic acid.
   D. citric acid.
   E. sodium bicarbonate.

_____ 32. The process by which glycogen is converted into glucose in the cells is:
   A. glycolysis.
   B. glycogenesis.
   C. glycogenolysis.
   D. gluconeogenesis.
   E. lipolysis.

_____ 33. The body's process of compensation for hypoperfusion is initiated by:
   A. glucose.
   B. oxygen.
   C. norepinephrine.
   D. pyruvic acid.
   E. cortisol.

_____ 34. The catecholamines epinephrine and norepinephrine are responsible during the body's response to hypoperfusion for:
   A. decreasing heart rate.
   B. decreasing cardiac contractile strength.
   C. arteriolar dilation.
   D. increasing blood pressure.
   E. decreasing blood volume.

_____ 35. During shock, the spleen may expel blood back into the circulatory system up to a volume of:
   A. 200 mL.
   B. 300 mL.
   C. 400 mL.
   D. 500 mL.
   E. 600 mL.

_____ 36. During hypoperfusion, the renin-angiotensin compensatory system:
   A. increases red blood cell production.
   B. causes the spleen to release blood.
   C. produces a potent vasoconstrictor.
   D. induces beneficial fluid shifts.
   E. reduces the production of lactic acid.

_____ 37. The stage of shock in which medical intervention is no longer effective is:
   A. compensated shock.
   B. decompensated shock.
   C. progressive shock.
   D. irreversible shock.
   E. septic shock.

_____ 38. During decompensated shock, which of the following is likely to occur?
   A. fluid shift from the interstitial spaces
   B. systemic alkalosis
   C. cardiac excitation
   D. dropping blood pressure
   E. all of the above

_____ 39. What type of shock is due to plasma loss from burns?
   A. cardiogenic
   B. hypovolemic
   C. neurogenic
   D. septic
   E. anaphylactic

_____ 40. What type of shock is due to a severe allergic reaction?
   A. cardiogenic
   B. hypovolemic
   C. neurogenic
   D. septic
   E. anaphylactic

_____ 41. Which type of shock results from infection that enters the bloodstream and is carried throughout the body?
   A. cardiogenic
   B. hypovolemic
   C. neurogenic
   D. septic
   E. anaphylactic

_____ 42. A relaxing of the blood vessel walls is the cause of which type of shock?
   A. cardiogenic
   B. hypovolemic
   C. neurogenic
   D. septic
   E. anaphylactic

_____ 43. The reason we are aware of multiple organ dysfunction syndrome (MODS) is that modern medicine is able to help patients survive the initial serious illness or injury.
   A. True
   B. False

_____ 44. The first evidence of MODS usually presents within:
   A. 12 hours.
   B. 24 hours.
   C. 72 hours.
   D. 7 to 10 days.
   E. 14 to 21 days.

_____ 45. Death from MODS usually occurs after:
   A. 24 hours.
   B. 48 hours.
   C. 72 hours.
   D. 14 days.
   E. 21 days.

Matching

Match the type of shock with the characteristic of its presentation.

Type of shock

A. cardiogenic

B. hypovolemic

C. neurogenic

D. septic

E. anaphylactic

Pathology or presentation

_____ 46. pulmonary edema

_____ 47. warm, red skin

_____ 48. itching and skin flushing

_____ 49. history of recent illness

_____ 50. hives

_____ 51. possible high fever

_____ 52. classic signs of shock

_____ 53. laryngeal edema

_____ 54. dry skin

_____ 55. history of diarrhea

Part 2: The Body's Defenses against Disease and Injury

Review of Chapter Objectives

After reading Part 2 of this chapter, you should be able to:

1. **Define the characteristics of the immune response.**　　　　　　　　　　pp. 271–273

   Foreign and invading cells or substances often have unique proteins on their surfaces called antigens. The immune system detects these antigens as being unlike those of the body's cells and initiates a response. This response uses antibodies to selectively control or destroy the foreign substance. As a result of the first contact with the foreign agent, the body develops a "memory" that produces a more rapid and effective response should the same antigen be recognized again. This response is called immunity.

   Immunity can be acquired or natural. Natural immunity is not generated by the immune response but is a genetically inhospitable environment for a particular organism—for example, human resistance to canine distemper. Active acquired immunity is that immunity gained from a response to an invading antigen and is long lasting. Passive immunity is acquired from an outside source such as an immunization or from maternal blood during gestation and is temporary.

The primary immune response occurs with the first exposure to an antigen and lags from 5 to 7 days after exposure. The secondary response occurs as the immune system is sensitized to the antigen by the first response. If it is again exposed to the antigen, it presents a more aggressive and faster response.

Humoral immunity is immunity resident in the blood and lymphatic fluid, primarily from B lymphocytes that produce antibodies. Cell-mediated immunity is immunity provided by T lymphocytes that recognize and directly attack the foreign antigen.

2. Discuss induction of the immune system. pp. 272–273

The immune system must be triggered or induced. This may occur due to the actions of antigens and immunogens, histocompatibility, and blood groupings.

Antigens that induce an immune response are called immunogens. Generally an antigen must be sufficiently foreign and sufficient in size, complexity, and number to generate an immune response.

Histocompatibility locus antigens are antigens that the body recognizes as either foreign or self. Those that are recognized as self (or non-foreign) do not generate an immune response, while those that are recognized as foreign (non-self) stimulate an immune response. It is extremely important to find compatible tissue for organ donation or tissue rejection may result.

Blood group antigens are associated with a different grouping of antigens than those associated with the histocompatibility response. The major blood group antigens consist of the Rh factor (present in about 85 percent of the population) and the A and B antigens associated with the ABO blood typing system.

3. Describe the inflammation response and its systemic manifestations. pp. 273–279

The inflammatory response is a swift, short-acting, nonspecific internal response to cellular injury from trauma or disease. It involves several plasma protein systems and provides four major functions. They are destroying and removing the unwanted substances, walling off the infected or inflamed area, stimulating the immune response, and promoting the healing process.

There are three major manifestations of the acute inflammatory response. They are fever, an increase in circulating white blood cells, and an increase in circulating plasma proteins. Fever is a result of fever-causing chemicals (endogenous pyrogens) released during phagocytosis and is caused by toxins released by bacteria or as a response to an antigen-antibody complex. The elevation in body temperature may make the environment less hospitable to the invading pathogen. Both the number of circulating white blood cells and plasma proteins increase as the body tries to defeat the infection.

The chronic inflammatory response is a response that lasts longer than 2 weeks. During chronic inflammation, the body tries to isolate the agent by forming a barrier around it. Sometimes this cavity is filled with a fluid mixture of cellular debris, dead white blood cells, and tissue fluid called pus.

4. Discuss the role of mast cells, the plasma protein system, and cellular components plus resolution and repair as part of the inflammation response. pp. 274–279

Mast Cells. Specialized cells called mast cells that resemble bags of granules are the chief activators of the inflammatory response. When injured, they initiate the inflammatory response by releasing their granules (degranulation) or by constructing substances that play important roles in the inflammatory response (synthesis).

Degranulation occurs as the mast cell is injured and releases vasoactive amines and chemotactic factors. The principal vasoactive amine is histamine, a potent agent that increases blood flow through the affected area and increases capillary permeability to permit fluid and white blood cells to migrate into the interstitial space. Chemotactic factors are agents that attract white blood cells to the site of inflammation.

Synthesis is the construction of leukotrienes and prostaglandins to enhance the inflammatory response. Leukotrienes have actions similar to histamine and chemotactic factors; however, they promote a slower and longer-lasting response. Prostaglandins cause increased perfusion and capillary permeability but limit the effects of histamine and reduce the release of enzymes from some white blood cells.

Plasma Protein Systems. In addition to the antigen-antibody system, there are three plasma protein systems that complement the inflammatory response system. They are the complement system, the coagulation system, and the kinin system.

The complement system is a complicated cascade system that is activated by antigen-antibody complexes, by products released by the invading bacteria, or by components of other plasma protein systems. The later portions of the cascade produce proteins that may coat the invading agent (opsonization), ingest the agent (phagocytosis), rupture the bacteria's cell membrane (lysis), cause the invading agents to clump together (agglutination), or neutralize the virus through actions similar to the degranulation of the mast cell. Complement proteins may also clog the tissues surrounding the infection and isolate it.

The coagulation or clotting system produces fibrin at the end of a clotting cascade. Fibrin is a sticky protein fiber that traps red blood cells to form a clot, prevents microorganism movement, increases vascular permeability, and produces some chemotactic substances.

The kinin system produces bradykinin, a protein that causes vasodilation, extravascular smooth muscle contraction, increased vascular permeability, and some chemotaxis.

Cellular components of the inflammatory response include the vascular response, increased capillary permeability, and exudation of white blood cells. The vascular response causes blood to flow more strongly into the injured area and helps push both plasma and white blood cells into the inflamed area. The increased capillary permeability is due to a constriction in the capillary wall cells that opens the spaces in between the cells and permits the large white blood cells to squeeze through (diapedesis). The white blood cells are phagocytes that engulf and digest invading cells and debris.

Resolution is the complete restoration of the structure and function of injured tissue. If the injury was more than minor and complete restoration is not possible, then repair will take place. Repair replaces original tissue with scar tissue.

5. Discuss hypersensitivity. pp. 279–280

Usually, hypersensitivity triggers an inflammation response that injures healthy tissue. There are four types of hypersensitivity that cause this destructive reaction. They are IgE-mediated reactions (type I), tissue-specific reactions (type II), immune complex-mediated reactions (type III), and cell-mediated reactions (type IV).

Type I reactions involve the immunoglobulin (antibody) IgE. These antibodies are created in great numbers with the first exposure to an antigen and are released with subsequent exposures, leading to a release of histamine and triggering of the inflammatory response. This results in skin flushing, itching, urticaria and edema, dyspnea, laryngeal edema, laryngospasm, bronchospasm, vasodilation and increased permeability, tachycardia, hypertension, nausea, vomiting, cramping and diarrhea, dizziness, headache, convulsions, and tearing. This type of reaction (anaphylactic) may be life-threatening.

Type II reactions are directed to specific types of tissue. The tissue is destroyed by either the complement cascade, which causes destruction of the target cell's membrane, by clearance of the target cell by macrophage action, by the antigen binding cytotoxic cells to the target cell, and finally by the antigen disabling receptor sites on the target cell.

Type III reactions are either localized or systemic reactions as the complement cascade system attracts neutrophils. They are unable to destroy the invading pathogen and release agents that destroy neighboring healthy cells.

Type IV reactions are activated directly by T cells and do not involve antibodies. The T cells activate other immune cells and attack antigen-bearing cells directly with toxins they produce.

6. Describe deficiencies in immunity and inflammation. pp. 280–282

Congenital or primary immunity deficiencies occur when the development of lymphocytes is impaired during fetal development. Differing immune deficiencies may develop depending upon whether T cells, B cells, or both are affected. In some cases just a small portion of the immune system is deficient and the body is unable to respond to one or a few antigens.

Acquired deficiencies occur after birth and do not result from genetic factors. Nutritional, iatrogenic (caused by medical care), trauma, and stress factors may also result in a decrease in the body's resistance to illness. A specific type of immune deficiency is acquired immune deficiency syndrome (AIDS). AIDS develops from an infection caused by human immunodeficiency virus (HIV). It carries its genetic information on RNA that converts into DNA when it invades a cell and then becomes part of the infected cell's genetic material. The virus may remain dormant for years until it becomes active and kills the host cell and infects other cells. It results in a pervasive invasion of the body's immune defenses.

7. **Describe homeostasis as a dynamic steady state.** p. 283

Homeostasis is often defined as a constant environment within the body and one that the body tries to maintain. In reality, this state is always changing due to turnover of body cells, to the aging process, to continuing body processes like synthesis and breakdown of all body substances, and to the effects of stressors. The body tries, however, to maintain a relatively constant environment.

8. **Describe neuroendocrine regulation.** pp. 274–286

When a psychologic stressor affects an individual, the sympathetic nervous system is stimulated and there is a release of catecholamines, cortisol, and other hormones.

Catecholamines (norepinephrine and epinephrine) are released when sympathetic nerve impulses (from the thoracic and lumbar portions of the spinal cord) stimulate the adrenal medulla. These catecholamines act on four different receptors: alpha 1, alpha 2, beta 1, and beta 2. Alpha 1 receptors cause peripheral vasoconstriction and mild bronchoconstriction and increase metabolism. Alpha 2 receptors mediate the actions of alpha 1 agents. Beta 1 receptors increase the heart rate, contractile strength, automaticity, and conductivity. Stimulation of beta 2 receptors causes vasodilation and bronchodilation.

Sympathetic stimulation also causes the adrenal cortex to produce a steroid hormone, cortisol. Cortisol stimulates the creation of glucose (gluconeogenesis) and limits glucose up-take by cells, increasing blood glucose levels. It also promotes the breakdown of proteins and lipids and acts as an immunosuppressant. While its effects do not support the inflammation and immune responses, cortisol ensures there are adequate energy sources and may help direct blood flow to critical organs during stress.

9. **Discuss the interrelationships between stress, coping, and illness.** pp. 286–288

The ability to cope with stress appears to have an impact on how effectively the body deals with disease. Positive coping mechanisms support the resolution of disease, while ineffective coping mechanisms exacerbate symptoms and the illness.

Content Self-Evaluation

MULTIPLE CHOICE

_____ 1. Which of the following are single-cell organisms consisting of cytoplasm surrounded by a rigid cell membrane?
   A. viruses
   B. bacteria
   C. fungi
   D. parasites
   E. prions

_____ 2. Which of the following are released by bacterial cells during their growth?
   A. antibiotics
   B. gram-negative material
   C. exotoxins
   D. endotoxins
   E. none of the above

_____ 3. The body's anatomical barrier against infection (the skin and linings of the respiratory and digestive systems) is considered:
   A. an external, specific barrier.
   B. an external, nonspecific barrier.
   C. an internal, specific barrier.
   D. an internal, nonspecific barrier.
   E. none of the above

_____ 4. The body's immune response against infection is considered:
   A. an external, specific response.
   B. an external, nonspecific response.
   C. an internal, specific response.
   D. an internal, nonspecific response.
   E. none of the above

_____ 5. The immune response to infection is more rapid than the inflammatory response and is not specific to the invading organism.
   A. True
   B. False

_____ 6. The proteins located on the surface of many substances that enter the body and are used during the immune response to identify foreign organisms are:
   A. antigens.
   B. antibodies.
   C. B cells.
   D. T cells.
   E. lymphocytes.

_____ 7. Which types of immunity refers to the body's initial response to exposure to an antigen?
   A. primary
   B. acquired
   C. natural
   D. secondary
   E. humoral

_____ 8. The type of immunity, resident in the blood, that produces antibodies and remembers a specific antigen is:
   A. cell-mediated.
   B. humoral.
   C. natural.
   D. primary.
   E. extrinsic.

_____ 9. Which of the following is NOT an essential characteristic of an antigen required to trigger an immune response?
   A. sufficient foreignness
   B. sufficient size
   C. sufficient complexity
   D. sufficient quantity
   E. sufficient lability

_____ 10. What percentage of the North American population has the Rh factor present in their blood?
   A. 15 percent
   B. 25 percent
   C. 45 percent
   D. 75 percent
   E. 85 percent

_____ 11. Under the ABO classification system, the universal blood donor is identified as having blood type:
   A. A.
   B. B.
   C. O.
   D. AB.
   E. B and O.

_____ 12. Individuals with which of the following blood types would have the A antibody?
   A. A
   B. B
   C. O
   D. AB
   E. B and O

_____ 13. Which of the following is NOT true of inflammatory response?
   A. It is of relatively short duration.
   B. It begins after 5 to 7 days.
   C. It involves many types of cells.
   D. It involves several protein systems.
   E. It is considered part of the body's immune system.

_____ 14. Which of the following is NOT a function of the inflammatory response?
   A. to destroy and remove unwanted substances
   B. to wall off the infected and inflamed area
   C. to stimulate the immune response
   D. to promote healing
   E. to agglutinate viruses

_____ 15. Degranulation by the mast cells occurs when the cell is stimulated by all of the following EXCEPT:
   A. physical injury.
   B. toxins.
   C. allergic reactions.
   D. histamines.
   E. venoms.

_____ 16. The attraction of white blood cells to the site of infection is called:
   A. synthesis.
   B. chemotaxis.
   C. allergy.
   D. the complement system.
   E. agglutination.

_____ 17. The action of histamine during the inflammatory response is to:
   A. increase capillary permeability.
   B. increase blood flow to the injured area.
   C. attack the invading cells.
   D. attract white blood cells.
   E. both A and B

_____ 18. Occasionally, when macrophages are unable to destroy foreign invaders, a granuloma will form to isolate the infection.
   A. True
   B. False

_____ 19. The best outcome from the wound healing process is:
   A. debridement.
   B. repair.
   C. resolution.
   D. scarring.
   E. granulation.

_____ 20. Which of the following describes a disturbance in the body's normal tolerance for self-antigens?
   A. allergy
   B. anaphylaxis
   C. autoimmunity
   D. isoimmunity
   E. granulation

_____ 21. Which of the following is a hypersensitivity response associated with antigens from another person?
   A. allergy
   B. anaphylaxis
   C. autoimmunity
   D. isoimmunity
   E. monoimmunity

_____ 22. The common allergic and anaphylactic responses are caused by which immunoglobulin (antibody)?
   A. IgM
   B. IgG
   C. IgA
   D. IgE
   E. IgD

_____ 23. Most cases of infection by the human immunodeficiency virus (HIV) in the United States result from:
   A. injection.
   B. droplet inhalation.
   C. skin contamination.
   D. body fluids during sexual intercourse.
   E. both A and D

_____ 24. A state of physical or psychological arousal to stimuli is:
   A. disease.
   B. homeostasis.
   C. stress.
   D. general adaptation syndrome.
   E. turnover.

_____ 25. The initial stage of the general adaptation syndrome in response to stress is:
   A. exhaustion.
   B. resistance.
   C. withdrawal.
   D. alarm.
   E. turnover.

_____ 26. The second stage of the general adaptation syndrome in response to stress is:
   A. exhaustion.
   B. resistance.
   C. withdrawal.
   D. alarm.
   E. turnover.

_____ 27. The final stage of the general adaptation syndrome in response to stress is:
   A. exhaustion.
   B. resistance.
   C. withdrawal.
   D. alarm.
   E. turnover.

_____ 28. During the initial stage of stress, which of the following is NOT likely to occur?
   A. tachycardia
   B. levels of circulating hormones returning to normal
   C. hypertension
   D. digestion slowing
   E. blood flow to skeletal muscles increasing

_____ 29. The interactions that contribute to the alteration of the immune system as an outcome of a stress response are called:
   A. general adaptation syndrome.
   B. homeostatic return.
   C. turnover response.
   D. stress-stressor combination.
   E. pyschoneuroimmunological regulation.

_____ 30. The continual synthesis and breakdown of body substances that results in homeostasis is:
   A. autocombustion.
   B. turnover.
   C. recycling.
   D. oxidation.
   E. plasmodynamics.

_____ 31. Catecholamines include which of the following hormones?
   A. endorphins
   B. epinephrine
   C. cortisol
   D. norepinephrine
   E. both B and D

_____ 32. The hormone released in the greatest quantity by the adrenal medulla is norepinephrine.
   A. True
   B. False

_____ 33. Stimulation of the alpha 1 receptors will cause:
   A. increased heart rate.
   B. inhibition of the effects of norepinephrine.
   C. vasoconstriction.
   D. bronchodilation.
   E. all of the above

_____ 34. Stimulation of the beta 2 receptors will cause:
   A. increased heart rate.
   B. inhibition of the effects of norepinephrine.
   C. vasoconstriction.
   D. bronchodilation.
   E. increase contractility.

_____ 35. Effective stress coping mechanisms have an apparent impact on how people deal with disease but do not effect the seriousness of the associated illness.
   A. True
   B. False

Chapter 5: Life-Span Development

Review of Chapter Objectives

After reading this chapter, you should be able to:

1. **Compare and contrast the physiological and psychosocial characteristics of the following life-span development stages.**

   Infant pp. 292–296

   Infancy is the period from birth to 1 year of age in which the vital signs are pulse rate 100 to 160, respiratory rate 30 to 60, systolic blood pressure 87 to 105, and body temperature of 98 to 100°F. The weight of the infant decreases immediately after birth and then increases, doubling birth weight after 4 to 6 months and tripling it after 9 to 12 months. Immediately after birth, the cardiovascular system changes dramatically from the maternal circulation, with the left ventricle increasing in strength throughout the first year. The infant airway is less stable than the adult's, and the infant is an obligate nasal breather and has delicate lung tissue that is prone to barotrauma. Acquired immunity from the mother somewhat protects the infant from 6 months up to about 1 year. The infant has well-developed reflexes including the startle (Moro), palmar grasp, rooting, and sucking reflexes, which usually disappear after the first few months. The infant's skull is not completely closed, and the openings (the fontanelles) may demonstrate dehydration when sunken. They close by 9 to 18 months.

   Psychosocially, the infant develops based upon instincts, drives, capacities, and interactions with the environment. Bonding occurs as the infant senses that his needs will be met by caregivers and develops attachments to family. The infant learns as caregivers gradually increase their expectations of the infant and child. In crisis, the infant will often follow a predictable sequence of responses: protest, despair, and withdrawal.

   Toddler and preschooler pp. 296–299

   The toddler is a child from 1 to 3 years of age with vital signs normally of a pulse rate of 80 to 110, respirations at 24 to 40, systolic blood pressure at 95 to 105, and temperature of 96.8 to 99.6°F. The preschooler is between 3 and 6 years of age and has vital signs of a pulse rate of 70 to 110, respirations of 22 to 34, a systolic blood pressure between 95 and 110, and a body temperature of 96.8 to 99.6°F. The toddler and preschooler gain about 2 kg in body weight per year. Their cardiovascular systems are better developed, and thermoregulation is more efficient than in infants. The lungs are increasing in surface area, yet rapid respirations will tire the child quickly. Passive immunity is lost, and the toddler and preschooler become more susceptible to minor respiratory and gastrointestinal infections, though they now begin to develop their own immunities.

   Psychosocially, the toddler and preschooler begin to use words and understand their meaning. By the age of 3 or 4 they have mastered the basics of language. They begin to understand cause and effect, develop separation anxiety, and engage in play-acting and magical thinking. They become progressively more influenced by peers and television. Divorce may have an important impact on their psychosocial development, because they may feel abandoned or responsible.

School-aged   pp. 298–299

The school-aged child is between 6 and 13 years old and has vital signs of a pulse rate of 65 to 110, respirations of 18 to 30, a systolic blood pressure of 97 to 112, and a body temperature of 98.6°F. As the vital signs continue to move toward normal adult values, the school-aged child grows at a rate of 6 cm and 3 kg per year. Brain function continues to increase, and primary teeth are replaced by permanent ones.

The school-aged child develops advanced decision-making skills and develops his own self-concept. Factors in this development include self-esteem, moral reasoning and judgment, and self-control.

Adolescent   pp. 299–300

The adolescent is between 13 and 19 years of age and has normal vital signs of a pulse rate of 60 to 90, respirations of 12 to 26, a systolic blood pressure of 112 to 128, and a body temperature of 98.6°F. The adolescent may experience a rapid growth spurt, with maximum growth occurring for the female by age 16 and by age 18 for the male. During this stage, children reach reproductive maturity. In females, the breasts enlarge and menstruation begins.

Adolescence is a time of great psychosocial change. The adolescent strives for autonomy, becomes interested in the opposite sex, and develops an individual identity. The development of logical, analytical, and abstract thinking continues, and the adolescent becomes disappointed when others, especially adults, do not live up to their personal code of ethics.

Early adult   pp. 300–301

The early adult years are between 19 and 40. During this stage of life, normal vital signs are a pulse rate of 60 to 100, respirations of 12 to 20, blood pressure of 120/80, and body temperature of 98.6°F. The body reaches peak performance between 19 and 26 years of age, then begins to slow. Spinal disks settle, leading to a loss in body height, and fatty tissues increase, leading to weight gain.

During this time period, most lifelong habits and routines develop and job stress is at its greatest. The family is also stressed by childbirth and the challenges it brings.

Middle-aged adult   p. 301

The middle-aged adult years are between 40 and 60. During this stage, normal vital signs include a pulse rate of 60 to 100, respirations of 12 to 20, a blood pressure of 120/90, and a body temperature of 98.6°F. During middle age, some degradation of vision and hearing occurs, and cardiovascular disease and cancer become health risks.

Middle-aged adults become concerned about the social clock and become more task oriented, aiming to accomplish their lifelong goals. They may experience the "empty-nest syndrome," in which the children leave home and parental responsibilities become much reduced. Financial commitments associated with elderly parents and young children may add stress.

Late-aged adult   pp. 301–305

The late-aged adult is older than 60 years and has vital signs that are dependent upon individual health status. The walls of the blood vessels thicken, increasing peripheral vascular resistance and reducing blood flow to the organs. The heart begins to show signs of disease of the valves, coronary arteries, electrical system, and the heart muscle itself. Blood volume decreases, as does the number of platelets and red blood cells. The respiratory surface area decreases, as does lung elasticity. The chest expands, and the chest wall stiffens. Respiratory workload increases, while efficiency decreases and coughing becomes less effective. The endocrine system works less efficiently, and glucose metabolism and insulin production decrease. The senses continue to deteriorate, including smell, eyesight, and hearing. Reaction time also diminishes.

Late-aged individuals are affected by concerns regarding housing, self-reliance, and financial burdens. They may be "forced" into retirement while they are still able to perform.

Content Self-Evaluation

MULTIPLE CHOICE

_____ 1. In which age group does normal body temperature become that found in adults?
   A. infant
   B. toddler
   C. preschooler
   D. school-aged
   E. adolescent

_____ 2. The toddler represents a child between the ages of:
   A. birth and 1 year.
   B. 1 and 3 years.
   C. 3 and 5 years.
   D. 6 and 12 years.
   E. 13 and 18 years.

_____ 3. The adolescent represents a child between the ages of:
   A. birth and one year.
   B. 1 and 3 years.
   C. 3 and 5 years.
   D. 6 and 12 years.
   E. 13 and 18 years.

_____ 4. Blood pressure generally rises with age.
   A. True
   B. False

_____ 5. The respiratory rate generally rises with age.
   A. True
   B. False

_____ 6. During the first week of life, the infant's weight is expected to:
   A. increase by 2 kg per week.
   B. decrease by 5 to 10 percent.
   C. double.
   D. triple.
   E. none of the above

_____ 7. When compared to the airway at any other stage of life, the infant's airway is:
   A. shorter.
   B. narrower.
   C. less stable.
   D. more easily obstructed.
   E. all of the above

_____ 8. The reflex sometimes referred to as the "startle reflex" is the:
   A. Moro reflex.
   B. palmar reflex.
   C. rooting reflex.
   D. sucking reflex.
   E. reflux reflex.

_____ 9. The anterior fontanelle closes between:
   A. 1 and 2 months.
   B. 2 and 4 months.
   C. 9 and 18 months.
   D. 1 and 2 years.
   E. none of the above

_____ 10. The process of learning used by children in which they build upon what they already know is called:
   A. bonding.
   B. secure attachment.
   C. scaffolding.
   D. benchmarking.
   E. modeling.

_____ 11. The toddler is very susceptible to minor respiratory and gastrointestinal infections.
   A. True
   B. False

_____ 12. The weight of the toddler's brain is approximately what percentage of the weight of the adult brain?
   A. 60 percent
   B. 70 percent
   C. 80 percent
   D. 90 percent
   E. 96 percent

_____ 13. Children begin to develop magical thinking at about:
   A. 1 to 2 years.
   B. 2 to 3 years.
   C. 3 to 4 years.
   D. 4 to 5 years.
   E. 5 to 6 years.

_____ 14. The school-aged child gains about how much weight per year?
   A. 1 kg
   B. 2 kg
   C. 3 kg
   D. 4 kg
   E. 5 kg

_____ 15. At what age does the female generally finish growing?
   A. 12
   B. 14
   C. 16
   D. 18
   E. 20

_____ 16. In late adolescence, the average male is taller and stronger than the average female.
   A. True
   B. False

_____ 17. Peak physical condition occurs among:
   A. the preschool-aged.
   B. the school-aged.
   C. adolescents.
   D. early adults.
   E. middle-aged adults.

_____ 18. The leading cause of death among early adults is:
   A. accidents.
   B. cardiovascular disease.
   C. cancer.
   D. respiratory disease.
   E. drug overdose.

_____ 19. The maximum life span for a human being is about:
   A. 76 years.
   B. 84 years.
   C. 96 years.
   D. 100 years.
   E. 120 years.

_____ 20. By the age of 80, the vessels of the cardiovascular system decrease their elasticity by about 50 percent.
   A. True
   B. False

_____ 21. During late adulthood, which of the following is expected?
   A. decreased blood volume
   B. decreased platelet count
   C. decreased number of red blood cells
   D. poor iron levels
   E. all of the above

_____ 22. Which of the following is NOT expected of the respiratory system during late adulthood?
   A. enlarged alveoli
   B. decreased airway diameter
   C. reduced lung surface area
   D. stiffening of the chest wall
   E. increased likelihood of respiratory disease

_____ 23. Which of the following is a likely result of tooth loss in the elderly?
   A. an increased swallowing time
   B. decreased peristalsis
   C. less-effective esophageal sphincter
   D. the swallowing of larger pieces of food
   E. all of the above

_____ 24. The individual in late adulthood is likely to be sensitive to loud noises and yet less able to hear indistinct speech or normal conversation in the presence of loud noise.
   A. True
   B. False

_____ 25. Arteriosclerotic heart disease is the major killer after age 40 in all age, sex, and racial groups.
   A. True
   B. False

MATCHING

Write the letter of the development stage in the space provided next to the characteristic most commonly associated with that age group.

A. Infant

B. Toddler

C. Preschooler

D. School-aged

E. Adolescent

F. Early adult

G. Middle-aged adult

H. Late-aged adult

_____ 26. Highest level of job stress

_____ 27. Concerned with "social clock"

_____ 28. Baby teeth begin to appear

_____ 29. Sexual maturity

_____ 30. Permanent teeth

_____ 31. Hearing loss for pure tones

_____ 32. Development of self-concept

_____ 33. Understanding of cause and effect

_____ 34. Hearing maturity

_____ 35. Loss of sucking and rooting reflexes

Chapter 6: General Principles of Pharmacology

Part 1: Basic Pharmacology

Review of Chapter Objectives

Because Chapter 6 is lengthy, it has been divided into parts to aid your study. Read the assigned textbook pages; then, progress through the objectives and self-evaluation materials as you would with other chapters. When you feel secure in your grasp of the content, proceed to the next part.

After reading Part 1 of this chapter, you should be able to:

1. **Describe important historical trends in pharmacology.** p. 309

   The use of herbs and minerals has been documented in the treatment of illness and injury since as early as 2000 B.C. Before that, the ancient Egyptians, Arabs, and Greeks probably passed formulations down through the generations by word of mouth. During the seventeenth and eighteenth centuries, tinctures of opium, coca, and digitalis were available, and the concept of inoculation with biologic extracts was developed by the late nineteenth century. By the end of that century, atropine, chloroform, codeine, ether, and morphine were in use. This past century has seen an explosion in the number and types of pharmaceuticals in use. As we begin the twenty-first century, recombinant DNA technology has produced human insulin and tissue plasma activator (tPA).

2. **Differentiate among the chemical, generic (nonproprietary), official (USP), and trade (proprietary) names of a drug.** pp. 309–310

   The chemical name of a drug represents its chemical composition and molecular structure. An example is 7-chloro-1,3-dihydro-1-methyl-5-phenyl-2H-1,4-benzodiazepine-2-one.

   The generic name of a drug is suggested by the original manufacturer and confirmed by the United States Adopted Name Council. An example, for which the chemical name is given above, is diazepam.

   The official name of a drug is established by the Federal Drug Administration when it is listed in the United States Pharmacopeia (USP). An example is diazepam, USP.

   The brand, trade, or proprietary name of a drug is the name given to the drug by a specific manufacturer. This name is a proper name and should be capitalized and may be followed by a trademark insignia. An example is Valium®, a brand name for diazepam.

3. **List the four main sources of drug products.** p. 310

   There are four main sources of drugs. They are plants, animals, minerals, and synthetic substances (laboratory).

4. List the authoritative sources for drug information. pp. 310–311

Drug inserts usually accompany prescription drugs and list information as required by the United States Food and Drug Administration.

The Physician's Desk Reference (PDR) is a compilation of materials supplied by drug manufacturers (usually the drug insert material). It also contains indexing and some drug photos.

Drug Information is a publication of the Society of Health System Pharmacists. It is an authoritative listing of virtually every drug used in the United States.

The Monthly Prescribing Reference is a periodic publication designed to keep physicians informed regarding the prescription of medications and which prescription drugs are used for which diseases.

The AMA Drug Evaluation is published by the American Medical Association and is a comprehensive listing of commonly used medications.

5. List legislative acts controlling drug use and abuse in the United States. pp. 311–313

The Pure Food and Drug Act of 1906 was enacted to improve the quality and labeling of drugs and named the United States Pharmacopeia as the country's official source for drug information.

The Harrison Narcotic Act of 1914 restricted the use of addictive drugs by controlling importation, manufacture, sale, and use of opium, cocaine, and their derivatives.

The Federal Food, Drug and Cosmetic Act of 1938 empowered the Food and Drug Administration (FDA) to establish and enforce standards for drugs.

In 1951, the Durham-Humphrey Amendments to the Federal Food, Drug and Cosmetic Act required pharmacists to have written or oral orders (prescriptions) for certain drugs and created a category of over-the-counter drugs.

The Comprehensive Drug Abuse Prevention and Control Act of 1970 repealed the Harrison Narcotics Act, established five schedules of controlled substances, and identified levels of control and required record keeping for each.

6. Differentiate among Schedule I, II, III, IV, and V substances and list examples of substances in each schedule. p. 312

Schedule I drugs include heroin, LSD, and mescaline drugs with a high potential for abuse and no medical indications. These drugs are used for research, analysis, and instruction only.

Schedule II drugs include opium, cocaine, morphine, codeine, oxycodone, methadone, and secobarbital. These drugs have a high potential for abuse and may lead to severe dependence, though they have some medical indications.

Schedule III drugs include opioids in limited amounts or combined with noncontrolled substances like Vicodin or Tylenol with codeine. These drugs have accepted medical indications.

Schedule IV drugs include diazepam, lorazepam, and phenobarbital. These are drugs of lower abuse potential compared to those in Schedule III and also have accepted medical indications.

Schedule V drugs include limited amounts of opioids. These drugs are often used for cough or diarrhea. They have less potential for abuse than Schedule IV drugs and have accepted medical indications.

7. Discuss standardization of drugs. p. 313

Drugs may contain the same active ingredient yet be far different in the way they are delivered to the body. To recognize this, an assay of the drug determines the amount and purity of the drug in the preparation. A bioassay determines the amount of drug that is available in a biological model and thereby establishes its bioequivalence, or relative therapeutic effectiveness compared with drugs with chemically equivalent compositions.

8. Discuss special considerations in drug treatment with regard to pregnant, pediatric, and geriatric patients. pp. 314–316

Pregnancy alters the mother's physiology and also adds a second party, the developing fetus, to the concerns regarding medication administration. The increased maternal heart rate, cardiac output, and blood volume can affect the onset and actions of many medications. Drugs may also alter fetal development and result in fetal injury, deformity, or death. During the third trimester, some drugs may pass through the placenta and affect the fetus directly.

Several anatomic and physiological differences between pediatric patients and adults result in differences in the ways drugs are absorbed and metabolized. Differences in gastric pH and emptying time and lower digestive enzyme levels in children change the way enteral medications are absorbed. A child's thinner skin causes topical agents to be absorbed more quickly. Lower plasma protein levels in children affect the availability of agents that usually bind to them. Higher water content in the neonate also affects drug absorption and distribution, as does the slower, then faster metabolism of the neonate and child, respectively. Organ maturity also affects drug metabolism and elimination. For children, drug administration is often guided by weight and in some cases guided by height (the Broselow tape).

With advancing age, the body's metabolism, gastric motility, decreased plasma proteins, reduced body fat and muscle mass, and depressed liver function all affect the absorption, metabolism, and elimination of drugs. Older patients are also likely to be on multiple medications for multiple diseases, thereby increasing the likelihood of adverse medication interactions.

9. **Discuss the paramedic's responsibilities and scope of management pertinent to the administration of medications.** pp. 313–314

There are six basic "rights" of drug administration that indicate the paramedic's essential responsibilities and practices. They are the right medication, the right dose, the right time, the right route, the right patient, and the right documentation.

The right medication. Ensure the medication is what is intended for the patient. Review your standing orders or, if an order is received from medical direction, repeat the order back to the physician so you are both clear on the medication, dose, route, and timing of the administration. Also examine the drug packaging to ensure it is the medication you wish to administer.

The right dose. Carefully calculate the dose (usually weight dependent) for the patient before you draw up the medication and again just before you administer it. Prehospital medications are usually packaged to accommodate a single administration. If the drug package you select has much more or less than you intend to use, recheck the packaging to ensure it is the right drug and right concentration and recheck your calculations to ensure the right dosage.

The right time. Usually prehospital medications are given rather rapidly and not on a schedule. Check the packaging and your protocols for administration rate and ensure you follow the sequencing, time intervals, and drip rates for emergency drugs.

The right route. While most emergency drugs are administered by the IV route, be aware of the alternate routes of drug administration, the drugs administered via those routes, and the circumstances requiring the use of those routes. With each medication administration, ensure you are using the right route.

The right patient. It is imperative to ensure that the patient is properly matched to medication. A patient-drug mismatch is an infrequent problem in prehospital care, but as EMS moves to the out-of-hospital environment, paramedics may be treating some patients on a routine basis. Always ensure that the medication order is for the patient you are attending.

The right documentation. Thoroughly document all aspects of patient care, including what drugs (medication, time, and route) were administered in what dosage.

10. **Review the specific anatomy and physiology pertinent to pharmacology.** pp. 316–326

Drugs modify or exploit the existing functions of cells; they do not confer any new properties. They also often have several sites of action throughout the body and must be thought of for their systemic actions. Drugs may cause their effects by binding to cell receptor sites, changing the physical properties of a cell, chemically combining with other chemicals, or altering a normal metabolic pathway.

The most common mechanism of action for drugs administered in the prehospital setting involves drugs that bind to receptor sites. These receptor sites are most commonly associated with the nervous system because this system is responsible for overall body control. Drugs frequently affect the receptors for pain and those of the autonomic nervous system, including the sympathetic and parasympathetic nervous systems. Autonomic effects include changes in the rate and strength of cardiac contraction, in the degree of peripheral vascular contraction (resistance), and in bronchoconstriction or dilation, to name just a few.

Other drugs act by changing the physical properties of the body, for example, by altering the osmolarity of the blood or by chemically combining with other substances to change the internal environment (as sodium bicarbonate combines with acids to make the blood more alkaline). Finally, some drugs alter a metabolic pathway to obtain their intended effect. Some anticancer drugs act in this way.

11. List and describe general properties of drugs. pp. 322–324

- Affinity is the force of attraction between the drug and the receptor site.
- Efficacy is the drug's ability to cause its expected effect.
- An agonist is a drug that causes the expected effect when bound to the receptor site.
- An antagonist is a drug that does not cause the expected effect when bound to the receptor site.
- An agonist-antagonist is a drug that binds to a receptor site, causing some expected effects and blocking others.
- A competitive antagonist is a drug that causes some effects as it binds to a receptor site but blocks the binding of another drug.
- A noncompetitive antagonist is a drug that binds to and deforms a receptor site so other drugs cannot bind there.

12. List and describe liquid and solid drug forms. pp. 321–322

Drugs come in many different forms. Solid drug forms include the following:

- Pills are drugs that are shaped spherically for easily swallowing.
- Powders are drugs simply in a powder form.
- Tablets are powders compressed into a disk-like form.
- Suppositories are drugs mixed with a wax-like base that melts at body temperature. They are usually inserted into the rectum or vagina.
- Capsules are gelatin containers filled with the drug powder or tiny pills. When the container dissolves, the drug is released into the gastrointestinal tract.

Liquid forms include the following:

- Solutions are drugs dissolved in a solvent, usually water- or oil-based.
- Tinctures are medications extracted using alcohol with some alcohol usually remaining.
- Suspensions are mixtures of a solvent and drug in which the solid portion will precipitate out.
- Emulsions are suspensions with an oily substance in the solvent that remains as globules even when mixed.
- Spirits are solutions of volatile drugs in alcohol.
- Elixirs are drugs mixed with alcohol and water, often with flavorings to improve taste.
- Syrups are solutions of sugar, water, and drugs.

13. List and differentiate routes of drug administration. pp. 320–321

Enteral routes deliver medications by absorption through the gastrointestinal tract. There are several routes of enteral administration. Oral routes are the most common for drug administration and are well suited for self-administration of medication. Naso- or orogastric tube administration uses either type of tube to direct medications into the stomach. Sublingual administration permits the drug to be absorbed by the capillaries under the tongue. Buccal (between the cheek and gum) absorption is similar to sublingual drug administration. Rectal administration is a route used for unconscious, vomiting, seizing, or uncooperative patients.

Routes outside the gastrointestinal tract are referred to as parenteral and typically use needles to inject medications into the circulatory system or tissues. With intravenous drug administration, a drug is injected directly into the veins, leading to rapid distribution of the medication. Endotracheal medication administration uses the endotracheal tube to place the medication into the lung field, where it is quickly absorbed by the bloodstream. Intraosseous administration directs medication into the medullary space of a long bone in the pediatric patient. Umbilical drug administration uses the umbilical artery or vein as an alternate IV site in the neonate. With intramuscular administration, the medication is injected into the muscle tissue, where it is rapidly absorbed by the bloodstream. Subcutaneous administration is just slightly slower than intramuscular administration. Transdermal administration is slightly slower than subcutaneous, and topical administration has the slowest absorption rate of all routes. With administration by inhalation/nebulization, a drug is introduced into the lung field, where it is absorbed. Nasal medications are introduced into the mucous membranes of the nose and are rapidly absorbed. With instillation, a drug is placed (topically) into a wound or the eye. Intradermal medications are delivered between dermal layers.

14. Differentiate between enteral and parenteral routes of drug administration.   pp. 320–321

Enteral routes of administration are those that direct drugs into the gastrointestinal system and include oral (PO), orogastric or nasogastric tube (OG/NG), sublingual (SL), buccal, and rectal. Parenteral routes are routes of administration outside the gastrointestinal tract and include intravenous (IV), endotracheal (ET), intraosseous (IO), umbilical, intramuscular (IM), subcutaneous (SQ), inhalation/nebulization, topical, transdermal, nasal, instillation, and intradermal.

15. Describe mechanisms of drug action.   pp. 322–324

How a drug interacts with the body to cause its effects is referred to as pharmacodynamics. Drugs induce their effects by binding to a receptor site, changing the physical properties of the body's cells, chemically combining with other substances, or altering a normal metabolic pathway.

16. List and differentiate the phases of drug activity, including the pharmaceutical, pharmacokinetic, and pharmacodynamic phases.   pp. 316–326

The pharmaceutical phase of drug activity addresses the drug's intrinsic characteristics such as how the drug dissolves or disintegrates once injected or ingested. Pharmacokinetics refers to the processes by which a drug is absorbed, distributed, biotransformed, and eliminated by the body. Pharmacodynamics is the mechanism (or mechanisms) by which a drug interacts with the body to accomplish its action.

17. Describe the processes called pharmacokinetics and pharmocodynamics, including theories of drug action, drug-response relationship, factors altering drug responses, predictable drug responses, iatrogenic drug responses, and unpredictable adverse drug responses.   pp. 316–326

There are two important elements of pharmacology: how drugs are transported into or out of the body (pharmacokinetics) and how drugs interact with the body to cause their effects (pharmacodynamics).

Pharmacokinetics examines the absorption, distribution, biotransformation, and elimination of drugs.

For a drug to perform its action, it must first reach its site of action, a process referred to as absorption. While some drugs affect target tissue directly (like antacids in the stomach), most must first find their way to the bloodstream. Drugs administered directly into a venous or arterial vessel are quickly transported to the heart, mixed with the blood, and distributed throughout the body. A drug injected into the muscle tissue and, to a somewhat lesser degree, into the subcutaneous tissue, is transported quickly to the bloodstream because of the more than adequate circulation in these tissues. However, shock and hypothermia may slow the process, while fever and hyperthermia may speed it. Oral medications must survive the gastric acidity and be somewhat lipid soluble to be transported across the intestinal membrane. The differing acid content of the digestive tract also impacts the dissociation of the drug into ions that are more difficult to move into the circulation. And finally, the drug's concentration affects its uptake by the bloodstream and, ultimately, its distribution. The end result of the absorption process is the concentration of the drug in the bloodstream and its availability for activation of the target tissue, called its bioavailability.

Once a drug enters the bloodstream, it must be carried throughout the body and to its site of action. The term for this process is distribution. Many factors affect the release and uptake of a drug by the body's cells. Some drugs bind to the plasma proteins of the blood and are released over a prolonged period of time. An increase in the blood's pH may increase the rate of release of the drug, or competition from other drugs for binding sites may cause more of a drug to become available. Distribution of some drugs is dependent upon their ability to cross the blood–brain or placental barriers. Other drugs are easily deposited in fatty tissue, bones, and teeth.

Once in the body, drugs are broken down into metabolites in a process called biotransformation. This process makes the drug more or less active and can make the drug more water soluble and easier to eliminate. Some drugs are totally metabolized, some are partially metabolized, while still others are not metabolized at all. The liver is responsible for most biotransformation, while the lungs, kidneys, and GI tract do some limited biotransformation.

Elimination is the excretion of the drug in urine, expired air, or in feces. Renal excretion is the major mechanism for eliminating drugs from the body. Drugs are eliminated as the blood pressure pushes and filters blood through kidney structures. This effect is enhanced by special cells that "pump" (active transport) some metabolites into the tubules. Kidney reabsorption also plays a part in drug excretion. Protein-soluble molecules and electrolytes are easily absorbed, but the uptake may be affected by the blood's pH.

A drug's effects on the body are referred to as pharmacodynamics. Drugs may cause their effects by binding on a receptor site, by changing physical properties, by chemically combining with other substances, or by altering a normal metabolic pathway.

Most drugs effect their actions by binding to receptor sites, especially those of the autonomic nervous system. The drug either inhibits or stimulates the cells or tissue. The force of attraction of a drug is referred to as its affinity. Affinity becomes important when different drugs compete for a site. The drug's efficacy is its ability to cause the expected response. Binding to a receptor site causes a change within the cell and induces the drug's effect. However, some drugs may establish a chain-reaction effect whereby other drugs are released and cause the desired effect. The number of receptor sites may change as the drug becomes available and uses them, thereby reducing the drug's continuing effect. Chemicals that bind to the receptor and cause the expected response are termed agonists. Antagonists bind to the site and do not cause the expected response. Some drugs have both properties. Often drugs compete for receptor site in a process called competitive antagonism, while a situation in which a drug attaches to a receptor, effectively locking out other drugs, is termed noncompetitive antagonism. Permanent binding to a receptor site is irreversible antagonism.

Drugs may also act by modifying the physical properties of a part of the body. For example, the drug mannitol changes the blood's osmolarity and increases urine output.

Some drugs chemically combine with other substances to cause their desired effect. For example, antacids interact with the hydrochloric acid in the stomach to reduce the pH.

Other drugs act by altering normal biologic processes and the metabolic pathways. Such drugs are used to treat cancers and viral infections.

The drug-response relationship is the relationship between a drug's pharmaceutical, pharmacokinetic, and pharmacodynamic properties. It most commonly relates to the blood plasma level of the drug. Other important factors include the speed of onset, duration of action, minimum effective concentration, and biologic half-life. Another very important factor in the drug-response relationship is the therapeutic index, or the ratio between the drug's lethal and effective doses.

Factors altering drug response include the patient's age, body mass, sex, pathologic state, genetic factors, and psychological factors as well as environmental considerations and the time of administration. These factors may increase or decrease the drug's ability to generate its desired effect.

Responses to drug administration may include unintended responses, or side effects. These are care-provider induced (iatrogenic) and include allergic reactions, idiosyncratic (unique to an individual) reactions, tolerance, cross tolerance, tachyphylaxis, cumulative effects, dependency, drug interactions, drug antagonisms, summation, synergistic reactions (a result greater than the expected additive result of two drugs administered together), potentiation, and interference. Some of these effects may be predictable and desired and some may be unexpected.

18. Differentiate among drug interactions. p. 326

Drugs have the potential to interact, cause, and alter the effects of other drugs taken by a patient. One drug may alter the effects of another by altering the rate of intestinal absorption, by competing for the same plasma protein binding site, by altering the other's metabolism and hence bioavailability, by causing an antagonistic or synergistic action at a receptor site, by altering the excretion rate of another drug through the kidneys, or by altering the electrolyte balance necessary for the other drug's actions.

19. Discuss considerations for storing and securing medications. p. 322

Temperature, humidity, ultraviolet radiation (sunlight), and time affect the potency of many drugs. It is important that they be stored under proper conditions and that they are rotated so they are utilized (or discarded) before their shelf life expires.

20. List the components of a drug profile by classification. p. 311

Names: The generic, trade, and sometimes the chemical names.
Classification: The broad group to which the drug belongs.
Mechanism of action: The way the drug causes it desired effects (its pharmacodynamics).
Indications: The conditions appropriate for the drug's administration.
Pharmacokinetics: How the drug is absorbed, distributed, and eliminated, including its onset and duration of action.
Side effects/adverse reactions: The drug's untoward or undesired effects.
Routes of administration: How the drug is given.
Contraindications: Conditions that make it inappropriate to administer a drug (including conditions in which administration is likely to cause a harmful outcome).
Dosage: The amount of drug that should be given.
How supplied: The typical concentrations and preparations of the drug.
Special considerations: How the drug may affect pregnant, pediatric, and geriatric patients.

Content Self-Evaluation

MULTIPLE CHOICE

_____ 1. The study of drugs and their interactions with the body is:
   A. pharmaceutics.
   B. pharmacokinetics.
   C. pharmacodynamics.
   D. pharmacology.
   E. pharmacopedia.

_____ 2. Which of the following types of drug names is 7 chloro-1,3-dihydro-1-methyl-5-phenyl-2H-1,4 benzodiazepine-2-one?
   A. chemical name
   B. generic name
   C. official name
   D. brand name
   E. common name

_____ 3. Which of the following types of drug names is diazepam?
   A. chemical name
   B. generic name
   C. official name
   D. brand name
   E. common name

_____ 4. Digitalis is an example of a drug derived from:
   A. a plant.
   B. an animal.
   C. a mineral.
   D. synthetic production.
   E. a lipid base.

_____ 5. Bovine insulin is an example of a drug derived from:
   A. a plant.
   B. an animal.
   C. a mineral.
   D. synthetic production.
   E. a lipid base.

_____ 6. The drug reference that presents manufacturer-provided drug information and some photos of drugs is the:
   A. EMS Guide to Drugs.
   B. Physician's Desk Reference.
   C. AMA Drug Evaluations.
   D. Monthly Prescribing Reference.
   E. all of the above

_____ 7. The broad group to which a drug belongs is its:
   A. indication.
   B. pharmacokinetics.
   C. classification.
   D. mechanism of action.
   E. none of the above

_____ 8. Conditions in which it is inappropriate to give a drug are referred to as its:
   A. mechanisms of action.
   B. indications.
   C. contraindications.
   D. side effects.
   E. special considerations.

_____ 9. Which of the following drugs is classified as a Schedule II controlled substance?
   A. heroin
   B. morphine
   C. codeine
   D. diazepam
   E. B and C

_____ 10. The assay of a drug in a preparation determines its:
   A. potency.
   B. amount and purity.
   C. effectiveness.
   D. availability in a biological model.
   E. effectiveness compared to other like drugs.

_____ 11. The bioequivalence of a drug in a preparation refers to its:
   A. potency.
   B. amount and purity.
   C. effectiveness.
   D. availability in a biological model.
   E. effectiveness compared to other like drugs.

_____ 12. Which of the following is NOT one of the six rights of medication administration?
   A. right dose
   B. right patient
   C. right documentation
   D. right time
   E. right mechanism

_____ 13. Dosages of many emergency drugs are based upon patient weight, so unit dose packaging may not contain the right amount for every patient.
   A. True
   B. False

_____ 14. Children are, for the most part, just small adults, so drug dosages just need to be reduced proportionally by weight.
   A. True
   B. False

_____ 15. Which of the following is NOT true regarding the newborn patient?
   A. The neonate has less gastric acid than an adult.
   B. The neonate has diminished blood plasma levels.
   C. The neonate has immature renal and hepatic systems.
   D. The neonate has less body water than an adult.
   E. The neonate has lower enzyme levels than an adult.

_____ 16. Drugs in which of the following FDA categories have demonstrated definite risks to the fetus?
   A. R
   B. A
   C. B
   D. C
   E. D

_____ 17. Which of the following is NOT true regarding the geriatric patient?
   A. The geriatric patient has decreased gastrointestinal motility.
   B. The geriatric patient has decreased body fat.
   C. The geriatric patient has decreased muscle mass.
   D. The geriatric patient is more likely to be disease free.
   E. The geriatric patient has decreased liver function.

_____ 18. Drugs do not confer any new properties on cells or tissues; they only modify or exploit existing functions.
   A. True
   B. False

_____ 19. Which of the following is NOT one of the four basic processes of pharmacokinetics?
   A. absorption
   B. distribution
   C. receptor binding
   D. biotransformation
   E. elimination

_____ 20. Which of the following represents an energy-consuming movement of ions against the concentration gradient?
   A. diffusion
   B. active transport
   C. osmosis
   D. filtration
   E. facilitated transport

_____ 21. Which of the following represents movement of molecules across a membrane from an area of higher pressure to an area of lower pressure?
   A. diffusion
   B. active transport
   C. osmosis
   D. filtration
   E. facilitated transport

_____ 22. The measure of the amount of a drug that is still active after it reaches the target organ is its:
   A. bioavailability.
   B. biotransformativity.
   C. metabolism.
   D. pro-drug effect.
   E. active distribution.

_____ 23. Which of the following is NOT a significant medium for elimination of drugs from the body?
   A. urine
   B. respiratory air
   C. feces
   D. sweat
   E. all are significant

_____ 24. Which of the following is NOT an enteral route of drug administration?
   A. oral
   B. umbilical
   C. buccal
   D. sublingual
   E. rectal

_____ 25. Which of the following is the preferred route for medication administration in most emergencies?
   A. intramuscular
   B. inhalation
   C. endotracheal
   D. intravenous
   E. subcutaneous

_____ 26. Drugs that are spherically shaped to be easy to swallow are:
   A. pills.
   B. suppositories.
   C. tablets.
   D. capsules.
   E. suspensions.

_____ 27. Drugs that are powders compressed into disks are:
   A. pills.
   B. suppositories.
   C. tablets.
   D. capsules.
   E. suspensions.

_____ 28. Preparations in which the solid does not dissolve in the solvent are:
   A. solutions.
   B. tinctures.
   C. suspensions.
   D. spirits.
   E. elixirs.

_____ 29. Preparations made with alcohol and water solvent, often with flavorings, are:
   A. solutions.
   B. tinctures.
   C. suspensions.
   D. spirits.
   E. elixirs.

_____ 30. Pharmacodynamics are best described as:
   A. interactions between drugs.
   B. the processes by which drugs are eliminated from the body.
   C. the effects of a drug on the body.
   D. the processes by which drugs bind to receptor sites.
   E. the process by which a drug is administered.

_____ 31. The location where a drug combines with a protein, resulting in a biochemical effect, is a(n):
   A. second messenger.
   B. antagonist.
   C. receptor.
   D. agonist.
   E. protein block.

_____ 32. A drug's ability to cause its expected response is referred to as its:
   A. affinity.
   B. efficacy.
   C. agonism.
   D. antagonism.
   E. equilibrium.

_____ 33. A chemical that binds to a receptor site but does not cause the expected effect is a(n):
   A. partial antagonist.
   B. competitive antagonist.
   C. agonist.
   D. antagonist.
   E. noncompetitive antagonist.

_____ 34. A chemical that binds to a receptor site causes the expected effect, and prevents other drugs from activating the receptor site is a(n):
   A. partial antagonist.
   B. competitive antagonist.
   C. agonist.
   D. antagonist.
   E. noncompetitive antagonist.

_____ 35. The drug morphine sulfate is an example of a(n):
   A. agonist-antagonist.
   B. competitive antagonist.
   C. agonist.
   D. antagonist.
   E. noncompetitive antagonist.

_____ 36. The drug nalbuphine (Nubain) is an example of a(n):
   A. agonist-antagonist.
   B. competitive antagonist.
   C. agonist.
   D. antagonist.
   E. noncompetitive antagonist.

_____ 37. A drug reaction that is unique to an individual is referred to as:
   A. idiosyncrasy.
   B. tachyphylaxis.
   C. antagonism.
   D. synergism.
   E. potentiation.

_____ 38. A drug reaction that is greater than expected from the administration of two drugs that have the same effect at the same time is referred to as:
   A. idiosyncrasy.
   B. tachyphylaxis.
   C. antagonism.
   D. synergism.
   E. potentiation.

_____ 39. The time span between when a drug drops below its minimum effective concentration and its complete elimination from the body is its:
   A. onset of action.
   B. duration of action.
   C. therapeutic index.
   D. biologic half-life.
   E. termination of action.

_____ 40. The ratio between a drug's lethal dose and its effective dose is its:
   A. onset of action.
   B. duration of action.
   C. therapeutic index.
   D. biologic half-life.
   E. termination of action.

Part 2: Drug Classifications

Review of Chapter Objectives

After reading Part 2 of this chapter, you should be able to:

1. Describe how drugs are classified. pp. 326–327

The Food and Drug Administration classifies a new drug using one-digit and one-letter designations. The numerical classification describes its origin: a new molecular drug, a new salt of a marketed drug, a new formulation or dosage, a new combination not previously marketed, a generic duplication of an existing drug, a new indication for an already marketed drug, and a drug on the market prior to the existence of the FDA. The letter classification identifies the treatment or therapeutic potential of a drug: an important therapeutic gain, a similarity to an existing drug or drugs, whether the drug is indicated in the treatment of AIDS and HIV disease, whether the drug has been developed to treat a severely debilitating or life-threatening disease, or whether the drug is an orphan drug (a drug developed for a relatively uncommon disease).

2. Review the specific anatomy and physiology pertinent to pharmacology with additional attention to autonomic pharmacology. pp. 327–370

Drugs affect many systems of the body including the central nervous system, the autonomic nervous system, the cardiovascular system, the respiratory system, the gastrointestinal system, and the endocrine system. Drugs are also used to treat infectious disease and inflammation.

Central Nervous System Pharmacology

The central nervous system consists of the brain and spinal column and all neurons that both originate and terminate within these structures. Since this system is responsible for conscious thought and affects many bodily functions, it is the target for many drugs used in medical care. These agents include analgesics, anesthetics, antianxiety, and sedative-hypnotic drugs, antiseizure and antiepileptic drugs, CNS stimulants, and psychotherapeutic drugs.

Analgesics are used to reduce the sensation of pain. These drugs include the opioid and nonopioid analgesics, adjunctive medications (to enhance the effects of the analgesics), and opioid agonists-antagonists. Agents that block the actions of analgesics, opioid antagonists, and in some cases analgesic antagonists are used in cases of overdose or to reverse or negate the undesired effects of analgesics.

Anesthetics are used to decrease the sensation of both touch and pain. Anesthetics may be given locally or systemically and in lower doses may produce a decreased sensation of pain while the patient may remain conscious. At higher doses, anesthetics generally induce unconsciousness.

Antianxiety and sedative-hypnotic drugs are used to reduce anxiety, induce amnesia, assist sleeping, and may be used as a part of a balanced approach to anesthesia. These drugs include the benzodiazepines, barbiturates, and alcohol. They decrease (depress) the central nervous system's response to stimuli.

Antiseizure and antiepileptic agents are used to prevent seizure activity and are often associated with undesirable side effects. Antiseizure agents generally act on the sodium and calcium channels in the neural membrane and include phenytoin, carbamazepine, valproic acid, and ethosuximide.

CNS stimulants are used to treat fatigue, drowsiness, narcolepsy, obesity, and attention deficit disorders. They cause their actions by either increasing the release and effectiveness of excitatory neurotransmitters or decreasing the release or effectiveness of inhibitory neurotransmitters. These agents include amphetamines, methylamphetamines, and methylxanthines.

Psychotherapeutic medications treat mental dysfunction, including schizophrenia, depression, and bipolar disorder. Schizophrenia is treated with neuroleptic (affecting the nerves) and antipsychotic drugs (phenothiazines and butyrophenones), which block numerous peripheral neuroreceptor sites. Antidepressants increase the availability, release, or effectiveness of norepinephrine and serotonin and are used to treat depression. These medications include the tricyclic antidepressants (TCAs), the selective serotonin reuptake inhibitors (SSRIs), and monoamine oxidase inhibitors (MAOIs). Bipolar disorder (manic depression) is manifested by dramatic mood swings and is treated with lithium.

Parkinson's disease is another central nervous system disorder caused by the destruction of dopamine-releasing neurons in the portion of the brain controlling fine motor movements. This disease is treated by stimulating the dopamine release (Sinemet) or with anticholinergic agents (benztropine).

Autonomic Nervous System Pharmacology

The autonomic nervous system is located within the peripheral nervous system and consists of the sympathetic (fight-or-flight) and parasympathetic (feed-and-breed) systems. These systems are antagonistic and provided control over body functions. The autonomic nervous system controls virtually every organ and body structure not under conscious control and is responsible for maintaining the internal human environment. The nerves of the two systems do not actually touch other nerves or target organs. Messages are carried through the small space between them (synapse) via chemical messengers (neurotransmitters). Acetylcholine is the neurotransmitter at the target organs of the parasympathetic nervous system, while norepinephrine is the neurotransmitter at the target organs for the sympathetic nervous system.

Stimulation of the parasympathetic nervous system causes pupillary constriction, digestive gland secretion, decreased cardiac rate and strength of contraction, bronchoconstriction, and increased digestive activity. Cholinergic (affecting the acetylcholine receptors) drugs stimulate the parasympathetic nervous system and produce salivation, lacrimation, urination, defecation, gastric motility, and emesis (signs suggested by the acronym SLUDGE). They cause their actions directly by acting on the receptor sites (bethanechol and pilocarpine) or indirectly by inhibiting the degradation of acetylcholine (neostigmine and physostigmine). Anticholenergic (parasympatholytic) drugs oppose the actions of acetylcholine and the parasympathetic nervous system. Atropine is the prototype anticholinergic drug, while scopolamine is used to treat motion sickness and ipratropium bromide (Atrovent) is inhaled to treat bronchoconstriction caused by asthma. Ganglionic blocking agents compete for the acetylcholine receptors at the ganglia and can effectively turn off the parasympathetic nervous system. Neuromuscular blocking agents produce a state of paralysis without inducing unconsciousness. Ganglionic stimulating agents (nicotine) stimulate the ganglia of both the parasympathetic and sympathetic nervous systems yet have no therapeutic purpose.

Stimulation of the sympathetic nervous system causes an increased heart rate and strength of contraction, bronchodilation, increased blood flow to the muscles, decreased blood flow to the skin and abdominal organs, release of glucose stores from the liver, increased energy production, decreased digestive activity, and the release of epinephrine and norepinephrine. Sympathetic receptors include four adrenergic receptors (alpha$_1$, alpha$_2$, beta$_1$, and beta$_2$) and dopaminergic receptors. Alpha$_1$ stimulation causes peripheral vasoconstriction, mild bronchoconstriction, and increased metabolism. Alpha$_2$ stimulation prevents the over-release of norepinephrine at the synapse. Beta$_1$ stimulation exclusively affects the heart and causes increased heart rate, cardiac contractile force, automaticity, and conduction. Beta$_2$ stimulation causes bronchodilation and selective vasodilation. Dopaminergic stimulation causes increased circulation to the kidneys, heart, and brain. Sympathomimetic (adrenergic) drugs stimulate the effects of the sympathetic nervous system, while sympatholytic drugs block the actions of the sympathetic nervous system. Alpha$_1$ drugs increase peripheral vascular resistance, preload, and blood pressure. Alpha$_1$ agonists are used to control blood pressure or to control injury due to the infiltration of an alpha$_1$ drug. Beta$_1$ drugs stimulate the heart and are primarily used in cardiac arrest or cardiogenic shock. Beta$_1$ antagonists are used to control blood pressure, suppress tachycardia, and reduce cardiac workload in angina. Beta$_2$ agonists are used to treat asthma.

Cardiovascular System Pharmacology

The cardiovascular system consists of the heart, blood vessels, and the blood. The heart is a four-chambered muscular organ that pumps most of the blood around the body. It is controlled by an intrinsic electrical system that coordinates cardiac muscular response and pumping action. The myocardium is unique in that it has the ability to generate an electrical impulse (automaticity) and conduct an impulse to surrounding tissue (conductivity). The heart muscle contracts and relaxes (depolarizes and repolarizes) as sodium, calcium, and potassium ions flow into and out of the cell.

Antidysrhythmic drugs are used to prevent or treat abnormal variations in the cardiac electrical cycle. Sodium channel blockers slow the influx of sodium back into the cell and, in effect, slow conduction through the atria and ventricles. Class IA sodium channel blockers (quinidine, procainamide, and disopyramide) slow repolarization, while class IB drugs (lidocaine, phenytoin, tocainide, mexiletine) speed repolarization and reduce automaticity in the ventricles. Class IC drugs (flecainide, propafenone) decrease conduction velocity through the atria, ventricles, bundle of His, and the Purkinje network and delay ventricular repolarization. Beta-blockers (propranolol, acebutolol, esmolol) are antagonistic to the beta 1 actions of the sympathetic nervous system. Since the beta receptors are attached to the calcium channels of the heart, these agents act in a manner very similar to the calcium channel blockers. Potassium channel blockers (bretylium, amiodarone) block the efflux of calcium; these agents prolong repolarization and the effective refractory period (the period before the myocardium can contract again). Calcium channel blockers (verapamil, diltiazem) decrease conductivity through the AV node and slow conduction of atrial flutter or fibrillation to the ventricles. Other antidysrhythmics include adenosine (a fast- and short-acting potassium and calcium blocker), digoxin (decreases SA node firing rate and conduction velocity through the AV node), and magnesium (effective in treating a polymorphic ventricular tachycardia—*torsade de pointes*).

Antihypertensive drugs manipulate peripheral vascular resistance, heart rate, or stroke volume to reduce blood pressure. Diuretics reduce the amount of circulating blood (and hence the cardiac preload and stroke volume) by increasing the urine output of the kidneys. They include loop diuretics (furosemide), thiazides (HydroDIURIL), potassium-sparing diuretics (spironolactone), and the osmotic diuretics (mannitol). Beta adrenergic antagonists (metoprolol) act by reducing the heart's rate and contractility as well as by reducing the release of hormones (renin) from the kidneys that ultimately cause vasoconstriction (through the renin-angiotensin-aldosterone system). Centrally acting adrenergic inhibitors (clonidine) stimulate alpha$_2$ receptors and inhibit the release of norepinephrine. Alpha$_1$ antagonists (prazosin, terazosin) competitively block the alpha 1 receptors, mediating sympathetic increases in peripheral vascular resistance. Finally, some drugs (labetalol, carvedilol) have combined alpha and beta antagonistic effects. Angiotensin converting enzyme (ACE) inhibitors (captopril, enalapril, lisinopril, enalaprilat) block the production of angiotensin II, a very potent vasoconstrictor, through the renin-angiotensin-aldosterone system.

Angiotensin II receptor antagonists act on the renin-angiotensin-aldosterone system by blocking the actions of angiotensin II at its receptor site. Calcium channel blockers (nifedipine) are also effective at controlling hypertension by selectively acting on the smooth muscles of the arterioles and reducing peripheral vascular resistance without reducing cardiac preload. Direct vasodilators (hydralazine, minoxidil, sodium nitroprusside) selectively dilate arterioles and decrease peripheral vascular resistance. Hypertension may also be controlled by agents that block the autonomic nervous system (trimethaphan) or with cardiac glycosides (digoxin, digitoxin) that affect the ion pumps of the myocardium and increase cardiac contraction strength but reduce heart rate.

Angina is treated with calcium channel blockers (verapamil, diltiazem, nifedipine) because they reduce cardiac workload and slow the heart rate. Organic nitrates (nitroglycerin, isosorbide, amyl nitrite) relax vascular smooth muscle, decreasing cardiac preload and workload, and, in Prinzmetal's angina, may increase coronary blood flow.

Three agents are used to prevent and break up blood clots that obstruct either the heart chambers or the blood vessels. Antiplatelet drugs (aspirin, dipyridamole, abciximab, ticlopidine) decrease the formation of platelet plugs during the clotting process. Anticoagulants (heparin, warfarin) interrupt the clotting cascade. Fibrinolytics (streptokinase, alteplase, reteplase, anistreplase) dissolve the fibrin mesh of clots and thereby help break apart clots after they form.

Antihyperlipidemic agents (lovastatin, simvastatin, cholestyramine) are used to reduce the level of low-density lipoproteins, a causative factor for coronary artery disease.

Respiratory System Pharmacology

The respiratory system is basically a pathway through which air travels in from the exterior to the air-exchange sacs, the alveoli, and then out again. Indications for pharmacologic intervention include asthma, rhinitis, and cough.

Asthma is a pathologic condition caused by an allergy to pet dander, dust, or mold that causes respiratory restriction or obstruction. The allergic response releases histamine, leukotrienes, and prostaglandins, producing immediate bronchoconstriction and then inflammation. Treatment includes beta$_2$ agonists (albuterol) to reduce bronchoconstriction and epinephrine for severe reactions not responding to beta$_2$ agonists. Anticholinergic agents (ipratropium) act along different pathways to the beta$_2$ agonists and may provide an additive effect in limiting bronchoconstriction. Glucocorticoids (beclomethasone, methylprednisolone, cromolyn) have antiinflammatory properties that reduce the amount of mucus and the edema in the airway and alveolar walls. Lastly, leukotriene antagonists (zileuton) block the formation of, or the receptors for leukotriene (zafirlukast). Leukotrienes are mediators released from mast cells that contribute powerfully to both bronchoconstriction and inflammation.

Rhinitis is the inflammation of the mucosa of the nasal cavity and may cause nasal congestion, itching, sneezing, and rhinorrhea (runny nose). Nasal decongestants (phenylephrine, pseudoephedrine, phenylpropanolamine) are alpha$_1$ agonists that reduce vasodilation and are given in mist or oral form. Antihistamines (alkylamines, ethanolamines, clemastine, phenothiazines, loratadine, cetirizine, fexofenadine) are used for more serious allergic reactions and block the action of histamine and thereby relieve bronchoconstriction, capillary permeability, and vasodilation. Cough suppressants (antitussive agents, both opioid and nonopioid) dull the cough reflex and are designed to treat unproductive coughing due to an irritated oropharynx. Expectorants are intended to increase the productivity of the cough while mucolytics make the mucus more watery and possibly more effective.

Gastrointestinal System Pharmacology

Drugs used to treat the gastrointestinal system are primarily for gastric ulcers, constipation, diarrhea, emesis, and to aid digestion. Peptic ulcer disease occurs as the balance between the protective coating of the stomach and its acidity is no longer maintained. The acid may then eat away at the intestinal lining and tissues underneath. The injury may result in internal hemorrhage. Peptic ulcer disease is treated with antibiotics (bismuth, metronidazole, amoxicillin, tetracycline) to treat the underlying cause and drugs (cimetidine, ranitidine, famotidine, nizatidine, omeprazole, lansoprazole, antacids, pirenzepine) that block or decrease the secretion of acid. Constipation is treated with bulk-forming (methylcellulose, psyllium), surfactant (docusate sodium), stimulant (phenolphthalein, bisacodyl), or osmotic (magnesium hydroxide) laxatives. Diarrhea is often caused by an underlying disease and is usually self-correcting. In severe cases, it is treated with antibiotics. Input from the inner ear, nose, and eyes or a response to anxiety or fear triggers the vomiting reflex (emesis), which can be useful for certain poisonings and overdoses (Ipecac). Antiemetics that reduce the vomiting reflex include serotonin antagonists (ondansetron), dopamine antagonists (phenothiazines, butyrophenones, metoclopramide), anticholenergics, and cannabinoids (dronabinol, nabilone). Finally, drugs used to aid ingestion are enzymes (pancreatin, pancrelipase) similar to endogenous enzymes found in the intestinal tract.

Endocrine System Pharmacology

The endocrine system provides the body with hormones essential to maintaining homeostasis and controlling overall body activity. It consists of the following glands: pituitary, pineal, thyroid, thymus, parathyroid, adrenal, pancreas, ovaries, and testes. These organs produce hormones that then circulate throughout the body and affect target organs. Drugs can affect the anterior and posterior pituitary, parathyroid and thyroid, adrenal, pancreas, and reproductive glands or simulate the hormones they produce.

The pituitary gland is made up of the anterior and posterior lobes and resides deep within the skull. The anterior pituitary gland releases hormones related to growth. Dwarfism results from a deficiency in growth hormone and is treated with somatrem and somatropin. Gigantism and acromegaly usually result from a tumor and are treated by surgical removal of the tumor or with the drug octreotide, which inhibits the release of the growth hormone. The posterior pituitary produces oxytocin and antidiuretic hormone (ADH). Oxytocin induces uterine contractions and precipitates delivery, while antidiuretic hormone increases water reabsorption in the kidneys and thereby regulates electrolyte balance, blood volume, and blood pressure. Diabetes insipidus is caused by inadequate circulating ADH and is treated with vasopressin, desmopressin, and lypressin.

The parathyroid gland regulates the levels of calcium and vitamin D. Chronic low calcium and vitamin D levels are treated with supplements, while high levels (usually due to tumors) are treated with surgical removal of all or part of the parathyroid gland.

The thyroid gland hormones play vital roles in growth, maturation, and metabolism. Child onset hyperthyroidism results in dwarfism and mental retardation, while adult onset hyperthyroidism manifests with a decreased metabolism, weight gain, fatigue, and bradycardia. Hypothyroidism is treated with levothyroxine, a synthetic analog of thyroxine, the major thyroid hormone. Goiters occur as a result of inadequate iodine in the diet and are treated with iodine supplements. Thyroid tumors often cause hyperthyroidism and are treated with surgery, radiation therapy, or the drug propylthiouracil or a combination of therapies.

The adrenal cortex secretes glucocorticoids that increase the glucose in the bloodstream, mineralocorticoids that regulate the salt–water balance, and androgens that regulate sexual development and maturity. Cushing's disease results in increased glucocorticoid secretion and hyperglycemia, obesity, hypertension, and electrolyte imbalances. It is usually treated surgically, with pharmacological intervention aimed at the symptoms; drugs used for this include antihypertensive agents (spironolactone), ACE inhibitors (captopril), and drugs that inhibit corticoid synthesis. Addison's disease is characterized by hyposecretion of corticoids and presents with hypoglycemia, emaciation, hypotension, hyperkalemia, and hyponatremia. It is treated with cortisone, hydrocortisone, and fludrocortisone.

The pancreas produces two hormones important to glucose metabolism. They are insulin and glucagon. Insulin is essential for the transport of glucose, potassium, and amino acids into the cells. It stimulates cell growth and division and converts glucose into glycogen in the liver and skeletal muscles. Glucagon increases blood glucose levels by promoting the synthesis of glucose from glycerol and amino acids and from breaking down glycogen into glucose. Diabetes is an inappropriate carbohydrate metabolism due to an inadequate release of insulin (Type I, juvenile onset) or a decreased responsiveness to insulin (Type II, adult onset). Oral hypoglycemic agents stimulate insulin release from the pancreas and are administered to the Type II diabetic. They are from four classes: sulfonylureas (tolbutamide, chlorpropamide, glipizide, glyburide), biguanides (metformin), alpha-glucosidase inhibitors (acarbose, miglitol), and thiazolidinediones (troglitazone). Pork, beef, or human insulin is injected subcutaneously daily for the Type I diabetic. Hyperglycemic agents (glucagon and diazoxide) act to increase blood glucose levels while 50 percent dextrose in water ($D_{50}W$) is an intravenous sugar solution intended to supply carbohydrates to the hypoglycemic patient.

The genitalia release hormones that regulate human sexuality and reproduction. In the female, the ovaries, ovarian follicles, and, during pregnancy, the placenta release these hormones. Drug therapy can supplement these hormones, provide contraception, stimulate or relax the pregnant uterus, or assist in fertility. Estrogen is administered post-menopause to reduce the risk of osteoporosis and coronary artery disease. It is also administered in delayed puberty. Progestins counteract the untoward effects of estrogen and are used to treat amenorrhea, endometriosis, and dysfunctional uterine hemorrhage. Estrogen and progestin (or progestin alone) are commonly used as contraceptives. Their side effects include a predisposition to thromboembolisms, hypertension, and uterine bleeding. Oxytocic agents (oxytocin) induce uterine contractions to induce or speed up labor, while tocolytics (terbutaline, ritodrine) relax the smooth muscle of the uterus and delay labor. Female infertility is treated with agents (clomiphene, urofollitropin, menotropin) that promote maturation of ovarian follicles. In the male, testosterone replacement therapy (testosterone enanthate, methyltestosterone, fluoxymesterone) is provided for deficiency or delayed puberty. An enlarged prostate is cared for with surgery or drug (finasteride) therapy. A recent drug, sildenafil, is used for erectile dysfunction and acts by relaxing vascular smooth muscle. However, in combination with nitrates, it may lead to decreased cardiac preload and profound hypotension.

Pharmacology of Infectious Disease

Infectious diseases are typically caused by bacteria, viruses, or fungi and are treated by antimicrobial drugs including antibiotics and antifungal, antiviral, and antiparasitic agents. Symptoms of microbial infection are treated with nonsteroidal antiinflammatory drugs (NSAIDs), and some diseases are treated prophylactically with serums and vaccines.

Antibiotics either kill the offending bacteria or decrease their ability to grow and reproduce. Penicillin, cephalosporin, and vancomycin act by inhibiting cell wall synthesis and causing the walls to rupture. Macrolide, aminoglycoside, and tetracycline antibiotics prevent cells from replicating.

Antifungal agents inhibit fungal growth (ketoconazole), while antiviral drugs act through various mechanisms (indinavir, acyclovir, zidovudine). Antiparasitic agents are used to treat malaria (chloroquine, mefloquine, quinine), amebiasis (paromomycin, metronidazole), and helminthiasis (mebendazole, niclosamide).

Other antimicrobials are used to treat diseases such as tuberculosis (isoniazid, refampin) and leprosy (dapsone, clofazimine).

Nonsteroidal antiinflammatory drugs (ketorolac, piroxicam, naproxen) limit the fever (antipyretics) and pain (analgesics) associated with headache, arthritis, dysmenorrhea, and orthopedic injuries.

3. **List and describe common prehospital medications, including indications, contraindications, side effects, routes of administration, and dosages.** pp. 327–370

   At the back of this workbook you will find a series of pages with drug cards. Each card contains the name/class, description, indications, contraindications, precautions, routes of administration, and dosages for a drug commonly used in prehospital emergency care. Detach the cards and begin to use them as flash cards. This will help you learn essential information about the drugs you will use during your career as a paramedic.

4. **Given several patient scenarios, identify medications likely to be prescribed and those that are likely a part of the prehospital treatment regimen.** pp. 327–370

   Prescribed Medications

   As you arrive at the side of and begin to assess and treat a patient, an important aspect of assessment will be to determine what medications the patient is taking (both prescribed and over-the-counter). Since many drugs are given for specific pathologies, the drugs prescribed may give you clues as to the patient's underlying problem. The general pathology classification and the drugs used to care for that pathology are listed below. As you progress through your training, and especially as you enter the medical emergencies portion of your training, the classification of pathologies and the drugs prescribed for such will become more specific and extensive.

Central Nervous System

Analgesics	Opioid agonists	opium, morphine
	Nonopioids	aspirin, NSAIDs, ibuprofen, acetaminophen
	Benzodiazepines	diazepam, lorazepam, midazolam
	Antihistamines	promethazine, caffeine
	Opioid agonist-antagonists	pentazocine, nalbuphine, butorphanol
Antianxiety	Benzodiazepines	diazepam, lorazepam, midazolam
	Barbiturates	phenobarbital
Antiseizure	Benzodiazepines	diazepam, lorazepam, midazolam
	Barbiturates	phenobarbital
	Hydantoins	phenytoin, fosphenytoin
	Succinimides	ethosuximide
	Miscellaneous	valproic acid
CNS stimulants	Amphetamines	amphetamine sulfate, methamphetamine, dextroamphetamine
	Methyphenidates	methylphenidate
	Methylxanthines	caffeine, aminophylline, theophylline
Antipsychotics	Phenothiazines	chlorpromazine
	Butyrophenones	haloperidol
	Miscellaneous	clozapine, risperidone
Antidepressant	TCAs	imipramine, amitriptyline, desipramine, nortriptyline
	SSRIs	fluoxetine, sertraline, paroxetine
	MAOIs	phenelzine
Bipolar disorder		lithium (bipolar disorder)
Parkinson's disease		levodopa, Sinemet, amantadine, bromocriptine
	MAOIs	selegiline
	Anticholinergics	benztropine, diphenhydramine

Autonomic Nervous System

Parasympathetic nervous system	Cholinergics	bethanechol, pilocarpine, neostigmine, physostigmine, echothiophate
	Anticholinergics	atropine, scopolamine, ipratropium bromide, dicyclomine, benztropine
Sympathetic nervous system	Adrenergics	norepinephrine, epinephrine, dopamine, dolbutamine, isoproterenol, ephedrine phenylephedrine, terbutaline
	Antiadrenergics	phenoxybenzamine, prazosin, phentolamine
	Beta-blockers	propranolol, metoprolol, atenolol
	Skeletal muscle relaxants	baclofen, cyclobenzaprine, carisoprodol dantrolene

Sense Organs

Eyes	Glaucoma	timolol, betaxolol, pilocarpine
	Diagnostic procedures	atropisol, scopolamine, phenylephrine
	Anesthetic	tetracaine
Ears	Antibiotics	chloramphenicol, gentamicin sulfate
	Wax removal	carbamide peroxide and glycerin

Cardiovascular System

Antidysrhythmics	Sodium channel blockers	quinidine, procainamide, disopyramide, lidocaine, phenytoin, mexiletine, flecainide, propafenone, moricine
	Beta-blockers	propranolol, esmolol
	Potassium channel blockers	bretylium, amiodarone
	Calcium channel blockers	verapamil, diltiazem
	Miscellaneous	adenosine, digoxin, magnesium
Diuretics	Loop	furosemide
	Thiazides	hydrochlorothiazide
	Potassium sparing	spironolactone
Antihypertensives	Adrenergic inhibitors	clonidine, methyldopa, reserpine, guanethidine, guanadrel, prazosin, terazosin, labetalol, carvedilol, nifedipine
	ACE inhibitors	captoril, enalapril, lisinopril
	Angiotension II antagonist	losartan
	Calcium channel blockers	nifedipine
	Vasodilators	hydralazine, minoxidil, sodium nitroprusside, trimethaphan, digoxin, digitoxin
	Antianginals	verapamil, diltiazem, nifedipine, nitroglycerin
Hemostatic agents	Antiplatelets	aspirin, dipyridamole, abciximab, ticlopidine
	Anticoagulants	heparin, warfarin
	Thrombolitics	streptokinase, alteplase, reteplase, anistreplase
	Antihyperlipidemics	lovastatin, simvastatin, cholestyramine

Respiratory System

Antiasthmatics	Beta$_2$ agents	albuterol, terbutaline
	Sympathomimetics	epinephrine, ephedrine, isoproterenol
	Methylxanthines	methylxanthine, theophylline, aminophylline
	Anticholinergics	ipratropium
	Glucocorticoids	methylprednisolone, cromolyn
	Leukotriene antagonists	zileuton, zafirlukast
Rhinitis and cough	Nasal decongestants	phenylephedrine, pseudoephedrine, phenylpropanolamine
	Antihistamines	
	Alkylamines	chlorpheniramine

	Ethanolamines	diphenhydramine, clemastine
	Phenothiazines	promethiazine, dimenhydrinate, loratadine, cetirizine, fexofenadine
	Cough suppressants antitussive	codeine, hydrocodone, dextromethorphan, diphenhydramine, benzonatate

Gastrointestinal System

Peptic ulcer disease	H$_2$ receptor agonists	cimetidine, ranitidine, famotidine, nizatidine
	Proton pump inhibitors	omeprazole, lansoprazole
	Antacids	aluminum, magnesium, calcium, or sodium compounds
	Anticholinergics	pirenzepine
Laxatives	Bulk-forming	methylcellulose, psyllium
	Surfactant	docusate sodium
	Stimulant	phenolphthalein, bisacodyl
	Osmotic	magnesium hydroxide
Antidiarrheal	Antibiotics	
Antiemetics	Serotonin antagonists	ondansetron
	Dopamine antagonists	
	Phenothiazines	prochlorperazine, promethazine
	Butyrophenones	haloperidol, droperidol
	Miscellaneous	metoclopramide
	Cannabinoids	dronabinol, nabilone
To aid digestion		pancreatin, pancrelipase

Endocrine System

Pituitary gland	Anterior pituitary	somatrem, somatropin, octreotide
	Posterior pituitary	vasopressin, desmopressin, lypressin
Parathyroid glands		calcium and vitamin D supplements
Thyroid gland		levothyroxine
Adrenal cortex	Cushing's disease	spironolactone, captopril
	Addison's disease	cortisone, hydrocortisone, fludrocortisone
Pancreas	Insulin	
	Oral hypoglycemics	
	Sulfonylureas	tolbutamide, chlorpropamide, glipizide, glyburide
	Biguanides	metformin
	Alpha-glucosidase inhibitors	acarbose, miglitol
	Thiazolidinediones	troglitazone
	Hyperglycemic agents	glucagon, diazoxide

Reproductive System

Female	Estrogen/Progestins	
	Oral contraceptives	
	Oxytocics	oxytocin, ergonovine
	Tocolytics	terbutaline, ritodrine
	Infertility agents	clomiphene, urofollitropin, menotropin
Male	Testosterone	enanthate, methyltestosterone, fluoxymesterone
	Enlarged prostate	finasteride
Sexual performance		levodopa, sildenafil

Cancer Drugs

	Antimetabolites	fluorouracil
	Alkylating agents	cyclophosphamide, mechlorethamine
	Mitotic inhibitors	vinblastine, vincristine

Infectious Disease

	Antibiotics	penicillin, cephalosporin, vancomycin
	Antifungals	ketoconazole
	Antivirals	acyclovir, zidovudine, indinavir
	Antiparasitics	
	Malaria	chloroquine, mefloquine, quinine
	Amebiasis	paromomycin, metronidazole
	Helminthiasis	mebendazole, niclosamide
	Antimicrobial	
	Tuberculosis	isoniazid, rifampin
	Leprosy	dapsone, clofazimine
	Nonsteroidal antiinflammatories	acetaminophen, ibuprofen, ketorolac, piroxicam, naproxen

Immune System

Immunosuppressants	azathioprine	
Immunomodulators	zidovudine, rotonavir, saquinavir	

Note that this is not a complete list of common prescription drugs. As you continue your studies and career as a paramedic, many prescription drugs will become familiar to you. It is also recommended that you obtain a small pocket book that lists common prescription drugs and the conditions for which they are normally prescribed.

Prehospital Medications

Indications for the drugs commonly used in prehospital emergency medical care are contained on the drug cards in at the end of this Workbook. Review them with special attention to the conditions in which each drug is used.

5. **Given various patient medications, assess the pathophysiology of a patient's condition by identifying classifications of drugs.** pp. 326–370

Within the discussion of the previous objective and throughout the text of this part of Chapter 6, drugs prescribed frequently for each common medical condition are noted. Finding one or more of these drugs with a patient might suggest preexisting medical conditions and, possibly, the underlying reason the patient called for your assistance. Whenever you find prescription drugs with a patient, you should determine what they were prescribed for and if the patient has been compliant with his or her drug administration. There are numerous pocket EMS drug guides that identify the most common prescription drugs by their various names and give the common reasons they are prescribed. If you are ever unsure of the nature and use of a patient's medication, contact your medical direction physician.

Content Self-Evaluation

MULTIPLE CHOICE

1. Drugs can be classified by:
   A. the body system they affect.
   B. the mechanism of their action.
   C. their indications.
   D. their source.
   E. all of the above

_____ 2. The drug that demonstrates the common properties of a class of drugs is called a:
   A. root drug.
   B. prototype drug.
   C. characteristic drug.
   D. primary drug.
   E. none of the above

_____ 3. Which of the following is NOT a division of the nervous system?
   A. central nervous system
   B. peripheral nervous system
   C. autonomic nervous system
   D. sympathetic nervous system
   E. antagonistic nervous system

_____ 4. Which nervous system controls motor functions?
   A. somatic
   B. autonomic
   C. sympathetic
   D. parasympathetic
   E. antagonistic

_____ 5. Which nervous system is responsible for the "feed-or-breed" response?
   A. somatic
   B. autonomic
   C. sympathetic
   D. parasympathetic
   E. antagonistic

_____ 6. A drug that relieves pain only is termed a(n):
   A. anesthetic.
   B. endorphin.
   C. analgesic.
   D. opioid.
   E. antimanic.

_____ 7. The prototype opioid drug is:
   A. heroin.
   B. morphine.
   C. aspirin.
   D. ibuprofen.
   E. acetaminophen.

_____ 8. Naloxone (Narcan) is the principal:
   A. non-opioid analgesic.
   B. opioid agonist.
   C. opioid antagonist.
   D. prehospital anesthetic.
   E. opioid agonist-antagonist.

_____ 9. Anesthetics, as a group, tend to cause which of the following?
   A. reconfigured sensation
   B. respiratory stimulation
   C. central nervous system depression
   D. cardiovascular stimulation
   E. endorphin stimulation

_____ 10. When using neuromuscular blocking agents, it is common to use antianxiety, amnesic, and analgesic agents as well.
   A. True
   B. False

_____ 11. Which of the following is the only anesthetic gas given in the prehospital setting?
   A. ether
   B. halothane
   C. enflurane
   D. nitrous oxide
   E. sodium pentothal

_____ 12. Sedative is a term that describes a drug that:
   A. decreases anxiety.
   B. deters sleep.
   C. reduces sensation.
   D. decreases pain sensation.
   E. is an opioid antagonist.

_____ 13. The antagonist for the benzodiazepines is:
   A. naloxone.
   B. flumazenil.
   C. thiopental.
   D. diazepam.
   E. midazolam.

CHAPTER 6 *General Principles of Pharmacology* 119

_____ 14. Amphetamines cause which of the following?
   A. release of epinephrine
   B. release of dopamine
   C. decreased wakefulness
   D. increased appetite
   E. weight gain

_____ 15. Caffeine is classified as a(n):
   A. methylxanthine.
   B. methylphenidate.
   C. amphetamine.
   D. opioid.
   E. endorphin.

_____ 16. The drug class used to care for patients with mental dysfunctions is:
   A. neuroleptic.
   B. psychotherapeutic.
   C. extrapyramidal.
   D. schizophrenic.
   E. antimanic.

_____ 17. It appears that dopamine, norepinephrine, and serotonin play a role in psychotic pathologies.
   A. True
   B. False

_____ 18. As a result of the extrapyramidal effects of antipsychotic drugs, these drugs are termed:
   A. Parkinsonian agents.
   B. extrapyramidogenics.
   C. neuroleptics.
   D. dopamine agonists.
   E. neurotransmitters.

_____ 19. The drug of choice for treating the extrapyramidal symptoms associated with antipsychotic drugs is:
   A. diazepam.
   B. furosemide.
   C. chlorpromazine.
   D. diphenhydramine.
   E. epinephrine.

_____ 20. Which of the following is NOT a sign or symptom of depression?
   A. weight loss
   B. weight gain
   C. sleep disturbances
   D. excessive energy
   E. inability to concentrate

_____ 21. Expected side effects of tricyclic antidepressants include all of the following EXCEPT:
   A. blurred vision.
   B. dry mouth.
   C. urinary retention.
   D. bradycardia.
   E. orthostatic hypotension.

_____ 22. Tricyclic antidepressants (TCAs) raise the seizure threshold and are effective antiseizure medications.
   A. True
   B. False

_____ 23. The drug of choice for the management of bipolar disorder is:
   A. valium.
   B. lithium.
   C. imipramine.
   D. phenelzine.
   E. morphine sulfate.

_____ 24. Parkinson's disease may present with which characteristic signs and symptoms?
   A. elation
   B. unsteady gait
   C. postural rigidity
   D. tachykinesia
   E. aggressiveness

_____ 25. Parkinson's disease is caused by a reduced number of presynaptic terminals that release dopamine.
   A. True
   B. False

_____ 26. Dopamine is given directly to the Parkinson's disease patient to help balance the dopamine-acetylcholine balance.
   A. True
   B. False

_____ 27. Which nervous system works in opposition to the parasympathetic nervous system?
   A. central
   B. sympathetic
   C. autonomic
   D. somatic
   E. antagonistic

_____ 28. The agents that transport impulses through the synapse between neurons and between nerve cells and the target organs are called:
   A. neuroeffectors.
   B. neurotransmitters.
   C. intrasynaptic agents.
   D. neuroleptic ions.
   E. transport cells.

_____ 29. The cholinergic neurotransmitter is:
   A. acetylcholine.
   B. epinephrine.
   C. norepinephrine.
   D. muscarinic antagonist.
   E. muscarinic agonist.

_____ 30. Which neurotransmitter serves both the sympathetic and parasympathetic nervous systems?
   A. acetylcholine
   B. epinephrine
   C. norepinephrine
   D. dopamine
   E. none of the above

_____ 31. A drug that stimulates the parasympathetic nervous system is called a(n):
   A. sympatholytic.
   B. sympathomimetic.
   C. parasympatholytic.
   D. parasympathomimetic.
   E. antiemetic.

_____ 32. A cholinergic drug is also which of the following?
   A. a sympatholytic
   B. a sympathomimetic
   C. a parasympatholytic
   D. a parasympathomimetic
   E. an antiemetic

_____ 33. The acronym that describes the effects of cholinergic stimulation is:
   A. SARIN.
   B. 2-PAM.
   C. SLUDGE.
   D. ALPHA.
   E. BETA.

_____ 34. The effects of cholinergic stimulation include all of the following EXCEPT:
   A. salivation.
   B. tachycardia.
   C. defecation.
   D. urination.
   E. emesis.

_____ 35. The prototype anticholenergic drug is:
   A. epinephrine.
   B. norepinephrine.
   C. acetylcholine.
   D. atropine.
   E. dopamine.

_____ 36. Neuromuscular blockade produces paralysis and amnesia to the event.
   A. True
   B. False

_____ 37. Which of the following is NOT an action caused by nicotine?
   A. tachycardia
   B. increased salivation
   C. vasoconstriction
   D. hypotension
   E. increased gastric secretion

_____ 38. Alpha₁ antagonist drugs are used almost exclusively to control hypertension.
  A. True
  B. False

_____ 39. What effect does alpha stimulation have on the heart?
  A. increases heart rate
  B. increases automaticity
  C. increases contractile strength
  D. increases oxygen consumption
  E. none of the above

_____ 40. Which type of drug decreases cardiac contractility and heart rate?
  A. beta₂ agonists
  B. beta₁ antagonists
  C. beta₁ agonists
  D. alpha₁ antagonists
  E. alpha₁ agonists

_____ 41. The prototype beta-blocker is:
  A. isoproterenol.
  B. dopamine.
  C. atropine.
  D. propranolol.
  E. none of the above.

_____ 42. Which of the following is NOT a naturally occurring catecholamine?
  A. dopamine
  B. epinephrine
  C. norepinephrine
  D. isoproterenol
  E. A and C

_____ 43. Which type of drug causes bronchodilation?
  A. beta₂ agonists
  B. beta₁ antagonists
  C. beta₁ agonists
  D. alpha₁ antagonists
  E. alpha₁ agonists

_____ 44. Beta-blockers and calcium channel blockers have similar effects on the heart.
  A. True
  B. False

_____ 45. Adenosine produces which of the following?
  A. facial pallor
  B. chest pain
  C. bronchodilation
  D. marked tachycardias
  E. all of the above

_____ 46. Hypertension affects about how many people in the United States?
  A. 10 million
  B. 25 million
  C. 50 million
  D. 100 million
  E. 250 million

_____ 47. Which of the following is an osmotic diuretic?
  A. hydrochlorothiazide
  B. furosemide
  C. potassium chloride
  D. mannitol
  E. spironolactone

_____ 48. The renin-angiotensin-aldosterone system performs what function?
  A. increasing hepatic function
  B. decreasing blood volume
  C. increasing vasoconstriction
  D. causing severe bronchoconstriction
  E. all of the above

_____ 49. Which of the following drug types is used in the treatment of hypertension?
  A. antihyperlipidemics
  B. glucocorticoids
  C. calcium channel blockers
  D. cardiac glycosides
  E. all of the above

_____ 50. Which of the following are actions caused by the administration of digoxin?
A. decreases intracellular sodium levels
B. decreases intracellular calcium
C. increases the strength of cardiac muscle contraction
D. increases ventricular engorgement during left heart failure
E. all of the above

_____ 51. The primary action of nitroglycerin in angina is to:
A. reduce preload.
B. reduce peripheral vascular resistance.
C. dilate the coronary arteries.
D. reduce the anginal pain.
E. increase blood pressure.

_____ 52. Thrombi are the primary pathologies for which of the following?
A. stroke
B. myocardial infarction
C. pulmonary embolism
D. hypertension
E. all of the above except D

_____ 53. Which of the following prevents thrombi by interrupting the clotting cascade?
A. antiplatelets
B. anticoagulants
C. fibrinolytics
D. hemostatic agents
E. all of the above

_____ 54. All of the following are used to treat or prevent thrombi EXCEPT:
A. antiplatelets.
B. antihyperlipidemic agents.
C. fibrinolytics
D. oral anticoagulants.
E. parenteral anticoagulants.

_____ 55. Warfarin is contraindicated in pregnant mothers because it is likely to cause:
A. uterine bleeding.
B. birth defects.
C. maternal hypertension.
D. vitamin K toxicity.
E. placenta previa.

_____ 56. Of the hemostatic agents, which can dissolve clots once they have formed?
A. aspirin
B. heparin
C. warfarin
D. streptokinase
E. thrombarin

_____ 57. Which of the following is of greatest help in reducing cholesterol levels in the blood?
A. low-density lipoproteins (LDL)
B. very low-density lipoproteins (VLDL)
C. high-density lipoproteins (HDL)
D. intermediate-density lipoproteins (IDL)
E. neutral-density lipoproteins (NDL)

_____ 58. Which of the events below occurs first in an asthma attack?
A. inflammatory response
B. mast cell rupture
C. release of histamine and leukotrienes
D. immediate bronchospasm
E. allergen binding to antibody on the mast cell

_____ 59. Which of the following groups is NOT used to treat asthma?
A. leukotriene antagonists
B. glucocorticoids
C. ganglionic blocking agents
D. methylxanthines
E. anticholinergics

_____ 60. Which of the following is the first line therapy for asthma?
A. selective beta$_2$ agonists
B. nonselective sympathomimetics
C. anticholinergics
D. glucocorticoids
E. leukotriene antagonists

_____ 61. Nasal decongestants act by which of the following actions?
    A. restricting histamine release
    B. blocking histamine action
    C. constricting nasal capillaries
    D. thinning nasal mucus
    E. all of the above

_____ 62. Histamine is a major agent in the severe anaphylactic reaction.
    A. True
    B. False

_____ 63. Antihistamine drugs are not indicated for asthma patients because they thicken bronchial secretions.
    A. True
    B. False

_____ 64. A drug that suppresses the urge to cough is a(n):
    A. expectorant.
    B. mucolytic.
    C. antitussive.
    D. surfactant.
    E. cannabinoid.

_____ 65. Most peptic ulcer disease is caused by:
    A. oversecretion of gastric acid.
    B. stress.
    C. alcohol consumption.
    D. decreased gastric circulation.
    E. a bacterium.

_____ 66. Which of the following is a type of laxative?
    A. bulk-forming
    B. osmotic
    C. surfactant
    D. stimulant
    E. all of the above

_____ 67. The drug chloramphenicol is used to treat what condition involving the ears?
    A. bacterial infections
    B. viral infections
    C. impacted wax
    D. inflammation and irritation
    E. all of the above

_____ 68. Which of the following drugs have ototoxic properties?
    A. aspirin
    B. other nonsteroidal anti-inflammatory drugs
    C. some antibiotics
    D. furosemide
    E. all of the above

_____ 69. The gland of the endocrine system that is regarded as the master gland is the:
    A. pituitary.
    B. thyroid.
    C. parathyroid.
    D. pancreas.
    E. adrenal.

_____ 70. The hormones produced by the thyroid play vital roles in growth, maturation, and:
    A. acromegaly.
    B. electrolyte balance.
    C. metabolism.
    D. gastric secretion regulation.
    E. all of the above

_____ 71. Goiters are typically caused by an insufficiency in:
    A. potassium.
    B. calcium.
    C. iodine.
    D. vitamin K.
    E. hemoglobin.

_____ 72. The adrenal cortex is responsible for the production of hormones for all the following purposes EXCEPT:
    A. to regulate salt balance.
    B. to regulate immunity.
    C. to regulate glucose production.
    D. to regulate water balance.
    E. to regulate sexual maturity.

_____ 73. The type of diabetes that typically manifests during childhood is:
   A. gestational.
   B. Type I.
   C. Type II.
   D. Type III.
   E. Type IV.

_____ 74. The pancreas secretes two hormones important to the regulation of glucose. They are insulin and:
   A. glucagon.
   B. glycogen.
   C. dextrose.
   D. cortisol.
   E. orinase.

_____ 75. Which of the following forms of insulin is not likely to cause an allergic reaction?
   A. lente
   B. pork
   C. beef
   D. recombinant
   E. bovine

_____ 76. The principal indication for estrogen replacement therapy in women is:
   A. postmenopause replacement.
   B. contraception.
   C. to delay childbirth.
   D. in delayed puberty.
   E. all of the above

_____ 77. Serious hypotension may occur in a patient who takes sildenafil when also taking:
   A. glucagon.
   B. nitrates.
   C. $D_{50}W$.
   D. antibiotics.
   E. thyroxine.

_____ 78. Antibiotics act by:
   A. killing the bacteria outright.
   B. creating antigens to deactivate the bacteria.
   C. engulfing the bacteria.
   D. decreasing the bacteria's growth rate.
   E. both A and D

_____ 79. The best age for vaccination against disease is:
   A. under 6 months.
   B. under 2 years.
   C. from 2 to 5 years.
   D. over 5 years of age.
   E. over 8 years of age.

_____ 80. The number associated with each B vitamin relates to:
   A. its order of discovery.
   B. its molecular size.
   C. its importance to the body.
   D. its point of absorption.
   E. none of the above

Chapter 7: Intravenous Access and Medication Administration

Part 1: Principles and Routes of Medication Administration

Review of Chapter Objectives

Because Chapter 7 is lengthy, it has been divided into parts to aid your study. Read the assigned textbook pages; then, progress through the objectives and self-evaluation materials as you would with other chapters. When you feel secure in your grasp of the content, proceed to the next part.

After reading Part 1 of this chapter, you should be able to:

1. Review the specific anatomy and physiology pertinent to medication administration.

pp. 378–405

Chapter 6 reviewed human anatomy as it pertains to the absorption, distribution, metabolization, and elimination of the drugs we use to treat disease and trauma. This chapter identifies the anatomy and physiology related to medication administration.

The percutaneous routes of drug administration include transdermal and mucous membrane administration. Transdermal administration permits drug absorption through the skin via topical application in which the medication is slowly and steadily absorbed. Mucous membrane administration methods include sublingual, buccal, ocular, nasal, and aural administration, in which a drug is given under the tongue, between the cheek and gum, in the eye, into the nose, or into the ear, respectively. Sublingual and buccal routes result in systemic absorption, while the remaining routes result in more local effects.

Pulmonary administration introduces a drug by nebulizer or metered dose inhaler or through an endotracheal tube. All three methods direct the drug to the lung tissue for action; however, endotracheal administration is an emergency route for systemic administration.

Enteral administration delivers a drug to the gastrointestinal tract, where it is absorbed. This is a relatively safe and simple route for drug administration and is the most common route for over-the-counter and prescription drug administration. The disadvantage of this route is that many factors can affect absorption including stress, diet, and metabolic rate. Liver function metabolizes some drugs, and a dysfunctional liver may alter the medication's metabolization or distribution. The enteral methods of administration include oral, gastric tube, and rectal administration. (Rectal administration is not subject to hepatic [liver] alteration.)

With parenteral administration, a drug is injected into the dermis (intradermal), the subcutaneous layer (subcutaneous), muscle (intramuscular), or veins (intravenous). The intradermal route provides little or no systemic absorption and is used for diagnostic testing and for the administration of local anesthetic. Subcutaneous injection promotes slow, sustained systemic absorption of a drug, while intramuscular injection permits systemic drug absorption at a moderate rate. Because intravenous drug administration injects the drug directly into the bloodstream, where it is directed to the heart, mixed with the returning venous blood, and then distributed systemically, it is the fastest parenteral administration route.

Anatomically, subcutaneous injections may be made into the skin regions over the deltoid muscle, the thighs, and, in some cases, the upper abdomen. Intramuscular injections may be given into the deltoid muscle, 2 inches below the acromial process; into the gluteal muscle, in the upper outer quadrant of the buttocks; into the anterolateral aspect of the thigh muscle (vastus lateralis); and into the central and lateral segment of the mid-thigh (rectus femoris).

2. Describe the indications, equipment needed, technique used, precautions, and general principles for the following:

All administration of medication requires the use of body substance isolation measures and medically clean techniques. The six rights of medication administration must be observed (see objective 5). With drug administration, you must watch carefully for the desired and adverse effects of the drug administration.

a. Inhalation routes of medication administration pp. 381–395

Pulmonary medications are administered via nebulizer, metered dose inhaler, and endotracheal tube. Drugs indicated for inhalation include those that cause bronchodilation, mucolytics, antibiotics, and topical steroids for respiratory emergencies, congestion, infection, and inflammation, respectively.

A nebulizer aerosolizes a small volume of liquid (or dissolved) medication using oxygen, which is then inhaled into the lungs and absorbed quickly. The device is assembled (mouth piece, medication reservoir, oxygen port, relief valve, and oxygen tubing and source), and 3 to 5 mL of solution (or a medication dissolved in 3 to 5 mL of sterile water) is placed in the medication reservoir. Oxygen is set to run at 5 to 8 liters per minute (without a humidifier), and the mouthpiece is placed in the patient's mouth. The patient should hold the nebulizer and inhale slowly and deeply with each breath, then hold the breath for 1 to 2 seconds before exhaling. The patient should continue doing this until the medication is gone (about 3 to 5 minutes). For nebulized medications to be effective, the patient must have an adequate tidal volume and respiratory rate, although nebulizers can be connected to an endotracheal tube during positive pressure ventilation.

Metered dose inhalers are frequently used in patients with COPD and asthma to deliver agents to induce bronchodilation. The device consists of a pressurized medication canister, plastic shell and mouthpiece, and possibly a spacer. The patient self-administers the drug by assembling the inhaler, shaking it for 2 to 5 seconds, inverting it, placing the mouthpiece in the mouth, and sealing the lips against the mouthpiece. Then, during the beginning of a deep inhalation, the patient presses the canister downward to release a dose of medication. A second dose may be necessary. Nebulizers are preferable to metered dose inhalers in acute respiratory emergencies because they administer the drug over more time and are less dependent on a single deep inspiration.

Endotracheal administration of a drug involves expressing the drug down the endotracheal tube (in a volume of 10 mL and from 2 to 2.5 times the normal intravenous dose). Narcan, atropine, lidocaine, and epinephrine can be administered this way in an emergency when IV access is not otherwise available. Once the drug is injected down the endotracheal tube, the ventilator provides several deep ventilations to deliver the drug to the pulmonary tissue.

b. Parenteral routes of medication administration pp. 390–405

Parenteral administration includes the routes utilizing needles to administer drugs into the tissues or vascular system—intradermal, subcutaneous, intramuscular, intravenous, and intraosseous routes. Begin the parenteral administration process by cleansing the patient's skin at the injection site with an antiseptic such as alcohol or a Betadine solution. The medication for injection is in solution and drawn up in a syringe, then injected with a needle (bevel up). For subcutaneous and intramuscular injection, consider injecting a 0.1-mL air bubble after the medication to limit leakage, and then massage the region to enhance absorption. Most emergency medications are injected via the intravenous route because of its rapid distribution throughout the body.

Intradermal drug administration calls for insertion of a 25- to 27-gauge needle at a 10° to 15° angle just into a segment of skin that is pulled taut. Slow injection of up to 1 mL of solution will create a small wheal of medication. Then remove the needle. Intradermal injection results in a very slow absorption rate greatly affected by local perfusion rates and is used for diagnostic testing and the administration of local anesthetics.

For subcutaneous administration, place a 24- to 26-gauge needle into a 1-inch "pinch" of the patient's skin at a 45° angle and inject no more than 1 mL of medication. The skin must be free of scarring, superficial nerves, blood vessels and tendons, tattoos, and bruising. Pulling the plunger back ensures that the needle is not in a blood vessel (aspiration of blood indicates a blood vessel entry). Subcutaneous injection may be given at many locations around the body, including the tissue under the tongue.

For intramuscular injections, use a 21- to 23-gauge needle inserted at a 90° angle into the deltoid (up to 2 mL), dorsal gluteal (up to 5 mL), vastus lateralis (up to 5 mL), or rectus femoris (up to 5 mL) muscle. Again, pulling back on the plunger ensures that the needle is not in a blood vessel. Intramuscular injection provides a predictable systemic absorption and is used for several prehospital drugs including glucagon and morphine. Careful placement of parenteral needles is important because of potential damage to nerves and arteries. Needles for intradermal, subcutaneous, and intramuscular injection are 3/8 to 1 inch in length.

c. **Percutaneous routes of medication administration** pp. 378–381

Transdermal drug administration is indicated for drugs that are readily absorbed through the skin; when slow, steady absorption is required; or for topical administration for local effects (antiinflammatories, bacteriostatics, and softening agents). Transdermal medications include lotions, creams, foams, wet dressings, adhesive-backed applications, and suppositories. The medication is applied to a clean, dry portion of skin according to the manufacturer's instructions. The medication is left for the required time and watched for the desired and adverse effects, and a dressing is placed over the application if necessary. Care must be taken not to get the drug on your skin and to watch for overdosing due to thin skin, increasing absorption rates, or for underdosing due to thick skin, scar tissue, or peripheral vascular disease, slowing absorption.

The mucous membrane route for drug administration permits drug absorption through the capillaries of the sublingual, buccal, ocular, nasal, or aural mucous membranes. With the sublingual route, a spray is applied or a tablet placed beneath the tongue, where the patient must let it dissolve and be absorbed. Nitroglycerin is a drug commonly administered via the sublingual route. With buccal administration a pill or other preparation is placed between the cheek and gum to permit absorption. Hormonal and enzyme preparations are commonly administered via the buccal route. Ocular administration involves one or both eyes. The patient lies supine or tips his head back and looks at the ceiling. The eyelid is pulled down and the droplet of a liquid medication (using an medicine dropper) or an ointment is placed into the conjunctival sac. Do not touch the eye or administer drugs directly on the eye unless specifically instructed to do so. Medications administered via this route include agents to treat eye pain, infection, or increased intraocular pressure or to lubricate the eyelid. Nasal administration involves the topical absorption of drops or sprays through the nasal mucosa for nasal congestion, hemorrhage, or infection. The patient is directed to blow his nose and tilt his head back. A medicine dropper or squeezable nebulizer expresses the drug into the nare(s), then the nare(s) is (are) held shut and/or the head is tilted forward to enhance the distribution of the medication. Aural administration is used to treat local infection or ear pain. Droplets or medicated gauze are placed into the affected ear while the patient lies supine with his head turned. The adult's pinna is pulled up and back, while the child's is pulled down and back to expose the auditory canal. Do not pack the canal tightly.

**d. Enteral routes of medication administration, including gastric tube
administration and rectal administration** pp. 385–390

Enteral drug administration includes oral, gastric tube, and rectal administration routes and results in drug absorption through the gastrointestinal tract. Medications administered this way (except the rectal route) are processed through the liver, affecting their metabolism and elimination.

Oral medications are introduced as capsules, tablets, pills, time-release capsules, elixirs, emulsions, lozenges, suspensions, or syrups introduced into the oral cavity and swallowed with 4 to 8 ounces of water. This is the most common method of over-the-counter and prescription drug administration because of its ease of administration.

Gastric tube administration introduces a drug down the naso- or orogastric tube and into the stomach. It is used when the patient has difficulty swallowing and in instances of overdose, trauma, upper gastrointestinal bleeding, or the need for nutritional support. Drugs in solid forms may be crushed (so as to move easily down the tube), mixed with water, and administered through the gastric tube, although such action will destroy the time-release action of coated drugs. When administering a drug via the gastric tube route, ensure proper placement by injecting air and auscultating over the epigastric area and by aspirating gastric contents through the tube. Flush the tube with 50 to 100 mL of saline, then prepare a volume of about 30 mL of medication (diluted to volume with normal saline) and administer the solution through the gastric tube. Follow administration with 50 to 100 mL of normal saline and clamp off the tube for about 30 minutes.

Rectal administration involves topical administration of a medication to the rectal mucosa and provides rapid predictable absorption. Use a syringe and 14-gauge needleless catheter (or small endotracheal tube) to introduce the medication into the rectum, then hold the buttocks closed to promote retention and absorption. A suppository is a soft, pliable form of drug that melts at body temperature and is inserted into the rectum for absorption. An enema is a liquid bolus of medication introduced through the rectum.

**3. Describe the indications, contraindications, side effects, dosages, and routes
of administration for medications commonly administered by paramedics.** pp. 378–405

There are many drugs used in the prehospital setting to care for the common medical and trauma emergencies. The Emergency Drug Cards at the back of this Workbook list many of these drugs, including the drug name/class, indications, contraindications, precautions, dosages, and routes of administration. Detach these cards and review them frequently to become familiar with the medications you will use during your prehospital patient care.

4. Discuss legal aspects affecting medication administration. pp. 376, 377

The administration of the wrong medication or withholding the right medication or providing it in the wrong dose or by the wrong route can have catastrophic consequences. Hence, medication administration is an area of paramedic practice where the paramedic is exposed to legal liability. You must ensure that you receive informed and expressed consent from the patient (when possible), provide medications in strict compliance with system protocols and the direction of on-line medical control, and follow proper administration techniques. Once a medication is administered, it is essential that you document the indication for the drug, any on-line authorization for the administration, the name of the person who delivered the drug, the drug name, dose, route time and rate of delivery, and the resulting patient response, whether positive or negative. These actions will go a long way to limiting your liability in drug administration.

**5. Discuss the "six rights" of drug administration and correlate
them with the principles of medication administration.** p. 375–376

There are basically six rights of drug administration. They are the right patient, the right drug, the right dose, the right time, the right route, and the right documentation.

The right patient. Ensure that the patient is the right person and properly matched to the medication. This is an infrequent problem in prehospital care, but as EMS moves to the out-of-hospital environment, we may be treating some patients on a routine basis. Ensure the medication order is for the patient you are attending.

The right drug. Ensure the drug is what is intended for the patient. Review your standing orders or, if the order is received from medical direction, repeat ("echo") the order back to the physician so you are both clear on the drug, dose, route, and timing of the order. Also examine the drug packaging to ensure that it contains the medication you wish to administer and that the medication is still sterile, has not expired, and is not contaminated or discolored.

The right dose. Carefully calculate the exact dose (usually weight dependent) for the patient before you draw up the medication and again just before you administer it. If the drug package you select has significantly more or less of the drug than you intend to use, recheck the packaging to ensure it is the right drug and right concentration, and recheck your calculations to ensure the right dosage. Never overdose or underdose your patient.

The right time. Usually prehospital medications are given rather rapidly and not on a schedule. Check the packaging and your protocols for administration rates and ensure that you follow the sequencing, time intervals between, and drip rates for emergency drugs.

The right route. Specific drugs require specific routes of administration. While most emergency drugs are administered by the IV route, be aware of alternate drug administration routes, the drugs that can be administered by those routes, and the circumstances requiring the use of those routes. With each medication administration, ensure you are using the right route.

The right documentation. Documentation of drug administration is of paramount importance. You must carefully record the patient's condition (the circumstances that require the drug's administration), the drug name, dose, and route of administration, and who administered the drug and at what time. It is also essential that you record the patient's response to the drug, whether good or bad.

6. Differentiate among the percutaneous routes of medication administration. pp. 378–381

The transdermal route of medication administration promotes slow, steady absorption of the drug across the dermis. Nitroglycerin is frequently administered for its systemic effects via this route, while lidocaine, antiinflammatories, and bacteriostatic solutions are administered for their local effects.

Sublingual drugs are absorbed through the mucous membranes beneath the tongue, where the medication is rapidly absorbed by the extensive vasculature there. Tablets or sprays are often used, and nitroglycerin is frequently administered this way in the emergency setting.

Buccal medications (usually tablets) are placed between the cheek and gums for absorption. Enzymes and hormonal preparations are also administered this way.

Ocular drug administration involves topical administration of a medication (usually drops or ointment) into one or both eyes. This route is typically used for treating eye pain or local infections, decreasing intraocular pressure, or lubrication of the eyelid.

Nasal medications are usually drops or sprays given through the nares to treat nasal congestion, hemorrhage, or infection.

Aural medications are delivered into the auditory canal using a medicine dropper (solution) or medicated gauze. These drugs are used to treat localized infection and ear pain.

7. Discuss medical asepsis and the differences between clean and sterile techniques. pp. 376–377

Medical asepsis describes a medical environment free of pathogens. The most aseptic environment is a sterile one, one free of all living organisms. However, in prehospital care we frequently cannot attain such a state. We utilize equipment and supplies that are sterile when packaged and then use medically clean techniques to reduce the risk of spreading infection. These techniques include the use of disinfectants to kill microorganisms on equipment and in the ambulance and of antiseptics to reduce the bacterial load on the patient's skin when we utilize procedures like venipuncture.

8. Describe uses of antiseptics and disinfectants. p. 377

Antiseptics are agents designed for topical use to destroy or inhibit pathogenic microorganisms already on living tissue. They are used to cleanse the skin before parenteral drug administration to prevent infection secondary to the needle stick.

Disinfectants are powerful agents that are toxic to living tissue. They are not designed for topical administration but for the direct cleaning of durable patient care equipment.

9. **Describe the use of body substance isolation (BSI) procedures when administering a medication.** p. 376

Any time there is the possibility of contact with body substances or patient wounds, you must use body substance isolation measures. Gloves, at a minimum, provide barrier protection to the caregiver from possibly infectious material at the scene and to the patient from the caregiver. Goggles and a mask also provide protection, as does hand washing after contact with a patient or possibly infected material.

10. **Describe disposal of contaminated items and sharps.** p. 377

Sharps and contaminated materials pose a risk for the spread of infection. Do not recap needles unless absolutely necessary and, in such instance, do so using only one hand. Used needles represent a real risk for introducing pathogens from the patient's blood into someone stuck with the needle. Dispose of all needles in a puncture-proof biohazard container. Ensure all medical waste is placed in a biohazardous waste bag and is not left at the scene. Follow your service's biohazard exposure plan should you receive a needle stick.

11. **Synthesize a pharmacologic management plan including medication administration.** pp. 375–405

As you care for patients with serious medical and trauma emergencies, you will often need to administer medications to them via the sublingual, oral, pulmonary, subcutaneous, intramuscular, intravenous, and interosseous routes. The procedures described in this chapter must become an integral part of your patient management skills.

The following objective, while not listed in the chapter, will help in your understanding of the chapter content.

*Supplemental Objective: Describe the equipment and procedures for preparing and drawing up a medication in anticipation of parenteral administration.

A syringe is a plastic, hollow, calibrated barrel into which fits a plunger that is used to draw up and administer very accurate volumes of a solution or liquid. Syringes range in size from 1 mL to 100 mL. A hypodermic needle is a hollow metal tube, one end of which is beveled and very sharp while the other end is equipped with an adapter to fit a syringe. Needles are measured in diameter or gauge from 14 (largest) to 27 (smallest) and vary in length from 3/8 to 1^1/$_2$ inch.

Medications come packaged for administration in glass ampules, single and multidose vials, nonconstituted vials, prefilled syringes, and premixed IV solutions. Ampules are sealed glass containers that must be broken to obtain the drug. A sterile gauze pad is wrapped around the ampule neck and the top is broken off. The needle from a syringe is placed within the ampule to draw out the necessary volume of solution. Single and multidose vials are glass containers with self-sealing rubber tops, usually protected with a metal cap. The cap is removed and the stopper cleansed with alcohol. A syringe is filled with a volume of air, equivalent to the desired volume of drug. The needle is inserted into the vial, the air is expressed inside, and the drug is withdrawn. The needle is then withdrawn from the vial, and the drug is ready for administration. Nonconstituted drug vials come either in the form of pairs of vials (the drug and solvent) that require you to introduce the solvent into the powdered drug vial or in specially designed vials (Mix-o-Vials) that permit mixing after you pop the seal between the drug and solvent. Once the drug is constituted, you withdraw it as from a standard vial. Preloaded syringes are vials containing the drug that screw into a syringe barrel and permit direct administration of the drug by pushing the vial barrel into the syringe. Intravenous premixed solutions for IV infusion come in bottles or plastic bags (plastic bags are used for prehospital administration). They contain a solution of drug and solvent for direct administration via an intravenous line with administration volume (and hence dose) controlled by setting the rate of administration.

Content Self-Evaluation

MULTIPLE CHOICE

_____ 1. Medication administration is an important part of the medical care provided by paramedics.
   A. True
   B. False

_____ 2. Which of the following is NOT one of the six rights of drug administration?
   A. the right dosage
   B. the right indication
   C. the right time
   D. the right documentation
   E. the right patient

_____ 3. The process you use to ensure you hear and correctly understand the medical direction physician's order to administer a medication is:
   A. protocol compliance.
   B. order confirmation with your partner.
   C. redundant physician orders.
   D. echoing the order back to the physician.
   E. asking the physician to repeat the order.

_____ 4. Which of the following must you know about the drugs you are authorized to administer?
   A. their usual dosages
   B. their contraindications
   C. their common side effects
   D. their routes of administration
   E. all of the above

_____ 5. When you administer drugs, which of the following body substance isolation measures should you always employ?
   A. gloves
   B. a mask
   C. goggles
   D. a gown
   E. A and D

_____ 6. The condition in which a medical environment is free of all pathogens is described as:
   A. asepsis.
   B. uncontaminated.
   C. medically clean.
   D. disinfection.
   E. none of the above

_____ 7. The environment that paramedics should strive to maintain while delivering prehospital emergency care is:
   A. aseptic.
   B. sterile.
   C. medically clean.
   D. disinfected.
   E. none of the above

_____ 8. To cleanse the site of a parenteral injection, you would use a(n):
   A. aseptic.
   B. disinfectant.
   C. detergent.
   D. antiseptic.
   E. dilutant.

_____ 9. When possible, you should recap needles:
   A. as a last resort.
   B. in a moving ambulance only.
   C. except in a moving ambulance.
   D. only when they have not been used on a patient.
   E. when directed by a physician.

©2007 Pearson Education, Inc.
Essentials of Paramedic Care, 2nd ed.

CHAPTER 7 *Intravenous Access* 133

_____ 10. Documentation regarding the administration of a drug should include all of the following EXCEPT the:
   A. time of administration.
   B. route of administration.
   C. class of drug administered.
   D. positive patient responses.
   E. negative patient responses.

_____ 11. Transdermal medications are provided in which of the following forms?
   A. ointments
   B. wet dressings
   C. foams
   D. lotions
   E. all of the above

_____ 12. Which of the following factors can decrease the absorption rate with transdermal medication administration?
   A. thin skin
   B. overdose
   C. penetrating solvents
   D. peripheral vascular disease
   E. all of the above

_____ 13. Which of the following is a common emergency drug administered sublingually?
   A. sodium bicarbonate
   B. epinephrine
   C. nitroglycerin
   D. aspirin
   E. magnesium

_____ 14. The route in which a drug is administered between the cheek and gum is:
   A. transdermal.
   B. sublingual.
   C. buccal.
   D. aural.
   E. inhalation.

_____ 15. Ocular medications are given for which conditions?
   A. eye pain
   B. eye infection
   C. increased intraocular pressure
   D. lubricating the eyelid
   E. all of the above

_____ 16. Ocular medications are most commonly administered:
   A. over the pupil.
   B. over the iris.
   C. over the sclera.
   D. into the conjunctival sac.
   E. all of the above

_____ 17. Nasal administration of medication is used frequently because of its rapid absorption rate and systemic effects.
   A. True
   B. False

_____ 18. The small volume nebulizer often used in prehospital emergency medical service administers what volume of medication?
   A. 1 to 2 mL
   B. 3 to 5 mL
   C. 5 to 10 mL
   D. 10 to 15 mL
   E. 15 to 20 mL

_____ 19. The small volume nebulizer's major advantage over the metered dose inhaler is that the patient does not need an adequate tidal volume for effective medication delivery.
   A. True
   B. False

_____ 20. The metered dose inhaler is activated to release its medication:
   A. just before the patient seals his lips to the mouthpiece.
   B. as the patient exhales.
   C. as the patient inhales.
   D. during both inhalation and exhalation.
   E. between inhalation and exhalation.

_____ 21. Nebulizers and metered dose inhalers are advantageous in respiratory emergencies because they deliver their medication to the exact site of action.
   A. True
   B. False

_____ 22. Endotracheal medication administration calls for drugs to be diluted to what volume?
   A. 1 mL   D. 5 mL
   B. 2 mL   E. 10 mL
   C. 3 mL

_____ 23. Which of the following drugs is NOT administered via the endotracheal route?
   A. meperidine   D. lidocaine
   B. naloxone   E. epinephrine
   C. atropine

_____ 24. Enteral medications are absorbed through the:
   A. liver.   D. portal system.
   B. gastrointestinal tract. E. accessory organs.
   C. mucous membranes.

_____ 25. Liver function is an important factor in the effectiveness of enteral drug administration.
   A. True
   B. False

_____ 26. When using a medicine cup to measure an oral dose of medication, you should use what aspect of fluid level to determine the fluid volume?
   A. the highest point of the meniscus
   B. the lowest point of the meniscus
   C. between the high and low point of the meniscus
   D. one calibration below the lowest level of the meniscus
   E. none of the above

_____ 27. The normal teaspoon holds about what volume of fluid?
   A. 2 mL   D. 10 mL
   B. 3 mL   E. 12 mL
   C. 5 mL

_____ 28. The advantage of rectal administration over the other enteral drug routes is that:
   A. the rectal route is easier to administer drugs through.
   B. there is no hepatic alteration of the drug.
   C. the rectal route can absorb more medication.
   D. rectal irritation is rare.
   E. all of the above

_____ 29. To inject a drug rectally you may use:
   A. a large catheter with needle removed.
   B. a special enema container with a rectal tip.
   C. a small endotracheal tube attached to a syringe.
   D. all of the above
   E. none of the above

_____ 30. A syringe should be chosen for drug administration that is slightly smaller than the volume of drug to be administered.
   A. True
   B. False

_____ 31. The smaller the gauge of a hypodermic needle, the smaller the diameter of its lumen.
   A. True
   B. False

_____ 32. What is the total dose of a drug contained in an ampule with 5 mL of a drug in a 0.3 mg/mL concentration?
   A. 0.3 mg
   B. 1.5 mg
   C. 5 mg
   D. 15 mg
   E. none of the above

_____ 33. Which of the following drug containers may contain multiple doses of a drug?
   A. vial
   B. ampule
   C. Mix-o-Vial
   D. preloaded syringe
   E. medicated solutions

_____ 34. Prior to drawing medication from a vial, you must first inject an equal volume of air into the vial.
   A. True
   B. False

_____ 35. Which of the following must be cleansed with an alcohol swab before the drug is withdrawn?
   A. vial
   B. ampule
   C. Mix-o-Vial
   D. preloaded syringe
   E. A and C

_____ 36. The drug route that calls for insertion of the needle at 10° to 15° is:
   A. intradermal.
   B. subcutaneous.
   C. intramuscular.
   D. intraosseous.
   E. none of the above

_____ 37. Which of the following is most likely to be an acceptable site for subcutaneous injection?
   A. forearms
   B. calves
   C. abdomen
   D. buttocks
   E. all of the above are acceptable

_____ 38. Through which of the following routes should you inject no more than 1 mL of a drug?
   A. intradermal
   B. subcutaneous
   C. intramuscular
   D. A and B
   E. all of the above

_____ 39. For intradermal and subcutaneous injections, the needle is inserted with the bevel down.
   A. True
   B. False

_____ 40. At which of the following intramuscular injection sites should you administer a maximum of 2 mL of a drug?
   A. deltoid
   B. gluteal
   C. vastus lateralis
   D. rectus femoris
   E. both B and C

_____ 41. When you pull back on the syringe plunger during subcutaneous or intramuscular injection and blood appears, you should:
   A. inject the drug.
   B. inject the drug followed by a small bubble of air.
   C. insert the needle 1 cm further.
   D. attempt the injection at another site.
   E. consider the appearance of blood insignificant.

_____ 42. The drug route that calls for use of a 21 to 23-gauge needle is:
   A. intradermal.
   B. subcutaneous.
   C. intramuscular.
   D. intraosseous.
   E. none of the above

_____ 43. The drug route that calls for use of a needle 3/8 to 1 inch long is:
   A. intradermal.
   B. subcutaneous.
   C. intramuscular.
   D. all of the above
   E. none of the above

_____ 44. The recommended angle of insertion for the needle when administering an intramuscular injection is:
   A. 10°.
   B. 15°.
   C. 45°.
   D. 90°.
   E. between 10° and 15°.

_____ 45. After injecting an intramuscular drug, massaging the site is contraindicated because it will slow absorption.
   A. True
   B. False

Part 2: Intravenous Access, Blood Sampling, and Intraosseous Infusion

Review of Chapter Objectives

After reading Part 2 of this chapter, you should be able to:

1. **Review the specific anatomy and physiology pertinent to medication administration.** pp. 405–442

   Various veins are found close to the surface of the skin and are relatively easy to locate because of their prominence, color, and/or feel. Common vessels used for peripheral venipuncture include those of the back of the hand, those of the arms, the vein of the antecubital fossa, and those of the feet and legs. An additional large vein available for catheter insertion is the external jugular vein on the lateral neck. The more distal veins should be used, when possible, as using a vein generally limits the use of veins distal to the site. Large veins must be used for blood administration, in the administration of some drugs, and in cases where large volumes of drugs must be administered. Central veins are not usually used in the prehospital setting because of the time needed to initiate the access, the difficulty in determining proper placement, and the incidence of complications.

   Intraosseous infusion directs the flow of fluid or a drug into the medullary space of a long bone, where it is available to the venous circulation. The tibia is the most frequent location of cannulation, with the proximal anterior and medial tibia just below the tibial tuberosity used for pediatric patients and the distal tibia just above the medial malleolus and just medial to the tibial crest for adults. A special needle is inserted through the compact bone and into the medullary space.

2. **Describe the indications, equipment needed, technique used, precautions, and general principles for the following:**

   a. Peripheral venous or external jugular cannulation pp. 405–431

   Peripheral venous access is the preferable route for medication administration in the emergency prehospital setting. Most emergency drugs are administered this way because it provides a direct route into the venous system, then to the heart, where the drug and blood are further mixed, and then to the body as distributed by the arterial system. Vascular access can be obtained using a steel needle with a beveled sharp edge. Most commonly, an over-the-needle catheter is advanced into the vein, with the needle then withdrawn, leaving the catheter to permit introduction of drugs or fluid or withdrawal of blood for diagnostic testing. The veins of the hands, arms, antecubital fossa, feet, and legs and the external jugular veins are common sites for intravenous cannulation.

The equipment used for intravenous therapy includes a venous constricting band to help engorge the veins; the needle for venipuncture; an antiseptic to cleanse the site; administration tubing to direct and control fluid administration from an IV bag or a syringe to draw up, then administer medication; tape or commercial devices to secure the intravenous catheter; and bacteriostatic ointment to protect the site from infection. An ideal location for venipuncture is free of injury and with relatively prominent veins. The caregiver should take appropriate body substance isolation measures before beginning the procedure. Then the venous constricting band is secured just proximal to the selected site and a vein is chosen. The area is cleansed with an alcohol or Betadine swab, using concentric circles moving outward from the selected site. An over-the-needle catheter is selected, with 14- to 18-gauge for blood, thick medications such as glucose, or fluid volume administration or a 20- to 22-gauge catheter for pediatric or geriatric patients or patients who do not need a larger catheter. The catheter is directed, bevel up, through the skin at an angle of 10° to 30° until a "pop" is felt or blood appears in the flash chamber. Once in the vein, the catheter is advanced an additional 0.5 cm and then the catheter is threaded into the vein. The needle is withdrawn, the constricting band is released, and the administration set or saline or heparin lock is attached. A small amount of fluid is run to ensure that the catheter is patent. Watch for edema around the site, which is suggestive of infiltration. Intravenous cannulation and infusion may result in local pain, infiltration, pyrogenic reactions, allergic reactions, catheter shear and embolism, inadvertent arterial puncture, circulatory overload, thrombophlebitis, thrombus formation, air embolism, and necrosis.

Fluid is infused through a venipuncture site to hydrate the patient or to keep the drug route open and quickly available. Most prehospital infusions use isotonic (same osmotic pressure as the plasma) solutions such as normal saline, 5 percent dextrose in water, or lactated Ringer's solution. These solutions flow through the administration set, where their rate of administration is regulated by adjusting the drip rate in a chamber. Most commonly 10 (macro) or 60 (micro) drops traveling through a drip chamber equal 1 milliliter. The administration set contains one or more injection ports to accommodate the administration of drugs or additional fluid administration. A special type of administration set is the measured volume administration set, which contains a calibrated chamber that will permit the discrete administration of a volume of fluid.

The external jugular vein is an alternate venous access site located on the lateral anterior neck. It is a large, easily found vein that permits venous access when other veins are collapsed due to hypovolemia or other vascular problems. It is close to the central circulation, so it provides almost immediate absorption of any drugs administered through it. The jugular vein can be engorged by placing digital pressure along the vein just above the clavical. External jugular cannulation is painful and risks damage to the airway or arterial structures in the neck.

b. Intraosseous needle placement and infusion   **pp. 435–442**

Intraosseous needle placement is indicated for the critical pediatric patient under 5 when you cannot establish other IV access sites or for the adult patient when you also cannot perform peripheral venous access because of disease or extreme hypovolemia. A special needle is introduced through the compact bone of the tibia and into the medullary space. There fluids or drugs are readily available for absorption and distribution by the venous system.

In the child, the needle is placed at 90° to the tibial plateau, just medial and about two finger widths below the tibial tuberosity (the anterior bump just below the patella). Don gloves and cleanse the site with an antiseptic swab. With a firm twisting motion, introduce the needle into the bone for a few centimeters until you feel a "pop" or reduced resistance. Remove the trocar, attach a syringe, and draw back on the syringe to aspirate bone marrow and blood. Rotate the plastic disk to engage the skin and secure the needle. Connect the IV fluid administration set and secure the needle with bulky dressings and tape. Adult or geriatric IO administration uses the flat tibial plate just two finger widths above the medial malleolus. IO infusion may result in bone fracture, infiltration, growth plate damage, pulmonary embolism, and the problems associated with venous cannulation. This site is not very effective for extensive fluid resuscitation in the adult.

c. Obtaining a blood sample   pp. 431–434

Blood composition, the presence of toxins, and blood gas levels are important values to determine for learning what is wrong with a patient. Since emergency care may alter these figures, it is sometimes important to draw blood in the prehospital setting. Blood is withdrawn from a vein through either a needle or catheter and is either placed directly in special containers (blood tubes) or into a syringe for distribution into the blood tubes. A large vein must be used, because the withdrawal of blood may collapse smaller veins. A needled vacutainer is introduced into an engorged vein and blood tubes are introduced, one at a time. The vacuum withdraws blood from the vein and into the tubes, which are then manually agitated to mix the blood with an anticoagulant (all but the red top tube). If a vacutainer is not available, 20 mL of blood may be drawn up in a syringe and distributed among the containers. It is important to fill the containers in order of red, blue, green, purple, and gray (as available), because they contain various anticoagulants and another order may cross-contaminate the blood.

Content Self-Evaluation

MULTIPLE CHOICE

1. Which of the following is an indication for intravenous administration?
   A. fluid replacement
   B. blood replacement
   C. drug administration
   D. need of blood for analysis
   E. all of the above

2. Both central venous and peripheral venous cannulation are common in prehospital care.
   A. True
   B. False

3. Which of the following is a likely site for intravenous cannulation?
   A. the hands
   B. the arms
   C. the legs
   D. the neck
   E. all of the above

4. Which of the following is NOT a central venous vessel?
   A. the internal jugular
   B. the subclavian
   C. the femoral
   D. the antecubital
   E. all of the above are central venous vessels

5. The solution that contains large proteins is a(n):
   A. colloid.
   B. crystalloid.
   C. isotonic.
   D. hypotonic.
   E. hypertonic.

6. The solution that contains an electrolyte concentration close to that of plasma is a(n):
   A. colloid.
   B. crystalloid.
   C. isotonic.
   D. hypotonic.
   E. hypertonic.

7. The solution that contains an electrolyte concentration greater than that of plasma is a(n):
   A. colloid.
   B. crystalloid.
   C. isotonic.
   D. hypotonic.
   E. hypertonic.

_____ 8. One example of a hypotonic solution is:
   A. normal saline.
   B. lactated Ringer's solution.
   C. plasmanate.
   D. 5 percent dextrose in water.
   E. dextran.

_____ 9. The most desirable replacement for blood lost during trauma is:
   A. normal saline.
   B. lactated Ringer's solution.
   C. plasmanate.
   D. 5 percent dextrose in water.
   E. none of the above

_____ 10. Which intravenous fluid bag would you discard?
   A. one that is cloudy
   B. one that is discolored
   C. one that is leaking
   D. one that is expired
   E. all of the above

_____ 11. For optimal fluid delivery, the drip chamber should be how full?
   A. 1/4
   B. 1/3
   C. 1/2
   D. 2/3
   E. none of the above

_____ 12. The administration set most appropriate for administration of intravenous solutions for fluid replacement is the:
   A. macrodrip administration set.
   B. microdrip administration set.
   C. measured volume administration set.
   D. blood tubing set.
   E. none of the above

_____ 13. The most common microdrip setting equaling 1 mL is:
   A. 10 gtts.
   B. 20 gtts.
   C. 45 gtts.
   D. 60 gtts.
   E. none of the above

_____ 14. The administration set most appropriate for administration of a very specific volume of intravenous solution or drug is the:
   A. macrodrip administration set.
   B. microdrip administration set.
   C. measured volume administration set.
   D. blood tubing set.
   E. none of the above

_____ 15. The major difference between blood tubing and a standard intravenous administration set is that blood tubing has a filter to remove clots and particulate matter.
   A. True
   B. False

_____ 16. Blood is not administered with fluids like lactated Ringer's solution because such solutions increase blood's potential for coagulation.
   A. True
   B. False

_____ 17. Many patients are prone to develop hypothermia during fluid administration.
   A. True
   B. False

_____ 18. The most common intravenous cannula used in the prehospital setting is the:
   A. over-the-needle.
   B. through-the-needle.
   C. hollow needle.
   D. angiocatheter.
   E. A and D

_____ 19. A needle gauge of 18 is smaller than a needle gauge of 22.
   A. True
   B. False

_____ 20. A venous constricting band should be left in place no longer than:
   A. 1 minute.
   B. 2 minutes.
   C. 3 minutes.
   D. 5 minutes.
   E. 10 minutes.

_____ 21. Leaving the constricting band on for too long is likely to cause:
   A. collapse of the vein.
   B. damage to the distal blood vessels.
   C. damage to the vessels under the band.
   D. changes in the distal venous blood.
   E. all of the above

_____ 22. When cleansing the site for intravenous cannulation, you should make one swipe over the intended site with a Betadine or alcohol swab.
   A. True
   B. False

_____ 23. The angle of insertion for intravenous cannulation is:
   A. 10°.
   B. 10° to 30°.
   C. 45°.
   D. 60°.
   E. 60° to 90°.

_____ 24. After you feel the "pop" associated with intravenous cannulation, you should:
   A. advance the catheter.
   B. advance the needle 0.5 cm, then advance the catheter.
   C. advance the needle 1 cm, then advance the catheter.
   D. advance the needle 2 cm, then advance the catheter.
   E. withdraw the needle, then advance the catheter.

_____ 25. You should consider using the external jugular vein as an IV access site only after you have exhausted other means of peripheral access or when the patient needs immediate fluid administration.
   A. True
   B. False

_____ 26. During external jugular vein cannulation, the patient's head should be:
   A. moved to the sniffing position.
   B. turned toward the side of access.
   C. turned away from the side of access.
   D. hyperextended.
   E. hyperflexed.

_____ 27. To fill the jugular access site and make the vessel easier to both locate and cannulate, you should:
   A. apply a venous constricting band, tightly.
   B. apply a venous constricting band, loosely.
   C. occlude the vein gently with a finger.
   D. perform the procedure without occluding the vein.
   E. have the patient take a deep breath and hold it.

_____ 28. When establishing an IV with blood tubing, you must be careful to:
   A. fill the drip chamber ⅓ full.
   B. completely cover the blood filter with blood.
   C. fill the set with normal saline first.
   D. fill the drip chamber ¾ full.
   E. both A and B above

_____ 29. Which of the following is a factor that may affect intravenous flow rates?
   A. failure to remove a venous constricting band
   B. edema at the access site
   C. the cannula tip up against a vein valve
   D. a clogged catheter
   E. all of the above

30. The complication of peripheral venous access in which a plastic embolus can form is:
    A. pyrogenic reaction.
    B. pain.
    C. thrombophlebitis.
    D. catheter shear.
    E. all of the above

31. The most common cause of catheter shear is:
    A. cannulating thick veins.
    B. cannulating underneath the constricting band.
    C. withdrawing the needle from within the catheter.
    D. withdrawing the catheter from the needle.
    E. faulty catheter construction.

32. If a blood clot appears to stop or slow intravenous fluid flow, forcefully inject a small amount of heparin into the catheter and continue the infusion.
    A. True
    B. False

33. You should change a large (500- to 1,000-mL) infusion bag when the volume remaining in the bag is:
    A. 10 mL.
    B. 20 mL.
    C. 30 mL.
    D. 50 mL.
    E. 100 mL.

34. If air becomes entrained in the administration set when you are changing an IV bag or bottle, you should:
    A. continue the infusion, because the volume of air is negligible.
    B. discard the set and use a new one.
    C. use a syringe placed between the bubbles and patient to withdraw the air.
    D. reverse the fluid flow until the bubbles enter the fluid bag or drip chamber.
    E. squeeze the tubing to push them into the drip chamber or bag.

35. Never administer an intravenous drug infusion as the primary IV line.
    A. True
    B. False

36. Which of the following is NOT true regarding infusion pumps?
    A. They deliver fluids under pressure.
    B. They are large and difficult to carry.
    C. Most pumps contain alarms for occlusion.
    D. Most pumps contain alarms for fluid source depletion.
    E. They deliver fluids at precise rates.

37. The reason venous blood sampling is important in the prehospital setting is that our interventions may alter the blood's composition or erase important information about it.
    A. True
    B. False

38. The color of the blood tube container that must be drawn first is:
    A. blue.
    B. red.
    C. green.
    D. purple.
    E. gray.

39. Drawing blood and injecting it into the blood tubes in the wrong order may result in:
    A. leaving the wrong volume of blood in a tube.
    B. cross-contamination of the blood with anticoagulants.
    C. depletion of the vacuum in the tubes at too early a stage.
    D. coagulation in the last tubes to be filled.
    E. all but C

_____ 40. Do not use a blood tube after its expiration date because the anticoagulant and vacuum may have become ineffective.
   A. True
   B. False

_____ 41. The device that accepts the blood tube to permit its filling is:
   A. the leur lock.
   B. the Huber needle.
   C. the vacutainer.
   D. the leur-sampling needle.
   E. either A or C

_____ 42. You should fill the blood tube to between a third and a half of its volume because the anticoagulant is measured for this amount of blood.
   A. True
   B. False

_____ 43. When using a syringe to fill your blood tubes, you should draw a volume of blood of about:
   A. 5 mL.
   B. 10 mL.
   C. 20 mL.
   D. 35 mL.
   E. 50 mL.

_____ 44. The complication from drawing blood in which red blood cells are destroyed is:
   A. hematocrit.
   B. hemoconcentration.
   C. hemolysis.
   D. hemotypsis.
   E. hematuria.

_____ 45. Hemoconcentration occurs during drawing blood:
   A. when the constricting band is left in place too long.
   B. when blood is drawn back through a needle that is too small.
   C. with premature mixing of the anticoagulant.
   D. with too vigorous a mixing of the blood and anticoagulant.
   E. with too forceful an aspiration of blood into the syringe.

_____ 46. When an IV catheter is withdrawn, place pressure on the venipuncture site with a sterile gauze pad for about 5 minutes.
   A. True
   B. False

_____ 47. The intraosseous site of infusion is most commonly used for which category of patient?
   A. geriatric patients
   B. cardiac patients
   C. children under 5 years of age
   D. patients with nonskeletal injuries
   E. all of the above

_____ 48. The proper site for intraosseous needle placement in the child is one to two finger widths:
   A. below and medial to the tibial tuberosity.
   B. below and lateral to the tibial tuberosity.
   C. above the medial malleolus.
   D. above the lateral malleolus.
   E. above and lateral to the tibial crest.

_____ 49. Confirmation that you are in the medullary space is achieved by:
   A. feeling the bone "pop."
   B. pushing the needle 2 to 4 mm.
   C. aspirating bone marrow and blood.
   D. feeling resistance to the twisting of insertion.
   E. none of the above

_____ 50. Complications of intraosseous cannulation include all of the following EXCEPT:
   A. pulmonary embolism.
   B. fracture.
   C. growth plate damage.
   D. aspiration of bone marrow.
   E. complete insertion.

Part 3: Medical Mathematics

Review of Chapter Objectives

After reading Part 3 of this chapter, you should be able to:

1. **Review mathematical equivalents.** pp. 442–444

   The basic units used for most of medicine are metric: the gram for weight, the liter for volume, and the meter for distance. The metric system is a decimal system that uses suffixes and prefixes to delineate larger and smaller quantities, most commonly kilo (1,000), milli (1/1000), and micro (1/1,000,000). Pharmacology math involves working with addition, subtraction, multiplication, and division as well as working extensively with ratios, fractions, and formulas.

2. **Differentiate temperature readings between the centigrade and Fahrenheit scales.** p. 444

   The centigrade (officially known as Celsius) scale graduates the temperature between the point at which ice melts and the point at which water boils into 100 degrees. The Fahrenheit scale graduates the range between the lowest temperature at which a salt-water mixture would remain a liquid (0 degrees) and the boiling point of water into 212 degrees. The Celsius scale is used in medicine, and the conversion between the two is demonstrated by the formulas below.

   $$°F = 9/5 \ °C + 32 \qquad °C = 5/9 \ (°F - 32)$$

3. **Discuss formulas as a basis for performing drug calculations.** pp. 444–449

   The major formula for determining the amount of a drug to be administered is as follows:

   $$\text{Volume to be administered} = \frac{\text{Volume on hand (desired dose)}}{\text{Dosage on hand}}$$

   The formula is mathematically manipulated so that the unknown element can be computed using the known values.

   Other elements of drug calculation call for determining the volume flowing through an intravenous administration set by monitoring the number of drops falling in a drip chamber per minute. Conversion is based upon the number of drops that equal one milliliter of fluid.

   $$\text{Drops/Minute} = \frac{\text{Volume on hand} \times \text{Drip factor} \times \text{Desired dose}}{\text{Dosage on hand}}$$

   You may also be required to convert pounds to kilograms (if the patient dosing is in weight of drug per kilogram of body weight). To do this you should know that:

   $$1 \text{ pound} = 2.2 \text{ kilograms}$$

   In some cases, it is important to administer a volume of medication over time, and the associated formula for such administration is:

   $$\text{Drops/Minute} = \frac{\text{Volume to be administered} \times \text{Drip factor}}{\text{Time in minutes}}$$

4. Describe how to perform mathematical conversions from the household system to the metric system. pp. 442–444

Weight. Weight conversion between household and metric measures is accomplished by dividing a weight in pounds by 2.2 to find the equivalent metric weight in kilograms. Conversely, if you know a weight in kilograms, multiply it by 2.2 to get the weight in pounds

$$kg = lbs/2.2 \qquad lbs = kg \times 2.2$$

Volume. Volume conversion between household and metric measures is based on the recognition that 1 quart is about equal to 1 liter, 1 cup to 250 milliliters, and so on.

Chapter 8: Airway Management and Ventilation

Review of Chapter Objectives

After reading this chapter, you should be able to:

1. **Describe the anatomy of the airway and the physiology of respiration. (see Chapter 3)**

2. **Explain the primary objective of airway maintenance.** p. 456

   The primary objective of airway maintenance is to keep the airway open and clear (patent) so that oxygen can be carried to and carbon dioxide carried away from the alveoli and the capillary beds of the pulmonary tissue.

3. **Identify commonly neglected prehospital skills related to the airway.** p. 469

   The manual maintenance of the airway, using the head-tilt/chin-lift or jaw thrust maneuver, is one of the most important but often neglected prehospital airway skills. Proper use of these techniques helps ensure an adequate airway early in the care process.

4. **Describe assessment of the airway and the respiratory system.** pp. 458–468

   Assessment of the airway is an integral part of both the initial assessment and the focused examination. During the initial assessment, the evaluation is directed at detecting any potentially life-threatening airway problems. If the patient is not conscious, alert, and demonstrating articulate speech, the airway and respiration are closely evaluated. The rate, depth, and symmetry of respiration are evaluated, as is the presence of any unusual respiratory sounds. During the focused exam, the emphasis is on the finer details of respiratory evaluation including skin color, auscultation of breath sounds, detection of abnormal breathing sounds, palpation of the thorax, and the use of pulse oximetry and/or capnography.

5. **Describe the modified forms of respiration and list the factors that affect respiratory rate and depth.** pp. 460–461

   Forms of respiration

   - Coughing—the forceful exhalation of a large volume of air to expel material from the airway.
   - Sneezing—sudden, forceful exhalation through the nose usually caused by nasal irritation.
   - Hiccoughing (hiccups)—sudden diaphragmatic spasm with spasmodic closure of the glottis that serves no useful purpose.
   - Sighing—slow, deep involuntary inspiration followed by a prolonged expiration that hyperinflates the lungs and expands collapsed alveoli.

- Grunting—forceful expiration against a partially closed epiglottis, usually an indication of respiratory distress.

Factors affecting respiratory rate and depth

- Kussmaul's respirations—deep, slow, or rapid gasping respirations commonly associated with diabetic ketoacidosis.
- Cheyne-Stokes respirations—progressively deeper, faster breathing alternating gradually with shallow, slower respirations indicating brainstem injury.
- Biot's respirations—irregular breathing pattern with sudden episodes of apnea indicating increased intracranial pressure.
- Central neurogenic hyperventilation—deep, rapid respirations indicating increased intracranial pressure.
- Agonal respirations—shallow, slow, or infrequent respirations indicating severe brain anoxia.

6. Discuss the methods for measuring oxygen and carbon dioxide in the blood and their prehospital use. pp. 462–468

Pulse oximetry is a noninvasive monitoring of the arterial oxygenation of the skin. It accurately reflects the oxygen delivery to the end organs, giving an ongoing evaluation of circulation and respiration. In prehospital care, the oximeter is quick and easy to use and provides an accurate and constant evaluation of the cardiorespiratory system.

Capnography is the noninvasive monitoring of exhaled CO_2 concentrations over time. It can be used to evaluate the initial and continuing placement of an endotracheal tube as well as the effectiveness of ventilations and CPR. The device can also monitor the patient's general condition and responses to medications. The real-time monitoring of $ETCO_2$ is rapidly becoming the standard of care in emergency medical services.

7. Define and explain the implications of partial airway obstruction with good and poor air exchange and complete airway obstruction. pp. 456–457

Obstruction of the airway by a foreign object or swelling may range from minor to complete. If the airway obstruction permits speech and coughing and you do not notice skin color changes, respiration is probably adequate and intervention may not be needed. However, if the patient has serious dyspnea, cannot speak or cough, is choking or gagging, and you notice skin color changes, intervention is necessary. Continued inadequate respiration will lead to increasing hypoxia. No air movement due to complete obstruction will rapidly lead to serious hypoxia and death.

8. Describe the common causes of upper airway obstruction, including:

- **the tongue** p. 457
  The most common cause of airway obstruction is the tongue. In the unconscious person or the supine patient, the lack of muscle tone allows the tongue to rest against the posterior pharynx and thereby obstruct the airway.
- **foreign body aspiration** pp. 457, 458
  Large, poorly chewed lumps of food and objects aspirated by children commonly account for airway obstruction. The victim will often grasp his or her throat, a universal distress signal.
- **laryngeal spasm** pp. 457–458
  The glottis is the smallest part of the airway and may be responsible for obstruction secondary to spasm. Spasm may be caused by stimulation by a foreign object as during endotracheal intubation.
- **laryngeal edema** pp. 457–458
  As the glottis is the narrowest part of the adult airway, swelling will rapidly reduce the airway lumen size and restrict breathing. Restriction and obstruction may be caused by anaphylaxis, epiglottitis, or the inhalation of toxic substances, superheated steam, or smoke.
- **trauma** p. 457
  Physical injury to the structures of the upper airway may result in loose objects such as the teeth, tissue, or clotted blood obstructing the airway. Further, blunt or penetrating trauma may result

in collapse of the airway due to fracture or displacement of the larynx or trachea. Soft-tissue swelling may also restrict the lumen of the airway.

9. **Describe complete airway obstruction maneuvers, including:**

   - **Heimlich maneuver** pp. 511–512

   The Heimlich maneuver involves a forceful upward and backward abdominal thrust using the hands placed halfway between the umbilicus and the xiphoid process. The increased abdominal and thoracic pressures help propel an obstruction up and out of the airway.

   - **removal with Magill forceps** pp. 511–512

   If basic life support measures fail to secure a patent airway, you may introduce a laryngoscope to visualize beyond the oral cavity. If you notice a foreign body obstructing the airway, you may then remove it using the Magill forceps.

10. **Describe causes of respiratory distress, including:**

    - **upper and lower airway obstruction** pp. 456–458

    Upper and lower airway obstructions range in severity from minor to complete obstructions and may be caused by the tongue, a foreign body, swelling, vomitus, blood, or teeth.

    - **inadequate ventilation** p. 458

    Insufficient minute volume compromises respiratory exchange and may be due to bronchospasm, rib fracture, hemo- or pneumothorax, drug overdose, airway obstruction, renal failure, or central nervous system injury.

    - **impairment of respiratory muscles** p. 458

    The respiratory muscles may be impaired by fatigue, central nervous system depression, or spinal injury.

    - **impairment of nervous system** p. 458

    Respiratory system control, provided by the central nervous system, may be depressed by drugs or by intracranial or spinal injury

11. **Explain the risk of infection to EMS providers associated with airway management and ventilation.** pp. 469, 525–526

    There are several diseases that can be transmitted by body fluids and airborne droplet transmission. The pocket mask reduces the contact with the patient and, if equipped with a one-way valve, lessens the exposure to droplet contamination.

12. **Describe manual airway maneuvers, including:**

    - **head-tilt/chin-lift maneuver** p. 469

    To execute the head-tilt/chin-lift airway maneuver, the rescuer places one hand on the patient's forehead, gently tilting the head back, while the other engages the mandible, displacing it anteriorly.

    - **jaw-thrust maneuver** pp. 469–470

    During the jaw-thrust (or the triple-airway maneuver), the rescuer places his fingers on the patient's lateral mandible, displacing it anteriorly while the thumbs displace it inferiorly. The maneuver may rotate the head and extend the neck. If spinal injury is suspected, the head should not be tilted backward (use the modified jaw-thrust).

    - **modified jaw-thrust maneuver** pp. 469–470

    The modified jaw-thrust (for the trauma patient) requires that the jaw-thrust maneuver be modified by manually securing the head in a neutral position while the mandible is displaced forward.

13. **Discuss the indications, contraindications, advantages, disadvantages, complications, special considerations, equipment, and techniques of the following:**

    - **upper airway and tracheobronchial suctioning** pp. 521–522

    Suctioning is the use of pressures that are less than atmospheric to draw fluids and semi-fluids out of the airway. It should be used any time it can effectively remove material from the airway.

Continuous suctioning should be avoided because it draws against the patient's ventilation attempts and generally interrupts artificial ventilation of the apneic patient. Suctioning can be provided by an electric or a mechanical device. Tracheobronchial suctioning passes a lubricated soft suction catheter down the endotracheal tube into the trachea or bronchi to remove secretions. Suction is applied for 10 to 15 seconds while the catheter is slowly turned and withdrawn.

- **nasogastric and orogastric tube insertion** pp. 522–523

Nasogastric tube insertion is recommended for the conscious patient, because it permits him or her to talk more easily, while the procedure is to be avoided when there is danger of skull fracture and further injury caused by the tube's placement. Both oral and nasal techniques may be used for gastric decompression when patient ventilation is restricted or there is danger of aspiration. The tube is measured for depth of insertion by measuring from the epigastrium to the angle of the jaw and then to the nares. Use a topical anesthetic spray, and then lubricate the distal tip and insert the tube through the nares and along the nasal floor or through the mouth along the midline. Advance the tube, encourage patient swallowing if possible, and then introduce 30 to 50 mL of air while listening over the epigastrium. The absence of gastric sounds and the inability to speak suggests tracheal placement and the need to reattempt insertion.

- **oropharyngeal and nasopharyngeal airway** pp. 471–474

The oropharyngeal airway is designed to maintain an airway by displacing the tongue anteriorly. It should not be used in conscious or semiconscious patients who have an intact gag reflex. Displace the tongue forward with a tongue blade and insert the airway along the base of the tongue. It may also be inserted by placing it, backward, into the oral cavity to the base of the tongue and then rotating it 180° and continuing the insertion. The oral or nasal airway should be used when ventilating the patient using any mechanical device.

The nasopharyngeal airway is inserted into the nasopharynx in the unconscious or semiconscious patient. It is a soft rubber tube that is lubricated and inserted posteriorly in the largest nostril (usually the left). It is indicated in the semiconscious patient or as the oral airway would be used. It should not be used in the patient with possible skull fracture.

- **ventilating a patient by mouth-to-mouth, mouth-to-nose, mouth-to-mask, one/two/three person bag-valve mask, flow-restricted oxygen-powered ventilation device, automatic transport ventilator** pp. 525–529

Ventilation by mouth-to-mouth or mouth-to-nose is an easy technique that requires no equipment, though it risks disease transmission. The rescuer seals his mouth over the patient's mouth or nose (or both with the small child or infant), closes the nostrils or mouth with his fingers, takes a deep breath, and inflates the patient's lungs. The procedure induces air with about 15 percent oxygen that will successfully sustain life. When possible, mouth-to-mask or bag-valve-mask ventilation is recommended.

The pocket mask is an adjunct to mouth-to-mouth ventilation that provides some protection against direct contact with the patient and the patient's exhaled air. It is simply sealed to the patient's face with the rescuer's hands and held in place during ventilation. It is recommended for use any time you would otherwise employ direct mouth-to-mouth ventilation. Some masks provide for supplemental oxygen administration that improves the percentage of oxygen provided to the patient.

Bag-valve-mask devices are mechanical devices that provide positive-pressure ventilation. The mask is sealed to the patient's face with one hand while the other hand squeezes the bag, pushing air into the patient's lungs. The device is best used for the intubated patient because the volume of air and the pressure delivered to the patient is low. If the patient is not intubated, the air exchange achieved by one person may not be enough to sustain life. With two or more persons, one rescuer seals the mask to the face and maintains head positioning while another uses both hands to squeeze the bag. Since the volume of the bag is limited, it is essential to obtain a good seal on the face when using the BVM. Any time the BVM is used, it should have the oxygen reservoir attached and oxygen flowing at 12 to 15 liters per minute.

Flow-restricted, oxygen-powered ventilation devices, sometimes called demand valve resuscitators, ventilate a patient with a flow of oxygen when a button or bar is pushed. They can be used with a face mask, EOA, EGTA, PtL airway, or endotracheal tube. They provide the patient with 100 percent oxygen. However, the pressures they use may cause gastric insufflation or lung tissue damage. They are not recommended for intubated or pediatric patients.

Automatic transport ventilators provide a patient with ventilation with 100 percent oxygen at a rate and volume determined by the user. Recent advances in technology make automatic ventilators compact and dependable for field use. They are not recommended for children under the age of 5 years and are dependent upon a good patient airway.

14. **Compare the ventilation techniques used for an adult patient to those used for pediatric patients, and describe special considerations in airway management and ventilation for the pediatric patient.** pp. 497–501, 527

During bag-valve-masking, one rescuer seals the mask to the face and thrusts the jaw anteriorly while the other rescuer compresses the bag. The small (450 mL) BVM is used for infants, while the standard pediatric BVM is adequate for children up to 8 years old. Ensure the mask seals well and that ventilation achieves good chest rise and breath sounds.

Endotracheal intubation of the pediatric patient is more difficult than for the adult for the following reasons; the airway structures are smaller and more flexible, the tongue is relatively larger, the epiglottis is floppier and rounder, the vocal folds are more difficult to visualize, and the narrowest part of the airway is the cricoid cartilage. A straight laryngoscope blade and uncuffed endotracheal tube are used for patients under 8 years of age. The tube is only introduced to 2 to 3 cm beyond the vocal cords (place the black glottic mark at the vocal cords). The procedure is more likely to produce vagal stimulation and may require atropine administration.

15. **Identify types of oxygen cylinders and pressure regulators, and explain safety considerations of oxygen storage and delivery, including steps for delivering oxygen from a cylinder and regulator.** pp. 523–524

Oxygen is commonly available in steel or aluminum cylinders of D (400 L), E (660 L), and M (3,450 L) sizes and is brought to administration pressures by a therapy regulator (50 psi) that allows for the administration of a liter/minute flow rate. Oxygen is a gas that easily supports combustion and should be used with caution near any ignition source or near grease. The pressure in the tank makes rupture an event that may produce serious injury, so tanks must be handled and stored carefully.

16. **Describe the indications, contraindications, advantages, disadvantages, complications, liter flow range, and concentration of delivered oxygen for the following supplemental oxygen delivery devices:** pp. 524–525

- **nasal cannula**
  The nasal cannula is a blind tube with ports to correspond to the patient's nostrils. Oxygen flows into the nares and the patient breathes enriched oxygen when breathing through the nose. The device delivers 24 to 44 percent oxygen with flows of 1 to 6 liters per minute. The nasal cannula is useful for the patient with anxiety regarding oxygen masks and for prolonged oxygen administration. It is of little benefit if the patient is not breathing through the nose unless the prongs are then placed facing into the mouth.
- **simple face mask**
  A simple face mask delivers oxygen into the mask in front of the patient's mouth and nose. The patient inhales 40 to 60 percent oxygen when the device receives an oxygen flow of 8 to 12 liters per minute. The simple oxygen face mask is useful for the routine administration of oxygen.
- **partial rebreather mask**
  The partial rebreather mask is indicated for patients needing moderate concentrations of oxygen. One-way disks limit mixing of oxygen with inspired air and help increase the oxygen concentration. Maximum oxygen flow is about 10 liters per minute.
- **nonrebreather mask**
  The nonrebreather mask consists of oxygen tubing and a face mask with a reservoir. Because of valves in the mask, oxygen flows into the reservoir while the patient exhales and into the patient from the input tubing and reservoir when the patient inhales. If the reservoir does not completely collapse (usually 10 to 15 liters per minute flow) on inspiration, oxygen delivery is between 80 percent and 95 percent.

- **Venturi mask**

  The Venturi mask is a high-flow oxygen mask that delivers very precise concentrations of oxygen. The oxygen concentration is generally low, with normal concentrations of 24, 28, 35, and 40 percent. It is often used to treat COPD patients who need supplemental oxygen but who may have respiratory drive problems with high-concentration oxygen.

17. **Describe the use, advantages, and disadvantages of an oxygen humidifier.**   **p. 525**

    Oxygen bubbles through sterile water to obtain humidification. Humidified oxygen administration benefits patients with croup, epiglottitis, or bronchiolitis or patients on long-term oxygen therapy.

18. **Describe the indications, contraindications, advantages, disadvantages, complications, equipment, and technique for the following:**

    - **endotracheal intubation by direct laryngoscopy**   **pp. 483–486**

      Endotracheal intubation is the method of choice for the patient who is unable to protect his airway. It may also be considered for the patient who is expected to lose the airway due to swelling, as may occur with inhalation injury or with a trauma patient or with one who is in need of assisted ventilation. The only contraindication to endotracheal intubation is the pediatric patient with possible epiglottitis, unless respirations are worsening. The procedure requires an endotracheal tube, a laryngoscope, and tape to secure the tube once in place. Once the patient is hyperventilated, the laryngoscope is inserted into the right side of the oral cavity, then moved to the left, displacing the tongue. It is negotiated down the airway until it engages the epiglottis (straight blade) or is negotiated into the vallecula. As the tongue and pharynx are lifted to visualize the glottic opening, the endotracheal tube is placed through the opening, then advanced 2 to 3 cm beyond. Placement is checked and then the cuff is inflated to seal the trachea.

    - **digital endotracheal intubation**   **pp. 489–491**

      Digital intubation is a blind intubation technique in which the endotracheal tube is guided into the glottis with the fingers of a hand inserted into the oral cavity. One hand is deeply inserted into the oral cavity, and one finger locates the epiglottis while the others direct the tube along its posterior surface and, hopefully, into the trachea. The technique is helpful in the trauma patient whose neck cannot be extended or the patient with a short neck, where visualization of the glottis is very difficult. The fingers of the rescuer must be protected with an oral airway, and great care must be used to ensure the endotracheal tube is correctly placed in the trachea.

    - **dual lumen airway**   **pp. 504–511**

      A dual lumen airway, like the Esophageal Tracheal CombiTube, has two lumens, or tubes. The device is inserted blindly through the mouth, and one lumen enters the trachea and the other enters the esophagus. After determining which tube has entered the trachea, the patient is ventilated through that tube. The dual lumen airway is easy to use and does not require special equipment. The device diminishes gastric distention and regurgitation and can be used on trauma patients because the neck can remain in the neutral position during insertion and ventilation. However, maintaining adequate mask seal is difficult, and the device cannot be used with pediatric patients or those with esophageal disease or caustic ingestions, or in conscious patients or those with a gag reflex.

    - **nasotracheal intubation**   **pp. 501–503**

      Nasotracheal intubation is a blind intubation technique that is recommended for spinal injury, clenched teeth, oral injuries and swelling, and obesity or arthritis preventing patient positioning in the sniffing position. The patient must be breathing and without nasal or basilar skull fractures. The endotracheal tube is inserted blindly into the largest nares and along the floor of the nasal cavity. Listen to the breath sounds, and once the breath sounds are heard clearly, advance the tube during the next inhalation. Carefully confirm proper tube placement. Once inserted, the tube can be secured more easily and the patient cannot bite or compress the tube.

    - **rapid-sequence intubation**   **pp. 494–497**

      Rapid-sequence intubation is indicated for a patient who has a gag reflex or is likely to fight any intubation attempt but who requires such a procedure. The procedure induces sedation, then muscle paralysis to permit easier intubation. The patient is ventilated while the medications take effect. The procedure requires that care providers continue ventilation during the entire time of paralysis and maintain the airway if endotracheal intubation is unsuccessful. Care must be taken to administer agents that do not cause hypotension and ICP increase in serious trauma patients.

- **endotracheal intubation using sedation** pp. 494–497

  To perform endotracheal intubation using sedation, the caregiver simply medicates the patient without employing a paralytic agent.

- **open cricothyrotomy** pp. 516–519

  Cricothyrotomy is an incision through the cricothyroid membrane to allow the passage of air. It is employed only when complete airway obstruction makes no other means of effectively ventilating the patient possible. The cricoid membrane is located (the first hard ring moving from the mid-trachea upward), then the membrane between it and the thyroid cartilage. The skin above the membrane is incised vertically with a scalpel and then the membrane is opened with a horizontal incision. A 6- or 7-mm endotracheal tube (or tracheostomy tube) is directed down the trachea, and the cuff is inflated. Complications of the open cricothyrotomy include severe hemorrhage, thyroid gland damage, damage to surrounding airway structures, subcutaneous emphysema, and incorrect tube placement.

- **needle cricothyrotomy (translaryngeal catheter ventilation)** pp. 512–516

  Percutaneous transtracheal catheter ventilation (or needle cricothyrotomy) is used only for severe, partial airway obstruction above the vocal cords that is not correctable by other methods. An over-the-needle catheter is inserted through the cricothyroid membrane with a syringe attached. Once the membrane is penetrated, air can be inspired into the syringe to confirm proper placement. The catheter is then directed caudally, the needle is withdrawn, and the catheter is attached to a high-pressure, high-volume oxygen line. High-pressure oxygen (50 psi) is passed through the large (14 ga or larger) catheter using special equipment and then is allowed to escape. Expiration should take twice as long as inflation. If the chest does not deflate, a second needle or an open cricothyrotomy may be needed.

- **extubation** p. 504

  Extubation is the removal of the endotracheal tube when a patient awakens and is intolerant of the endotracheal tube. Removal calls for the deflation of the cuff and withdrawal of the tube during expiration or a cough. Laryngospasm may occur with the withdrawal of the endotracheal tube.

19. Describe the use of cricoid pressure during intubation. pp. 470–471, 483, 484

Cricoid pressure or Sellick's maneuver places posteriorly directed pressure on the cricoid cartilage, compressing the esophagus and preventing vomit from entering the pharynx. The procedure also may move the structures of the airway so they may be more easily viewed during intubation attempts. Once applied, Sellick's procedure must be maintained until the endotracheal tube is placed, as early release may permit emesis to enter the pharynx. Do not apply excessive pressure, as doing so may obstruct the trachea.

20. Discuss the precautions that should be taken when intubating the trauma patient. pp. 492, 493

The trauma patient may have sustained spinal injury: All airway care must be provided with limited (if any) movement of the head and neck. In addition to the cervical collar, the head should be held in a neutral position manually by an EMT while intubation is attempted. Oro- or nasotracheal intubation, lighted stylet intubation, or digital techniques may be attempted.

21. Discuss agents used for sedation and rapid-sequence intubation. pp. 494–497

Midazolam, diazepam, etomidate, ketamine, sodium thiopental, propofol, and fentanyl are used to sedate patients as the first step of rapid-sequence intubation. Then paralytics such as succinylcholine, vecuronium, atracurium, and pancuronium are used to relax the skeletal muscles and permit endotracheal intubation. The drugs atropine and lidocaine may also be used as part of the rapid-sequence intubation regimen.

22. **Discuss methods to confirm correct placement of the endotracheal tube.** pp. 486–489

Verify and document at least three of the following: visualization of the tube passing through the vocal cords, the presence of bilateral breath sounds, absence of breath sounds over the epigastrium, positive end-tidal CO_2 change, verification of placement by an esophageal detector device, condensation in the endotracheal tube, absence of vomitus within the endotracheal tube, and the absence of vocal sounds once the tube is in place. It is highly recommended that the patient's chest be auscultated for bilateral breath sounds to ensure the endotracheal tube has not been introduced too far and into the right mainstem bronchus.

Content Self-Evaluation

MULTIPLE CHOICE

_____ 1. Which of the following is the most common cause of upper airway obstruction?
   A. the tongue
   B. foreign bodies
   C. trauma
   D. laryngeal swelling
   E. aspiration of blood or vomitus

_____ 2. All of the following conditions may cause reduced inspiratory volumes EXCEPT:
   A. pneumothorax.
   B. asthma.
   C. high inspired oxygen concentrations.
   D. respiratory muscle paralysis.
   E. emphysema.

_____ 3. The normal respiratory rate for an adult at rest is:
   A. 8 to 12.
   B. 12 to 20.
   C. 18 to 24.
   D. 24 to 32.
   E. 40 to 60.

_____ 4. Which of the following is a breathing pattern associated with flail chest?
   A. abdominal breathing
   B. paradoxical breathing
   C. diaphragmatic breathing
   D. intercostal retraction
   E. both A and C

_____ 5. It is unlikely that a patient will have significant hypoxia and not display cyanosis.
   A. True
   B. False

_____ 6. Which modified form of respiration is designed to expand alveoli that may have collapsed during periods of inactivity or rest?
   A. coughing
   B. sneezing
   C. hiccoughing
   D. grunting
   E. sighing

_____ 7. The respiratory pattern that presents with deep and rapid respirations is:
   A. apneustic respirations.
   B. Cheyne-Stokes respirations.
   C. Biot's respirations.
   D. central neurogenic hyperventilation.
   E. agonal respirations.

_____ 8. Stridor is most commonly associated with:
   A. laryngeal constriction or edema.
   B. the tongue blocking the airway.
   C. narrowing of the bronchioles.
   D. fluids within the airway.
   E. foreign bodies in the lower airway.

_____ 9. The feeling of flexibility or stiffness associated with the lungs and ventilation is:
   A. back pressure.
   B. resiliency.
   C. compliance.
   D. effusion.
   E. Hering-Breuer reflex.

_____ 10. The absence of CO₂ in exhaled air, as identified by the end-expiratory CO₂ detector, suggests:
   A. ventilation is not deep enough.
   B. ventilations are not occurring fast enough.
   C. the endotracheal tube may be in the esophagus.
   D. the oxygen percentage of inspired air is insufficient.
   E. all of the above

_____ 11. The normal partial pressure of CO₂ in exhaled air is:
   A. 5 mmHg
   B. 25 mmHg
   C. 38 mmHg
   D. 45 mmHg
   E. 86 mmHg

_____ 12. The disposable device that records the level of exhaled CO₂ using pH-sensitive chemically impregnated paper is a:
   A. capnometer.
   B. capnograph.
   C. capnogram.
   D. colormetric device.
   E. nonwaveform ETCO₂ device.

_____ 13. If the end-tidal CO₂ detector becomes contaminated with gastric contents, further readings may be unreliable.
   A. True
   B. False

_____ 14. When perfusion decreases, the ETCO₂ level reflects cardiac output and coronary perfusion pressure.
   A. True
   B. False

_____ 15. The value of capnography is that it can assess which of the following?
   A. the effectiveness of CPR
   B. proper initial endotracheal tube placement
   C. continuing proper endotracheal tube placement
   D. patient responses to medications
   E. all of the above

_____ 16. In the head-tilt/chin-lift maneuver, the fingers under the chin should apply a firm pressure to ensure the jaw remains closed.
   A. True
   B. False

_____ 17. The intent behind employing Sellick's maneuver is to:
   A. displace the diaphragm.
   B. increase venous return.
   C. prevent regurgitation.
   D. clear an airway obstruction.
   E. increase blood flow to the brain.

_____ 18. Which of the following is an advantage of the nasopharyngeal airway over the oropharyngeal airway?
   A. It has a larger diameter.
   B. It is easier to insert.
   C. It is blocked less frequently by vomitus.
   D. It does not stimulate the gag reflex as strongly.
   E. It can be used with a BVM.

_____ 19. Insertion of the nasopharyngeal airway directs the soft rubber tube:
   A. directly up and into the nostril.
   B. directly along the floor of the nasal cavity.
   C. into the left nostril, most frequently.
   D. laterally along the side of the nasal cavity.
   E. directly into the vallecula space.

20. The airway adjunct that acts primarily by displacing the tongue forward is the:
    A. oropharyngeal airway.
    B. PtL airway.
    C. endotracheal tube.
    D. nasopharyngeal airway.
    E. esophageal gastric tube airway.

21. The preferred technique of insertion for the oropharyngeal airway in pediatric patients calls for inserting the airway using a tongue blade without rotating the device.
    A. True
    B. False

22. The airway technique preferred for use with the patient who is unconscious is:
    A. the oropharyngeal airway.
    B. the nasopharyngeal airway.
    C. endotracheal intubation.
    D. nasotracheal intubation.
    E. dual lumen airway.

23. The light of the laryngoscope should be a bright yellow and flicker slightly when pressure is placed on the blade.
    A. True
    B. False

24. The tip of the curve of the Macintosh laryngoscope blade is designed to fit into the:
    A. nasopharynx.
    B. glottic opening.
    C. vallecula.
    D. arytenoid fossa.
    E. epiglottis.

25. The laryngoscope blade considered to be best designed for intubation of the infant is:
    A. the Macintosh blade.
    B. the curved blade.
    C. the straight blade.
    D. either B or C
    E. none of the above

26. The pilot balloon of the endotracheal tube should be very firm to ensure there is a good seal between the tube and the interior of the trachea.
    A. True
    B. False

27. The major purpose for using a malleable stylet during endotracheal intubation is to:
    A. maintain a preset curve in the tube.
    B. keep the tube's lumen open.
    C. stiffen the tube so it can be pushed through the glottis.
    D. prevent foreign matter from entering the tube.
    E. all of the above

28. Which of the following is NOT an indication for endotracheal intubation?
    A. respiratory arrest
    B. cardiac arrest
    C. inability to protect the airway
    D. obstruction due to foreign object, swelling, or burns
    E. severe epiglottitis

29. Which of the following is a likely occurrence when using an endotracheal intubation to secure the airway?
    A. Gastric distention is more likely.
    B. Complete airway control is achieved.
    C. The tracheal suctioning becomes more complicated.
    D. Medications can no longer be introduced into the trachea.
    E. It makes obtaining a good mask seal more difficult.

_____ 30. When using the laryngoscope to visualize the glottis, it is best to use the teeth as a fulcrum to increase your ability to lift the tissue.
   A. True
   B. False

_____ 31. To reduce the risk of hypoxia, limit attempts at intubation to no more than:
   A. 15 seconds.
   B. 30 seconds.
   C. 45 seconds.
   D. 60 seconds.
   E. 80 seconds.

_____ 32. Which of the following is NOT an indication of esophageal intubation?
   A. absence of chest rise with ventilation
   B. gurgling sound over the epigastrium
   C. a falling pulse oximetry reading
   D. skin color turning pink
   E. increasing resistance to ventilatory effort

_____ 33. Upon placing the endotracheal tube, you hear very faint breath sounds and some gurgling over the epigastric region. You should next:
   A. advance the tube slightly.
   B. withdraw the tube slightly.
   C. inflate the cuff and auscultate again.
   D. ventilate more forcibly.
   E. remove the tube and re-intubate.

_____ 34. Upon placing the endotracheal tube in a patient, you determine that you can only auscultate breath sounds on the right side. You should next:
   A. withdraw the tube a few centimeters.
   B. withdraw the tube completely.
   C. pass the tube a few centimeters further.
   D. secure the tube and ventilate more aggressively.
   E. check the mask seal.

_____ 35. The purpose of the cuff on the end of the endotracheal tube is to:
   A. help guide the tube to its proper location.
   B. prevent dislodging of the tube after it is correctly placed.
   C. seal the airway.
   D. center the tube in the trachea.
   E. widen the opening of the vocal cords.

_____ 36. What volume of air is used to inflate the cuff of an endotracheal tube?
   A. 2 to 4 mL
   B. 4 to 6 mL
   C. 5 to 10 mL
   D. 10 to 15 mL
   E. 15 to 25 mL

_____ 37. Confirmation of proper endotracheal tube placement is achieved by:
   A. visualizing the tube passing through the glottis.
   B. hearing clear and bilaterally equal breath sounds.
   C. noting the absence of gastric sounds with ventilation.
   D. observing condensation on the endotracheal tube with exhalation.
   E. any three of the above

_____ 38. Which of the following is NOT a standard procedure when performing endotracheal intubation using the transillumination technique?
   A. cutting the tube to 35 to 37 cm
   B. conforming the stylet and tube to a "hockey-stick" configuration
   C. placing the stylet in the ETT and locking the ETT in place at its proximal end
   D. lifting the patient's tongue and jaw forward with your fingers
   E. advancing the tube/stylet into the mouth and advancing it into the hypopharynx

_____ 39. The pattern of light that indicates that the lighted stylet is in the proper position to advance the endotracheal tube when performing transillumination intubation is:
   A. a very dim and diffuse light.
   B. a circle of light at the Adam's apple.
   C. a light on either side of the Adam's apple.
   D. absent light in the neck.
   E. a bright light above the Adam's apple.

_____ 40. Digital intubation may be indicated in all of the following EXCEPT:
   A. an unconscious trauma patient with suspected C-spine injury.
   B. a patient with facial injuries that distort the anatomy.
   C. an unconscious patient with a gag reflex.
   D. an entrapped patient who cannot be properly positioned.
   E. a patient with copious amounts of blood or other fluids remaining in the airway.

_____ 41. Indications for rapid-sequence intubation include which of the following?
   A. impending respiratory failure
   B. acute disorder threatening the airway
   C. altered mental status with risk of aspiration
   D. Glasgow coma scale of 8 or less
   E. all of the above

_____ 42. Which of the following is NOT a paralytic agent used for rapid-sequence intubation?
   A. succinylcholine   D. atracurium
   B. midazolam   E. pancuronium
   C. vecuronium

_____ 43. The duration of action of succinylcholine (Anectine) is approximately:
   A. 1 to 2 minutes.   D. 4 to 6 minutes.
   B. 2 to 3 minutes.   E. 10 to 15 minutes.
   C. 3 to 5 minutes.

_____ 44. If you cannot intubate the patient who has been paralyzed, the patient has no definitive airway.
   A. True
   B. False

_____ 45. The reason the succinylcholine is used in prehospital care is that it:
   A. is fast acting and of short duration.
   B. is the easiest to administer.
   C. does not cause muscle fasciculations.
   D. can be used with massive crush injuries.
   E. has a half-life of 30 minutes.

_____ 46. It is essential that an adult patient be premedicated with vecuronium prior to the administration of succinylcholine because fasciculations are otherwise likely to cause musculoskeletal trauma.
   A. True
   B. False

_____ 47. In the intubation of children under 8 years old, it is recommended that the paramedic use:
   A. a cuffed endotracheal tube and a straight laryngoscope blade.
   B. an uncuffed endotracheal tube and a straight laryngoscope blade.
   C. a cuffed endotracheal tube and a curved laryngoscope blade.
   D. an uncuffed endotracheal tube and a curved laryngoscope blade.
   E. an uncuffed endotracheal tube and digital technique.

_____ 48. Because of the anterior location of the glottic opening, it is essential to use a stylet with the endotracheal tube during pediatric intubation.
   A. True
   B. False

_____ 49. Which of the following is NOT an advantage of nasotracheal intubation?
   A. It is well tolerated by a semiconscious patient.
   B. It is easier and quicker to perform than orotracheal intubation.
   C. It can be performed without displacing the patient's head.
   D. The tube cannot be bitten.
   E. The tube can be easily anchored.

_____ 50. Which of the following is NOT required for blind nasotracheal intubation?
   A. a neutral or slightly extended neck
   B. a generally quiet environment
   C. a strong, malleable stylet
   D. a patient who is breathing
   E. a preoxygenated patient

_____ 51. The primary danger associated with extubation is:
   A. laryngospasm.
   B. aspiration.
   C. fasciculations.
   D. tracheal damage.
   E. vomiting.

_____ 52. The major disadvantage to the use of the Esophageal Tracheal CombiTube is that:
   A. the trachea is not isolated.
   B. the tube must be in the trachea.
   C. it is associated with gastric distension and vomiting.
   D. it cannot be used in the trauma patient.
   E. it is somewhat time-consuming to insert.

_____ 53. Which of the following are features of the PtL airway?
   A. It can be inserted blindly.
   B. It can seal off the nasal and oral cavities.
   C. The patient can be ventilated regardless of whether the tube is in the trachea or esophagus.
   D. It can be inserted without moving the cervical spine.
   E. all of the above

_____ 54. The only indication for the use of a needle cricothyrotomy is the inability to establish an airway by any other means.
   A. True
   B. False

_____ 55. An advantage to the use of a needle cricothyrotomy is that subsequent ventilation of the patient requires no special or additional equipment.
   A. True
   B. False

_____ 56. The open cricothyrotomy should not be performed on the patient under 12 years of age because the cricothyroid membrane is small and underdeveloped.
   A. True
   B. False

_____ 57. Which of the following is a part of suctioning the stoma patient?
   A. preoxygenating with 100 percent oxygen
   B. injecting 3 mL of saline
   C. inserting the catheter until resistance is met
   D. withdrawing the catheter while the patient exhales or coughs
   E. all of the above

_____ 58. Which of the following is NOT indicated when suctioning through the endotracheal tube?
   A. Insert the catheter until you meet resistance.
   B. Suction only during insertion.
   C. Pre-oxygenate the patient.
   D. Rotate the suction catheter while suctioning.
   E. Suction no longer than 10 to 15 seconds.

_____ 59. Nasogastric tube placement is indicated in a patient:
   A. with facial fractures.
   B. with a possible basilar skull fracture.
   C. who is awake.
   D. for whom a relatively large gastric tube is indicated.
   E. all of the above

_____ 60. Which of the devices listed below delivers the highest concentration of oxygen to the patient?
   A. nasal cannula
   B. simple face mask
   C. nonrebreather mask
   D. Venturi mask
   E. A and D

_____ 61. Which of the devices below delivers the most controlled concentration of oxygen to a patient?
   A. nasal cannula
   B. simple face mask
   C. nonrebreather mask
   D. Venturi mask
   E. B and C

_____ 62. The bag-valve mask with an oxygen supply attached and oxygen flowing at 15 L per minute delivers what percentage of oxygen to the patient?
   A. 21 percent
   B. 40 to 60 percent
   C. 60 to 70 percent
   D. 90 to 95 percent
   E. 99.9 percent

_____ 63. One rescuer bag-valve-masking is difficult to perform effectively because:
   A. it is difficult to maintain proper airway positioning.
   B. it is difficult to maintain mask seal.
   C. it is difficult to squeeze the bag.
   D. all of the above
   E. none of the above

_____ 64. Hazards of using the demand valve to ventilate a patient include all of the following EXCEPT:
   A. oxygen toxicity.
   B. gastric distention.
   C. pulmonary barotrauma.
   D. pneumothorax.
   E. subcutaneous emphysema.

_____ 65. Which of the following is NOT an advantage of automatic ventilators?
   A. They free a rescuer when the patient is not breathing.
   B. They are convenient and easy to use.
   C. They are dependable.
   D. They can be used on children younger than age 5.
   E. They are lightweight and tolerant to temperature extremes.

Chapter 9: Therapeutic Communications

Review of Chapter Objectives

After reading this chapter, you should be able to:

1. **Define communication.** p. 533

   Communication is the exchange of information through the use of common symbols—written, spoken, or of other kinds. The basic elements of communication include a sender, an encoded message, a receiver, and feedback. The sender encodes a written, spoken, signed, or other message to the receiver. The receiver decodes the message to derive his interpretation of the content. He then provides feedback to the sender. If, because of the feedback, the sender believes the communication was accurately received, the communication was successful.

2. **Identify internal and external factors that affect an interview.** pp. 533–535, 539–540

   There are several reasons why communications can be ineffective or fail. They include prejudice, lack of empathy or understanding, lack of (or a perceived invasion of) privacy, or internal or external distractions. If the sender, receiver, or both are subject to these influences, the communication is likely to be ineffective. On the other hand, trust and rapport between sender and receiver can facilitate communication.

3. **Identify strategies for developing rapport with the patient.** p. 534

   Developing rapport with a patient is dependent upon truly feeling empathy for the patient and observing several principles of good interpersonal communication. Use your patient's name frequently with the proper form of address (Mr., Ms., or Mrs.). Use a professional but compassionate tone of voice and explain what you are doing and why, and be honest about what is happening. Keep a kind, calming, and caring facial expression, use the appropriate style of communication, and listen carefully to what your patient says.

   Using the following techniques can provide feedback to your interviewee and thus help develop rapport:

   - Silence gives your patient time to gather his thoughts and complete his answer.
   - Reflection, your echoing of the patient's response, assures you understand the interviewee's answer.
   - Facilitation encourages the patient to make further responses.
   - Empathy is using your body language and your speech to assure the patient you are interested and concerned.
   - Clarification involves asking the interviewee to explain answers you don't understand.
   - Confrontation is a technique in which you ask direct questions about confusing or contradictory statements by the patient.
   - Interpretation is a statement of your understanding of the events and circumstances of which the interviewee has offered an explanation.

- Explanation is a technique in which you share objective information you gather with the interviewee.
- Summarization is your brief review of all the pertinent information you have gathered from the interviewee.

4. Discuss open-ended and closed questions. pp. 537–538

Open-ended questions provide the patient with the opportunity to respond to your question with an unguided, spontaneous answer. An example is "What happened to cause you to call for an ambulance?" or "Describe what you had for lunch." Closed, or direct, questions guide the patient to an answer of yes or no or some other short response. The question does not allow for an explanation of the circumstance. Examples of closed or direct questions are "Do you have any chest pain?" and "Does it hurt to breathe?"

5. Discuss common errors made when interviewing patients. pp. 539–540

Common errors associated with interviewing include providing false assurance, giving inappropriate advice, using authority inappropriately, using avoidance language, improperly distancing yourself from the interviewee, using professional jargon, talking instead of listening, interrupting the interviewee, and using questioning language that implies guilt (using "why" questions).

6. Identify the nonverbal skills used in patient interviewing. pp. 535–536

Distance

The distance at which you place yourself from the patient during the interview process is an important tool in making the patient comfortable and in defining your role as a caregiver. The closer you come to the patient, the more personal and intimate your conversation. However, unwanted entry into someone's personal space can be perceived as threatening.

Relative level

The relative difference between a caregiver's eye level and the patient's is important. When the caregiver's eye level is above the patient's, it reflects a state of authority; an eye level equal with the patient's indicates equality; while an eye level below the patient's indicates a willingness to let the patient have some control over the interview. Each position has advantages and disadvantages when interviewing the emergency patient.

Stance

A closed stance (arms crossed, fists clenched, and the body square to the patient) suggests disinterest, discomfort, fear, or anger. An open stance (open hands, relaxed muscles, and a nodding head) suggests comfort, interest, and confidence.

Eye contact

Eye contact with a patient suggests interest and an entry into the patient's personal space. It is a powerful communication tool and a way to convey the caregiver's empathy with the patient.

Touching

Touching is also a way to communicate empathy and concern. Like eye contact, however, it can be threatening when not used in the right circumstances.

7. Identify interview methods used to assess mental status. p. 538

By carefully watching the patient's body language and attending to his verbal and nonverbal responses to questioning, you can assess his level of responsiveness and his ability to concentrate. Be especially watchful of speech and how the patient phrases sentences and articulates. Also note how well he answers questions and the appropriateness of questions he asks.

8. Discuss strategies for interviewing a patient who is not motivated to talk. pp. 535, 538, 540

Be sure the patient understands your questions and why you are asking them. Use the feedback techniques explained in objective 3. Take the time to develop rapport and trust with the patient and to communicate your empathy toward his situation. Assure there is no language barrier and that you and the patient are isolated so that information given is confidential. Provide supportive feedback to encourage freer communication. If information is unavailable from the patient, ask family or bystanders to help provide it.

9. Describe the use of, and differentiate between, facilitation, reflection, clarification, empathetic responses, confrontation, and interpretation. p. 539

There are several feedback techniques to use during an interview, including:

Facilitation—encouraging the speaker to provide more information
Clarification—asking the speaker to help you understand confusing parts of his or her response
Empathetic responses—showing you understand the patient
Confrontation—focusing the speaker on a particular part of his or her response
Interpretation—relating your interpretation of the speaker's information

10. Differentiate strategies used for interviewing hostile and cooperative patients. pp. 538, 543

The uncooperative patient is one who simply does not want to help with, participate in, or permit your assessment or care for him. A hostile patient displays anger and may be a risk to you. Work carefully to establish rapport with each type, but recognize that the hostile patient may endanger you and your crew. Always maintain distance from the hostile patient and have an escape route ready should a threat of violence become an attempt.

11. Summarize developmental considerations that influence patient interviewing. pp. 540–542

Your interviewing techniques must be flexible to accommodate the developmental considerations that influence patient assessment and care. Be patient, understanding, and empathetic and listen carefully to what the patient says. Adjust your interviewing technique, intensity, eye contact, eye level, touch, and stance to meet the needs of your patient. Be simple and straightforward with young children, and build a good rapport with their caregivers, as they are the ones the children look to for guidance. With age, children become more objective, realistic, trusting, and cooperative. With the elderly, show respect and appreciate the difficulties preexisting diseases and reduced hearing and eyesight can have on their ability to understand what is happening to them.

12. Define the unique interviewing techniques for patients with special needs. pp. 540–543

Patients with special needs include children, the elderly, patients with sensory impairments, and those with language or cultural considerations. Generally an empathetic and calm approach to any of these patients will be helpful, combined with special strategies for each group.

Effective interviewing techniques depend on a child's age, as they grow quickly from infancy to childhood, to adolescence, and to adulthood. Begin by talking with and establishing a rapport with the child's caregivers (parents and family) and gradually approach the patient. Keep your eye level close to the child's and speak choosing your words carefully so the patient can understand and is not threatened. Explain what you are doing and why, being honest and truthful. Build trust and use a toy to distract younger children from their symptoms and your intrusion into their personal space.

Elderly patients require respect, the proper form of address, slower explanations, and patience. Take along their living assists—eyeglasses, hearing aids, and so on—if you must transport them, and always respect their dignity.

Sensory impairment can make communication more difficult and requires careful explanations of what is going to happen to the patient and why. Guide the sightless patient with an arm and provide written or signed communication for the hearing impaired. If the patient can lip read, assure your face is illuminated and facing directly toward him when you speak.

Language and cultural barriers are obstacles to effective communication that can only be overcome with patience and compassion. Do not judge a patient's values or try to impose yours on him. Use an interpreter (family member or sibling) and phrase questions and statements carefully, addressing both the patient and interpreter. Recognize that eye contact and personal distances may mean different things in different cultures. Respect cultural folk medicines and beliefs.

13. **Discuss cross-cultural interviewing considerations.** pp. 542–543

    When interviewing across cultures, be patient, understanding, and empathetic. Understand the differences in how the culture perceives eye contact and personal distances and resist making judgments due to stereotyping. Respect folk medicine practices and beliefs.

14. **Given several preprogrammed simulated patients, provide a patient interview using therapeutic communication.** pp. 533–543

    During every day of your career as a paramedic, you will attend patients and their families to determine what is wrong with the patient and then to provide care. These encounters will, from time to time, be with patients who do not trust you, do not understand you, are threatened by you, are frightened by you, or do not understand what is happening to them. They present a challenge to good communication that you must overcome to extract information from them and begin your care. The impression you leave with these patients is the impression they will carry of the emergency medical service system until they again call on the system for assistance. During your classroom, practical, and clinical experience, work to develop your interviewing skills, especially with troublesome patients, so you present a good image to the people who use our services.

Content Self-Evaluation

Multiple Choice

_____ 1. Creating a message is also known as:
   A. alliterating.
   B. encoding.
   C. receiving.
   D. interpreting.
   E. drafting.

_____ 2. Empathy is the identification with and understanding of another's situation, feelings, and motives.
   A. True
   B. False

_____ 3. Which of the following represents an example of an external distraction to communication?
   A. lack of empathy
   B. prejudice
   C. loud music
   D. thinking about family or the job
   E. all of the above

_____ 4. Which of the following is NOT one of the elements necessary for a paramedic to make a good first impression?
   A. clean, neat uniform
   B. arrogant demeanor
   C. interested and caring facial expression
   D. consideration for the patient
   E. good personal hygiene

_____ 5. Which of the following techniques is NOT considered to be a way to build patient trust and rapport?
   A. using your patient's name
   B. explaining what you are doing and why
   C. addressing your patient as "honey" or "sweetie"
   D. modulating your voice
   E. using an appropriate style of communication

_____ 6. The interpersonal zone that extends 4 to 12 feet from the patient is:
   A. the intimate zone.
   B. personal distance.
   C. social distance.
   D. public distance.
   E. none of the above

_____ 7. Which of a caregiver's eye levels imparts authority and may intimidate the patient?
   A. one higher than the patient's eye level
   B. one lower than the patient's eye level
   C. one on the same level with the patient's
   D. both A and B
   E. both B and C

_____ 8. Sunglasses often help reduce the intimidation of eye contact and should be kept on when possible.
   A. True
   B. False

_____ 9. Closed questions direct the patient and elicit very specific responses; since this is not desired during an interview, these questions should be avoided at all costs.
   A. True
   B. False

_____ 10. The listening and feedback technique in which the interviewer encourages the speaker to provide more information is:
   A. summarization.
   B. explanation.
   C. reflection.
   D. clarification.
   E. facilitation.

_____ 11. Common errors made when interviewing patients include all of the following EXCEPT:
   A. using professional jargon.
   B. echoing back the patient's statements as part of the reflection technique.
   C. inappropriate distancing.
   D. inappropriate advice.
   E. providing false assurances.

_____ 12. Interrupting a patient to guide him to the information you need is both a useful tool in the interview process and a good listening skill.
   A. True
   B. False

_____ 13. A difficult patient interview may stem from which of the following?
   A. a disease process
   B. fear
   C. language differences
   D. cultural differences
   E. all of the above

_____ 14. When treating a child, you must also consider treating the caregivers since they may be upset and concerned.
   A. True
   B. False

_____ 15. The viewing of one's own life as more desirable or acceptable or best is:
   A. ethnicity.
   B. cultural diversity.
   C. ethnocentrism.
   D. cultural imposition.
   E. cultural arrogance.

Essentials of Paramedic Care

Division 2

Patient Assessment

History Taking

Review of Chapter Objectives

With each chapter of the Workbook, we identify the objectives and the important elements of the text content. You should review these items and refer to the pages listed if any points are not clear.

After reading this chapter, you should be able to:

1. **Describe the techniques of history taking.** pp. 547–550

    For successful history taking, establish a rapport with the patient to gain his confidence and to set the stage for investigation of the chief complaint and medical history. Factors that will help in establishing rapport include:

    - Well-groomed initial appearance
    - Positive body language
    - Good eye contact with the patient
    - Professional demeanor
    - Demonstration of interest in the patient

    Your introduction should convey your interest in helping the patient and begin the two-way communication. It should convey your care and compassion for the patient and begin to build his trust in you.

    Once you have introduced yourself and established your intent to help the patient, begin your questioning. Determine the formal chief complaint and investigate the current and past medical history. Pose questions in a way the patient understands, using terminology and the English language at the patient's level of comprehension.

    Questioning frequently involves asking the patient personal, and possibly embarrassing, questions. At such times, ask these questions in a sensitive, nonthreatening way. "Ease into" the discussion of sensitive topics and use questions that are nonjudgmental. You may suggest to the patient that the issue of concern to him is common to many people in our society. Practice in questioning will help you develop the most effective approach. Be prepared to explain that the answers to questions are used for the patient's care and are not communicated beyond the necessary care providers.

2. **Describe the structure, purpose, and how to obtain a comprehensive health history.** pp. 547–561

    The comprehensive health history establishes a relationship between you and the patient and draws out pertinent information about the patient's medical history. This information may explain the current problem or guide further care in either the prehospital or in-hospital settings. The comprehensive patient history is gained by investigative questioning of the patient about past and current medical problems, including the chief complaint, the present illness (OPQRST-ASPN), the past medical history, current health status, and a review of systems.

3. List the components of a comprehensive history of an adult patient. pp. 550–561

The comprehensive patient history includes the following:

- Preliminary data (age, race, sex, and so on)
- The chief complaint
- The present illness or problem (including investigation of onset, provocation, quality, region/radiation, severity, time, as well as associated symptoms and pertinent negatives—OPQRST-ASPN)
- Past medical history (including the patient's general health, childhood and adult illnesses, psychiatric illness, serious accidents or injuries, and surgeries and hospitalizations)
- Current health status (including patient medications; allergies; use of tobacco, alcohol, and drugs; diet; recent screening tests and immunizations; exercise; leisure and sleep patterns; and environmental hazard/safety measures, family history, and psychosocial history)
- A review of systems (including, as appropriate, general physical information; skin; head, eyes, ears, nose, throat (HEENT); respiratory; cardiac; gastrointestinal; urinary; genital; peripheral vascular; musculoskeletal; neurologic; hematologic; endocrine; psychiatric)

The following objectives, while not listed in the chapter, will help in your understanding of the chapter content.

*Supplemental Objective: Describe the review of systems and explain how it assists in identifying the patient's primary medical problem.

The review of systems is an examination of each body system during the patient history. It is performed to rule out or further investigate medical problems and to assure that pertinent information is not overlooked during the assessment. Systems examined include:

- Skin
- Head, eyes, ears, nose, throat (HEENT)
- Respiratory
- Cardiac
- Gastrointestinal
- Urinary
- Genital
- Peripheral vascular
- Musculoskeletal
- Neurologic
- Hematologic
- Endocrine
- Psychiatric

*Supplemental Objective: Identify techniques for working with patients with special challenges.

- **Silent patient.** Be patient yourself. Speak reassuringly. Gently shake the patient. Consider a neurologic problem.
- **Overly talkative patient.** Focus the patient on the important areas. Summarize what he or she says. Be patient.
- **Numerous symptoms.** Be more clear in questioning; suspect an emotional problem.
- **Anxious patient.** Encourage free conversation and reassure the patient.
- **Patient needing reassurance.** Ask about his anxieties. Offer emotional support.
- **Anger and hostility.** Accept the patient's responses without becoming defensive or angry.
- **Intoxicated patient.** Be friendly and nonjudgmental. Listen to what the patient says, not how he says it. Make your safety and scene safety priorities.
- **Crying patient.** Be patient. Accept the crying as a natural venting of emotions and be supportive.

- **Depression.** Recognize the condition as a serious medical problem. Ask the patient whether he has had suicidal thoughts.
- **Sexually attractive or seductive patient.** Maintain a professional relationship. Try to have a partner present.
- **Confusing behaviors or histories.** Suspect mental illness, dementia, or delirium. Pay careful attention to the patient's mental status. Be reassuring.
- **Patient of limited intelligence.** Try to evaluate the patient's mental abilities. Show genuine interest and establish a positive relationship. Elicit what information you can.
- **Language barriers.** Seek out an interpreter. Be aware that important information is likely to be lost in translation.
- **Patient with hearing problems.** Speak to the patient's best ear. If he reads lips, position yourself directly in front of him in good lighting, and speak slowly in a low-pitched voice. Consider writing your questions.
- **Patient who is blind or has limited vision.** Identify yourself immediately and explain why you are there. Explain what you are doing before you do it.
- **Family and friends.** If gaining pertinent information directly from the patient is difficult, talk to family members or friends on the scene.

Content Self-Evaluation

Each of the chapters in this Workbook includes a short content review. The questions are designed to test your ability to remember what you read. At the end of this Workbook, you can find the answers to the questions as well as the pages where the topic of the question was discussed in the text. If you answer the question incorrectly or are unsure of the answer, review the pages listed.

MULTIPLE CHOICE

_____ 1. In the majority of medical cases, the basis of the paramedic's field diagnosis is the:
   A. chief complaint.
   B. index of suspicion.
   C. mechanism of injury.
   D. patient history.
   E. vital signs.

_____ 2. Always accept information from previous caregivers gratefully, but briefly reconfirm it with the patient.
   A. True
   B. False

_____ 3. Always use appropriate language during the interview to establish a closer, more trusting relationship.
   A. True
   B. False

_____ 4. It is best to form a prearranged list of specific questions to assure you cover all bases while interviewing your patient.
   A. True
   B. False

_____ 5. The process of encouraging the patient to provide details about his condition is called:
   A. empathy.
   B. confrontation.
   C. reflection.
   D. clarification.
   E. facilitation.

_____ 6. The reason (pain, discomfort, or dysfunction) that the patient or other person summons emergency medical services is termed the:
   A. primary problem.
   B. chief complaint.
   C. nature of the illness.
   D. mechanism of injury.
   E. none of the above

_____ 7. The underlying cause of the patient's pain, discomfort, or dysfunction is called the:
   A. primary problem.
   B. chief complaint.
   C. nature of the illness.
   D. mechanism of injury.
   E. none of the above

_____ 8. Any activity that alleviates a patient's symptoms would fit under which element of the OPQRST-ASPN mnemonic for the history of the current illness?
   A. O
   B. P
   C. Q
   D. R
   E. S

_____ 9. Which of the following is an important part of the past medical history?
   A. radiation of the pain
   B. last oral intake
   C. surgeries or hospitalizations
   D. quality of the pain
   E. all of the above

_____ 10. A medication not taken as prescribed may account for medical problems due to which of the following?
   A. overmedication
   B. undermedication
   C. allergic reaction
   D. untoward reaction
   E. all of the above

_____ 11. Allergies should be expected for all of the following EXCEPT:
   A. the "caine" family.
   B. tetanus toxoid.
   C. glucose.
   D. narcotics.
   E. both A and B

_____ 12. A patient who has smoked 21 packs of cigarettes a week for 10 years has a pack history of:
   A. 21 pack/years.
   B. 70 pack/years.
   C. 7 pack/years.
   D. 30 pack/years.
   E. 10 pack/years.

_____ 13. Which of the following is NOT a system examined during the review of systems?
   A. skin
   B. lymphatic system
   C. musculoskeletal system
   D. hematologic system
   E. endocrine system

_____ 14. Which step below would you attempt with the patient who suddenly goes silent?
   A. Stay calm and observe for nonverbal clues.
   B. Arrange for air medical transport.
   C. Terminate the interview immediately.
   D. Attempt to walk the patient back and forth a few times.
   E. Rapidly provide oral glucose.

_____ 15. Crying is a form of venting emotional stress; be patient and provide a patient who is crying with supportive remarks.
   A. True
   B. False

MATCHING

Classify each question or statement under the OPQRST category that best applies by writing the letter of the category in the space provided.

O. Onset
P. Provocation/palliation
Q. Quality
R. Region/radiation
S. Severity
T. Time

_____ 16. How does this compare to the worst pain you have ever felt?
_____ 17. Does rest lessen your pain?
_____ 18. Point to where you feel pain.
_____ 19. Does this pain feel crushing in nature?
_____ 20. Does deep breathing increase the pain?
_____ 21. Did this pain begin suddenly or gradually?
_____ 22. Where does this pain travel to?
_____ 23. When did the first symptoms begin?
_____ 24. Describe how the pain feels.
_____ 25. Were you walking or running when this pain first began?

Chapter 11

Physical Exam Techniques

Part 1, pp. 566–604

Review of Chapter Objectives

Because Chapter 11 is lengthy, it has been divided into sections to aid your study. Read the assigned text pages, then progress through the objectives and self-evaluation materials as you would with other chapters. When you feel secure in your grasp of the content, proceed to the next section.

After reading this section of the chapter, you should be able to:

1. Define and describe the techniques of inspection, palpation, percussion, auscultation.
pp. 566–569

Inspection is the process of informed observation, viewing the patient for anatomical shape, coloration, and movement. It is the least invasive examination tool, yet may provide the most patient information.

Palpation is the use of touch to gather information regarding size, shape, position, temperature, moisture, texture, movement, and response to pressure. The fingertips are most sensitive, while the palm best evaluates vibration and the back of the hand, temperature.

Percussion is the production of a vibration in tissue to elicit sounds. These sounds—dull, resonant, hyperresonant, tympanic, and flat—identify the nature of the tissue underneath. The vibration is generated by striking the first knuckle of a finger placed against the area to be percussed with the fingertip of the other hand.

Auscultation is listening for sounds within the body, most frequently with a stethoscope. The intensity, pitch, duration, quality, and timing of sounds in the patient's lungs, heart, blood vessels, and intestines are compared against normal sounds.

2. Describe the evaluation of mental status.
pp. 629–632

See Workbook, Section III of this chapter.

3. Evaluate the importance of a general survey.
pp. 576–584

The general survey is the first part of the comprehensive exam. It is made up of your evaluation of the patient's appearance—including level of consciousness, expression, state of health, general characteristics (weight, height, and so on.), posturing, dress, grooming, and so on—the vital signs, and additional assessments such as pulse oximetry, cardiac monitoring, and blood glucose determination. The survey helps you form a general impression of your patient's health.

©2007 Pearson Education, Inc.
Essentials of Paramedic Care, 2nd ed.

4. **Describe the examination of the following body regions, differentiate between normal and abnormal findings, and define the significance of abnormal findings:**

Skin, hair, and nails   pp. 585–590

Observe the skin carefully for color, especially in the nail beds, lips, conjunctiva, and mucous membranes of the mouth. Pink skin reflects good oxygenation, while pale skin reflects poor blood flow from hypovolemia, hypothermia, compensatory shock, or anemia. A bluish-colored skin, cyanosis, suggests blood is low in oxygen. A yellow sclera or general discoloration, jaundice, is due to liver failure. Other skin observations may include petechiae, small round, flat purplish spots caused by capillary bleeding from a variety of etiologies, and ecchymosis, a larger, black-and-blue discoloration that is often the result of trauma or bleeding disorders. Moisture, temperature, texture, mobility, and turgor are also evaluated. Skin lesions are disruptions in normal tissue that may take on almost any shape, color, or arrangement.

Inspect and palpate the hair to determine color, quality, distribution, quantity, and texture and inspect and palpate the scalp for scaling, lesions, redness, lumps, or tenderness. Generalized hair loss may reflect chemotherapy; failure to develop normal hair patterns may be caused by a pituitary or hormonal problem; and unusual facial hair in women suggests a hormonal imbalance. Mild scalp flaking suggests dandruff; heavy scaling, psoriasis; and greasy scaling, seborrheic dermatitis. Lice eggs (nits) may be found firmly attached to the hair shafts. Normal hair texture is smooth and soft in Caucasians; in people of African descent, the texture is coarser. Dry, brittle, or fragile hair is abnormal.

Inspect the finger nails and toenails for color. Note any discolorations, lesions, ridging, grooves, depressions, or pitting. Depressions suggest systemic disease. Compress the nail and bed to determine its adherence and look for nail hygiene. Any boggyness suggests cardiorespiratory disease.

Head, scalp, and skull   pp. 590, 592

Observe and palpate the skull and facial region for symmetry, smoothness, wounds, bleeding, size, and general contour. Examine the hair and scalp as described above. Check the eyes for bilateral periorbital and mastoid ecchymosis, "raccoon eyes" and "Battle's sign," respectively. They suggest basilar skull fracture and occur an hour or so after injury. Palpate the facial region for crepitation, false motion, or instability suggesting fracture. Evaluate the temporomandibular joint for pain, tenderness, swelling, and range of motion. Have the patient open and close his mouth and jut and retract his jaw. Any loss of normal function suggests injury.

Eyes, ears, nose, mouth, and pharynx   pp. 590–603

Examine for visual acuity as described below (objective 5), then evaluate for peripheral vision. While the patient faces you, have him look at your nose while you extend your arms, bend your elbows and wiggle the fingers. If he notices the fingers moving in all four directions (up, down, left, and right) for each eye, his peripheral vision is grossly normal. Inspect the eyes for symmetry, shape, inflammation, swelling, misalignment (disconjugate gaze), lesions, and contour. Examine the eyelids, open and closed, for swelling, discoloration, droop (ptosis), styes, and lash positioning. Observe the tearing or dryness of the eyes. Gently retract the lower eyelid while asking the patient to look through a range of motion. Examine the sclera for signs of irritation, cloudiness, yellow discoloration (jaundice), any nodules, swelling, discharge, or hemorrhage into the scleral tissue. With an oblique light source, inspect the cornea for opacities. Inspect the size, shape, symmetry, and reactivity of the pupils. Note the pupils' direct and consensual response to increased light intensity. A sluggish pupil suggests pressure on CN-III; bilateral sluggishness suggests global hypoxia or depressant drug action. Constricted pupils suggest opiate overdose, while dilated and fixed pupils reflect brain anoxia. Ask the patient to focus on your finger close at hand, then move the hand to his nose, then away. The eyes should converge, while the pupils should constrict slightly. Then have him follow your finger as you move it through an "H" pattern. The eyes should move smoothly together. Nystagmus is a jerky movement at the distal extremes of ocular movement. Gently touch the cornea with a strand of cotton. The patient should respond with a blink. Using an ophthalmoscope, look into the eye's anterior chamber for signs of blood (hyphema), cells, or pus (hypopyon), and check the cornea for lacerations, abrasions, cataracts, papilledema (from increased ICP), vascular occlusions, and retinal hemorrhage.

Examine the ears by looking for symmetry from in front of the patient, then examine each ear separately. Examine the external portion (auricle) for shape, size, landmarks, and position on the head. Examine the surrounding area for deformities, lesions, tenderness, and erythema. Pull the helix upward and outward, press on the tragus and on the mastoid process and note any discomfort or pain suggesting otitis or mastoiditis. Some pain may be associated with toothache, a cold, sore throat, or cervical spine injury. Inspect the ear canal for discharge (pus, mucus, blood, or cerebral spinal fluid [CSF]) and inflammation. Trauma can account for blood, mucus, and CSF in the ear canal. Check hearing acuity by covering one ear and whispering, then speaking into the other. Hearing loss may be accounted for by trauma, accumulation of debris (often cerumen), tympanic membrane rupture, drug use, and prolonged exposure to loud noise. Visualize the inner canal with the otoscope. With the largest speculum that will fit the canal, turn the patient's head away from you, pull the auricle slightly up and backward, and insert the otoscope. Inspect for wax (cerumen), discharge, redness, lesions, perforations, and foreign bodies. Then focus on the tympanic membrane. It should be a translucent pearly gray. Color changes suggest fluid behind the eardrum or infection. Also check for bulging, protractions, or perforations.

Visualize the patient's nose from the front and sides to determine any asymmetry, deviation, tenderness, flaring, or abnormal color. Tilt your patient's head back slightly and examine the nostrils. Insert the otoscope and check for deviation of the septum and perforations. Examine the nasal mucosa for color, and the color, consistency, and quantity of drainage. Rhinitis (a runny nose) suggests seasonal allergies; a thick yellow discharge, infection; and blood, epistaxis from trauma or a septal defect. Test each side of the nose for patency by occluding the other side during a breath. There is normally some difference in patency between the sides. Palpate the frontal sinuses for swelling and tenderness.

Begin assessment of the mouth by observing the lips for color and condition. They should be pink, smooth, symmetrical, and without lesions, swelling, lumps, cracks, or scaliness. Using a bright light and tongue blade, examine the oral mucosa for color, lesions, white patches, or fissures. The mucosa should be pinkish-red, smooth, and moist. The gums should be pink with clearly defined margins around the teeth. The teeth should be well formed and straight. If the gums are swollen, bleed easily, and are separated from the teeth, suspect periodontal disease. Ask the patient to stick his tongue out and note its velvety surface. Hold the tongue with a 2 × 2-gauze pad and inspect all sides and the bottom. All surfaces should be pink and smooth. Then examine the pharynx and have the patient say "aaaahhh" while you hold the tongue down with a tongue blade. Watch the movement of the uvula and the coloration and condition of the palatine tonsils and posterior pharynx. Look for any pus, swelling, ulcers, or drainage. Also notice any odors including alcohol, feces (bowel obstruction), acetone (diabetic ketoacidosis), gastric contents, coffee-grounds-like material (gastric hemorrhage), pink-tinged sputum (pulmonary edema), or the smell of bitter almonds (cyanide poisoning).

Neck   pp. 603–604

Inspect your patient's neck for symmetry and visible masses. Note any deformity, deviations, tugging, scars, gland enlargement, or visible lymph nodes. Examine for any open wounds and cover them with an occlusive dressing. Examine the jugular veins for distention while the patient is seated upright and at a 45° incline. Palpate the trachea to assure it is in line. Palpate the thyroid while the patient swallows to assure it is small, smooth, and without nodules. Palpate each lymph node to determine size, shape, tenderness, consistency, and mobility. *Tender, swollen, and mobile nodes suggest inflammation from infection, while hard and fixed ones suggest malignancy.*

See Workbook, Parts 2 and 3 of this chapter for additional review of objective 4.

5. Describe the assessment of visual acuity.   pp. 590–592

Visual acuity is the ability to read detail. A wall chart with lines of progressively smaller letters is placed at 20 feet from the patient. He then reads to the smallest line in which he can recognize at least one half the letters. The result is recorded as the distance from the chart and the distance at which a person with normal sight could distinguish the letters, 20/20 for normal or 20/60 for someone who reads what is normally read at 60 feet.

6. Explain the rationale for the use of an ophthalmoscope and otoscope. pp. 575, 593–596, 597–599

The ophthalmoscope is a light source and a series of lenses that permit you to examine the interior of the patient's eyes. It allows you to examine the retina, blood vessels, and optic nerve at the back of the posterior chamber of the eye.

The otoscope is a light source and a magnifying lens that permits examination of a patient's ears and nose. It allows you to examine the external auditory canal and the tympanic membrane for trauma, irritation, or infection.

See Workbook, Part 2 of this chapter for review of objectives 7 and 8.

9. Differentiate the percussion notes and their characteristics. pp. 567–568

Percussion provides three basic sounds; dull, resonant, and hyperresonant. Dull reflects a density and is a medium-pitched thud. It is usually caused by a dense organ (like the liver) or fluid, like blood, underneath. Resonant sounds are generally associated with a less dense tissue, like the lungs, and are lower-pitched and longer lasting sounds. Hyperresonant sounds reflect air, or air under pressure, and are the lowest-pitched sounds and the ones that diminish in volume most slowly.

The following objectives, while not listed in the chapter, will help in your understanding of the chapter content.

10. Describe special examination techniques related to the assessment of the chest. pp. 605–609

Pulse is the wave of pressure generated by the heart as it expels blood into the arterial system. It is measured by palpating a distal artery (or auscultated during blood pressure determination) and is evaluated for rate, rhythm, and quality (strength). The normal pulse is strong, regular, and has a rate of between 60 and 80 beats per minute.

Respiration is the movement of air through the airway and into and out of the lungs. It is evaluated by observing and/or feeling chest excursion and listening to air movement. The rate, effort, and quality (depth and pattern) of respirations are determined. Normal respiration moves a tidal volume of 500 mL at a rate of 12 to 20 times per minute with symmetrical chest wall movement.

Blood pressure is the force of blood against the arterial wall during the cardiac-pulse cycle. It is measured using a sphygmomanometer (blood pressure cuff) and stethoscope. The maximum or systolic blood pressure—the reading obtained when the ventricles contract, the lower or diastolic blood pressure—the reading obtained when the ventricles relax, and the difference between them, the pulse pressure, are evaluated. The systolic pressure is usually between 100 and 135, and the diastolic, between 60 and 80.

Temperature is the body core temperature and is the product of heat-creating metabolism and body heat loss. It is measured by a glass or electronic thermometer placed in the axilla, mouth, or rectum. Normal body temperature is 98.6°F (37°C).

11. Describe the auscultation of the chest, heart, and abdomen. pp. 606–613

Pulse oximetry is the noninvasive measurement of oxygen saturation in the tissue of a distal extremity. It provides a real-time evaluation of oxygen delivery to the distal circulation. Normal readings are between 96 and 100 percent. Readings below this reflect problems with either respiration or circulation and demand intervention.

Capnography is the real-time evaluation of carbon dioxide in exhaled air. There are two types of end-tidal CO_2 monitors: small, disposable colormetric devices that change color in the presence of carbon dioxide and electronic devices that provide either a light indicating a minimum CO_2 content or a digital or wave-form display giving the concentration. Both devices are used to confirm proper endotracheal tube placement.

Cardiac monitoring uses electronics to display the electrical activity of the heart. The monitor shows an electronic or paper tracing of the heart's activity, either a normal rhythm, a dysrhythmia, or no activity—asystole. This information is essential to identifying when to shock the heart back to a normal rhythm or to treat it through the use of medication.

Blood glucose determination is performed by using a glucometer, a small electronic device that evaluates the color of a blood-stained reagent strip. The glucose level can rule out or identify hypoglycemia in a patient with a lowered level of consciousness or in the known diabetic.

Content Self-Evaluation

MULTIPLE CHOICE

_____ 1. Of the physical examination techniques used in prehospital care, which is the least invasive?
   A. inspection
   B. auscultation
   C. palpation
   D. percussion
   E. C and D

_____ 2. "Crackles" would be found using which of the following assessment techniques?
   A. palpation
   B. auscultation
   C. inspection
   D. percussion
   E. none of the above

_____ 3. "Tenderness" would be discovered using which of the following assessment techniques?
   A. palpation
   B. auscultation
   C. inspection
   D. percussion
   E. none of the above

_____ 4. Which of the following techniques should be performed first during the physical examination?
   A. palpation
   B. auscultation
   C. inspection
   D. percussion
   E. none of the above

_____ 5. Which part of the hands and fingers is best suited to evaluate tissue consistency?
   A. tips of the fingers
   B. pads of the fingers
   C. palm of the hand
   D. back of the hands or fingers
   E. none of the above

_____ 6. Which part of the hands and fingers is best suited to evaluate vibration?
   A. tips of the fingers
   B. pads of the fingers
   C. palm of the hand
   D. back of the hands or fingers
   E. none of the above

_____ 7. Noticing areas of warmth during palpation might reflect an injury before significant edema and discoloration develop.
   A. True
   B. False

_____ 8. The booming sound produced by percussing an air-filled region is:
   A. hyperresonance.
   B. dull.
   C. resonance.
   D. flat.
   E. none of the above

_____ 9. The only region where you perform auscultation as other than the last step of assessment is the:
   A. anterior thorax.
   B. neck.
   C. abdomen.
   D. peripheral arteries.
   E. posterior thorax.

_____ 10. A heart rate above 100 is known as a:
   A. bradycardia.
   B. tachycardia.
   C. hypercardia.
   D. tachypnea.
   E. bradypnea.

_____ 11. One likely cause of bradycardia is:
   A. fever.
   B. pain.
   C. parasympathetic stimulation.
   D. fear.
   E. blood loss.

_____ 12. Which of the following is NOT an aspect of pulse evaluation?
    A. volume
    B. rhythm
    C. quality
    D. rate
    E. none of the above

_____ 13. Normal exhalation is:
    A. an active process involving accessory muscles.
    B. an active process involving the diaphragm and intercostal muscles.
    C. active in its early stages and passive in later stages.
    D. passive in its early stages and active in later stages.
    E. a passive process.

_____ 14. For a patient with an airway obstruction, exhalation is likely to be:
    A. an active process involving accessory muscles.
    B. an active process involving only the diaphragm and intercostal muscles.
    C. active in its early stages and passive in later stages.
    D. passive in its early stages and active in later stages.
    E. a passive process.

_____ 15. The amount of air a patient moves into and out of his lungs in one breath is the:
    A. normal volume.
    B. respiratory volume.
    C. residual volume.
    D. tidal volume.
    E. minute volume.

_____ 16. The pressure of the blood within the blood vessels while the ventricles are relaxing is the:
    A. Korotkoff blood pressure.
    B. systolic blood pressure.
    C. diastolic blood pressure.
    D. asystolic blood pressure.
    E. atrial blood pressure.

_____ 17. The diastolic blood pressure represents a measure of:
    A. systemic vascular resistance.
    B. the cardiac output.
    C. the viscosity of the blood.
    D. the strength of ventricular contraction.
    E. relative blood volume.

_____ 18. Which of the following are likely to influence a patient's blood pressure?
    A. anxiety
    B. position (lying, sitting, standing)
    C. recent smoking
    D. eating
    E. all of the above

_____ 19. Generally, hypertension in a healthy adult is any blood pressure higher than:
    A. 120/80.
    B. 140/90.
    C. 160/90.
    D. 180/100.
    E. 200/100.

_____ 20. What is the pulse pressure in a patient with the following vital signs: pulse 82 and strong; respirations 14 and full; and blood pressure 144/96?
    A. 14
    B. 40
    C. 48
    D. 96
    E. 120

_____ 21. In the tilt test, what vital sign change is a positive sign of hypovolemia?
    A. blood pressure drops by 10 to 20 mmHg
    B. blood pressure rises by 10 to 20 mmHg
    C. pulse rate drops by 10 to 20 beats per minute
    D. pulse rate rises by 10 to 20 beats per minute
    E. either A or D

_____ 22. Hyperthermia can result from all of the following EXCEPT:
    A. high environmental temperatures.
    B. infections.
    C. reduced metabolic activity.
    D. drugs.
    E. increases in metabolic activity.

_____ 23. What technique of stethoscope use best transmits low-pitched sound to the ear?
　　　　A. light pressure on the diaphragm　　D. light pressure on the bell
　　　　B. firm pressure on the diaphragm　　E. strong pressure on the bell
　　　　C. moderate pressure on the bell

_____ 24. The bell of a stethoscope is best for listening to the sounds of:
　　　　A. blood vessel bruits.　　D. the lung.
　　　　B. the blood pressure.　　E. none of the above
　　　　C. the heart.

_____ 25. Which of the following is NOT a characteristic of a good stethoscope?
　　　　A. thick, heavy tubing　　D. a bell with a rubber-ring edge
　　　　B. long tubing (70 to 100 cm)　　E. all of the above
　　　　C. snug-fitting earpieces

_____ 26. Generally, each narrow line on a sphygmomanometer represents what pressure difference?
　　　　A. 1 mmHg　　D. 5 mmHg
　　　　B. 2 mmHg　　E. 10 mmHg
　　　　C. 4 mmHg

_____ 27. If a patient has a regular and strong pulse, you should determine the pulse rate by assessing the number of beats in:
　　　　A. two minutes and dividing by 2.
　　　　B. three minutes.
　　　　C. 30 seconds and multiplying by 2.
　　　　D. 15 seconds and multiplying by 4.
　　　　E. 10 seconds and multiplying by 5.

_____ 28. Use of which of the following pulse points is recommended with a small child?
　　　　A. radial　　D. popliteal
　　　　B. brachial　　E. dorsalis pedis
　　　　C. carotid

_____ 29. It is important to attempt to evaluate your patient's respiratory rate and volume without his being aware of it.
　　　　A. True
　　　　B. False

_____ 30. The proper position of the patient's arm when taking the blood pressure is:
　　　　A. arm slightly flexed.　　D. clothing removed from the upper arm.
　　　　B. palm up.　　E. all of the above
　　　　C. fingers relaxed.

_____ 31. The sphygmomanometer should be inflated to what level beyond the point at which the patient's radial pulse disappears?
　　　　A. 10 mmHg　　D. 40 mmHg
　　　　B. 20 mmHg　　E. between B and C
　　　　C. 30 mmHg

_____ 32. The first blood pressure reading is the systolic blood pressure.
　　　　A. True
　　　　B. False

_____ 33. When using the oral glass thermometer, it should be left in the mouth for what period of time?
　　　　A. 30 to 45 seconds　　D. 2 minutes
　　　　B. 30 to 60 seconds　　E. 3 to 4 minutes
　　　　C. 1 to 2 minutes

_____ 34. The normal patient oxygen saturation without supplemental oxygen at sea level should be:
   A. between 90 to 95 percent.
   B. below 95 percent.
   C. 100 percent.
   D. 96 to 100 percent.
   E. below 90 percent.

_____ 35. A patient suffering from carbon monoxide poisoning will likely have a pulse oximetry reading that is:
   A. accurate.
   B. falsely high.
   C. falsely low.
   D. erratic and inaccurate.
   E. unreadable.

_____ 36. The ECG of a cardiac monitor can tell you all of the following EXCEPT:
   A. the heart rate.
   B. the sequence of cardiac events.
   C. the timing of cardiac events.
   D. the pumping ability of the heart.
   E. both A and C

_____ 37. Evaluation of the skin involves evaluating its:
   A. moisture.
   B. temperature.
   C. turgor.
   D. color.
   E. all of the above

_____ 38. Pale skin is least likely to be caused by which of the following?
   A. increased deoxyhemoglobin
   B. a cold environment
   C. shock compensation
   D. anemia
   E. hypovolemic shock

_____ 39. Which of the following skin discolorations represents a yellow hue?
   A. cyanosis
   B. jaundice
   C. eccyhmosis
   D. erythema
   E. pallor

_____ 40. A heavy scaling of the skin under the hair is:
   A. dandruff.
   B. nits.
   C. seborrheic dermatitis.
   D. psoriasis.
   E. none of the above

_____ 41. The blueish discoloration around the orbits of the eyes, suggestive of a basilar skull fracture, is called:
   A. "raccon eyes."
   B. "Battle's sign."
   C. periorbital ecchymosis.
   D. retroauricular ecchymosis.
   E. either A or C

_____ 42. The characteristic of the unaffected eye responding to stimuli in the affected eye is:
   A. consensual response.
   B. direct response.
   C. simultaneous response.
   D. ipsilateral response.
   E. none of the above

_____ 43. About 20 percent of the population have a noticeable difference in the size of the pupils, a condition called:
   A. hyphema.
   B. anisocoria.
   C. glaucoma.
   D. hypopyon.
   E. none of the above

_____ 44. Otorrhea is a discharge from the ear that may contain:
   A. pus.
   B. mucus.
   C. blood.
   D. cerebrospinal fluid.
   E. all of the above

_____ 45. The term for a common nosebleed is:
   A. epistaxis.
   B. otorrhea.
   C. rhinorrhea.
   D. rhinitis.
   E. none of the above

Part 2, pp. 605–626

Review of Chapter Objectives

After reading this section of the chapter, you should be able to:

4. **Describe the examination of the following body regions, differentiate between normal and abnormal findings, and define the significance of abnormal findings (continued):**

   Thorax (anterior and posterior)   pp. 605–609

   To assess the chest, you need a stethoscope with a bell and diaphragm. Expose the entire thorax with consideration for the patient's dignity and modesty, and inspect, palpate, percuss, and auscultate. Compare findings from one side of the chest to the other and from posterior to anterior. Look for general shape and symmetry as well as for the rate and pattern of breathing. Observe for retractions and the use of accessory muscles (suggestive of airway obstruction or restriction), and palpate for deformities, tenderness, crepitus (suggestive of rib fracture), and abnormal chest excursion (suggestive of flail chest or spinal injury). Feel for vibrations associated with air movement and speech. Percuss the chest for dullness (hemothorax, pleural effusion, or pneumonia), resonance, and hyperresonance (pneumothorax or tension pneumothorax). Finally, auscultate the lung lobes for normal breath sounds, crackles (pulmonary edema), wheezes (asthma), rhonchi, stridor (airway obstruction), and pleural friction rubs.

   Arterial pulse including rate, rhythm, and amplitude   pp. 609–612

   Locate a soft and pulsing carotid artery in the neck, just lateral to the cricoid cartilage to avoid pressure on the carotid sinus. Carefully press down until the pulse wave just lifts your finger off the artery. Determine the rate and carefully evaluate for regularity. Irregularity may be caused by dysrhythmia, while variation in strength may be due to such phenomena as pulsus paradoxus, increasing strength with exhalation and decreasing with inhalation. Also note any thrills (humming or vibration) and listen with the stethoscope for bruits (sounds of turbulent flow).

   Jugular venous pressure and pulsations   pp. 609–612

   Examine the anterior neck and locate the jugular veins. Position your patient with his head elevated 30° and turned away from you. Look for pulsation just above the suprasternal notch. Identify the highest point of pulsation and measure the distance from the sternal angle. The highest point of pulsation is usually between 1 and 2 cm from the sternal angle. (Distension when the patient is elevated at higher angles may reflect tension pneumothorax or pericardial tamponade, while flat veins at lower angles may suggest hypovolemia.)

   Abdomen   pp. 612–615

   Question your patient regarding any pain, tenderness or unusual feeling, and recent bowel and bladder function. Carefully inspect the area for scars, dilated veins, stretch marks, rashes, lesions, and pigmentation changes. Discoloration around the umbilicus (Cullen's sign) or over the flanks (Grey Turner's sign) suggest intraabdominal hemorrhage. Assess the size and shape of the abdomen, determining whether it is scaphoid (concave), flat, round, or distended, and look for any bulges or hernias. Ascites result in bulges in the flanks and across the abdomen suggesting congestive heart or liver failure, while suprapubic bulges suggest a full bladder or pregnant uterus. Look also for any masses, palpations, or peristalsis. A slight vascular pulsing is normal, but excessive movement suggests an aneurysm. Auscultate and percuss as described earlier. Then depress each quadrant gently and release. Look for patient expression or muscle guarding suggestive of injury or peritonitis.

Male and female genitalia p. 615

Assure patient privacy, a warm environment, and patient modesty during the exam; also be sure the patient has emptied his or her bladder before beginning. Expose only those body areas that you must, and explain what you are going to do before you do it. Inspect the genitalia for development and maturity. Visually inspect the mons pubis, labia, and perineum of the female patient for swelling, lesions, or irritation suggestive of a sebaceous cyst or sexually transmitted disease. Check the hair bases for small red maculopapules suggestive of lice. Retract the labia and inspect the inner labia and urethral opening. Examine for a white curdy discharge (fungal infection) or yellow-green discharge (bacterial infection). For the male, inspect the penis and testicles, noting inflammation and lesions suggestive of sexually transmitted disease. Check for lice and examine the glans for degeneration, inflammation, or discharge. Yellow discharge is reflective of gonorrhea.

Anus and rectum pp. 615–616

Position your patient on his or her left side with legs flexed and buttocks near the edge of the stretcher. Be sensitive to the patient's feelings and drape or cover any areas not being observed. With a gloved hand, spread the buttocks apart and examine the area for lumps, ulcers, inflammations, rashes, or lesions. Palpate any areas carefully, noting inflammation or tenderness. If appropriate, obtain a fecal sample for testing.

Musculoskeletal system pp. 616–625

Advancing age causes changes in the musculoskeletal system including shortening and increased curvature of the spine, a reduction in muscle mass and strength, and a reduction in the range of motion. Observe the patient's general posture, build, and muscular development as well as the movement of the extremities, gait, and position at rest. Then inspect all regions of the body for deformities, symmetry and symmetrical movement, joint structure, and swelling, nodules, or inflammation. Deformities are often related to misaligned articulating bones, dislocations, or subluxations. Impaired movement is usually related to arthritis; nodules related to rheumatic fever or rheumatoid arthritis; and redness related to gout, rheumatic fever, or arthritis. Compare dissimilar joints to determine what structures might be affected. Assess range of motion by moving the limb, ask the patient to move the limb, and then ask the patient to move the limb against resistance. Note any asymmetry and inequality between active and passive motion. Also examine for crepitation (a grating vibration or sound) that may suggest arthritis, an inflamed joint, or a fracture. Avoid manipulating a deformed or painful joint. Perform a physical exam on each joint, moving it through its normal range of motion and noting any deformities, limited or resistant movement, tenderness, and swelling.

7. **Describe the survey of respiration.** pp. 570–572, 605–609

The survey of the chest assesses the thorax and respiration by inspection, palpation, percussion, and auscultation. Compare findings side to side and anterior to back. Visualize and auscultate the five lung lobes during your exam. Examine the patient's respiration, looking for increased inspiratory or expiratory time or any sounds indicating upper or lower airway obstruction. Examine the chest for symmetry and symmetry of motion and any retraction or any anterior-posterior dimension abnormality. Also feel for any unusual vibrations associated with speech. Percuss the chest and note any hyperresonance or dullness. Listen through the stethoscope for lung sounds over each lobe and note any crackles or wheezes. Identify the respiratory rate and volume of each breath and determine the minute volume.

8. **Describe percussion of the chest.** pp. 567–568, 606, 607, 609

Percuss both the anterior and posterior chest surfaces, examining for resonant (normal), hyperresonant (air-filled pneumothorax or tension pneumothorax), or dull sounds (fluid-filled hemothorax). Percuss both sides symmetrically from the apex to the base at 5 cm intervals, avoiding the scapula. Determine the boundaries of any hyperresonance or dullness.

See Workbook, Part 1 of this chapter for review of objective 9.

10. **Describe special examination techniques related to the assessment of the chest.**

    ### Chest excursion pp. 605–609
    Place your hands at the 10th intercostal space with the fingers spread and feel for the chest excursion as the patient breathes deeply. Your hand should move equally about 3 to 5 cm with each breath.

    ### Fremitus
    Place a cupped hand against the chest wall at various locations and feel for vibrations while the patient says "ninety-nine" or "one-on-one." These vibrations should be equal throughout the chest. Note any enhanced, decreased, or absent fremitus.

    ### Diaphragm excursion
    Percuss the border of the rib cage for the dullness of the diaphragm during quiet breathing. Then mark the highest and lowest movement during respiration. Repeat the process on the other side of the chest. This excursion should be about 6 cm and equal on each side.

11. **Describe the auscultation of the chest, heart, and abdomen.**

    ### Chest pp. 606–613
    Have your patient breathe more deeply and slowly than normal with an open mouth. Using the stethoscope's disk, auscultate each side of the chest from the apex to the base every 5 cm, listening at each location for one full breath.

    ### Heart pp. 606–613
    Using the diaphragm of the stethoscope, listen for heart sounds at the 2nd through 5th intercostal spaces at both sternal borders and at the point of maximum impulse (PMI). Repeat the process using the bell of the stethoscope to discern lower-pitched sounds.

    ### Abdomen pp. 606–613
    Using the stethoscope's disk, auscultate each abdominal quadrant for at least 30 seconds to 1 minute.

12. **Distinguish between normal and abnormal auscultation findings of the chest, heart, and abdomen and explain their significance.**

    ### Chest pp. 606–613
    Normal breath sounds are the quiet sounds (almost low-pitched sighs) of air moving. Abnormal breath sounds are termed adventitious, and include the following. Any crackles (a light crackling, popping, nonmusical sound) suggest fluid in the smaller airways. Late inspiratory crackles suggest heart failure or interstitial lung disease, while early crackles suggest heart failure or chronic bronchitis. Wheezes (more musical notes) denote obstruction of the smaller airways. The closer they appear to inspiration, the more serious the obstruction is. Stridor is a high-pitched, loud inspiratory wheeze reflective of laryngeal or tracheal obstruction. Grating or squeaking sounds describe pleural friction rubs and occur as the pleural layers become inflamed, then rub together. You may also listen for sound transmission while the patient speaks. Bronchophony occurs when you hear the words "ninety-nine" abnormally clearly through the stethoscope, a suggestion that blood, fluid, or a tumor has replaced normal tissue. Assess for whispered pectoriloquy by asking the patient to whisper "ninety-nine"; unusually clear sounds indicate an abnormal condition. Egophony occurs when you can hear the sound of long "e" as "a" when vocal resonance is abnormally increased.

    ### Heart pp. 606–613
    The normal heart produces a "lub-dub" sound heard through the disk of the stethoscope with each cardiac contraction. The "lub" and "dub" may split when valves close out of sync; "la-lub-dub" reflects an S_1 split while "lub-da-dub" is an S_2 split. S_2 splitting is normal in children and young adults, though abnormal in older adults if expiratory or persistent splitting occurs. S_3 splitting produces a "lub-dub-dee" cadence like the word "Kentucky." It occurs commonly in children and young adults, but reflects blood filling a dilated ventricle and may suggest ventricular failure in the

patient over 30. The S₄ heart sound is the "dee" sound of "dee-lub-dub" with a cadence similar to the word "Tennessee." It develops from vibrations as the atrium pushes blood into a ventricle that resists filling, suggestive of heart failure.

Abdomen pp. 606–613

Normal bowel sounds consist of a variety of high-pitched gurgles and clicks that occur every 5 to 15 seconds. More frequent activity suggests an increase in bowel motility and especially loud and prolonged gurgling sounds (borborygmi) indicate hyperperistalsis. Decreased or absent sounds suggest a paralytic ileus or peritonitis. You may also hear swishing sounds (bruit) over the major vessels suggesting vascular defect such as aneurysm or stenosis.

13. **Describe special techniques of the cardiovascular examination.**

    Inspection for signs of cardiovascular insufficiency pp. 609–612

    Examine the extremities for signs of insufficiency including pallor, delayed capillary refill, temperature variation, and dependent edema. Then assess the carotid arteries for pulse strength, rate, and rhythm. Does the rate or strength vary with respirations? Do you feel thrills (feel a humming sensation)? If so, auscultate for bruits.

    Jugular vein distention pp. 609–612

    Position the patient supine with the head elevated 30° and turned away from the side being assessed. Look for pulsations of the external jugular vein on either side of the trachea just before it passes behind the manubrium. Locate the highest point of pulsation and measure the distance from the sternal angle. Normal venous pressure distends the vein above the clavicle between 1 to 2 cm. Examine both jugulars for symmetrical pulsing and distention.

    Point of maximum impulse (PMI) pp. 609–612

    Have the patient lie comfortably with his head elevated 30°. Inspect and palpate the chest for the apical impulse or the PMI. It is normally at the 5th intercostal space, mid-clavicular line. In muscular or obese patients, you may need to percuss the point (dull vs. resonant).

Content Self-Evaluation

MULTIPLE CHOICE

_____ 1. A likely location to notice retraction during forced inspiration is:
   A. the suprasternal notch.
   B. the intercostal spaces.
   C. the supraclavicular space.
   D. all of the above
   E. none of the above

_____ 2. The type of motion associated with a free segment of the chest where the segment moves opposite to the rest of the chest during breathing is:
   A. symbiotic.
   B. paradoxical.
   C. antagonistic.
   D. retractive.
   E. traumatic.

_____ 3. During the palpation of the chest, you should feel for which of the following?
   A. tenderness
   B. deformities
   C. depressions
   D. asymmetry
   E. all of the above

_____ 4. During the check for chest excursion, the distance between your thumbs should increase by what amount during the patient's inspiration?
   A. 2 cm
   B. 3 to 5 cm
   C. 5 to 6 cm
   D. 10 to 12 cm
   E. the hands should not move

_____ 5. Increased tactile fremitus suggests which of the following conditions?
   A. pneumonia
   B. pneumothorax
   C. pleural effusion
   D. emphysema
   E. all of the above

_____ 6. Which condition is most likely to cause an area of the lung that is dull to percussion?
   A. pneumothorax
   B. tension pneumothorax
   C. hemothorax
   D. pericardial tamponade
   E. friction rubs

_____ 7. Light popping, nonmusical sounds heard in the chest during inspiration are known as:
   A. rhonchi.
   B. stridor.
   C. crackles.
   D. wheezes.
   E. none of the above

_____ 8. Hearing words transmitted clearly as you auscultate the chest with the stethoscope is a normal finding called bronchophony.
   A. True
   B. False

_____ 9. The "lub" of the heart sounds represents which event of the cardiac cycle?
   A. ejection of blood from the ventricles
   B. ventricular contraction
   C. ventricular filling
   D. closing of the aortic and pulmonic valves
   E. closing of the tricuspid and mitral valves

_____ 10. An eccyhmotic discoloration over the umbilicus is:
   A. Grey Turner's sign.
   B. borborygmi.
   C. Hering-Breuer sign.
   D. Cullen's sign.
   E. none of the above

_____ 11. Auscultation of high-pitched gurgles and clicks every 5 to 15 seconds in the abdomen indicates:
   A. borborygmi.
   B. increased bowel motility.
   C. absent bowel sounds.
   D. normal bowel sounds.
   E. ascites.

_____ 12. The sound or feeling caused by unlubricated bone ends rubbing together is:
   A. palpable fremitus.
   B. crepitation.
   C. bruit.
   D. friction rub.
   E. the pooh-pooh sign.

_____ 13. Carpal tunnel syndrome involves which nerve?
   A. brachial
   B. median
   C. radial
   D. ulnar
   E. olecranon

_____ 14. A lateral curvature of the spine is:
   A. lordosis.
   B. scoliosis.
   C. kyphosis.
   D. spina bifida.
   E. none of the above

_____ 15. Tenderness at a vertebral process and in the surrounding musculature of the lumbar spine is most likely due to:
   A. vertebral process fracture.
   B. ligamentous injury.
   C. paravertebral muscular spasm.
   D. herniated intervertebral disk.
   E. none of the above

Part 3, pp. 629–650

Review of Chapter Objectives

After reading this section of the chapter, you should be able to:

2. **Describe the evaluation of mental status.**   **pp. 629–632**

    The evaluation of the mental status begins with your interview. The evaluation permits you to determine your patient's level of responsiveness, general appearance, behavior, and speech. You specifically look at his appearance and behavior, speech and language skills, mood, thought and perception, insight and judgment, and memory and attention.

4. **Describe the examination of the following body regions, differentiate between normal and abnormal findings, and define the significance of abnormal findings (continued):**

    Heart and blood vessels   **pp. 609–612**
    Examine the cardiovascular function by inspecting for skin pallor or other signs suggestive of arterial insufficiency or occlusion. Then evaluate carotid and peripheral pulses for rate, rhythm, and quality as well as the jugular vein for signs of distension (JVD). A heart rate above 100 is tachycardia and may be related to excitement and stress or shock while a heart rate below 60 (bradycardia) may be related to an athlete's state of conditioning or head injury. Excessive JVD suggests right heart failure or cardiac tamponade, while abnormally low distension may suggest hypovolemia. Auscultate the heart sounds either side of the sternum at the 2nd intercostal space and the left side of the sternum at the 5th intercostal space. Variations of the normal "lub-dub" suggest cardiac abnormalities, although some variant sounds may be normal in children and young adults.

    Peripheral vascular system   **pp. 625, 627–629**
    Examine the upper, then the lower extremities, and compare them, one to another, for the following: size, symmetry, swelling, venous congestion, skin and nail bed color, temperature, skin texture, and turgor. Yellow brittle nails, swollen digit ends (clubbing), or poor nail bed color suggest chronic arterial insufficiency. Assess the distal circulation, noting the strength, rate, and regularity of the pulse and comparing pulses bilaterally. If you have difficulty palpating a pulse or can't find one, palpate a more proximal site. Feel the spongy compliance of the vessels, note their coloration, and examine for inflammation along the vein, indicative of deep vein thrombosis. Gently feel for edema and pitting edema in each distal extremity.

    Nervous system   **pp. 629–642**
    To evaluate mental status and speech, examine your patient's appearance and behavior, speech and language, mood, thoughts and perceptions, and memory and attention. Observe the patient's appearance and behavior, level of consciousness, posture and motor behavior, appropriateness of dress, grooming and personal hygiene, and the patient's facial expression. Note any abnormal speech pattern and observe the patient's attitude toward you and others expressed both verbally and nonverbally. Note any excessive emotion or lack of emotion. Assess the patient's thoughts and perceptions. Are they realistic and socially acceptable? Question for any visions, voices, perceived odors, or feelings about things that are not there. Examine the patient's insights and judgments to determine if he knows what is happening. Assess the patient's memory and attention and determine his orientation to time, place, and person (sometimes considered as person and own person). Then test immediate, recent, and remote memory. Any deviation from a normal and expected response is to be noted and suggests illness or psychiatric problem.

        Begin the examination of the motor system by observing the patient for symmetry, deformities, and involuntary movements. Tremors or fasiculations while the patient is at rest suggest Parkinson's disease, while their occurrence during motion suggests postural tremor. Determine muscle bulk, which is classified as normal, atrophy, hypertrophy, or pseudotrophy (bulk without strength as in muscular dystrophy). Unilateral hand atrophy suggests median or ulnar nerve paralysis. Check tone by moving a relaxed limb through a range of motion. Describe any flaccidity or rigidity and then examine muscle strength starting with grip strength and continuing through all limbs. Again note any asymmetry (the patient's dominant side should be slightly stronger). Observe the patient's gait and have him walk a straight line (heel to toe). Any ataxia suggests cerebellar disease, loss of position sense, or intoxication. Also have the patient walk on his toes, then heels, hop on each foot, and then do a shallow knee bend. Perform a Romberg test (have him stand with his feet together and eyes closed for 20 to 30 seconds). Any excessive sway (a positive Romberg test) suggests ataxia from loss of position sense, while inability to maintain balance with eyes open represents cerebellar ataxia. Ask the patient to hold his arms straight out in front with his palms up and eyes closed. Pronation suggests mild hemiparesis, drifting sideways or upward suggests loss of positional sense. Ask your patient to perform various rapid alternating movements and observe for smoothness, speed, and rhythm. The dominant side should perform best, and any slow, irregular, or clumsy movements suggest cerebellar or extrapyramidal disease. Have your patient touch his thumb rapidly with the tip of the index finger, place his hand on his thigh and rapidly alternate from palm up to down, and assess for point-to-point testing (touch his nose, then your index finger several times rapidly, or, for the legs, have him touch heel to knee, then run it down the shin). Any jerking, difficulty in performing the task, or tremors suggest cerebellar disease. For position testing, have the patient perform the leg test with his eyes closed.

Evaluate the sensory system by testing sensations of pain, light touch, temperature, position, vibration, and discrimination. Compare responses bilaterally and from distal to proximal, then associate any deficit discovered with the dermatome it represents. Test superficial and deep tendon reflexes and note a dulled (cord or lower neuron damage) or hyperactive response (upper neuron disease).

Cranial nerves pp. 632–635

CN-I is checked by evaluating the ability to sense odors in each nostril.
CN-II is checked by testing for visual acuity and field of view.
CN-III is checked by examining pupillary direct and consensual response.
CN-III, IV, and VI are checked by testing for smooth and unrestricted extraocular motion.
CN-V is checked by testing the masseter muscle strength and sensation on the forehead, cheek, chin, and cornea.
CN-VII is checked by examining the patient's face during conversations, looking for any asymmetry, eyelid droop, or abnormal movements.
CN-VIII is checked by evaluating for hearing and balance (with his eyes closed).
CN-IX and X are checked by evaluating speech, swallowing, saying "aaahhh," and the gag reflex.
CN-XI is checked by testing trapezius and sternocleidomastoid muscles at rest and by evaluating head turning and shoulder raising.
CN-XII is checked by evaluating speech and having the patient extend his tongue outward.

Any deviation from a normally expected response is a reason to suspect a cranial nerve injury.

14. Describe the general guidelines of recording examination information. p. 647

Use a standard format to organize the information. Use appropriate medical terminology and language. Present your findings legibly, accurately, and truthfully, remembering that your record will become a legal document. Include all data discovered in your assessment.

The standard organization for medical documentation is the S (Subjective), O (Objective), A (Assessment), and P (Plan) format (SOAP format):

Subjective information is what your patient or others tell you, including the chief complaint and the past and present medical history.
Objective information is that which you observe or determine during the scene size-up, initial assessment, focused history and physical exam, detailed assessment, and ongoing assessments.
Assessment summarizes the findings to suggest a field diagnosis.
Plan is the further diagnosis, treatment, and patient education you intend to offer.

15. **Discuss the examination considerations for an infant or child.** pp. 642–647

Children are not small adults, but patients with special physiological and psychological differences. In general, remain calm and confident, establish a rapport with the parents, and have them help with the exam. Provide positive feedback to both the child and parents.

The transition from newborn to adulthood is a continuum of development, both physically and emotionally. When assessing pediatric patients, keep the following differences from adults in mind:

The bones of the skull do not close until about 18 months and joints remain cartilaginous until 5 years.

The child's airway is narrow and will be more quickly and severely obstructed than the adult's.

Instead of listening for verbal complaints, note the child's eyes, expression, and the degree of activity it takes to distract him from the problem as an indication of its seriousness.

Rib fractures are rare due to the cartilaginous nature of the ribs, though the tissue underneath is more prone to injury.

The liver and spleen are proportionally large and are more subject to injury.

Children are more likely to experience bone injury rather than ligament and tendon injury.

Normal vital signs for children will change through the stages of their development.

Content Self-Evaluation

MULTIPLE CHOICE

_____ 1. A normal pulse quality would be reported as:
   A. 0.
   B. 1+.
   C. 2+.
   D. 3+.
   E. 4+.

_____ 2. Which of the following is NOT a sign of proximal arterial occlusion?
   A. thrills
   B. pulse deficit
   C. cold limb
   D. poor color in the fingertips
   E. slow capillary refill

_____ 3. Pitting edema that depresses 1/2 to 1 inch is reported as:
   A. 0.
   B. 1+.
   C. 2+.
   D. 3+.
   E. 4+.

_____ 4. The pitting of edema will usually disappear within how many seconds after the release of pressure?
   A. 2
   B. 4
   C. 6
   D. 8
   E. 10

_____ 5. A complete neurological exam includes which of the following areas?
   A. cranial nerves
   B. motor system
   C. reflexes
   D. sensory system
   E. all of the above

_____ 6. A patient who is drowsy but answers questions is considered to be:
   A. lethargic.
   B. obtunded.
   C. stuporous.
   D. comatose.
   E. none of the above

_____ 7. Normal speech is:
   A. inflected.
   B. clear and strong.
   C. fluent and articulate.
   D. varies in volume.
   E. all of the above

_____ 8. The term *dysphonia* refers to which of the following?
   A. defective speech caused by motor deficits
   B. voice changes due to vocal cord problems
   C. defective language due to neurologic problem
   D. voice changes due to aging
   E. none of the above

_____ 9. The term *aphasia* refers to which of the following?
   A. defective speech caused by motor deficits
   B. voice changes due to vocal cord problems
   C. defective language due to a neurologic problem
   D. voice changes due to aging
   E. none of the above

_____ 10. Which of the following is one of the three basic grades of memory:
   A. intermediate.
   B. verifiable.
   C. redux.
   D. remote.
   E. retrograde.

_____ 11. A question about a patient's wife's birthday tests which of the following types of memory?
   A. intermediate
   B. verifiable
   C. redux
   D. remote
   E. retrograde

_____ 12. During the test of extraocular eye movement you should trace which figure in front of your patient's eyes?
   A. an "X"
   B. an "H"
   C. a "+"
   D. a large "O"
   E. any of the above

_____ 13. Stimulation for a blink by touching the eye's surface with fine cotton fibers tests which of the following?
   A. corneal reflex
   B. ptosis
   C. EOM
   D. the trigeminal nerve
   E. none of the above

_____ 14. When a person loses his sense of balance, which cranial nerve has most likely been injured?
   A. equilibrial
   B. glossopharyngeal
   C. acoustic
   D. vagus
   E. accessory

_____ 15. Damage to CN-12 will cause the tongue to deviate in which manner?
   A. downward
   B. upward
   C. toward the side of injury
   D. away from the side of injury
   E. furrow and curve upward

_____ 16. The twitching of small muscle fibers is:
   A. spasm.
   B. tics.
   C. tremors.
   D. fasciculations.
   E. atrophy.

_____ 17. In cases of muscular dystrophy, the patient's muscles:
   A. increase in size.
   B. decrease in size.
   C. increase in strength.
   D. decrease in strength.
   E. both A and D

_____ 18. During your testing of a patient's muscle strength, you notice one side to be slightly stronger than the other. This is a normal finding.
   A. True
   B. False

_____ 19. Which of the following procedures describes the Romberg test? Have the patient:
   A. walk heel-to-toe in a straight line.
   B. stand with eyes closed for 20 to 30 seconds.
   C. walk across the room and turn and walk back again.
   D. do a shallow knee bend on each leg in turn.
   E. walk first on his heels, then toes.

_____ 20. An area of skin innervated by a specific peripheral nerve root is a(n):
   A. afferent region.   D. dermatome.
   B. sensory topographic region.   E. both A and C
   C. myotome.

_____ 21. The score on the muscle strength scale that describes a patient able to perform active movement against gravity is:
   A. 5.   D. 2.
   B. 4.   E. 1.
   C. 3.

_____ 22. To assess the sensory system, you must test for:
   A. pain.   D. dermatome.
   B. light touch.   E. A, B, and C
   C. temperature.

_____ 23. Babinski's response is positive when the sole of the foot is stroked and:
   A. the big toe plantar flexes while other toes dorsiflex.
   B. the big toe plantar flexes while other toes fan out.
   C. the big toe dorsiflexes while other toes fan out.
   D. the big toe dorsiflexes while other toes plantar flex.
   E. all toes plantar flex.

_____ 24. In caring for the ill or injured child, it is important to be which of the following?
   A. confident   D. calm
   B. direct   E. all of the above
   C. honest

_____ 25. Which of the following is NOT recommended as part of the assessment and care for an ill or injured child?
   A. Separate the patient from the parents if possible.
   B. Give the patient a toy or object to play with.
   C. Elicit a parent's help in obtaining a history.
   D. Perform invasive procedures late in the assessment if possible.
   E. Provide feedback and reassurance.

_____ 26. The soft spots in the skull, called fontanelles, close at about what age?
   A. 6 months   D. 24 months
   B. 12 months   E. 30 months
   C. 18 months

_____ 27. Bulging along the sutures of the skull of a young child suggests which of the following?
   A. dehydration
   B. reduced venous pressure in the jugular veins
   C. decreased arterial pressure
   D. arterial blockage to the cerebrum
   E. none of the above

_____ 28. Because the tissue of the child's upper airway is so flexible, injuries, infections, or minor obstructions do not adversely affect it as seriously as they would an adult's.
   A. True
   B. False

_____ 29. Which of the following statements regarding the chest of an infant or small child is FALSE?
   A. Children have a less mobile mediastinum than adults.
   B. The chest is rather elastic.
   C. The chest is rather flexible.
   D. Chest fractures are less likely.
   E. The chest is comprised of more cartilage than the adult's.

_____ 30. Because of the structure of the thoracic cage, the child is less likely to develop tension pneumothorax than the adult.
   A. True
   B. False

_____ 31. The normal respiratory rate for an infant is:
   A. 30 to 50 breaths per minute.
   B. 30 to 60 breaths per minute.
   C. 24 to 40 breaths per minute.
   D. 22 to 34 breaths per minute.
   E. 18 to 30 breaths per minute.

_____ 32. The normal systolic blood pressure for the newborn is:
   A. 60 to 90.
   B. 87 to 105.
   C. 95 to 105.
   D. 95 to 110.
   E. 112 to 128.

_____ 33. Which of the following is NOT true regarding the abdomen of the child?
   A. The liver is proportionally larger than the adult's.
   B. The spleen is proportionally larger than the adult's.
   C. The abdominal muscles provide less protection than the adult's.
   D. The abdomen rarely bulges at the end of inspiration.
   E. Inguinal hernias are common in young children.

_____ 34. Which of the following statements is true regarding the recording of examination findings?
   A. The patient care report is only as good as the accuracy, detail, and depth you provide.
   B. The patient chart is a legal document.
   C. The absence of an expected sign in a patient may be just as important as its presence.
   D. The universally accepted organization for recording patient information is SOAP.
   E. all of the above

_____ 35. The patient's chief complaint is recorded under which element of the SOAP documentation format?
   A. S
   B. O
   C. A
   D. P
   E. none of the above

Chapter 12

Patient Assessment in the Field

Part 1, pp. 654–673

Review of Chapter Objectives

Because Chapter 12 is lengthy, it has been divided into sections to aid your study. Read the assigned text pages, then progress through the objectives and self-evaluation materials as you would with other chapters. When you feel secure in your grasp of the content, proceed to the next section.

After reading this section of the chapter, you should be able to:

1. **Recognize hazards/potential hazards associated with the medical and trauma scene.** pp. 654–660

    During the scene size-up, you must examine the scene before you arrive at the patient's side. It is a time to evaluate and prepare for hazards including blood, fluids, airborne pathogens, and other conditions that may threaten your life or health. These conditions include the hazards of fire, structural collapse, traffic, unstable surfaces, electricity, broken glass, or jagged metal. Hazardous materials can involve chemical spills, radiation, and toxic environments. Finally, scene hazards can also include violent, disturbed, or unruly bystanders or patients. These hazards are not limited to the trauma scene but may be found at many medical scenes as well.

2. **Identify unsafe scenes and describe methods for making them safe.** pp. 654–660

    Your responsibility at the emergency scene is to recognize hazards including fire, structural collapse, traffic, unstable surfaces, electricity, broken glass, jagged metal, and hazardous materials and then act appropriately to protect yourself, other rescuers, and your patient. Unless you are specially trained and equipped to handle a specific hazard, do not enter the scene. In most cases, you will rely on the fire department, rescue service, police department, power company, hazmat team, or other specially trained personnel to secure the scene before you enter. If there is ever a question of whether a scene is safe or unsafe, do not enter the scene.

3. **Discuss common mechanisms of injury/nature of illness.** pp. 662–663

    Trauma is induced by a mechanism of injury through which forces enter the body and do physical harm. Common mechanisms include blunt trauma—for example, vehicle crashes (auto, recreational, watercraft, and bicycle), pedestrian versus vehicle impacts, falls—and penetrating trauma—for example, gunshot and knife wounds. Medical problems have a related cause called the nature of the illness. The scene can provide evidence as to the nature of the illness. Examples include the presence of nebulizers, which suggest asthma, drug paraphernalia, which suggest overdose, and medications, which suggest preexisting cardiac or other problems.

4. **Predict patterns of injury based on mechanism of injury.** pp. 662–663, 673–675

Analyze the strength, direction, and nature of the forces expressed to the patient during the incident. This analysis will suggest the probable type of injury, the organs involved, and the seriousness of injury. In a vehicle crash, for example, such things as a broken windshield, a bent steering wheel, an intrusion into the passenger compartment, and the use of restraints by occupants can suggest potential injuries and their severity. Types of injuries can also be predicted for each type of vehicle crash—frontal, lateral, rear-end, rotational, and rollover. The analysis of the accident can lead to your anticipation of possible injuries, or an index of suspicion.

5. **Discuss the reason for identifying the total number of patients at the scene.** p. 661

Determining the number of patients at a scene is important to assure that the needed resources are summoned to the scene and that every patient is cared for. At each and every scene, you should ask yourself, "Could there be others who are injured or ill?" While at the trauma scene it is common to find a patient wandering among the bystanders, the medical scene can have "hidden patients," too. The wife of a cardiac arrest patient, for example, may herself become a patient because of the emotional stress of the incident. Knowing the number of patients can help you gauge whether on-scene resources are adequate or whether you need to request that additional units and manpower be dispatched to the scene. The earlier this request is made, the quicker those resources will arrive.

6. **Organize the management of a scene following size-up.** pp. 654–660

The management of the scene following the scene size-up includes requesting both the appropriate units and personnel to manage scene hazards and the appropriate number and care levels of ambulances and personnel to treat the patients. You must also take the necessary steps to assure overall scene safety and to protect yourself, the patient, other scene personnel, and bystanders. The scene size-up also prepares you to manage the care of the patient by helping you recognize the mechanism of injury and anticipate injuries (index of suspicion) or by recognizing the nature of the illness.

7. **Explain the reasons for identifying the need for additional help or assistance during the scene size-up.** pp. 654, 656–660

Multiple patients at the emergency scene can rapidly overwhelm your ability to provide effective care. If you wait until you are at a patient's side before calling for additional help, you may be distracted from making the call and delay an effective response. In cases where the number of patients far outstrips your ability to provide care, you may need to initiate a mass casualty response.

8. **Summarize the reasons for forming a general impression of the patient.** pp. 664–665

The initial general impression of your patient takes into account the patient's age, gender, race, and other factors that will help you determine the seriousness of the problem and establish your priorities for patient care and transport. As you learn more about the patient through the initial assessment and the focused history and physical assessment, you will refine and improve on the accuracy and depth of the general impression. As you develop your general impression of the patient early in the assessment process, you can also begin to establish a rapport with him or her, explaining why you are there, what will be happening to him or her, and giving the patient the opportunity to refuse care.

9. **Discuss methods of assessing mental status/levels of consciousness in the adult, infant, and child patient.** pp. 665–666

Initially determine the patient's mental status by categorizing him according to the AVPU system. Using this method, the patient is classified either Alert, responsive to Verbal stimuli, responsive to Painful stimuli, or Unresponsive. You can further refine the evaluation by questioning the patient to determine orientation to place, time, and person and by differentiating his or her response to pain into purposeful and purposeless movement and decerebrate and decorticate posturing. An alert response for the infant or child is difficult to assess because of that patient's limited speech capabilities. Evaluate pediatric patients for activity and curiosity, being aware that the quiet child is often a seriously ill or injured one.

10. **Discuss methods of assessing and securing the airway in the adult, child, and infant patient.** pp. 666–667

The patient who is speaking clearly (or the child or infant who is crying loudly) has a patent airway. For other patients, position your head at the patient's mouth and look, listen, and feel for air moving through the airway. If you detect no movement, open the airway by using either the jaw-thrust (in patients with trauma and suspected spine injury) or the head-tilt/chin-lift. Suction any fluids from the airway and remove obstructions using the Heimlich maneuver or laryngoscopy with Magill forceps. Secure the airway, as needed, with an oral or nasal airway, endotracheal intubation, or creation of a needle or surgical airway. When you have a pediatric patient, be sure to position the head and neck properly (using slight extension and padding under the shoulders), taking account of the differences in the pediatric anatomy. Also, reduce the size of the airways, laryngoscope blades, and endotracheal tubes you use with these patients.

11. **State reasons for cervical spine management for the trauma patient.** pp. 664–665

The spinal cord is the major communication distribution and collection conduit for the central nervous system. It is protected by the spinal column, the bony and flexible structure that runs from the base of the skull to just below the pelvis. If the column is injured, it may become unstable and permit injury to the spinal cord. Because injuries to the cord have such serious consequences, you should immobilize the spine early in your assessment and care to protect this essential communication pathway. Its immobilization will not harm the patient, while uncontrolled movement can cause permanent spinal cord injury.

12. **Analyze a scene to determine if spinal precautions are required.** pp. 664–665, 673–675

Your examination of the scene and the analysis of the mechanism of injury will suggest or rule out the potential for spinal injury. The patient with a significant mechanism of injury—severe vehicle crash, fall from a height, injury causing a major long-bone fracture, or any injury or mechanism of injury that suggests the body was subjected to significant trauma forces—has a likelihood of spinal fracture and requires spinal precautions.

13. **Describe methods for assessing respiration in the adult, child, and infant patient.** pp. 667–668

If your patient is speaking clearly (or if an infant or child patient is crying loudly), presume the airway is clear. Otherwise, listen for the sounds of airway restriction or obstruction, such as gurgling, stridor, or wheezes. If airway sounds are absent, place your ear at the patient's mouth while you listen, watch, and feel for air movement through it. If there is any doubt about airway patency, position the head with the jaw-thrust or head-tilt/chin-lift. With a child, do not hyperextend the neck as this may block the airway. You may have to place padding behind the shoulders of a small child or infant to maintain proper head positioning.

14. **Describe the methods used to locate and assess a pulse in an adult, child, and infant patient.** pp. 668–671

Use the pads of your fingers and apply gentle, increasing pressure until you feel a strong pulsing over the radial artery in the adult and brachial artery in the small child or infant. If the radial or brachial pulse cannot be felt, check the carotid or, in the infant, the apical pulse. An adult radial pulse generally suggests a blood pressure of at least 80 mmHg, while a carotid pulse suggests a systolic blood pressure of at least 60 mmHg. Pulse rates usually decrease with age from a high of 100 to 180 in the infant to 60 to 100 in the adult. The pulse should be strong and regular.

15. **Discuss the need for assessing the patient for external bleeding.** pp. 669–670

   The patient with the potential for external hemorrhage must be assessed to determine both the nature and the extent of the blood loss. Any significant external hemorrhage must be halted and the amount of loss approximated to help prevent hypovolemia and to determine what effects the loss will have on the patient's body.

16. **Describe normal and abnormal findings when assessing skin color, temperature, and condition.** p. 669

   Normal skin is warm, moist, and pink in color (in light-skinned people), reflecting good perfusion. The body's compensation for shock results in vasoconstriction, which produces mottled, cyanotic, pale or ashen skin color, and skin that is cool to the touch. Capillary refill times may exceed 3 seconds, though this may be due to a number of preexisting conditions in adults.

17. **Explain the reason and process for prioritizing a patient for care and transport.** pp. 669, 672–673

   At the conclusion of the initial assessment, you must determine your patient's priority, which will indicate how to proceed with assessment, care, and transport. With a seriously ill or injured patient, perform a rapid head-to-toe assessment. With a stable medical or trauma patient, perform a focused history and physical exam. You will also need to determine the priority for transport—either immediate transport with care rendered en route or with most care provided at the scene followed by transport.

18. **Use the findings of the initial assessment to determine the patient's perfusion status.** pp. 668–672

   The initial assessment provides you with a general impression of the patient, a determination of the patient's mental status, and an evaluation of the airway, breathing, and circulation. This information indicates the status of the patient's respiration/oxygenation and circulation. It also indicates the patient's level of consciousness and the perfusion of the body's most important end-organ, the brain.

Content Self-Evaluation

MULTIPLE CHOICE

_____ 1. As a paramedic, you will certainly never perform a comprehensive history and physical exam in the acute setting.
   A. True
   B. False

_____ 2. Which component of the trauma patient assessment process will be performed during patient transport?
   A. scene survey
   B. initial assessment
   C. focused history and physical exam
   D. detailed physical exam
   E. ongoing assessment

_____ 3. After the scene size-up and if necessary, you should inform the dispatcher of:
   A. the nature of the medical or trauma emergency.
   B. what resources you need.
   C. the phone number at which you can be reached.
   D. what actions you and your crew are taking.
   E. all of the above except C

_____ 4. Which of the following is NOT a component of the scene size-up?
   A. body substance isolation
   B. general impression of the patient
   C. location of all patients
   D. mechanism of injury/nature of the illness analysis
   E. scene safety

_____ 5. Which of the following body substance isolation devices will you employ with every patient you treat?
   A. latex or vinyl gloves
   B. protective eyewear
   E. face mask
   D. gown
   E. both B and C

_____ 6. Whenever you plan to intubate a patient, you should wear:
   A. latex or vinyl gloves and a gown.
   B. protective eyewear, a gown, and a face mask.
   C. latex or vinyl gloves, protective eyewear, and a face mask.
   D. protective eyewear and a gown.
   E. latex or vinyl gloves.

_____ 7. The HEPA respirator is designed to filter out which of the following pathogens that may be encountered when providing prehospital emergency care?
   A. tuberculosis
   B. small pox
   C. anthrax
   D. the flu
   E. tetanus toxoid

_____ 8. The intent of the safety analysis portion of the scene survey is to assure the safety of:
   A. the patient.
   B. bystanders.
   C. fellow responders.
   D. yourself.
   E. all of the above

_____ 9. To properly handle a scene safety issue, you must be:
   A. properly trained.
   B. properly equipped.
   C. properly clothed.
   D. prepared to attempt rescue procedures in which you have not been trained.
   E. A, B, and C above

_____ 10. Potential hazards to rule out before entering the scene include all of the following EXCEPT:
   A. fire.
   B. electrocution.
   C. contamination with blood.
   D. structural collapse.
   E. broken glass and jagged metal.

_____ 11. When called to a shooting or domestic disturbance, until the police arrive and secure the scene you should remain:
   A. a few blocks away.
   B. outside the residence.
   C. just down the street.
   D. at the door but don't enter.
   E. either B or C

_____ 12. At which of the following incidents would you NOT expect to discover more than one patient in your scene size-up?
   A. a two-car accident
   B. a carbon monoxide poisoning in a home
   C. a car crash in which a child seat and diaper bag are visible
   D. a fall out of a tree
   E. a hazardous materials spill in a high school chemistry lab

_____ 13. You should delay the call for additional ambulances until you begin your initial assessment because you will not have enough information to determine the needs of the scene until then.
A. True
B. False

_____ 14. The two important functions that must begin immediately in the mass casualty situation are:
A. triage and incident management.
B. rescue and triage.
C. firefighting and rescue.
D. incident management and extrication.
E. incident management and scene isolation.

_____ 15. The responsibilities of incident management at a disaster scene include all of the following EXCEPT:
A. performing a scene size-up.
B. triaging initial patients for care.
C. determining the need for additional resources.
D. radioing for additional equipment and personnel.
E. directing incoming crews.

_____ 16. The responsibilities of the triage person at the disaster scene include all of the following EXCEPT:
A. determining a patient's priority for immediate transport.
B. determining a patient's priority for delayed transport.
C. performing simple, but lifesaving procedures.
D. providing intensive care on salvageable patients.
E. all of the above

_____ 17. The mechanism of injury analysis examines:
A. body locations affected.
B. strength of the crash forces.
C. direction of the crash forces.
D. nature of the crash forces.
E. all of the above

_____ 18. The index of suspicion is best defined as:
A. patient priority for care based on the MOI.
B. anticipation of the nature of forces involved in an accident.
C. prediction of injuries based upon the MOI.
D. prediction of degree of injury based on the patient's appearance.
E. none of the above

_____ 19. The nature of the illness is determined from information you receive from:
A. the patient.
B. the patient's family.
C. bystanders.
D. scene clues.
E. all of the above

_____ 20. The initial assessment includes all of the following EXCEPT:
A. forming a general impression of the patient.
B. stabilizing the cervical spine as needed.
C. immobilizing of fractures.
D. assessing the airway.
E. assessing the circulation.

_____ 21. The general patient impression is based upon all of the following EXCEPT:
A. blood pressure.
B. mechanism of injury.
C. chief complaint.
D. the environment.
E. your instincts.

_____ 22. Which of the following is NOT a purpose served by your initial introduction to the patient?
   A. identifying yourself
   B. identifying your reason for being there
   C. establishing your level of training
   D. giving the patient an opportunity to refuse care
   E. obtaining informed consent

_____ 23. During the initial assessment, the cervical spine should be stabilized:
   A. after the airway is established.
   B. just before you attempt artificial ventilation.
   C. immediately, if suggested by the MOI.
   D. after the circulation check.
   E. as the last step of the initial assessment.

_____ 24. Which of the following conditions does NOT normally cause an altered mental status?
   A. eupnea   D. poisoning
   B. drug overdose   E. sepsis
   C. head injury

_____ 25. A patient who only moves his arm when firmly pinched between the thumb and first finger and shows no other responses will be classified as which of the following under the AVPU system?
   A. A
   B. V
   C. P
   D. U
   E. cannot be determined with the information at hand

_____ 26. A patient who is disoriented and confused would be classified as which of the following under the AVPU system?
   A. A
   B. V
   C. P
   D. U
   E. cannot be determined with the information at hand

_____ 27. Stridor can usually be caused by all of the following EXCEPT:
   A. infection.   D. severe swelling.
   B. gastric distress.   E. allergic reaction.
   C. foreign body.

_____ 28. For stridor that is caused by respiratory burns, the care procedure most likely to maintain the airway is:
   A. suctioning.
   B. blow-by oxygen and a quiet ride to the hospital.
   C. a surgical airway.
   D. early endotracheal intubation.
   E. vasoconstrictor medications.

_____ 29. A patient with abnormally deep respirations is said to be:
   A. hyperpneic.   D. bradypneic.
   B. tachypneic.   E. hypopneic.
   C. eupneic.

_____ 30. The presence of a radial pulse suggests that the systolic blood pressure is at least:
   A. 60 mmHg.   D. 100 mmHg.
   B. 70 mmHg.   E. 120 mmHg.
   C. 80 mmHg.

LISTING

List the components of patient assessment in the field.

31. _____

32. _____

33. _____

34. _____

35. _____

Part 2, pp. 673–703

Review of Chapter Objectives

After reading this section of the chapter, you should be able to:

19. Describe orthostatic vital signs and evaluate their usefulness in assessing a patient in shock. pp. 688–689

The test for orthostatic vital signs, also called the tilt test, evaluates vital signs (blood pressure and pulse rate) before and after moving the patient from the supine to the seated, or from seated to the full standing position. If after 30 to 60 seconds either the blood pressure drops by more than 10 mmHg or the pulse rate rises by more than 10, consider the test positive and suspect hypovolemia. (Note that the change in pulse rate is the more sensitive indicator.) Do not use this test when other indicators of shock are present as it places stress on the cardiovascular system.

20. Describe the medical patient physical examination. pp. 685–689

The medical patient physical exam evaluates the head, ears, eyes, nose, and throat (HEENT); chest; abdomen; pelvis; extremities; posterior surface; and vital signs discretely, looking for illness or disease signs. The exam may be modified to meet the specific patient complaints of chest pain, respiratory distress, altered mental status, and acute abdomen. The medical patient exam may also include the results of pulse oximetry as well as cardiac and glucose level monitoring.

21. Differentiate between the assessment for unresponsive, altered mental status and alert medical patients. pp. 683–691

Responsive and unresponsive medical patients are examined in much different fashions. The responsive patient can provide information regarding his or her chief complaint, history of the present illness, past medical history, and current health status. This information, along with a physical exam focused on the areas of expected signs, provides the information necessary to make a field diagnosis.

The unresponsive patient cannot provide this information, and the caregiver must garner it from family and bystanders and through a more intensive and comprehensive physical examination.

The patient with an altered mental status is assessed like the unresponsive patient, though some information may be obtained from the patient. The information may not be reliable, hence the need for a more comprehensive physical exam.

22. Discuss the reasons for reconsidering the mechanism of injury. pp. 673–675

After the initial and rapid trauma assessments or focused history and physical exam, you have gathered enough information about your patient to determine if the mechanism of injury (and your resulting index of suspicion for associated injuries) agrees with your assessment findings. If they do, maintain your priority for care and transport. If they do not agree, reevaluate your index of suspicion and the physical findings and possibly adjust your patient's priority. If you do alter your patient's priority, always err on the side of precaution.

23. Recite examples and explain why patients should receive a rapid trauma assessment. p. 675

Every patient with a significant mechanism of injury, an altered level of consciousness, or multiple body-system traumas should receive the rapid trauma assessment. These patients are likely to have serious internal injuries and/or hemorrhage. However, the signs and symptoms of serious injury and shock are often hidden by other, more gruesome or painful injuries or by the body's compensatory mechanisms. Without maintaining a high index of suspicion for serious injury and evaluating the patient via the rapid trauma assessment, you are likely to overlook the patient with serious and life-threatening injury.

24. Describe the trauma patient physical examination. pp. 675–682

The physical assessment of the trauma patient begins during the initial assessment with the check of the ABCs and then branches to either the rapid trauma assessment or focused history and physical exam. The patient with a serious mechanism of injury, altered mental status, or multi-system trauma receives a rapid trauma assessment, a fast, systematic physical exam evaluating body regions where serious or life-threatening problems are likely to occur. This assessment is a rapid evaluation of the critical structures and regions of the head (HEENT), neck, chest, abdomen, pelvis, extremities, posterior body, and vital signs. The patient with isolated trauma has an assessment directed at the areas of expected injury or patient complaint.

25. Describe the elements of the rapid trauma assessment and discuss their evaluation. pp. 675–682

Each region of the body is inspected, palpated, and, as appropriate, auscultated and percussed to identify the signs of injury (DCAP-BTLS and crepitus). For each region, the specific assessment considerations include the following:

Evaluate the head for any signs of serious bleeding and deformity from skull fracture. Also check for discharge from the ears and nose, for the stability of the facial bones, and for the patency of the airway.

Evaluate the neck for lacerations involving the major blood vessels and serious hemorrhage and possible air embolism. Examine the jugular veins for abnormal distention and palpate the position and any unusual motion of the trachea. Also examine for subcutaneous emphysema and then any evidence of spinal trauma.

Evaluate the chest for signs of respiratory distress, including use of accessory muscles and retractions, and any signs of open wounds. Also observe the motion of the chest. Chest excursion should be bilaterally equal and symmetrical. Palpate for signs of clavicular or costal fracture and subcutaneous emphysema. Erythema may be present, but the frank ecchymotic discoloration of a contusion takes time to develop. Auscultate the lungs at the mid-axillary line for bilaterally equal breath sounds.

Evaluate the abdomen for exaggerated abdominal wall motion, and inspect and palpate for signs of injury, noting rigidity, guarding, tenderness, and rebound tenderness.

Evaluate the pelvis for signs of injury and apply pressure directed posteriorly and medially to the iliac crests and pressure directed posteriorly to the symphysis pubis to check for pelvic instability.

Evaluate the extremities for signs of injury, distal circulation, and innervation.

Evaluate the posterior body for signs of injury, and be especially watchful for potential signs of spinal injury.

Evaluate vital signs, first to establish a baseline, and then to obtain other readings to compare to that baseline. Evaluate direct pupil response to light during the rapid trauma assessment, but evaluate the other pupillary responses during more specific and directed evaluation.

Gather a patient history while you perform the rapid trauma assessment. This should include the elements of the SAMPLE assessment (Signs/Symptoms, Allergies, Medications, Past medical history, Last oral intake, and Events preceding the incident).

26. Identify cases when the rapid assessment is suspended to provide patient care. p. 675

The rapid trauma assessment is interrupted to provide patient care whenever you identify any life-threatening condition that can be quickly addressed. Just as you would suction the airway when you find it full of fluids during the initial assessment, you might provide pleural decompression during the rapid trauma assessment when you notice a developing tension pneumothorax. You might also administer oxygen to a patient who begins to display dyspnea and accessory muscle use during your chest examination. Other examples might include employing the PASG for the patient with the early signs of shock compensation and an unstable pelvic fracture found during the pelvic assessment or immediate provision of spinal immobilization upon noticing a neurologic deficit during the extremity exam.

27. Discuss the reason for performing a focused history and physical exam. pp. 673, 682, 683–684

The focused history and physical exam is the third step (following the scene size-up and initial assessment) of the patient assessment process. It is an assessment directed at the areas where the signs of serious injury or illness are expected. It also draws upon a quick history to identify information supporting a specific diagnosis and elements critical to the continued care of the patient. The focused history and physical exam takes you quickly toward determining the nature of the illness or the existence of serious and specific injuries. It is performed in different ways for trauma patients with significant injuries or mechanisms of injury, trauma patients with isolated injuries, responsive medical patients, and unresponsive medical patients.

28. Describe when and why a detailed physical examination is necessary. p. 692

The detailed assessment is a combination of a detailed history and a comprehensive physical exam either to identify or to learn more about the effects of an illness or injury on the body. It, in its entirety, is employed only when all other assessment and care procedures have been performed, most likely during transport to the hospital and then only for patients with serious trauma or disease. Since the seriously ill or injured patients require constant care, this assessment is rarely performed in the prehospital setting. However, portions of the detailed physical exam are frequently employed to examine specific body regions, looking for expected signs of illness or injury.

29. Discuss the components of the detailed physical examination. pp. 692–698

The detailed physical exam involves a comprehensive evaluation of each body region using the skills of inspection, palpation, auscultation, and percussion. It begins at the head and progresses downward to the extremities and includes the following:

Head. Inspect and palpate for any skull or facial asymmetry, deformity, instability, tenderness, unusual warmth, or crepitus. Look for the development of Battle's sign and periorbital ecchymosis.
Eyes. Carefully inspect the eye for shape, size, coloration, and foreign bodies as well as pupillary equality, light reactivity, consensual movement, and visual acuity.
Ears. Examine the external ear for signs of injury and the ear canal for hemorrhage or discharge.
Nose and sinuses. Palpate the external aspect of the nose and examine the nares for signs of injury, hemorrhage, discharge, and flaring. The nasal mucosa is rich in vasculature and may bleed heavily.
Mouth and pharynx. Examine the oral cavity for signs of injury and the potential for airway compromise. Notice any fluids or odors and examine tongue movement for signs of cranial nerve injury.
Neck. Briefly inspect the neck for signs of injury with special attention to open wounds and possible severe hemorrhage and air embolism. Palpate the trachea to identify any unusual movement and examine for jugular vein distention.

Chest and lungs. Observe the patient's breathing for symmetrical chest movement and respiratory pattern. Note any accessory muscle use, and auscultate and percuss for unusual findings. Look for signs of injury, and palpate for crepitus and tenderness.

Cardiovascular system. Look to the skin for pallor, and palpate a pulse for rate, rhythm, and strength. Auscultate for heart sounds, and locate the point of maximal impulse.

Abdomen. Inspect and palpate for signs of injury and rebound tenderness, rigidity, and guarding.

Pelvis. Observe the area, then place medial and posterior pressure on the iliac crests and posterior pressure on the symphysis pubis.

Genitalia. As needed, examine these organs for hemorrhage and, in the male, priapism.

Anus and rectum. If hemorrhage is present, inspect the anus and rectum and apply direct pressure to halt bleeding.

Peripheral vascular system. Inspect all four extremities, observing and palpating for signs of injury and skin color, moisture, temperature, and capillary refill to assure distal circulation.

Musculoskeletal system. Palpate the musculature of the extremities, feeling for differences in muscle tone and the flexibility and the active and passive range of motion in joints.

Nervous system. Evaluate the nervous system by examining the following:

- **Mental status and speech.** Assess the patient's level of consciousness and orientation and compare these findings to earlier ones. Note speech patterns and the patient's appropriateness of dress and actions.
- **Cranial nerves.** Test the discrete cranial nerves that have not already been tested.
- **Motor system.** Inspect the patient's general body structure, positioning, muscular development, and coordination.
- **Sensory system.** Test for ability to sense pain, touch, position, temperature, and vibration over the extremities, and as necessary, the dermatomes.
- **Reflexes.** Test deep tendon reflexes with a reflex hammer, noting heightened or diminished responses. Test superficial abdominal reflexes and plantar response.

Vital signs. Repeat the evaluation of the vital signs including blood pressure, pulse, respiration, temperature, and pupillary response.

30. Explain what additional care is provided while performing the detailed physical exam. pp. 692–698

Since the complete detailed physical exam is an elective assessment, any time a significant sign of injury or the patient's condition suggests a care step, perform that step. The same principle applies when a portion of the comprehensive physical exam is performed on a discrete body region as a part of the focused history and physical exam.

31. Distinguish between the detailed physical exam that is performed on a trauma patient and that of the medical patient. pp. 692–698

The detailed physical exam for the trauma patient focuses evaluation on the areas where signs of injury are expected based upon the mechanism of injury analysis or the patient's complaints (for example, examination for signs of anterior chest injury when an auto steering wheel is deformed). The detailed physical exam for the medical patient is directed to the areas of patient complaint as well as those areas where the signs of an expected illness might be found (for example, an examination for pitting edema in the dependent areas with the congestive heart failure patient). The history component of the assessment also differs with trauma and medical patients. With the trauma patient, you may gather an abbreviated (SAMPLE) history, while with the medical patient, you may perform a more in-depth history evaluation as described in Chapter 10, "History Taking."

32. Differentiate between patients requiring a detailed physical exam and those who do not. p. 692

The patients who receive a complete detailed physical exam are patients with serious medical or trauma injuries. They receive the detailed physical exam during transport to the hospital after other important care measures have been employed. They represent a very small percentage of patients that you will treat because seriously ill or injured patients often require almost continuous care. Portions of the detailed exam will, however, be performed on many patients, and these portions will be directed at a body region where signs of injury or illness are expected. Patients receiving portions of the detailed exam include those with isolated injuries and those patients with stable medical problems. Seriously ill or injured patients may receive a detailed exam aimed at discovering significant signs of the pathology generally associated with cardiac, respiratory, vascular, abdominal, musculoskeletal, or nervous system problems.

33. Discuss the rationale for repeating the initial assessment as part of the ongoing assessment. pp. 698–699, 700

The initial assessment, with its examination of mental status and evaluation of the airway, breathing, and circulation, contains crucial elements of continuing patient assessment. These components of the initial assessment can quickly tell you when the patient is suffering from a life-threatening or serious problem and can help you monitor the patient's need for care. For this reason, these components are an integral part of any ongoing assessment.

34. Describe the components of the ongoing assessment. pp. 698–701

The components of the ongoing assessment include reassessment of the pertinent elements of the initial assessment, focused history and physical exam or rapid trauma assessment, and vital signs and include:

Mental status. Quickly reevaluate the patient's mental status to determine AVPU status or level of orientation.
Airway patency/breathing rate and quality. Perform a quick check of airway patency and breathing rate, volume, and quality to assure respiration is adequate.
Pulse rate and quality. Quickly reevaluate the pulse rate, strength, and regularity to assure they remain within normal limits.
Skin condition. Quickly check the skin for moisture, temperature, and capillary refill to monitor distal perfusion.
Vital signs. Reassess blood pressure and temperature (along with pulse and respiration) and compare to baseline findings to determine whether the patient's condition is improving, deteriorating, or remaining the same.
Focused assessment. Quickly reevaluate the signs of injury/illness to identify any changes. This may include reevaluating pertinent negatives to rule out an evolving problem.
Effects of interventions. Repeat the ongoing assessment soon after any major intervention to determine the intervention's impact on the patient's condition.
Transport priorities. Based upon the findings of the ongoing assessment, either confirm or modify the patient's priority for care and transport.

35. Describe trending of assessment components. pp. 698–701

Trending of the elements of the ongoing assessment—comparing of sequential findings—will suggest whether your patient's condition is improving, deteriorating, or remaining the same. This information prompts you to modify your priorities for patient care and transport, and may ultimately cause you to modify your field diagnosis.

36. Discuss medical identification devices/systems. p. 680

Examine the patient's wrists, ankles, and neck for medical alert jewelry reflecting preexisting medical conditions such as diabetes, epilepsy, allergies, use of medications, and the like. Also check the wallet or purse for such information. This information may help you and the emergency department in prescribing care for the patient.

37. **Given several preprogrammed and moulaged medical and trauma patients, provide the appropriate scene survey, initial assessment, focused assessment, detailed assessment, and ongoing assessments.** pp. 653–701

During your classroom, clinical, and field training, you will assess real and simulated patients and develop management plans for them. Use the information presented in this text chapter, the information on patient assessment in the field presented by your instructors, and the guidance given by your clinical and field preceptors to develop good patient assessment skills. Continue to refine these skills once your training ends and you begin your career as a paramedic.

Content Self-Evaluation

MULTIPLE CHOICE

_____ 1. The focused history and physical exam is conducted differently for the four different categories of patients. Which of the following is NOT one of those categories?
   A. responsive medical patient
   B. unresponsive medical patient
   C. pediatric patient with altered consciousness
   D. trauma patient with an isolated injury
   E. trauma patient with a significant mechanism of injury

_____ 2. Which of the following is NOT a mechanism of injury that calls for rapid transport to the trauma center?
   A. ejection from a vehicle
   B. vehicle rollover
   C. severe vehicle deformity in a high-speed crash
   D. fall from less than 20 feet
   E. bicycle collision with loss of consciousness

_____ 3. The decision to provide rapid transport of a patient to the trauma center is predicated upon either the mechanism of injury or the:
   A. blood pressure reading.
   B. physical signs of trauma.
   C. pulse oximetry reading.
   D. ongoing assessments.
   E. none of the above

_____ 4. If you arrive at your patient's side only moments after the accident, he or she may not have lost enough blood to demonstrate the signs of shock.
   A. True
   B. False

_____ 5. Which of the following body regions is examined during the rapid trauma assessment?
   A. head
   B. neck
   C. pelvis
   D. thorax
   E. all of the above

_____ 6. The "B" of DCAP-BTLS stands for:
   A. burns.
   B. bumps.
   C. blemishes.
   D. bilateral injury.
   E. bruises.

_____ 7. Which of the following is NOT represented within the DCAP-BTLS mnemonic?
   A. contusions
   B. abrasions
   C. burns
   D. crepitus
   E. swelling

_____ 8. Scalp wounds tend to bleed heavily because:
   A. there is a lack of a protective vasospasm mechanism.
   B. the hair helps continue the blood loss.
   C. the close proximity of the skull permits blood to flow quickly outward.
   D. direct pressure is difficult to apply.
   E. both A and C

_____ 9. Subcutaneous emphysema is best described as:
   A. a grating sensation.
   B. air trapped under the skin.
   C. air leaking from the respiratory system.
   D. retraction of the tissues between the ribs.
   E. fluid accumulation just beneath the skin.

_____ 10. Suprasternal and intercostal retractions are caused by:
   A. tension pneumothorax.   D. flail chest.
   B. subcutaneous emphysema.   E. either B or D
   C. airway obstruction or restriction.

_____ 11. To assure adequate air exchange for the patient with a flail chest, you should:
   A. perform a needle decompression.
   B. assist ventilations with a BVM and oxygen.
   C. apply oxygen only.
   D. perform an endotracheal intubation.
   E. cover the wound with an occlusive dressing.

_____ 12. When assessing the pelvis for possible fracture, you should apply:
   A. anterior pressure on the iliac crests.
   B. lateral pressure on the symphysis pubis.
   C. firm pressure on the lower abdomen.
   D. medial and posterior pressure on the iliac crests.
   E. pressure to move the hips to the flexed position.

_____ 13. Your finding that a patient is able to move a limb, but the limb is cool, pale, and without a pulse is consistent with:
   A. neurologic compromise.
   B. vascular compromise.
   C. both a vascular and neurologic compromise.
   D. spinal injury.
   E. peripheral nerve root injury.

_____ 14. The "A" of the SAMPLE history stands for:
   A. alcohol consumption.   D. allergies.
   B. adverse reactions.   E. none of the above
   C. attitude.

_____ 15. With a patient who has a crushing injury to his index finger received when it was caught in a closing door, which form of patient assessment would be most reasonable?
   A. the rapid trauma assessment and a quick history
   B. the rapid trauma assessment and a detailed history
   C. a quick history and a physical exam focused on the injury
   D. a detailed patient history and a physical exam focused on the injury
   E. a detailed physical exam

_____ 16. While gathering the history of a chest pain patient, you will likely:
   A. attach a cardiac monitor.   D. start an IV, if appropriate.
   B. administer oxygen.   E. all of the above
   C. take vital signs.

_____ 17. The pain or discomfort that caused the patient to call you to his or her side is called the:
  A. presenting problem.
  B. differential diagnosis.
  C. field diagnosis.
  D. chief complaint.
  E. present illness.

_____ 18. A patient statement that "deep breathing makes my chest hurt" represents which element of the OPQRST-ASPN mnemonic for investigation of the chief complaint?
  A. O
  B. P
  C. R
  D. S
  E. PN

_____ 19. The jugular veins in a patient with normal cardiovascular function remain full or distended up to which of the following degrees of patient tilt?
  A. 15°
  B. 30°
  C. 45°
  D. 60°
  E. 90°

_____ 20. If you hear bilateral crackles on inspiration when auscultating a patient's chest, you should suspect:
  A. congestive heart failure.
  B. bronchospasm.
  C. asthma.
  D. chronic obstructive pulmonary disease.
  E. all of the above

_____ 21. In a patient who displays hyperresonance to percussion, you should suspect:
  A. pleural effusion.
  B. pulmonary edema.
  C. pneumonia.
  D. emphysema.
  E. none of the above

_____ 22. Examine a patient for unusual pulsation of the descending aorta:
  A. just right of the umbilicus.
  B. just left of the umbilicus.
  C. along a line from the umbilicus to the middle symphysis pubis.
  D. just beneath the zyphoid process.
  E. anywhere in the abdomen.

_____ 23. Accumulation of fluid within the abdominal cavity is common in patients with:
  A. hypovolemia.
  B. aortic aneurysm.
  C. emphysema.
  D. gastric ulcer disease.
  E. cirrhosis of the liver.

_____ 24. A patient in whom unequal pupils are a normal condition displays:
  A. Cullen's sign.
  B. anisocoria.
  C. consensual response.
  D. accommodation.
  E. Bell's palsy.

_____ 25. Vital signs provide the assessing paramedic with:
  A. a window into what is happening with the patient.
  B. an objective capsule of the patient's clinical status.
  C. possible indications of severe illness.
  D. possible indications of the need to intervene.
  E. all of the above

_____ 26. A pulse oximetry reading of 88 percent would indicate the need for:
  A. aggressive airway and ventilatory care.
  B. only the administration of blow-by oxygen.
  C. only some repositioning of the patient's head.
  D. no care at this point.
  E. careful monitoring of the patient for further deterioration.

_____ 27. The type of patient most likely to receive the most comprehensive assessment is:
   A. the severe trauma patient.
   B. the minor trauma patient.
   C. the responsive medical patient.
   D. the unresponsive medical patient.
   E. both A and D

_____ 28. Paramedics employ the complete detailed physical assessment at the scene:
   A. rarely.
   B. occasionally.
   C. frequently.
   D. rarely in trauma patients, frequently in medical patients.
   E. frequently in trauma patients, rarely in medical patients.

_____ 29. Reflexes not likely to be tested during the detailed physical exam are the:
   A. clavicular.
   B. biceps.
   C. triceps.
   D. Achilles.
   E. abdominal plantar.

_____ 30. Serial ongoing assessments will facilitate:
   A. reassessment of the patient.
   B. revision of the field diagnosis.
   C. changes in the management plan.
   D. documentation of the effects of interventions.
   E. all of the above

Clinical Decision Making

Review of Chapter Objectives

After reading this chapter, you should be able to:

1. **Compare the factors influencing medical care in the out-of-hospital environment to other medical settings.** p. 706

   Most health care providers function in very controlled and supportive environments. The paramedic carries out the skills of other health care providers, but he often does so in hostile and adverse conditions. Paramedics perform assessments, form field diagnoses, and devise and employ patient management plans at the scenes of emergencies in spite of poor weather, limited ambient light, limited diagnostic equipment, and few support personnel. The paramedic also must perform these skills under extreme constraints of time and often without on-scene consultation and supervision.

2. **Differentiate between critical life-threatening, potentially life-threatening, and non-life-threatening patient presentations.** p. 706

   Critical life-threatening presentations include major multisystem trauma, devastating single system trauma, end-stage disease presentations, and acute presentations of chronic disease. These patients may present with airway, breathing, neurological, or circulatory (shock) problems and demand aggressive resuscitation.

   Potential life-threatening presentations include serious multisystem trauma and multiple disease etiologies. Patient presentation generally includes moderate to serious distress. The care required is sometimes invasive but generally supportive.

   Non-life-threatening presentations are isolated and uncomplicated minor injuries or illness. The patient is stable without serious signs or symptoms or the need for aggressive intervention.

3. **Evaluate the benefits and shortfalls of protocols, standing orders, and patient care algorithms.** pp. 706–707

   Protocols are written guidelines identifying the specific management of various medical and trauma patient problems. They may also be developed for special situations such as physician-on-the-scene, radio failure, and termination of resuscitation. They provide a standard care approach for patients with "classical" presentations. They do not apply to all patients or to patients who present with multiple problems and should not be adhered to so rigidly as to limit performance in unusual circumstances.

   Standing orders are protocols that a paramedic can perform before direct on-line communication with a medical direction physician. They speed emergency care but may not address the atypical patient.

Patient care algorithms are flowcharts with lines, arrows, and boxes that outline appropriate care measures based on patient presentation or response to care. They are generally useful guides and encourage uniform patient care, but again, they do not adequately address the atypical patient.

4. **Define the components, stages, and sequences of the critical thinking process for paramedics.** pp. 708–714

   Components of critical thinking include the following:

   Knowledge and Abilities
   Knowledge and abilities comprise the first component of critical thinking. Your knowledge of prehospital emergency care is the basis for your decisions in the field. This knowledge comes from your classroom, clinical, and field experience. It is used to sort out your patient's presentation to determine the likely cause of the problem and to select the appropriate care skills. Your abilities are the technical skills you employ to assess or care for a patient.

   Useful Thinking Styles

   - **Reflective versus Impulsive Situation Analysis.** Reflective analysis refers to taking time to deliberately and analytically contemplate possible patient care, as might occur with unknown medical illness. Impulsive analysis refers to the immediate response that the paramedic must provide in a life-threatening situation, as might be required with decompensating shock or cardiac arrest.
   - **Divergent versus Convergent Data Processing.** Divergent data processing considers all aspects of a situation before arriving at a solution and is most useful with complex situations. Convergent data processing focuses narrowly on the most important aspects of a situation and is best suited for uncomplicated situations that require little reflection.
   - **Anticipatory versus Reactive Decision Making.** With anticipatory decision making, you respond to what you think may happen to your patient. With reactive decision making, you provide a care modality once the patient presents with a symptom.

   Thinking under Pressure
   Thinking under pressure is a difficult but frequent challenge of prehospital emergency medicine. The "fight-or-flight" response may diminish your ability to think critically to such an extent that you are only able to respond at the pseudo-instinctive level, with preplanned and practiced responses (like the mental checklist) that are performed almost without thought. One example of a mental checklist includes the following steps:

   Scan the situation by standing back and looking for subtle clues to the patient's complaint or problem.
   Stop and think of both the possible benefits and side effects of each of your care interventions.
   Decide and act by executing your chosen care plan with confidence and authority.
   Maintain control of the scene, patient care, and your own emotions, even under the stress of a chaotic scene.
   Reevaluate your patient's signs and symptoms and your associated care plan and make changes as the situation changes.

5. **Apply the fundamental elements of critical thinking for paramedics.** pp. 711–714

   - **Form a concept.** Gather enough information from your first view of the patient and scene size-up to form a general impression of the patient's condition and the likely cause.
   - **Interpret the data.** Perform the patient assessment and analyze the results in light of your previous assessment and care experience. Form a field diagnosis.
   - **Apply the principles.** With the field diagnosis in mind, devise a management plan to care for the patient according to your protocols, standing orders, and patient care algorithms.
   - **Evaluate.** Through frequent ongoing assessments, reassess the patient's condition and the effects of your interventions.
   - **Reflect.** After the call, critique your call with the emergency department staff and your crew to determine what steps might be improved and add this call to your experience base.

6. Describe the effects of the "fight-or-flight" response and its positive and negative effects on a paramedic's decision making. p. 710

The "fight-or-flight" response is the intense activation of the sympathetic branch of the autonomic nervous system. Secretion of the system's major hormone, epinephrine, causes an increase in heart rate and cardiac output. It raises respiratory rate and volume, directs blood to the skeletal muscles, dilates the pupils (for distant vision), and increases hearing perception. However, the increased epinephrine may diminish critical thinking ability and concentration, impairing your ability to perform well in an emergency unless you raise your assessment and care skills to a pseudo-instinctive level, at which point acting under the pressure of an emergency becomes second nature.

7. Summarize the "six Rs" of putting it all together. pp. 713–714

- **Read the patient.** Observe, palpate, auscultate, smell, and listen to the patient for signs and symptoms. Assure the ABCs and obtain a set of vital signs.
- **Read the scene.** Observe the scene or general environment for clues to the mechanism of injury or nature of the illness.
- **React.** Address the priorities of care from the ABCs to other critical, then serious, then minor problems and care priorities.
- **Reevaluate.** Conduct frequent ongoing assessments to identify any changes caused either by the disease or by your interventions.
- **Revise the management plan.** Based on the ongoing assessments, revise your management plan to best serve your patient's changing condition.
- **Review performance.** At the end of every response, critique the performance of your crew and identify ways to improve future responses.

8. Given several preprogrammed and moulaged trauma and medical patients, demonstrate clinical decision making. pp. 705–714

With your classroom, clinical, and field experience, you will assess and develop a management plan for the real and simulated patients you attend. Use the information presented in this text chapter, the information on clinical decision making presented by your instructors, and the guidance given by your clinical and field preceptors to develop good clinical decision-making skills. Continue to refine these skills once your training ends and you begin your career as a paramedic.

Content Self-Evaluation

MULTIPLE CHOICE

_____ 1. Which of the following terms best describes the first paramedics of the 1970s?
   A. field technician
   B. prehospital emergency care practitioner
   C. orderly
   D. field attendant
   E. field aide

_____ 2. The term describing the severity of a patient's condition is:
   A. multiparity.
   B. epiphysis.
   C. tonicity.
   D. acuity.
   E. declivity.

_____ 3. The paramedic's final determination of the patient's most likely primary problem is know as the:
   A. field diagnosis.
   B. differential field diagnosis.
   C. chief complaint.
   D. improvisation.
   E. standing order.

_____ 4. Which of the following is NOT a level of patient acuity?
   A. life-threatening condition
   B. non-life-threatening condition
   C. potential non-life-threatening condition
   D. potential life-threatening condition
   E. both A and B

_____ 5. Which patient acuity level presents the greatest challenge to the paramedic's critical thinking skills?
   A. life-threatening condition
   B. non-life-threatening condition
   C. potential non-life-threatening condition
   D. potential life-threatening condition
   E. B and C equally

_____ 6. Which of the following terms represents a flowchart of patient care procedures?
   A. protocol
   B. standing order
   C. algorithm
   D. special care enhancement
   E. proviso

_____ 7. A policy of administering nitroglycerin to a cardiac chest pain patient is an example of a(n):
   A. protocol.
   B. standing order.
   C. algorithm.
   D. special care enhancement.
   E. proviso.

_____ 8. A policy by which nitroglycerin can be administered to a cardiac chest pain patient without a physician's order is an example of a(n):
   A. protocol.
   B. standing order.
   C. algorithm.
   D. special enhancement.
   E. proviso.

_____ 9. The major disadvantage to the use of protocols and standing orders is that they:
   A. apply only to atypical patients.
   B. often do not permit the paramedic to adapt to a patient's unique presentation.
   C. only cover multiple disease etiologies.
   D. address only patients with vague presentations.
   E. none of the above

_____ 10. In the case where a particular protocol does not seem to fit the patient presentation, you should contact the medical direction physician for advice and direction regarding your patient's care.
   A. True
   B. False

_____ 11. The data-processing style that focuses on the most important aspect of a critical situation is:
   A. reflective.
   B. impulsive.
   C. divergent.
   D. convergent.
   E. anticipatory.

_____ 12. The style of situation analysis that causes you to respond instinctively to a situation rather than to think about it is:
   A. reflective.
   B. impulsive.
   C. divergent.
   D. convergent.
   E. anticipatory.

_____ 13. One way to remain in control in otherwise extremely stressful situations is to learn to perform technical skills at a pseudo-instinctive level.
   A. True
   B. False

_____ 14. Which of the following is NOT a step in the critical decision-making process?
   A. forming a concept
   B. interpreting the data
   C. applying the principles
   D. evaluating the result
   E. evaluating the interventions

_____ 15. Which of the following is NOT an element of the six "Rs" of critical decision making?
   A. reading the scene
   B. researching the management plan
   C. reacting
   D. reading the patient
   E. reevaluating

MATCHING

Write the letter of the step in the critical decision-making process in the space provided next to the emergency response action appropriate for that step.

A. Form a concept.

B. Interpret the data.

C. Apply the principles.

D. Evaluate.

E. Reflect.

_____ 16. Field diagnosis

_____ 17. Provide ongoing assessment

_____ 18. Perform the focused physical exam

_____ 19. Pulse oximetry

_____ 20. Follow standing orders

_____ 21. Differential diagnosis

_____ 22. Assess MS-ABCs

_____ 23. Employ protocols

_____ 24. Determine the initial vital signs

_____ 25. Determine if treatment is improving the patient's condition

Chapter 14

Communications

Review of Chapter Objectives

After reading this chapter, you should be able to:

1. **Identify the role and importance of verbal, written, and electronic communications in the provision of EMS.** pp. 718–719, 726–730

   EMS is a team endeavor that requires effective communications among the various participants in the response and patient care. This communication is between you and the emergency dispatcher, the patient, his family, bystanders, other emergency response personnel, such as police, fire, and rescue personnel, and health care professionals from physicians' offices, clinics, and emergency departments, and finally with the medical direction physician. These communications, be they oral, written, or electronic, establish the key links that assure the best patient outcome.

2. **Describe the phases of communications necessary to complete a typical EMS response.**

   Detection and citizen access pp. 720–726
   This marks the initial entry point into the emergency service system at which a party identifies that an emergency exists and then requests EMS assistance through a universal entry number such as 911 or some other mechanism.

   Call taking p. 724
   This is the stage of EMS response in which a call taker questions the caller about the reported emergency in order to identify its exact location, determine the nature of the call, and initiate an appropriate response.

   Emergency response p. 724
   This phase includes the activities occurring from the moment a dispatcher requests a response by an EMS unit until the call concludes with the unit back in service. It includes various radio, face-to-face, and written communications among the dispatcher, emergency response crews, the patient, family and bystanders, and health care professionals, including the medical direction physician.

   Prearrival instructions pp. 724–725
   These are a series of predetermined, medically approved instructions given by the dispatcher to the caller to help the caller provide some patient support until EMS personnel arrive.

   Call coordination and incident recording p. 725
   These terms refer to the interactions between the dispatcher and the responding units that assure an efficient and appropriate response. Call coordinating, for example, might involve changing the mode of response and the number and type of responding units. Incident recording refers to the

logging of times associated with various response activities and the tape recording of communications associated with the call.

Discussion with medical direction   pp. 720–726

This is the opportunity for the care provider to describe the patient he or she is caring for and to obtain approval from the medical direction physician to initiate invasive or advanced life support procedures. Communication with medical direction also permits the emergency department to prepare for the patient's arrival.

Transfer communications   pp. 720–726

These are the communications that occur between the first responder and the paramedic or as the patient is delivered to the emergency department. They are intended to communicate the results of the assessment, the care given, and the patient's response to care prior to the arrival of the paramedic or on arrival at the emergency department.

3. List factors that impede and enhance effective verbal and written communications.   pp. 718–719

The factors impacting effective verbal or written communications are either semantic (dealing with the meaning of words) or technical (hardware).

In the area of semantics, the use of standard codes and plain English in verbal communications enhances good and clear communications, while use of nonstandard codes and jargon may confuse it. The same holds true for written communication. Nonstandard abbreviations and subjective, sloppy, incomplete, or illegible documentation leads to confusion and miscommunication. Complete, objective, legible, and efficient documentation leads to an efficient transfer of information. A well-designed prehospital care report makes written communication easier.

In the technical area, a well-designed and maintained radio or phone communications system will go a long way in assuring good and dependable communications. Improperly maintained or operated radios will, on the other hand, likely provide only intermittent and poor-quality communication.

4. Explain the value of data collection during an EMS response.   pp. 718–719, 730

The written call report is a record that includes the patient's name and address, scene location, agency responding, crew on board, and the times associated with response, arrival, and transport to a care facility. It also contains the results of the assessment and care of the patient. This administrative information can be used to bill for services and improve EMS system efficiency, by quality assurance/improvement committees to improve system performance, and by educators and researchers to identify what the system is doing and the impacts of its interventions. Finally, the call report becomes a legal record of the incident and the EMS care provided or offered.

5. Recognize the legal status of verbal, written, and electronic communications related to an EMS response.   pp. 718–719, 732–733

The legal guidelines that apply to verbal and written communication in emergency medical service also apply to electronic communications. The information in these communications is considered confidential and must only be released in approved circumstances. The reports must be objective and not demean, libel, or slander another person. Any such action is accountable in a court of law.

6. Identify current technology used to collect and exchange patient and/or scene information electronically.   pp. 726–730

Cellular phones today provide duplex communications directly from the patient's side to the emergency department. These lightweight and versatile devices enhance EMS-to-physician communications and permit excellent ECG transmission. The only disadvantages to cell phones are user fees and unreliability at peak times.

Another electronic aid to dispatch is the facsimile or fax machine. It permits dispatch to send hard copy to the responding unit's station, assuring that elements of the address and nature of the dispatch are communicated accurately.

Computers are also increasing the efficiency of the dispatch system by recording times and system action in real time and making data recovery and research much easier.

Other new technologies that may affect prehospital care include: the electronic touch pad, which allows rapid recording of patient information; the handheld computer, which uses a pen-based system to log patient information and times associated with the emergency response and care; electronic transmission of diagnostic information (including pulse oximetry, 12-lead ECG, blood sugar, and end-expiratory CO_2 monitoring) provided directly to the emergency department, which may change the degree and number of field interventions permitted. In the future, voice recognition software may make real-time narrative recording of patient evaluation and interventions at the emergency scene and during transport a reality.

7. **Identify the various components of the EMS communications system and describe their function and use.** pp. 717–718, 720–726

The Emergency Medical Dispatcher (EMD) is the person who takes the call for assistance, dispatches the appropriate units, monitors the call's progress, and assures that the pertinent response data is recorded. He or she may guide the caller through initial emergency care using prearrival instructions.

The patient, his family, and bystanders are responsible for detecting the emergency, accessing the emergency response system, and relaying information about the cause and nature of the emergency to EMS system personnel. Since they are not trained in emergency medical communication, the responsibility of assuring good communications falls on the members of the EMS system.

Personnel from other responding agencies such as the police, fire service, rescue, and other ambulance services are also individuals who provide information important to assuring proper EMS response, and their input must be taken into account to assure scene coordination and optimum utilization of resources.

Health care professionals (aides, nurses, physician assistants, nurse practitioners, and physicians) at clinics, physicians' offices, and emergency departments are important people in the EMS system. They can provide invaluable information about the patient and the care he or she has had or should receive.

Finally, the medical director and medical direction physicians are significant resources for the prehospital emergency care provider. They are the individuals who extend their licenses to paramedics, thereby permitting them to practice prehospital care. These physicians also represent a body of knowledge of emergency medicine that may be tapped while paramedics are at the scene, en route with a patient, or at the emergency department for guidance regarding patient care.

8. **Identify and differentiate among the following communications systems:**

Simplex p. 727

This refers to a radio or communication system that uses only one frequency and allows only one unit to transmit at a time. With this type of communication, one party must wait until the speaking party completes his message before beginning to speak.

Duplex p. 727

This is a radio or communication system that uses two frequencies for each channel, thus permitting two units to transmit and listen at the same time. This is similar to telephone communication, where one party can interrupt the other.

Multiplex p. 727

This is a duplex system with an additional capability of transmitting data, like an ECG strip, simultaneously with voice.

Trunked   p. 728
These are computer-controlled systems that pool all radio frequencies and assign transmissions to unused frequencies to assure the most efficient use of available communications channels.

Digital communications   p. 728
These systems translate analog sounds into digital code for transmissions that are less prone to interference and are more compact than analog (normal voice) communications. This type of a system can be enhanced with devices like the mobile data terminal, which displays information such as street addresses, and can prompt the responder to send information like "arrived."

Cellular telephone   pp. 728–729
These are part of a multiplex radio-telephone system tied to a computer that uses radio towers to transmit signals in regions called cells. The technology is inexpensive but can accrue substantial monthly charges; the transmissions may be interrupted by certain geographic features; and heavy use at peak times may limit access to the system.

Facsimile   p. 729
These devices transmit and receive printed information through telephone or wireless communication systems. Such a machine might give a responding unit a printout of the nature and street address of the call or, possibly, detailed medical information about it.

Computer   p. 729
The use of these devices in EMS is expanding rapidly. They are already helping to analyze data for review of calls and dispatches. Portable input devices, such as the touch pad and handheld computer, are being developed to permit recording of emergency response events in the field. In the future, paramedics may use computers with voice recognition software to complete prehospital care reports without paper.

9. **Describe the functions and responsibilities of the Federal Communications Commission.**   pp. 732–733

   The Federal Communications Commission (FCC) controls and regulates all nongovernmental communications in the United States. It assigns broadcast frequencies and has set aside several frequencies within each radio bandwidth for emergency medical services. The commission also establishes technical standards for radio equipment, licenses and regulates people who repair radios, monitors frequencies for appropriate usage, and checks base stations and dispatch centers for appropriate licenses and records.

10. **Describe the role of emergency medical dispatch and the importance of prearrival instructions in a typical EMS response.**   pp. 732–733

    The Emergency Medical Dispatcher (EMD) is the first person in the EMS system who communicates with the scene and possibly the patient. He or she begins and coordinates the EMS response and communications and assures data regarding the call are recorded. He or she also provides prearrival instructions to callers—for example, how to perform mouth-to-mouth artificial ventilation on an apneic patient—so that emergency care can begin as early as possible, thus helping to maintain the victim until trained prehospital personnel can arrive.

11. **List appropriate caller information gathered by the Emergency Medical Dispatcher.**   p. 724

    The information that is gathered by the EMD to determine the response priority and that is then communicated to the appropriate responding EMS service includes:

    - Caller's name
    - Call-back number

- Location or address of the event
- Nature of the call
- Any additional information necessary to prioritize the call

12. Describe the structure and importance of verbal patient information communication to the hospital and medical direction. pp. 730–732

The verbal patient report to hospital personnel and the medical direction physician is essential to assure the efficient transfer and continuity of care. It consists of the following:

- Information identifying the care provider and level of training
- Patient identification information (name, age, sex, and so on)
- Subjective patient data (chief complaint, additional symptoms, past history, and so on)
- Objective patient data (vital signs, pulse oximetry readings, and so on)
- Plan for care of patient

For the trauma patient, the information and order of presentation is the same, although the subjective and objective information are modified to include mechanism of injury and suspected injuries.

13. Diagram a basic communications system. pp. 718–719

Basic communication is the process of exchanging information between individuals. A model for a communications system should start with an idea, followed by the encoding of that idea into useful language, sending the encoded message via a medium (direct voice, radio, or written), having another person receive and decode the message, and ultimately, receiving feedback from the original message.

14. Given several narrative patient scenarios, organize a verbal radio report for electronic transmission to medical direction. pp. 717–733

During your classroom, clinical, and field training, you will communicate with various elements of the EMS system, including dispatchers, patients, family members, bystanders, other EMS and scene personnel, and health care professionals, including medical direction physicians. Use the information presented in this text chapter, the information on communication presented by your instructors, and the guidance given by your clinical and field preceptors to develop good communication skills. Continue to refine these skills once your training ends and you begin your career as a paramedic.

Content Self-Evaluation

MULTIPLE CHOICE

_____ 1. Essential participants in communications within the EMS system include:
   A. the emergency medical dispatcher.
   B. the patient, his family, or bystanders.
   C. other responders, including police, fire, and other ambulance personnel.
   D. health care providers, including nurses, physicians, and medical direction physicians.
   E. all of the above

_____ 2. In general, the use of codes decreases the radio time and increases the recipient's understanding of the message, which has led many EMS systems to adopt extensive use of codes for their communications.
   A. True
   B. False

_____ 3. A radio band is a:
   A. series of radios that communicate one with another.
   B. pair of radio frequencies used for multiplexing.
   C. range of radio frequencies.
   D. pair of radio frequencies used for duplexing.
   E. none of the above

_____ 4. Use of proper terminology in both written and verbal communications will:
   A. decrease the length of communications.
   B. increase the accuracy of communications.
   C. increase the clarity of communications.
   D. reduce the ambiguity in communications.
   E. all of the above

_____ 5. Features of the enhanced 911 center include all of the following EXCEPT:
   A. display of the caller's location.
   B. display of the caller's phone number.
   C. immediate call-back ability.
   D. a system of physician/ambulance interface.
   E. both B and C

_____ 6. The answering center for emergency calls that then transfers them to the appropriate agency for dispatch is the:
   A. enhanced 911 center.
   B. PSAP.
   C. GPS.
   D. Emergency Routing Center.
   E. none of the above

_____ 7. Most current wireless phones do not provide the PSAP with the phone's location and call-back number.
   A. True
   B. False

_____ 8. Which system below may identify the exact location of a wireless phone?
   A. geographic triangulation
   B. landline induction
   C. global positioning system
   D. either A or C
   E. none of the above

_____ 9. Terrestrial-based triangulation of a wireless phone's location is dependent on which of the following?
   A. signal strength
   B. height of the wireless phone antenna
   C. three towers receiving the signal
   D. the proximity of the PSAP
   E. both A and C

_____ 10. The Enhanced 911 center may soon be notified of a vehicle collision, the forces involved, and its location through which of the following technological enhancements?
   A. ANI
   B. ALI
   C. CAN
   D. PSAP
   E. none of the above

_____ 11. In the future, which of the following may be communicated to the dispatch center from a vehicle involved in a collision?
   A. the exact location of the incident
   B. a change in velocity of the collision
   C. the vehicle identification number
   D. the crash-worthiness rating of the vehicle involved
   E. all of the above

_____ 12. The system that uses standardized caller questioning to determine the level and type of response is:
   A. priority dispatching.
   B. system status management.
   C. enhanced emergency medical dispatch.
   D. prearrival instructions packaging.
   E. dispatch triage.

_____ 13. The role of the modern-day Emergency Medical Dispatcher includes:
   A. priority dispatching.
   B. prearrival instructions.
   C. call coordinating.
   D. incident recording.
   E. all of the above

_____ 14. The report that occurs as you transfer patient responsibilities to the emergency department staff must include:
   A. chief complaint.
   B. assessment findings.
   C. care rendered.
   D. results of care.
   E. all of the above

_____ 15. A radio system that transmits and receives on the same frequency is called:
   A. simplex.
   B. duplex.
   C. triplex.
   D. multiplex.
   E. none of the above

_____ 16. Which radio transmission design permits the receiver to interrupt the caller while the caller is talking?
   A. simplex
   B. duplex
   C. multiplex
   D. trunking
   E. none of the above

_____ 17. The radio system that uses a computer to determine and assign available frequencies is called:
   A. simplex.
   B. duplex.
   C. multiplex.
   D. trunking.
   E. none of the above

_____ 18. Advantages of cellular communications in EMS include all of the following EXCEPT:
   A. duplex capability.
   B. allowing direct physician/patient communication.
   C. ability to handle an unlimited number of calls.
   D. reduced on-line times.
   E. transmission of better ECG signals.

_____ 19. One of the paramedic's most important skills is gathering essential patient information, organizing it, and communicating it to the medical direction physician.
   A. True
   B. False

_____ 20. A standard format for transmitting patient information assures all of the following EXCEPT:
   A. communication efficiency.
   B. physician assimilation of patient condition information.
   C. completeness of medical information.
   D. easier use of multiplex signals.
   E. both A and C

_____ 21. All of the following are appropriate for good EMS communications EXCEPT:
   A. speaking close to the microphone.
   B. speaking across or directly into the microphone.
   C. talking in a normal tone of voice.
   D. speaking without emotion.
   E. taking time to explain everything in detail.

_____ 22. It is important to press the microphone button for one second before speaking.
   A. True
   B. False

_____ 23. If the portable radio you are using is unable to transmit well from your location, attempt to:
   A. move to higher ground.
   B. touch the antenna to something metal.
   C. move towards a window or away from structural steel.
   D. both A and C
   E. none of the above

_____ 24. The major difference between the medical and trauma patient reports is that the trauma format provides a description of the mechanism of injury and identifies suspected injuries.
   A. True
   B. False

_____ 25. The Federal Communications Commission is responsible for all of the following below EXCEPT:
   A. assigning and licensing radio frequencies.
   B. establishing technical standards for radio equipment.
   C. assuring the proper use of medical terminology in radio communications.
   D. monitoring radio frequencies for proper use.
   E. spot-checking radio base stations for proper licensing and records.

Chapter 15

Documentation

Review of Chapter Objectives

After reading this chapter, you should be able to:

1. **Identify the general principles regarding the importance of EMS documentation and ways in which documents are used.** pp. 736–738

   The principal EMS document, the prehospital care report (PCR), is the sole permanent written documentation of the response, assessment, care, and transport offered during an emergency call. It is a medical document conveying details of medical care and patient history that remains a part of the patient record as well as a legal document that may be reviewed in a court of law. The PCR may also be reviewed by medical direction to determine the appropriateness of your actions during the call and used by your service to bill the patient for services. Lastly, the PCR may be used by researchers to determine the effectiveness of care measures in improving patient outcomes.

2. **Identify and properly use medical terminology, medical abbreviations, and acronyms.** pp. 738, 740–743

   Medical terminology is the very precise and exact wording used to describe the human body and injuries or illnesses. Proper use of this terminology turns the PCR into a medical document. However, if terms are misspelled or misused, they may distract from the document and confuse the reader about the patient's condition and the care he either has had or should receive. Carry a pocket dictionary, and only use words when you are sure of both their spelling and usage. The same holds true of medical abbreviations. They must be applied properly and have the same meaning to both the writer and reader. EMS systems should use a standardized set of abbreviations and acronyms to assure good and efficient documentation.

3. **Explain the role of documentation in agency reimbursement.** p. 737

   Good documentation is essential for ambulance agencies that bill for services they provide. The PCR provides the name and address of the patient as well as the nature and circumstances of injury and illness. It also includes the care and transport provided. Without this information, the service may not be able to obtain reimbursement for services rendered and, ultimately, to afford to provide the vehicle, equipment, and personnel necessary to provide prehospital emergency care.

4. **Identify and eliminate extraneous or nonprofessional information.** pp. 747–748

   The ambulance call should be documented in a brief and professional way. The PCR describing it may be scrutinized by hospital staff, the medical direction physician, quality improvement committees, supervisors, lawyers, and the news media. Any derogatory comments, jargon, slang, biased statements, irrelevant opinions, or libelous statements will distract from the seriousness of the document and from acceptance of the preparer's professionalism.

5. Describe the differences between subjective and objective elements of documentation. pp. 748–749

Subjective information is information that you obtain from others or is your opinion that is not based on observable facts. It includes the patient's, family's, or bystander's description of the chief complaint and symptoms, medical history, and nature of the illness or mechanism of injury.

Objective information is information you obtain through direct observation, palpation, auscultation, percussion, or diagnostic evaluation of your patient. It includes the vital signs and the results of the physical exam, including such things as glucose level determination and ECG monitor and pulse oximeter readings.

6. Evaluate a finished document for errors and omissions and proper use and spelling of abbreviations and acronyms. pp. 745, 747–748

The PCR must contain all information obtainable and necessary for describing the patient's condition recorded in a clearly legible way. The report must be written so that another health care provider can easily understand what is being said and can mentally picture the scene, the patient presentation, the care rendered, and the transport offered by the initial providers. In many cases, what to include in the PCR is a judgment decision made by the care provider, though the report must contain an accurate description of the patient's medical or trauma problem and an accurate and complete history. Correct spelling and use of medical terms is essential and reflects the knowledge of the care provider. Proper use of abbreviations and acronyms can help make the PCR more concise; their improper use, however, may produce ambiguity, confusion, and misunderstanding in readers. Reread the finished PCR and check it carefully before submitting it.

7. Evaluate the confidential nature of an EMS report. p. 756

Confidentiality is a patient right and breaching it can result in severe consequences. Do not discuss or share patient or call information with anyone not involved in the care of the patient. The only exceptions—as necessary—are administration, which may need information for billing; police agencies carrying out a criminal investigation; requests for the information under subpoena from a court; and quality assurance committees that may need the information (with the patient's name blocked out) for system review and improvement or for research.

8. Describe the potential consequences of illegible, incomplete, or inaccurate documentation. pp. 745, 747–748

A legible, complete, and accurate PCR is essential to call documentation. The information in it must be easy to read thanks to both good penmanship and conscientious attention to detail. The report must describe all the pertinent information gathered at the scene and en route to the hospital as well as all actions taken by you and others in the care of the patient. Failure to create a thorough, readable PCR reduces the information available to other caregivers and may reduce their ability to provide effective care. The document you produce also reflects on your ability to provide assessment and care and your professionalism in general.

9. Describe the special documentation considerations concerning patient refusal of care and/or transport. pp. 753–754

Be careful in the documentation of a patient who refuses care and/or transport. While a conscious and mentally competent patient has the right to refuse care, his doing so may pose legal problems for care providers. Document the nature and severity of the patient's injuries, any care you offered, any care he refused, and document carefully the assessment criteria you used to determine the patient was capable of making the decision to refuse care or transport. Also document the patient's reasons for refusing care and your efforts to convince him to change his mind. If possible, have the refusal of care and your explanation to the patient of the consequences of care refusal signed by the patient and witnessed by family or bystanders or police. Advise the patient to seek other medical help, like his family physician, and to call EMS again if he changes his mind or his condition worsens.

10. Demonstrate how to properly record direct patient or bystander comments. p. 744

Direct statements by patients and bystanders must be recorded exactly as they were made and the key phrases placed in quotation marks. Treating the information this way is highly important because it identifies that the information is directly from the source, not an interpretation. Identify clearly the source of any quotation you include in a PCR.

11. Describe the special considerations concerning mass casualty incident documentation. p. 755

Often a mass casualty situation calls for an atypical EMS response and unusual documentation procedures. Care providers rarely stay with a patient from the beginning to the end of prehospital care, and the time spent at a patient's side is very much at a premium. Hence, documentation must be efficient and incremental. Document your assessment findings and any interventions you perform at the patient's side quickly and clearly. Many agencies or systems have their own forms such as triage tags that simplify the documentation procedure.

12. Demonstrate proper document revision and correction. p. 747

Everyone makes mistakes during a health care career and during the process of care documentation. When this happens, it is essential to make corrections in such a way that there is no appearance of impropriety. If an error is made, draw a single line through the error and enter the correction and your initials. If the error is noted after the report is turned in, write a narrative addendum explaining both the nature of the error and the needed correction and assure that the addendum is included with all copies of the PCR. Correct errors as soon as possible after they are discovered.

13. Given a prehospital care report form and a narrative patient care scenario, record all pertinent administrative information using a consistent format; identify and record the pertinent, reportable clinical data for each patient; correct errors and omissions, using proper procedures; and note and record "pertinent negative" clinical findings. pp. 736–756

During your classroom, clinical, and field training, you will complete various reports, including prehospital care reports, on the real and simulated patients you attend. Use the information presented in this text chapter, the information on documentation presented by your instructors, and the guidance given by your clinical and field preceptors to develop good documentation skills. Continue to refine these skills once your training ends and you begin your career as a paramedic.

Content Self-Evaluation

MULTIPLE CHOICE

1. The prehospital care report is likely to be reviewed by which of the following?
   A. researchers
   B. EMS administrators
   C. lawyers
   D. medical professionals
   E. all of the above

_____ 2. Which of the following is NOT an appropriate purpose for reviewing a prehospital care report?
   A. to identify a chronological account of the patient's mental status
   B. to learn about what calls other paramedics had
   C. to help detect patient improvement or deterioration
   D. to identify what bystanders and family may have said at the scene
   E. to determine baseline assessment findings

_____ 3. The prehospital care report may yield information that the quality improvement committee may use to identify problems with individual paramedics or with the EMS system.
   A. True
   B. False

_____ 4. The prehospital care report should contain all of the following EXCEPT:
   A. a description of your patient's condition when you arrived.
   B. your opinions about the patient's attitude or social/economic situation.
   C. a description of your patient's condition after interventions.
   D. the medical status of your patient upon arrival at the emergency department.
   E. response time to the call.

_____ 5. If you have doubts about the spelling of a term when completing a PCR, use a phonetically close spelling; doing this may still convey the right meaning and will not reflect poorly on your professionalism.
   A. True
   B. False

_____ 6. Which of the following is NOT a time commonly recorded on the prehospital care report?
   A. call received
   B. dispatch time
   C. arrival at the patient's side
   D. arrival at the scene
   E. departure from the scene

_____ 7. Since your watch, the dispatch clock, and other timing devices are not often synchronized, it is important to record all times on the PCR care report from one clock or watch when possible or to indicate when different clocks are used.
   A. True
   B. False

_____ 8. Which of the following is NOT an example of a pertinent negative?
   A. no shortness of breath in a myocardial infarction patient
   B. no history of epilepsy in seizing patient
   C. clear breath sounds in a congestive heart failure patient
   D. a blood pressure of 90/60
   E. no jugular vein distention in a congestive heart failure patient

_____ 9. The recommended way of indicating the exact words spoken by a patient or bystander is to:
   A. underline the passage.
   B. draw one line through the center of the word or passage.
   C. begin and end the passage with quotation marks.
   D. place the passage in parentheses.
   E. none of the above

_____ 10. All of the following describe good documentation EXCEPT:
   A. complete.
   B. altered.
   C. accurate.
   D. objective.
   E. legible.

_____ 11. The PCR is created by the paramedic as a personal record of what happened at the scene and during transport and thus its legibility to others is not important.
   A. True
   B. False

_____ 12. The benefit of check boxes on a prehospital care report is that they:
   A. assure common information is recorded for every call.
   B. eliminate the need for a patient narrative.
   C. address every chief complaint.
   D. speed the completion of the narrative.
   E. all of the above

_____ 13. When should the prehospital care report be completed?
   A. at the end of the day
   B. at the end of your duty shift
   C. once back at quarters
   D. shortly after leaving the hospital
   E. upon or shortly after transferring patient care at the hospital

_____ 14. Whenever possible, have all members of your crew read or reread the prehospital care report before you submit it.
   A. True
   B. False

_____ 15. What is the best way to add additional information to the prehospital care report after it has been submitted to the hospital?
   A. Search and make changes on all copies.
   B. Change only the original report.
   C. Create an addendum and add it to all reports.
   D. Never add additional material to the report once distributed.
   E. Send a memorandum to medical control.

_____ 16. Use of professional jargon in the PCR is an indicator of the writer's professionalism.
   A. True
   B. False

_____ 17. Which of the following is the best example of a subjective and possibly libelous statement?
   A. "The patient smelled of beer."
   B. "The patient walked with a staggering gait."
   C. "The patient used abusive language and spoke with slurred speech."
   D. "The patient was drunk and obnoxious."
   E. None of the above is a potentially libelous statement.

_____ 18. Which of the following is a part of the subjective patient information?
   A. chief complaint
   B. past medical history
   C. history of the current medical problem
   D. patient's description of what happened
   E. all of the above

_____ 19. The portion of your narrative report that contains your general impression of the patient is the:
   A. subjective narrative.
   B. objective narrative.
   C. assessment/management plan.
   D. SOAP plan.
   E. none of the above

_____ 20. You should document a pediatric assessment in head-to-toe order, even though you may have performed it from toe-to-head.
   A. True
   B. False

_____ 21. Which of the following is true about the body systems method of assessment?
   A. It focuses on body systems rather than body areas.
   B. It usually addresses only the system(s) affected.
   C. It is best suited to screening and preadmission exams.
   D. It can be a comprehensive approach to documentation.
   E. all of the above

_____ 22. The term that describes what you believe to be the patient's most likely problem is the:
   A. definitive assessment.   D. field diagnosis.
   B. clinical diagnosis.   E. none of the above
   C. assessment object.

_____ 23. The management portion of your documentation should include which of the following?
   A. any interventions
   B. the results of ongoing assessments
   C. any changes in the patient's condition
   D. the patient's condition when care is transferred at the emergency department
   E. all of the above

_____ 24. Which of the following is NOT a part of the subjective information recorded on the PCR?
   A. vital signs   D. chief complaint
   B. past medical history   E. none of the above
   C. review of systems

_____ 25. Which of the following are elements of the objective information recorded on the PCR?
   A. your general impression of the patient
   B. the results of any diagnostic tests
   C. the results of the physical exam
   D. vital signs
   E. all of the above

_____ 26. Which of the following formats records the chief complaint, history, assessment, treatment, and transport information in that order?
   A. SOAP format   D. Call Incident format
   B. CHART format   E. none of the above
   C. Patient Management format

_____ 27. The most significant feature of the patient management format of documentation is that it:
   A. documents the chronological sequence of events and actions.
   B. focuses exclusively on assessment findings.
   C. uses a free-flowing narrative style.
   D. is most frequently used for patients with minor injuries/problems.
   E. none of the above

_____ 28. The call incident format for documenting an emergency response is best suited for which type of patient?
   A. the unresponsive medical patient
   B. the responsive medical patient
   C. the trauma patient with no significant mechanism of injury
   D. the trauma patient with a significant mechanism of injury
   E. both B and C

_____ 29. In obtaining a patient refusal against medical advice, it is important to:
   A. determine that the patient is alert, oriented, and competent to make the decision.
   B. clearly explain to the patient the risks of not receiving care.
   C. try to convince the patient to obtain care.
   D. explain that if the condition worsens the patient should call for the ambulance or otherwise seek immediate care.
   E. all of the above

_____ 30. If your ambulance call is canceled en route to the scene, you should:
   A. simply return to base.
   B. write canceled on the front of the PCR.
   C. note the canceling authority and time of cancellation on the PCR.
   D. secure the name of the patient as well as any other information.
   E. none of the above

MATCHING

Write the letter of the word or phrase in the space provided next to the appropriate abbreviation.

A. shortness of breath
B. acute myocardial infarction
C. positive end-expiratory pressure
D. normal sinus rhythm
E. nausea/vomiting
F. do not resuscitate
G. breath sounds/blood sugar
H. premature ventricular contraction
I. not applicable
J. nitroglycerin
K. intraosseous
L. weight
M. sexually transmitted disease

N. against medical advice
O. congestive heart failure
P. chief complaint
Q. left lower quadrant
R. electrocardiogram
S. to keep open
T. central nervous system
U. intracranial pressure
V. jugular vein distention
W. treatment
X. motor vehicle crash
Y. year old

_____ 31. CC
_____ 32. y/o
_____ 33. wt
_____ 34. CNS
_____ 35. SOB
_____ 36. n/v
_____ 37. AMI
_____ 38. CHF
_____ 39. ICP
_____ 40. MVC
_____ 41. STD
_____ 42. NTG
_____ 43. LLQ

_____ 44. BS
_____ 45. ECG
_____ 46. JVD
_____ 47. n/a
_____ 48. AMA
_____ 49. DNR
_____ 50. PEEP
_____ 51. Tx
_____ 52. IO
_____ 53. TKO
_____ 54. NSR
_____ 55. PVC

Essentials of Paramedic Care

Division 3

Trauma Emergencies

Chapter 16

Trauma and Trauma Systems

Review of Chapter Objectives

With each chapter of the Workbook, we identify the objectives and the important elements of the text content. You should review these items and refer to the pages listed if any points are not clear.

After reading this chapter, you should be able to:

1. **Describe the prevalence and significance of trauma.** pp. 761–762

   Trauma is the fourth most common cause of mortality and the number one killer for persons under the age of 44. It accounts for about 150,000 deaths per year and may be the most expensive medical problem of society today. Traumas can be divided into those caused by blunt and penetrating injury mechanisms, with only 10 percent of all trauma patients experiencing life-threatening injuries and the need for the services of the trauma center/system.

2. **List the components of a comprehensive trauma system.** pp. 762–764

   The trauma system consists of a state-level agency that coordinates regional trauma systems. The regional systems consist of regional, area, and community trauma centers and, in some cases, other facilities designated and dedicated to the care of trauma patients. The trauma system also consists of injury prevention, provider education, data registry, and quality assurance programs.

3. **Identify the characteristics of community, area, and regional trauma centers.** pp. 762–763

   - **Community or Level III Trauma Center.** This is a general hospital with a commitment to provide resources and staff training specific to the care of trauma patients. Such centers are generally located in rural areas and will stabilize the more serious trauma patients, and then transport them to higher-level trauma centers.
   - **Area or Level II Trauma Center.** This is a facility with an increased commitment to trauma patient care including 24-hour surgery. A Level II center can handle all but the most critical and specialty trauma patients.
   - **Regional or Level I Trauma Center.** This is a facility, usually a university teaching hospital, that is staffed and equipped to handle all types of serious trauma 24 hours a day and 7 days a week, as well as to support and oversee the regional trauma system.

   In some areas there is a Level IV trauma facility, which receives trauma patients and stabilizes them for transport to a higher-level facility.

©2007 Pearson Education, Inc.
Essentials of Paramedic Care, 2nd ed.

4. Identify the trauma triage criteria and apply them to narrative descriptions of trauma patients.   pp. 764–766

Trauma triage criteria include a listing of mechanisms of injury and physical findings suggestive of serious injury. The criteria identify patients likely to benefit from the care offered by the Level I or II trauma center. They include:

Mechanism of Injury

- Falls greater than 20 feet (three times the victim's height)
- Pedestrian/bicyclist versus auto collisions
- Motorcycle accidents (over 20 MPH)
- Ejections from vehicles
- Severe vehicle impacts
- Rollovers with serious impact
- Death of another vehicle occupant
- Prolonged extrications

Physical Findings

- Revised Trauma Score less than 11
- Pediatric Trauma Score less than 9
- Glasgow Coma Scale less than 14
- Systolic blood pressure less than 90
- Pulse greater than 120 or less than 50
- Penetrating trauma (nonextremity)
- Multiple proximal long-bone fractures
- Flail chest
- Pelvic fractures
- Limb paralysis
- Respiratory rate greater than 29 or less than 10
- Airway or facial burns
- Burns greater than 15 percent body surface area (BSA)

5. Describe how trauma emergencies differ from medical emergencies in the scene size-up, assessment, prehospital emergency care, and transport.   pp. 764–766

Scene size-up of the trauma incident differs from that with the medical emergency in that it is usually associated with more numerous scene hazards and involves an analysis of the mechanism of injury, using the evidence of impact to suggest possible injuries (the index of suspicion).

Assessment employs an initial assessment examining the risk of spinal injury, a quick mental status check, and an evaluation of airway, breathing, and circulation (ABCs), followed by a rapid trauma assessment looking to the head and torso and any sites of potential serious injury suggested by the index of suspicion or patient complaint.

Prehospital care and transport of the trauma patient is designed to provide expedient and supportive care and rapid transport of the patient to the trauma center or other appropriate facility.

6. Explain the "Golden Hour" concept, and describe how it applies to prehospital emergency medical service.   pp. 765–766

Research has demonstrated that the seriously injured trauma patient has an increasing chance for survival as the time from the injury to surgical intervention is reduced. Practically, this time should be as short as possible, ideally less than one hour. This "Golden Hour" concept directs prehospital care providers to reduce on-scene and transport times by expeditious assessment and care at the scene and by the use of air medical transport when appropriate and available.

7. **Explain the value of air medical service in trauma patient care and transport.** pp. 765–766

Air medical transport can move the trauma patient more quickly and along a direct line from the crash scene to the trauma center, thereby reducing transport time and increasing the likelihood that the patient will reach definitive care expeditiously.

Content Self-Evaluation

MULTIPLE CHOICE

_____ 1. Auto accidents account for how many deaths each year?
   A. 12,000
   B. 24,000
   C. 44,000
   D. 68,000
   E. 150,000

_____ 2. Although trauma poses a serious threat to life, its presentation often masks the patient's true condition.
   A. True
   B. False

_____ 3. Some 90 percent of all trauma patients do not have serious, life-endangering injuries.
   A. True
   B. False

_____ 4. Trauma triage criteria are mechanisms of injury or physical signs exhibited by the patient that suggest serious injury.
   A. True
   B. False

_____ 5. The legislation that led to the development of today's Emergency Medical Services system was the:
   A. Trauma Care Systems Planning and Development Act of 1970.
   B. Consolidated Emergency Services Act of 1971.
   C. Highway Safety Act of 1966.
   D. Trauma Systems Act of 1963.
   E. National Readiness Act of 1960.

_____ 6. The trauma system is predicated on the principle that serious trauma is:
   A. a frequent occurrence.
   B. usually a medical emergency.
   C. inevitable.
   D. a surgical disease.
   E. fatal if the patient is not seen by a qualified physician in less than 30 minutes.

_____ 7. A Level I trauma center is usually a(n):
   A. community hospital.
   B. teaching hospital with resources available full-time for emergency cases.
   C. emergency department with 24-hour service.
   D. nonemergency health care facility.
   E. stabilizing and transport facility.

_____ 8. The small community hospital or health care facility in a remote area, designated as a receiving facility for trauma, is Level:
   A. I.
   B. II.
   C. III.
   D. IV.
   E. V.

_____ 9. Specialty centers may also be designated for provision of which of the following special services?
   A. pediatric trauma center
   B. burn center
   C. neurocenter
   D. hyperbaric center
   E. all of the above

_____ 10. The period of time between the occurrence of serious injury and surgery suggested as a goal for prehospital care providers is the:
   A. Platinum 10 minutes.
   B. Golden Hour.
   C. trauma time differential.
   D. bleed-out equation.
   E. critical differential.

_____ 11. In applying trauma triage criteria, it is best to err on the side of precaution.
   A. True
   B. False

_____ 12. Trauma triage criteria are designed to over-triage trauma patients to ensure those with more subtle injuries are not missed.
   A. True
   B. False

_____ 13. The reduction in the incidence and seriousness of trauma in recent years can be credited to:
   A. better highway design.
   B. better auto design.
   C. use of auto restraint systems.
   D. development of injury prevention programs.
   E. all of the above

_____ 14. The standardized data retrieval system used to evaluate and improve the trauma system is the:
   A. prehospital care report system.
   B. trauma triage system.
   C. trauma registry.
   D. trauma quality improvement program.
   E. CISD.

_____ 15. Quality Improvement is a significant method of assessing system quality and providing for its improvement.
   A. True
   B. False

Chapter 17

Blunt Trauma

Review of Chapter Objectives

After reading this chapter, you should be able to:

1. **Identify, and explain by example, the laws of inertia and conservation of energy.** pp. 771–772

   Inertia is the tendency for objects at rest or in motion to remain so unless acted upon by an outside force. In some cases, that force is the energy exchange that causes trauma. For example, a bullet will continue its travel until it exchanges all its energy with the tissue it strikes.

   Conservation of energy is the physical law explaining that energy is not lost but changes form in the auto or other impact. An example is the deformity in the auto when it impacts a tree.

2. **Define kinetic energy and force as they relate to trauma.** pp. 772–773

   Kinetic energy is the energy any moving object possesses. This energy is the potential to do harm if it is distributed to a victim.

   Force is the exchange of energy from one object to another. It is determined by an object's mass (weight) and the rate of velocity change (acceleration or deceleration). This force induces injury.

3. **Compare and contrast the types of vehicle impacts and their expected injuries.** pp. 774–777, 779–790

   There are basically five types of vehicle impacts—frontal, lateral, rotational, rear-end, or rollover impacts. There are four events within each impact. First, the vehicle impacts the object and quickly comes to rest. Then, the vehicle occupant impacts the vehicle interior and comes to rest. Meanwhile, various organs and structures within the occupant's body collide with one another, causing compression and stretching and injury. In the fourth event, objects within the vehicle may continue their forward motion until they impact the slowed or stopped occupant. In some instances, secondary vehicle impacts occur; these are impacts that may subject the injured occupant to additional acceleration, deceleration, and injury.

   Frontal impact is the most common type of auto collision, although it also offers the most structural protection for the occupant. The front crumple zones of the auto absorb energy and the restraints—seat belts and airbags—provide additional protection. The anterior surface of the victim impacts the steering wheel, dash, windshield, and/or firewall resulting in chest, abdominal, head, and neck injuries as well as knee, femur, and hip fractures.

   Lateral impacts occur without the benefit of the front crumple zones, thereby permitting transmission of more energy directly to the occupant. The occupant is turned 90 degrees to the impact, resulting in fractures of the hip, femur, shoulder girdle, clavicle, and lateral ribs. Internal injury may result to the aorta and spleen on the driver's side or liver on the passenger's side. An unbelted occupant may impact the other occupant, causing further injury.

Rotational impacts result from oblique contact between vehicles, spinning as well as slowing the autos. This mediates the deceleration and reduces the expected injury. Injury patterns resemble a mix of those associated with frontal and lateral patterns, though the severity is generally reduced.

Rear-end impacts push the auto, auto seat, and finally the occupant forward. The body is well protected, though the head may remain stationary while the shoulders move rapidly forward. The result may be hyperextension of the head and neck and cervical spine injury. Once the vehicle begins deceleration, other injuries may occur as the body contacts the dash, steering wheel, or windshield if the occupant is unbelted.

Rollovers occur as the roadway elevation changes or a vehicle with a high center of gravity becomes unstable around a turn. The vehicle impacts the ground as it turns, exposing the occupants to multiple impacts in places where the vehicle interior may be not designed to absorb such impacts. The result may be serious injuries to anywhere on the body or ejection of the occupants. Restraints greatly reduce the incidence of injury and ejection, while ejection greatly increases the chance of occupant death.

4. Discuss the benefits of auto restraint and motorcycle helmet use. pp. 777–779, 788

Lap belts and shoulder straps control the deceleration of the vehicle occupant during a crash, slowing them with the auto. The result is a great reduction in injuries and deaths. However, when improperly worn, serious injuries may result. Shoulder straps alone may account for serious neck injury while the lap belt worn too high may injure the spine and abdomen.

Airbags inflate explosively during an impact and provide a cushion of gas as the occupant impacts the steering wheel, dash, or vehicle side. This slows the impact, reduces the deceleration rate, and reduces injuries. The airbag may entrap the driver's fingers and result in fractures or may impact a small driver or passenger who is seated close to the device and result in facial injury.

Child safety seats provide much needed protection for infants and small children for whom normal restraints do not work adequately by themselves because of the children's rapidly changing anatomical dimensions. The seat faces rearward for infants and very small children, then should be turned to face forward as the child grows. This positioning permits the seat belt to provide restraint, similar to that provided for the adult. Child safety seats should not be positioned in front of airbag restraint systems because inflation of those devices may push the rear-facing child forcibly into the seat.

Motorcycle helmet use can significantly reduce the incidence and severity of head injury, the greatest cause of motorcycle crash death. Helmets do not, however, reduce the incidence of spinal injury.

5. Describe the mechanisms of injury associated with falls, crush injuries, and sports injuries. pp. 796–799

Falls are a release of stored gravitational energy resulting in an impact between the body and the ground or other surface. Injuries occur at the point of impact and along the pathway of transmitted energy, resulting in soft tissue, skeletal, and internal trauma.

Crush injuries are injuries caused by heavy objects or machinery entrapping and damaging an extremity. The resulting wound restricts blood flow and allows the accumulation of toxins. When the pressure is removed, blood flow may move the toxins into the central circulation and hemorrhage from many disrupted blood vessels at the wound site may be hard to control.

Sports injuries are commonly the result of direct trauma, fatigue, or exertion. They often result in injury to muscles, ligaments, and tendons and to the long bones. Special consideration must be given to protecting such an injury from further aggravation until it can be seen by a physician.

6. Identify the common blast injuries and any special considerations regarding their assessment and proper care. pp. 790–796

The blast injury process results in five distinct mechanisms of injury—pressure injury, penetrating objects, personnel displacement, structural collapse, and burns.

Pressure injury occurs as the pressure wave moves outward, rapidly compressing, then decompressing anything in its path. A victim is impacted by the wave and air-filled body spaces such as the lungs, auditory canals, sinuses, and bowels may be damaged. Hearing loss is the most frequent result of pressure injury, though lung injury is most serious and life-threatening. The pressure change may damage or rupture alveoli resulting in dyspnea, pulmonary edema, pneumothorax, or air embolism. Care includes provision of high-flow oxygen, gentle positive-pressure ventilation, and rapid transport. The hearing loss patient needs careful reassurance and simple instruction.

Penetrating objects may be the bomb casing or debris put in motion by the pressure of the explosion. They may impale or enter the body, resulting in hemorrhage and internal injury. Care specific to the resulting injury should be provided, and any hemorrhage controlled by direct pressure. Any impaled object should be immobilized and the patient given rapid transport to the trauma center.

Personnel displacement occurs as the pressure wave and blast wind propel the victim through the air and he or she then impacts the ground or other surface. Blunt and penetrating trauma may result, and such injuries are cared for following standard procedures.

Collapse of a structure after a blast may entrap victims under debris and result in crush and pressure injuries. The collapse may make victims hard to locate and then extricate. Further, the nature of the crush-type wounds may make control of hemorrhage difficult, while the release of a long-entrapped extremity may be dangerous as the toxins that accumulated when circulation is disrupted are distributed to the central circulation.

Burns may result directly from the explosion or as a result of secondary combustion of debris or clothing. Generally the initial explosion will cause only superficial damage because of the short duration of the heat release and the fluid nature of the body. However, incendiary agents and burning debris or clothing may result in severe full-thickness burns.

7. **Identify and explain any special assessment and care considerations for patients with blunt trauma.** pp. 779–799

Blunt injury patients must be carefully assessed because the signs of serious internal injury may be hidden or absent. Careful analysis of the mechanism of injury and the development of an index of suspicion for serious injury may be the only way to anticipate the true seriousness of the injuries.

8. **Given several preprogrammed and moulaged blunt trauma patients, provide the appropriate scene size-up, initial assessment, rapid trauma or focused physical exam and history, detailed exam, and ongoing assessment and provide appropriate patient care and transportation.** pp. 771–799

During your training as an EMT-Paramedic, you will participate in many classroom practice sessions involving simulated patients. You will also spend some time in the emergency departments of local hospitals as well as in advanced-level ambulances gaining clinical experience. During these times, use your knowledge of the mechanisms of blunt trauma to help you assess and care for the simulated or real patients you attend.

Content Self-Evaluation

MULTIPLE CHOICE

_____ 1. The study of trauma is related to a branch of physics called:
   A. kinetics.
   B. velocity.
   C. ballistics.
   D. inertia.
   E. heuristics.

_____ 2. The anticipation of injuries based upon the analysis of the collision mechanism is referred to as the:
   A. mechanism of injury.
   B. index of suspicion.
   C. trauma triage criteria.
   D. mortality potential.
   E. RTS.

_____ 3. Penetrating trauma is the most common type of trauma associated with patient mortality.
   A. True
   B. False

_____ 4. The tendency of an object to remain at rest or remain in motion unless acted upon by an external force is:
   A. kinetics.
   B. velocity.
   C. ballistics.
   D. inertia.
   E. deceleration.

_____ 5. Two autos accelerate from a stop sign to a speed of 30 miles per hour, the first one by normal acceleration and the second when it was struck from behind by another vehicle. Assuming that both vehicles have the same weight, which vehicle gained the most kinetic energy?
   A. the vehicle in normal acceleration
   B. the vehicle struck from behind
   C. both vehicles gained the same kinetic energy
   D. cannot be determined since the kinetic energy is not known
   E. cannot be determined since the force is not known

_____ 6. Which of the following is an example of energy dissipation from an auto accident?
   A. sound of the impact
   B. bending of the structural steel
   C. heating of the compressed steel
   D. internal injury to the occupant
   E. all of the above

_____ 7. Which of the following increases the kinetic energy of an object most quickly?
   A. the temperature of the object
   B. increasing object speed
   C. decreasing object speed
   D. increasing object mass
   E. decreasing object mass

_____ 8. Blunt trauma may cause:
   A. rupture of the bowel.
   B. bursting of the alveoli.
   C. crushing of blood vessels.
   D. contusion of the liver or kidneys.
   E. all of the above.

_____ 9. Which of the following is a common cause of blunt trauma?
   A. auto collisions
   B. falls
   C. sports injuries
   D. pedestrian impacts
   E. all of the above

_____ 10. In which order do the events of an auto collision usually occur?
   A. body collision, vehicle collision, organ collision, secondary collisions
   B. organ collision, vehicle collision, body collision, secondary collisions
   C. vehicle collision, secondary collisions, body collision, organ collision
   D. vehicle collision, body collision, organ collision, secondary collisions
   E. body collision, vehicle collision, secondary collisions, organ collision

_____ 11. The major effect of the seat belt during the auto collision is to slow the passenger with the auto.
   A. True
   B. False

_____ 12. A supplemental restraint system (SRS) refers to which of the following?
   A. shoulder belts
   B. airbags
   C. lap belts
   D. child seats
   E. all of the above

_____ 13. Which of the following restraint systems is likely to induce hand fractures?
   A. shoulder belts
   B. passenger airbags
   C. driver-side airbags
   D. child seats
   E. lap belts

_____ 14. While less convenient than a child carrier, holding a child in the arms is relatively safe except in the most severe of crashes.
   A. True
   B. False

_____ 15. The type of auto impact that occurs most frequently in rural areas is:
   A. lateral.
   B. rotational.
   C. frontal.
   D. rear-end.
   E. rollover.

_____ 16. Which type of auto impact occurs most frequently in the urban setting?
   A. lateral
   B. rotational
   C. frontal
   D. rear-end
   E. rollover

_____ 17. The down-and-under pathway is most commonly associated with which type of auto collision?
   A. lateral
   B. rotational
   C. frontal
   D. rear-end
   E. rollover

_____ 18. When analyzing the lateral impact injury mechanism, you must assign a higher index of suspicion for serious life-threatening injury than with other types of impact.
   A. True
   B. False

_____ 19. Which of the following injuries are associated with significant lateral impact?
   A. aortic aneurysms
   B. clavicular fractures
   C. pelvic fractures
   D. vertebral fractures
   E. all of the above

_____ 20. With rotational impacts, the seriousness of injury is often less than vehicle damage would suggest.
   A. True
   B. False

_____ 21. The most common injury associated with the rear-end impact is to the:
   A. abdomen.
   B. pelvis.
   C. aorta.
   D. femur.
   E. neck.

_____ 22. Which of the following is a hazard commonly associated with auto collisions?
   A. hot liquids
   B. caustic substances
   C. downed power lines
   D. sharp glass or metal edges
   E. all of the above

_____ 23. With modern vehicle construction that incorporates crumple zones, you can dependably use the amount of vehicular damage to approximate the patient injuries inside.
   A. True
   B. False

_____ 24. In fatal collisions, about what percentage of the drivers are legally intoxicated?
   A. 10 percent
   B. 20 percent
   C. 35 percent
   D. 50 percent
   E. 83 percent

_____ 25. The most common body area associated with vehicular mortality is the:
   A. head.
   B. chest.
   C. abdomen.
   D. extremities.
   E. spine.

_____ 26. In motorcycle accidents, the highest index of suspicion for injury should be directed at the:
   A. neck.
   B. pelvis.
   C. head.
   D. femurs.
   E. extremities.

_____ 27. Use of a helmet in a motorcycle crash reduces the incidence of neck injury by about:
   A. 25 percent.
   B. 35 percent.
   C. 58 percent.
   D. 75 percent.
   E. does not impact neck injury incidence

_____ 28. In an auto versus child pedestrian accident, you would expect the victim to turn toward the impact.
   A. True
   B. False

_____ 29. In addition to the danger of trauma, the boating collision patient is also likely to suffer possible hypothermia and near-drowning.
   A. True
   B. False

_____ 30. Which of the mechanisms below can cause patient injury in a blast?
   A. the pressure wave
   B. flying debris
   C. the patient being thrown into objects
   D. heat
   E. all of the above

_____ 31. Underwater detonation of an explosive generally increases its lethal range by:
   A. 10 percent.
   B. 25 percent.
   C. 100 percent.
   D. 300 percent.
   E. 500 percent.

_____ 32. A victim's orientation to the blast does not effect the nature and severity of the injuries he or she sustains from an explosion.
   A. True
   B. False

_____ 33. The arrow-shaped projectiles in military-type explosives that are designed to extend the injury power of a bomb are called:
   A. ordinance.
   B. casing material.
   C. flechettes.
   D. oatmeal.
   E. granulation.

_____ 34. When victims are within a structure that contains an explosion, like a building, the effects of the blast are concentrated and the severity of the expected injuries increases.
   A. True
   B. False

_____ 35. Which of the following are secondary blast injuries?
   A. heat injuries
   B. pressure injuries
   C. projectile injuries
   D. injuries caused by structural collapse
   E. both A and B

_____ 36. If you suspect that a blast was a terrorist act, you should be cautious of secondary explosive devices intended to injure rescue personnel.
   A. True
   B. False

_____ 37. The most serious and common traumas associated with explosions affect the:
   A. heart.
   B. bowel.
   C. auditory canal.
   D. lungs.
   E. brain.

_____ 38. When ventilating the victim of a severe blast, you should use forceful deep ventilations with the bag-valve mask, as doing this will ensure good chest expansion.
   A. True
   B. False

_____ 39. Severe injury is generally associated with a fall from:
   A. three times the patient's own height.
   B. twice the patient's own height.
   C. greater than 12 feet.
   D. more than 6 feet.
   E. none of the above

_____ 40. Sports injuries are frequently associated with:
   A. fatigue.
   B. extreme exertion.
   C. compression.
   D. rotation.
   E. all of the above

Chapter 18

Penetrating Trauma

Review of Chapter Objectives

After reading this chapter, you should be able to:

1. **Explain the energy exchange process between a penetrating object or projectile and the object it strikes.** pp. 803–806

   The kinetic energy of a bullet is dependent upon its mass and even more so on its velocity according to the kinetic energy formula ($KE = m \times v^2/2$). This energy is distributed to the body tissues in the form of damage as the bullet slows. Due to the semifluid nature of body tissue, the passage of a bullet causes injury as the bullet directly strikes tissue and contuses and tears it and as it sets the tissue in motion outward and away from the bullet's path (cavitation). The faster the bullet and the larger its presenting surface (profile), the more rapid the exchange of energy and the resulting injury.

2. **Determine the effects that profile, yaw, tumble, expansion, and fragmentation have on projectile energy transfer.** pp. 804–806

   The rate of projectile energy exchange and the seriousness of resulting injury are dependent upon the rate of energy exchange. That rate is directly related to the bullet's presenting surface or profile. The larger the bullet's caliber (diameter), the greater its profile, the more rapid its exchange of energy with body tissue, and the greater the damage it causes. Yaw (swinging around the axis of the projectile's travel), tumble, expansion, and fragmentation all lead to a greater area of the bullet striking tissue than simply its profile, and hence these factors increase the damaging power of a bullet.

3. **Describe elements of the ballistic injury process including direct injury, cavitation, temporary cavity, permanent cavity, and zone of injury.** pp. 804–806, 809–811

   As a penetrating object enters the body it disrupts the tissue it contacts by tearing it, displacing it from its path, and causing direct injury. As the object's velocity increases, the rate of energy exchange increases and the rate of tissue displacement increases. A bullet's speed is so great that the bullet's passage sets the semifluid body tissue in motion away from the bullet's path. This creates a cavity behind and to the side of the projectile pathway. This cavitation further stretches and tears tissue as it creates a temporary cavity. The natural elasticity of injured tissue and the adjoining tissue closes the cavity, but an area of disrupted tissue remains (the permanent cavity). The zone of injury is the region along and surrounding the bullet track where tissue has been disrupted due to direct injury or to the stretching and tearing of cavitation.

4. Identify the relative effects a penetrating object or projectile has when striking various body regions and tissues. pp. 811–816

The passage of a bullet (and its cavitational wave) has varying effects depending on the elasticity (resiliency) and density of the tissue the bullet strikes. Connective tissue is very resilient, stretches easily, and will somewhat resist cavitational injury. Solid organs are generally very dense and much less resilient than connective tissue. They do not withstand the force generated by the cavitational wave as well as connective tissue, and the resulting injury can be expected to be much greater. Hollow organs are resilient when not distended with fluid; if an organ is full, however, the cavitational wave may cause the organ to rupture. Direct injury can also perforate an organ and permit spillage of its contents into surrounding tissue. Lung tissue is both very resilient and air filled. The tiny air pockets (the alveoli) absorb the energy of the bullet's passage and limit lung injury. On the other hand, bone is extremely dense and inelastic. Direct contact with a bullet or, in some cases, just the cavitational wave may shatter the bone and drive fragments into surrounding tissue. Slow-moving penetrating objects do not produce a cavitational wave, and injury from them is limited to the pathway of the object.

The passage of a bullet and its associated injury are related to the bullet's path of travel and, specifically, to the body region it passes through. Extremity wounds are by far the most common, yet due to the limited major body structures in the extremities, they rarely result in life-threatening injury. If the projectile strikes the bone, however, the dramatic exchange of energy may cause great tissue disruption and vascular injury, which can result in severe hemorrhage. Abdominal penetration most commonly affects the bowel, which is reasonably tolerant of the cavitational wave. However, the upper abdomen contains the liver, pancreas, and spleen, solid organs that are subject to severe injury from direct injury and cavitation. Penetrating chest trauma may affect the lungs, heart and great vessels, esophagus, trachea, and diaphragm. The lung is rather resilient to penetrating injury, while the heart and great vessels may perforate or rupture with rapid exsanguination ensuing. Tracheal tears may result in airway compromise, while esophageal tears may release gastric contents into the mediastinum with potentially deadly results. Large penetrations of the thoracic wall may permit air to move in and out (sucking or open pneumothorax) or may open the airway internally to permit air to enter the pleural space (closed pneumothorax). Neck injuries may permit severe hemorrhage, disrupt the trachea, or allow air to enter the jugular veins and embolize the lungs. Head injuries may disrupt the airway or may penetrate the cranium and cause extensive, rarely survivable, injury to the brain.

5. Anticipate the injury types and the extent of damage associated with high-velocity/high-energy projectiles, such as rifle bullets; with medium-energy/medium-velocity projectiles such as handgun and shotgun bullets, slugs, or pellets; and with low-energy/ low-velocity penetrating objects, such as knives and arrows. pp. 806–809

High-velocity/high-energy projectiles (rifle bullets) are likely to cause the most extensive injury because they have the potential to impart the most kinetic energy to the patient. Their rapid energy exchange causes the greatest cavitational wave and is most likely to produce bullet deformity and fragmentation. These characteristics cause more severe tissue damage to a greater area. The effects of these projectiles can be further enhanced if the bullet hits bone and causes it to shatter, creating additional projectiles that are driven into adjoining tissue.

Medium-velocity/medium-energy projectiles (from handguns) are likely to cause only moderate injury beyond the direct pathway of the bullet as their reduced energy does not usually cause the bullet deformity, fragmentation, and extensive cavitation waves seen with rifle projectiles. The shotgun is a particularly lethal weapon at close range because its medium-energy projectiles are numerous and their numbers cause many direct injury pathways.

Low-velocity/low-energy penetrating objects are commonly knives, arrows, ice picks, and other objects traveling at low speeds. They generally cause only direct injury along the path of their travel. They may, however, be moved about, once inserted, and either left in place or withdrawn.

6. **Identify important elements of the scene size-up associated with shootings or stabbings.** pp. 816–817

Penetrating trauma, especially when associated with shootings or stabbings, presents the danger of violence directed toward others (other rescuers, bystanders, your patient, and you). It is essential that you approach the scene with great caution and ensure that the police have secured it before you approach or enter. Penetrating trauma also calls for gloves as minimum BSI precaution, with goggles and gown required for spurting hemorrhage, airway management, or massive blood contamination. During the scene size-up, you should evaluate the mechanism of injury including the type of weapon, caliber, distance, and angle between the shooter and the victim, and the number of shots fired and patient impacts.

7. **Identify and explain any special assessment and care considerations for patients with penetrating trauma.** pp. 817–818

In assessing the patient with penetrating trauma you must anticipate the projectile or penetrating object's pathway and the structures it is likely to have injured. The exit wound from a projectile may help you better approximate the wounding potential, and remember that the bullet may have been deflected along its course and damaged or completely missed critical structures. Always suspect and treat for the worst-case scenario. Be especially wary of injuries to the head, chest, and abdomen as wounds to these regions often have lethal outcomes. Cover all open wounds that enter the thorax or neck with occlusive dressings and be watchful for the development of dyspnea due to pneumothorax, tension pneumothorax, or pulmonary emboli. Be prepared to provide aggressive fluid resuscitation, but understand that doing so may dislodge forming clots and increase the rate of internal hemorrhage. Stabilize any impaled objects and only remove them when it is required to ensure a patent airway, to perform CPR, or to transport the patient.

8. **Given several preprogrammed and moulaged penetrating trauma patients, provide the appropriate scene size-up, initial assessment, rapid trauma or focused physical exam and history, detailed exam, and ongoing assessment and provide appropriate patient care and transportation.** pp. 803–818

During your training as an EMT-Paramedic you will participate in many classroom practice sessions involving simulated patients. You will also spend some time in the emergency departments of local hospitals as well as in advanced-level ambulances gaining clinical experience. During these times, use your knowledge of the mechanisms of penetrating trauma to help you assess and care for the simulated or real patients you attend.

Content Self-Evaluation

MULTIPLE CHOICE

_____ 1. Approximately what number of deaths are attributable to shootings each year?
   A. 25,000
   B. 28,000
   C. 44,000
   D. 50,000
   E. 100,000

_____ 2. An object traveling at twice the speed of another object of the same weight has:
   A. twice the kinetic energy.
   B. three times the kinetic energy.
   C. four times the kinetic energy.
   D. eight times the kinetic energy.
   E. ten times the kinetic energy.

_____ 3. Wounds from rifle bullets are considered two to four times more lethal than handgun bullets.
   A. True
   B. False

_____ 4. The curved tract a bullet follows during flight is called its:
   A. ballistics.
   B. cavitation.
   C. trajectory.
   D. yaw.
   E. parabola.

_____ 5. The surface of a projectile that exchanges energy with the object struck is its:
   A. caliber.
   B. profile.
   C. drag.
   D. yaw.
   E. expansion factor.

_____ 6. When a rifle bullet hits tissue, normally it will:
   A. continue without tumbling.
   B. tumble once, then travel nose first.
   C. tumble quickly, then slowly rotate.
   D. wobble but not tumble.
   E. tumble 180 degrees then continue.

_____ 7. While handgun bullets are made of relatively soft lead, their kinetic energy is generally not sufficient to cause significant deformity.
   A. True
   B. False

_____ 8. Civilian hunting ammunition is designed to deform and will frequently fragment when striking soft tissue.
   A. True
   B. False

_____ 9. Which of the following statements accurately describes a rifle bullet in contrast to a handgun bullet?
   A. It is a heavier projectile.
   B. It travels at a greater velocity.
   C. It is more likely to deform.
   D. It is more likely to fragment.
   E. all of the above

_____ 10. The shotgun is limited in range and accuracy; however, injuries it inflicts at close range can be very severe or lethal.
   A. True
   B. False

_____ 11. Which element of the projectile injury process is related to the actual damage caused as the bullet contacts tissue?
   A. direct injury
   B. pressure wave
   C. temporary cavity
   D. permanent cavity
   E. zone of injury

_____ 12. The movement of tissue away from the bullet's path as it passes through the body is a result of:
   A. direct injury.
   B. the pressure wave.
   C. a temporary cavity.
   D. fragmentation.
   E. referred injury.

_____ 13. The passage of a projectile through the body results in a region where tissues are disrupted and not functioning normally that is known as the:
   A. direct injury.
   B. pressure wave.
   C. temporary cavity.
   D. permanent cavity.
   E. zone of injury.

_____ 14. The temporary cavity formed as a high-velocity/high-energy bullet passes may be how large?
   A. 12 times the projectile's profile
   B. 14 times the projectile's profile
   C. 16 times the projectile's profile
   D. 100 times the projectile's profile
   E. rarely more than the projectile's profile

_____ 15. The tissue structure that is very resilient, yet dense, and usually sustains limited damage with the passage of a projectile is:
   A. a solid organ.
   B. a hollow organ.
   C. connective tissue.
   D. bone.
   E. a lung.

_____ 16. The tissue structure that is likely to rupture and spill its contents when struck by a projectile is:
   A. a solid organ.
   B. a hollow organ.
   C. connective tissue.
   D. bone.
   E. a lung.

_____ 17. Penetrating wounds to the extremities account for about 70 percent of all penetrating wounds yet account for less than 10 percent of fatalities related to this injury mechanism.
   A. True
   B. False

_____ 18. The abdominal organ most tolerant to the compression caused by a cavitational wave is the:
   A. bowel.
   B. liver.
   C. spleen.
   D. kidney.
   E. pancreas.

_____ 19. Because of the pressure-driven dynamics of respiration, any bullet wound to the chest is likely to seriously compromise breathing.
   A. True
   B. False

_____ 20. The body region in which a penetrating wound has the greatest likelihood of drawing air into the venous system is the:
   A. abdomen.
   B. thorax.
   C. head.
   D. neck.
   E. none of the above

_____ 21. Which of the following is NOT associated with an entrance wound?
   A. tattooing
   B. a small ridge of discoloration around the wound
   C. a blown outward appearance
   D. subcutaneous emphysema
   E. propellant residue on the surrounding tissue

_____ 22. The entrance wound is more likely to reflect the actual damaging potential of the projectile than the exit wound.
   A. True
   B. False

_____ 23. Which of the following information should you gain through the scene size-up, if possible?
   A. the gun caliber
   B. the angle of the gun to the victim
   C. the type of gun used
   D. assurance that no other weapons are involved
   E. all of the above

_____ 24. As you care for a patient at a potential crime scene, actions you take to help preserve evidence should include:
   A. cutting through, not around bullet or knife holes in clothing.
   B. moving what you can away from the patient.
   C. removing obviously dead patients from the scene as quickly as possible.
   D. disturbing only the items necessary to provide patient care.
   E. all of the above

_____ 25. Frothy blood at a bullet exit or entrance wound suggests a(n):
   A. simple pneumothorax.
   B. open pneumothorax.
   C. tension pneumothorax.
   D. pericardial tamponade.
   E. mediastinum injury.

Chapter 19

Hemorrhage and Shock

Review of Chapter Objectives

After reading this chapter, you should be able to:

1. **Describe the epidemiology, including the morbidity/mortality and prevention strategies, for shock and hemorrhage.** pp. 829–831, 837–841

   Shock is the transitional stage between normal physiological function of the body and death. It is the underlying killer of all trauma patients and is prevented using the strategies described for each of the types of trauma addressed by the following seven chapters. Hemorrhage is loss of the body's precious medium, blood, and is a common cause of shock and death in the trauma patient. Strategies to prevent hemorrhage are those designed to prevent trauma as discussed in the next seven chapters.

2. **Discuss the anatomy, physiology, and pathophysiology of the cardiovascular system.** (see Chapters 3 and 4)

   The cardiovascular system is a closed system of interconnected tubes (blood vessels) that direct blood to the essential organs and tissues of the body. Arteries distribute blood to the various organs and tissues of the body. Arterioles determine the amount of blood perfusing the tissue of an organ and together constrict and increase peripheral vascular resistance or dilate and reduce peripheral vascular resistance. Progressive vasoconstriction can help maintain blood pressure and circulation to the most critical organs as the body loses blood during hemorrhage or fluid during other forms of shock. The venous system collects blood and returns it to the heart. It contains about 64 percent of the total blood volume and, when constricted, can return a relatively great volume (up to 1 liter) to the active circulation.

   The cardiovascular system is powered by the central pump, the heart. It circulates the blood and, against the peripheral vascular resistance, drives the blood pressure. Its output is a factor of preload (the blood delivered to it by the venous system), stroke volume (the amount of blood ejected into the aorta with each contraction), rate, and afterload (the peripheral vascular resistance). The heart can help compensate for blood loss by attempting to maintain cardiac output by increasing its stroke volume (which is hard to do in hypovolemic states) or by increasing its rate.

   Finally, the cardiovascular system contains a precious fluid, blood. Blood provides oxygen and nutrients to the body cells and removes carbon dioxide and waste products of metabolism. Blood also contains clotting factors that will occlude blood vessels if they are torn or disrupted.

   The central nervous system provides control of the cardiovascular system using baroreceptors in the carotid arteries and aortic arch to sense fluctuations in blood pressure. It will maintain blood pressure by increasing heart rate, cardiac preload, and peripheral vascular resistance. Hormones from the kidneys and elsewhere help control blood volume and electrolytes as well as the production of erythrocytes.

3. Define shock based on aerobic and anaerobic metabolism. (see Chapter 4)

Cells are the elemental building blocks of the body and ultimately carry out all body functions. They derive their energy from a two-step process. The first step, called glycolysis, requires no oxygen (anaerobic) and generates a small amount of energy. The second step, called the citric acid or Krebs cycle, requires oxygen (aerobic) and generates about 95 percent of the cell's energy. In shock, which is inadequate tissue perfusion that does not adequately supply the cells with oxygen, the cells produce energy in an inefficient way and toxins accumulate.

4. Describe the body's physiological response to changes in blood volume, blood pressure, and perfusion. pp. 837–841

Increased peripheral resistance is caused by the constriction of the arterioles and provides two mechanisms that combat shock. The arterioles constrict and maintain the blood pressure, and they divert blood to only the critical organs. This reduction in perfusion to the less-critical organs results in the increased capillary refill time and the cool, clammy, and ashen skin often associated with shock states. It also results in reduced pulse pressure and weak pulses.

Venous constriction compensates for some blood loss and helps maintain cardiac preload. Since the veins account for 64 percent of the blood volume, this is reasonably effective in minor to moderate blood loss.

As the cardiac preload drops, the heart rate increases in an attempt to maintain cardiac output and blood pressure. In the presence of significantly reduced preload, this may not be effective.

Peripheral vascular shunting directs the blood away from the skin, conserves body heat, and reduces fluid loss through evaporation. It also redirects blood to more critical areas.

Fluid shifts are the result of drawing fluid from the interstitial and cellular spaces. Fluid moves into the vascular space. While this is a slow mechanism, it can provide the vascular system with several liters of fluid.

5. Describe the effects of decreased perfusion at the capillary level. pp. 838–839

Decreased capillary perfusion limits the amount of oxygen and nutrients delivered to the body cells. It usually causes the release of histamine that, in turn, causes precapillary sphincter dilation and an increase in perfusion. However, in shock states this is not effective, and the cells must revert to anaerobic metabolism while the by-products of metabolism accumulate and the available oxygen is exhausted. Carbon dioxide, metabolic acids, and other waste products accumulate while body cells begin to die.

6. Discuss the cellular ischemic, capillary stagnation, and capillary washout phases related to hemorrhagic shock. pp. 838–839

- **Cellular ischemia.** As shock ensues, decreased perfusion, first to the noncritical organs, then to all organs, diminishes blood flow through the microcirculation. At the cellular level this diminishes the supply of oxygen and nutrients to the cells and restricts the removal of carbon dioxide and the waste products of metabolism. The cells quickly exhaust their supply of oxygen and begin to use anaerobic metabolism as their sole source of energy to remain alive. This produces an accumulation of pyruvic acid, which in turn converts to lactic acid and the cells become more acidotic. As cells begin to die, their decomposition releases even more toxins that then begin to affect other cells.
- **Capillary stagnation.** With diminished capillary flow, coupled with the increasingly hypoxic and acidic environment caused by the ischemic cells, the red blood cells become sticky and clump together. They form columns of coagulated erythrocytes called rouleaux that either block the capillary to further flow of blood or will wash out and cause microemboli.
- **Capillary washout.** The toxic environment of the ischemic tissue associated with severe shock finally causes the post-capillary sphincters to dilate and release the hypoxic and acidotic blood

as well as the rouleaux into the venous circulation. As this washout becomes extensive, it further reduces the effectiveness of the cardiovascular system and the body moves quickly toward irreversible shock.

7. **Discuss the various types and degrees of shock and hemorrhage.** pp. 829–831, 837–841

Hemorrhage can be divided into four stages as a patient moves through compensated, decompensated, and irreversible shock.

Stage 1 blood loss is a loss of up to 15 percent of the patient's blood volume. It generally presents with some nervousness, cool skin, and slight pallor. It is difficult to detect as the body compensates well for blood loss in this range.

Stage 2 blood loss is a loss of up to 25 percent of the patient's blood volume. Signs and symptoms become more apparent as the body finds it more difficult to compensate for the loss. The patient may display thirst, anxiety, restlessness, and cool and clammy skin.

Stage 3 blood loss is a loss of up to 35 percent of the patient's blood volume. It presents with the signs of stage 2 blood loss and air hunger, dyspnea, and severe thirst. Survival is unlikely without immediate intervention.

Stage 4 blood loss is a blood loss in excess of 35 percent of the patient's blood volume. The patient begins to display a deathlike appearance with pulses disappearing and respirations becoming very shallow and ineffective. The patient becomes very lethargic and then unconscious and survival becomes unlikely.

8. **Predict shock and hemorrhage based on mechanism of injury.** pp. 832, 841–842

Shock due to internal blood loss can be a very silent killer if not recognized and the patient brought to definitive care (surgery) quickly. Severe blunt and deep penetrating trauma can induce internal hemorrhage that is both difficult to identify and treat. If you wait until the frank signs of shock appear, too much time may have passed for care to be effective. Hence, it is very important to both analyze the mechanism of injury to anticipate shock and to recognize the very early signs of shock.

A large hematoma may account for up to 500 mL of blood loss, while fractures of the humerus or tibia/fibula may account for 500 to 750 mL. Femoral fractures may account for up to 1,500 mL of blood, while pelvic fractures often involve hemorrhage of up to 2,000 mL. Internal hemorrhage into the chest or abdomen may contribute even greater losses. In penetrating or severe blunt trauma to the chest or abdomen, suspect the development of shock. Also suspect the rapid development of shock in the patient who begins to display the early signs of shock (an increasing pulse rate, decreasing pulse pressure, and anxiety and restlessness) very quickly after the trauma event.

9. **Identify the need for intervention and transport of the patient with hemorrhage or shock.** pp. 831–834, 841–843

Hemorrhage and shock are progressive pathologies that eventually become irreversible. To be effective in care, we must carefully assess our patients for the earliest of signs and intervene with rapid transport to a facility that can rapidly provide surgical intervention (to halt the internal bleeding). We also must immediately halt any external hemorrhage and provide supplemental high-flow, high-concentration oxygen. Intravenous fluids may be run to replace volume, but care must be used to prevent increased internal hemorrhage and hemodilution.

10. **Discuss the assessment findings and management of internal and external hemorrhage and shock.** pp. 831–834, 841–843

Tachycardia is a compensatory cardiac action to maintain cardiac output when a reduced preload is present. A weak pulse reflects a narrowing pulse pressure and increasing peripheral vascular resistance to maintain systolic blood pressure. Cool, clammy skin is due to the redirection of blood to more critical organs than the skin. Ashen, pale skin may present due to hypoxia and peripheral vasoconstriction. Agitation, restlessness, and reduced level of consciousness occurs as the brain receives a reduced flow of oxygenated blood. The hypoxia causes the defense mechanisms of agitation and restlessness, followed by a noticeable reduction in the level of consciousness. Dull, lackluster eyes occur secondary to low perfusion and hypoxic states. Rapid, shallow respiration may occur as shock progresses, the respiratory muscles tire in the hypoxic state, and respiratory effort becomes less efficient. Dropping oxygen saturation may also provide evidence to support developing shock. As the peripheral circulation slows, the readings may drop or become erratic. Falling blood pressure heralds the progression from compensated to decompensated shock. As a late sign, it should not be used to determine the presence of shock.

External hemorrhage must be controlled by direct pressure. If direct pressure alone does not work, use elevation, pressure points or, as a last resort, the tourniquet, to stop the hemorrhage. If all sites of hemorrhage are controlled and you can rule out internal hemorrhage, provide fluid resuscitation to return the blood pressure and vital signs to normal.

Should the mechanism of injury or any early development of shock signs or symptoms suggest internal hemorrhage or external hemorrhage cannot be controlled, transport should be expedited and care initiated immediately. Provide high-flow, high-concentration oxygen and ventilatory support as needed and infuse fluids to maintain the blood pressure just below 100 mmHg, ensuring it does not drop below 50 mmHg.

11. **Differentiate between the administration rate and volume of IV fluid in patients with controlled versus uncontrolled hemorrhage.** pp. 844–846

If hemorrhage has been controlled (as with external hemorrhage), then fluid resuscitation can be aimed at returning the blood pressure and other vital signs toward normal. However, if the hemorrhage is internal, and especially if it involves the chest, abdomen, or pelvis, great care must be exercised not to enhance the hemorrhage or excessively dilute the remaining blood. Resuscitation is generally aimed at stabilizing the blood pressure somewhere just below 80 mmHg and preventing it from dropping below 50 mmHg. To maintain these parameters, lactated Ringer's solution (preferred) or normal saline should be run rapidly through trauma or blood tubing and large-bore short catheters. Pressure infusers may be necessary as the blood pressure begins to fall below 50 mmHg. Usually prehospital care is limited to between 1 and 3 liters of crystalloid.

12. **Relate pulse pressure and orthostatic vital sign changes to perfusion status.** pp. 834, 843

Pulse pressure is the difference between the systolic and diastolic blood pressures and is responsible for the pulse. It is a relative measure of the effectiveness of cardiac output against peripheral vascular resistance. One of the early signs of shock is a decreasing pulse pressure, occurring as cardiac output begins to fall and the body increases peripheral vascular resistance in an attempt to maintain blood pressure.

Normally the body can maintain blood pressure and perfusion despite rapid changes from one position to another. However, in hypovolemia the body is already in a state of compensation so it becomes more difficult to maintain the pulse rate and blood pressure as someone moves from a supine to a seated or a standing position. If hypovolemic compensation exists, this movement will cause an increase in pulse rate and a drop in systolic blood pressure (usually by 20 points or more).

13. **Define and differentiate between compensated and decompensated hemorrhagic shock.** pp. 839–840

Compensated shock is a state in which the body is effectively compensating for fluid loss, or other shock-inducing pathology, and is able to maintain blood pressure and critical organ perfusion. If the original problem is not corrected or reversed, compensated shock may progress to decompensated shock.

Decompensated shock is a state in which the cardiovascular system cannot maintain critical circulation and begins to fail. Hypoxia affects the blood vessels and heart so they cannot maintain blood pressure and circulation.

Irreversible shock is a state of shock in which the human system is so damaged that it cannot be resuscitated. Once this stage of shock sets in the patient will die, even if resuscitation efforts restore a pulse and blood pressure.

14. **Discuss the pathophysiological changes, assessment findings, and management associated with compensated and decompensated shock.** pp. 839–840

   As the body experiences a stressor that induces shock, the cardiovascular system is quick to compensate. The venous system constricts to maintain a full vascular system and preload. The heart rate increases to maintain cardiac output, and the arterioles constrict, increasing peripheral vascular resistance to maintain blood pressure (the pressure of perfusion). As these actions become significant, the patient becomes anxious and slightly tachycardic, and the skin becomes cool and pale (circulation is shunted from the skin to more vital organs). With increasing blood loss, the compensation becomes more significant, and thirst, a rapid, weak pulse, and restlessness become apparent. These signs become more apparent as greater compensation is required to maintain the blood pressure. When the body reaches the limits of its compensation and it can no longer maintain the blood pressure, BP drops precipitously, circulation all but stops, and the patient moves very quickly into irreversible shock.

   Care for the shock patient includes high-flow, high-concentration oxygen, hemorrhage control, and fluid resuscitation to maintain vital signs when hemorrhage is controlled, with a stable blood pressure just below 100 mmHg (88 mmHg may be optimal with continuing hemorrhage), or use aggressive fluid resuscitation if the blood pressure drops below 50 mmHg.

15. **Identify the need for intervention and transport of patients with compensated and decompensated shock.** pp. 841–849

   The body's ability to compensate for shock is limited. While it can maintain blood pressure, the compensation is not without cost. As the arterioles constrict, they deny blood flow to some organs and the arterioles use energy and tire. The venous vessels tire as they constrict to reduce the volume of the vascular system. If compensation is significant or prolonged, the body may move into decompensation, especially if the hemorrhage is not controlled. Most serious internal hemorrhage can only be halted with surgical intervention, most commonly at a trauma center. In the time between our recognition of shock and arrival at the trauma center, we can help the body with its compensation by providing oxygen and fluid resuscitation.

16. **Differentiate among normotensive, hypotensive, or profoundly hypotensive patients.** pp. 841–849

   A normotensive patient is one who has a systolic blood pressure of at least 100 mmHg. Hypotension is the patient with a blood pressure of less than 100 mmHg, while a blood pressure of less than 50 mmHg is considered profound hypotension. However, these figures apply to the young healthy adult and must be adjusted to the norms for the patient you are treating. (For example, a small young female may normally have a blood pressure below 100 mmHg and may not need fluid resuscitation.)

17. **Describe differences in administration of intravenous fluid in the normotensive, hypotensive, or profoundly hypotensive patients.** pp. 844–846

   Administration of intravenous fluids in the normotensive patient without hypovolemia permits the rapid administration of medications and may be indicated when hypovolemia is anticipated (the burn patient). In the patient who is in compensated shock and maintains a relatively normal systolic blood pressure, fluid resuscitation is indicated if hemorrhage is controlled. If the hemorrhage is internal and cannot be controlled in the field, aggressive fluid resuscitation may lead to increased internal hemorrhage and hemodilution making perfusion and clotting less effective. Generally, the administration of intravenous fluids in the normotensive patient is limited.

   In the patient who is hypotensive (BP < 100 mmHg), intravenous fluids are administered to maintain, not increase, the blood pressure. Here again aggressive fluid resuscitation would dilute the blood and decrease the effectiveness of perfusion and clotting. An increase in blood pressure would also likely break apart clots that are reducing the internal hemorrhage.

In the patient who is profoundly hypotensive (absent pulses and you are unable to determine a blood pressure, or it is < 50 mmHg), aggressive fluid resuscitation is indicated. Here the consequences of severe hypoperfusion outweigh the risks of further hemorrhage.

18. **Discuss the physiologic changes associated with application and inflation of the pneumatic anti-shock garment (PASG).** pp. 846–847

The pneumatic anti-shock garment (PASG) is an air bladder that circumferentially applies pressure to the lower extremities and abdomen. In theory, it compresses the venous blood vessels, returning some blood to the critical circulation, and compresses the arteries, increasing peripheral vascular resistance. These actions increase circulating blood volume and blood pressure, which should help the patient in shock. However, in some cases of shock, this may increase the rate of internal hemorrhage and may disrupt the clotting mechanisms that are restricting blood loss associated with internal injury.

19. **Discuss the indications and contraindications for the application and inflation of the PASG.** pp. 846–847

The PASG is indicated for any patient who displays internal or external hemorrhage in the lower abdomen, pelvis, or lower extremities. It is recommended for the stabilization of any pelvic fracture and may be helpful with bilateral femoral fractures with the signs and symptoms of shock.

The PASG should not be used in the patient who is experiencing pulmonary edema or has a head or penetrating chest injury. It should be used with caution on any patient who is experiencing dyspnea as it may increase intraabdominal pressure and restrict the movement of the diaphragm. The abdominal section should not be employed if the patient is in the third trimester of pregnancy, has an abdominal evisceration, or an impaled object in the abdomen.

Prior to application of the PASG, the patient's blood pressure, pulse rate and strength, and level of consciousness should be assessed and recorded. The abdomen, lower back, and lower extremities should be visualized to ensure that no sharp debris that could harm either the patient or the garment is present.

20. **Given several preprogrammed and moulaged hemorrhage and shock patients, provide the appropriate scene size-up, initial assessment, rapid trauma or focused physical exam and history, detailed exam, and ongoing assessment and provide appropriate patient care and transportation.** pp. 822–849

During your training as an EMT-Paramedic you will participate in many classroom practice sessions involving simulated patients. You will also spend some time in the emergency departments of local hospitals as well as in advanced-level ambulances gaining clinical experience. During these times, use your knowledge of hemorrhage and shock to help you assess and care for the simulated or real patients you attend.

Content Self-Evaluation

MULTIPLE CHOICE

1. Which of the following types of hemorrhage is characterized by bright red blood?
   A. capillary bleeding
   B. venous bleeding
   C. arterial bleeding
   D. both A and C
   E. both A and B

2. Which of the following types of hemorrhage is characterized by dark red blood?
   A. capillary bleeding
   B. venous bleeding
   C. arterial bleeding
   D. both A and C
   E. none of the above

_____ 3. Which of the following is NOT a stage in the clotting process?
   A. intrinsic phase
   B. vascular phase
   C. platelet phase
   D. coagulation phase
   E. all of the above

_____ 4. Which of the following represents the phase of clotting where blood cells are trapped in fibrin strands?
   A. intrinsic phase
   B. vascular phase
   C. platelet phase
   D. coagulation phase
   E. marrow phase

_____ 5. The coagulation process normally takes about what length of time?
   A. 1 to 2 minutes
   B. 3 to 4 minutes
   C. 4 to 6 minutes
   D. 7 to 10 minutes
   E. 10 to 12 minutes

_____ 6. Cleanly and transversely cut blood vessels tend to bleed very heavily.
   A. True
   B. False

_____ 7. Which of the following is likely to adversely affect the clotting process?
   A. aggressive fluid resuscitation
   B. hypothermia
   C. movement at the site of injury
   D. drugs such as aspirin
   E. all of the above

_____ 8. Bleeding from capillary or venous wounds is easy to halt because the pressure driving the hemorrhage is limited.
   A. True
   B. False

_____ 9. Fractures of the femur can account for a blood loss:
   A. from 500 to 750 mL.
   B. up to 1,500 mL.
   C. in excess of 2,000 mL.
   D. less than 500 mL.
   E. in excess of 2,500 mL.

_____ 10. In which stage of hemorrhage does the patient first display ineffective respiration?
   A. the first stage
   B. the second stage
   C. the third stage
   D. the fourth stage
   E. the terminal stage

_____ 11. The intravascular fluid accounts for what percentage of the total body water?
   A. 7 percent
   B. 15 percent
   C. 35 percent
   D. 45 percent
   E. 75 percent

_____ 12. In which stage of hemorrhage does the patient first display thirst?
   A. the first stage
   B. the second stage
   C. the third stage
   D. the fourth stage
   E. none of the above

_____ 13. In which stage of hemorrhage does the patient first display air hunger?
   A. the first stage
   B. the second stage
   C. the third stage
   D. the fourth stage
   E. none of the above

_____ 14. Which of the following react differently to blood loss than the normal, healthy adult?
   A. pregnant women
   B. athletes
   C. the elderly
   D. children
   E. all of the above

_____ 15. The late pregnancy female is likely to have a blood volume:
   A. much less than normal.
   B. slightly less than normal.
   C. slightly greater than normal.
   D. much greater than normal.
   E. that is normal and does not change with pregnancy.

_____ 16. Obese patients are likely to have a blood volume:
   A. much less than normal.   D. much greater than normal.
   B. slightly less than normal.   E. none of the above
   C. slightly greater than normal.

_____ 17. The risk of transmitting disease to your trauma patient is probably much greater than the risk of obtaining a disease from him.
   A. True
   B. False

_____ 18. The sooner the signs and symptoms of shock appear in your patient, the greater the hemorrhage rate and the likelihood that the patient will move into the later stages of shock.
   A. True
   B. False

19. Fractures of the pelvis can account for a blood loss:
   A. from 500 to 750 mL.
   B. up to 1,500 mL.
   C. in excess of 2,000 mL.
   D. up to 500 mL.
   E. of none because the pelvis does not bleed.

_____ 20. A black, tarry stool is called:
   A. hemoptysis.   D. hematochezia.
   B. melena.   E. ebony stool.
   C. hematuria.

_____ 21. A positive tilt test demonstrating orthostatic hypotension is positive when:
   A. the blood pressure rises by at least 20 mmHg.
   B. the blood pressure falls by at least 20 mmHg.
   C. the pulse rate rises by at least 20 beats per minute.
   D. the pulse rate falls by at least 20 beats per minute.
   E. both B and C

_____ 22. For the patient in compensated shock, you should perform an ongoing assessment:
   A. every 5 minutes.
   B. every 15 minutes.
   C. after every major intervention.
   D. after noting any change in signs or symptoms.
   E. all except B

_____ 23. Which of the following is a technique used to help control hemorrhage?
   A. direct pressure   D. limb splinting
   B. elevation   E. all of the above
   C. pressure points

_____ 24. When using a blood pressure cuff as a tourniquet, you should inflate the blood pressure cuff:
   A. until the bleeding slows.
   B. to the diastolic blood pressure.
   C. to the systolic blood pressure.
   D. to 30 mmHg above the systolic blood pressure.
   E. none of the above

_____ 25. Which of the following is NOT a pulse pressure point?
   A. the brachial artery
   B. the carotid artery
   C. the femoral artery
   D. the popliteal artery
   E. the radial artery

_____ 26. The column of coagulated erythrocytes caused by capillary stagnation is called:
   A. ischemia.
   B. rouleaux.
   C. capillary washout.
   D. hydrostatic reflux.
   E. compensated reflux.

_____ 27. Which list places the stages of shock in the order of their occurrence.
   A. irreversible, decompensated, compensated
   B. compensated, decompensated, irreversible
   C. compensated, irreversible, decompensated
   D. decompensated, irreversible, compensated
   E. decompensated, compensated, irreversible

_____ 28. Which stage of shock ends with a precipitous drop in blood pressure?
   A. compensated
   B. decompensated
   C. irreversible
   D. hypovolemic
   E. none of the above

_____ 29. Which of the following does NOT occur during the compensated stage of shock?
   A. increasing pulse rate
   B. decreasing pulse strength
   C. decreasing systolic blood pressure
   D. skin becomes cool and clammy
   E. the patient experiences thirst and weakness

_____ 30. Once the patient becomes profoundly unconscious and loses his vital signs, he moves into irreversible shock.
   A. True
   B. False

_____ 31. Which of the following suggests shock?
   A. a pulse rate above 100 in the adult
   B. a pulse rate above 140 in the school-age child
   C. a pulse rate above 160 in the preschooler
   D. a pulse rate above 180 in the infant
   E. all of the above

_____ 32. When using a pulse oximeter, you should use oxygen and ventilation to keep the reading above which oxygen saturation value?
   A. 45 percent
   B. 80 percent
   C. 85 percent
   D. 95 percent
   E. 99 percent

_____ 33. The color, temperature, and general appearance of the skin can indicate shock before there are changes in the blood pressure.
   A. True
   B. False

_____ 34. During assessment you note that the patient's lower extremities and lower abdomen are warm and pink while the upper extremities, thorax, and upper abdomen are cool and clammy. This presentation is consistent with which type of shock?
   A. hypovolemic
   B. neurogenic
   C. obstructive
   D. cardiogenic
   E. respiratory

_____ 35. Which of the following may be an indication to employ overdrive respiration?
   A. severe rib fractures
   B. flail chest
   C. diaphragmatic respirations
   D. head injury
   E. all of the above

_____ 36. Which of these fluid replacement choices would be most desirable for the patient who is losing blood through internal bleeding?
   A. packed red blood cells
   B. fresh frozen plasma
   C. whole blood
   D. colloids
   E. crystalloids

_____ 37. Most of the solutions used in prehospital care for infusion are:
   A. hypotonic colloids.
   B. isotonic colloids.
   C. hypertonic colloids.
   D. hypotonic crystalloids.
   E. isotonic crystalloids.

_____ 38. Which of the following characteristics of a catheter will ensure that fluids run rapidly through it?
   A. short length, small lumen
   B. short length, large lumen
   C. long length, small lumen
   D. long length, large lumen
   E. large lumen and either long or short length

_____ 39. In the patient that has internal bleeding and hypovolemia, the objective blood pressure to maintain by PASG and fluid infusions is:
   A. 120 mmHg.
   B. 80 mmHg.
   C. 50 mmHg.
   D. below 50 mmHg.
   E. at a steady level.

_____ 40. The PASG may return what volume of blood to the central circulation?
   A. 250 mL
   B. 500 mL
   C. 750 mL
   D. 1,000 mL
   E. none at all

Chapter 20

Soft-Tissue Trauma

Review of Chapter Objectives

After reading this chapter, you should be able to:

1. **Describe the incidence, morbidity, and mortality of soft-tissue injuries.** p. 854

   Soft tissue injuries are by far the most prevalent type of injuries to occur, accounting for over 10 million visits to the emergency department yearly. Any mechanism of injury affecting the human system must first penetrate the skin and then the soft tissues to injure any organ. However, soft-tissue injuries rarely by themselves threaten life. Open injuries to the skin may permit pathogens to enter and infection to develop, and significant wounds may cause cosmetic and, to some degree, functional disruption of the skin. Injuries to the skin may also permit significant hemorrhage.

2. **Describe the anatomy and physiology of the integumentary system, including epidermis, dermis, and subcutaneous tissue.** (see Chapter 3)

   The integumentary system is the largest body organ, accounting for about 16 percent of weight. It provides the outer barrier for the body and protects it against environmental extremes, fluid loss, and pathogen invasion. The three-layer structure consists of:

   a. **Epidermis**
      The epidermis is the most superficial layer of the skin and consists of numerous layers of dead or dying cells. The epidermis provides a flexible covering for the skin and a barrier to fluid loss, absorption, and the entrance of pathogens.
   b. **Dermis**
      The dermis is the true skin. It is made up of connective tissue and houses the sensory nerve endings, many of the specialized skin cells that produce sweat, oil, and so forth, and the upper-level capillary beds that allow for the conduction of heat to the body's surface.
   c. **Subcutaneous tissue**
      The subcutaneous layer, although not a true part of the skin, works in concert with the skin to insulate the body from heat loss and the effects of trauma. It consists of connective and adipose (fatty) tissues.

3. **Identify the skin tension lines of the body.** pp. 857–858

   The skin is a flexible cover for the body and as such is firmly connected to some parts of the anatomy while at other locations it is somewhat mobile. Its elasticity permits a wide range of motion by the musculoskeletal system while maintaining its own integrity. This elasticity creates tension along lines (called skin tension lines) that will cause a wound to gape or remain somewhat closed based upon its orientation to the skin tension lines. Please see the illustration (Figure 20-6) on page 858 of the textbook.

4. Predict soft-tissue injuries based on mechanism of injury. pp. 872–874

Blunt trauma is most likely to produce closed soft-tissue injury such as a contusion or hematoma, especially when the tissue is trapped between the force and skeletal structures like the ribs or skull. Crush injury occurs as the soft tissue is trapped in machinery or under a very heavy object. Penetrating trauma occurs as an object passes through the soft tissues, introducing pathogens to the body's interior and creating the risk of infection. Penetrating injury is likely to produce lacerations, incisions, and punctures as well as internal hemorrhage. Shear and tearing injuries may result in avulsions or amputation.

5. Discuss blunt and penetrating trauma. pp. 854–860

Blunt trauma is a kinetic force spread out over a relatively large surface area and directed at the body. It is most likely to induce injuries that do not break the skin, including contusions, and internal hemorrhage between the fascia, or hematomas. The stretching forces caused by blunt trauma, if significant enough, may cause a tear in the skin (laceration) and an open wound. Compression-type injuries can cause crushing wounds where the tissues and blood vessels and nerves are crushed, stretched, and torn.

Penetrating trauma, depending upon its exact mechanism, may cause a laceration (a jagged cut), an incision (a very precise or surgical cut), or a puncture (a deep wound with an opening that closes). Tearing or shear forces may cause an avulsion (a tearing away of skin), or an amputation (a complete severance or tearing away of a digit or limb). Scraping forces may abrade away the upper layers of skin and produce an abrasion.

6. Discuss the pathophysiology of soft-tissue injuries. pp. 854–860

Soft-tissue injuries either damage blood vessels and the structure of the soft tissue (blunt trauma) or open the envelope of the skin (penetrating trauma) and may permit pathogens to enter and blood to escape. Blunt trauma includes contusions, hematomas, and crush injuries. Penetrating trauma includes abrasions, lacerations, incisions, punctures, impaled objects, avulsions, and amputations. Soft-tissue wounds may also present with hemorrhage, either capillary (oozing), venous (flowing), or arterial (spurting). The hemorrhage may be external or internal. Once injured, the soft tissue has the ability to heal itself through hemostasis, inflammation, epithelialization, neovascularization, and collagen synthesis. It also is able, through the recruitment of blood cells (phagocytes), to combat invading pathogens and prevent or combat infection. Infection risk is increased with preexisting diseases like COPD or with diseases that compromise the immune system like HIV infection and AIDS. Use of medications like the NSAIDs also affects infection risk. The contamination introduced into the wound, the wound location (distal extremities), and the nature of the wound (puncture, crush, and avulsion) also have an impact on the risk of infection.

7. Differentiate among the following types of soft-tissue injuries:

  a. Closed pp. 855–856
  i. Contusion
    A contusion is a closed wound caused by blunt trauma that damages small blood vessels. The blood vessels leak, and the affected area becomes edematous. The contusion is characterized by swelling, pain, and, later on, discoloration. Since the wound is closed, the danger of infection is remote.
  ii. Hematoma
    The hematoma is a blunt soft-tissue injury in which blood vessels (larger than capillaries) are damaged and leak into the fascia, causing a pocket of blood. Large hematomas may accumulate up to 500 mL of blood.
  iii. Crush injuries
    Crush injuries occur as the soft tissues are trapped between a compressing force and an unyielding object and extensive injury occurs. The injury disrupts blood vessels, nerves,

muscle, connective tissue, bone, and possibly internal organs. Such an injury often provides a challenge to management because there is often serious bleeding from numerous sources and the nature of the wound makes the bleeding hard to control. Open crush injuries are frequently associated with severe infection.

b. Open pp. 857–860

i. **Abrasions**

An abrasion is a scraping away of the upper layers of the skin. It will normally present with capillary bleeding, and since the wound is open and may involve an extended surface, it can be associated with infection.

ii. **Lacerations**

Laceration is the most common open wound. It is a tear into the layers of the skin and, sometimes, deeper. A laceration can involve blood vessels, muscles, connective tissue, and other underlying structures. Since it is an open wound, it carries with it the danger of infection and external hemorrhage.

iii. **Incisions**

The incision is a very smooth laceration made by a surgical or other sharp instrument. It is otherwise a laceration.

iv. **Avulsions**

An avulsion is a partial tearing away of the skin and soft tissues. It is commonly associated with blunt skull trauma, animal bites, or machinery accidents. The degloving injury is a form of avulsion.

v. **Impaled objects**

An impaled object is any object that enters and then is lodged within the soft or other tissue. While its entry poses an infection risk, removing the object risks increased hemorrhage because the impaled object may be tamponading blood loss. Removal may also cause further harm if the object is irregular in shape.

vi. **Amputations**

An amputation is the partial or complete severance of a body part. The injury usually results in the complete loss of the limb distal to the site of severance; however, the severed limb can sometimes be successfully reattached or its tissue may be used for grafting to extend the length and usefulness of the remaining limb.

vii. **Punctures**

Punctures are penetrating wounds into the skin where the nature of the wound (deep and narrow) encourages closure. Pathogens driven into the wound by the mechanism find a hypoxic environment and may thrive in the injured tissue, resulting in serious infection.

8. Discuss the assessment and management of open and closed soft-tissue injuries. pp. 871–888

In the prehospital setting, the assessment of soft-tissue injuries is straightforward. In fact, soft-tissue injuries may be the only physical indications of serious internal injuries underneath. The assessment of these internal injuries is only complicated because the discoloration normally associated with them takes a few hours to develop. Examine the skin for any deformity, discoloration, or variation in temperature. Visualize any noted wound and determine its nature and extent. Be able to describe it (as it will be covered by a dressing and bandaging) to the attending physician upon your arrival at the emergency department.

The management of a soft-tissue wound is simply accomplished by meeting three objectives: immobilizing the wound site, keeping the wound clean (as sterile as possible), and controlling any hemorrhage. Immobilization will assist the clotting and healing processes. Keeping the wound sterile will reduce the bacterial load and reduce the risk and severity of infection. Controlling the hemorrhage with the use of direct pressure will limit blood loss and speed the repair cycle. In most circumstances, direct pressure effectively controls hemorrhage. Occasionally both direct pressure and elevation of the limb may be necessary. In severe cases of hemorrhage, the use of pressure points will be needed in addition to direct pressure and elevation. In extreme cases, such as severe crush injury, a tourniquet may be needed.

9. **Discuss the incidence, morbidity, and mortality of crush injuries.** pp. 856, 884–886

Crush injury is an infrequent mechanism that often results in severe soft-tissue damage. The extensive nature of the injury predisposes it to infection, which can be severe. Entrapment of a limb or body region may lead to crush syndrome in which a prolonged lack of circulation leads to the breakdown of muscle tissues and to rhabdomyolysis. Reperfusion of the affected region then transports myoglobin to the kidneys, threatening renal failure, and potassium to the heart, causing dysrhythmias or sudden death.

10. **Define the following conditions:**

   a. **Crush injury** pp. 856, 867–868, 884–886

   Crush injury occurs when a part of the body is trapped between a force and an object resisting it. Such injuries may occur as a limb is trapped in machinery, under a car as a jack releases, or in a building collapse. The injury disrupts the soft, connective, vascular, and nervous tissue and may injure internal organs.

   b. **Crush syndrome** pp. 856, 868, 884–886

   Crush syndrome occurs as a body part is trapped for more than 4 hours. The reduced or absent circulation within the trapped part does not permit the supply of oxygen and nutrients nor does it allow removal of carbon dioxide and waste products. The tissues become hypoxic and acidotic, and waste products accumulate. Upon release of the entrapping pressure, these toxins are returned to the central circulation with very severe effects. Fluid from the blood also flows into the injured tissue, resulting in a significant contribution to hypovolemia.

   c. **Compartment syndrome** pp. 866–867, 886

   Compartment syndrome occurs as edema increases the pressure within a fascial compartment of the body. The pressure restricts venous flow from the extremity, capillary flow through the affected portion of the limb, and arterial return to the central circulation. The result of untreated compartment syndrome is often loss of some of the muscle mass and possibly the shortening of the muscle mass.

11. **Discuss the mechanisms of injury, assessment findings, and management of crush injuries.** pp. 856, 867–868, 884–886

Crush injuries occur as soft tissues are trapped between two forces. The result is damage to the soft tissues, blood vessels, nerves, muscles, and bones. The limb or region that is crushed may appear normal or may be quite disfigured. Distal sensation and circulation may be disrupted, and the wound may not bleed at all or hemorrhage severely with no distinct site of hemorrhage. The limb may also feel hard and "boardlike" as hypoxia and acidosis cause the muscles to contract. Management of crush injury follows routine soft-tissue injury care with special emphasis on hemorrhage control (use of a tourniquet may be necessary), keeping the wound clean (as the crush injury is at increased risk for infection), and elevating the limb (to enhance venous return and distal circulation).

12. **Discuss the effects of reperfusion and rhabdomyolysis on the body.** pp. 868, 885–886

As a limb or other body region is compressed for more than 4 hours, the lack of circulation causes a destruction of muscle tissue (rhabdomyolysis). This destruction releases a protein, myoglobin; phosphate; potassium; and lactic and uric acids. When compression is released, reperfusion returns these toxins to the central circulation. Myoglobin clogs the tubules of the kidneys, especially when the patient is in hypovolemic shock. This may result in renal failure and, ultimately, death. More immediate, however, is the effect of the release of electrolytes on the heart. That release may result in dysrhythmias or sudden death. Other effects of reperfusion include calcification of the vasculature or of nervous tissue and increased cellular and systemic acidosis as restored circulation permits the production of uric acid.

13. **Discuss the pathophysiology, assessment, and care of hemorrhage associated with soft-tissue injuries, including:**

   a. **Capillary bleeding**   pp. 861, 875–878

   Capillary bleeding oozes from the wound and usually continues for a few minutes as the capillaries do not have the musculature to constrict as do the arteries and veins. The hemorrhage is usually minimal and can easily be controlled with the application of a dressing and minimal pressure.

   b. **Venous bleeding**   pp. 861, 875–878

   Venous hemorrhage may be extensive as the volume flowing through the vessels is equivalent to the amount flowing through arteries, though the pressure of flow is much less. Venous hemorrhage is limited as the injured vessel constricts and clotting mechanisms are usually effective. Simple direct pressure will easily stop most venous hemorrhage.

   c. **Arterial bleeding**   pp. 861, 875–878

   Arterial hemorrhage is powered by the blood pressure and, if the wound is open, may spurt bright red blood. The musculature of the arterial vessels will constrict to limit hemorrhage, but bleeding will likely still be heavy. Direct pressure must be applied to the bleeding site to effectively control it; in some cases, use of elevation and pressure points will be necessary.

   Basically, hemorrhage can be controlled by employing direct pressure, elevation, proximal arterial pressure, and, if all else fails, a tourniquet.

   Direct pressure is a very effective first-line technique for the control of hemorrhage. Since hemorrhage is powered by blood pressure, digital pressure at the site of blood loss should easily stop most blood loss.

   Elevation can be used to complement direct pressure. Elevating an extremity decreases the blood pressure to the limb, and the hemorrhage may be easier to control. Use elevation only for wounds on otherwise uninjured limbs, and only after direct pressure alone has proved ineffective.

   Use of a pressure point is an adjunct to both direct pressure and elevation. A proximal artery is located and compressed, reducing the pressure of the hemorrhage. Use of pressure points can be very helpful in the crush wound where the exact location of blood loss is difficult to locate.

   The tourniquet is the last technique to be used in attempts to control hemorrhage. A limb is circumferentially compressed above the systolic pressure under a wide band, such as a blood pressure cuff. If a lower pressure is used, the wound will bleed more severely. The tourniquet carries with it the additional hazard of permitting toxins to accumulate in the unoxygenated limb. These toxins endanger the future use of the limb and, when released into the central circulation, the patient's life.

14. **Describe and identify the indications for and application of the following dressings and bandages:**   pp. 869–871

   a. **Sterile/nonsterile dressing**

   Sterile dressings are used for wound care as it is important to reduce the amount of contamination at a wound site to reduce the risk of infection.

   b. **Occlusive/nonocclusive dressing**

   Most dressings are nonocclusive, which means they permit both blood and air to travel through them in at least a limited way. Occlusive dressings do not permit the flow of either fluid or air and are useful in sealing a chest or neck wound to prevent the aspiration of air or covering a moist dressing on an abdominal evisceration to prevent its drying.

   c. **Adherent/nonadherent dressing**

   Adherent dressings support the clotting mechanisms; however, as they are removed, they will dislodge the forming clots. Most dressings are specially treated to be nonadherent to reduce reinjury when they are removed from a wound.

   d. **Absorbent/nonabsorbent dressing**

   Most dressings used to treat wounds are absorbent, and they will soak up blood and other fluids. Nonabsorbent dressings absorb little or no fluid and are used to seal wound sites when a barrier to leaking is desired, for example, with the clear membranes that are used to cover venipuncture sites.

e. Wet/dry dressing
Wet dressings may provide a medium for the movement of infectious agents and are not frequently used in prehospital care. They may be used for abdominal eviscerations and burns.

f. Self-adherent roller bandage
The self-adherent roller bandage is soft, gauze-like material that molds to the contours of the body and is effective in holding dressings in place. As its stretch is limited, it does not pose the danger of increasing the bandaging pressure with each wrap as do some other bandaging materials.

g. Gauze bandage
Gauze bandaging is a self-adherent material that does not stretch and may increase the pressure beneath the bandage with consecutive wraps or with edema and swelling from the wound.

h. Adhesive bandage
An adhesive bandage is a strong gauze, paper, or plastic material backed with an adhesive. It can effectively secure small dressings to the skin where circumferential wrapping is impractical. It is inelastic and will not accommodate edema or swelling.

i. Elastic bandage
An elastic bandage is made of fabric that stretches easily. It conforms well to body contours but will increase the pressure applied with each wrap of the bandage. These bandages are often used to help strengthen a joint or apply pressure to reduce edema but should be used with great care, if at all, in the prehospital setting.

15. Predict the possible complications of an improperly applied dressing or bandage.
pp. 869–871, 881–882

Improper application of a dressing may include use of the wrong dressing for the injury or the application of the right dressing in an incorrect manner. Use of a nonocclusive dressing with an open chest wound may permit air to enter the thorax, increasing the severity of a pneumothorax, or use of such a dressing for a neck wound may permit air to enter the jugular vein, creating pulmonary emboli. Use of dry dressings with an abdominal evisceration may permit tissues to dry, adding additional injury, while use of wet dressings in other circumstances provides a route for infection of wounds. Adherent dressings may facilitate natural clotting but may dislodge clots and reinstitute hemorrhage as they are removed. If a dressing is too large for the wound, it may not permit application of adequate direct pressure to arrest hemorrhage. If a dressing is too small, it may become lost in the wound and again not provide a focused direct pressure to stop hemorrhage.

Improperly applied bandaging may either be insufficient to immobilize the dressing or to protect it from catching on items during care and transport. It may be too tight, restricting edema and swelling and compressing the soft tissues beneath, which can cause reduced or absent blood flow to the distal extremity. In such a case, the bandaging acts as a venous tourniquet and may actually increase the rate of hemorrhage as it increases the venous pressure. On the other hand, a bandage that is too loose may not maintain adequate direct pressure to stop bleeding or may not hold the dressing securely to the injury site.

16. Discuss the process of wound healing, including:

a. Hemostasis
pp. 862–863

Hemostasis is the process by which the body tries to restrict or halt blood loss. It begins with the constriction of the injured blood vessel wall to reduce the rate of hemorrhage. The injured tissue of the vessel wall and the platelets become sticky. The platelets then aggregate to further occlude the lumen. Finally, the clotting cascade produces fibrin strands that trap erythrocytes and form a more durable clot to halt all but the most severe hemorrhage.

b. Inflammation
p. 863

Cells damaged by trauma or invading pathogens signal the body to recruit white blood cells (phagocytes) to the injury site. These cells engulf or attack the membranes of the foreign agents. The by-products of this action cause the mast cells to release histamine, which dilates precapillary vessels and increases capillary permeability. Fluid and oxygen flows into the region resulting in an increase in temperature and edema.

c. Epithelialization p. 863

The stratum germinativum cells of the epidermis create an expanding layer of cells over the wound edges. This layer eventually joins almost unnoticeably, or, if the wound is too large, a region of collagen may show through (scar tissue).

d. Neovascularization p. 863

Neovascularization occurs as the capillaries surrounding the wound extend into the new tissue and begin to provide the new tissue with circulation. These new vessels are very delicate and prone to injury and tend to bleed easily.

e. Collagen synthesis p. 864

Collagen synthesis is the building of new connective tissue (collagen) in the wound through the actions of the fibroblasts. Collagen binds the wound margins together and strengthens the healing wound. The early repair is not as good as new but by the fourth month the wound tissue is about 60 percent of the original tissue's strength.

17. Discuss the assessment and management of wound healing. pp. 861–868

Wound healing is most commonly complicated by movement of the injury site or by infection. Injuries affecting joints, other locations associated with movement, or regions with poor circulation are most prone to improper wound healing. Immobilization can help the process. Infection is a common complication of open soft-tissue injuries and results in delayed or incomplete wound healing. Wound healing is best managed by keeping the site immobilized (within reason) and keeping the site as sterile as possible, with frequent dressing changes. In some cases, wound drainage may help remove the products of pathogen breakdown and enhance the recovery and healing process.

18. Discuss the pathophysiology, assessment, and management of wound infection. pp. 864–866

Next to hemorrhage, infection is the most common complication of open soft-tissue wounds. It occurs as pathogens are introduced into the wound site and grow, usually in the damaged, warm, and hypoxic tissues. The most common infectious agents are of the Staphylococcus and Streptococcus bacterial families. It takes a few days for the bacteria to grow to the numbers necessary for the development of significant signs and symptoms. Consequently, infection is not usually seen during emergency care. The site of infection is generally swollen, reddened, and warm to the touch. A foul-smelling collection of white blood cells, dead bacteria, and cellular debris (pus) may drain from the wound, and visible red streaks (lymphangitis) may extend from the wound margins toward the trunk. The patient may complain of fever and malaise. The management of an infected wound includes keeping the wound clean, permitting it to drain, and administering antibiotics.

19. Formulate treatment priorities for patients with soft-tissue injuries in conjunction with:

a. Airway/face/neck trauma pp. 886–887

Soft-tissue injury to the face and neck generally heals well due to the more than adequate circulation in the area. However, these wounds, due to their prominence, deserve special attention because of their cosmetic implications. They also deserve special concern because of the potential danger to the airway. First, ensure that the airway is patent and not in danger of being obstructed from either hemorrhage or swelling. Intubate early, possibly with rapid sequence intubation, to ensure the airway remains patent. In the most severe cases, cricothyrotomy (needle or surgical) may be necessary. If there are any open wounds to the neck, ensure they are covered with occlusive dressings to prevent the passage of air into the jugular veins.

b. Thoracic trauma (open/closed) pp. 887–888

Anticipate internal chest injury associated with superficial soft-tissue injuries to the thorax and cover any significant open wounds with occlusive dressings sealed on three sides. Auscultate the chest frequently to monitor respiratory exchange and anticipate progressive chest pathologies, increasing edema, or pneumothorax. Also anticipate associated internal hemorrhage and abdominal injuries and move quickly to transport the patient to a trauma center.

c. **Abdominal trauma** p. 888

In cases of abdominal trauma, consider the possibility of internal injury and dress all open wounds. Anticipate internal hemorrhage and move quickly to transport the patient to a trauma center. Cover any abdominal eviscerations with moistened sterile dressings, and then cover with occlusive dressings.

20. **Given several preprogrammed and moulaged soft-tissue trauma patients, provide the appropriate scene size-up, initial assessment, rapid trauma or focused physical exam and history, detailed exam, and ongoing assessment and provide appropriate patient care and transportation.** pp. 854–888

During your training as an EMT-Paramedic you will participate in many classroom practice sessions involving simulated patients. You will also spend some time in the emergency departments of local hospitals as well as in advanced-level ambulances gaining clinical experience. During these times, use your knowledge of soft-tissue injuries to help you assess and care for the simulated or real patients you attend.

Content Self-Evaluation

MULTIPLE CHOICE

_____ 1. About what percentage of soft-tissue wounds become infected, with a significant resultant morbidity?
   A. 2 percent
   B. 7 percent
   C. 15 percent
   D. 50 percent
   E. 75 percent

_____ 2. Which of the following types of wounds are unlikely to heal well?
   A. wounds that gape
   B. wound associated with static tension lines
   C. wounds associated with dynamic tension lines
   D. wounds perpendicular to tension lines
   E. all except B

_____ 3. The type of wound characterized by erythema usually seen during the prehospital setting is the:
   A. abrasion.
   B. contusion.
   C. laceration.
   D. incision.
   E. avulsion.

_____ 4. Which of the following wounds is not considered open?
   A. laceration
   B. abrasion
   C. contusion
   D. puncture
   E. avulsion

_____ 5. Which of the following wound types is characterized as a very clean, open wound?
   A. abrasion
   B. contusion
   C. laceration
   D. incision
   E. avulsion

_____ 6. Crush injuries usually involve injury to:
   A. blood vessels.
   B. nerves.
   C. bones.
   D. internal structures.
   E. all of the above

_____ 7. Which of the following is NOT usually considered an open wound?
   A. abrasion
   B. crush injury
   C. incision
   D. degloving injury
   E. avulsion

_____ 8. The wound that poses the greatest risk for serious infection is the:
   A. puncture.
   B. laceration.
   C. contusion.
   D. incision.
   E. hematoma.

_____ 9. The injury in which the skin is pulled off a finger, hand, or extremity by farm or industrial machinery is called a(n):
   A. amputation.
   B. incision.
   C. complete laceration.
   D. degloving injury.
   E. transection.

_____ 10. Amputations that occur cleanly are likely to be associated with severe hemorrhage.
   A. True
   B. False

_____ 11. The natural tendency of the body to maintain its normal environment and function is called:
   A. anemia.
   B. homeostasis.
   C. hemostasis.
   D. coagulation.
   E. metabolism.

_____ 12. When torn or cut, the muscles in the capillaries constrict, thereby limiting hemorrhage.
   A. True
   B. False

_____ 13. The agents that recruit cells responsible for the inflammatory response are called:
   A. macrophages.
   B. lymphocytes.
   C. chemotactic factors.
   D. granulocytes.
   E. fibroblasts.

_____ 14. The cells that attack invading pathogens directly or through an antibody response include all except:
   A. macrophages.
   B. lymphocytes.
   C. white blood cells.
   D. granulocytes.
   E. fibroblasts.

_____ 15. The stage of the healing process in which the phagocytes and lymphocytes are most active is:
   A. inflammation.
   B. epithelialization.
   C. neovascularization.
   D. collagen synthesis.
   E. none of the above

_____ 16. Regenerated skin, after about four months, is about how strong as compared to the original skin?
   A. 20 percent
   B. 30 percent
   C. 40 percent
   D. 50 percent
   E. 60 percent

_____ 17. Infection usually appears how long after the initial wound?
   A. 12 to 24 hours
   B. 1 to 2 days
   C. 2 to 3 days
   D. 4 to 6 days
   E. 7 to 10 days

_____ 18. Which of the following is an infection risk factor with soft-tissue wounds?
  A. advancing age
  B. crush injury
  C. NSAIDs use
  D. cat bites
  E. all of the above

_____ 19. Closing wounds with staples or sutures increases the risk of infection.
  A. True
  B. False

_____ 20. It is common practice to provide tetanus boosters if the patient's last booster was over:
  A. 1 year ago.
  B. 2 years ago.
  C. 3 years ago.
  D. 4 years ago.
  E. 5 years ago.

_____ 21. Which of the following can interfere with normal clotting?
  A. aspirin
  B. warfarin
  C. streptokinase
  D. penicillin
  E. all of the above

_____ 22. The location at greatest risk for compartment syndrome is the:
  A. calf.
  B. thigh.
  C. forearm.
  D. arm.
  E. ankle.

_____ 23. The excessive growth of scar tissue within the boundaries of the wound is called:
  A. hypertrophic scar formation.
  B. keloid scar formation.
  C. anatropic scar formation.
  D. residual scar formation.
  E. regressive scar formation.

_____ 24. A patient is not likely to experience injury, even when immobilized for a long period on a long spine board, PASG, or rigid splint.
  A. True
  B. False

_____ 25. The nature of crush injury produces an injury area that is an excellent growth medium for infection.
  A. True
  B. False

_____ 26. A crush injury that produces crush syndrome usually requires what minimum time of entrapment?
  A. 1 hour
  B. 2 hours
  C. 4 hours
  D. 6 hours
  E. 10 hours

_____ 27. Which of the following is likely with the release of entrapment in the patient suffering crush syndrome?
  A. kidney failure
  B. cardiac dysrhythmias
  C. hypovolemia
  D. abnormal vascular calcifications
  E. all of the above

_____ 28. The type of dressing that prevents the movement of fluid or air through the dressing is:
  A. sterile.
  B. nonadherent.
  C. absorbent.
  D. occlusive.
  E. nonocclusive.

_____ 29. The bandages that increase pressure beneath the bandage with each consecutive wrap are:
   A. elastic bandages.
   B. self-adherent roller bandages.
   C. gauze bandages.
   D. adhesive bandages.
   E. triangular bandages.

_____ 30. Not only is the skin the first body organ to experience trauma, it is often the only one to display the signs of injury.
   A. True
   B. False

_____ 31. Which of the following are important factors to consider in the assessment and management of external hemorrhage?
   A. type of bleeding
   B. rate of hemorrhage
   C. volume of blood lost
   D. stopping further hemorrhage
   E. all of the above

_____ 32. Which of the following is one of the primary objectives of bandaging?
   A. neat appearance
   B. hemorrhage control
   C. allowing easy movement of the wound
   D. debridement
   E. aeration

_____ 33. Insufficient tourniquet pressure may increase the rate and volume of hemorrhage.
   A. True
   B. False

_____ 34. The restoration of circulation once a tourniquet is released may cause which of the following?
   A. shock
   B. hypovolemia
   C. lethal dysrhythmias
   D. renal failure
   E. all of the above

_____ 35. After bandaging a patient's severely hemorrhaging forearm wound, you notice that the limb is cool, capillary refill is slowed, and the radial pulse cannot be found. You should:
   A. apply more dressing material and increase the pressure.
   B. leave the bandage as it is.
   C. loosen the bandage.
   D. elevate the extremity and assess circulation again.
   E. remove the bandage.

_____ 36. To alleviate pain associated with soft-tissue injury, you should administer morphine sulfate:
   A. 10 mg IV.
   B. 2 mg every 5 minutes titrated to pain relief.
   C. 5 mg every 5 minutes titrated to pain relief.
   D. 10 mg every 10 minutes times 2.
   E. 20 mg every 5 minutes titrated to pain relief.

_____ 37. With a large and gaping wound to the neck, use a(n):
   A. large absorbent dressing.
   B. large nonadherent dressing.
   C. occlusive dressing.
   D. nonabsorbent dressing.
   E. triangular bandage.

_____ 38. The type of dressing recommended for blood and fluid leaking from the auditory canal is a(n):
   A. nonocclusive dressing.
   B. nonadherent dressing.
   C. occlusive dressing.
   D. gauze dressing.
   E. wet dressing.

_____ 39. Which of the following is NOT a distal sign that a circumferential bandage is too tight?
   A. diaphoresis
   B. pallor
   C. loss of pulses
   D. tingling
   E. swelling

_____ 40. You find a patient who has suffered a finger amputation. You should keep the amputated part:
   A. warm and dry.
   B. warm and moist.
   C. cool and dry.
   D. cool and moist.
   E. packed in ice.

_____ 41. If the amputated part cannot be immediately located, wait only a few minutes at the scene as its transport with the patient is extremely important.
   A. True
   B. False

_____ 42. In which of the following situations is removal of an impaled object allowed or required?
   A. The object obstructs the airway.
   B. The object prevents performance of CPR.
   C. The object is impaled in the cheek.
   D. The object is impaled in the chest of a trauma patient who needs resuscitation.
   E. all of the above

_____ 43. Care for the patient with crush syndrome includes:
   A. rapid transport.
   B. fluid resuscitation.
   C. diuresis.
   D. possibly systemic alkalinization.
   E. all of the above

_____ 44. The most ideal fluid for the resuscitation of the crush syndrome patient, prior to extrication, is:
   A. hetastarch.
   B. normal saline.
   C. sodium bicarbonate.
   D. 5 percent dextrose in 1/2 normal saline.
   E. Dextran.

_____ 45. It is recommended that you infuse what volume of fluid to the crush syndrome patient per hour of entrapment?
   A. 10 mL/kg/hr
   B. 20 mL/kg/hr
   C. 30 mL/kg/hr
   D. 50 mL/kg/hr
   E. 100 mL/kg/hr

_____ 46. Sudden cardiac arrest care after extrication of the entrapped patient with crush syndrome should include the routine cardiac drugs and:
   A. potassium for hypokalemia.
   B. calcium chloride for hypokalemia.
   C. sodium bicarbonate for hypokalemia.
   D. dopamine for low blood pressure.
   E. none of the above

_____ 47. The most prominent symptom of compartment syndrome is:
   A. pain out of proportion to physical findings with the injury.
   B. reduced or absent distal pulses.
   C. increased skin tension in the affected limb.
   D. paresthesia.
   E. paresis.

_____ 48. Compartment syndrome is most likely to occur:
   A. immediately after injury.
   B. within 2 hours of injury.
   C. within 3 hours of injury.
   D. within 4 hours of injury.
   E. 6 to 8 hours after injury.

_____ 49. The most effective treatment in the prehospital setting for compartment syndrome is:
   A. a fasciectomy.
   B. the application of cold packs.
   C. elevation of the extremity.
   D. massaging the extremity.
   E. none of the above

_____ 50. A wound involving which of the following requires transport?
   A. nerves
   B. blood vessels
   C. tendons
   D. ligaments
   E. all of the above

Burns

Review of Chapter Objectives

After reading this chapter, you should be able to:

1. **Describe the anatomy and physiology of the skin and remaining human anatomy as they pertain to thermal burn injuries.** (see Chapter 3)

   The skin or integumentary system is the largest organ of the body and consists of three layers, the epidermis, the dermis, and the subcutaneous layer. It functions as the outer barrier of the body and protects it against environmental extremes and pathogens. The outermost layer is the epidermis, a layer of dead or dying cells that provides a barrier to fluid loss, absorption, and the entrance of pathogens. The dermis is the true skin. It houses the sensory nerve endings, many of the specialized skin cells that produce sweat, oil, and so on, and the upper-level capillary beds that allow for the conduction of heat to the body's surface. The subcutaneous layer, although not a true part of the skin, works in concert with the skin to insulate the body from heat loss and the effects of trauma.

2. **Describe the epidemiology, including incidence, mortality, morbidity, and risk factors for thermal burn injuries as well as strategies to prevent such injuries.** p. 892

   The incidence of burn injury has been declining over the past few decades but still accounts for over 1 million burn injuries and over 50,000 hospitalizations each year. Those at greatest risk are the very young, the elderly, the infirm, and those exposed to occupational risk (firefighters, chemical workers, and so on). Burns are the second leading cause of death for children under 12 and the fourth leading cause of trauma death.

   Much of the decline in burn injury and death is attributable to better building codes, improved construction techniques, and the use of smoke detectors. Educational programs that teach children not to play with matches or lighters and that instruct the family to turn the water heater down to below 120°F have also helped reduce burn morbidity and mortality.

3. **Describe the local and systemic complications of a thermal burn injury.** pp. 893–894, 904–906

   Thermal burn injury results as the rate of molecular movement in a cell increases, causing the cell membranes and proteins to denature. This causes a progressive injury as the heat penetrates deeper and deeper through the skin and into the body's interior. At the local level, the injury disrupts the envelope of the body, permitting fluid to leak from the capillaries into the tissue and evaporate, resulting in dehydration and cooling. Serious circumferential burns may form an eschar and constrict, restricting ventilation or circulation to a distal extremity.

The systemic effects of serious burns include severe dehydration and infection. Fluid is drawn to the injured tissue as it becomes edematous and then may evaporate in great quantities as the skin loses its ability to contain fluids. Infection can be massive and can quickly and easily overwhelm the body's immune system. The products of cell destruction from the burn process may enter the bloodstream and damage the tubules of the kidneys, resulting in failure. Organ failure due to burn byproducts may also affect the liver and the heart's electrical system. Lastly, the burn injury and the associated evaporation of fluid may cool the body more rapidly than it can create heat. The result is a lowering of body temperature, hypothermia.

4. Identify and describe the depth classifications of burn injuries, including superficial burns, partial-thickness burns, and full-thickness burns. pp. 902–903

Superficial (first-degree) burns involve only the upper layers of the epidermis and dermis. The effects are limited to an irritation of the upper sensory tissues with some pain, minor edema, and erythema.

Partial-thickness (second-degree) burns penetrate slightly deeper than first-degree burns and cause blistering, erythema, swelling, and pain. Since the cells that reproduce the skin's upper layers are still alive, complete regeneration is expected.

Full-thickness (third-degree) burns penetrate the entire dermis, causing extensive destruction. The burned area may display a variety of appearances and colors, the site is anesthetic, and healing is prolonged. Third-degree burns may involve not only the skin, but also underlying tissues and organs. (Organ and other tissue involvement is sometimes called fourth-degree burn.)

5. Describe and apply the "rule of nines" and the "rule of palms" methods for determining body surface area percentage of a burn injury. pp. 903–904

The "rule of nines" approximates the body surface area burned by assigning each body region 9 percent of the total. These regions include: each upper extremity, the anterior of each lower extremity, the posterior of each lower extremity, the anterior of the abdomen, the anterior thorax, the upper back, the lower back, and the entire head and neck. The remaining 1 percent is assigned to the genitalia. For children, the head is given 18 percent, and the lower extremities are assigned 13 1/2 percent each.

The "rule of palms" method of approximating burn surface area assumes the victim's palm surface (excluding the fingers) is equivalent to 1 percent of the total body surface area. The care provider then estimates the burn surface area by determining the number of palmar surfaces it would take to cover the wound.

6. Identify and describe the severity of a burn including a minor burn, a moderate burn, and a critical burn. pp. 909–912

Minor burns are those that are superficial and cover less than 50 percent of the body surface area (BSA), partial-thickness burns covering less than 15 percent of the BSA, or full-thickness burns involving less than 2 percent of the body surface area.

Moderate burns are classified as superficial burns over more than 50 percent of the BSA, partial-thickness burns covering less then 30 percent of the BSA; or full-thickness burns covering less than 10 percent of the BSA.

Critical burns are those partial-thickness burns covering more than 30 percent of the BSA, full-thickness burns over 10 percent of the BSA, and any significant inhalation injury. Critical burns also include any burns that involve any partial or full-thickness burn to the hands, feet, genitalia, joints, or face.

7. Describe the effects age and preexisting conditions have on burn severity and a patient's prognosis. pp. 905–906, 910–911

Burn patients who are very young, very old, or have a significant preexisting disease are at increased risk for the systemic problems associated with burn injury. They cannot tolerate massive fluid losses often associated with burns because they have smaller fluid reserves and they cannot effectively fight the ensuing massive infection commonly associated with large burns. They should be considered one step closer to critical than consideration of their burn type and BSA would normally place them.

8. Discuss complications of burn injuries caused by trauma, blast injuries, airway compromise, respiratory compromise, and child abuse. pp. 901–902, 906–909, 914–915

Traumatic injury, in the presence of burn injury, is a complicating factor that interferes with the burn healing process and may exacerbate hypovolemia. Any time these injuries coexist, the patient should be considered a higher priority than either injury would suggest, and the paramedic must care for both conditions.

Blast mechanisms produce injury through thermal burns, the pressure wave, projectile impact, and structural collapse (crush) mechanisms. When burns coexist with these other injuries, the patient priority for care and transport must be elevated at least one priority level and all injuries must be cared for. Again, the patient will have to heal from multiple injuries, making the recovery process more difficult.

Airway and respiratory compromise associated with burn injury is an extremely serious complication. The airway must be secured early, possibly with rapid sequence intubation, and adequate ventilation with supplemental oxygen ensured. Swelling of the upper or lower airway may rapidly occlude it, preventing both ventilation and intubation. In extreme circumstances, cricothyrotomy may be required. Also be watchful for carbon monoxide poisoning as it can reduce the effectiveness of oxygen transport without overt signs.

Burns associated with child abuse often result from scalding water immersion, open flame burns, or cigarette-type injuries. The child presents with a history of a burn that does not make sense, such as stove burns when he or she cannot yet reach the stove, multiple circular burns (cigarettes), or burns isolated to the buttocks, which occur as the child lifts his or her legs during attempts at immersion in hot water.

9. Describe thermal burn management including considerations for airway and ventilation, circulation, pharmacological and nonpharmacological measures, transport decisions, and psychological support/communication strategies. pp. 906–915

The management of the burn patient is a rather complicated, multifaceted process. The first consideration is to extinguish the fire to ensure the burn does not continue. If necessary, use water from a low-pressure hose and remove all jewelry, leather, nylon, or other material that may continue to smolder or hold heat and continue to burn the patient. Also consider removing any restrictive jewelry or clothing, as such an item may act as tourniquet, restricting distal blood flow as the burn region swells.

Then assess and ensure that the airway remains adequate. With any history suggestive of an inhalation burn or injury, carefully assess and monitor the airway for any signs of restriction. If they are found, move to protect the airway with rapid sequence intubation early, before the progressive airway swelling prevents intubation or significantly restricts the size of the endotracheal tube you can introduce. Small and painful burns may be covered with wet dressings to occlude airflow and reduce the pain; however, any extensive burn should be covered with a sterile dry dressing to prevent body cooling and the introduction of pathogens through the dressing.

Resuscitation for extensive burns must include large volumes of prehospital fluid (0.5 mL/kg × BSA), as burns often account for massive fluid loss into and through the burn. The patient must also be kept warm because by their nature burns account for rapid heat loss.

Any burns on opposing tissue, such as between the fingers and toes, should be separated by nonadherent dressings, as the burned surfaces are likely to adhere firmly together and cause further damage when they are pulled apart. In painful burns consider morphine, in 2 mg increments, for pain relief as long as there is no evidence of hypotension or respiratory depression.

Watch for any constriction from eschar formation that may reduce or halt distal circulation or restrict respiration. Medical direction may request a surgical incision to relieve the pressure (an escharotomy).

Any burn patient with serious injury should be transported to the burn center where he or she can receive the specialized treatment needed. Also ensure that the burn patient receives therapeutic communication while you are at the scene and during transport. The burn injury is very painful and the appearance can be very frightening. Constantly talk with the patient. Try to distract him or her from the injury, and monitor level of consciousness and anxiety level throughout your care and transport.

10. Describe special considerations for a pediatric patient with a burn injury and describe the criteria for determining pediatric burn severity. pp. 903–904, 905–906, 910–911

To determine the severity of a burn for a pediatric patient, you must first examine the depth of burn (superficial, partial, or full-thickness) and then determine the BSA affected. With children the head is given a greater percentage of BSA (18 percent) and the legs are given less (13½ percent). (Please note that there are several more specific methods to determine BSA for children that better take into account their changing anatomy, but they are more complicated and age- and size-specific and harder to use.) Once the BSA and depth of burn are determined, the pediatric patient is assigned a level of severity one place higher than that for the adult. Any serious burn to the airway, face, joint, hand, foot, or any circumferential burn is considered serious or critical as is the pediatric burn patient with another preexisting disease or traumatic injury.

11. Describe the specific epidemiologies, mechanisms of injury, pathophysiologies, and severity assessments for inhalation, chemical, and electrical burn injuries and for radiation exposure. pp. 914–921

Inhalation injuries are commonly associated with burn injuries and endanger the airway. They are caused by the inhalation of hot air or flame, which cause limited damage, by superheated steam, which results in much more significant thermal damage, or by the inhalation of toxic products of combustion, which results in chemical burns. Inhalation injury can also involve carbon monoxide poisoning and the absorption of chemicals through the alveoli and systemic poisoning. Any sign of respiratory involvement during the burn assessment process is reason to consider early and aggressive airway care and rapid transport.

Chemical burn injury is most frequently found in the industrial setting and is frequently associated with the effects of strong acids or alkalis. Both mechanisms destroy cell membranes as they penetrate deeper and deeper. The nature of the wounding process is somewhat self-limiting, though alkali burns tend to penetrate more deeply. Any chemical burn that disrupts the skin should be considered serious.

Electrical burn injuries are infrequent but can be very serious. As electricity passes through body tissue, resistance creates heat energy and damage to the cell membranes. The blood vessels and nerve pathways are especially sensitive to electrical injury. The heat produced can be extremely high and cause severe and deeply internal burn injury, depending upon the voltage and current levels involved. Any electrical burn that causes external injury or any passage of significant electrical current through the body is reason to consider the patient a high priority for transport, even if no overt signs of injury exist. Electrical injury can also affect the muscles of respiration and induce hypoxia or anoxia if the current remains. Electrical disturbances can also affect the heart, producing dysrhythmias. A special electrical injury is the lightning strike. Extremely high voltage can cause extensive internal injury, though often the current passes over the exterior of the body, resulting in limited damage. Resuscitation of the patient struck by lightning should be prolonged as this mechanism of injury may permit survival after lengthy resuscitation.

Radiation exposure is a relatively rare injury process caused by the passage of radiation energy through body cells. The radiation changes the structure of molecules and may cause cells to die, dysfunction, or reproduce dysfunctional cells. Radiation hazards cannot be seen, heard, or felt, yet they can cause both immediate and long-term health problems and death. The objective of rescue and care is to limit the exposure for both the patient and rescuer. Radiation exposure is cumulative. The less time in an area of hazard, the less effect radiation will have on the human body. The greater the distance from a radiation source, the less strength and potential it has to cause damage. Radiation levels are diminished as the particles travel through dense objects. By placing more mass between the source and patient and rescuers, the exposure is reduced. Since it is very difficult to determine the extent of exposure, gather what information you can and transport the patient for further evaluation.

12. Discuss special considerations that impact the assessment, management, and prognosis of patients with inhalation, chemical, and electrical burn injuries and with exposure to radiation. pp. 914–921

When assessing an inhalation injury, you should examine the mechanism of injury to identify any unconsciousness or confinement during fire or any history of explosive steam expansion and inhalation. Study the patient carefully for signs of facial burns, carbonaceous sputum, or any hoarseness. Should there be any reason to suspect inhalation injury, monitor the airway very carefully and consider oxygen therapy and early intubation (RSI) as needed. The airway tissues can swell quickly and result in serious airway restriction or complete obstruction.

Chemical burn injury is indicated by the signs or history of such exposure and should begin with an identification of the agent and type of exposure. Remove contaminated clothing and dispose of it properly. The site of exposure should be irrigated with copious amounts of cool water and, once the chemical is completely removed, covered with a dry sterile dressing. Special consideration should be given to contact with phenol (soluble in alcohol), dry lime (brush off before irrigation), sodium metal (cover with oil to prevent combustion), and riot control agents (emotional support). The prognosis for a serious chemical burn is related to the agent, length of exposure to it, and depth of damage. These injuries are often severe and will leave damaged or scar tissue behind.

With an electrical burn injury, direct your assessment to seeking out and examining entrance and exit wounds and to trying to determine the voltage and current of the source. The wounds should be covered with dry sterile dressings and the patient monitored for dysrhythmias. Even if the entrance and exit wounds seem minor, consider this patient for rapid transport as the internal injury may be extensive.

Radiation is invisible and otherwise undetectable by human senses. When radiation exposure is suspected, ensure that you and the patient remain as remote from the source (distance) with as much matter as possible between you and the source (shielding) and that you spend as little time close to the source as possible. Attention to these factors will reduce the amount of radiologic exposure for both you and the patient. Assessment of the patient exposed to a radiation source is very difficult because the signs of injury are delayed except in cases of extreme exposure. Any suggestion of exposure to radiation merits examination at the emergency department and assessment of the risk by specially trained experts in the field. Limited radiation exposure does not often result in medical problems, but more severe doses may cause sterility or, later in life, cancer. Extensive exposure may cause severe illness or death.

13. Differentiate between supraglottic and subglottic inhalation burn injuries. pp. 901–902

A supraglottic inhalation burn is a thermal injury to the mucosa above the glottic opening. It is a significant burn because the tissue is very vascular and will swell very quickly and extensively. Because of the moist environment and the vascular nature of the tissue, it takes great heat energy to cause burn injury. When such injury occurs, however, the associated swelling can quickly threaten the airway.

Subglottic (or infraglottic) inhalation burns occur much less frequently because the moist supraglottic tissue absorbs the heat energy and the glottis will likely close to prevent the injury from penetrating more deeply. However, superheated steam, as is produced when a stream of water hits a particularly hot portion of a fire, has the heat energy to carry the burning process to the subglottic region. There, airway burns are extremely critical, as even slight tissue swelling will restrict the airway.

Special consideration should also be given to the toxic nature of the hot gasses inhaled during the inhalation burn. Modern construction materials and the widespread use of synthetics are products that release toxic agents when they burn (cyanide, arsenic, hydrogen sulfide, and others). Often these agents will combine with the moisture of the airway and form caustic compounds that induce chemical burns of the airway, or they may be absorbed into the bloodstream, causing systemic poisoning. The risk for inhalation injury increases with a history of unconsciousness or with being within a confined space during a fire.

14. Describe the special considerations for a chemical burn injury to the eye. p. 919

Chemicals introduced onto the surface of the eye threaten to damage the delicate corneal surface. It is imperative that you consider these injuries when chemicals are splashed and that the eye is irrigated for up to 20 minutes. Irrigation may be accomplished by running normal saline through an administration set into the corner of the eye and directed away from the other eye if it is not affected. If both eyes are involved, a nasal cannula may be helpful in directing fluid flow to both eyes simultaneously. Be alert for contact lenses, as they may trap chemicals under their surface and prevent effective irrigation.

15. Given several preprogrammed, simulated thermal, inhalation, electrical, and chemical burn injury and radiation exposure patients, provide the appropriate scene size-up, initial assessment, rapid trauma or focused physical exam and history, detailed exam, and ongoing assessment and provide appropriate patient care and transportation. pp. 892–921

During your training as an EMT-Paramedic you will participate in many classroom practice sessions involving simulated patients. You will also spend some time in the emergency departments of local hospitals as well as in advanced-level ambulances gaining clinical experience. During these times, use your knowledge of burn trauma to help you assess and care for the simulated or real patients you attend.

Content Self-Evaluation

MULTIPLE CHOICE

_____ 1. The incidence of burn injury has been on the decline over the past decade.
   A. True
   B. False

_____ 2. A preventative action that will reduce the incidence of scalding injuries is:
   A. use of childproof faucets.
   B. education of children on the dangers of hot water.
   C. placing caution stickers on water faucets.
   D. lowering the water heater temperature to 120°F.
   E. none of the above

_____ 3. Burns result from the disruption of the proteins found in cell membranes.
   A. True
   B. False

_____ 4. The area of a burn that suffers the most damage is generally the:
   A. zone of hyperemia.   D. zone of coagulation.
   B. zone of denaturing.   E. zone of most resistance.
   C. zone of stasis.

_____ 5. The theory of burns that explains the burning process is:
   A. the thermal hypothesis.
   B. Jackson's theory of thermal wounds.
   C. the Phaseal discussion of burns.
   D. the hypermetabolism dynamic.
   E. none of the above

_____ 6. The order in which the phases of the body's response to a burn would normally be expected to occur is:
   A. emergent, fluid shift, hypermetabolic
   B. fluid shift, hypermetabolic, emergent
   C. fluid shift, emergent, hypermetabolic
   D. hypermetabolic, fluid shift, emergent
   E. emergent, hypermetabolic, fluid shift

_____ 7. Which of the following skin types has the greatest resistance to the passage of electrical current?
   A. mucous membranes
   B. wet skin
   C. calluses
   D. the skin on the inside of the arm
   E. the skin on the inside of the thigh

_____ 8. Electrical injury is likely to cause which of the following?
   A. serious injury where the electricity enters the body
   B. serious injury where the electricity exits the body
   C. damage to nerves
   D. damage to blood vessels
   E. all of the above

_____ 9. Prolonged contact with alternating current may result in respiratory paralysis.
   A. True
   B. False

_____ 10. Chemical burns involving strong alkalis are likely to be deep due to coagulation necrosis.
   A. True
   B. False

_____ 11. Burns due to strong acids are likely to be less deep than burns due to strong alkalis because they produce liquefaction necrosis.
   A. True
   B. False

_____ 12. Which of the following radiation types is least powerful?
   A. neutron
   B. alpha
   C. gamma
   D. beta
   E. delta

_____ 13. Which of the following radiation types is the most powerful type of ionizing radiation?
   A. lambda
   B. alpha
   C. gamma
   D. beta
   E. delta

_____ 14. Which of the following is a type of radiation present only inside nuclear reactors and bombs?
   A. neutron
   B. alpha
   C. gamma
   D. beta
   E. delta

_____ 15. To protect themselves from radiation exposure, EMS personnel should:
   A. limit the duration of exposure.
   B. increase the shielding from exposure.
   C. increase the distance from the source.
   D. ensure that the patient is decontaminated.
   E. all of the above

_____ 16. The radiation dose that is lethal to about 50 percent of those exposed is:
   A. 0.2 Gray.
   B. 100 rads.
   C. 1 Gray.
   D. 4.5 Grays.
   E. 200 rads.

_____ 17. As radiation exposure increases, the signs of exposure become less evident and only reappear later in the course of the disease.
   A. True
   B. False

_____ 18. Which of the following is commonly associated with inhalation injury?
   A. carbon monoxide poisoning
   B. toxic inhalation
   C. supraglottic injury
   D. subglottic injury
   E. all of the above

_____ 19. Which type of circumstance is most likely to cause subglottic thermal burn injury?
   A. inhalation of hot air
   B. inhalation of flame
   C. inhalation of superheated steam
   D. standing in a burn environment
   E. inhalation of toxic substances

_____ 20. What percentage of burn patients who die have associated airway burn injury?
   A. 20 percent
   B. 35 percent
   C. 50 percent
   D. 60 percent
   E. 80 percent

_____ 21. The burn characterized by erythema, pain, and blistering is the:
   A. superficial burn.
   B. partial-thickness burn.
   C. full-thickness burn.
   D. electrical burn.
   E. chemical burn.

_____ 22. The burn characterized by discoloration and lack of pain is the:
   A. superficial burn.
   B. partial-thickness burn.
   C. full-thickness burn.
   D. electrical burn.
   E. chemical burn.

_____ 23. An adult has received burns to the entire anterior chest and to the entire left upper extremity, circumferentially. Using the rule of nines, the percentage of body surface (BSA) area involved is:
   A. 9 percent.
   B. 18 percent.
   C. 27 percent.
   D. 36 percent.
   E. 48 percent.

_____ 24. A child has received burns to the entire left lower extremity and the genitals. Using the rule of nines, the percentage of the body surface area involved is:
   A. 9 percent.
   B. 10 percent.
   C. 14 1/2 percent.
   D. 19 percent.
   E. 21 1/2 percent.

_____ 25. An adult has received burns to the entire left lower extremity and the genitals. Using the rule of nines, the percentage of the body surface area involved is:
   A. 9 percent.
   B. 10 percent.
   C. 18 percent.
   D. 19 percent.
   E. 21 percent.

_____ 26. A child receives burns to his entire head and neck and upper back. What percentage of body surface area is involved?
   A. 9 percent
   B. 10 percent
   C. 18 percent
   D. 19 percent
   E. 27 percent

_____ 27. Which of the following systemic complications should you suspect with all serious burns?
   A. hypothermia
   B. hypovolemia
   C. infection
   D. eschar formation
   E. all of the above

_____ 28. Which of the following conditions would increase the impact a burn has on a patient?
   A. being very young
   B. being very old
   C. having the flu
   D. emphysema
   E. all of the above

_____ 29. Which of the following should NOT be removed from any burned area of a patient?
   A. nylon clothing such as a windbreaker
   B. small pieces of burned fabric lodged in the wound
   C. shoes and socks
   D. rings, watches, and other articles of jewelry
   E. leather belts

_____ 30. When considering intubation of the patient with suspected airway injury due to inhalation of the byproducts of combustion, you should have a supply of several smaller than normal endotracheal tubes ready.
   A. True
   B. False

_____ 31. In severe inhalation injury due to airway burns it may be necessary to perform a cricothyrotomy to secure an adequate airway.
   A. True
   B. False

_____ 32. High-flow oxygen therapy is very helpful in cases of carbon monoxide poisoning because it will then be carried in sufficient quantities in the plasma to maintain life.
   A. True
   B. False

_____ 33. Your assessment reveals an area of burn that is reddened, painful, and just beginning to display blisters. What burn classification would you give this burn?
   A. superficial burn
   B. partial-thickness burn
   C. full-thickness burn
   D. first-degree burn
   E. A or D

_____ 34. The patient you are attending has her entire left upper extremity seriously burned. The forearm and hand are very painful and reddened, while the upper arm is relatively painless and a dark red color. What percentage of the BSA and burn depth would you assign this patient?
   A. 9 percent full-thickness burn
   B. 9 percent partial-thickness burn
   C. 4½ percent full-thickness burn
   D. 4½ percent partial-thickness burn
   E. 4½ percent partial-thickness and 4½ percent full-thickness burn

_____ 35. Your assessment reveals a burn patient with superficial burns to 27 percent of the body. To which classification of burn severity would you assign her?
   A. minor
   B. moderate
   C. serious
   D. critical
   E. none of the above

_____ 36. Your assessment reveals a burn patient with full-thickness burns to the entire left thigh and calf. What classification of burn severity would you assign him?
   A. minor
   B. moderate
   C. serious
   D. critical
   E. none of the above

_____ 37. Your assessment reveals a burn patient with partial-thickness burns to all of both lower extremities. What classification of burn severity would you assign her?
   A. minor
   B. moderate
   C. serious
   D. critical
   E. none of the above

_____ 38. Your assessment reveals a burn patient with partial-thickness burns to her entire lower extremities and a suspected femur fracture. What classification of burn severity would you assign her?
   A. minor
   B. moderate
   C. serious
   D. critical
   E. none of the above

_____ 39. Cool water immersion may reduce the depth and significance of small burns if applied within:
   A. 1 to 2 minutes.
   B. 2 to 4 minutes.
   C. 4 to 5 minutes.
   D. 10 minutes.
   E. 20 minutes.

_____ 40. The patient with any full-thickness burn should be considered for administration of tetanus toxoid as the wound is an open one.
   A. True
   B. False

_____ 41. In general, moderate to severe burns should be covered with:
   A. moist occlusive dressings.
   B. dry sterile dressings.
   C. cool water immersion.
   D. plastic wrap covered by a soft dressing.
   E. warm water immersion.

_____ 42. Adjacent full-thickness burns, such as those affecting the fingers and toes, should be held together without dressings to ensure rapid healing.
   A. True
   B. False

_____ 43. The Parkland formula for fluid administration calls for administration of 4 mL of fluid to a patient multiplied by the patient's BSA involved. What other factor(s) determines the total fluid administered in the first 24 hours?
   A. patient's age
   B. patient's weight
   C. depth of burns
   D. age of the patient
   E. all of the above

_____ 44. Which of the following is the preferred fluid for resuscitation of the severely burned patient?
   A. normal saline
   B. ½ normal saline
   C. dextrose 5 percent in water
   D. lactated Ringer's solution
   E. dextrose 5 percent in normal saline

_____ 45. Which of the following drugs may be given to the patient with severe burns in the prehospital setting?
   A. ipratropium
   B. morphine
   C. epinephrine
   D. furosemide
   E. haloperidol

_____ 46. Which of the following may be appropriate when a forming eschar is restricting distal blood flow to an extremity?
   A. elevating the extremity
   B. incising the eschar to relieve the pressure
   C. wrapping the extremity in dry sterile dressings
   D. administering morphine
   E. immersing the limb in cold water

_____ 47. A patient was found unconscious in a burning mobile home. Your assessment discovers severe dyspnea, no airway restriction, chest pain, altered mental status, and some seizure activity. What condition would you suspect?
   A. carbon monoxide poisoning
   B. cyanide poisoning
   C. chemical burns to the lungs
   D. hypoxia due to inhalation of oxygen-deprived air
   E. superheated steam inhalation

_____ 48. If an IV line is not yet established in a patient with suspected cyanide poisoning, you should administer which of the following?
   A. amyl nitrate
   B. sodium nitrate
   C. sodium thiosulfide
   D. haloperidol
   E. ipratropium

_____ 49. In addition to the entrance and exit wounds normally expected with the passage of electrical current through the human body, the paramedic should expect:
   A. ventricular fibrillation.
   B. cardiac irritability.
   C. internal damage.
   D. smoldering clothing.
   E. all of the above

_____ 50. In the United States, lightning strikes hit about how many people per year?
   A. 25
   B. 50
   C. 100
   D. 300
   E. 500

_____ 51. The patient who is unresponsive, apneic, and pulseless due to a lightning strike is not a likely candidate for successful resuscitation.
   A. True
   B. False

_____ 52. In general, caustic chemical contamination should be cared for by:
   A. dry sterile dressings.
   B. chemical antidotes.
   C. rigorous scrubbing.
   D. cool water irrigation.
   E. rapid transport.

_____ 53. The chemical phenol is soluble in:
   A. water.
   B. dry lime.
   C. normal saline.
   D. ammonia.
   E. none of the above

_____ 54. Which chemical agent reacts vigorously with water?
   A. phenol
   B. bleach
   C. sodium
   D. riot control agents
   E. ammonia

_____ 55. Known antidotes and neutralizers for chemical contamination and burns will reduce the injury caused by the agent if administered immediately.
   A. True
   B. False

_____ 56. How long should you irrigate a patient's eye contaminated with chemicals of an unknown nature?
   A. less than 2 minutes
   B. up to 5 minutes
   C. up to 15 minutes
   D. up to 20 minutes
   E. none of the above

_____ 57. When chemicals are splashed into the eye of the patient wearing contact lenses, the contact should be removed to ensure irrigation will remove all of the agent.
   A. True
   B. False

_____ 58. If the source of radiation cannot be contained or moved away from the patient:
   A. the patient should be brought to you.
   B. care should be offered by you in protective gear.
   C. care should be offered by specialists in protective gear.
   D. care should be offered by the highest-ranking officer.
   E. A or C

_____ 59. Which action can be used to reduce rescuer exposure to a radiation source?
   A. increase the distance from the source
   B. decrease the time exposed to the source
   C. increase the shielding between the rescuer and source
   D. protect against inhalation of contaminated dust
   E. all of the above

_____ 60. Once exposed to a significant radiation source, the patient will become a source of radiation that the rescuer must then protect him- or herself against. No amount of decontamination will reduce this danger.
   A. True
   B. False

Musculoskeletal Trauma

Review of Chapter Objectives

After reading this chapter, you should be able to:

1. **Describe the incidence, morbidity, and mortality of musculoskeletal injuries.**

   p. 925

   In trauma, musculoskeletal injuries are second in frequency only to soft-tissue injuries. They account for millions of injuries ranging from strains to fractures and dislocations and are rarely, by themselves, life-threatening. However, significant musculoskeletal injuries are found in 80 percent of patients who suffer multisystem trauma and may account for significant disability.

2. **Discuss the anatomy and physiology of the muscular and skeletal systems.**

   (see Chapter 3)

   The skeletal system is a living body system that protects vital organs, acts as a storehouse for body salts and other materials needed for metabolism, produces erythrocytes, permits us to have an upright stature, and permits us to move with relative ease through the environment. The skeletal system consists of the axial and appendicular skeletons.

   The common long bone consists of a diaphysis, metaphysis, and epiphysis. The diaphysis is the hollow skeletal shaft of the long bone and contains the yellow bone marrow. It is covered by the periosteum, which contains sensory nerve fibers and initiates the bone repair cycle. The metaphysis is the transitional region between the diaphysis and the epiphysis. In this region, the thin layer of compact bone of the diaphysis shaft becomes the honeycomb of the weight-bearing epiphyseal region. The epiphysis is the articular end of the bone. Through the widening of the metaphysis and the cancellous bone underneath, the weight-bearing, articular surface distributes support over a large surface area.

   Bones join at an area called a joint, where they move together to permit articulation. The actual surface of movement is the articular surface and is covered with cartilage, a smooth, shock-absorbing surface that allows free movement between the two ends of the adjoining bones. It is the actual joint surface. The joint is held together with ligaments, which are bands of connective tissue attaching bones to each other. These bands encapsulate the joint and allow some stretch, while holding the articulating bones firmly together.

   Muscles make up most of the body's mass, are the driving power behind body motion, and also provide most of the body's heat energy. They only have the ability to contract with force; hence, they are usually paired with one opposing the motion of the other. Muscles are usually attached by strong connective tissue called tendons. The point of attachment that remains stationary with muscle contraction is the origin, while the point of attachment that moves is the insertion.

3. **Predict injuries based on the mechanism of injury, including:** pp. 926–931, 933

   - **Direct.** Direct injury can be caused by blunt or penetrating mechanisms that deliver kinetic energy to the location of injury and may account for fractures, dislocations, muscle contusions, strains, sprains, subluxations, or combinations of the above.
   - **Indirect.** Indirect injuries are injuries that occur as energy is transmitted along the musculoskeletal system to a point of weakness. For example: A person falls forward and braces the fall on an outstretched arm. The energy is transmitted up the extremity to the clavicle, where a fracture occurs. Another example is the football player whose cleated shoe remains stationary while contact with an opposing player turns his body, resulting in an injury to the ligament of the knee.
   - **Pathologic.** Pathologic injury results from tumors of the periosteum, bone, articular cartilage, ligaments, tendons, or muscles. Diseases that affect the musculoskeletal structures may also cause injuries as may radiation treatment. Bones or joint structures injured in this way are not likely to heal well.

4. **Discuss the types of musculoskeletal injuries, including:**

   - **Fractures (open and closed)** pp. 928–931
   A fracture is a break in the continuity of the bone. It may present with pain, false motion, angulation, and, possibly, an open wound.
   - **Dislocations/fractures** pp. 927–928
   A dislocation is a displacement of one of the bones of a joint from the joint capsule. The area is noticeably deformed, the limb is usually fixed in position, and the injury is very painful. Due to the proximity of blood vessels and nerves, there is a concern for involvement of these structures and loss of distal circulation and sensation. A fracture is a disruption in the continuity of a bone. In a closed fracture, bone ends do not penetrate the skin. In an open fracture, they do. Other types of fractures include hairline, impacted, transverse, oblique, comminuted, spiral, fatigue, greenstick, and epiphyseal. Fractures may also occur in the proximity of joints and present in a similar fashion with similar dangers.
   - **Sprains** p. 928
   A sprain is the tearing of the ligaments of a joint. The injury produces pain, swelling, and discoloration with time. Since the injury has damaged the joint's integrity, further exertion may cause joint failure. A subluxation is a transitional injury between the sprain and dislocation. The ligaments have been stretched and do not provide a stable joint. The range of motion may be limited and the site is very painful.
   - **Strains** p. 927
   A strain is an overstretching of a muscle body that produces pain. The muscle fibers have been damaged; however, there is usually no internal hemorrhage or associated discoloration.

5. **Describe the six "Ps" of musculoskeletal injury assessment.** p. 935

   - **Pain.** The patient with musculoskeletal injury may report pain, pain on touch (tenderness), or pain on movement of the injured limb.
   - **Pallor.** The skin at the injury site and distal to it may be pale or flushed and capillary refill may be delayed.
   - **Paralysis.** The patient may be unable to move the limb and/or may have diminished strength distal to the injury.
   - **Paresthesia.** The patient may complain of numbness or tingling or may have limited or no sensation distal to the injury.
   - **Pressure.** The patient may complain of a sensation of pressure at the site of injury or palpation may detect a greater skin tone and tissue rigidity at the injury site.
   - **Pulses.** The distal pulses may be diminished or absent distal to the injury site.

6. List the primary signs and symptoms of extremity trauma. pp. 933–937

The primary signs of extremity trauma include pain, mechanism of injury, deformity (angulation or swelling), soft-tissue injuries (suggesting injury beneath), unusual limb placement, inequality in limb length, and the inability of the patient to bear weight or use the extremity.

7. List other signs and symptoms that can indicate less obvious extremity injury. pp. 935–937

In addition to the six "Ps" of musculoskeletal injury, the injury may demonstrate instability of the joint or limb, inequality of sensation or limb strength, crepitus (a grating sensation), unusual motion, abnormal muscle tone, and unusual regions of warmth or coolness.

8. Discuss the need for assessment of pulses, motor function, and sensation before and after splinting. p. 940

It is essential to monitor distal pulses, sensation, and motor function during the splinting process. You need to first determine a baseline to ensure that the distal function of the limb is intact before you begin the process. If an initial deficit is found, minor movement of the limb may restore it. Once the process is complete, and frequently thereafter, you need to ensure that the splint does not constrict the limb too forcibly, restricting distal blood flow. The check will also ensure that venous return is adequate and that the nerves remain uncompressed and functional.

9. Identify the circumstances requiring rapid intervention and transport when dealing with musculoskeletal injuries. pp. 933–934

Because musculoskeletal injuries are not often associated with life-threatening injuries, they by themselves do not frequently require rapid intervention and transport. However, when the distal circulation or innervation is interrupted by the injury, immediate intervention and rapid transport may be indicated. If a distal pulse or nervous function deficit is noted, you may try to gently manipulate the injury site to restore pulse or function (this includes dislocation reduction in some circumstances). It is also imperative to bring the patient to the emergency department quickly if your attempts to correct the circulation or nervous problem are unsuccessful.

10. Discuss the general guidelines for splinting. pp. 938–942

Once any patient life threats and serious injuries have been cared for, splinting may take place. The injury is assessed as are the distal pulse, sensation, and motor function. Any open wound is covered with a sterile dressing and the limb is positioned for splinting, as long as the injury is no closer than 3 inches from a joint. Provide any movement for limb positioning with gentle in-line traction unless the movement significantly increases pain or resistance is felt. Choose a device (long padded board splint, air splint, traction splint, and so on) that accommodates the limb and secure it to immobilize the joint above and the joint below the injury. Secure the splint from the distal to the proximal end to ensure the best venous return and check distal circulation, sensation, and motor function in the limb at the end of the splinting process. Joint injuries are generally immobilized as found unless there is distal pulse, sensation, or motor function deficit. Then an attempt to align the injury may be indicated.

11. Explain the benefits of the application of cold and heat for musculoskeletal injuries. pp. 944–945

The application of cold to a musculoskeletal injury in the few hours after the injury constricts the vasculature and limits edema. This ensures better circulation through the limb after the injury, especially if splinting is employed. Heat applied after 48 hours will increase the circulation to the injury site and speed the healing process.

12. Describe age-associated changes in the bones. p. 931

As bones develop in the fetus they are almost exclusively cartilaginous in nature. This makes them extremely flexible but not very rigid. With the newborn and infants, the cartilage begins to fill with salt deposits and becomes stronger and more rigid. It is, however, still very flexible and one reason infants have a hard time standing and holding their heads up. Bones lengthen from the epiphyseal plate near the bone ends, an area where fracture may disrupt the growth process. With increasing age, children's bones become more rigid, but they are prone to fractures like the greenstick, breaking and splintering on one side but not breaking completely. By the late teen years, the bone tissue reaches its maximum strength. As an adult reaches 40 years of age, bone degeneration begins. The bones become less flexible and more prone to fracture. They also heal more slowly. With advancing age and continuing bone degeneration, fractures may occur with normal stresses and lead to falls.

13. Discuss the pathophysiology, assessment findings, and management of open and closed fractures.   **pp. 928–931, 933–948**

Fractures are generally traumatic events that disrupt the structure of the bone. They may be a result of blunt trauma such as a fall or an auto collision or of penetrating trauma as when a bullet slams into a rib. Assessment will reveal a patient who complains of pain and the inability to use the extremity. Physical assessment will reveal angulation, swelling, deformity, and false motion (where joint-like motion is unexpected). Distally, the limb may display pallor, coolness, diminished or absent pulses, reduced sensation or motor function, and may be shortened when compared to the opposing limb. By definition, there will be an open wound associated with an open fracture, though it may be caused by the offending force causing the fracture or by one or more of the fractured bone ends penetrating the skin. Management includes covering any open wound with a sterile dressing and then gently aligning the bone with traction and immobilizing it and the joints above and below the injury with a splinting device.

14. Discuss the relationship between the volume of hemorrhage and open or closed fractures.   **pp. 934, 945–946**

Fractures alone, whether open or closed, do not often account for severe and continued blood loss with the exception of pelvic and femoral fractures. Pelvic fractures may account for more than 2,000 mL of blood loss and femoral fractures, up to 1,500 mL. Tibial/fibular and humeral fractures may account for 500 mL of loss, and other fractures and dislocations for less. These losses do contribute to hypovolemia and shock in the multisystem trauma patient. Closed fractures have limited blood loss because of fascial containment of the hemorrhage, with the exception of the pelvis, where lack of any fascial compartment helps account for the severe hemorrhage associated with that injury. Open wounds may permit blood to be lost externally in excess of the numbers above, but hemorrhage control techniques should easily control that loss.

15. Discuss the indications and contraindications for use of the pneumatic anti-shock garment (PASG) in the management of fractures.   **pp. 945–946**

Use of the PASG is indicated in fractures of the pelvis because of its ability to immobilize the pelvis and lower extremities and its ability to apply pressure to the abdomen and lower extremities, thereby limiting the blood loss associated with such injuries. The pelvic sling and long board is an acceptable pelvic splint. The PASG may also be indicated in the stabilization of the patient with bilateral femur fracture for the same reasons. Contraindications include any isolated femur fracture because the traction splint provides preferred immobilization. The PASG should not be used with hip dislocations and for any fractures more distal than 3 inches above the knee.

16. Describe the special considerations involved in femur fracture management.   **pp. 945–947**

The femur is the largest long bone of the body and its fracture requires great energy, resulting in a serious and very traumatic injury. The injury is generally very painful, causing the large muscles of the thigh to contract and naturally splint the site. This action pushes the broken femur ends into the muscles of the thigh, increasing the pain and causing further muscle spasm. The result is a serious and progressing injury. Gentle traction can prevent further damage and pain from the femur movement and then relax the muscle masses, allowing the femur ends to move back to a more anatomic position. This enhances blood flow through the limb and reduces soft-tissue injury caused by the overriding bones. Gentle traction is applied manually and then is maintained by a traction splint device.

17. Discuss the pathophysiology, assessment findings, and management of dislocations.   **pp. 928, 948–949, 949–950, 951**

Dislocations are forceful events that displace the bone ends from their proper location within a joint by stretching or tearing ligaments. The patient will complain of pain and the inability to use the joint, while you will notice deformity of the joint and unusual limb placement. Dislocations are usually immobilized as they are found unless the pulse, sensation, or motor function distal to the injury is disrupted or the time from injury to care at the emergency department will be long. Then attempts made at dislocation reduction may be made.

18. Discuss the out-of-hospital management of dislocations/fractures, including splinting and realignment.   **pp. 942–952**

The objective of dislocation and fracture care is splinting to prevent further injury during transport to the emergency department. A splint should be chosen for ease in application, ability to immobilize the fracture or dislocation site (and the joint above and below), and patient comfort. The limb should be aligned to ensure adequate immobilization with the splint by bringing the distal limb in line (using gentle traction) with the proximal limb. The movement continues until the limb is aligned, you meet resistance, or the patient experiences a significant increase in pain. The devices below should be utilized only if they can accomplish the goals of splinting effectively.

Pelvis—PASG, long spine board with pelvic sling
Hip—long spine board, orthopedic stretcher
Femur—traction splint
Knee—padded board splints
Tibia and fibula—padded board splints, air splint
Ankle—pillow splint, padded board splint, air splint
Foot—pillow splint, padded board splint, air splint, conforming splint
Shoulder—sling and swathe
Humerus—cuff and collar sling and swathe
Elbow—padded board splint
Radius and ulna—padded board splint, air splint
Wrist—padded board splint, air splint
Hand—padded board splint, conforming splint, air splint
Finger—conforming splint, padded board splint

19. Explain the importance of manipulating a knee dislocation/fracture with an absent distal pulse.   **pp. 949–950**

The absence of distal pulses secondary to a fracture or dislocation may be due to associated pressure on the artery due to bone displacement. Gentle, controlled manipulation may move the bones enough to reestablish the distal circulation and ensure that the distal tissues receive adequate perfusion during the remaining care and transport.

20. Describe the procedure for reduction of a shoulder, finger, or ankle dislocation/fracture.   **pp. 950, 951, 952**

The general process for dislocation reduction is to use increasing traction to move the bone ends apart (distraction) and then toward a normal anatomic position. The pull is slowly increased over about 3 minutes or until you feel the bone ends "pop" into position and see the limb assume a more normal anatomic appearance. The distal circulation, sensation, and motor function are examined before and after the procedure to ensure that distal function remains normal. Generally, reduction is not attempted unless there is serious neurovascular compromise. If the procedure does not produce relocation in a few minutes, splint the limb as is and transport.

Shoulder dislocations are most commonly anterior (hollow or squared-off shoulder) or posterior (elbow and forearm held off the chest). Place a strap across the chest and under the arm and have a rescuer pull traction against the traction you pull along the arm while you draw the arm somewhat away from the chest (abduction). Some rotation along the axis of the humerus (by rotating the elbow) may facilitate reduction. For the less-common inferior dislocation, have one rescuer stabilize the chest while you flex the elbow and apply a firm traction along the axis of the humerus. Gently rotate the humerus externally.

Finger dislocations are relatively common and most often displace posteriorly. Grasp the finger and apply firm distal traction, distracting the two bone ends and moving the finger toward the normal anatomic position.

Ankle dislocations present with the ankle turned outward (lateral), the foot pointing upward (anterior), and the foot pointing downward (posterior). With the anterior dislocation, grasp the toe and heel and rotate the foot toward a normal orientation. With the anterior dislocation, move the foot posteriorly, while with posterior dislocations, move the foot anteriorly.

21. Discuss the pathophysiology, assessment findings, and management of sprains, strains, and tendon injuries. pp. 927, 928, 952

Sprains generally result from the movement of a joint beyond its normal range of motion while the ligaments holding it together are stretched or torn. The patient will complain of a mechanism of injury and pain at the joint that usually increases with any attempt to move it or put weight on it. Management is centered around immobilizing the site and transporting the patient to rule out fracture (by X-ray).

Strains are overexertion injuries to the muscles where muscle fibers are torn. The particular muscle is sore, and pain will increase with attempts to use it. Care is centered around rest and reduced use of the muscle until the body can heal it.

Tendon injuries include tears or ruptures of the tendons, or the tendons may pull loose from their skeletal attachments. Injury is usually due to overexertion or to severe blunt or penetrating trauma. Care is usually directed at immobilizing the patient's affected limb in the position of function (neutral positioning) and transporting for assessment and possible surgical repair at the emergency department.

22. Differentiate among musculoskeletal injuries based on the assessment findings and history. pp. 933–938

It is very difficult to differentiate between muscle, joint, and long-bone injuries in the prehospital setting. Hence, treat any suspected musculoskeletal injury found within 3 inches of a joint as a dislocation, splinting it as it is found unless there is a distal neurovascular deficit. In that case, reduction may be considered. Injuries affecting the limbs and more than 3 inches from the joint are considered fractures and are brought into alignment using gentle distal traction unless there is a great increase in pain or you meet resistance.

23. Given several preprogrammed and moulaged musculoskeletal trauma patients, provide the appropriate scene size-up, initial assessment, rapid trauma or focused physical exam and history, detailed exam, and ongoing assessment and provide appropriate patient care and transportation. pp. 925–955

During your training as an EMT-Paramedic you will participate in many classroom practice sessions involving simulated patients. You will also spend some time in the emergency departments of local hospitals as well as in advanced-level ambulances gaining clinical experience. During these times, use your knowledge of musculoskeletal trauma to help you assess and care for the simulated or real patients you attend.

Content Self-Evaluation

MULTIPLE CHOICE

_____ 1. Musculoskeletal injuries can include injury to:
   A. bones.
   B. tendons.
   C. ligaments.
   D. muscles.
   E. all of the above

_____ 2. Contusion can account for significant fluid loss into the more massive muscles of the body.
   A. True
   B. False

_____ 3. A specific sign associated with compartment syndrome is:
   A. deep pain.
   B. absent distal pulses.
   C. pain on passive extension.
   D. absent distal sensation.
   E. diaphoresis.

_____ 4. The condition in which exercise draws down the supply of oxygen and energy reserves and metabolic waste products accumulate, limiting the ability of a muscle group to perform is called:
   A. cramp.
   B. fatigue.
   C. strain.
   D. sprain.
   E. spasm.

_____ 5. The tissue that is normally damaged in a sprain is the:
   A. tendon.
   B. ligament.
   C. muscle.
   D. articular cartilage.
   E. epiphyseal plate.

_____ 6. The overstretching of a muscle that presents with pain is a:
   A. strain.
   B. sprain.
   C. cramp.
   D. spasm.
   E. subluxation.

_____ 7. Which of the following fractures is relatively stable?
   A. hairline
   B. impacted
   C. transverse
   D. comminuted
   E. both A and B

_____ 8. Which of the following fractures is most likely to be open?
   A. fibula
   B. tibia
   C. femur
   D. humerus
   E. ulna

_____ 9. In serious long-bone fractures, especially those that are manipulated after injury, there is the possibility of fat embolizing and becoming lodged in the lungs.
   A. True
   B. False

_____ 10. Which of the following types of fractures is likely to occur only in the pediatric patient?
   A. greenstick
   B. oblique
   C. transverse
   D. comminuted
   E. spiral

_____ 11. The bones of the elderly are likely to be:
   A. less flexible.
   B. more brittle.
   C. more easily fractured.
   D. more slow to heal.
   E. all of the above

_____ 12. The dislocation, or fracture in the area of a joint, is generally less significant than the long-bone shaft fracture because it does not have as high an incidence of vascular and nervous injury.
   A. True
   B. False

_____ 13. The energy and degree of manipulation needed to cause further injury after a bone has broken is much less than was initially needed to cause the fracture.
   A. True
   B. False

_____ 14. The growth of bone that comes after a fracture and encapsulates the fracture site is called the:
   A. epiphyseal outgrowth.
   B. periosteum.
   C. callus.
   D. natural splinting.
   E. comminution.

_____ 15. Which of the following is caused by a build-up of uric acid crystals in the joints?
   A. gout
   B. rheumatoid arthritis
   C. osteoarthritis
   D. bursitis
   E. tendinitis

_____ 16. An inflammation of the small synovial sacs that reduce friction and cushion tendons from trauma is:
   A. gout.
   B. rheumatoid arthritis.
   C. osteoarthritis.
   D. bursitis.
   E. tendinitis.

_____ 17. Which of the following is an indication for the use of PASG in the patient with skeletal injury?
   A. pelvic fracture
   B. serious tibial fracture
   C. femur fracture
   D. hip dislocation
   E. both A and D

_____ 18. With which of the fractures below should you consider immediate transport of the patient because of possible internal blood loss?
   A. humerus
   B. femur
   C. tibia
   D. pelvis.
   E. both B and D

_____ 19. When assessing a limb for possible fracture, you should examine distally for:
   A. sensation.
   B. motor strength.
   C. circulation.
   D. crepitus.
   E. all of the above

_____ 20. A patient complains of a "pins and needles" sensation between the webs of his toes and a serious crushing-type injury has caused his calf to feel "almost board hard." What injury would you suspect?
   A. tibial fracture
   B. muscular contusion
   C. compartment syndrome
   D. tendinitis
   E. subluxation

_____ 21. An elderly patient who has suffered a fracture due to bone degeneration is expected to experience what level of pain when compared to a traumatic fracture?
   A. about the same
   B. more pain
   C. less pain
   D. no pain at all
   E. extreme pain

_____ 22. As the effects of the fight-or-flight response wear off, the symptoms of fracture will become less evident.
   A. True
   B. False

_____ 23. It is essential to tell the patient that limb alignment will cause some increased pain, as this will help maintain his or her confidence in you.
    A. True
    B. False

_____ 24. In general, long-bone shaft fractures should be splinted:
    A. aligned, except if resistance is experienced.
    B. as found.
    C. extended, except if resistance is experienced.
    D. flexed, except if resistance is experienced.
    E. none of the above

_____ 25. Do not attempt realignment of any fracture within 3 inches of a joint.
    A. True
    B. False

_____ 26. Which of the following limb positions is ideal for the immobilization of most extremity injuries?
    A. extended
    B. flexed
    C. hyperextended
    D. hyperflexed
    E. neutral

_____ 27. Ascending to altitude in a helicopter will cause the pressure in the air splint to:
    A. increase.
    B. decrease.
    C. remain the same.
    D. become less uniform.
    E. become more uniform.

_____ 28. The traction splint is designed to splint which musculoskeletal injury?
    A. knee dislocation
    B. hip dislocation
    C. pelvic fracture
    D. femur fracture
    E. all of the above

_____ 29. Which of the following is a disadvantage of the vacuum splint when applying it to splint fractures?
    A. It is difficult to apply.
    B. It is bulky and heavy.
    C. It shrinks during application.
    D. It takes more than two rescuers to apply.
    E. all of the above

_____ 30. Align a seriously angulated long-bone fracture unless:
    A. there is an absent distal pulse.
    B. there is absent sensation.
    C. both sensation and pulses are intact.
    D. you meet with resistance.
    E. you feel crepitus.

_____ 31. If after moving a limb to alignment you notice the distal pulse is absent, you should:
    A. splint the limb, as is.
    B. gently move the limb to restore the pulse.
    C. return the limb to the original positioning.
    D. elevate the limb and then splint it.
    E. splint and apply an ice pack.

_____ 32. With joint injury you should not move the limb around, even to restore circulation or sensation.
    A. True
    B. False

_____ 33. Early reduction of a dislocation usually results in which of the following?
    A. less stress on the ligaments
    B. less stress on the joint structure
    C. better distal circulation
    D. better distal sensation
    E. all of the above

_____ 34. Signs that a reduction of a dislocation has been effective include:
   A. feeling a "pop."
   B. patient reports of less pain.
   C. greater mobility in the joint.
   D. less deformity of the joint.
   E. all of the above

_____ 35. Heat may be applied to a muscular injury:
   A. immediately.
   B. after 1 hour.
   C. after 24 hours.
   D. after 48 hours.
   E. not at all.

_____ 36. The splinting device recommended for a painful and isolated fracture of the femur is:
   A. the vacuum splint.
   B. the PASG.
   C. the spine board and padding.
   D. long padded board splints.
   E. none of the above

_____ 37. The splinting device recommended for a painful and isolated fracture of the tibia is the:
   A. traction splint.
   B. PASG.
   C. long spine board and padding.
   D. padded board splint.
   E. sling and swathe.

_____ 38. The splinting device recommended for an isolated fracture of the humerus is the:
   A. traction splint.
   B. sling and swathe.
   C. air splint.
   D. padded board splint.
   E. both B and D

_____ 39. The fracture of the forearm close to the wrist that presents with the "silver fork" deformity is called:
   A. Richardson's fracture.
   B. Colles' fracture.
   C. Volkman's contracture.
   D. Blundot's inversion.
   E. none of the above

_____ 40. An anterior hip dislocation normally presents with the:
   A. foot turned outward.
   B. foot turned inward.
   C. knee flexed.
   D. knee turned outward.
   E. knee turned inward.

_____ 41. In general, anterior dislocations of the knee can be reduced in the prehospital setting.
   A. True
   B. False

_____ 42. Which of the following is NOT a sign of patellar dislocation?
   A. knee in the flexed position
   B. significant joint deformity
   C. the extremity drops at the knee
   D. lateral displacement of the patella
   E. none of the above

_____ 43. If a patient presents with an ankle deformed with the foot turned outward, you would suspect which type of ankle dislocation?
   A. anterior
   B. posterior
   C. lateral
   D. medial
   E. inferior

_____ 44. If a patient presents with an ankle deformed with the foot pointing upward, you should suspect which type of ankle dislocation?
   A. anterior
   B. posterior
   C. lateral
   D. medial
   E. inferior

_____ 45. When a patient's shoulder appears "squared-off," the patient complains of severe pain, and she cannot move her arm, you should suspect what type of shoulder dislocation?
   A. anterior
   B. inferior
   C. superior
   D. posterior
   E. lateral

_____ 46. The elbow dislocation is a simple injury but one that it is essential to reduce in the field.
   A. True
   B. False

_____ 47. Which of the following injuries can be adequately splinted by using the short padded board splint, placing the hand in the position of function, and slinging and swathing the extremity?
   A. radial fractures
   B. ulnar fractures
   C. wrist fractures
   D. finger fractures
   E. all of the above

_____ 48. Nitrous oxide in the prehospital setting:
   A. is nonexplosive.
   B. diffuses easily into air-filled spaces.
   C. reduces the perception of pain.
   D. all of the above
   E. can be self-administered.

_____ 49. Which of the following is NOT an analgesic that is used to control the pain of musculoskeletal injuries?
   A. meperidine
   B. nalbuphine
   C. none of the above
   D. morphine
   E. Astramorph

_____ 50. The "I" within the acronym RICE used by athletic trainers stands for:
   A. immobilization.
   B. ice for the first 48 hours.
   C. instability.
   D. intensity of pain.
   E. both A and B

Chapter 23: Head, Facial, and Neck Trauma

Review of Chapter Objectives

After reading this chapter, you should be able to:

1. **Describe the incidence, morbidity, and mortality of head, facial, and neck injuries.** pp. 959–960

    Approximately 4 million people experience significant head trauma each year, with 1 in 10 requiring hospitalization. Head trauma is the most common cause of trauma death, being especially lethal in auto collisions. Gunshot wounds to the head are less frequent but have a mortality of 75 to 80 percent. The population most at risk for head injury is the male between 15 and 24 years of age, infants and young children, and the elderly.

2. **Explain head and facial anatomy and physiology.** (see Chapter 3)

    Several layers of soft, connective, and skeletal tissues protect the brain. These include the scalp, the cranium, and the meninges. The scalp is a thick and vascular layer of tissue that is strong and flexible and able to absorb tremendous kinetic energy. Beneath it are several layers of connective and muscular fascia that further protect the skull and its contents and that are only connected to the skull on a limited basis. This permits the scalp to move with glancing blows and further protect the cranium.

    The skull consists of numerous bones, fused together at fixed joints called sutures. These bones form a container for the brain called the cranium. The cranium is made up of three layers of bone, two thin layers of compact bone separated by a layer of cancellous bone. This construction makes the cranium both light and very strong. This vault for the brain is fixed in volume and does not accommodate any expansion of its contents. However, in the newborn and infant, the skull is more cartilaginous and more flexible, with two open areas, the anterior and posterior fontanelles. These spaces close by 18 months.

    The meninges are three layers of tissue—the dura mater, the arachnoid, and the pia mater—that provide further protection for the brain. The dura mater is a tough, fibrous layer that lines the interior of the skull and spinal foramen and is continuous with the inner periosteum of the cranium. The pia mater is a delicate membrane covering the convolutions of the brain and spinal cord. The arachnoid is a weblike structure between the dura mater and pia mater. The cerebrospinal fluid fills the subarachnoid space and "floats" the brain and spinal cord to help absorb the energy of trauma.

    The brain occupies about 80 percent of the volume of the cranium and is made up of the cerebrum, cerebellum, and brainstem. The cerebrum occupies most of the cranial vault and is the center of consciousness, personality, speech, motor control, and perception. It is separated into right and left hemispheres by the falx cerebri, extending inward from the anterior, superior, and posterior central skull. The cerebellum sits beneath the posterior half of the cerebrum and is responsible for fine-tuning muscular control and for balance and muscle tone. It is separated from the cerebrum by the tentorium cerebelli, a fibrous sheath that runs transverse to the falx cerebri along the base of the cerebrum. The brainstem runs anterior to the cerebellum and central and inferior to the cerebrum. It consists of the hypothalamus, thalamus, pons, and medulla oblongata. The brainstem controls the endocrine system and most primary body functions including respiration, cardiac activity, temperature, and blood pressure.

The face, consisting of several bones covered with soft tissue, protects the special sense organs of sight, smell, hearing, balance, and taste and forms and protects the upper airway and the beginning of the alimentary canal. The brow ridge (a portion of the frontal bone), the nasal bones, and the zygoma form the eye sockets and protect the eyes. The upper jaw (the maxilla) and the moveable lower jaw (mandible) provide the skeletal structures that form the opening of the mouth. Cavities within this region (sinuses) help to provide shape to the face without increasing the weight of the head. The nasal cavity provides an extended surface to warm, humidify, and cleanse incoming air. The oral cavity houses the tongue and teeth and accommodates the early physical and chemical breakdown of food.

3. **Differentiate between the following types of facial injuries, highlighting the defining characteristics of each:**

   a. **Eye** pp. 975–977

   The eye is a globe filled with a crystal-clear fluid (vitreous humor) that focuses light through a lens onto light-sensitive tissue, the retina. The amount of light entering the eye is determined by the size of the opening, the pupil (as controlled by the iris). The delicate surface of the eye is covered by the cornea (over the pupil and iris) and the conjunctiva (over the white portion of the eyeball, called the sclera). The eye is well protected from most blunt trauma by the skeletal structures of the brow ridge, zygomatic arch, and nasal bones. Blunt trauma may induce hyphema (blood filling the anterior chamber), subconjunctival hemorrhage (a blood-red discoloration of the sclera), and retinal detachment. Penetrating trauma or severe blunt trauma may directly injure the eye or entrap the small muscles that control it.

   b. **Ear** pp. 974–975

   The external portion of the ear is the pinna, a cartilaginous structure covered by skin and only minimally supplied with circulation. A natural opening into the skull, the external auditory canal channels sound to the tympanum, where it and then the ossicles (the three bones of hearing) are set in motion. The ossicles vibrate the window of the cochlea, stimulating this organ of hearing to send impulses to the brain. The inner ear also houses the semicircular canals, which serve as an organ sensing head movement and balance. The pinna is easily injured, bleeds minimally, and heals poorly. Injury to the internal structures of the ear occurs very infrequently but may be caused by pressure differentials as with the blast overpressures of an explosion, with the unequalized pressure associated with diving, or with direct insertion of an object into the ear canal.

   c. **Nose** pp. 973–974

   The nasal cavity is a pair of hollows formed by the junctures of the ethmoid, nasal, and maxillary bones. The external openings of the nose are the nares, formed by the nasal cartilage and anterior soft tissues. Frontal impact may fracture the nasal cartilage or bones, and severe Le Fort–type fractures may disrupt the nasal region. Since the area has a significant blood supply to warm incoming air, hemorrhage (epistaxis) can be heavy.

   d. **Throat** pp. 977–978

   The throat or pharynx may be injured with lower facial or upper neck injury through either blunt or penetrating mechanisms. This region is made up of predominantly soft tissue and gains some support from the structure of the jaw and hyoid bones. Injury may fracture these bones, reducing the structural integrity of the region, or may damage soft tissues, resulting in massive swelling that threatens the airway. Any serious injury to this region is likely to endanger the airway.

e. Mouth   **p. 973**

The mouth, or oral cavity, is made up of the upper and lower jaws, the hard and soft palates (superiorly), and the musculature and connective tissue in the base of the tongue. Fracture of the mandible and, to a lesser degree, the maxilla may reduce the structural integrity of the cavity and endanger its patency as a part of the airway. Injury may also result in severe soft-tissue swelling, hemorrhage, and in some cases, the loss of teeth.

4. Predict head, facial, and other related injuries based on mechanism of injury.   **pp. 960–961**

Injuries to the head, face, and neck occur secondary to blunt or penetrating mechanisms. The most common cause of serious and blunt head trauma is the auto collision; other common mechanisms include falls, acts of violence, and, occasionally, sport-related activities. The neck is well protected both anteriorly and laterally, but it still may be impacted as the neck strikes the steering wheel or when the shoulder strap alone restrains movement of a vehicle's occupant. Penetrating injury is not as common as blunt injury but can still endanger life. Penetrating injuries to the cranium can be devastating to the brain tissue and are frequently not survivable, especially those injuries caused by high-energy gunshot wounds. Gunshot wounds to the face can also be life-threatening as they may compromise the airway and distort facial and airway features.

5. Differentiate between facial injuries based on the assessment and history.   **pp. 972–977**

The greatest dangers from skeletal or soft-tissue injury to the face are related to endangering of the airway, injury to the sensory organs housed and protected there, and damage to the cosmetic appearances of the region. The region is also very vascular and prone to serious blood loss. Facial fractures are classified according to the Le Fort criteria, with Le Fort I fractures relating to simple maxillary fractures, Le Fort II to fractures extending into the nasal bones, and Le Fort III to fractures involving the facial region all the way up to the brow ridge. These fractures are usually due to serious blunt trauma.

6. Explain the pathophysiology, assessment, and management for patients with eye, ear, nose, throat, and mouth injuries.   **pp. 972–997**

Eye injury may be due to blunt trauma and includes hyphema (blood in the eye's anterior chamber), conjunctival hemorrhage, or retinal detachment (the patient complaining of a curtain across part of the field of view). Severe blunt injury may cause orbital fracture, making it appear as though the eye was avulsed, or may entrap the ocular muscles and limit eye movement. Management includes covering both eyes with a paper cup over any protruding tissue or impaled object and bandaging. The patient must also be calmed and reassured because these injuries are very anxiety provoking. Penetrating eye trauma not only injures the delicate ocular tissue but also risks the loss of either aqueous or vitreous humors.

Ear injury most commonly affects the pinna and is due to glancing blows. Infrequently the internal organs of hearing and balance are damaged due to objects inserted into the ear or from dramatic pressure changes caused by explosions or diving injuries. External injury is cared for with dressing and bandaging, while with any internal injury the ear is covered with gauze to permit the drainage of any fluids from the external auditory canal.

Nasal injury can involve the nasal cartilage and bones and cause fractures or dislocations. Hemorrhage in this area (epistaxis) can be very heavy. If possible, the patient's head should be brought forward to ensure that blood from the nasal cavity drains outward and not down the throat, which could irritate the stomach and increase the likelihood of vomiting.

Injuries to the oral cavity are related to fractures of the mandible and associated soft-tissue destruction. Penetrating trauma, especially that produced by high-speed projectiles, can cause severe injury to the structures and tissues of the facial region and result in serious hemorrhage and danger to the patency of the airway. The airway should be maintained with suctioning, oral or nasal airway insertion, or with rapid sequence intubation, if necessary.

Pharyngeal injury is associated with serious risk of soft-tissue swelling and airway compromise. Use suction to remove fluids and consider early intubation because progressive swelling will restrict the airway and make later attempts at intubation more difficult.

7. Explain anatomy and relate physiology of the CNS to head injuries. pp. 966–972

The brain occupies 80 percent of the volume of the cranial vault. The brain consists of three major components: the cerebrum, the cerebellum, and the brainstem. The cerebrum is the center for conscious thought, perception, and motor control and is the largest structure within the cranium. The cerebellum fine-tunes muscle movement and is responsible for muscle tone. The brainstem is made up of the thalamus, the hypothalamus, the pons, and the medulla oblongata. It is responsible for control of the vital signs and for consciousness. The central nervous system tissue is very delicate; very dependent upon adequate perfusion and a constant supply of oxygen, glucose, and thiamine; and easily injured by the forces of trauma. The contents of the cranium are protected by the scalp, the cranium, and the meninges. They are bathed in cerebrospinal fluid that floats them in a near-weightless environment.

8. Distinguish between facial, head, and brain injury. pp. 961–977

Facial injury involves the soft or skeletal structures of the face, including the facial bones and mandible, the nasal cavity, the oral cavity, and the soft tissues covering the region. Their injury threatens the airway and the patient's cosmetic appearance. Serious facial injury is also suggestive of head and brain injury.

Head injury suggests that serious blunt or penetrating forces were expressed to the head with the potential for intracranial injury. Head injury involves damage to the scalp or cranium. It may also include brain (or intracranial) injury.

Brain injury is injury to the cerebrum, cerebellum, or brainstem. It may be caused by blunt trauma, either injuring tissue and blood vessels at the point of impact (coup injury) or injuring tissue and blood vessels away from the point of impact (contrecoup injury). Injury may also occur with an expanding lesion, as with epidural or subdural hematoma, with extensive cerebral edema that causes an increase in intracranial pressure, with a decrease in intracranial perfusion, and possibly with physical brain damage from pressure and displacement secondary to hemorrhage or edema.

9. Explain the pathophysiology of head/brain injuries. pp. 960–972

Brain injury either is direct, related to the initial insult, or indirect, related to progressive pathologies secondary to the insult such as developing tissue irritation, inflammation, edema, hemorrhage, and physical displacement or by hypoxia. Direct injuries can be either coup or contrecoup in origin and include both the focal and diffuse injuries.

Focal injuries include cerebral contusion, which produces confusion and some local swelling, and intracranial hemorrhage, which produces hemorrhage as an arterial vessel above the dura mater ruptures and leads to a quickly evolving accumulation of blood and pressure (epidural hematoma) or as a venous vessel beneath the arachnoid membrane ruptures and produces a more gradual hemorrhage and buildup of pressure (subdural hematoma). Hemorrhage may also occur within the tissue of the brain (intracerebral hemorrhage) leading to a small accumulation of blood and some associated irritation, edema, and increase in intracranial pressure.

Diffuse injuries include the concussion (a mild or moderate diffuse axonal injury) and moderate and severe axonal injuries. These injuries are common and, with increasing severity, increasingly impair neurologic function and decrease the potential for return to a neurologically intact state. Diffuse injuries contuse, tear, shear, or stretch the brain tissue and cause injury that is often distributed throughout the brain.

Indirect injuries result as pressure displaces, compresses, or restricts the blood flow to regions of the brain. This secondary-type injury may induce hypoxia or ischemia that damages brain cells, causing inflammation and resulting in edema and further increases in ICP.

10. Explain the concept of increasing intracranial pressure (ICP). pp. 969–970

The cranium is a rigid container with a fixed volume. It is full and each of its contents (cerebrum, cerebellum, brainstem, cerebrospinal fluid, and blood) occupies a component of the volume. Within this container, there is a limited constant pressure, the intracranial pressure. This pressure rarely exceeds 10 mmHg and at such a low level does not restrict cerebral blood flow. However, if one of the cranial residents increases its volume (vascular, as with hematoma, or the cerebrum itself, as with edema), another resident will have to decrease its volume or a pressure increase will result. During increasing ICP, some of the venous blood will leave the cranium, and then some cerebrospinal fluid will move to the spinal cord. These compensatory mechanisms work rather well, but the volume they can compensate for is limited. If expansion continues, the intracranial pressure (ICP) begins to rise. As it does, the difference between the intracranial pressure (ICP) and the mean arterial pressure (MAP) falls. This is the pressure driving cerebral perfusion (cerebral perfusion pressure, CPP). If CPP drops below 50 mmHg, cerebral perfusion pressure is not adequate to perfuse the brain. The body will increase the blood pressure in an attempt to maintain cerebral perfusion (autoregulation), but this only increases the edema or hemorrhage in a progressively worsening cycle.

11. Explain the effect of increased and decreased carbon dioxide on ICP. pp. 969–970

Increased carbon dioxide concentrations in the blood cause the cerebral arteries to dilate and thereby provide better circulation to the contents of the cranium. This, however, can increase the intracranial pressure and increase any damage occurring due to a preexisting elevated intracranial pressure.

Decreased carbon dioxide causes vasoconstriction in the cerebral arteries and limits blood flow to the brain. If the blood CO_2 levels are reduced excessively, this will seriously limit cerebral blood flow and cause further injury to the patient who is already suffering from reduced cerebral blood flow (as with increased intracranial pressure).

12. Define and explain the process involved with each of the levels of increasing ICP. pp. 969–970

The damage caused by increasing intracranial pressure (ICP) is progressive and limits cerebral perfusion. Normal intracranial pressure is very minimal and does not interfere with perfusion. However, as an injury (edema or an accumulation of blood) expands, it compresses the contents of the cranium. This compresses the veins and forces some venous blood from the cranium. If the pressure continues to rise, the pressure begins to move cerebrospinal fluid from the cranium (and into the spinal cord). If the pressure rise continues, arteries are compressed and cerebral blood flow suffers. This reduced circulation through the cerebrum causes a rise in the systemic blood pressure (autoregulation). This increases the cerebral blood flow but also increases the rate of intracranial hemorrhage and further increases the ICP. The result is a rapid rise in ICP, a reduction in cerebral blood flow, and cerebral hypoxia.

13. Relate assessment findings associated with head/brain injuries to the pathophysiologic process. pp. 961–972

The most noticeable findings of brain injury are associated with the vital signs and include increasing blood pressure, erratic respirations (Cheyne-Stokes, Kussmaul's, central neurologic hyperventilation, or ataxic respirations), and a slowing pulse. These things are known collectively as Cushing's triad. These signs indicate severe injury to the medulla oblongata, possibly due to its herniation into the foramen magnum. Eye signs, such as one pupil dilating and becoming unresponsive, are due to pressure on the oculomotor nerve as it is compressed against the tentorium. Such a sign is usually related to injury on the same (ipsilateral) side. The patient frequently demonstrates a reduced level of orientation or responsiveness and a Glasgow Coma Scale score of less than 15. The patient may also display retrograde or anterograde amnesia. These are generalized signs related to either diffuse axonal injury or increased intracranial pressure.

14. Classify head injuries (mild, moderate, severe) according to assessment findings. pp. 966–970

Head injuries are classified according to the Glasgow Coma Scale. Those patients who score from 13 to 15 are considered to have received a mild injury, those from 9 to 12, a moderate injury, and those with a score of 8 or below are considered to have a severe head injury. Any change in the level of consciousness or orientation or any personality changes are signs of at least a mild head injury. Any finding that suggests the pulse rate is slowing, the respirations are becoming more erratic, and the blood pressure is rising due to head injury should be considered to indicate that the patient has a severe injury. The patient with the signs of a mild or moderate head injury must be watched very carefully because these pathologies frequently progress to more severe injuries.

15. **Identify the need for rapid intervention and transport of the patient with a head/brain injury.** pp. 978, 984

The pathologic processes at work in the patient with serious head injury are completely internal and cannot be repaired or stabilized in the field. High-flow oxygen administration and adequate ventilation (not hyperventilation) will ensure the best cerebral oxygenation without blowing off too much CO_2. Ensuring good cardiovascular function and maintaining blood pressure are essential. In some systems, medications are also used to reduce cerebral edema in the field. However, often the only definitive way to correct the problems affecting the patient with serious head trauma is surgical intervention. For this reason, care for head injury patients focuses on bringing them quickly to a center capable of neurosurgical intervention.

16. **Describe and explain the general management of the head/brain injury patient, including pharmacological and nonpharmacological treatment.** pp. 985–996

The general management of the patient with recognized or suspected head injury begins with immobilization of the cervical spine to ensure no aggravation of any spinal injury. This manual immobilization is maintained and augmented by the application of a cervical collar, until the immobilization is continued by mechanical immobilization with a vest-type device or long spine board. The airway and adequate ventilation must be ensured. High-flow, high-concentration oxygen is the first-line drug for the patient with head injury. Ventilate with full breaths at about 10 ventilations per minute (20 BPM for the child and 25 BPM for the infant) to ensure end-tidal CO_2 remains at 35 to 40 mmHg for most patients and 30 to 35 mmHg for patients with suspected herniation. Intubation may be attempted early using rapid sequence intubation with vecuronium as the paralytic of choice because succinylcholine may cause an increase in ICP. Sedatives are indicated to premedicate the patient for the RSI procedure. Atropine will reduce airway secretions and may also reduce vagal stimulation and any increase in ICP that would otherwise occur during intubation attempts.

17. **Analyze the relationship between carbon dioxide concentration in the blood and management of the airway in the head/brain injured patient.** pp. 969–970

In general, the higher the level of carbon dioxide in the blood, the greater the need to ventilate the patient. However, very low levels of carbon dioxide cause cerebral vasodilation, which may lead to a more rapidly increasing intracranial pressure. The objective of airway and respiratory care for the head injury patient is to ensure a patent airway and good respiratory exchange without blowing off too much CO_2. This generally means that a patient should be ventilated with full breaths at 10 times per minute. Adjust volume of breaths to maintain an $ETCO_2$ of between 35 to 40 mmHg. For patients with signs of herniation, ventilate at 20 breaths per minute and maintain an $ETCO_2$ of 30 to 35 mmHg.

18. **Explain the pathophysiology, assessment, and management of a patient with:**

   a. **Scalp injury** pp. 961–962, 980–981, 985–996

   Scalp injuries tend to bleed heavily because their blood vessels do not constrict as well as those elsewhere on the body. This type of hemorrhage is easy to control because of the firm skull beneath, except when skull fracture is suspected. In that case, use distal pressure points and controlled direct pressure to stop any serious bleeding. Glancing injuries may expose the skull and flap the scalp over on itself. Remove any gross contaminants and cover the exposed surfaces with a sterile dressing. These injuries will heal very well due to the more than adequate blood supply they receive.

b. Skull fracture pp. 962–965, 980–981, 985–996

Skull fractures are skeletal injuries that usually heal uneventfully. The greatest concern is for the possible damage within the cranium. Skull fracture is anticipated by the mechanism of injury and should be suspected if fluids are draining out of the nose or ears. The retroauricular or bilateral periorbital ecchymoses associated with basilar skull fracture are not frequently seen in the prehospital setting because they take hours to develop. Immobilize the potentially fractured skull carefully and cover the ears and nose with gauze to ensure free outward movement of any cerebrospinal fluid.

c. Cerebral contusion pp. 966–967, 985–996

The cerebral contusion is usually due to direct head trauma and may be the result of coup or contrecoup injury mechanisms. The patient may experience regional related neurologic deficits that resolve with time. This patient should be suspected of severe but more slowly progressive injury and watched very carefully. Administer oxygen and transport quickly.

d. Intracranial hemorrhage (including epidural, subdural, subarachnoid, and intracerebral hemorrhage) pp. 967–968, 985–996

Intracranial hemorrhage (be it epidural, subdural, subarachnoid [a subset of subdural], or intracerebral) is a progressive injury mechanism that occurs as blood accumulates, displaces brain tissue, and raises intracranial pressure or as bleeding irritates brain tissue, initiates an inflammatory response, and causes cerebral edema and an increase in intracranial pressure. Patients with intracranial hemorrhage will display progressively deteriorating levels of orientation and consciousness and a history of serious head trauma. The elderly and chronic alcoholics may have an increased incidence of brain injury due to a reduced cerebral mass and more room for the brain to move within the cranium during head trauma. Intracranial hemorrhage management includes oxygen, airway management, ensuring adequate ventilation, ensuring adequate blood pressure, and rapid transport. Rapid sequence intubation may be necessary, and mannitol may relieve some of the edema associated with the injury and ease the increased intracranial pressure.

e. Axonal injury (including concussion and moderate and severe diffuse axonal injury) pp. 968, 985–996

Diffuse axonal injury may be anticipated by the mechanism of injury and by observation of any signs of diminished or deteriorating levels of orientation and consciousness. Care is directed at oxygen administration, airway management, ensuring adequate ventilation, ensuring adequate blood pressure, and rapid transport. In severe cases, rapid sequence intubation may be necessary, and mannitol may relieve some of the edema associated with the injury and ease the increased intracranial pressure.

f. Facial injury pp. 972–977, 985–996

Facial injury may be anticipated by the mechanism of injury or recognized by soft-tissue injuries to or structural deformities of the region. Care is directed at maintaining the airway, protecting the eyes, and controlling any significant blood loss.

g. Neck injury pp. 977–978, 982, 985–996

Neck injury is anticipated by the mechanism of injury and by a quick evaluation of the region. The spine is immobilized manually, a cervical collar is applied, and eventually manual immobilization is replaced with the mechanical immobilization of the vest-type immobilization device or the long spine board. Open soft-tissue injuries are covered with sterile dressings (or occlusive dressings if the injury is significant) and the airway is assessed to ensure that it is not at risk.

19. Develop a management plan for the removal of a helmet for a head-injured patient. p. 979

A helmet is carefully removed using techniques that limit the movement of the cervical spine and head. Full-face helmets provide the greatest challenge to removal, and to deal with them you should employ the techniques described in Chapter 24, "Spinal Trauma," Division 3.

20. Differentiate between the types of head/brain injuries based on the assessment and history. pp. 960–985

The pathologies of head injury will either make your patient get worse or better. Contusion and mild diffuse axonal injuries are likely to improve with time. However, as diffuse axonal injury gets more severe, the chances for recovery lessen and associated edema will likely increase the ICP and cause progressive neurologic deficit. Patients with intracranial hemorrhage (epidural and subdural) and intracerebral hemorrhage are likely to deteriorate with time. Epidural hemorrhage patients will show decreasing levels of consciousness and then the signs of increasing intracranial hemorrhage (eye signs, increasing systolic blood pressure, slowing and strengthening pulse, and erratic respirations). Patients with subdural and intracerebral hemorrhage will take longer to display these signs and may not do so in the prehospital setting. Be advised, however, that one injury may be superimposed upon another. The concussion may render a patient unconscious and permit him to awaken, experience a lucid interval, and then deteriorate due to a developing epidural hematoma.

21. **Given several preprogrammed and moulaged head, face, and neck trauma patients, provide the appropriate scene size-up, initial assessment, rapid trauma or focused physical exam and history, detailed exam, and ongoing assessment and provide appropriate patient care and transportation.** pp. 959–997

During your training as an EMT-Paramedic you will participate in many classroom practice sessions involving simulated patients. You will also spend some time in the emergency departments of local hospitals as well as in advanced-level ambulances gaining clinical experience. During these times, use your knowledge of head, facial, and neck trauma to help you assess and care for the simulated or real patients you attend.

Content Self-Evaluation

MULTIPLE CHOICE

_____ 1. The most common cause of trauma-related death is due to injury to the:
   A. head.
   B. thorax.
   C. abdomen.
   D. pelvis.
   E. extremities.

_____ 2. What percentage of penetrating wounds to the cranium result in mortality?
   A. 30 to 40 percent
   B. 40 to 50 percent
   C. 65 to 70 percent
   D. 75 to 80 percent
   E. 90 to 95 percent

_____ 3. Scalp wounds may present in a manner that confounds assessment.
   A. True
   B. False

_____ 4. Serious scalp injury is unlikely to produce hypovolemia and shock as the arteries there frequently constrict and effectively limit blood loss.
   A. True
   B. False

_____ 5. Which of the following statements is NOT true of scalp wounds?
   A. They pose a risk of meningeal infection.
   B. Wounds there tend to heal very well.
   C. Wounds there tend to bleed heavily.
   D. Contusions there swell outward noticeably.
   E. Avulsion of the scalp is not a likely injury.

_____ 6. The most common type of skull fracture is:
   A. depressed.
   B. basilar.
   C. linear.
   D. comminuted.
   E. spiral.

_____ 7. The type of skull fracture most often associated with high-velocity bullet entry is:
   A. depressed.
   B. basilar.
   C. linear.
   D. comminuted.
   E. spiral.

_____ 8. It is common for the paramedic to observe either Battle's sign or bilateral periorbital ecchymosis in the patient who has just sustained a basilar skull fracture.
   A. True
   B. False

_____ 9. The discoloration found around both eyes due to basilar skull fracture is:
   A. retroauricular ecchymosis.
   B. bilateral periorbital ecchymosis.
   C. Cullen's sign.
   D. the halo sign.
   E. Gray's sign.

_____ 10. Blood and CSF draining from the ear may display a:
   A. speckled appearance.
   B. concentric lighter yellow circle.
   C. congealed mass.
   D. greenish discoloration.
   E. none of the above

_____ 11. A cranial fracture, by itself, is a skeletal injury that will heal with time; it is the injury underneath that is of most concern.
   A. True
   B. False

_____ 12. The type of injury that causes damage to the brain on the side opposite the impact is called:
   A. coup.
   B. subdural hematoma.
   C. subluxation.
   D. contrecoup.
   E. concussion.

_____ 13. Which of the following is considered a focal injury?
   A. cerebral contusion
   B. epidural hematoma
   C. subdural hematoma
   D. intracerebral hemorrhage
   E. all of the above

_____ 14. Which of the following injuries is most likely to cause the patient to deteriorate rapidly?
   A. cerebral contusion
   B. epidural hematoma
   C. subdural hematoma
   D. intracerebral hemorrhage
   E. concussion

_____ 15. Which of the following is an injury with venous bleeding into the arachnoid space?
   A. cerebral contusion
   B. epidural hematoma
   C. subdural hematoma
   D. intracerebral hemorrhage
   E. concussion

_____ 16. The injury that classically presents with unconsciousness immediately after the accident followed by a lucid interval and then a decreasing level of consciousness is most likely a(n):
   A. concussion.
   B. epidural hematoma.
   C. subdural hematoma.
   D. cerebral hemorrhage.
   E. both A and B

_____ 17. Which of the following head injuries would you NOT expect to get worse with time?
   A. intracerebral hemorrhage
   B. subdural hematoma
   C. concussion
   D. epidural hematoma
   E. intracranial hemorrhage

_____ 18. Indirect brain injury occurs as a result of, but after, initial injury.
   A. True
   B. False

_____ 19. As intracranial hemorrhage begins, it first displaces which occupant of the cranium?
A. cerebrospinal fluid
B. venous blood
C. arterial blood
D. oxygen
E. the pia mater

_____ 20. Perfusion through the cerebrum is a factor of intracranial pressure and:
A. systolic blood pressure.
B. diastolic blood pressure.
C. mean arterial pressure.
D. cerebral perfusion pressure.
E. none of the above

_____ 21. High levels of carbon dioxide in the blood will cause which of the following?
A. hyperventilation
B. cerebral artery constriction
C. cerebral artery dilation
D. hypertension
E. none of the above

_____ 22. Vomiting, changes in the level of consciousness, and pupillary dilation result from herniation of the upper brainstem through the:
A. tentorium incisura.
B. foramen magnum.
C. falx cerebri.
D. transverse sinus.
E. tentorium cerebelli.

_____ 23. Cushing's triad includes which of the following?
A. erratic respirations
B. increasing blood pressure
C. slowing heart rate
D. A and B
E. A, B, and C

_____ 24. Which of the following respiratory patterns is NOT indicative of brain injury?
A. eupnea
B. ataxic respirations
C. central neurogenic hyperventilation
D. Cheyne-Stokes respirations
E. agonal respirations

_____ 25. In the presence of intracranial pressure, the fontanelles of the infant will:
A. withdraw.
B. become stiff.
C. bulge.
D. pulsate.
E. atrophy.

_____ 26. Increasing intracranial pressure is likely to cause pupillary dilation on the ipsilateral side.
A. True
B. False

_____ 27. With facial trauma, lower airway obstruction is more likely due to blood than other fluids or physical obstruction.
A. True
B. False

_____ 28. According to the Le Fort criteria, a fracture involving just the maxilla and limited instability is classified as:
A. Le Fort I.
B. Le Fort II.
C. Le Fort III.
D. Le Fort IV.
E. Le Fort V.

_____ 29. Which type of Le Fort fracture is likely to result in cerebrospinal fluid leakage?
A. Le Fort I
B. Le Fort III
C. Le Fort IV
D. Le Fort V
E. none of the above

_____ 30. Which of the following statements is TRUE regarding injuries to the pinna of the ear?
A. They hemorrhage severely.
B. Hemorrhage is difficult to control.
C. Hemorrhage is limited.
D. Wounds there do not heal very well.
E. both C and D

_____ 31. Which of the following mechanisms is likely to injure the tympanum?
   A. basilar skull fracture
   B. an explosion
   C. diving injury
   D. an object forced into the ear
   E. all of the above

_____ 32. The collection of blood in front of a patient's pupil and iris due to blunt trauma is called a(n):
   A. hyphema.
   B. retinal detachment.
   C. aniscoria.
   D. anterior chamber hematoma.
   E. sub-conjunctival hemorrhage.

_____ 33. A sudden and painless loss of sight is most likely a(n):
   A. hyphema.
   B. retinal detachment.
   C. acute retinal artery occlusion.
   D. anterior chamber hematoma.
   E. sub-conjunctival hemorrhage.

_____ 34. Blood vessel injury in the neck region carries with it the hazards of all of the following EXCEPT:
   A. severe venous hemorrhage.
   B. severe arterial hemorrhage.
   C. development of subcutaneous emphysema.
   D. air aspiration.
   E. pulmonary emboli.

_____ 35. The patient with a suspected brain injury should be ventilated with full breaths:
   A. 8 to 10 times per minute.
   B. 12 to 20 times per minute.
   C. 20 to 24 times per minute.
   D. 24 to 30 times per minute.
   E. 30 to 36 times per minute.

_____ 36. Which of the following is a probable sign of increasing intracranial pressure?
   A. decreasing pulse strength
   B. weakening pulse strength
   C. slowing pulse rate
   D. increasing pulse strength
   E. both C and D

_____ 37. The major reason for allowing fluid to drain from the nose or ear is that:
   A. it may speed the rise of intracranial pressure
   B. its flow will prevent pathogens from entering the meninges
   C. it is impossible to stop the flow anyway
   D. regeneration of CSF is beneficial to the healing process
   E. none of the above

_____ 38. When light intensity changes in one eye and both respond, this response is called:
   A. diplopia.
   B. aniscoria.
   C. consensual reactivity.
   D. synergism.
   E. photophobia.

_____ 39. Any significant open wound to the anterior or lateral neck should be covered with a(n):
   A. wet dressing.
   B. occlusive dressing.
   C. nonadherent dressing.
   D. adherent dressing.
   E. pressure dressing.

_____ 40. When a patient reports of sensitivity to light, this is an example of:
   A. diplopia.
   B. aniscoria.
   C. consensual reactivity.
   D. synergism.
   E. photophobia.

_____ 41. During your assessment you determine that the patient exhibits confused speech, follows simple commands, and opens his eyes on his own. What Glasgow Coma Scale value would you assign?
   A. 15
   B. 14
   C. 12
   D. 10
   E. 7

_____ 42. A patient who responds only to pain by withdrawing, mutters incomprehensible words when shouted at loudly, and opens his eyes only to pain is given what Glasgow Coma Scale score?
   A. 14
   B. 12
   C. 10
   D. 8
   E. 6

_____ 43. Which of the following could be considered a component of Cushing's triad?
   A. Cheyne-Stokes respirations
   B. decreasing pulse rate
   C. increasing blood pressure
   D. ataxic respirations
   E. all of the above

_____ 44. The head injury patient may vomit without warning and the vomiting may be projectile in nature.
   A. True
   B. False

_____ 45. If the head injury patient is found without any other suspected injuries, what positioning would be best for her?
   A. the Trendelenburg position
   B. with the head of the spine board elevated 30 degrees
   C. left lateral recumbent position
   D. immobilized completely and rolled to her side
   E. none of the above

_____ 46. Which of the following airway techniques is NOT acceptable for the patient with suspected basilar skull fracture?
   A. nasopharyngeal airway insertion
   B. directed intubation
   C. digital intubation
   D. orotracheal intubation
   E. rapid sequence intubation

_____ 47. The process of inserting an endotracheal tube increases the intracranial pressure and should only be done by the care provider most experienced in the procedure.
   A. True
   B. False

_____ 48. Which of the following is an acceptable method for confirming endotracheal tube placement in the head injury patient?
   A. use of an end-tidal CO_2 monitor
   B. use of a pulse oximeter
   C. observing bilaterally equal chest rise
   D. good and bilaterally equal breath sounds
   E. all of the above

_____ 49. For adequate ventilation through a needle cricothyrotomy, you must use a demand valve ventilator.
   A. True
   B. False

_____ 50. When locating the cricoid cartilage, either for Sellick's maneuver or the cricothyrotomy, it is the first hard rigid ring you feel as you move your fingers up the trachea from the suprasternal notch.
   A. True
   B. False

_____ 51. Ventilation of the head injury patient should be guided by capnography to maintain a CO_2 level of:
   A. 10 to 20 mmHg.
   B. 20 to 30 mmHg.
   C. 30 to 40 mmHg.
   D. more than 50 mmHg.
   E. 40 to 50 mmHg.

_____ 52. Care for the patient with increasing intracranial pressure must NOT include aggressive fluid resuscitation, even if the patient's blood pressure drops below 60 mmHg.
   A. True
   B. False

_____ 53. In the head injury patient you must keep the blood pressure above:
   A. 50 mmHg.
   B. 60 mmHg.
   C. 90 mmHg.
   D. 120 mmHg.
   E. none of the above

_____ 54. Which of the following drugs is the first-line diuretic in the treatment of head injury?
   A. oxygen
   B. mannitol
   C. Furosemide
   D. succinylcholine
   E. morphine

_____ 55. Which of the following paralytics increases ICP and should be used with caution, if at all, in head injury patients?
   A. diazepam
   B. mannitol
   C. Vecuronium
   D. succinylcholine
   E. midazolam

_____ 56. It is recommended to administer diazepam by adding it first to the plastic IV bag as this ensures a uniform administration.
   A. True
   B. False

_____ 57. Which of the following drugs will reverse the effects of diazepam and midazolam?
   A. narcan
   B. flumazenil
   C. Atropine
   D. thiamine
   E. none of the above

_____ 58. Which of the following actions of atropine make it a desirable adjunct to rapid sequence intubation?
   A. It reduces vagal stimulation.
   B. It reduces airway secretions.
   C. It reduces fasciculations.
   D. It helps maintain heart rate during intubation.
   E. all of the above

_____ 59. Dextrose is administered to the head injury patient:
   A. routinely.
   B. for hyperglycemia only.
   C. for hypoglycemia only.
   D. for suspected diabetes or alcoholism.
   E. with hetastarch.

_____ 60. Dislodged teeth from a patient should be:
   A. wrapped in gauze soaked in water.
   B. wrapped in gauze soaked in sterile saline.
   C. wrapped in dry gauze.
   D. kept dry but cool.
   E. replaced immediately.

Spinal Trauma

Review of Chapter Objectives

After reading this chapter, you should be able to:

1. **Describe the incidence, morbidity, and mortality of spinal injuries in the trauma patient.** p. 1001

   Spinal cord injuries account for over 15,000 permanent injuries, occurring most frequently in males aged from 16 to 30. Auto collisions account for almost half of the injuries, while falls, penetrating injuries, and sports-related injuries also contribute significantly to the toll. Spinal cord injuries are especially devastating because they affect the very specialized tissue of the central nervous system, which has relatively little ability to repair itself, and because the cord is the major communication conduit of the body. Injury often results in permanent loss of function below the lesion.

2. **Describe the anatomy and physiology of spinal structures and structures related to the spine, including:** (see Chapter 3)

   a. **Cervical spine**
   The cervical spine is the vertebral column between the cranium and the thorax. It consists of seven irregular bones held firmly together by ligaments that both support the weight of the head and permit its motion while protecting the delicate spinal cord that runs through the central portion of these bones.

   b. **Thoracic spine**
   The thoracic vertebral column consists of 12 thoracic vertebrae, one corresponding to each rib pair. Like the cervical spine, it consists of irregular bones held firmly together by ligaments that support the weight of the head and neck and permit its motion while protecting the delicate spinal cord that runs through the central portion of these bones.

   c. **Lumbar spine**
   The lumbar spine consists of five lumbar vertebrae with massive vertebral bodies to support the weight of the head, neck, and thorax. Here the spinal cord ends at the juncture between L-1 and L-2 and nerve roots fill the spinal foramen from L-2 into the sacral spine.

   d. **Sacrum**
   The sacrum consists of five sacral vertebrae that are fused into a single plate that forms the posterior portion of the pelvis. The upper body balances on the sacrum, which connects with the pelvis at a fixed joint, the sacroiliac joint.

   e. **Coccyx**
   The coccygeal region of the spine consists of three to five fused vertebrae that form the remnant of a tail.

   f. **Spinal cord**
   The spinal cord is a component of the central nervous system consisting of very specialized nervous system cells that do not repair themselves very well. The cord is the body's major

communications conduit, sending motor commands to the body and returning sensory information to the brain.

- **g. Nerve tracts**

  The nerve tracts are pathways within the spinal cord for impulses from distinct areas and with distinct sensory or motor functions. The two major types of nerve tracts are ascending tracts, those that carry sensory information to the brain, and descending tracts, those that carry motor commands to the body.

- **h. Dermatomes**

  The dermatomes are distinct regions of the body's surface that are sensed by specific peripheral nerve roots. For example, the collar region is sensed by C-3, the nipple line is sensed by T-4, the umbilicus is sensed by T-10, and the lateral (little) toe is sensed by S-1. These landmarks are useful in denoting where the loss of sensation occurs, secondary to spinal injury.

3. **Predict spinal injuries based on mechanism of injury.** pp. 1001–1004

Most spinal trauma is related to extremes of motion. These include extension/flexion, lateral bending, rotation, and axial loading/distraction. These types of movement place stresses on the vertebral column that stretch and injure the ligaments, fracture the vertebral elements, rupture the intervertebral disks, and dislocate the vertebra. While these are all connective or skeletal tissue injuries, they threaten the protective function served by the vertebral column and endanger the spinal cord. The injury mechanism itself or further movement of the vertebral column may cause the skeletal elements to compress, contuse, lacerate, sever, or stretch the cord, resulting in neurologic injury and a deficit below the level of injury.

A frontal impact injury mechanism is likely to cause axial loading and a crushing-type injury to the spine as well as flexion injury (as may occur in the auto or diving incidents). Lateral impact auto collisions are likely to cause lateral bending injury, while rear-end impacts are likely to cause extension, then flexion injury. Hangings may cause distraction injury. Rotational injuries may occur during sporting events.

Penetrating injury is a direct type of injury that disrupts the connective and skeletal structure of the vertebral column and may directly involve the spinal cord. Deep and powerful knife injuries and bullet wounds are the most common mechanisms of this injury.

4. **Describe the pathophysiology of spinal injuries.** pp. 1004–1007

The spinal cord, like all central nervous system tissue, is extremely specialized and delicate and does not repair itself well, if at all. The spinal cord may be injured in much the same way as the brain by mechanisms including concussion, contusion, compression, laceration, hemorrhage, and transection. The concussion is a jarring that momentarily disrupts the cord function. Contusion results in some damage and bleeding into the cord but will likely repair itself. Compression may occur due to vertebral body displacement or as a result of cord edema; it deprives portions of the cord of blood, and ischemic damage may result. The degree of injury and its permanence is related to the amount of compression and the length of time the compression remains. Laceration occurs as bony fragments are driven into the cord and damage it. If the injury is severe, the injury is probably permanent. Hemorrhage into the cord results in compression and irritation of the cord tissue as blood crosses the blood–brain barrier. The injury may also restrict blood flow to a portion of the cord, extending the injury. Transection is a partial or complete severance of the cord with its function lost, for the most part, below the lesion.

5. **Identify the need for rapid intervention and transport of the patient with spinal injuries.** pp. 1007–1012

The need for rapid intervention and transport of the spinal injury patient must take into account the key element of prehospital care, which is immobilizing the vertebral column to restrict motion and any further injury. Once injured, the vertebral column can no longer protect the spinal cord from injury and, in fact, becomes the source of probable injury with manipulation. It is imperative that the head be brought to the neutral position and maintained there until the injury heals, it is corrected surgically, or X-rays and CT scans rule out injury. This means that once spinal injury is suspected, the patient remains immobilized until delivered to the emergency department.

6. **Describe the pathophysiology of traumatic spinal injury related to:**

- **Spinal shock** p. 1006

  Spinal shock is a transient form of neurogenic shock due to a temporary injury to the spinal cord. It results as the brain loses control over body functions including vasoconstriction, motor control, and sensory perception below the level of injury.

- **Neurogenic shock** p. 1006

  Neurogenic shock is a more permanent result of cord injury resulting in loss of control over body functions including vasoconstriction, motor control, and sensory perception below the level of injury. The injury results in an inability to control peripheral vascular resistance and blood pressure.

- **Quadriplegia/paraplegia** p. 1005

  The loss of neurologic control over the lower extremities (paraplegia) and the loss of control over all four limbs (quadriplegia) is related to the location of the spinal cord lesion. The higher the injury along the vertebral column, the more of the body is affected. These injuries are related to the distribution of the dermatomes for sensation and myotomes for motor control. Injuries at or below the thoracic spine (T-3) involve the lower extremities (paraplegia), while injuries above this level affect all four extremities (quadriplegia).

- **Incomplete and complete cord injury** pp. 1005–1006

  Injury to the spinal cord can result from the mechanisms discussed earlier. A complete cord injury completely severs the spinal cord, and the potential to send and receive nerve impulses below the site of the injury is lost. Results may include, depending on the site of injury, incontinence, paraplegia, quadriplegia, and partial or complete respiratory paralysis.

  With incomplete cord injury, the spinal cord is only partially severed. There is potential for recovery of function.

- **Cord syndromes**

  There are three common types of incomplete cord syndrome:

  —**Central cord syndrome** p. 1006

  Central cord syndrome is related to hyperextension-type injuries and is often associated with a preexisting disease like arthritis that narrows the spinal foramen. It usually results in motor weakness of the upper extremities and in some cases loss of bladder control. The prognosis for at least some recovery for the central cord syndrome is the best of all the cord syndromes.

  —**Anterior cord syndrome** p. 1005

  Anterior cord syndrome is due to damage caused by bone fragments or pressure on the arteries that perfuse the anterior portion of the cord. The affected limbs are likely only to retain motion, vibration, and positional sensation with motor and other perceptions lost.

  —**Brown-Séquard syndrome** p. 1006

  Brown-Séquard syndrome is most often caused by a penetrating injury that affects one side of the cord (hemitransection). Sensory and motor loss is noted on the ipsilateral side, while pain and temperature sensation is lost on the contralateral side. The injury is rare but often associated with some recovery.

7. **Describe the assessment findings associated with and management for traumatic spinal injuries.** pp. 1007–1027

The primary assessment finding used to determine the need for spinal precautions is the mechanism of injury. Vertebral column injury may present with only minimal signs and symptoms of injury, often overshadowed by more painful injuries. Failure to immobilize the spine early during assessment and care may lead to vertebral column movement and damage to the spinal cord.

The signs and symptoms of spinal injury include pain or tenderness along the spinal column, any neurologic deficit, especially if it corresponds to the dermatomes and is bilateral, including any deficits in sensation to touch, temperature, motion, vibration, and so on. Any loss in the ability to move (paralysis) or muscular strength (paresis) is suggestive of spinal cord injury. Special signs associated with spinal injury include an involuntary erection of the penis (priapism), loss of bowel and bladder control, and diaphragmatic breathing.

8. **Describe the various types of helmets and their purposes.** p. 1019

Helmets are made for use in contact sports, bicycling, skateboarding, in-line skating, and motorcycling. Some helmets are partial and can be easily removed at the accident scene. Other helmets (football, for example) completely enclose the head and may be difficult to remove at the accident scene and may pose immobilization problems for prehospital caregivers. It must be remembered that, while helmets offer some protection for the head, they have not been proven to reduce spinal injuries.

9. **Relate the priorities of care to factors determining the need for helmet removal in various field situations including sports-related incidents.** pp. 1019–1020

Remember that while a helmet provides some protection for head injury, it does not necessarily protect the spine. Take immobilization precautions if the mechanism of injury suggests the potential for spinal injury. If the patient can be fully immobilized with the helmet on, it can be left in place. However, you must remove a helmet if the helmet does not immobilize the patient's head, if the helmet cannot be securely immobilized to the long spine board, if it prevents airway care, or if it prevents assessment of anticipated injuries. The helmet should also be removed if you anticipate development of airway or breathing problems. Always be sure that helmet removal will not cause further injuries.

Procedures for helmet removal will vary with the type of helmet. The prime consideration is to continue to maintain manual spinal immobilization of the patient throughout whatever procedure is used and then to ensure that the patient receives proper mechanical immobilization once the helmet is removed.

10. **Given several preprogrammed and moulaged spinal trauma patients, provide the appropriate scene size-up, initial assessment, rapid trauma or focused physical exam and history, detailed exam, and ongoing assessment and provide appropriate patient care and transportation.** pp. 1001–1027

During your training as an EMT-Paramedic you will participate in many classroom practice sessions involving simulated patients. You will also spend some time in the emergency departments of local hospitals as well as in advanced-level ambulances gaining clinical experience. During these times, use your knowledge of spinal trauma to help you assess and care for the simulated or real patients you attend.

Content Self-Evaluation

MULTIPLE CHOICE

_____ 1. Which of the following motions is likely to result from hanging?
   A. extension
   B. flexion
   C. lateral bending
   D. axial loading
   E. distraction

_____ 2. Spinal cord injury can occur without injury to the vertebral column or its associated ligaments.
   A. True
   B. False

_____ 3. The region that accounts for more than half of spinal cord injuries is the:
   A. cervical spine.
   B. thoracic spine.
   C. lumbar spine.
   D. sacral spine.
   E. coccygeal spine.

_____ 4. A spinal cord concussion is likely to produce residual deficit.
   A. True
   B. False

_____ 5. The region of the vertebral column in which the spinal cord ends is the:
   A. cervical.
   B. thoracic.
   C. lumbar.
   D. sacral.
   E. coccygeal.

_____ 6. Spinal shock is a temporary form of neurogenic shock.
   A. True
   B. False

_____ 7. Which of the following is a sign associated with neurogenic shock?
   A. priapism
   B. decreased heart rate
   C. decreased peripheral vascular resistance
   D. warm skin below the injury
   E. all of the above

_____ 8. Which of the following is associated with the resolution of shock due to cord injury and results in hypertension?
   A. autonomic hyperreflexia syndrome
   B. neurogenic shock
   C. spinal shock
   D. central cord syndrome
   E. both B and D

_____ 9. Which of the following is NOT a mechanism of injury likely to cause spinal injury?
   A. fall from over three times the patient's height
   B. high-speed motor vehicle crash
   C. serious blunt trauma above the shoulders
   D. penetrating trauma directed to the lateral thorax
   E. penetrating trauma directed to the spine

_____ 10. Helmets reduce the incidence of both head and spine injury.
   A. True
   B. False

_____ 11. Oral intubation is generally more difficult in the patient who requires spinal precautions because the landmarks are more difficult to visualize.
   A. True
   B. False

_____ 12. During the initial assessment, you should be aware that exaggerated abdominal movement and limited chest excursions often suggest:
   A. airway obstruction.
   B. the need to reposition the head and neck.
   C. diaphragmatic breathing.
   D. neurogenic shock.
   E. cardiac contusion.

_____ 13. The pulse rate in the patient with spinal injury is likely to be:
   A. fast.
   B. very fast.
   C. slow.
   D. very slow.
   E. normal.

_____ 14. The "hold-up" positioning of the arms is due to injury at or around:
   A. C-3.
   B. T-1.
   C. T-4.
   D. T-10.
   E. S-1.

_____ 15. Which of the following is indicative of spinal injury?
   A. increased heart rate
   B. increasing blood pressure
   C. excessive chest expansion
   D. a normal body temperature
   E. none of the above

_____ 16. Proper immobilization of the patient with spinal injury should include placing a blanket roll under the knees.
   A. True
   B. False

_____ 17. The most ideal position for the adult head during spinal immobilization is:
   A. 1 to 2 inches above the spine board.
   B. level with the spine board.
   C. with padding under the shoulders and the head on the spine board.
   D. with the head slightly extended and level with the board.
   E. none of the above

_____ 18. Which of the following is a contraindication to continuing to move the head and spine toward the neutral, in-line position?
   A. You meet with significant resistance.
   B. Your patient complains of a significant increase in pain.
   C. You notice gross deformity along the spine.
   D. You notice an increase in the signs of neurologic injury.
   E. all of the above

_____ 19. Some gentle axial traction on the head will make cervical immobilization more effective.
   A. True
   B. False

_____ 20. The ideal position for the small adult's or large child's head during spinal immobilization is:
   A. 1 to 2 inches above the spine board.
   B. level with the spine board (ground level).
   C. with padding under the shoulders and the head on the spine board.
   D. with the head slightly extended and level with the board.
   E. none of the above

_____ 21. The standing takedown for the patient with spinal injuries requires a minimum of how many care providers?
   A. two
   B. three
   C. four
   D. five
   E. no less than six

_____ 22. Under which of the following circumstances should a helmet be removed from a patient?
   A. The head is not immobilized within the helmet.
   B. The helmet prevents airway maintenance.
   C. You cannot secure the helmet firmly to the long spine board.
   D. You anticipate breathing problems.
   E. all of the above

_____ 23. A four-count cadence is preferable for moves as it better signals care providers when the move starts.
   A. True
   B. False

_____ 24. Orthopedic stretchers are not rigid enough to be used for spinal immobilization by themselves.
   A. True
   B. False

_____ 25. The vest-type immobilization device is meant to permit rescuers to move the patient from a seated to a supine position in an auto crash by rotating the buttocks on the seat, then tilting the patient to the supine position.
   A. True
   B. False

_____ 26. Which of the following circumstances would not automatically merit employment of rapid extrication techniques?
   A. toxic fumes
   B. an auto collision
   C. an immediate threat of fire
   D. rising water
   E. none of the above

_____ 27. Once you immobilize the body to the long spine board, you can then secure the head to it.
   A. True
   B. False

_____ 28. Which of the following is routinely used in the prehospital setting for the treatment of spine injuries?
   A. mannitol
   B. methylprednisolone
   C. dexamethasone
   D. furosemide
   E. none of the above

_____ 29. If a suspected spinally injured patient does not respond to fluid resuscitation, which drug would you consider?
   A. methylprednisolone
   B. atropine
   C. furosemide
   D. dopamine
   E. diazepam

_____ 30. To address bradycardia in the suspected spinally injured patient, which drug would you consider?
   A. methylprednisolone
   B. atropine
   C. furosemide
   D. dopamine
   E. diazepam

Chapter 25

Thoracic Trauma

Review of Chapter Objectives

After reading this chapter, you should be able to:

1. **Describe the incidence, morbidity, and mortality of thoracic injuries in the trauma patient.** pp. 1031–1032

   Chest trauma accounts for about 25 percent of vehicular mortality and is second only to head trauma as a reason for death in the auto accident. Heart and great vessel injuries are the most common cause of death from blunt trauma. Penetrating trauma to the chest also results in significant mortality with heart and great vessel injuries, again, accounting for the greatest mortality. Modern auto and highway design, the speed at which the chest trauma patient arrives at the trauma center, and newer surgical techniques have significantly reduced chest trauma mortality in the last decade.

2. **Discuss the anatomy and physiology of the thoracic organs and structures.** (see Chapter 3)

   The ribs, thoracic spine, sternum, and diaphragm define the structure of the thoracic cage. The skeletal components allow the cage to expand as the ribs are lifted upward and outward by contraction of the intercostal muscles, and the intrathoracic volume further expands as the diaphragm contracts and moves downward. The net action of this muscle movement is to increase the volume of the thoracic cage and to reduce its internal pressure. Air from the environment moves through the airway into the alveoli to equalize this pressure, and inspiration occurs. The intercostal muscles relax and the thorax settles, while the diaphragm rises back into the thorax and the volume of the cavity decreases. This increases the intrathoracic pressure, and air rushes out to equalize with the environment. This is expiration. The pleura, two serous membranes, seal the lungs to the interior of the thoracic cage during this action and ensure that the lungs expand and contract with the changing volume of the thoracic cavity. The lungs have exceptional circulation, with capillary beds surrounding the alveoli to ensure a free exchange of oxygen and carbon dioxide between the alveolar air and the bloodstream.

   The lungs fill all but the central portion of the chest cavity and are found on either side of the central structure, called the mediastinum. The mediastinum contains the heart, trachea, esophagus, major blood vessels, and several nerve pathways. The heart is located in the left central chest and is the major pumping element of the cardiovascular system. The inferior and superior vena cavae collect blood from the lower extremities and abdomen and the upper extremities, head, and neck, respectively, and return it to the heart. The pulmonary arteries and veins carry blood to and from the lungs respectively, and the aorta distributes the cardiac output to the systemic circulation. The trachea enters the mediastinum just beneath the manubrium and bifurcates at the carina into the left and right mainstem bronchi. The esophagus enters the mediastinum just behind the trachea and exits through the diaphragm.

3. **Predict thoracic injuries based on mechanism of injury.** pp. 1032–1034

As in other regions of the body, thoracic trauma results from either blunt or penetrating mechanisms of injury. Blunt trauma may result from deceleration (as in an auto crash), crushing mechanism (as in a building collapse), or pressure injury (as with an explosion). Deceleration frequently causes the "paper bag" syndrome, lung and cardiac contusions, rib fractures, and vascular injuries. Crushing mechanisms may cause traumatic asphyxia and vascular damage and restrict respiratory excursion. Blast mechanisms may cause lung injuries or vascular tears.

Penetrating trauma may involve any structure within the thorax, although injury to the heart and great vessels is most likely to be lethal. Lung tissue is rather resilient and suffers limited injury with a bullet's passage, while the heart and great vessels are damaged explosively, especially if engorged with blood at the time of the bullet's impact. Slower velocity penetrating objects result in damage that is limited to the actual pathway of the object.

4. **Discuss the pathophysiology of, assessment findings with, and the management and need for rapid intervention and transport of the patient with chest wall injuries, including:**

   a. **Rib fracture** pp. 1035–1036, 1054–1055

   Blunt or penetrating trauma induces a fracture and possible associated injury underneath. The fracture itself is of only limited concern; however, the pain from such an injury may limit chest excursion and suggests more serious injury beneath. Care is directed to administering oxygen, considering the possibility of underlying injury, and supplying pain medication to ensure respirations are not limited by pain. These injuries do not by themselves require immediate intervention or transport.

   b. **Flail segment** pp. 1037–1038, 1055

   A flail segment is the result of several ribs (three or more) broken in numerous (two or more) places. This creates a rib segment that is free to move independently from the rest of the thorax. This paradoxical motion greatly decreases the efficiency of respiration as air that would be exhaled moves to the region under the flail segment and then returns to the unaffected lung with inspiration. Care includes seeing that the section is stabilized, the patient is given oxygen, possibly using overdrive ventilation. Consider the flail chest patient a candidate for rapid transport. Because of the severity of forces required to compromise the chest wall with this injury and the likelihood of serious underlying injury, this patient is given a high priority for care and transport.

   c. **Sternal fracture** pp. 1036–1037

   As with the flail chest patient, suspect the patient with sternal fracture of having serious internal injury. The kinetic forces necessary to fracture the sternum are likely to injure and contuse the heart and other structures of the mediastinum. The patient will have a history of blunt chest trauma and may complain of chest pain similar to that of a myocardial infarction. Administer oxygen, monitor the heart with an ECG, and watch the patient very carefully for any signs of myocardial or great vessel injury. This patient is a candidate for rapid transport.

5. **Discuss the pathophysiology of, assessment findings with, and management and need for rapid intervention and transport of the patient with injury to the lung, including:**

   a. **Simple pneumothorax** pp. 1038–1039

   A simple or closed pneumothorax is an injury caused by either blunt or penetrating trauma that opens the airway to the pleural space. Air accumulates within the space and displaces the lung, resulting in less-effective respirations and reduced oxygenation of the blood. This patient has a history of trauma and progressive dyspnea. Oxygen is administered and the patient is observed for progression to tension pneumothorax.

   b. **Open pneumothorax** pp. 1039–1040, 1055–1056

   Open pneumothorax is like simple pneumothorax, though in this case the injury penetrates the thoracic wall. The injury must be significantly large in order for air to move preferentially through the wound. The patient will have an open chest wound and dyspnea. Care includes sealing the wound on three sides to prevent further progress of the pneumothorax, oxygen administration, and monitoring the patient for the development of tension pneumothorax.

   c. **Tension pneumothorax**   pp. 1040–1041, 1056–1057

   Tension pneumothorax is a pneumothorax created under the mechanisms associated with simple or open pneumothorax that progresses because of a valve-like injury site. The valve permits air to enter the pleural space but not exit. This results in a progressive lung collapse, followed by increasing pressure that displaces the mediastinum and restricts venous return to the heart. The patient has a trauma history and progressive dyspnea that becomes very severe. The patient may also display subcutaneous emphysema and distended jugular veins. Care is directed at decompressing the thorax with the insertion of a catheter into the second intercostal space, providing oxygen, and monitoring the patient for a recurring tension pneumothorax.

   d. **Hemothorax**   pp. 1041–1042, 1057

   A hemothorax is a collection of blood in the pleural space. It may occur with or without pneumothorax. Hemothorax will generally become a hypovolemic problem before it seriously endangers respiration because the amount of fluid loss necessary to restrict respiration is great. The patient may experience dyspnea and the signs and symptoms of hypovolemic compensation (shock). Provide the patient with shock care, oxygen, fluid replacement, and rapid transport.

   e. **Hemopneumothorax**   pp. 1041–1042

   A hemopneumothorax is simply the existence of blood loss into the pleura and an accumulation of air there as well. Its presentation includes the signs and symptoms associated with both of these pathologies. Care is directed at oxygen administration and rapid transport.

   f. **Pulmonary contusion**   pp. 1042–1043

   Pulmonary contusion is a blunt trauma injury to the tissue of the lung resulting in edema and stiffening of the lung tissue. This reduces the efficiency of air exchange and causes an increased workload associated with respiration. If the region involved is limited, the patient may only experience very mild dyspnea. If the area is extensive, the patient may experience severe dyspnea. Care is centered around ensuring good oxygenation, including overdrive ventilation when indicated, and rapid transport.

6. **Discuss the pathophysiology of, findings of assessment with, and management and need for rapid intervention and transport of the patient with myocardial injuries, including:**

   a. **Myocardial contusion**   pp. 1043–1044, 1057–1058

   Myocardial contusion is simply a contusion to the myocardium, usually related to blunt anterior chest trauma. The patient will present with myocardial-infarction-like pain and possible dysrhythmias. Care is directed at oxygen therapy, cardiac medications as indicated, and rapid transport.

   b. **Pericardial tamponade**   pp. 1044–1045, 1058

   Pericardial tamponade is usually related to penetrating trauma in which a wound permits blood from within the heart to enter the pericardium. It progressively fills the pericardium and restricts ventricular filling. The cardiac output drops and circulation is severely restricted. The patient will present with a penetrating trauma mechanism and will move quickly into shock, and possibly, sudden death. Care is insertion of a needle into the pericardial sac and the withdrawal of fluid. Any patient suspected of this injury requires immediate transport to the closest hospital.

   c. **Myocardial rupture**   p. 1046

   Myocardial rupture is often associated with high-velocity penetrating trauma. The bullet's passage through the engorged heart causes the blood to move outward from the bullet's path (cavitation) explosively. The heart wall tears, and the patient hemorrhages extensively as cardiac output ceases. The patient will display the signs of sudden death and no resuscitation efforts will be successful.

7. **Discuss the pathophysiology of, findings of assessment with, and management and need for rapid intervention and transport of the patient with vascular injuries, including injuries to:**

   a. Aorta pp. 1046–1047, 1058

   Aortic aneurysm is a ballooning of the aorta as blunt trauma shears open the tunica intima and tunica media. Blood under systolic pressure enters the injury site and begins to dissect the vessel, causing it to balloon like a tire's inner tube. The patient will have a history of blunt trauma and complain of a tearing central chest pain that may radiate into the back. Care is centered around gentle but rapid transport to the trauma center. Oxygen is administered and fluid infusion should be very minimal.

   A rupture or penetrating injury to the aorta results in almost immediate death as the vessel is very large and contains great pressure. The patient will have a history of penetrating or severe blunt chest trauma and display the signs of shock and move quickly to decompensation and death. Care is directed to oxygen administration, shock management, and rapid transport to the trauma center.

   b. Vena cava p. 1047

   Injury to the vena cava is only slightly less severe than aortic injury since the vessels carry the same volume of fluid, but under different pressures (less for the vena cava). The progression of injury is just slightly slower with injury to the vena cava, though the result of injury is probably the same. In the field, it may be difficult to determine the exact blood vessel involved in a penetrating injury to the chest.

   c. Pulmonary arteries/veins p. 1047

   As with aortic and vena caval injuries, the patient will have a history of penetrating or severe blunt trauma and the signs and symptoms of hypovolemia and shock. Care is directed at helping the body compensate for shock, some fluid resuscitation, and rapid transport.

8. **Discuss the pathophysiology of, findings of assessment with, and management and need for rapid intervention and transport of patients with diaphragmatic, esophageal, and tracheobronchial injuries.** pp. 1047–1048, 1058

   Diaphragmatic injury is usually due to severe compression of the abdomen during blunt abdominal trauma or due to penetrating trauma along the border of the rib cage. Remember that the diaphragm is a dynamic muscle that moves up and down with respiration. Injury may result in less-effective respiration and/or the movement of abdominal organs into the chest cavity, most commonly the bowel. The injury may present similarly to tension pneumothorax as the abdominal contents displace the lung tissue. Bowel sounds may also be heard in the chest, though it usually takes too much time to decipher these sounds. Care is directed at treating shock and dyspnea with rapid transport indicated.

   Esophageal injury does not usually present with acute symptoms other than a history of penetrating trauma to the central chest. Perforation may permit food, drink, or gastric contents to enter the mediastinum, where it either forms an excellent medium for infection (with gastric contents) or damages some of the structures within. The result is serious damage to some of the most important structures within the chest and a significant mortality rate. The patient with such injury will present with penetrating injury to the region and care is directed toward other, more immediately important pathologies. Nevertheless, suspect esophageal injury and communicate that suspicion to the attending physician.

   Tracheobronchial injuries are usually related to penetrating trauma to the upper mediastinum, and they open the major airways to the mediastinum. The injuries permit air to enter the mediastinum and possibly the neck. The patient will have dyspnea (possibly severe) and may have subcutaneous emphysema. Positive-pressure ventilation may make matters worse as air is then actively "pushed" into the mediastinal space. The patient may also experience pneumothorax and tension pneumothorax.

9. **Discuss the pathophysiology of, findings of assessment with, and management and need for rapid intervention and transport of the patient with traumatic asphyxia.** pp. 1048, 1058

Traumatic asphyxia is a crushing-type injury in which the crushing mechanism remains in place and restricts both respiration and venous return to the central circulation. The patient may display bulging eyes, petechial hemorrhage, and red or blue skin above the level of compression. The injury may damage many internal blood vessels but tamponades hemorrhage because of the continuing compression. Once the compression is released, profound hypovolemia may occur and the patient may demonstrate the signs and symptoms of serious internal injury. Care is directed at oxygen administration, ventilation, fluid resuscitation, and rapid transport to the trauma center.

10. **Differentiate between thoracic injuries based on the assessment and history.** pp. 1048–1053

Anterior blunt trauma is most likely to cause rib fracture, pulmonary contusion, closed pneumothorax ("paper bag" syndrome) (possibly progressing to tension pneumothorax), and myocardial contusion. Sharp pain suggests rib fracture, while dull pain suggests pulmonary or myocardial contusion. Dyspnea may be present in all circumstances but will likely be progressive and become severe with pulmonary contusion or pneumothorax. Lateral impact may cause traumatic aortic aneurysm with tearing chest pain, possibly radiating to the back. Crushing injury may cause traumatic asphyxia and display with a discolored upper body and severe shock at the pressure release.

Penetrating trauma may induce an open pneumothorax but is more likely to cause closed pneumothorax unless there is a very large entrance wound. Injury to the great vessels and heart may cause immediate exsanguination, while heart injury may lead to pericardial tamponade. Penetrating trauma to the central chest may perforate any mediastinal structure, including the trachea or esophagus. Rapid hypovolemia and shock suggest great vessel or heart injury, while progressively increasing dyspnea suggests tension pneumothorax. Severe dyspnea, absent breath sounds on the ipsilateral side, and distended jugular veins confirm a probable diagnosis of tension pneumothorax. Any penetration of the thorax with possible entry into the mediastinum should suggest esophageal or tracheal injury.

11. **Given several preprogrammed and moulaged thoracic trauma patients, provide the appropriate scene size-up, initial assessment, rapid trauma or focused physical exam and history, detailed exam, and ongoing assessment, and provide appropriate patient care and transportation.** pp. 1031–1058

During your training as an EMT-Paramedic you will participate in many classroom practice sessions involving simulated patients. You will also spend some time in the emergency departments of local hospitals as well as in advanced-level ambulances gaining clinical experience. During these times, use your knowledge of thoracic trauma to help you assess and care for the simulated or real patients you attend.

Content Self-Evaluation

MULTIPLE CHOICE

1. Which of the following is NOT likely to be associated with blunt trauma?
    A. pericardial tamponade
    B. pneumothorax (paper bag syndrome)
    C. traumatic asphyxia
    D. aortic aneurysm
    E. myocardial contusion

_____ 2. Which of the following is NOT likely to be associated with penetrating trauma?
   A. open pneumothorax
   B. esophageal disruption
   C. traumatic asphyxia
   D. cavitational lung injury
   E. comminuted fracture of the ribs

_____ 3. Rib fracture is found in about what percentage of significant chest trauma?
   A. 10 percent
   B. 25 percent
   C. 35 percent
   D. 50 percent
   E. 65 percent

_____ 4. Which ribs are fractured the most frequently?
   A. ribs 1 and 3
   B. ribs 4 through 8
   C. ribs 7 through 9
   D. ribs 8 through 11
   E. ribs 9 through 12

_____ 5. Which rib group, when fractured, results in up to 30 percent incidence of serious associated internal injury?
   A. ribs 1 and 3
   B. ribs 4 through 8
   C. ribs 7 through 9
   D. ribs 9 through 12
   E. both A and D

_____ 6. Which of the following groups is more likely to experience internal injury without rib fracture?
   A. the pediatric patient
   B. the adult male patient
   C. the elderly male patient
   D. the elderly female patient
   E. the adult female patient

_____ 7. Which of the following are associated with rib fracture?
   A. local pain
   B. crepitus
   C. limited chest excursion
   D. hemothorax
   E. all of the above

_____ 8. Which of the following is most frequently associated with sternal fracture?
   A. hemothorax
   B. myocardial contusion
   C. esophageal injury
   D. simple pneumothorax
   E. open pneumothorax

_____ 9. Air from under the flail segment in flail chest does which of the following?
   A. moves out from under the segment during expiration
   B. moves toward the mediastinum during expiration
   C. does not move with the segment
   D. moves out from under the segment during inspiration
   E. none of the above

_____ 10. As the pain of the flail chest increases with time, the amount of paradoxical movement will decrease due to muscular splinting.
   A. True
   B. False

_____ 11. Simple pneumothorax is associated with what percentage of serious thoracic trauma?
   A. 5
   B. 10 to 30
   C. 25 to 50
   D. 60
   E. more than 75

_____ 12. The condition in which a part of the chest wall moves in opposition to the rest of the chest due to numerous rib fractures is called:
   A. pneumothorax.
   B. tension pneumothorax.
   C. hemothorax.
   D. atelectasis.
   E. none of the above

_____ 13. The chest injury that causes the patient to experience increasing dyspnea because of an open or closed pneumothorax that has a valve-like function and allows intrathoracic pressure to increase is referred to as:
   A. subcutaneous emphysema.
   B. traumatic asphyxia.
   C. hyperbaric mediastinal displacement.
   D. tension pneumothorax.
   E. flail chest.

_____ 14. For a significant amount of air to move through an open wound to create an open pneumothorax, the wound opening must be:
   A. just large enough to permit air passage.
   B. two-thirds the size of the tracheal opening.
   C. the size of the trachea.
   D. about the size of a hunting rifle bullet.
   E. larger than the trachea.

_____ 15. Which of the following is a very late sign of tension pneumothorax?
   A. head and neck petechiae
   B. intercostal bulging
   C. a narrowing pulse pressure
   D. tracheal deviation away from the injury
   E. distended jugular veins

_____ 16. Each hemithorax can hold up to what volume of blood from a hemothorax?
   A. 500 mL
   B. 750 mL
   C. 1,500 mL
   D. 3,000 mL
   E. 4,500 mL

_____ 17. Which of the following statements is NOT true regarding hemothorax?
   A. Hemorrhage into the thorax is more severe due to decreased pressure there.
   B. Serious hemothorax may displace an entire lung and has a 75 percent mortality rate.
   C. Hemothorax often occurs with pneumothorax.
   D. Hemothorax rarely occurs with simple rib fractures.
   E. none of the above

_____ 18. Distant or absent breath sounds heard during auscultation of the chest and the signs of shock are suggestive of which pathology?
   A. pneumothorax
   B. tension pneumothorax
   C. aortic aneurysm
   D. pulmonary contusion
   E. hemothorax

_____ 19. Which of the following problems would most likely result in a chest area that was dull to percussion?
   A. pneumothorax
   B. tension pneumothorax
   C. hemothorax
   D. subcutaneous pneumothorax
   E. pericardial tamponade

_____ 20. Your patient has received chest trauma yet did not initially present with crackles. However, as the assessment continues, they are heard in both the lower lung fields. This condition is most likely a result of which of the following?
   A. pulmonary contusion
   B. hemothorax
   C. pneumothorax
   D. aortic aneurysm
   E. pericardial tamponade

_____ 21. Extensive pulmonary contusions may account for blood losses up to 1,500 mL.
   A. True
   B. False

_____ 22. The most common cause of myocardial contusion is:
   A. blunt anterior chest trauma.
   B. blunt lateral chest trauma.
   C. penetrating anterior chest trauma.
   D. blunt posterior chest trauma.
   E. the pressure wave of an explosion.

_____ 23. A patient presents with the signs of shock, jugular vein distention, distant heart sounds, and a narrowing pulse pressure. The lung fields are clear. Which condition is most likely the cause?
   A. tension pneumothorax
   B. hemothorax
   C. traumatic asphyxia
   D. pericardial tamponade
   E. atelectasis

_____ 24. Pericardial tamponade occurs with what frequency in serious chest trauma patients?
   A. less than 2 percent of the time
   B. 10 percent of the time
   C. 20 percent of the time
   D. 25 percent of the time
   E. 30 to 45 percent of the time

_____ 25. Which of the following is a sign of pericardial tamponade?
   A. pulsus paradoxus
   B. a narrowing pulse pressure
   C. distended jugular veins
   D. hypotension
   E. all of the above

_____ 26. The patient with pericardial tamponade may be in hypovolemic shock due to the volume of blood lost into the pericardial sac.
   A. True
   B. False

_____ 27. A decrease in jugular vein distention during inspiration is known as:
   A. Beck's triad.
   B. pulsus paradoxus.
   C. Cushing's reflex.
   D. Kussmaul's sign.
   E. electrical alternans.

_____ 28. If the chamber of the heart is significantly damaged yet does not rupture immediately, it is likely to rupture in around two weeks.
   A. True
   B. False

_____ 29. Your patient was involved in a lateral impact auto accident. The car is greatly deformed, though the patient does not have many signs of injury. During your assessment, he complains of a tearing sensation in his central chest and numbness in his left upper extremity. Your highest index of suspicion of injury is for:
   A. traumatic asphyxia.
   B. pulmonary contusion.
   C. aortic aneurysm.
   D. myocardial contusion.
   E. pericardial tamponade.

_____ 30. What percentage of patients with traumatic aortic aneurysm survive the initial impact and injury?
   A. as high as 10 percent
   B. as high as 20 percent
   C. 50 percent
   D. 70 percent
   E. 73 percent

_____ 31. In a patient with a history of blunt lateral trauma and a suspected traumatic aortic aneurysm, which signs or symptoms would you expect to find?
   A. severe tearing chest pain
   B. pulse deficit between extremities
   C. reduced pulse strength in the lower extremities
   D. hypertension
   E. all of the above

_____ 32. A harsh systolic murmur is heard over the central chest. This is suggestive of which pathology?
　　A. pneumothorax
　　B. tension pneumothorax
　　C. traumatic aortic aneurysm
　　D. pulmonary contusion
　　E. hemothorax

_____ 33. The right side is the site of most diaphragmatic ruptures as most assailants are right-handed.
　　A. True
　　B. False

_____ 34. The traumatic diaphragmatic rupture is likely to present like which of the following thoracic injuries?
　　A. tension pneumothorax
　　B. pulmonary contusion
　　C. aortic aneurysm
　　D. pericardial tamponade
　　E. esophageal injury

_____ 35. The two major problems associated with traumatic asphyxia are restriction of chest excursion and:
　　A. distortion of the airway.
　　B. restriction of venous return.
　　C. atelectasis.
　　D. hemorrhage during the compression.
　　E. massive strokes.

_____ 36. The classic signs of traumatic asphyxia include which of the following?
　　A. bulging eyes
　　B. conjunctival hemorrhage
　　C. petechiae of the head and neck
　　D. dark red or purple appearance of the head and neck
　　E. all of the above

_____ 37. Serious penetrating trauma will likely require which of the following body substance isolation procedures?
　　A. gloves
　　B. face shield
　　C. gown
　　D. mask
　　E. all of the above

_____ 38. During your assessment of a supine patient with blunt chest trauma, you notice slight jugular vein distention. With no other signs of injury, this suggests which of the following?
　　A. a normal patient
　　B. pericardial tamponade
　　C. tension pneumothorax
　　D. traumatic asphyxia
　　E. B, C, and D

_____ 39. Crackles heard during auscultation of the chest are suggestive of which pathology?
　　A. pneumothorax
　　B. tension pneumothorax
　　C. aortic aneurysm
　　D. pulmonary contusion
　　E. hemothorax

_____ 40. Hyperresonance heard during percussion of the chest is suggestive of which pathology?
　　A. pneumothorax
　　B. tension pneumothorax
　　C. hemothorax
　　D. pulmonary contusion
　　E. both A and B

_____ 41. Which of the following thoracic structures takes the least energy to fracture and often results in a more common, yet less serious, thoracic injury?
　　A. ribs 1 through 3
　　B. ribs 4 through 8
　　C. ribs 9 through 12
　　D. the sternum
　　E. the manubrium

_____ 42. A patient who displays subcutaneous emphysema is most likely to have which of the conditions listed below?
   A. traumatic asphyxia
   B. tension pneumothorax
   C. the paper bag syndrome
   D. pulmonary contusion
   E. cardiac contusion

_____ 43. Overdrive ventilation (bag-valve-masking) of the patient with flail chest will cause the flail segment to move with, rather than in opposition to, the chest wall.
   A. True
   B. False

_____ 44. Which of the following is an indication for the use of IV infusion?
   A. diaphragmatic rupture
   B. penetrating chest injury
   C. chest trauma with a blood pressure below 80
   D. chest trauma with a blood pressure below 50
   E. suspected pericardial tamponade

_____ 45. Meperidine, diazepam, or morphine sulfate may be given to the minor rib fracture patient to reduce pain and increase respiratory excursion.
   A. True
   B. False

_____ 46. The patient who is suspected of a flail chest or other thoracic cage injury, without suspected spine injury, should be positioned:
   A. on the uninjured side.
   B. on the injured side.
   C. supine with legs elevated.
   D. on the left lateral side.
   E. on the right lateral side.

_____ 47. The open pneumothorax should be cared for using which of the following techniques?
   A. Pack the wound with a sterile dressing.
   B. Cover the wound with an occlusive dressing and tape securely.
   C. Cover the wound with an occlusive dressing, taped on three sides.
   D. Attempt to close the wound with a hemostat and then cover with a sterile dressing.
   E. Cover the wound loosely with a sterile dressing.

_____ 48. Which location is recommended for prehospital pleural decompression?
   A. second intercostal space, midclavicular line
   B. fifth intercostal space, midclavicular line
   C. fifth intercostal space, midaxillary line
   D. A and B
   E. A and C

_____ 49. A few minutes after you have inserted a needle and decompressed a tension pneumothorax, you notice that a patient's dyspnea is getting worse and breath sounds on the injured side are becoming diminished. Which action would you take?
   A. Insert a second needle.
   B. Remove the dressing.
   C. Provide overdrive ventilation.
   D. Consider nitrous oxide administration.
   E. all of the above

_____ 50. A patient is trapped in a wrecked auto for about half an hour and is suspected of having traumatic asphyxia. Care should include which of the following?
   A. two large-bore IVs
   B. normal saline or lactated Ringer's solution
   C. fluids run rapidly
   D. consideration of sodium bicarbonate
   E. all of the above

Abdominal Trauma

Review of Chapter Objectives

After reading this chapter, you should be able to:

1. **Describe the epidemiology, including morbidity/mortality, for patients with abdominal trauma as well as prevention strategies to avoid the injuries.** p. 1062

   While serious abdominal trauma accounts for some mortality, it ranks behind head and chest trauma as a region associated with trauma deaths. Rapid transport to the trauma center and modern surgical techniques have accounted for a great decrease in abdominal trauma mortality and morbidity, but it still remains a serious consideration during trauma assessment and care. Highway and vehicle design and the proper use of restraints have reduced abdominal injuries greatly, however, and more correct use of seat belts by greater numbers of the population can lead to continuing decreases in both the incidence and severity of abdominal injury.

2. **Apply the epidemiologic principles to develop prevention strategies for abdominal injuries.** p. 1062

   The current major causes of abdominal injury are improper seat belt use and violence. Education programs designed to promote the use and proper application of seat belts and programs to reduce unintentional or deliberate injuries resulting from handguns can help further reduce abdominal injury.

3. **Describe the anatomy and physiology of the abdominal organs and structures.** (see Chapter 3)

   The abdomen is one of the body's largest cavities, bounded superiorly by the diaphragm, laterally by the flank muscles, inferiorly by the pelvis, posteriorly by the spine and back muscles, and anteriorly by the abdominal muscles. Since most of its border is soft tissue, it is rather unprotected from injury. The abdomen contains the continuous, muscular tube of digestion, the alimentary canal. It enters the abdomen through the hiatus of the diaphragm as the esophagus. It joins the stomach, an organ that physically mixes the food with gastric juices and then sends it out and into the small bowel. The first portion of the bowel, the duodenum, mixes the digesting food with bile (a byproduct of the liver) and pancreatic juices and then begins the process of absorption. The remainder of the small bowel draws the nutrients from the food.

   As the digesting food enters the large bowel, it is mixed with bacteria, releasing water and any remaining nutrients. They are absorbed, and the material is pushed by peristalsis to the rectum, awaiting defecation. The bowel is a thin vascular tube that drains its blood supply through the liver for detoxification, where some nutrients are stored and others added to the circulation.

The liver is a large solid organ found in the right upper quadrant, just below the diaphragm. The pancreas is a delicate organ found in the lower aspect of the upper left quadrant with a portion of it extending into the right upper quadrant. In addition to digestive juices, it manufactures insulin and glucagon. The kidneys are found deep within the flanks and filter blood to remove excess water and electrolytes. They are very vascular organs that excrete urine into the ureters through which the urine then travels to the bladder. The bladder (in the central pelvic space) rids the body of urine through the urethra. The spleen is an organ of the immune system and is very delicate and vascular, residing in the left upper quadrant.

The abdominal cavity is lined with a serous membrane, the peritoneum. It covers the anterior abdominal organs and a double-layer sheath of it forms the omentum, which covers the anterior surface of the abdomen. The bowel is slung from the posterior wall of the abdomen by connective tissue called the mesentery that also provides perfusion to the bowel. The abdominal aorta and inferior vena cava run along the spinal column and branch frequently to serve the abdominal organs.

4. Predict abdominal injuries based on blunt and penetrating mechanisms of injury. pp. 1062–1069

Blunt trauma compresses, shears, or decelerates the various organs and structures within the abdomen resulting in rupture of the hollow organs, fracture or tearing of the solid organs, or tearing or severance of the abdominal vasculature. The spleen is the most frequently injured organ with the liver the second most commonly injured structure. The bowel, kidneys, and diaphragm are also common recipients of blunt injury.

Penetrating injury to the abdomen may involve low- and high-velocity objects. Bullets disrupt a larger cylinder of tissue with their passage and are especially damaging to hollow organs filled with fluid and to the extremely dense and delicate solid organs of the abdomen. Mortality is about ten times greater with high-energy bullets than with stab-type wounds. The liver is affected more frequently than the bowel, with the spleen, kidneys, and pancreas injured in descending order of frequency. A special category of penetrating injury is the shotgun blast. At short range (under 3 yards), the projectiles have tremendous energy and create numerous tracts of serious injury.

5. Describe open and closed abdominal injuries. pp. 1062–1065

Open wounds to the abdomen may be very small, such as those caused by a bullet or knife, or large enough to permit abdominal contents to protrude (an evisceration). Bullet wounds may cause injury beyond their direct path through cavitation and are especially harmful to the solid organs (liver, spleen, kidneys, pancreas) or to the stomach and intestinal tract when full of fluid. Shotgun blasts, especially if delivered from less than 9 feet, are extremely damaging because the many small projectiles still have significant kinetic energy and have not yet spread out to disperse their energy.

Blunt (closed) injuries may compress the internal organs of the abdomen between the offending object and the spine or posterior abdominal wall or between other organs. The force may shear solid organs and their vascular attachments or may directly cause organ fracture and hemorrhage or the spillage of organ contents or both. Hollow organs may rupture and spill their contents into the abdominal cavity. Severe abdominal compression may rupture the diaphragm and push abdominal organs into the thorax.

6. Identify the need for rapid intervention and transport of the patient with abdominal injuries based on assessment findings. pp. 1069–1074

The abdomen, for the most part, is bound by connective and muscle tissue rather than the skeletal structures found protecting the skull and thorax. This permits an easier transmission of traumatic forces to the internal organs and frequent injury. The abdomen also does not show the dramatic signs and symptoms of injury seen elsewhere, again because of the lack of rigid skeletal protection. Hence, it is important to carefully assess the abdominal cavity, looking for any sign of trauma (such as erythema), and to question the patient about pain or other abdominal symptoms. Gastric, duodenal, and pancreatic contents and, to a lesser degree, blood and bacteria irritate the abdominal lining (the peritoneum) only after the passage of time, which again limits the signs and symptoms of serious abdominal injury visible during prehospital care.

7. **Explain the pathophysiology of solid and hollow organ injuries, abdominal vascular injuries, pelvic fractures, and other abdominal injuries.** pp. 1065–1069

Solid Organ Injuries

The spleen is well protected, although it is very delicate and not contained within a strong capsule. It frequently ruptures and bleeds heavily. The liver is a very dense and vascular organ in the right upper quadrant just behind the lower border of the rib cage. It is contained within a strong capsule, although it can be lacerated during severe deceleration by its restraining ligament (the ligamentum teres). The kidneys are well protected both by their location deep within the flank and by strong capsules. The pancreas is located in the lower portion of the left upper quadrant, extending just into the right quadrant. It is more delicate than either the liver or kidneys even though it lies deep within the central abdomen. When injured, it may hemorrhage and release pancreatic juices into the abdomen.

Hollow Organ Injuries

Hollow organs include the stomach, small and large bowel, rectum, gallbladder, urinary bladder, and pregnant uterus. Compression may contuse them or cause them to rupture while penetrating injury may perforate them. The gallbladder, stomach, and first part of the small bowel may release digestive juices that will chemically irritate and damage the abdominal structures. Injury can cause the rest of the bowel to release material high in bacterial load that can induce infection. The rupture of the urinary bladder will release blood and urine into the abdomen. Injury to the abdomen may cause blood in emesis (hematemesis), blood in the stool (hematochezia), or blood in the urine (hematuria).

Abdominal Vascular Injuries

The major vascular structures of the abdomen include the abdominal aorta, the inferior vena cava, and many arteries branching to the abdominal organs. These vessels may be injured by blunt trauma, though penetrating trauma is a far more frequent cause of injury. The abdomen does not develop an internal pressure against hemorrhage as do the muscles and other solid regions of the body, and bleeding may continue unabated while the accumulation of blood is difficult to recognize.

Pelvic Fractures

Pelvic fractures are addressed in Chapter 22, "Musculoskeletal Trauma," Division 3. However, remember that pelvic fracture can cause injury to the bladder, genitalia, and rectum, and to some very large blood vessels with serious associated hemorrhage.

Other Abdominal Organ Injuries

Other injuries include injuries to the mesentery and peritoneum. The mesentery supports the bowel and may be injured, most commonly at points of fixation like the ileocecal or duodenal/jejunal junctures. Hemorrhage here is often contained by the peritoneum. Peritoneal injury is generally related to irritation either by chemical action (most rapid) or by bacterial contamination (12 to 24 hours).

8. **Describe the assessment findings associated with and the management of solid and hollow organ injuries, abdominal vascular injuries, pelvic fractures, and other abdominal injuries.** pp. 1069–1077

Injury to the abdominal contents is difficult to ascertain because the signs and symptoms of injury are often diffuse and around 30 percent of patients with serious abdominal injury have no clear signs or symptoms of injury. During assessment, you should seek to discover what evidence of injury exists and what it suggests about the injury's precise nature and location. Pay attention to pain, tenderness, and rebound tenderness in each quadrant and note any thirst or other signs of hypovolemia and shock.

The management of the patient with suspected abdominal trauma is basically supportive with airway maintenance, oxygen, ventilation as needed, and fluid resuscitation. Establish large-bore IVs but do not run fluids aggressively unless the blood pressure drops below 80 mmHg. Use of the PASG may be helpful, especially if the blood pressure drops below 50 mmHg. Cover any evisceration with a sterile dressing soaked in normal saline and cover that with an occlusive dressing to prevent evaporation. As with all hypovolemia patients, keep the patient warm and provide rapid transport.

9. **Differentiate between abdominal injuries based on the assessment and history.** pp. 1069–1075

As mentioned earlier, 30 percent of patients with serious abdominal injury present without signs and symptoms. Many others present with diffuse signs and symptoms, making it very hard to differentiate among the different abdominal pathologies. Try to relate the mechanism of injury or any patient complaints to the anatomic region involved and the specific organs found there. For example, left flank trauma and pain may suggest splenic injury, while right upper quadrant injury and pain may suggest liver pathology.

Penetrating abdominal trauma will present with an entrance wound and, possibly, an exit wound. It may also manifest with the signs and symptoms of blunt abdominal trauma due to the same mechanisms. Evisceration will be evident by the protrusion of bowel from an open wound involving the abdominal wall.

Blunt abdominal trauma may be recognized by abdominal tenderness, rebound tenderness, pain, or a pulsing mass. It may involve any of the abdominal or retroperitoneal organs. Signs will be superficial such as contusions or, more likely, erythema. Symptoms may result from the injury or from blood, body fluids, or bacteria (causing delayed pain) in the peritoneal cavity.

10. **Given several preprogrammed and moulaged abdominal trauma patients, provide the appropriate scene size-up, initial assessment, rapid trauma or focused physical exam and history, detailed exam, and ongoing assessment, and provide appropriate patient care and transportation.** pp. 1062–1077

During your training as an EMT-Paramedic you will participate in many classroom practice sessions involving simulated patients. You will also spend some time in the emergency departments of local hospitals as well as in advanced-level ambulances gaining clinical experience. During these times, use your knowledge of abdominal trauma to help you assess and care for the simulated or real patients you attend.

Content Self-Evaluation

MULTIPLE CHOICE

_____ 1. Due to the anatomy of the abdomen, injury to its contents often presents with limited signs and symptoms.
   A. True
   B. False

_____ 2. Bullets cause an abdominal wound mortality rate that is about equal to that caused by slow-moving penetrating objects.
   A. True
   B. False

_____ 3. What percentage of the time does a penetrating mechanism injure the liver?
   A. 50 percent   D. 20 percent
   B. 40 percent   E. 10 percent
   C. 30 percent

_____ 4. What percentage of the time does a blunt mechanism injure the liver?
   A. 50 percent
   B. 40 percent
   C. 30 percent
   D. 20 percent
   E. 10 percent

_____ 5. Which of the following organs is most frequently damaged during blunt abdominal trauma?
   A. the small bowel
   B. the liver
   C. the spleen
   D. the kidneys
   E. the pancreas

_____ 6. The abdomen is the area for greatest concern when the patient is exposed to severe blast forces.
   A. True
   B. False

_____ 7. Penetration of the abdominal wall resulting in protrusion of the abdominal contents is called:
   A. peristalsis.
   B. chyme.
   C. peritonitis.
   D. emulsification.
   E. evisceration.

_____ 8. The abdominal organs, with deep expiration, move as far up into the thorax as:
   A. the xiphoid process.
   B. the tips of the floating ribs.
   C. the nipple line.
   D. the seventh intercostal space.
   E. none of the above

_____ 9. The term describing frank blood in the stool is:
   A. hematochezia.
   B. hematemesis.
   C. hemoptysis.
   D. hematuria.
   E. hematocrit.

_____ 10. The organ most likely to be injured by left flank blunt trauma is:
   A. the small bowel.
   B. the liver.
   C. the spleen.
   D. the kidneys.
   E. the pancreas.

_____ 11. The organ that is likely to be injured in severe deceleration as its ligament restrains, then lacerates it is:
   A. the small bowel.
   B. the liver.
   C. the spleen.
   D. the kidneys.
   E. the pancreas.

_____ 12. Most abdominal vascular injuries are associated with penetrating trauma.
   A. True
   B. False

_____ 13. Hemorrhage into the abdomen is of serious concern because it:
   A. quickly puts pressure on internal organs.
   B. limits respirations.
   C. rapidly affects the heart.
   D. may trigger a vagal response, slowing the heart.
   E. none of the above

_____ 14. Blunt injury to the mesentery often occurs at:
   A. the gastric-duodenal juncture.
   B. the duodenal-jejunal juncture.
   C. the jejunal-ileal juncture.
   D. the ileocecal juncture.
   E. both B and D

_____ 15. How long does it take bacteria to grow in sufficient numbers to irritate the peritoneum?
   A. 2 to 4 hours
   B. 4 to 6 hours
   C. 6 to 8 hours
   D. 8 to 10 hours
   E. over 12 hours

_____ 16. The number one killer of pregnant females is:
   A. heart attack.
   B. ectopic pregnancy.
   C. allergic reactions.
   D. trauma.
   E. stroke.

_____ 17. Unrestrained pregnant occupants in vehicles are how many more times likely to suffer fetal mortality in an auto collision than their belted counterparts?
   A. two
   B. three
   C. four
   D. five
   E. six

_____ 18. The late-term pregnant female is at increased risk for vomiting and aspiration.
   A. True
   B. False

_____ 19. Supine positioning of the mother may cause hypotension due to:
   A. compression of the inferior vena cava.
   B. increased circulation to the uterus.
   C. increased intraabdominal pressure.
   D. decreased intraabdominal pressure.
   E. Kussmaul's respirations.

_____ 20. It may take a maternal blood loss of what percentage before the heart rate begins to increase in the late-term pregnancy?
   A. 10 to 15 percent
   B. 15 to 20 percent
   C. 20 to 25 percent
   D. 25 to 30 percent
   E. 30 to 35 percent

_____ 21. Due to the flexibility of the pediatric thorax, which injury is more likely to occur with blunt trauma?
   A. liver injury
   B. spleen injury
   C. kidney injury
   D. all of the above
   E. none of the above

_____ 22. Children may not show signs of blood loss until they have lost what percentage of their volume?
   A. 25 percent
   B. 35 percent
   C. 45 percent
   D. over 50 percent
   E. over 65 percent

_____ 23. What percentage of patients with abdominal injury do not present with any signs or symptoms?
   A. 10 percent
   B. 20 percent
   C. 30 percent
   D. 40 percent
   E. 50 percent

_____ 24. The signs of abdominal trauma may become less specific due to the progression of peritonitis.
   A. True
   B. False

_____ 25. Blunt injury to the right flank region is likely to cause which of the following?
   A. splenic injury
   B. kidney injury
   C. bowel injury
   D. bladder injury
   E. colon injury

_____ 26. Thirst may be one of the few symptoms of abdominal injury as internal hemorrhage loss draws down the body's blood volume.
A. True
B. False

_____ 27. Hemorrhage into the abdomen may account for how much blood loss before it becomes noticeable?
A. 500 mL
B. 750 mL
C. 1,000 mL
D. 1,500 mL
E. 2,500 mL

_____ 28. The major reason auscultation of bowel and other abdominal sounds is not recommended in the field is because:
A. the sounds are not clear.
B. the sounds do not rule out injury.
C. the lack of sounds does not confirm injury.
D. it takes too long to assess bowel sounds adequately.
E. B, C, and D

_____ 29. Prehospital administration of IV fluid should be limited to:
A. 1,000 mL.
B. 2,000 mL.
C. 3,000 mL.
D. 4,000 mL.
E. 5,000 mL.

_____ 30. Care for the abdominal evisceration includes use of which of the following?
A. a dry adherent dressing
B. a dry nonadherent dressing
C. a sterile dressing moistened with normal saline
D. an occlusive dressing
E. a sterile cotton gauze dressing

_____ 31. At what blood pressure would you consider applying the PASG in the presence of an abdominal evisceration?
A. 120 mmHg
B. 100 mmHg
C. 90 mmHg
D. 60 mmHg
E. 30 mmHg

_____ 32. Which position is indicated for the late pregnancy patient?
A. supine
B. right lateral recumbent
C. with the head elevated 30 degrees
D. left lateral recumbent
E. Trendelenburg

_____ 33. Unless the blood pressure is less than 50 mmHg, use of the PASG is contraindicated in:
A. geriatric patients.
B. patients with low blood pressure.
C. tuberculosis patients.
D. abdominal evisceration patients.
E. diabetic patients.

_____ 34. Aggressive fluid resuscitation may aggravate the relative anemia associated with late-term pregnancy.
A. True
B. False

_____ 35. Use of the PASG may be beneficial for the patient in early (first-term) pregnancy.
A. True
B. False

Essentials of Paramedic Care

Division 4

Medical Emergencies

Chapter 27

Pulmonology

Review of Chapter Objectives

With each chapter of the Workbook, we identify the objectives and the important elements of the text content. You should review these items and refer to the pages listed if any points are not clear.

After reading this chapter, you should be able to:

1. **Discuss the epidemiology of pulmonary diseases and pulmonary conditions.**   p. 1081

   Respiratory emergencies are among the most common EMS calls—up to 28 percent, according to one study. Respiratory emergencies lead to over 200,000 deaths per year. Because of the frequency of such calls, it is critical that you be knowledgeable about diseases that affect the respiratory system.

2. **Identify and describe the function of the structures located in the upper and lower airway.**   (see Chapter 3)

   The airway is functionally divided into the upper airway and the lower airway. The upper airway is comprised of the nasal cavity, pharynx, and larynx. The lower airway is comprised of the trachea, bronchi, alveoli, and lungs. The ability to take in oxygen and excrete carbon dioxide via the airway is essential to life. Therefore, it is critical that you be able to identify and understand the function of each structure of the airway and of the airway as a whole.

3. **Discuss the physiology of ventilation and respiration.**   pp. 1081–1084; see Chapter 3

   The major function of the respiratory system is the exchange of gases between the person and the environment. Three processes allow the gas exchange to take place: ventilation, diffusion, and perfusion. Ventilation is the movement of air in and out of the lungs. Diffusion is the movement of gases between the lungs and the pulmonary capillaries (oxygen from the lungs into the bloodstream; waste carbon dioxide from the bloodstream into the lungs) as well as between the systemic capillaries and the body tissues (oxygen from the bloodstream into the cells; waste carbon dioxide from the cells into the bloodstream). Perfusion is the circulation of blood through the capillaries. Adequate perfusion is critical to adequate gas exchange in the lungs and body tissues. These three processes—ventilation, diffusion, and perfusion—together provide for respiration.

4. **Identify common pathological events that affect the pulmonary system.**   pp. 1084–1086

   Any disease state that affects the pulmonary system will ultimately disrupt ventilation, diffusion, or perfusion, or a combination of these processes. Ventilation may be disrupted by diseases that cause obstruction of any part of the airway, disrupt the normal function of the chest wall, or impair the nervous system's control of breathing. Diffusion can be disrupted by a change in concentration of atmospheric oxygen or by any disease that affects the structure or patency of

©2007 Pearson Education, Inc.
Essentials of Paramedic Care, 2nd ed.

alveoli, the thickness of the respiratory membrane, or the permeability of the capillaries. Perfusion will be affected by any disease that limits blood flow through the lungs and the body or reduces the volume of the oxygen-carrying red blood cells or hemoglobin. Understanding how different diseases and conditions may affect the processes of respiration is important to your ability to choose appropriate emergency care for a respiratory emergency.

5. **Compare various airway and ventilation techniques used in the management of pulmonary diseases.** pp. 1098–1118

   Two principles govern the overall management of respiratory emergencies. (1) Give first priority to the airway. (2) Always provide oxygen to patients with respiratory distress or the possibility of hypoxia, including those with chronic obstructive pulmonary disease (COPD).

6. **Review the use of equipment utilized during the physical examination of patients with complaints associated with respiratory diseases and conditions.** pp. 1091–1092, 1093–1098

   You should be familiar with the use of equipment that is available for physical examination of patients with respiratory complaints. Equipment includes the stethoscope, the pulse oximeter, handheld devices for measuring peak expiratory flow rate (PEFR), and capnography.

7. **Identify the epidemiology, anatomy, physiology, pathophysiology, assessment findings, and management (including prehospital medications) for the following respiratory diseases and conditions:**

   a. **Adult respiratory distress syndrome** pp. 1100–1101

   Adult respiratory distress syndrome (ARDS) is characterized by pulmonary edema caused by fluid accumulation in the interstitial spaces in the lungs. The mortality rate is 70 percent. ARDS occurs as a result of increased vascular permeability and decreased fluid removal from the lungs. A variety of lung insults can cause this inability to maintain proper fluid balance, including sepsis, pneumonia, inhalation injuries, emboli, tumors, and others noted in the text chapter. ARDS interferes with diffusion, causing hypoxia. In addition to evaluating the degree of the patient's respiratory distress, assessment is aimed at discovering symptoms and history that point to the underlying condition. Prehospital management is supportive (oxygen supplementation is essential to compensate for diffusion defects); in-hospital care is aimed at treatment of the underlying condition.

   b. **Bronchial asthma** pp. 1101–1102, 1105–1108

   Asthma is an obstructive lung disease that causes abnormal ventilation. While deaths from other respiratory diseases are decreasing, deaths from asthma have been on the increase, with 50 percent of those deaths occurring before the patient reaches the hospital. Asthma is thought to be caused by a combination of genetic predisposition and environmental triggers that differ from individual to individual. These include allergens, cold air, exercise, stress, and certain medications. Exposure to a trigger causes release of histamine, which, in turn, causes both bronchial constriction and capillary leakage that leads to bronchial edema. The result is a significant decrease in expiratory airflow, which is the essence of an "asthma attack." In the early phase of an attack, inhaled bronchodilator medications such as albuterol will help. In the late phase, inflammation sets in and antiinflammatory drugs are required to alleviate the condition. Assessment must focus first on evaluation and support of the airway and breathing. Most patients will report a history of asthma. The physical exam should focus on the chest and neck to assess breathing effort. The respiratory rate is the most critical of the vital signs. EMS systems should also be able to measure the peak expiratory flow rate. Treatment is aimed at correction of hypoxia (oxygen administration) and relief of bronchospasm and inflammation. A special case is status asthmaticus—a severe, prolonged attack that does not respond to bronchodilators. It is a serious emergency requiring prompt recognition, treatment, and transport. Another special case is asthma in children, which is treated much as for adults but with altered medication dosages and some special medications.

c. Chronic bronchitis   pp. 1101–1102, 1104–1105

Chronic bronchitis is classified, along with emphysema, as a chronic obstructive pulmonary disease (COPD). COPD affects 25 percent of adults, with chronic bronchitis affecting one in five adult males. Chronic bronchitis reduces ventilation as a result of increased mucus production that blocks airway passages. It is often caused by cigarette smoking but also occurs in nonsmokers. There may be a history of frequent respiratory infections. Chronic bronchitis is usually associated with a productive cough and copious sputum. Patients tend to be overweight and often become cyanotic, so they are sometimes called "blue bloaters." Auscultation of the airway often reveals rhonchi due to mucus occlusion. The goals of treatment are relief of hypoxia and reversal of bronchoconstriction. Because these patients may be dependent on a hypoxic respiratory drive (low oxygen levels stimulate respiration), respiratory effort may become depressed when oxygen is administered. Needed oxygen should not be withheld, but the patient's respirations must be carefully monitored. IV fluids may help loosen mucous congestion. Medical direction may also order administration of a bronchodilator, such as albuterol, metaproterenol, or ipratropium bromide, and may also recommend corticosteroid administration.

d. Emphysema   pp. 1101–1104

Like chronic bronchitis, emphysema is classified as a chronic obstructive pulmonary disease (COPD). Alveolar walls are destroyed by exposure to noxious substances such as cigarette smoke or other environmental toxins. The disease also causes destruction of the walls of the small bronchioles, which contributes to a trapping of air in the lungs. The result is a decrease in both ventilation and diffusion. Patients tend to breathe through pursed lips, which creates a positive pressure that helps to prevent alveolar collapse. A developing decrease in PaO_2 leads to a compensatory increase in red blood cell production (polycythemia). Emphysema patients are more susceptible to acute respiratory infections and cardiac dysrhythmias. They become dependent on bronchodilators and corticosteroids and, in the final stages, supplemental oxygen. In contrast to chronic bronchitis sufferers, emphysema patients often lose weight and seldom have a cough except early in the morning. Because of the habit of breathing through pursed lips and the color produced by polycythemia, they are sometimes called "pink puffers." Clubbed fingers are common. Auscultation may reveal diminished breath sounds and, at times, wheezes and crackles. There may also be signs of right-sided heart disease. As a result of severe respiratory impairment, COPD patients may exhibit confusion, agitation, somnolence, one-to-two-word dyspnea, and use of accessory muscles to assist respiration.

e. Pneumonia   pp. 1109–1110

Pneumonia, or lung infection, is a leading cause of death in the elderly and those with HIV infection and is the fifth leading cause of death in the United States overall. It is an infection most commonly caused by bacterial or viral agents, rarely by fungal and other pathogens. Risk factors center on conditions that cause a defect in mucous production or ciliary action that weaken the body's natural defenses against invaders of the respiratory system. Common signs and symptoms include an ill appearance, fever and shaking chills, a productive cough, and sputum. Many cases involve pleuritic chest pain. Auscultation usually reveals crackles in the involved lung segments, or sometimes wheezes or crackles, and occasionally egophony (change in spoken "E" sound to "A"). Percussion produces dullness over the affected areas. Some forms of pneumonia do not produce these distinctive symptoms, presenting instead with systemic complaints such as headache, malaise, fatigue, muscle aches, sore throat, nausea, vomiting, and diarrhea. Diagnosis in the field is unlikely and treatment is supportive. Place the patient in a comfortable position and administer high-flow oxygen. In severe cases, ventilatory assistance and possibly endotracheal intubation may be necessary. Medical direction may recommend administration of a beta agonist. Antipyretics may be given to reduce a high fever.

f. Pulmonary edema   pp. 1100–1101

Pulmonary edema (fluid in the interstitial spaces of the lungs) is often associated with ineffective cardiac pumping action, as in left-sided ventricular heart disease. (Pulmonary edema associated with heart disease is discussed in Chapter 28, "Cardiology.") Noncardiogenic pulmonary edema was discussed above under the objective for adult respiratory distress syndrome (ARDS).

g. Pulmonary thromboembolism pp. 1114–1116

A pulmonary embolism is a blood clot (thrombus) that lodges in an artery in the lungs. One in five cases of sudden death is caused by pulmonary thromboembolism. It is a life-threatening condition because it can significantly reduce pulmonary blood flow (perfusion), causing hypoxemia (lack of oxygen in the blood). Immobilization, such as recent surgery, a long-bone fracture, or being bedridden, increases the risk of developing an embolism. Other risk factors for clot formation include pregnancy, oral birth control medications, cancer, and sickle cell anemia. The classic symptom of pulmonary embolism is a sudden onset of severe dyspnea, which may or may not be accompanied by pleuritic pain. The physical exam may reveal other signs including labored breathing, tachypnea, and tachycardia. In severe cases, there may be signs of right-sided heart failure, including jugular vein distention and possibly falling blood pressure. Auscultation may reveal no significant findings. In 50 percent of cases, examination of the extremities will reveal signs suggesting deep venous thrombosis (warm, swollen extremity with a thick cord palpated along the medial thigh and pain on palpation or when extending the calf). Because a large embolism may cause cardiac arrest, be prepared to perform resuscitation. Primary care is aimed at support of the airway, breathing, and circulation. As necessary, assist ventilations and provide supplemental oxygen. Endotracheal intubation may be required. Establish IV access, monitor vital signs and cardiac rhythms, and transport expeditiously to a facility that can care for the patient's critical needs.

h. Neoplasms of the lung pp. 1112–1113

Lung cancer (neoplasms, literally "new growths" or tumors) is the leading cause of cancer-related death in the United States in both men and women. The primary problems are disruption of diffusion and, if the bronchioles are involved, of ventilation as well. The primary risk factor is cigarette smoking. Inhalation of other environmental toxins is also a risk factor. Less commonly, lung cancer can result from the spread of cancer from another part of the body. EMS calls to patients with lung cancer may involve a variety of complaints related to the disease, including cough, hoarseness, chest pain, and bloody sputum. There may be fever, chills, and chest pain if the patient has developed pneumonia. There can be weakness, numbness of the arm, shoulder pain, and difficulty swallowing. The physical exam may reveal weight loss, crackles, wheezes, rhonchi, and diminished breath sounds in the affected lung. There may be venous distention of the arms and neck. Your primary responsibility is to identify and address signs of respiratory distress. Assist ventilation and administer supplemental oxygen as needed. Establish IV access and consult medical direction about possible administration of bronchodilators and corticosteroids. Transport, but be alert for any DNR (do not resuscitate) orders.

i. Upper respiratory infections pp. 1108–1109

Infections of the upper airways of the respiratory tract are among the most common infectious conditions for which patients seek medical assistance, and you will see them in the field. Even though these infections are rarely life-threatening, they can produce considerable discomfort. At-home management is usually symptomatic, with treatment for pain and fever, as needed, as well as appropriate antibiotic therapy if the infection is bacterial. However, a URI in a person with preexisting pulmonary disease can trigger severe problems and you should pay particularly close attention to airway and ventilation in patients with asthma or COPD. Be sure to monitor the condition with pulse oximetry, capnography, and ECG during transport to a treatment facility.

j. Spontaneous pneumothorax p. 1116

Spontaneous pneumothorax, which occurs in the absence of trauma, is a relatively common condition, occurring in roughly 18 persons per 100,000 population. It is relatively likely to recur as well (with 50 percent recurrence rate at 2 years). Significant risk factors include male gender; age 20 to 40 years; tall, thin stature; and history of cigarette smoking. Presentation is marked by sudden onset pleuritic chest or shoulder pain, often precipitated by a bout of coughing or by heavy lifting. The loss of negative pressure in the affected hemithorax prevents proper chest expansion, and the patient may report dyspnea. In individuals who do NOT have significant underlying pulmonary disease, a pneumothorax of up to 15 to 20 percent of the chest cavity can be tolerated fairly well. Monitor symptoms and pulse oximetry readings during transport. Be especially attentive in your ongoing assessment of patients who require positive-pressure ventilation. These patients are at higher risk for development of tension pneumothorax, which is marked by increasing resistance to ventilation, along with hypoxia, cyanosis, and possible hypotension. Examination will reveal tracheal deviation away from the affected side of the chest and distention of the jugular vein. Needle decompression of a tension pneumothorax may be required.

k. Hyperventilation syndrome   pp. 1116–1117

Hyperventilation, with rapid breathing, chest pain, and numbness in the extremities, is often associated with anxiety, and it is called hyperventilation syndrome in this setting. However, you should remember that a number of significant and common medical conditions can cause hyperventilation, including cardiovascular and pulmonary conditions such as acute myocardial infarction and pulmonary thromboembolism, sepsis, pregnancy, liver failure, and several metabolic and neurologic disorders. Be conservative and consider hyperventilation to be a sign of a serious medical problem until proven otherwise. Management centers on reassurance and assisting the patient to consciously decrease the rate and depth of breathing (maneuvers that will increase PCO_2).

*Supplemental objective: Severe acute respiratory syndrome (SARS)   pp. 1111–1112

Severe acute respiratory syndrome is rapidly progressing respiratory distress caused by a virus similar to that responsible for the common cold. Transmission occurs through droplets as the patient coughs or sneezes and these droplets contact the membranes of the mouth, nose, or eyes. Incubation takes from 2 to 7 days and the patient is considered contagious as long as they display symptoms. Signs and symptoms associated with SARS include rhinorrhea, chills, muscle aches, headache, diarrhea, and the signs of serious respiratory distress—dyspnea, cough, cyanosis, and hypoxia. Management of the SARS patient includes PPE, high-flow/high-volume oxygen, pulse oximetry monitoring, and respiratory assistance and endotracheal intubation, as needed. Initiate intravenous fluid administration to assure adequate hydration and consider a nebulized bronchodilator if wheezing is present.

*This objective is in addition to the listed DOT objectives.

8. **Given several preprogrammed patients with nontraumatic pulmonary problems, provide the appropriate assessment, prehospital care, and transport.**   pp. 1081–1118

During your training as an EMT-Paramedic you will participate in many classroom sessions involving simulated patients. You will also spend some time in the emergency departments of local hospitals as well as in advanced-level ambulances gaining clinical experience. During these times, use your knowledge of pulmonary disease to help you assess and care for the simulated or real patients you attend.

Content Self-Evaluation

MULTIPLE CHOICE

_____ 1. Which of the following is considered an intrinsic risk factor for respiratory disease?
     A. smokestack pollutants   D. cigarette smoking
     B. polluted water   E. stress
     C. genetic predisposition

_____ 2. The three processes that allow gas exchange to occur in the lungs and body tissues are:
     A. ventilation, diffusion, perfusion.
     B. inspiration, expiration, ventilation.
     C. resistance, compliance, perfusion.
     D. ventilation, inspiration, expiration.
     E. inspiration, compliance, diffusion.

_____ 3. The mechanical process of moving air in and out of the lungs is:
     A. ventilation.   D. inspiration.
     B. diffusion.   E. inhalation.
     E. perfusion.

_____ 4. The process by which gases move between the alveoli and the pulmonary capillaries is:
   A. infusion.
   B. perfusion.
   C. respiration.
   D. diffusion.
   E. permeation.

_____ 5. Lung perfusion is dependent on three factors—adequate blood volume, efficient pumping by the heart, and intact:
   A. alveoli.
   B. respiratory membrane.
   C. bronchioles.
   D. goblet cells.
   E. pulmonary capillaries.

_____ 6. Any of the following can disrupt ventilation EXCEPT:
   A. obstruction of the upper airway.
   B. obstruction of the lower airway.
   C. blockage of the pulmonary arteries.
   D. impairment of normal function of the chest wall.
   E. abnormalities of the nervous system's control of breathing.

_____ 7. Which of the following abnormal breathing patterns is characterized by long, deep breaths that are stopped during the inspiratory phase and separated by periods of apnea?
   A. ataxic (Biot's) respirations (seen with increased intracranial pressure)
   B. central neurogenic hyperventilation (seen with stroke or brainstem injury)
   C. Kussmaul's respirations (seen with metabolic acidosis)
   D. apneustic respirations (seen with stroke or severe central nervous system disease)
   E. Cheyne-Stokes respirations (seen with terminal illness or brain injury)

_____ 8. Which of the following is NOT likely to cause hypoxia (a supply of oxygen inadequate to meet the needs of the body's cells)?
   A. ascension to a high altitude
   B. esophageal ulceration
   C. black lung disease
   D. left-sided heart failure
   E. asbestos inhalation

_____ 9. Pulmonary shunting results from:
   A. alveolar collapse.
   B. blockage of pulmonary capillaries.
   C. bronchoconstriction.
   D. excess mucous production.
   E. airway obstruction.

_____ 10. The most important action when you arrive on scene and discover that a hazardous material is present is to:
   A. have supplemental oxygen available.
   B. assure your own safety.
   C. search for additional patients.
   D. put on self-contained breathing apparatus.
   E. call for a hazardous materials team.

_____ 11. You are dispatched to a patient with difficulty breathing. Which of the following should be part of the scene size-up?
   A. Establish a patent airway.
   B. Look for clues to the possible cause.
   C. Evaluate AVPU mental status.
   D. Determine respiration rate.
   E. Ready the oxygenation equipment.

_____ 12. The patient with SARS is considered contagious during which time period?
   A. while the patient displays signs and symptoms
   B. for 2 to 7 days after contact
   C. for 10 to 14 days after contact
   D. for 2 to 7 days after symptoms first appear
   E. for 10 to 14 days after symptoms first appear

_____ 13. Which of the following is NOT a classic sign of respiratory distress?
A. pursed lips
B. tracheal tugging
C. diaphoresis
D. nasal flaring
E. cyanosis

_____ 14. Which of the following is TRUE with regard to assessing the airway?
A. Noisy breathing usually indicates a complete obstruction.
B. Obstructed breathing is not always noisy breathing.
C. If the airway is blocked, artificial respiration must be started immediately.
D. If the airway is blocked, endotracheal intubation must be established.
E. If the airway is open, the patient is breathing.

_____ 15. Which of the following is the MOST ominous sign of possible life-threatening respiratory distress?
A. altered mental status
B. audible stridor
C. one- to two-word dyspnea
D. tachycardia
E. use of accessory muscles

_____ 16. Orthopnea is:
A. dizziness when rising from a supine position.
B. dyspnea that occurs while lying supine.
C. short attacks of dyspnea that interrupt sleep.
D. apnea that occurs while in an upright position.
E. pleuritic pain that occurs during breathing.

_____ 17. Many respiratory complaints result from worsening of a long-standing disease the patient knows he has and can tell you about during the history. All of the following are such long-term respiratory diseases EXCEPT:
A. pneumonia.
B. asthma.
C. emphysema.
D. lung cancer.
E. chronic bronchitis.

_____ 18. Which of the following medications would be of LEAST significance if found in the home of a patient with a respiratory complaint?
A. oxygen
B. bronchodilator
C. vitamin C tablets
D. corticosteroid
E. antibiotic

_____ 19. Allergic reaction to a medication may be the cause of a respiratory complaint.
A. True
B. False

_____ 20. A patient with significant respiratory distress may breathe through pursed lips. Breathing through pursed lips helps to:
A. prevent tracheal collapse.
B. force air past a bronchial obstruction.
C. bring up excess mucus.
D. close the epiglottis.
E. keep the alveoli open.

_____ 21. Pink or bloody sputum is commonly seen with any of the following EXCEPT:
A. pulmonary edema.
B. lung cancer.
C. tuberculosis.
D. allergic reaction.
E. bronchial infection.

_____ 22. Asymmetrical chest movement is most likely to be found during:
A. auscultation.
B. capnometry.
C. oximetry.
D. inspection.
E. percussion.

_____ 23. Subcutaneous emphysema is most likely to be found during:
   A. oximetry.
   B. percussion.
   C. capnometry.
   D. palpation.
   E. inspection.

_____ 24. Wheezing is most likely to be detected during:
   A. oximetry.
   B. auscultation.
   C. percussion.
   D. capnometry.
   E. palpation.

_____ 25. Rattling sounds in the larger airways associated with excess mucus are called:
   A. stridor.
   B. wheezing.
   C. crackles.
   D. snoring.
   E. rhonchi.

_____ 26. A harsh, high-pitched sound heard on inspiration, associated with upper airway obstruction, is called:
   A. snoring.
   B. stridor.
   C. crackles.
   D. rhonchi.
   E. rales.

_____ 27. In general, tachycardia is a nonspecific finding seen, for example, with fear, anxiety, or fever. In a patient with a respiratory complaint, however, tachycardia may also indicate:
   A. hypothermia.
   B. hypertrophy.
   C. hypotension.
   D. hyperopia.
   E. hypoxia.

_____ 28. Drugs that may cause an elevation in both heart rate and blood pressure include:
   A. diuretics such as furosemide.
   B. analgesics such as morphine sulfate.
   C. tranquilizers such as diazepam.
   D. sympathomimetics such as albuterol.
   E. beta blockers such as labetalol.

_____ 29. An elevated respiratory rate in a patient with dyspnea is most likely caused by:
   A. bradycardia.
   B. dysuria.
   C. hypoxia.
   D. anemia.
   E. tachycardia.

_____ 30. Which of the following measures end-expiratory carbon dioxide?
   A. spirometry
   B. sphygmomanometry
   C. capnometry
   D. oximetry
   E. tomography

_____ 31. Two conditions in which respiration is frequently dependent on hypoxic respiratory drive and use of supplemental oxygen may induce respiratory depression are:
   A. asthma and pneumonia.
   B. spontaneous pneumothorax and pneumonia.
   C. asthma and emphysema.
   D. asthma and adult respiratory distress syndrome.
   E. chronic bronchitis and emphysema.

_____ 32. The pulmonary edema characteristic of adult respiratory distress syndrome (ARDS) is caused by:
   A. left-sided cardiac ventricular failure.
   B. right-sided cardiac ventricular failure.
   C. accumulation of fluid in the pulmonary interstitial spaces.
   D. obstruction of pulmonary capillaries by thrombi.
   E. chronic constriction of terminal airways and alveoli.

_____ 33. Factors that commonly cause acute aggravation of symptoms due to chronic obstructive pulmonary disease (COPD) include all of the following EXCEPT:
   A. progression of lung cancer.
   B. exertion, including heavy lifting and exercise.
   C. allergens such as foods and dust.
   D. tobacco smoke.
   E. occupational airborne pollutants such as chemical fumes.

_____ 34. Common physical attributes of a person with emphysema include all of the following EXCEPT:
   A. chronic cough.
   B. barrel chest.
   C. clubbing of the fingers.
   D. pinkish tone to skin.
   E. thin build.

_____ 35. Common physical attributes of a person with chronic bronchitis include all of the following EXCEPT:
   A. chronic cough.
   B. thin build.
   C. bluish, cyanotic tone to skin.
   D. cough producing large amounts of sputum.
   E. ankle edema.

_____ 36. The epidemiology of asthma includes all of the following EXCEPT:
   A. an increase in mortality rate over the past decade.
   B. the death rate in whites that is roughly twice that in blacks.
   C. it is a common disorder in both males and females.
   D. mortality change seen mostly in persons over age 45 years.
   E. half of asthma deaths occur in the prehospital setting.

_____ 37. Medications commonly used by persons with asthma include all of the following EXCEPT:
   A. beta agonists administered via inhaler.
   B. oral doses of aspirin.
   C. anticholinergics administered via inhaler.
   D. oral doses of corticosteroid.
   E. cromolyn sodium administered via inhaler.

_____ 38. The chief management goals for an acute asthma attack involve improvement in:
   A. blood pH (acidosis), hypoxia, and wheezing.
   B. hypoxia, bronchospasm, and wheezing.
   C. blood pH (acidosis), hypoxia, and local inflammation.
   D. hypoxia, bronchospasm, and local inflammation.
   E. hypoxia, wheezing, and local inflammation.

_____ 39. Be prepared for which of the following when caring for a patient with status asthmaticus?
   A. respiratory acidosis with electrolyte imbalance
   B. dehydration with early signs of renal failure
   C. respiratory depression when administered supplemental oxygen
   D. respiratory arrest requiring endotracheal intubation
   E. tracheal inflammation causing airway obstruction

_____ 40. Upper respiratory infections can affect all of the following EXCEPT:
   A. the sinuses.
   B. the lungs.
   C. the middle ear.
   D. the nose.
   E. the pharynx.

_____ 41. Pleuritic chest pain associated with pneumonia is:
   A. dull and aching in character.
   B. sharp or tearing in character.
   C. cramplike and hard to localize.
   D. likely to radiate to the jaw or left arm.
   E. only present on deep inspiration.

_____ 42. Major risk factors for pneumonia are HIV infection, very young or very old, and immunosuppressive therapy.
   A. True
   B. False

_____ 43. Standard management of lung cancer includes all of the following EXCEPT:
   A. checking for instructions such as DNR (do not resuscitate) orders.
   B. placement of ECG leads for cardiac monitoring.
   C. administration of supplemental oxygen.
   D. airway and ventilatory support as needed.
   E. emotional support of patient and family.

_____ 44. Roughly one in five cases of sudden death is due to pulmonary emboli.
   A. True
   B. False

_____ 45. The mortality rate for pulmonary emboli is greater than 50 percent.
   A. True
   B. False

_____ 46. Risk factors for pulmonary emboli include all of the following EXCEPT:
   A. obesity.
   B. pregnancy.
   C. prolonged immobilization.
   D. deep venous thrombophlebitis.
   E. use of oral contraceptives, especially in smokers.

_____ 47. The ventilation-perfusion mismatch characteristic of pulmonary embolism is due to loss of blood flow to a ventilated segment of lung tissue.
   A. True
   B. False

_____ 48. Common physical findings in pulmonary embolism include all of the following EXCEPT:
   A. evidence suggestive of deep venous thrombosis.
   B. labored, painful breathing.
   C. tachypnea and tachycardia.
   D. cardiac dysrythmias.
   E. normal chest auscultation.

_____ 49. Which of the following statements about spontaneous pneumothorax is FALSE?
   A. Most patients have acute onset pain in the chest or shoulder region.
   B. Onset of pain often follows coughing or heavy lifting.
   C. Spontaneous pneumothorax is much more common in women than in men.
   D. Spontaneous pneumothorax is more common among smokers and persons with COPD.
   E. Supplemental oxygen is sufficient therapy for the majority of patients with spontaneous pneumothorax.

_____ 50. The respiratory alkalosis of hyperventilation syndrome often results in:
   A. cramping of the muscles of the hands and feet.
   B. slowing of cardiac electrical conduction, causing bradycardia.
   C. cramping of facial muscles causing characteristic grimace.
   D. one of several cardiac dysrhythmias.
   E. altered mental status, specifically, lethargy and depression.

_____ 51. Respiratory emergencies due to central nervous system (CNS) dysfunction are relatively rare.
   A. True
   B. False

_____ 52. Numerous peripheral nervous system conditions can cause respiratory compromise, including the diseases of polio and amyotrophic lateral sclerosis, as well as Guillian-Barré syndrome.
   A. True
   B. False

_____ 53. The processes of ventilation, diffusion, and perfusion allow gas exchange to occur efficiently in the lungs and other body tissues. The derangement in pulmonary embolism is principally of:
   A. ventilation.
   B. diffusion.
   C. perfusion.
   D. a combination of ventilation and diffusion.
   E. a combination of diffusion and perfusion.

_____ 54. Carbon monoxide exposure is potentially life-threatening because carbon monoxide displaces oxygen from hemoglobin in red blood cells.
   A. True
   B. False

_____ 55. The most common auscultation finding in a patient with pneumonia is:
   A. stridor over the involved segment.
   B. decreased or absent breath sounds over the involved segment.
   C. expiratory wheezing over the involved segment.
   D. crackles (rales) over the involved segment.
   E. pleural friction rub over the involved segment.

MATCHING

Match each respiratory emergency with its key prehospital management steps by writing the letter of the steps in the space provided next to the emergency.

_____ 56. adult respiratory distress syndrome (ARDS)

_____ 57. chronic obstructive pulmonary disease (COPD), either emphysema or chronic bronchitis

_____ 58. asthma

_____ 59. childhood epiglottitis

_____ 60. lung cancer

_____ 61. inhalation of a toxic substance

_____ 62. pulmonary embolism

A. correct hypoxia, reverse bronchospasm, and reduce inflammation

B. ensure safety of rescue personnel, remove patient for transport, maintain open airway, and deliver humidified, high-concentration oxygen

C. maintain airway and ventilation as needed, deliver oxygen, establish IV access, cardiac monitoring, and pulse oximetry and transport to facility for care of underlying condition

D. maintain airway, ventilation, and circulation as needed, deliver oxygen, establish IV access, cardiac monitoring, and pulse oximetry and check extremities during transport to appropriate facility

E. maintain airway and ventilation as needed with exception that examination of the throat should be avoided

F. relieve hypoxia, reverse bronchoconstriction, assist ventilations as needed

G. deliver oxygen, support ventilation as allowed by orders or advance directive, correct hypoxia as possible, and provide emotional support

Cardiology

Part 1: Cardiovascular Anatomy and Physiology, ECG Monitoring, and Dysrhythmia Analysis

Review of Chapter Objectives

Because Chapter 28 is lengthy, it has been divided into two parts to aid in your study. Read the assigned text pages, then progress through the objectives and self-evaluation materials as you would with other chapters. When you feel secure in your grasp of the content, proceed to the next part.

After reading Part 1 of this chapter, you should be able to:

1. **Describe the incidence, morbidity, and mortality of cardiovascular disease.** p. 1126

   Cardiovascular disease (CVD) is serious and extremely common, with more than 60 million Americans affected. Morbidity is considerable: An American has a nonfatal heart attack (myocardial infarction, MI) roughly every 29 seconds. Coronary heart disease (CHD), one type of CVD, is the single largest killer of Americans and Canadians. Roughly 466,000 Americans die annually from CHD, half of them before reaching a hospital. Many deaths from CHD are sudden and involve lethal cardiac dysrhythmias. Many deaths from MI occur within the first 24 hours, frequently within the first hour.

2. **Discuss prevention strategies that may reduce the morbidity and mortality of cardiovascular disease.** p. 1126

   There are two public health prevention strategies. The first is to educate people about the risk factors for CVD and encourage lifestyle modifications to minimize the potential impact of risk factors. The second strategy is to teach signs and symptoms of a heart attack so patients can receive medical intervention as soon as possible. As you will see, the likelihood of success with fibrinolytic therapy for a heart attack in evolution (treatment with a clot-buster drug to dissolve the clot causing myocardial ischemia/hypoxia) is highest when care is instituted very early in the course of the attack.

3. **Identify the risk factors most predisposing to coronary artery disease.** p. 1126

   Factors proven to increase the risk of CVD include (1) smoking, (2) older age, (3) family history of cardiac disease, (4) hypertension, (5) hypercholesterolemia, (6) diabetes mellitus, (7) cocaine use, and (8) male gender. Factors that are thought to increase risk include (1) diet, (2) obesity, (3) oral contraceptives, (4) sedentary lifestyle, (5) Type A personality (competitive and aggressive), and (6) psychosocial tension (stress).

4. Describe the anatomy of the heart, including the position in the thoracic cavity, layers of the heart, chambers of the heart, and location and function of cardiac valves. pp. 1127–1128; see Chapter 3

The adult heart is roughly the size of a clenched fist, and it lies in the center of the mediastinum posterior to the sternum and anterior to the spine. Roughly two thirds of the heart lies to the left of midline, with roughly one third to the right. The bottom of the heart, the apex, lies just above the diaphragm, whereas the top of the heart, or base, lies at roughly the level of the second rib. The heart's connections with the great vessels are at the base. The heart is made up of three tissue layers: The innermost is the endocardium, which has the same type of cells as the endothelial lining of blood vessels and is continuous with the linings of the vessels entering and leaving the heart. The thickest layer is the middle layer of muscle cells, the myocardium. These unique muscle cells physically resemble skeletal muscle but have electrical properties similar to smooth muscle cells. The outermost layer of the heart is the pericardium, a protective sac made of connective tissue arranged in two layers, the visceral pericardium (also called the epicardium) and the parietal pericardium. Normally, about 25 mL of pericardial fluid is contained between the two layers of pericardium, and the heart moves freely within the pericardial sac.

The heart is made up of two side-by-side pumps, the left side and the right side. Each side has an upper chamber, the atrium, which receives blood, and a lower chamber, the ventricle, which pumps blood into other blood vessels. The atria are separated by an interatrial septum, and the ventricles are separated by an interventricular septum. The atrial walls are thin in contrast with the ventricular walls, and almost all of the heart's pumping force is generated by the ventricles. The left ventricle, which pumps blood into the aorta, has a much thicker wall than the right ventricle, which pumps blood into the pulmonary artery (see Figure 28-1 and Figure 28-2).

The heart contains two sets of valves that help to keep blood flowing properly through the chambers and into the aorta and pulmonary artery: The atrioventricular valves lie between each atrium and ventricle. The left atrioventricular valve is called the mitral valve, and it has two characteristic leaflets. The right atrioventricular valve is called the tricuspid valve, and it has three characteristic leaflets. When the papillary muscles that connect the valves to the walls of the heart relax, the leaflets open and blood flows from the atria into the ventricles. Special fibers called the chordae tendoneae connect the leaflets of a valve to the papillary muscles, and these fibers prevent the leaflets from prolapsing back into the atrium when the valve is open. The semilunar valves lie between the ventricles and the artery into which each empties. The left semilunar valve, or aortic valve, lies between the left ventricle and the aorta. The right semilunar valve, or pulmonic valve, lies between the right ventricle and the pulmonary artery. When these valves open, blood flows in a one-way path from the ventricles into the arteries, and backflow into the ventricles is prevented.

The superior and inferior vena cavae carry deoxygenated blood from the body to the right atrium. Blood flows through the right atrium and ventricle before entering the pulmonary artery, which carries it to the lungs. Oxygenated blood leaves the lungs through the pulmonary veins and enters the left atrium. The left ventricle pumps the blood into the aorta, which feeds the oxygenated blood into peripheral arteries to flow to the rest of the body. Pressure within the heart is markedly higher on the left than on the right because resistance to flow is higher in the peripheral circulation than it is in the pulmonary circulation. Consequently, the myocardium of the left ventricle thickens as an infant ages to the point that the adult left ventricle is markedly thicker than the right.

5. Identify the major structures of the vascular system, the factors affecting venous return, the components of cardiac output, and the phases of the cardiac cycle. pp. 1128–1130; see Chapter 3

In the pulmonary circulation, blood enters the lungs via the pulmonary arteries and their smaller branches, the arterioles. It eventually flows through capillaries that form networks over alveoli, and gas exchange (movement of oxygen into the blood and carbon dioxide from the blood) takes place here. The oxygenated blood then flows into the pulmonary venules and larger pulmonary veins and enters the left atrium. The peripheral circulation begins with the aorta, which receives oxygenated blood from the left ventricle. The aorta has numerous branches. These arteries and the smaller arterioles ensure oxygenated blood flows to all parts of the body. Oxygenated blood eventually enters capillary beds and oxygen exchange between blood and tissues occurs. Deoxygenated blood enters smaller venules, which empty into the larger veins that return blood to the right atrium. Gas exchange occurs in capillaries because their walls are only one cell thick. This same cell layer, the endothelium, is the innermost layer of arteries and veins.

Although the heart acts effectively as two side-by-side pumps, the contraction of the myocardium takes place as if the heart is one unit. The two atria contract at the same time, and the ventricles contract together. The atrioventricular valves open and close together, as do the two semilunar valves. The sequence of events that occurs between the end of one ventricular contraction and the next is called the cardiac cycle. Diastole, or relaxation phase, is the first part of the cycle. During diastole, blood enters the ventricles through the mitral and tricuspid valves. The aortic and pulmonic valves are closed, so the ventricles fill and no blood flows into the great vessels. During systole, the second phase, the heart contracts. First, the atria contract quickly, pumping the last of their blood into the ventricles. Then, when the pressure within the ventricles becomes greater than the pressure in the aorta and pulmonary artery, the semilunar valves open, the ventricles contract, and blood is pumped into the great arteries. This same pressure event closes the atrioventricular valves, eliminating backflow through the heart.

Under normal conditions, about two thirds of the blood in the left ventricle at the end of diastole is pumped into the aorta during systole. This ratio of blood pumped to blood contained is called the cardiac ejection fraction. The amount of blood pumped by the left ventricle in one contraction is called the stroke volume, and it varies between roughly 60 and 100 mL, with an average of 70 mL. Cardiac output is defined as the amount of blood pumped in one minute. It is a function of stroke volume and heart rate: stroke volume (mL/beat) × heart rate (beats/minute) = cardiac output (mL/minute). Under average conditions, the heart rate is 60–100 bpm. Thus, average cardiac output = 70 mL × 70 bpm = 4,900 mL/minute, or almost 5L every minute.

6. Define preload, afterload, and left ventricular end-diastolic pressure and relate each to the pathophysiology of heart failure. **(see Chapter 3)**

Stroke volume (the volume of blood pumped in one heartbeat) depends on three factors: preload, cardiac contractility, and afterload. The heart can only pump out the blood it receives during diastole. The pressure filling the ventricle at the end of diastole is termed preload and determines how well the ventricle will fill. Starling's law states that as the stretch on cardiac muscle increases (that is, as preload increases), the greater will be the force of the subsequent contraction. When preload increases, contraction pressure increases. Because the major factor determining preload is venous return from the body (or the lungs), the greater the venous return, the greater the preload and the greater the ventricular contraction pressure. Obviously, this only applies to a range of normal return volumes. If an excessive volume flows into the atrium, the atrium will become overly stretched and eventually weaken. For the left ventricle, which pumps blood to the body (including the vital brain, myocardium, and kidneys), preload is determined by venous return from the lungs. Afterload is the pressure against which the ventricles must contract to pump blood into the aorta and pulmonary arteries. An increase in afterload (peripheral resistance) decreases stroke volume. Conversely, a decrease in afterload eases the work of the ventricles and increases stroke volume.

Cardiac output (the amount of blood pumped into the aorta per minute) depends on left ventricular end-diastolic volume, myocardial contractility, and peripheral vascular resistance as measured at the origin of the aorta. Heart failure, the inability of the left ventricle to pump a physiologically adequate supply of blood, can result from a preload (ventricular end-diastolic volume) that is too low to allow effective pumping (a clinical example is shock), a reduction in cardiac contractility such that effective pumping is impossible (a clinical example is loss of myocardium through one or more MIs), or a significant increase in systemic vascular resistance (hypertension). In many cases, more than one factor (preload, contractility, afterload) may be chronically disturbed.

**7. Identify the arterial blood supply to any given area of
the myocardium.** p. 1128; see Chapter 3

The left coronary artery supplies the left ventricle, the interventricular septum, part of the right ventricle, and the heart's electrical conduction system. It has two main branches, the anterior descending artery and the circumflex artery. The right coronary artery supplies a portion of the right atrium and ventricle and part of the conduction system. It has two main branches, the posterior descending artery and the marginal artery. (Note that anatomic variants do exist.) There are normally numerous anastomoses, or connections, among the coronary arteries and their branches. Most of the blood drains from the coronary circulation through the anterior great cardiac vein and the lateral marginal veins into the coronary sinus. The right coronary artery empties directly into the right atrium via smaller cardiac veins.

**8. Compare and contrast the coronary arterial distribution to the major
portions of the cardiac conduction system.** p. 1128; see Chapter 3

Objective 7 explains the distribution of blood through the coronary artery system.

The pacemaker cells (those with the highest level of automaticity, and thus the drivers for all of the other conductive cells) are generally in the sinoatrial (SA) node, which is located high in the right atrium (an area supplied by the right coronary artery). One branch of the conduction system leads to the left atrium. Most of the conductive cells run in one of the internodal atrial pathways through the right atrial wall to meet at the atrioventricular (AV) node. The left coronary artery typically supplies these tissues.

The conduction system then passes through the bundle of His into the interventricular septum, where the right and left bundle branches become apparent as feeders of conduction branches into the walls of the right and left ventricles (see Figure 28-3). The right bundle branch delivers the electrical impulse to the apex of the right ventricle. From there, the fibers of the Purkinje system spread it across the myocardium. The interventricular septum is typically supplied by the left coronary artery, as are the conduction fibers in the wall of the left ventricle. Some fibers in the right ventricular wall may be supplied by the right coronary artery.

**9. Identify the structure and course of all divisions and subdivisions
of the cardiac conduction system.** pp. 1129–1130; see Chapter 3

The cardiac conduction system, which carries the electrical impulse that causes depolarization and contraction of myocardial cells, is shown in Figure 3-93. The pacemaker cells are normally found in the sinoatrial (SA) node, which is located high in the right atrium, and this is the usual origin of the electrical impulse that triggers each heartbeat. Several internodal atrial pathways carry the impulse from the SA node through the wall of the right atrium to the atrioventricular (AV) node. The impulse is carried to the left atrium via another pathway. At the AV junction, the conduction of the impulse is slowed (which allows adequate time for the ventricles to fill). The impulse moves from the AV junction via the AV fibers to the bundle of His, located high in the interventricular septum. The impulse then moves down the right and left bundle branches. The right bundle branch delivers the impulse to the apex of the right ventricle, and the fibers of the Purkinje system deliver it from there across the myocardium. The left bundle branch delivers the impulse to the thicker myocardium of the left ventricle. The left bundle branch does so via the anterior and posterior fascicles, both of which eventually terminate in the Purkinje system. Repolarization, which electrically readies the myocardial cells for the next heartbeat, proceeds in the opposite direction.

**10. Identify and describe how the heart's pacemaking control, rate,
and rhythm are determined.** p. 1130; see Chapter 3

The cells with the highest degree of automaticity act as the heart's pacemakers, and these cells are usually found in the SA node, located high in the right atrium. On average, these cells generate impulses at the rate of 60–100 bpm. The cells of the AV node typically generate impulses at the lower rate of 40–60 bpm, and the cells of the Purkinje system, which also demonstrate automaticity, fire at roughly 15–40 bpm. Impulses generated in the SA node and conducted normally through the heart produce the ECG patterns characteristic of normal atrial rhythm.

Heart rate is controlled in part by the nervous system, and this level of control enables the heart rate to accommodate the increased body oxygen need characteristic of exertion or stress. Regulation of heart rate by the autonomic nervous system is discussed in detail in objective 17.

11. Explain the physiological basis of conduction delay in the AV node. (see Chapter 3)

Not all fibers within the cardiac conduction system are the same size or absolutely alike in conduction properties. The fibers in the AV junction conduct impulses more slowly than most other conduction fibers, delaying the arrival of the electrical impulse in the AV node. Conduction within the AV node itself is also slower, and the cumulative effect is a delay that allows the ventricles time to fill properly before they contract, pumping blood out of the heart.

12. Define the functional properties of cardiac muscle. (see Chapter 3)

The heart is made up of three groups of cardiac muscle fibers: atrial, ventricular, and specialized excitatory and conductive fibers. Atrial and ventricular cardiac muscle is striated in the same way that skeletal muscle is structured, and contraction is much the same except for one notable difference. Cardiac muscle has unique structures called intercalated discs that physically connect muscle fibers and enable extremely swift conduction of impulses from fiber to fiber (with a speed approximately 400 times that of a normal cell membrane). This uniquely rapid conduction of an impulse among muscle fibers enables cardiac muscle to function effectively as a single contractile unit. This collective functional unit is termed a syncytium. The heart has two syncytia, the atrial syncytium and the ventricular syncytium. The atria contract together in a superior to inferior direction, expelling blood into the ventricles. The ventricles contract together in an inferior to superior direction, pumping blood into the pulmonary arteries and aorta. The syncytia are separated physically and physiologically by the fibrous structure that supports the atrioventricular valves. The only normal route for impulse conduction from the atria to the ventricles is through the AV node.

Thus, the syncytial myocardial cells have the functional properties of excitability (they can respond to an electrical stimulus), conductivity (they can send an impulse to an adjoining cell), and contractility (they respond to an electrical impulse by contracting).

The even more specialized myocardial cells of the conduction system have the same properties plus an additional one, automaticity. The conductive fibers show excitability and contractility similar to those of other myocardial cells. They have an even higher degree of conductivity, which enables them to transmit an impulse so quickly that it triggers syncytial myocardium to contract in a unified manner. Their unique property is automaticity: They have the ability to depolarize without any external stimulation. This property, which is also called self-excitability, is the basis for electrical initiation of each heartbeat. The conductive cells with the highest degree of automaticity (normally those in the SA node) act as the pacemaker for the whole cardiac unit.

13. Define the events comprising electrical potential. (see Chapter 3)

Impulse conduction and subsequent muscle fiber contraction are based functionally on depolarization of cells that maintain an electrical resting potential in the unstimulated state. Cardiac muscle cells (atrial, ventricular, and excitatory/conductive) expend energy to maintain a difference between the ion concentrations in the cell and those in the extracellular fluid. Pumps in the cell membrane expel sodium ions (Na^+) from the inside of the cell, making the inside of the cell more negatively charged than the surrounding extracellular fluid. This negative resting potential can be measured, and it is typically about -90 mV for a myocardial cell.

14. List the most important ions involved in myocardial action potential and their primary function in this process. (see Chapter 3)

The three most important ions in cardiac function are potassium, sodium, and calcium. Proper amounts of potassium in the extracellular fluid and sodium in the internal cellular environment are vital to establish and maintain the resting potential. Extracellular concentration of calcium ions is vital for excitation of the cardiac contractile process.

15. Describe the events involved in the steps from excitation to contraction of cardiac muscle fibers. p. 1130; see Chapter 3

Impulse conduction and subsequent muscle fiber contraction are based functionally on depolarization of cells that maintain an electrical resting potential in the unstimulated state and are described in objective 13 above.

When a myocardial cell is stimulated by an electrical impulse, the membrane opens to ions. As Na$^+$ ions rush into the cell, the internal charge actually becomes positive relative to the outside environment—with a potential of roughly +20 mV—a change of 110 mV. The rapid influx of Na$^+$ ions and resultant change of membrane polarity is termed the action potential. During this same period when the membrane is permeable to ions, there is also a slower influx of Ca^{++} ions, which further increases the positive charge within the myocardial cell. After depolarization (the switch from a negative to a positive internal electrical potential) is complete, the syncytial muscle contracts as a unit. Just as rapidly (in a fraction of a second), the membrane pumps become active again, expel the excess ions, and reestablish the resting potential through repolarization of the membrane (reestablishment of the resting, negative potential).

16. Describe the clinical significance of Starling's law. (see Chapter 3)

Starling's law states that as the stretch on cardiac muscle increases (that is, as preload increases), the greater will be the force of the subsequent contraction. When preload increases, contraction pressure increases. Because the major factor determining preload is venous return from the body (or the lungs), the greater the venous return, the greater the preload and the greater the ventricular contraction pressure. If an excessive volume flows into the atrium, the atrium will become overly stretched and eventually weaken. For the left ventricle, which pumps blood to the body (including the vital brain, myocardium, and kidneys), preload is determined by venous return from the lungs.

17. Identify the structures of the autonomic nervous system and their effect on heart rate, rhythm, and contractility. (see Chapter 3)

The sympathetic and parasympathetic components of the autonomic nervous system act in opposition to each other, and the balance of their effects regulates heart function. The sympathetic nervous system innervates the heart through the cardiac plexus of nerves, which is located at the base of the heart. Its neurotransmitter, norepinephrine, acts to increase heart rate and cardiac contractility. There are two types of receptors in the sympathetic nervous system. Alpha receptors are found mostly in the peripheral blood vessels, where they modulate vasoconstriction. The beta1 receptors are mostly found within the heart; they are responsible for the increase in heart rate and contractility with sympathetic stimulation. (Beta$_2$ receptors are chiefly in the lungs and peripheral blood vessels, and their stimulation results in bronchodilation and vasodilation.) Parasympathetic innervation of the heart is through the vagus nerve (cranial nerve X). Its neurotransmitter is acetylcholine, and parasympathetic stimulation of the heart (most of the vagus nerve fibers end in the atria, although some innervate the upper ventricles) results in slowed heart rate and slowed atrioventricular conduction.

18. Define and give examples of positive and negative inotropism, chronotropism, and dromotropism. (see Chapter 3)

Inotropy refers to the strength of myocardial contraction. Sympathetic nervous stimulation acts as a positive inotropic agent, one that increases cardiac contractility. Parasympathetic stimulation, by acting as an opposite to sympathetic activity, acts as a negative inotropic agent. Chronotropy refers to heart rate (chronos = time). A positive chronotropic agent increases heart rate, whereas a negative chronotropic agent decreases heart rate. Sympathetic nervous stimulation acts as a positive chronotropic agent, whereas parasympathetic stimulation acts as a negative chronotropic agent. Dromotropy refers to the rate of impulse conduction. A positive dromotropic agent increases conduction speed, whereas a negative dromotropic agent slows impulse conduction.

19. Discuss the pathophysiology of cardiac disease and injury. pp. 1142–1185

Adequate heart function depends on adequate venous return and other vascular factors, as well as the intrinsic factors of myocardial health and function and adequacy of the electrical conduction system. Hypertension, atherosclerosis, and diabetes are risk factors for cardiac disease because they damage blood vessels, including the coronary arteries. Impaired perfusion of the myocardium (particularly the left ventricle responsible for cardiac output to the body) can lead to ischemia or MI. If infarction occurs, the amount of functional myocardium decreases, and this can ultimately lead to a decrease in cardiac output dependent on the area involved and the amount of myocardium lost.

There are innate disorders of the electrical conduction system, including developmental variants such as the accessory pathways that can make dysrhythmias more likely (such as Wolff-Parkinson-White syndrome). In addition, ischemia or infarction of the fibers of the conduction system can also make development of dysrhythmias more likely, including some (such as the tachycardias and the ventricular dysrhythmias) that can impair cardiac output to some degree or be directly life-threatening by precluding any adequacy of cardiac output (namely, ventricular fibrillation).

External agents that can harm cardiac function and possibly damage cardiac tissue include drugs. In some cases, drugs used to treat cardiac dysfunction can cause different cardiac problems.

20. Explain the purpose of ECG monitoring and its limitations. p. 1130

The electrocardiogram (electro = electrical, cardio = heart, gram = record) visualizes the heart's electrical activity as recorded from skin-surface electrodes. The heart is the largest generator of electrical energy in the body, and this is conducted through the body to the skin. An ECG machine records changes in current as a positive impulse (shown on the machine or on a paper printout as an upward deflection), a negative impulse (shown as a downward deflection), or no change (a flat, isoelectric line). The pattern shown over time is a chronological record of the heart's electrical activity, and it is called a rhythm strip.

The ECG in no way assesses the contractility of the myocardium or the pumping ability of the left ventricle, only the electrical activity in the different regions of the heart. There are other limitations of ECG monitoring. Artifacts may occur on the tracing, deflections that do NOT reflect the electrical activity of the heart. Artifacts may be due to a variety of causes, including muscle tremor, shivering, movements by the patient, loose electrodes, interference at the 60-hertz range, and machine malfunction. It is important that you be able to recognize artifacts and try to eliminate them from the tracing.

21. Correlate the electrophysiological and hemodynamic events occurring throughout the entire cardiac cycle with the various ECG waveforms, segments, and intervals. pp. 1134–1141

The components of an ECG tracing reflect the electrical changes in the heart with each impulse conducted through the heart (Figure 28-7):

- **P wave.** This first component of the ECG reflects atrial depolarization. On Lead II, it appears as a positive, rounded wave that comes before the QRS complex. Normally, this correlates hemodynamically with the opening of the AV valves and atrial contraction, which completes the filling of the ventricles with blood.
- **QRS complex.** This second component of the ECG reflects ventricular depolarization. The Q wave is the initial negative deflection after the P wave; the R wave is the first positive deflection after the P wave; and the S wave is the first negative deflection after the R wave. You should note that not all three waves need be present, and the shape of the QRS complex can vary among individuals. Normally, this correlates hemodynamically with the opening of the semilunar valves and ventricular contraction, pumping blood into the pulmonary arteries and aorta.
- **T wave.** The T wave, which follows the QRS complex, reflects repolarization of the ventricles. It is normally positive in Lead II, rounded, and moves in the same direction as the QRS complex. This is the correlate of ventricular relaxation after contraction.
- **U wave.** A U wave is an occasional finding; when it occurs, it follows the T wave and is usually positive in deflection. U waves are normal in some individuals. You should note that it reflects electrolyte abnormalities in other patients.

In addition, three time intervals and a segment of the ECG reading also have clinical significance:

- **P-R interval (called PRI or P-Q interval, PQI).** The P-R interval is the distance from the beginning of the P wave (the beginning of atrial depolarization) to the beginning of the QRS complex (the beginning of ventricular depolarization). It represents the time taken to send the impulse from the atria to the ventricles (the delay at the AV junction and node). The R wave is absent in some individuals, and in these patients you will see a P-Q interval instead. The terms PRI and PQI are used interchangeably.

- **QRS interval.** The QRS interval is the distance from the first deflection of the QRS complex to the last, and it represents the time necessary for ventricular depolarization and onset of ventricular contraction.
- **Q-T interval.** This is the distance from the beginning of the Q wave to the beginning of the T wave, and it represents the total duration of ventricular depolarization. The duration of the Q-T interval normally has an inverse relationship with heart rate. At increased heart rates (tachycardia), the Q-T interval is generally shortened. With bradycardia, Q-T interval is generally lengthened.
- **S-T segment.** This is the distance from the S wave to the beginning of the T wave, and generally it is isoelectric. In some states such as myocardial ischemia, this segment may be either elevated or depressed.

22. Identify how heart rates, durations, and amplitudes may be determined from ECG recordings. pp. 1134–1141

ECG graph paper is standardized such that paper always moves across the recording stylus at 22 mm/sec. (Each small box represents 0.04 second, and each large box is equivalent to five small boxes, or 0.20 second.) ECG paper also has time interval markings at the top of the paper, with marks placed at 3-second intervals (or 15 large boxes, 15 × 0.20 = 3.0 seconds).

Three methods exist for quickly establishing heart rate. First, if a patient has a regular rhythm, you can take the number of heartbeats in 6 seconds, multiply by 10, and get rate in beats per minute (bpm). Second, you can measure the R-R interval (also in a patient with a regular rhythm) in seconds, divide into 60, and you have heart rate per minute. If the R-R interval is 0.65 second, 60 ÷ 0.65 = 92 bpm. (Other methods using the R-R interval are described on text page 00.) The triplicate method, also useful only in the case of a regular rhythm, requires you to find an R wave that falls on a dark line bordering a large box. You can then assign numbers corresponding to heart rate to the next six dark lines to the right: This equates to 300, 150, 100, 75, 60, and 50 bpm. The number corresponding to the dark line closest to the peak of the next R wave is a rough estimate of heart rate. Last, you can use a commercial heart rate calculator ruler. If you prefer this method, make sure you are comfortable with at least one alternative method that does not require a physical aid!

The same standardization of time allows you to calculate the durations of the physiologically important intervals in the ECG tracing: Normal P-R interval duration is 0.12–0.20 sec; QRS interval duration is 0.08–0.12 sec; and Q-T interval is 0.33–0.42 sec. A prolonged P-R interval is one that lasts longer than 0.20 second and represents an extended delay in the AV node. A prolonged Q-T interval is one longer than 0.42 second and is thought to be related to an increased risk of certain ventricular dysrhythmias and sudden death.

The amplitude of deflections is also standardized: When a machine is properly calibrated, an amplitude of two large boxes represents 1.0 mV.

23. Relate the cardiac surfaces or areas represented by the ECG leads. pp. 1131–1132, 1140

A pair of electrodes constitutes a lead. In hospital settings, a specific 12-lead configuration is standard for ECGs. In the field, a 3-lead system is often used, although one lead is adequate for detection of life-threatening dysrhythmias.

A 3-lead configuration uses leads I, II, and III, and it shows three axes of the heart (Figure 28-4):

- Lead I (bipolar placed on a limb: positive = left arm, negative = right arm), axis 0° (parallel to collarbones)
- Lead II (bipolar placed on a limb: positive = left leg, negative = right arm), axis 60° (right atrium downward toward apex)
- Lead III (bipolar placed on a limb: positive = left leg, negative = left arm), axis 120° (left atrium downward toward apex)

Addition of three unipolar (also termed augmented) leads adds additional axes of view:

- aVR (augmented/unipolar on right arm), axis 210°
- aVL (augmented/unipolar on left arm), axis −30°
- aVF (augmented/unipolar on left foot), axis 90°

Normal recordings from the augmented leads are similar to those for leads I, II, and III except that the deflections for aVR are inverted. The inversion is because the axis is negative, that is, it points upward toward the base of the heart instead of downward toward the apex.

The six precordial (chest) leads permit a view of the horizontal plane of the heart, which makes it possible to distinguish activity in different parts of the left ventricle and in the septum. They are designated V_1–V_6; the letter V identifies them as unipolar leads.

The deflections are primarily downward for leads V_1 and V_2 because the leads are nearer the base of the heart than the apex, and thus they reflect the direction of electronegativity during depolarization. Deflections are primarily upward for leads V_4, V_5, and V_6 because they are nearer the apex, and thus they are in the direction of electropositivity during depolarization.

Table 28-2 (text page 1141) summarizes the portions of the heart examined by each set of leads:

- Leads I and aVL evaluate activity in the left side of the heart in a vertical plane.
- Leads II, III, and aVF evaluate activity in the inferior (diaphragmatic) side of the heart.
- Lead aVR evaluates activity in the right side of the heart in a vertical plane.
- Leads V_1 and V_2 evaluate activity in the right ventricle.
- Leads V_3 and V_4 evaluate activity in the interventricular septum and the anterior wall of the left ventricle.
- Leads V_5 and V_6 evaluate activity in the anterior and lateral walls of the left ventricle.

Overall, leads V_1–V_4 view the anterior surface of the heart, and leads I and aVL view the lateral surface of the heart. Leads II, III, and aVF view the inferior surface of the heart. Abnormal activity in a given set of leads, particularly in combination with a clinical picture consistent with acute myocardial infarction, can allow earlier identification and intervention in the ischemia-infarction process.

Lead II gives the best view of the ECG waves, and it best depicts the conduction system's activity. In single-lead systems, the lead used is generally lead II or a lead called modified chest lead 1 (MCL_1). This chapter, as well as the remainder of the text, uses lead II as its monitor lead. A monitor lead can provide (1) the rate of heartbeat, (2) the regularity of heartbeat, and (3) the time for conduction of impulse throughout various parts of the heart.

A monitor lead CANNOT provide (1) the presence or location of infarct, (2) the axis deviation or chamber enlargement, (3) the right-to-left differences in conduction or impulse formation, and (4) the quality or presence of pumping action.

24. Differentiate among the primary mechanisms responsible for producing cardiac dysrhythmias. pp. 1140, 1142–1185

Major causes of cardiac dysrhythmias include the following: (1) myocardial ischemia; (2) necrosis or infarction; (3) autonomic nervous system imbalance; (4) distention of the heart chambers (especially the atria, secondary to congestive heart failure); (5) blood gas abnormalities, including hypoxia and abnormal pH; (6) electrolyte imbalances (primarily calcium, potassium, and magnesium); (7) trauma to the myocardium (namely, cardiac contusion); (8) drug effects and drug toxicity; (9) electrocution; (10) hypothermia; (11) CNS damage; (12) idiopathic events; (13) normal occurrences.

Note that dysrhythmias in a healthy heart are of little significance.

25. Describe a systematic approach to the analysis and interpretation of cardiac dysrhythmias. pp. 1141–1185

The following characterize normal sinus rhythm: (1) heart rate between 60 and 100 bpm; (2) regular rhythm, with constant P-P and R-R intervals; (3) P waves that are normal in shape, upright, and appear only before each QRS complex; (4) P-R interval that is constant and lasting 0.12–0.20 second; and (5) QRS complex with normal shape and duration less than 0.12 second. Any deviation from the normal electrical rhythm constitutes a dysrhythmia. The term arrhythmia is properly reserved for states in which there is no cardiac electrical activity.

Dysrhythmias can be approached in a number of ways, including nature of origin (namely, changes in automaticity versus disturbances in conduction), magnitude (major versus minor), severity (life-threatening versus non-life-threatening), and site (or location) of origin. This book classifies dysrhythmias into six categories by origin: (1) dysrhythmias originating in the SA node; (2) dysrhythmias originating in the atria; (3) dysrhythmias originating within the AV junction; (4) dysrhythmias sustained or originating in the AV junction; (5) dysrhythmias originating in the ventricles; (6) dysrhythmias resulting from disorders of conduction.

26. Describe the dysrhythmias originating in the sinus node, the AV junction, the atria, and the ventricles. pp. 1144–1185

Sinus Node

Sinus bradycardia results from slowing of impulse generation in the SA node and may be due to increased parasympathetic (vagal) tone, intrinsic disease of the SA node, drug effects (typically digitalis, propranolol [a beta-blocker], or quinidine), or it may be found as a normal finding in a healthy, well-conditioned person.

Sinus bradycardia on the ECG: rate less than 60 bpm, rhythm regular, pacemaker site SA node, P waves upright and normal in shape, P-R interval normal in duration and constant, QRS complex normal in duration.

Clinical significance occurs when decreased heart rate causes decreased cardiac output, hypotension, angina, or CNS symptoms; this is especially likely when rate is less than 50 bpm. Slow heart rate may also lead to atrial ectopic or ventricular ectopic rhythms. However, in a healthy athlete, sinus bradycardia may have no clinical significance.

Sinus tachycardia results from an increased rate of SA node discharge, and it may result from any of the following: exercise, fever, anxiety, hypovolemia, anemia, pump failure, increased sympathetic tone, hypoxia, or hyperthyroidism.

Sinus tachycardia on the ECG: rate greater than 100 bpm, rhythm regular, pacemaker site SA node, P waves upright and normal in shape, P-R interval normal, and QRS complex normal in duration.

Clinical significance occurs when sinus tachycardia is a compensatory mechanism for decreased stroke volume. If the rate is greater than 140 bpm, cardiac output may fall because ventricular filling time is inadequate. Very rapid rates increase myocardial oxygen demand and may precipitate ischemia or even infarct in diseased hearts. Prolonged sinus tachycardia accompanying acute myocardial infarction (AMI) is often an ominous finding suggesting cardiogenic shock.

Sinus dysrhythmia often results from a variation of the R-R interval. It may be a normal finding sometimes related to the respiratory cycle and changes in intrathoracic pressure. Pathologically, sinus dysrhythmia can be caused by increased parasympathetic (vagal) tone.

Sinus dysrhythmia on the ECG: rate 60–100 bpm and varying with respiration, rhythm irregular, pacemaker site SA node, P waves upright and normal in shape, P-R interval normal, and QRS complex normal.

Clinical significance is minimal. Sinus dysrhythmia is a normal variant, particularly in the young and the aged.

Sinus arrest occurs when the SA node fails to discharge an impulse, resulting in short periods of cardiac standstill. This standstill can persist until pacemaker cells lower in the conductive system discharge (generating escape beats) or until the sinus node resumes discharge. Sinus arrest can result from ischemia of the SA node, digitalis toxicity, excessive parasympathetic (vagal) tone, or degenerative fibrotic disease.

Sinus arrest on the ECG: rate is normal to slow, depending on the frequency and duration of the arrest, rhythm is irregular, pacemaker site is the SA node, P waves are upright and normal in shape, P-R interval and QRS complex are normal.

Clinical significance is that frequent or prolonged episodes may compromise cardiac output, resulting in syncope or other problems. There is always the danger of complete loss of SA node activity. Usually, an escape rhythm develops; cardiac standstill, however, may result.

AV Junction

Dysrhythmias originating in the atrioventricular (AV) junction may be due to malfunction in the junctional cells themselves or due to a slowing or blockage in conduction of an impulse from the atria to the ventricles through the AV junction. The group of dysrhythmias termed atrioventricular (AV) blocks originate within the AV junction, and they can be due to either pathology within the AV junctional tissue or to a physiological block such as atrial fibrillation.

First-degree AV block actually involves a delay in conduction at the level of the AV node rather than a complete blockage. Thus, first-degree AV block is not a rhythm itself but a condition imposed on an underlying rhythm; you must be able to establish the underlying rhythm. Although first-degree AV block can occur in a healthy heart, it is most commonly due to ischemia at the AV junction.

First-degree AV block on the ECG: rate dependent upon underlying rhythm, rhythm usually regular although it can be slightly irregular, pacemaker site either SA node or atrial, P waves normal, P-R interval longer than 0.20 sec (this is diagnostic), and QRS complex usually less than 0.12 second, but may be bizarre in shape if conductive system disease exists in the ventricles.

Clinical significance lies not in first-degree block, which is usually no danger itself, but rather in the possibility that the observed AV block may precede development of a more advanced block.

Type I second-degree AV block (also termed second-degree Mobitz I or Wenckebach) represents an intermittent block at the AV node. The characteristic cyclic pattern features progressively longer P-R intervals followed by a completely blocked impulse. The cycle is repetitive, and the P-P interval remains constant. The ratio of conducted to nonconducted impulses (seen as P waves to QRS complexes) is commonly 5:4, 4:3, 3:2, or 2:1. The pattern may be either constant or variable. Although this type of AV block occurs in healthy hearts, it is most common with ischemia at the AV junction. Additional causes include increased parasympathetic (vagal) tone and drug effect.

Type I second-degree AV block on the ECG: atrial rate is unaffected, whereas ventricular rate may be either normal or slowed. Atrial rhythm is typically regular, whereas ventricular rhythm is irregular because of the nonconducted beats, pacemaker site may be either in SA node or atria, P waves are normal, but the P waves for nonconducted impulses are not followed by QRS complexes. P-R interval becomes progressively longer until the QRS complex is dropped, then the cycle repeats. The QRS complex is usually shorter than 0.12 second but may be bizarre in shape if conductive system disease exists in the ventricles.

Clinical significance lies in decreased cardiac output if beats are frequently dropped; symptoms include syncope and angina. Note that this block may occur as a transient phenomenon immediately after an inferior wall MI.

Type II second-degree AV block is also called second-degree Mobitz II or infranodal block. This is also an intermittent block, but it is characterized by P waves that are not conducted to the ventricles without any change in length of the P-R interval before a beat is dropped. The ratio of conduction (P waves to QRS complexes) is commonly 4:1, 3:1, or 2:1, and the ratio may either be constant or vary. A 2:1 Mobitz II block is often indistinguishable from a 2:1 Mobitz I block. Type II second-degree block is usually associated with acute MI and septal necrosis.

Type II second-degree AV block presentation on the ECG: atrial rate is unaffected, whereas ventricular rate is usually bradycardic. Rhythm may be regular or irregular, dependent on whether conduction ratio is constant or variable. Pacemaker site is in the SA node or atria. P waves are normal, although some P waves are not followed by QRS complexes. The P-R interval is constant for conducted beats, but may be longer than 0.21 second. QRS complex may be normal, although it is often longer than 0.12 second because of the abnormal depolarization sequence.

Clinical significance is in the possibility of decreased cardiac output. Because this block is often associated with cell necrosis secondary to MI, it is considered more serious than Mobitz I. Many Mobitz II blocks develop into full AV blocks.

Third-degree AV block, or complete block, is characterized by the absence of conduction between the atria and ventricles due to complete electrical block at or below the AV node. In this case, the atria and ventricles pace independently of each other. The sinus node frequently functions normally, depolarizing the atrial syncytium, whereas an escape pacemaker below the atria paces the ventricular syncytium. Third-degree block can occur with acute MI, digitalis toxicity, or degeneration of the conductive system as can occur in the elderly.

Third-degree AV block on the ECG: Atrial rate is unaffected. Ventricular rate is 40–60 bpm if escape pacemaker is junctional, less than 40 bpm if pacemaker is lower in the ventricles. Both the atrial and ventricular rhythms are usually regular. Pacemaker site is typically SA node for atria, AV junction or ventricular for ventricles. P waves are normal but show no relationship to QRS complexes, often falling within the T wave and QRS complex. There is no relationship between the P waves and R waves. The QRS complex is longer than 0.12 second if the pacemaker is ventricular and less than 0.12 second if pacemaker is junctional.

Clinical significance lies in severe compromise of cardiac output due to decreased ventricular contraction rate and loss of coordinated atrial kick.

A third group of dysrhythmias can originate in the AV junction or AV node, and these include premature junctional contractions, junctional escape complexes and junctional rhythms, accelerated junctional rhythm, and paroxysmal junctional tachycardia. All four of these dysrhythmias share some ECG features: (1) There are inverted P waves on lead II resulting from the retrograde depolarization of the atria. The P wave's relation to QRS depolarization depends on the relative timing of atrial and ventricular depolarization. The P wave can appear first if the atria depolarize first, or the QRS can come first if the ventricles depolarize first. If all chambers depolarize at the same time, the P wave and QRS complex can be superimposed, which effectively masks the P wave. P-R interval is less than 0.12 second, and there is normal duration of the QRS complex.

Premature junctional contractions (PJCs) result from a single impulse originating in the AV node that occurs before the next expected sinus beat; thus, the beat is considered "premature." A PJC causes a compensatory pause when the SA node discharges before the premature impulse reaches it. A PJC is associated with a noncompensatory pause if the premature impulse depolarizes the sinus node and interrupts the heart's normal cadence. PJCs can result from a number of conditions, including use of alcohol, tobacco, or caffeine, sympathomimetic drugs, ischemic heart disease, hypoxia, digitalis toxicity, or from no apparent cause (idiopathic).

PJC presentation on the ECG: Rate and rhythm depend on underlying rhythm, and rhythm is usually regular except for the PJC. Pacemaker site is an ectopic focus in the AV junction. P waves are inverted and may appear before or after the QRS complex. P-R interval is less than 0.12 second if P wave occurs before QRS and is actually an R-P interval if P wave follows QRS complex. QRS complex itself is usually normal, although it may be longer than 0.12 second if the PJC is conducted through the partially refractory ventricles.

Clinical significance of isolated PJCs is minimal. Frequent PJCs suggest organic heart disease and may be precursors of other junctional dysrhythmias.

A junctional escape beat, or a junctional escape rhythm, is a dysrhythmia that results when the primary pacemaker, usually the SA node, is slower than that of the AV node. The AV node becomes the pacemaker, generally discharging at its typical 40–60 bpm. This is a compensatory mechanism that prevents cardiac standstill. Junctional escape has several etiologies, including increased vagal tone, which can result in SA node slowing, pathological SA node discharge, or heart block.

Junctional escape rhythm presentation on the ECG: Rate is typically 40–60 bpm, rhythm irregular in single junctional escape complex or regular in junctional escape rhythm. Pacemaker site is the AV node. P waves are inverted and may have any relationship to the QRS complex. P-R interval is less than 0.12 second if P wave occurs before QRS and is actually an R-P interval if P wave follows QRS complex. QRS complex is generally normal, although it may be greater than 0.12 second.

Clinical significance is decreased cardiac output due to slowed heart rate, with associated risk for precipitation of angina, syncope, or other problems. If rate is fairly rapid, rhythm may be well tolerated.

Accelerated junctional rhythms result from increased automaticity in the AV junction, causing the AV junction to discharge faster than its intrinsic rate. If the rate is fast enough, it will override the SA node. Accelerated junctional rhythm is not fast enough to qualify as tachycardia; however, it is considered accelerated because it is much faster than the typical junctional rate. A common cause is ischemia of the AV junction.

Accelerated junctional rhythm on ECG: Rate is 60–100 bpm, rhythm is regular, and pacemaker site is AV junction. P waves are inverted and may have any relationship with the QRS complex. P-R interval is less than 0.12 second if P wave occurs before QRS and is actually an R-P interval if P wave follows QRS complex. QRS complex is normal.

Clinical significance lies in the possible cause of ischemia, which can precipitate other, much less well-tolerated dysrhythmias.

Paroxysmal junctional tachycardia (PJT) develops when rapid AV junctional depolarization overrides the SA node. It often occurs in paroxysms (sudden episodes), which may last minutes or hours before terminating abruptly. It may be due to increased automaticity of a single AV nodal focus or by a reentry phenomenon at the AV node. PJT is often more appropriately called paroxysmal supraventricular tachycardia (PSVT) because the rapid rate may make it indistinguishable from paroxysmal atrial tachycardia. PJT may occur at any age and may or may not be related to underlying heart disease. Stress, overexertion, tobacco, and caffeine may precipitate it. However, it is frequently associated with underlying atherosclerotic heart disease (ASHD) and rheumatic heart disease. PJT rarely occurs with MI. It can occur with accessory pathway conduction such as Wolff-Parkinson-White syndrome.

PJT on the ECG: Rate is 100–180 bpm, with characteristically regular rhythm except at onset and termination of paroxysm. Pacemaker site is AV junction. If present, P waves are inverted and may have any relationship with the QRS complex. Turning up the speed of the ECG recording to 55 mm/sec spreads out the complex and may aid in identifying P waves. P-R interval is less than 0.12 second if P wave occurs before QRS complex and is actually an R-P interval if P wave follows QRS complex. QRS complex is normal.

Clinical significance in younger patients with good cardiac reserve is minimal for a short time, and the patient usually perceives the PJT as palpitations. However, rapid rate decreases ventricular filling time and thus markedly decreases cardiac output. The reduced diastolic phase of the cardiac cycle can also compromise coronary artery perfusion. PJT can precipitate angina, hypotension, or congestive heart failure.

Atria

Dysrhythmias can also originate in atrial tissue outside the SA node or in the internodal pathways.

Atrial tachycardia, also called ectopic tachycardia or wandering pacemaker, is the passive transfer of pacemaker sites from the SA node to other latent sites in the atria or AV junction. Often more than one pacemaker site is present, causing variation in the R-R interval and P wave morphology. Atrial tachycardia can arise as a variant of sinus dysrhythmia, as a normal phenomenon in the very young or aged, or as part of ischemic heart disease or atrial dilation.

Atrial tachycardia on the ECG: Rate is usually normal, and rhythm is slightly irregular. Pacemaker site varies among SA node, atrial tissue, and AV junction. P wave morphology changes from beat to beat (as pacemaker site changes), or there may be no P waves present. P-R interval varies. It may be less than 0.12 second, normal, or longer than 0.20 second. QRS complex is normal.

Clinical significance is minimal because there are usually no detrimental effects. Occasionally, atrial tachycardia may precede other atrial dysrhythmias such as atrial fibrillation, and sometimes it may signal digitalis toxicity.

Multifocal atrial tachycardia (MAT) is usually found in acutely ill patients, and about 60 percent of them will have significant pulmonary disease. Certain medications used for pulmonary indications (such as theophylline) may worsen the dysrhythmia. At least three different P waves are noted, indicating the various ectopic foci. MAT can result from pulmonary disease, metabolic disorders (namely, hypokalemia), ischemic heart disease, or occur after recent surgery.

Multifocal atrial tachycardia on the ECG: Rate is greater than 100 bpm, and rhythm is irregular. Pacemaker sites are ectopic sites in the atria. There are organized, discrete nonsinus P waves with at least three different forms. P-R interval varies, and the duration of the QRS complex may be less than 0.12 second, normal, or longer than 0.20 second, dependent on the AV node's refractory status when the ectopic impulse reaches it.

Clinical significance lies in the fact most affected patients are acutely ill; this dysrhythmia may indicate a serious underlying medical illness.

Premature atrial contractions (PACs) result from a single electrical impulse originating in the atria outside the SA node, which in turn causes a premature depolarization before the next expected SA impulse. Because the premature impulse depolarizes the atrial syncytium and the SA node, there is a noncompensatory pause in the underlying rhythm. PACs may result from use of caffeine, tobacco, or alcohol, use of sympathomimetic drugs, ischemic heart disease, hypoxia, digitalis toxicity, or no apparent cause (idiopathic).

PACs on the ECG: Rate and rhythm depend on underlying rhythm, with rhythm generally regular except for PAC. Pacemaker site is an ectopic focus in the atria. The P wave of the PAC is different than the P waves of the underlying rhythm. It occurs earlier than the next expected P wave and may be masked by the preceding T wave. The P-R interval is usually normal, although it may vary with the location of the ectopic focus. Foci near the SA node have a P-R interval of 0.12 second or longer, whereas ectopic foci near the AV node have an interval of 0.12 second or less. The QRS complex is usually normal, although duration may exceed 0.12 second if the PAC is abnormally conducted through the partially refractory ventricles. If the ventricles are refractory and do not depolarize, there will not be a QRS complex.

Clinical significance is slight for isolated PACs. However, frequent PACs may indicate organic heart disease and may precede other atrial dysrhythmias.

Paroxysmal supraventricular tachycardia (PSVT) occurs when rapid atrial depolarization overrides the SA node; this often occurs in a sudden onset paroxysm that may last minutes to hours before terminating abruptly. It may be caused by increased automaticity of a single atrial focus or by reentry at the AV node. PSVT may occur at any age and often is not associated with underlying heart disease. It may be precipitated by stress, overexertion, tobacco, or caffeine. It frequently is associated with underlying atherosclerotic cardiovascular disease and rheumatic heart disease. PSVT is rare in patients with MI; it can occur in patients with Wolff-Parkinson-White syndrome.

PSVT on the ECG: Rate is 150–250 bpm, and rhythm is usually regular except at onset and termination of paroxysm. Pacemaker site is in the atria outside the SA node. The atrial P waves vary slightly from the sinus P waves. The atrial P wave may be impossible to see, especially when rate is rapid. Turning up the speed of the machine to 50 mm/sec spreads out the complex and may help in identifying P waves. The P-R interval is usually normal, although it may vary with location of the ectopic focus. Ectopic pacemakers near the SA node have intervals close to 0.12 second, whereas foci near the AV node have intervals of 0.12 second or less. The QRS complex is normal.

Clinical significance is less in younger patients with good cardiac reserve, who may tolerate PSVT well for short periods. Patients often perceive PSVT as palpitations. Rapid rates are associated with decreased cardiac output due to inadequate ventricular filling time. The shortened diastolic phase of the cardiac cycle can compromise coronary artery perfusion. PSVT may precipitate angina, hypotension, or congestive heart failure.

Atrial flutter results from a rapid atrial reentry circuit and an AV node that physiologically cannot conduct all impulses through to the ventricles. The AV junction may allow impulses in a 1:1, 2:1, 3:1, or 4:1 ratio or greater, resulting in a discrepancy between atrial and ventricular rates. AV block may be consistent or variable. Atrial flutter may occur in normal hearts but is usually associated with organic disease. Atrial dilation with congestive heart failure is a cause of atrial flutter. MI is only rarely a cause.

Atrial flutter on the ECG: Atrial rate is 250–350 bpm, with ventricular rate dependent on ratio of AV conduction. Atrial rhythm is regular; ventricular rhythm may be regular or irregular if block is variable. Pacemaker sites are in the atria outside the SA node. Rather than a P wave, F (flutter) waves are present, which resemble sawteeth or a picket-fence pattern. This pattern may be difficult to identify in a 2:1 flutter. However, if the ventricular rate is 150 bpm, suspect 2:1 flutter. The P-R interval is usually constant but may vary, and the QRS complex is normal.

Clinical significance depends on ventricular rate. Flutter with normal ventricular rates is generally well tolerated. Rapid ventricular rates may compromise cardiac output and result in symptoms. Atrial flutter often occurs in conjunction with atrial fibrillation and is then termed atrial fib-flutter.

Atrial fibrillation results from multiple areas of reentry within the atria or from multiple ectopic foci bombarding an AV node that physiologically cannot handle all the incoming impulses. AV conduction is random and highly variable. Atrial fibrillation may be chronic and is often associated with underlying heart disease, such as rheumatic or atherosclerotic heart disease or congestive heart failure. Atrial dilation occurs with congestive heart failure and often causes atrial fibrillation.

Atrial fibrillation on the ECG: Atrial rate is approximately 350–750 bpm, and ventricular rate is highly variable depending on conduction through the AV node. Rhythm is irregularly irregular. Pacemaker sites are numerous ectopic foci in the atria. P waves are not discernible. Fibrillation (f) waves are present, indicating chaotic atrial activity. There is no P-R interval, but the QRS complex is normal.

Clinical significance is in loss of atrial contraction with atrial kick, thus reducing cardiac output 20 to 25 percent. There is frequently a pulse deficit between the apical and peripheral pulse rates. If rate of ventricular response is normal, as often occurs in patients on digitalis, the rhythm may be well tolerated. If the ventricular rate is less than 60 bpm, cardiac output may fall. Suspect digitalis toxicity in patients with atrial fibrillation and a ventricular rate less than 60 bpm. If ventricular response is rapid and coupled with loss of atrial kick, cardiovascular compromise may occur with hypotension, angina, infarct, congestive heart failure, or shock.

Patients with accessory pathways such as those with Wolff-Parkinson-White who develop atrial flutter or atrial fibrillation present special concerns. Verapamil, which decreases conduction through the AV node and may shorten the refractory period of the accessory path, may precipitate either ventricular tachycardia or ventricular fibrillation.

Ventricles

Dysrhythmias originating in the ventricles are associated with many causes, including ischemia, hypoxia, and certain medications. The location of the pacemaker site dictates the shape of the QRS complex.

A ventricular escape beat (ventricular escape rhythm or idioventricular rhythm) results when impulses from higher pacemakers fail to reach the ventricles or when the discharge rate of higher pacemakers falls to less than that of the ventricles (normally 15–40 bpm). Ventricular escape rhythms are compensatory mechanisms that prevent cardiac standstill. There are several etiologies, including slowing of supraventricular pacemaker sites or high-degree AV block. They are frequently the first organized rhythms seen following successful defibrillation.

Ventricular escape rhythms on ECG: Rate is generally 15–40 bpm or less, with irregular rhythm in a single ventricular escape complex. Escape rhythm is usually regular unless the pacemaker site is low in the ventricular conduction system. The pacemaker site is the ventricles, and there are no P waves and no P-R intervals. The QRS complex is longer than 0.12 second and bizarre in shape.

Clinical significance lies in decreased cardiac output secondary to slow heart rate. Ventricular escape rhythms are a safety mechanism that you should NOT suppress. Escape rhythms may be either perfusing or nonperfusing.

Accelerated idioventricular rhythm, a subtype of ventricular escape rhythm, is an abnormally wide ventricular dysrhythmia typically associated with an acute MI. The rate is usually 60–110 bpm, and the patient does not require treatment unless hemodynamic instability is present, in which case the ventricular focus should be treated with atropine or overdrive pacing. The principal goal is treatment of the underlying MI.

Premature ventricular contraction (PVC) is a single ectopic impulse arising in a focus in either ventricle that occurs before the next expected beat in the underlying rhythm. PVCs may result from increased automaticity in the ectopic cell or by a reentry mechanism. The alteration in ventricular depolarization results in a wide and bizarre QRS complex and may, in addition, cause the T wave to deflect in the direction opposite to the QRS complex. Because PVCs normally do not depolarize the SA node and interrupt its rhythm, these ectopic beats lead to a fully compensatory pause. Occasionally, a PVC is interpolated between two sinus beats without causing any disturbance in the underlying rhythm. If more than one PVC is observed, it may be possible to distinguish whether there is one (unifocal) or multiple (multifocal) ectopic foci. PVCs with the same morphology imply the same focus. If the coupling interval (the distance between the preceding beat and the PVC) is constant for multiple PVCs, then the PVCs are probably unifocal. PVCs often occur in cluster patterns, including bigeminy (where every other beat is a PVC), trigeminy (where every third beat is a PVC), and quadrigeminy (where every fourth beat is a PVC). Repetitive PVCs are a pattern of two or more PVCs without a normal (sinus) beat between them, and they typically occur as couplets or triplets. More than three consecutive PVCs are often considered ventricular tachycardia. Causes of PVCs include myocardial ischemia, increased sympathetic tone, hypoxia, acid–base disturbances, electrolyte imbalances, normal variation, and idiopathic cases.

PVCs on the ECG: Rate depends on underlying rhythm and rate of PVCs, rhythm of PVCs interrupts regularity of underlying rhythm and is occasionally irregular, and pacemaker site is within a ventricle. P waves are absent; however, a normal sinus P wave may appear before a PVC. There is thus no P-R interval. The QRS complex of the PVC is longer than 0.12 second and bizarre in morphology.

Clinical significance may be slight in patients without heart disease, who sense the PVC as a skipped beat. In patients with myocardial ischemia, PVCs may suggest ventricular irritability and may precede lethal ventricular dysrhythmias. PVCs are often classified as benign or malignant. Malignant PVCs show at least one of five traits: (1) more than six PVCs/minute; (2) R on T phenomenon; (3) couplets or runs of ventricular tachycardia; (4) multifocal in nature; and (5) associated chest pain. Because the ventricles do not fill properly with most PVCs, you will usually not feel a pulse during the PVCs themselves. Grades 0–5 on the Lown system equate the combination of malignant PVC traits to a numerical score. Grade 0 has no PVCs, whereas Grade 4 has repetitive PVCs (couplets or triplets) and Grade 5 shows R on T phenomenon.

Treatment is indicated for patients with a prior history of heart disease or symptoms or if the PVCs are malignant.

Ventricular tachycardia (VT) consists of three or more consecutive ventricular complexes at a rate of 100 bpm or higher. This rhythm overrides the heart's normal pacemaker, and thus the atria and ventricles are asynchronous. In monomorphic VT all complexes appear the same, whereas in polymorphic VT the complexes appear in different sizes and shapes. The causes for VT are the same as for PVCs.

VT on the ECG: Rate is roughly 100–250 bpm, with regular or slightly irregular rhythm, and pacemaker site in a ventricle. If P waves are present, they are not associated with the QRS complexes. There is no P-R interval, and the QRS complex is longer than 0.12 second and bizarre in morphology.

Clinical significance lies in the poor stroke volume and rapid rate associated with VT, which may cause severe compromise in cardiac output and coronary artery perfusion. Always remember that VT may deteriorate into ventricular fibrillation. Treatment type depends on whether VT is perfusing or nonperfusing.

Ventricular fibrillation is a chaotic ventricular rhythm that usually results from many reentry circuits within the ventricles. There is no ventricular depolarization or contraction. Although many causes have been identified, it is notable that most result from advanced coronary artery disease.

Ventricular fibrillation on ECG: There is no organized rate or rhythm, and P waves are usually absent. P-R interval is absent, as are QRS complexes. The pacemaker sites are numerous ectopic foci within the ventricles.

Clinical significance is the lethal nature of this dysrhythmia due to lack of cardiac output or organized electrical pattern within the heart.

Asystole is cardiac standstill marked by absence of all cardiac electrical activity. Asystole may be the primary event in cardiac arrest; it is usually associated with massive MI, ischemia, and necrosis. It may result from heart block when no escape pacemaker takes over, and asystole is often the final outcome of ventricular fibrillation.

Asystole on the ECG: There is no electrical activity with complete absence of P waves, QRS complexes, and T waves.

The likelihood of successful resuscitation is very low.

Artificial pacemaker rhythm results from regular cardiac stimulation by an electrode implanted in the heart and connected to a power source. Demand pacemakers represent an escape rhythm. Ventricular pacemakers stimulate only the right ventricle, resulting in an idioventricular-type rhythm. Dual-chambered pacemakers (also called AV sequential pacemakers) stimulate the atria and then the ventricles. Pacemakers are typically implanted in patients who have chronic high-grade heart block or sick sinus syndrome or who have had episodes of severe symptomatic bradycardia.

Pacemakers on the ECG: Rate varies with the preset rate of the pacemaker. Rhythm is regular if the heart is paced constantly, whereas rhythm is irregular if pacing is on demand. Pacemaker site depends on electrode placement. Ventricular pacemakers will not produce a P wave. Any sinus P waves seen are unrelated to the paced QRS complexes. Dual-chambered pacemakers produce a P wave behind each atrial spike. The spike is an artifact caused by each firing of the pacemaker, and it may be an upward or downward deflection. QRS complexes are usually longer than 0.12 second and bizarre in morphology, and they often resemble those of ventricular escape rhythms. A QRS complex should follow each pacemaker spike. When this occurs, the pacemaker is said to be "capturing" the ventricles. With demand pacemakers, some natural QRS complexes may appear, and these will not be associated with any spike.

27. Describe the process and pitfalls of differentiating wide QRS complex tachycardias. pp. 1174–1176

Ventricular tachycardia (VT) is the paradigm of a tachycardia with a wide, frequently bizarre QRS complex. In the discussion under objective 26, you learned that nonperfusing VT requires immediate treatment in order to restore tissue oxygenation. Drugs that may be useful include lidocaine, procainamide, or amiodarone. Synchronized cardioversion is generally the next alternative treatment. In cases with chest pain, dyspnea, or systolic BP less than 90 mmHg, synchronized cardioversion is indicated as the immediate treatment. Torsade de pointes, a subtype of VT, is commonly caused by certain antidysrhythmic drugs, including procainamide and amiodarone. Thus, prompt recognition of torsade de pointes—before initiating any treatment—is vital because you do NOT want to use the antidysrhythmics normally used for VT.

When you look at your initial rhythm strip, the QRS complexes of VT are relatively uniform in appearance and amplitude (check Figure 28-40). In contrast, the QRS complexes of torsade de pointes characteristically are not uniform in appearance and amplitude. Instead (as shown in Figure 28-41), the QRS complexes are wide and change in amplitude over the span of several complexes. The span of complexes also tends to vary roughly around a central point. Look at Figure 28-41, and draw a line joining the peaks of the upward deflections and another line connecting the lowest points of the downward deflections. You will see that the two lines almost form a "fish" shape that has its ends at a central point and that the strip shows one such large shape after another. This is the twisting about a point that is implicit in the French torsade de pointes. Another characteristic on ECG is a Q-T interval lengthened to 600 milliseconds or more during the breaks between the twisting spans of widened QRS complexes.

28. Describe the conditions of pulseless electrical activity. pp. 1182–1183

Pulseless electrical activity (PEA, also called electrical mechanical dissociation) means that electrical complexes are present on ECG, but there are no accompanying cardiac contractions. This is the paradigm of the situation in which you should treat the patient rather than the monitor. The ECG may show normal sinus rhythm, but your patient will be pulseless. Underlying conditions that can result in PEA and their general treatment (dependent on local protocol) include (1) hypovolemia/fluid resuscitation; (2) cardiac tamponade/pericardiocentesis; (3) tension pneumothorax/needle thoracostomy; (4) hypoxemia/intubation and oxygen; and (5) acidosis/sodium bicarbonate, as well as massive pulmonary embolism and rupture of the ventricular wall.

29. Describe the phenomena of reentry, aberration, and accessory pathways. pp. 1143–1144, 1153, 1184–1185

Reentry (of an impulse) occurs when two branches of a conduction pathway are altered by a pathologic process such that conduction is slowed in one branch and a unidirectional block is caused in the other. In this case, a normal anterograde depolarizing impulse travels slowly through the branch with slowed conduction and is blocked in the other. After the impulse travels through the branch with slowed conduction, it enters the branch with the block and is then conducted in the opposite retrograde direction back toward the source of the impulse. Because this tissue is no longer refractory, it is depolarized by the returning impulse (the one with retrograde directionality). This reentry of an impulse back into the pathway of origin can result in rapid rhythms such as paroxysmal supraventricular tachycardia or atrial fibrillation.

Aberration, or aberrant conduction, reflects conduction of an impulse through the heart's conductive system in abnormal fashion. Aberrant conduction reflects a single supraventricular beat that is conducted through the ventricles in a delayed manner. In bundle branch block (either the right or left bundle can be affected), all supraventricular impulses traveling through the affected branch are delayed. If both branches are affected, third-degree heart block exists. Note that the impulses in these cases arise above the level of the ventricles, unlike the pure ventricular rhythms. In incomplete bundle branch block, the QRS complex will be normal. In complete bundle branch block, there will be a widened QRS complex on the ECG, and this may cause confusion as to whether the rhythm is supraventricular or ventricular in origin. Although there are exceptions, you can use the following guidelines to try to distinguish bundle branch block from a pure ventricular rhythm: (1) a changing bundle branch block suggests SVT with aberrancy; (2) a trial of carotid sinus massage may slow conduction through the AV node and terminate a reentrant SVT or slow conduction of other supraventricular dysrhythmias, whereas it will have no effect on ventricular dysrhythmias; (3) AV block (AV dissociation) indicates ventricular origin; (4) a full compensatory pause, usually seen after a ventricular beat, indicates ventricular tachycardia (VT); (5) fusion beats suggest VT as well; and (6) a QRS duration of longer than 0.14 second usually indicates VT.

An accessory pathway is an extra conduction pathway within the conduction system. In Wolff-Parkinson-White syndrome (WPW), the extra conduction pathway is the bundle of Kent, a pathway that is between the atria and ventricles. The presence of this extra (or accessory) pathway means that the depolarizing impulse effectively bypasses the AV node, shortening the P-R interval and prolonging the QRS complex. Although most patients with the syndrome are asymptomatic, WPW is associated with a high incidence of tachydysrhythmias, usually through a reentry phenomenon. WPW is also referred to as a preexcitation syndrome because the ventricles are electrically excited before the impulse can arrive via the AV node. Although it is not always present on ECG monitoring, a delta wave (a slur on the upstroke of the QRS complex) is indicative of WPW.

30. **Identify the ECG changes characteristically produced by electrolyte imbalances and specify their clinical implications.** p. 1185

You should always suspect hyperkalemia in patients with a history of renal failure who are on dialysis because potassium tends to be retained in the body. On an ECG, an early sign of hyperkalemia is tall, peaked T waves in the precordial leads. As the blood level rises higher, conduction decreases and the P-R and Q-T intervals increase in length. At very high potassium levels, an idioventricular rhythm may develop and eventually become a classic sine wave. In hypokalemia, the opposite ion disturbance, prominent U waves occur. Very low blood potassium levels can cause a widened QRS complex.

Clinically, hyperkalemia causes the heart to dilate and become flaccid and heart rate slows. Elevation of blood potassium to two to three times the normal value can cause so much heart weakness and abnormalities in rhythm that death may ensue.

31. **Identify patient situations where ECG rhythm analysis is indicated.** pp. 1142–1185

You will have specific guidelines for ECG monitoring. They will include direct medical cardiac causes such as history of heart disease, MI, or dysrhythmia, as well as any current evidence of dysrhythmia or hemodynamic instability or patient complaints suggestive of angina or acute MI. They will also cover traumatic causes (chest injury that may involve the heart or lungs) and evidence suggesting inadequate oxygenation in the body (such as altered level of consciousness) that may reflect cardiovascular compromise. Last, you may have guidelines recommending monitoring in some metabolic situations (such as hypothermia). Remember that you always treat the patient, not the ECG.

32. **Recognize the ECG changes that may reflect evidence of myocardial ischemia and injury and their limitations.** p. 1140

Changes in the S-T segment are usually looked for as evidence of myocardial ischemia or acute MI. Ischemic tissue produces abnormalities such as S-T segment depression (the norm is an isoelectric line) or an inverted T wave, with inversion usually symmetrical. Tissue injury, which occurs next in the early phase of an MI, may elevate the S-T segment. Finally, as tissue dies a significant Q wave develops. (Such a Q wave is at least one small square wide, lasting 0.04 second or more, or is more than one third the height of the QRS complex.) Q waves may also indicate extensive transient ischemia. It is often difficult to interpret an ECG without knowledge of the patient's baseline ECG, and this is particularly true in patients with history of cardiac disease such as prior MI.

33. Correlate abnormal ECG findings with clinical interpretation. pp. 1142–1185

See objectives 26–28, 30, 32, and 35. You may also find a J wave (or Osborn wave) on ECG monitoring. This wave is a slow, positive, rounded deflection at the end of the QRS complex that accompanies hypothermia. Other ECG changes seen with hypothermia include T wave inversion, P-R, QRS, or Q-T prolongation, sinus bradycardia, atrial flutter or fibrillation, AV block, PVCs, ventricular fibrillation, or asystole.

34. Identify the major mechanical, pharmacological, and electrical therapeutic objectives in the treatment of the patient with any dysrhythmia. pp. 1142–1185

The descriptions of dysrhythmias, their clinical significance, and ECG findings associated with them are given in objective 26. Treatments for the conditions are discussed below.

- **Sinus bradycardia.** The overall goal of treatment is satisfactory heart rate, with subsequently adequate cardiac output and blood pressure and decreased risk of more dangerous dysrhythmias. Thus, treatment is based on symptoms, and no treatment may be needed unless hypotension or ventricular irritability is present. If treatment is needed, give a 0.5 mg bolus atropine sulfate, and repeat every 3 to 5 minutes until rate is satisfactory or you have given 3.0 mg atropine. If atropine fails, consider transcutaneous cardiac pacing (TCP), if available.
- **Sinus tachycardia.** Treatment is directed at the underlying cause. Hypovolemia, fever, anemia, or other cause should be corrected. The overall goal is to reduce heart rate to a level compatible with adequate ventricular filling time, with supports in place to maintain an adequate stroke volume.
- **Sinus dysrhythmia.** Sinus dysrhythmia is a normal variant, particularly in the young and aged. Treatment is thus typically not required.
- **Sinus arrest.** If the patient is extremely bradycardic or symptomatic, give a 0.5 mg bolus atropine sulfate. The goal of pharmacologic therapy is to bring rate up to a level where symptoms are eliminated because cardiac output is adequate.
- **First-degree AV block.** Treatment is generally restricted to observation unless heart rate drops significantly. If possible, avoid administration of any drug that will further slow AV conduction, such as lidocaine and procainamide. The goal of treatment, if needed, is to preserve or improve AV conduction, eliminating the risk of development of a higher degree of heart block. When necessary, treatment may be needed to increase heart rate to a level compatible with adequate cardiac output.
- **Type I second-degree AV block (also termed second-degree Mobitz I or Wenckebach).** Treatment is generally restricted to observation. If possible, you want to avoid administration of any drug that will further slow AV conduction, such as lidocaine and procainamide. If heart rate falls and the patient becomes symptomatic, give 0.5 mg atropine IV. Repeat every 3 to 5 minutes until rate is satisfactory or you have given 3.0 mg of atropine. If atropine fails, consider TCP if available. Overall goal is preservation or improvement of AV conduction and maintenance of a heart rate associated with adequate cardiac output.
- **Type II second-degree AV block (also called second-degree Mobitz II or infranodal block).** Definitive treatment is pacemaker insertion to preserve a normal rhythm and adequate cardiac output. In the prehospital setting, give medications if needed to stabilize the patient. Use caution in giving atropine to patients with second-degree Mobitz II blocks because the atropine may increase atrial rate but also worsen the AV nodal block. Consider TCP if available. If the patient remains symptomatic, do not delay application of TCP while waiting for IV access or time for atropine to take affect.
- **Third-degree AV block.** Definitive treatment is pacemaker insertion to preserve adequate cardiac output. In the prehospital setting, give medications if needed to stabilize patient. Use caution in giving atropine to patients with third-degree blocks because the atropine may increase atrial rate but also worsen the AV nodal block. Consider TCP if available. If the patient remains

symptomatic, do not delay application of TCP while waiting for IV access or time for atropine to take affect. NEVER use lidocaine to treat third-degree block with ventricular escape beats.

- **Premature junctional contractions (PJCs).** Treatment is restricted to observation if the patient is asymptomatic.
- **Junctional escape rhythm.** Treatment in the field is generally restricted to observation (as patients are asymptomatic); however, care is needed if hypotension or ventricular irritability is present. If needed, give 0.5 mg bolus atropine, and repeat every 3 to 5 minutes until rate is satisfactory or you've given 3.0 mg atropine. If atropine fails, consider TCP if available. Overall goal is preservation of cardiac output and blood pressure and prevention of more dangerous ventricular dysrhythmias.
- **Accelerated junctional rhythm.** Treatment goal is to correct ischemia.
- **Paroxysmal junctional tachycardia (PJT).** Treatment in the patient who is not tolerating PJT, as evidenced by hemodynamic instability, consists of the following sequence of steps. (1) Vagal maneuvers. (2) Therapy with adenosine (Adenocard). (3) Electrical therapy with synchronized cardioversion if ventricular rate is higher than 150 bpm or patient is hemodynamically unstable. If time allows, use presedation. Apply synchronized DC countershock of 100 joules. Remember that DC countershock is contraindicated if digitalis toxicity is suspected. The overall goal is to reach a heart rate compatible with adequate ventricular filling time and good cardiac output, as well as to ensure adequate coronary artery perfusion.
- **Atrial tachycardia.** Treatment options for symptomatic patients include consideration of adenosine or verapamil to lower heart rate and prevent other dysrhythmias, including atrial fibrillation.
- **Multifocal atrial tachycardia.** Treatment of the underlying medical condition usually resolves the dysrhythmia. Specific antidysrhythmic therapy is usually not needed.
- **Premature atrial contractions (PACs).** Treatment for the symptomatic patient is oxygen via nonrebreather mask and establishment of IV access, along with consultation with medical direction. Field goal is to maintain tissue oxygenation and prepare for possible development of other, more clinically significant dysrhythmias.
- **Paroxysmal supraventricular tachycardia (PSVT).** Treatment for patients who are not tolerating the rapid heart rate, as evidenced by hemodynamic instability, should consist of the following series of techniques: (1) Vagal maneuvers. Note that carotid sinus massage should not be done in patients with carotid bruits or known cerebrovascular or carotid artery disease. (2) Pharmacological therapy with adenosine IV. If this fails and patient has normal blood pressure and a narrow QRS complex, consider use of verapamil if no contraindications exist. (3) Electrical therapy with synchronized cardioversion. DC countershock is contraindicated when digitalis toxicity is suspected. The overall goal is attainment of heart rate compatible with adequate cardiac output and coronary perfusion.
- **Atrial flutter.** Treatment is indicated for cases with rapid ventricular rates and hemodynamic compromise. Immediate cardioversion is indicated in unstable patients. Occasionally, you may use pharmacological therapy with stable patients, especially if the rapid ventricular rate is causing congestive heart failure. Several medications slow ventricular rate, including diltiazem (Cardizem), verapamil, digitalis, beta-blockers, procainamide, and quinidine. Procainamide and quinidine are often used to convert back to sinus rhythm. Consult local medical direction for protocol specifics.
- **Atrial fibrillation.** Prehospital treatment is necessary when rapid ventricular rates with hemodynamic instability occur. Electrical therapy with immediate cardioversion is required in unstable patients—persons with heart rates greater than 150 bpm and associated chest pain, dyspnea, decreased level of consciousness, or hypotension. Pharmacological therapy may be useful, especially when rapid heart rate is causing congestive heart failure. Drugs that may be used include diltiazem, verapamil, digitalis, beta-blockers, procainamide, and quinidine. Atrial fibrillation is a documented risk factor for stroke because atrial dilation allows for stagnation of blood and development of clots. You may wish to consider administration of an anticoagulant. Consult medical direction for specifics of possible pharmacological options. Immediate treatment goal is improvement of cardiac output. (Ultimate goal is adjustment of digitalis level, if toxicity is cause.)

Patients with accessory pathways such as those with Wolff-Parkinson-White who develop atrial flutter or atrial fibrillation present special concerns. Verapamil, which decreases conduction through the AV node and may shorten the refractory period of the accessory path, may precipitate either ventricular tachycardia or ventricular fibrillation.

- **Ventricular escape rhythms.** Treatment depends on whether the rhythm is perfusing or not. If perfusing, the goal is to increase heart rate with atropine or, if it fails, TCP if available. With a nonperfusing rhythm, follow your pulseless electrical activity (PEA) protocol, including airway stabilization and CPR and IV epinephrine. Direct treatment is aimed at the primary problem, such as hypovolemia, hypoxia, cardiac tamponade, acidosis, or other. Consider a fluid challenge.
- **Accelerated idioventricular rhythm.** This is a subtype of ventricular escape rhythm and is an abnormally wide ventricular dysrhythmia typically associated with an acute MI. The rate is usually 60–110 bpm, and the patient does not require treatment unless hemodynamic instability is present, in which case the ventricular focus should be treated with atropine or overdrive pacing. The principal goal is treatment of the underlying MI.
- **Premature ventricular contractions (PVCs).** Treatment is indicated for patients with a prior history of heart disease or symptoms or if the PVCs are malignant. Administer oxygen and establish IV access. If the patient is symptomatic, give lidocaine at a dose of 1.0–1.5 mg/kg body weight. Give an additional bolus of 0.5–0.75 mg/kg every 5 to 10 minutes as needed until a total of 3.0 mg/kg has been reached. If PVCs are effectively suppressed, start a lidocaine drip at a rate of 2–4 mg/minute. Reduce dose in appropriate patients, and consider procainamide or bretylium if the ceiling dose of lidocaine has been reached or the patient is allergic to lidocaine. Overall goal is adequate ventricular filling and cardiac output and prevention of ventricular tachycardia or ventricular fibrillation.
- **Ventricular tachycardia (VT).** Treatment type depends on whether VT is perfusing or nonperfusing. If there is a pulse (perfusing VT), give oxygen and place an IV line. Give lidocaine IV at 1.0–1.5 mg/kg and additional doses of 0.5–0.75 mg/kg up to a total of 3.0 mg/kg. If unsuccessful, try procainamide or amiodarone as a second-line agent. Instability (namely, chest pain, dyspnea, or systolic BP less than 90 mmHg) calls for synchronized cardioversion. If you note instability at the outset of treatment, such as falling blood pressure or altered level of consciousness, initiate cardioversion immediately after starting oxygen and an IV. If there is no pulse (nonperfusing VT), treat as for ventricular fibrillation. Treatment goals are to maintain adequacy of cardiac output and coronary artery perfusion and to prevent ventricular fibrillation.
- **Ventricular fibrillation.** Treatment of ventricular fibrillation and nonperfusing VT is the same: Initiate CPR and follow with DC countershock at 200 joules. If unsuccessful, repeat at 200–300 joules; if still unsuccessful, try at 360 joules. Subsequent to countershock, control airway and establish IV access. Epinephrine 1:10,000 is the drug of first choice; give every 3 to 5 minutes as needed. If unsuccessful, consider second-line agents such as lidocaine, bretylium, amiodarone, procainamide, or even magnesium sulfate.
- **Asystole (or cardiac standstill).** Treatment is CPR, airway management, oxygenation, and medication. If there is any doubt of an underlying rhythm, attempt defibrillation.

35. Describe artifacts that may cause confusion when evaluating the ECG of a patient with a pacemaker. pp. 1131, 1179, 1181–1182

ECG findings for patients with pacemakers are given in objective 26.

Note that any patient who has a demand pacemaker may have normal ECG sequences when the pacemaker has not been activated. There will not be any spikes during this time period, only when the pacemaker has been activated. In contrast, patients with a fixed-rate pacemaker will always have spike artifacts because the pacemaker is continually firing at its preset rate.

36. List the possible complications of pacing. pp. 1181–1182

Possible problems with pacemakers include the following: (1) The battery fails. If batteries fail before they are replaced, pacing stops and the patient's underlying rhythm returns. (2) The pacemaker runs away. In this case (rarely seen with newer pacemakers), the pacemaker discharges at a rapid rate rather than the preset rate. In the older pacemakers, this is most likely to be seen when the battery runs low. Newer models avoid this possible problem by gradually increasing rate as the battery runs low. (3) Failure of a demand pacemaker to shut down when the innate rate exceeds the preset rate. When this happens, the heart's pacemaker and the artificial pacemaker compete, with both pacing the myocardium. If a paced beat falls during the relative refractory period, it can precipitate ventricular fibrillation. (4) Failure to capture. In this instance, battery failure or displacement of the pacemaker lead results in pacemaker discharge (with resultant ECG spike) that does not lead to depolarization of the myocardium (thus there is no QRS complex following the spike). Bradycardia often is seen.

37. List the causes and implications of pacemaker failure.   pp. 1181–1182

As seen in objective 36, battery failure, although unlikely, is probably the most common cause of pacemaker dysfunction or failure. Displacement of the discharge lead can also lead to pacemaker failure. In these cases, the patient's underlying rhythm is usually seen, and it is often bradycardic and sufficiently low in cardiac output to cause symptoms (or the pacemaker would not have been implanted). In other patients, asystole can occur when a fixed-rate pacemaker fails.

The failure of a demand pacemaker to shut down (a different way in which pacemaker function is lost) may lead to ventricular fibrillation if a paced beat occurs while the myocardium is in absolute or relative refractory state.

38. Identify additional hazards that interfere with artificial pacemaker function.   pp. 1181–1182

You should always examine unconscious patients for evidence of a pacemaker: Batteries, for instance, are often palpable under the skin (commonly in the axillary or shoulder region). You can treat bradydysrhythmias, asystole, and ventricular fibrillation in patients with failed pacemakers as you would in other patients, but you must be careful not to discharge defibrillation paddles directly over the battery pack.

39. Recognize the complications of artificial pacemakers as evidenced on an ECG.   pp. 1181–1182

See objective 35.

Content Self-Evaluation

MULTIPLE CHOICE

_____ 1. Each year, how many people in the United States die from coronary heart disease (CHD)?
   A. 144,000
   B. 225,000
   C. 466, 000
   D. 1 million
   E. 1.3 million

_____ 2. Which of the following is a risk factor for cardiovascular and coronary heart disease?
   A. obesity
   B. oral contraceptive use
   C. cocaine use
   D. family history
   E. all of the above

_____ 3. From innermost to outermost, the three tissue layers of the heart are:
   A. the endocardium, the pericardium, and the myocardium.
   B. the endocardium, the myocardium, and the syncytium.
   C. the endocardium, the myocardium, and the pericardium.
   D. the myocardium, the epicardium, and the pericardium.
   E. the epicardium, the myocardium, and the endocardium.

_____ 4. The apex of the heart is the location where the great vessels connect to the heart.
   A. True
   B. False

_____ 5. The heart valve located between the right atrium and ventricle is the:
    A. mitral.
    B. tricuspid.
    C. aortic.
    D. pulmonic.
    E. semilunar.

_____ 6. Which of the following blood vessels carries oxygenated blood?
    A. pulmonary vein
    B. superior vena cava
    C. aorta
    D. pulmonary artery
    E. both A and C

_____ 7. The blood supply to the left ventricle, interventricular septum, part of the right ventricle, and the heart's conduction system comes from the two branches of the left coronary artery, which are the:
    A. anterior descending artery and the circumflex artery.
    B. anterior descending artery and the posterior descending artery.
    C. circumflex artery and the posterior descending artery.
    D. circumflex artery and the marginal artery.
    E. marginal artery and the posterior descending artery.

_____ 8. The tunica adventicia is which layer of the artery?
    A. the inner endothelial layer
    B. the muscular middle layer
    C. the fibrous covering layer
    D. a ligamentous intermediate layer
    E. none of the above

_____ 9. The normal cardiac output is approximately what volume?
    A. 500 mL
    B. 1,200 mL
    C. 2,400 mL
    D. 5,000 mL
    E. 6,000 mL

_____ 10. Stimulation of the heart by the sympathetic nervous system results in:
    A. negative inotropic and chronotropic effects.
    B. negative chronotropic and dromotropic effects.
    C. positive chronotropic and dromotropic effects.
    D. positive inotropic and chronotropic effects.
    E. positive inotropic and dromotropic effects.

_____ 11. The cardiac conductive cells have which of the following properties?
    A. excitability
    B. conductivity
    C. automaticity
    D. contractility
    E. all of the above

_____ 12. Which of the following is an important property of cardiac tissue?
    A. automaticity
    B. conductivity
    C. excitability
    D. contractility
    E. all of the above

_____ 13. All of the following can cause an artifact on ECG EXCEPT:
    A. a diaphoretic patient.
    B. an enlarged heart.
    C. movement by the patient.
    D. shivering by the patient.
    E. loose electrodes.

_____ 14. Which of the following is NOT an electrode location used for the bipolar leads?
    A. right leg
    B. left leg
    C. right arm
    D. left arm
    E. all of the above are used

_____ 15. A single monitoring lead cannot identify which of the following?
    A. presence of an infarct
    B. location of an infarct
    C. axis deviation information
    D. quality of pumping actions
    E. all of the above

_____ 16. The smallest box on the ECG paper represents what period of time?
   A. 0.02 seconds
   B. 0.04 seconds
   C. 0.10 seconds
   D. 0.20 seconds
   E. 0.25 seconds

_____ 17. Which of the following represents the first (generally) positive deflection (on lead II) of the ECG?
   A. the P wave
   B. the QRS complex
   C. the T wave
   D. the U wave
   E. the P-R interval

_____ 18. Which element of the ECG is normally between 0.8 and 0.12 seconds in duration?
   A. the P wave
   B. the P-R interval
   C. the QRS interval
   D. the S-T segment
   E. the T wave

_____ 19. A prolonged Q-T interval is longer than 0.38 second.
   A. True
   B. False

_____ 20. Which of the following is not a criteria for ECG rhythm strip analysis?
   A. memorize the rules for each rhythm
   B. always be consistent and analytical
   C. identify the dysrhythmia by its similarity to established rules
   D. use the eyeball approach for the initial analysis
   E. analyze a given rhythm strip according to a specific formula

_____ 21. In your analysis of a dysrhythmia you determine there is no relationship among R-R intervals. You would classify this dysrhythmia as:
   A. regular.
   B. occasionally irregular.
   C. irregularly irregular.
   D. regularly irregular.
   E. reciprocating.

_____ 22. Common causes of dysrhythmias include all of the following EXCEPT:
   A. myocardial ischemia or infarction.
   B. electrolyte and pH disturbances.
   C. CNS or autonomic nervous system damage.
   D. drug effects.
   E. hyperthermia.

_____ 23. In the bradycardia algorithm, the first drug in the intervention sequence is:
   A. procainamide.
   B. epinephrine.
   C. atropine.
   D. isoproterenol.
   E. dopamine.

_____ 24. Which of the following dysrhythmias has an R-R interval that often varies with respiration?
   A. sinus arrest
   B. paroxsysmal supraventricular tachycardia
   C. sinus dysrhythmia
   D. sinus bradycardia
   E. sinus tachycardia

_____ 25. Of the atrial dysrhythmias listed below, which is often an indication of serious underlying medical disease?
   A. atrial tachycardia
   B. atrial flutter
   C. premature atrial contractions (PACs)
   D. multifocal atrial tachycardia (MAT)
   E. paroxysmal supraventricular tachycardia (PSVT)

_____ 26. Which of the following dysrhythmias has a characteristic sawtooth-shaped P wave?
   A. atrial flutter
   B. atrial fibrillation
   C. ventricular fibrillation
   D. Mobitz I second-degree block
   E. Mobitz II second-degree block

_____ 27. Which of the following dysrhythmias is rhythm irregularly irregular?
   A. atrial flutter
   B. atrial fibrillation
   C. paroxysmal supraventricular tachycardia
   D. sinus dysrhythmia
   E. all of the above

_____ 28. The diagnostic finding for first-degree AV block on ECG is:
   A. the presence of some QRS complexes not preceded by a P wave.
   B. a P-R interval longer than 0.20 second.
   C. a QRS complex widened to longer than 0.12 second.
   D. an R-T interval widened for those beats with an initial P wave.
   E. the presence of some P waves without following QRS complexes.

_____ 29. The chief difference between Type I and Type II second-degree AV block is the pattern of lengthening P-R interval before the blocked impulse in Type I second-degree AV block.
   A. True
   B. False

_____ 30. All of the following statements about third-degree AV block are true EXCEPT:
   A. the atrial rate is unaffected, and ventricular rate depends on site of ventricular pacemaker.
   B. P waves are normal but show no relationship to the QRS complex.
   C. there is an absence of conduction between the atria and the ventricles.
   D. both atrial and ventricular rhythms are usually regular.
   E. QRS complexes are always normal in length.

_____ 31. Never use lidocaine to treat third-degree heart block in patients with ventricular escape beats.
   A. True
   B. False

_____ 32. All of the following statements about ECG findings for dysrhythmias originating in the AV junction are true EXCEPT:
   A. P-R interval is less than 0.12 second.
   B. P waves are inverted in Lead II.
   C. T waves are blunted and widened.
   D. QRS complexes are normal in duration.
   E. P waves are masked if atrial depolarization occurs during ventricular depolarization.

_____ 33. Caffeine, tobacco, alcohol, and sympathomimetic drugs are common causes of:
   A. junctional escape rhythms.
   B. accelerated junctional rhythm.
   C. paroxysmal junctional tachycardia.
   D. premature junctional contractions.
   E. junctional bradycardia.

_____ 34. Which of the following may precipitate paroxysmal junctional tachycardia?
   A. smoking
   B. caffeine
   C. stress
   D. overexertion
   E. all of the above

_____ 35. All of the following statements about dysrhythmias originating in the ventricles are true EXCEPT:
   A. ischemia, hypoxia, and drug effects are common causes.
   B. T waves are blunted and widened.
   C. P waves are absent.
   D. the pacemaker site determines QRS morphology.
   E. QRS complexes are 0.12 second or longer in duration.

_____ 36. Which of the following is indicated in the treatment of symptomatic paroxysmal junctional tachycardia?
   A. lidocaine
   B. adenosine
   C. vagal maneuvers
   D. syncronized cardioversion
   E. all but A

_____ 37. The treatment of choice for ventricular escape rhythms is lidocaine.
   A. True
   B. False

_____ 38. Possible characteristics of malignant PVCs include all EXCEPT:
   A. R on T phenomenon.
   B. couplets or longer runs of ventricular tachycardia.
   C. two PVCs per minute.
   D. multifocal origin within the ventricles.
   E. accompanying chest pain.

_____ 39. Torsades de pointes varies in both cause and ECG appearance from other forms of:
   A. ventricular escape rhythm.
   B. accelerated idioventricular rhythm.
   C. ventricular fibrillation.
   D. premature ventricular contraction.
   E. ventricular tachycardia.

_____ 40. Nonperfusing ventricular tachycardia and ventricular fibrillation are treated identically, including initiation of CPR followed by:
   A. epinephrine 1:10,000 IV bolus.
   B. adenosine IV bolus.
   C. transcutaneous cardiac pacing (TCP).
   D. DC countershock at 360 joules.
   E. atropine IV bolus.

_____ 41. The first DC countershock for a patient in ventricular fibrillation is at what energy level (or biphasic equivalent)?
   A. 100 joules
   B. 200 joules
   C. 300 loules
   D. 360 joules
   E. Shock is not indicated.

_____ 42. You are attending a patient and apply ECG electrodes to note a rhythm with a dramatic spike preceding each bizarre but regular QRS complex (at a rate of 70 bpm). What is the likely cause of this rhythm?
   A. monitor failure
   B. a low battery
   C. The monitor is set on cardioversion mode.
   D. The patient has a pacemaker.
   E. a wandering atrial pacemaker

_____ 43. Often placing a magnet over a pacemaker will cause it to fire 70 times per minute.
   A. True
   B. False

_____ 44. Which of the following is a possible cause of PEA?
   A. hypovolemia
   B. tension pneumothorax
   C. massive pulmonary embolism
   D. cardiac tamponade
   E. all of the above

_____ 45. Which of the following is an ECG disturbance you might expect with a patient who is experiencing hypothermia?
   A. a J or Osborn wave
   B. T wave inversion
   C. PR interval prolongation
   D. atrial flutter
   E. all of the above

MATCHING

Write the letter of the definition or description regarding cardiac function in the space provided next to the term to which it applies. The same description or definition may be used more than once or not at all.

_____ 46. cardiac cycle

_____ 47. diastole

_____ 48. systole

_____ 49. ejection fraction

_____ 50. preload

_____ 51. afterload

_____ 52. cardiac output

_____ 53. stroke volume

A. the ratio of blood pumped from the ventricle compared with the amount contained at the end of diastole

B. the series of events between the end of a cardiac contraction to the end of the next

C. the resistance against which the heart must pump

D. the phase of the cardiac cycle during which the heart contracts

E. the amount of blood pumped by the ventricle during one cardiac contraction

F. the amount of blood pumped by the ventricle during one minute

G. the phase of the cardiac cycle during which the heart muscle is relaxed

H. the end-diastolic volume in the ventricle

I. the phase of the cardiac cycle during which blood enters the coronary arteries

Write the letter of innate rate of impulse discharge in beats per minute (bpm) in the space provided next to the part of the cardiac conduction system to which it applies.

_____ 54. Purkinje system

_____ 55. AV node

_____ 56. SA node

A. 60–100 bpm

B. 15–40 bpm

C. 40–60 bpm

Special Project:

Dysrhythmia Recognition

It is helpful to employ a systematic approach to the analysis of dysrhythmias. The following order of analysis may help you consistently and accurately identify dysrhythmias.

Regularity—Determine if the rate is regular, slightly irregular, regularly irregular, or irregularly irregular.
Rate—Determine the overall and underlying rate of the QRS complexes.
P wave—Determine if P waves are present and whether they are upright and rounded.

PRI—Determine the length of the P-R interval if it is consistent.
QRS complex—Determine the width of the QRS Complex and its general shape.

Once you have evaluated the above criteria, use them to help you determine the rhythm or dysrhythmia on the next 27 sample rhythm strips.

Rhythm 1

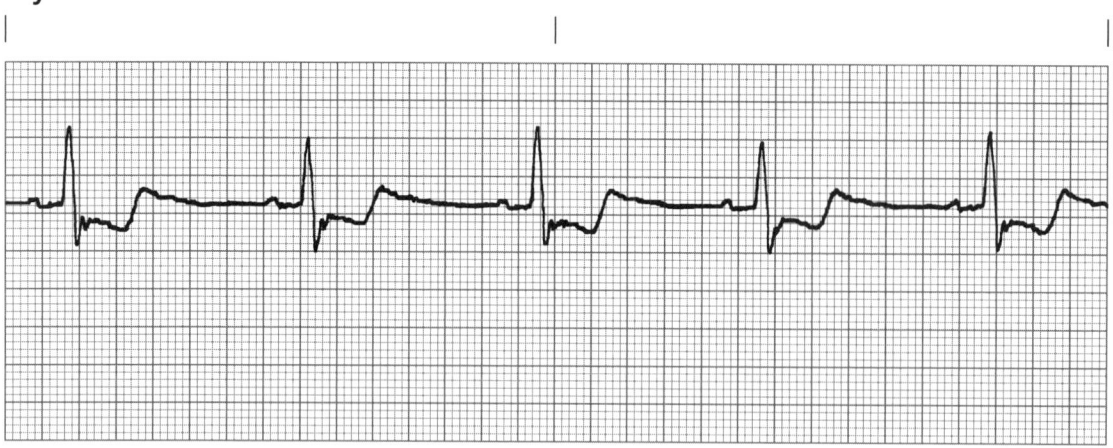

Regularity: _____   Rate: _____   P-Waves: _____
PRI: _____   QRS: _____   Interp: _____

Rhythm 2

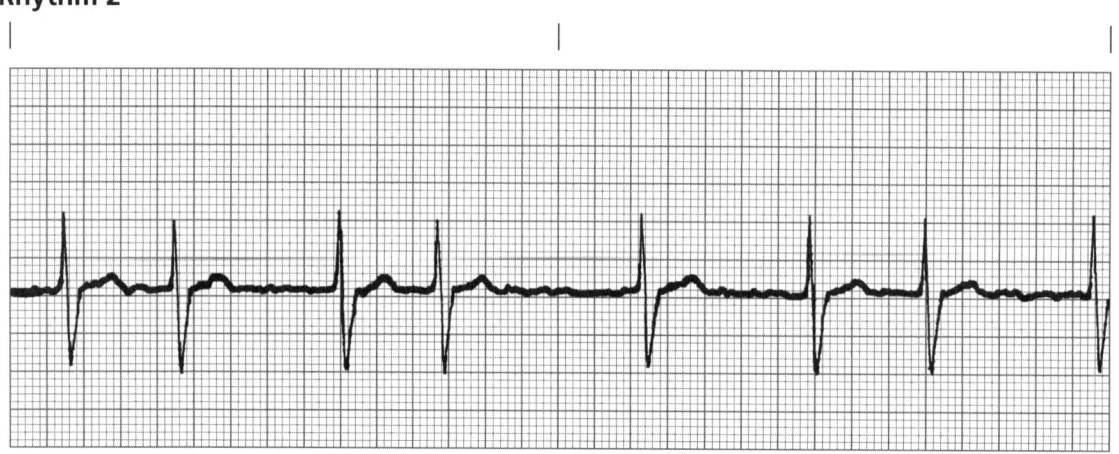

Regularity: _____   Rate: _____   P-Waves: _____
PRI: _____   QRS: _____   Interp: _____

These strips originally appeared in *Basic Arrhythmias*, 6th edition, by Gail Walraven (© 2006 Prentice Hall Health).

Rhythm 3

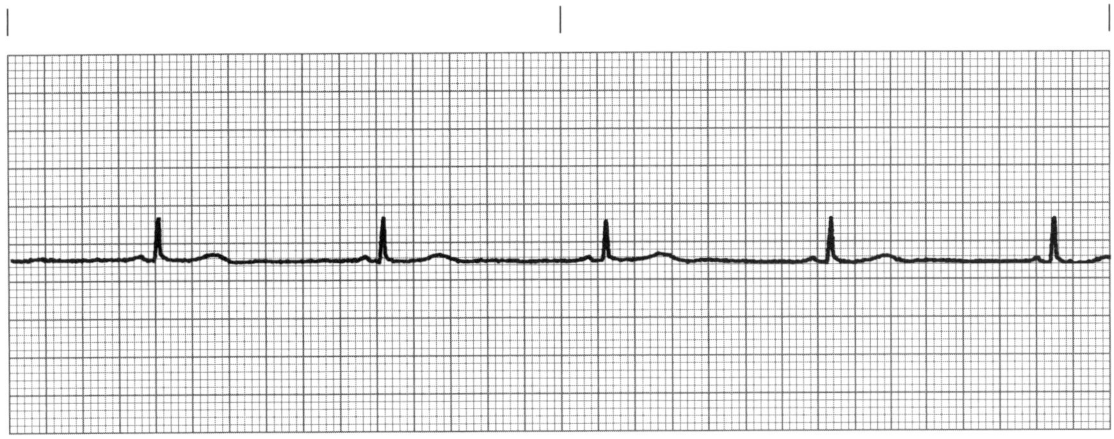

Regularity: _____ Rate: _____ P-Waves: _____
PRI: _____ QRS: _____ Interp: _____

Rhythm 4

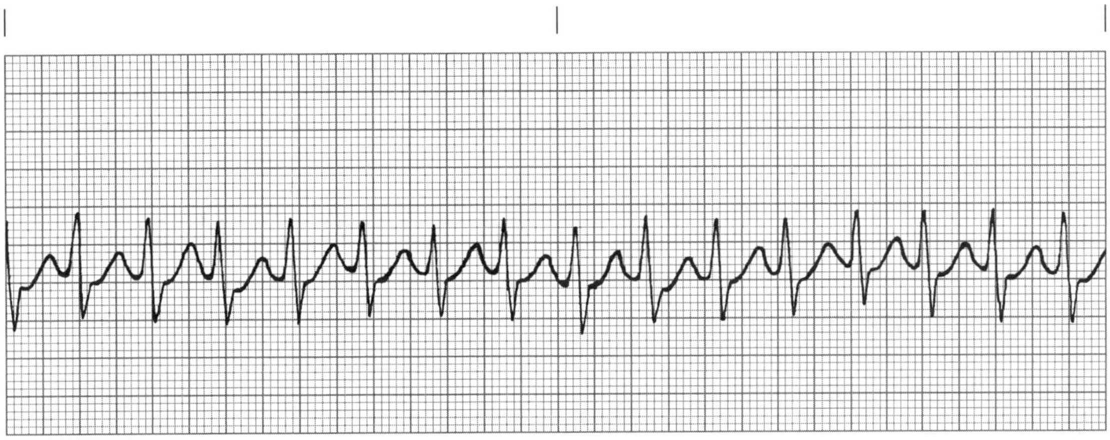

Regularity: _____ Rate: _____ P-Waves: _____
PRI: _____ QRS: _____ Interp: _____

Rhythm 5

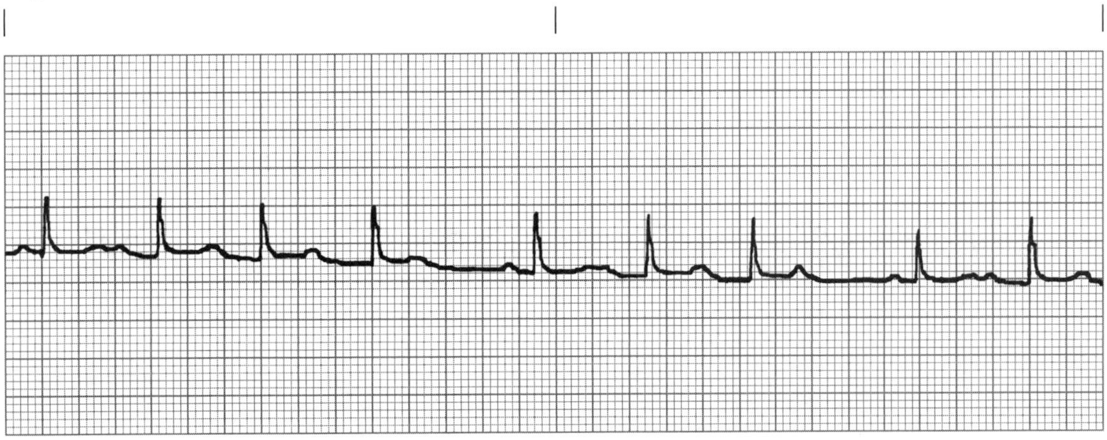

Regularity: _____ Rate: _____ P-Waves: _____
PRI: _____ QRS: _____ Interp: _____

Medical Emergencies

Rhythm 6

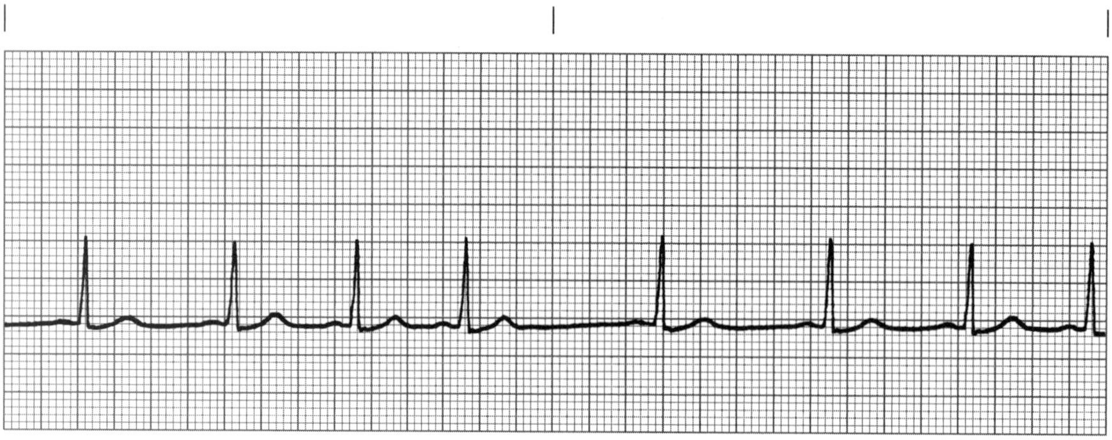

Regularity: _____ Rate: _____ P-Waves: _____
PRI: _____ QRS: _____ Interp: _____

Rhythm 7

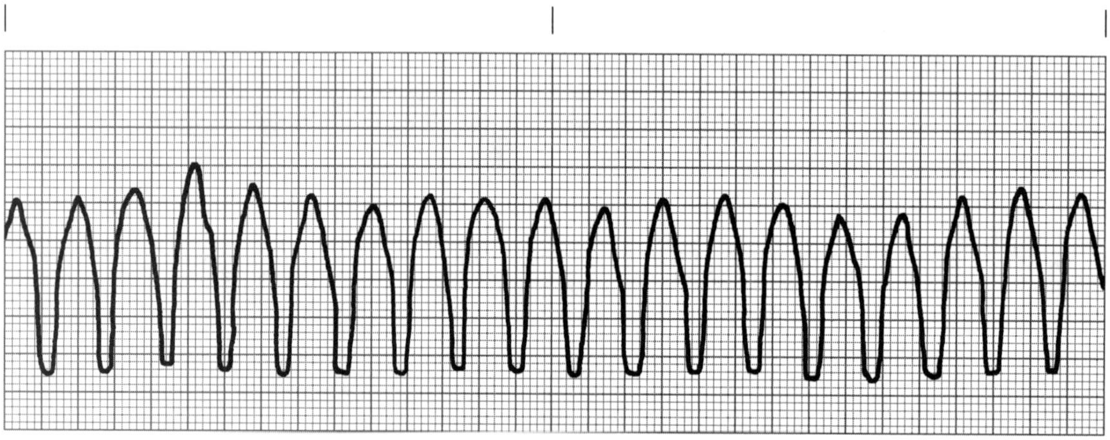

Regularity: _____ Rate: _____ P-Waves: _____
PRI: _____ QRS: _____ Interp: _____

Rhythm 8

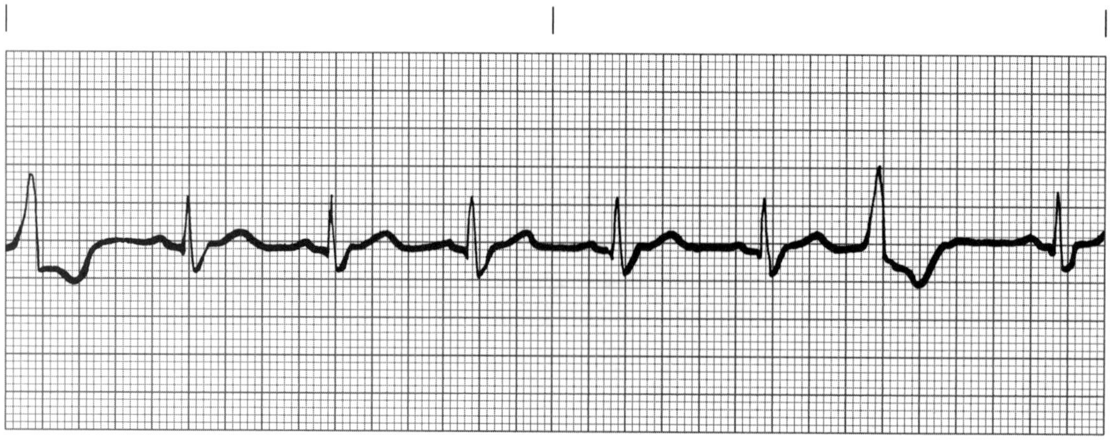

Regularity: _____ Rate: _____ P-Waves: _____
PRI: _____ QRS: _____ Interp: _____

Rhythm 9

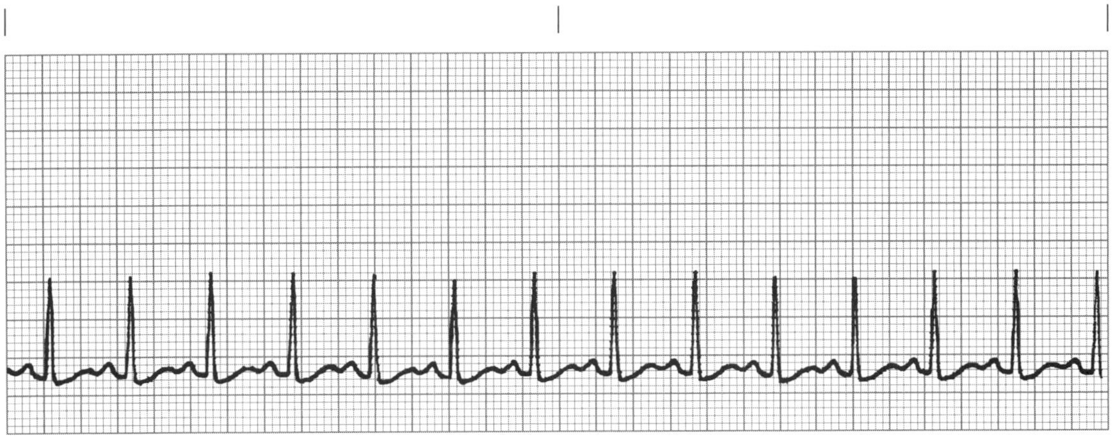

Regularity: _____ Rate: _____ P-Waves: _____
PRI: _____ QRS: _____ Interp: _____

Rhythm 10

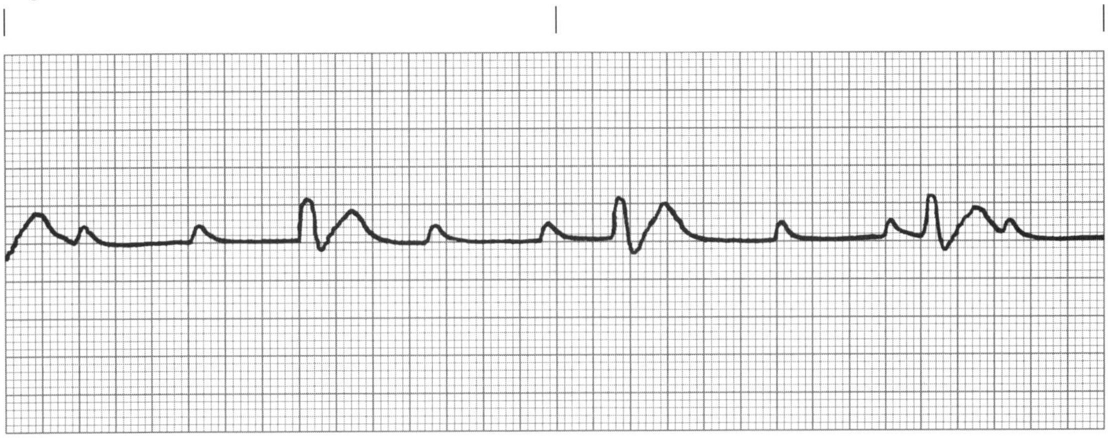

Regularity: _____ Rate: _____ P-Waves: _____
PRI: _____ QRS: _____ Interp: _____

Rhythm 11

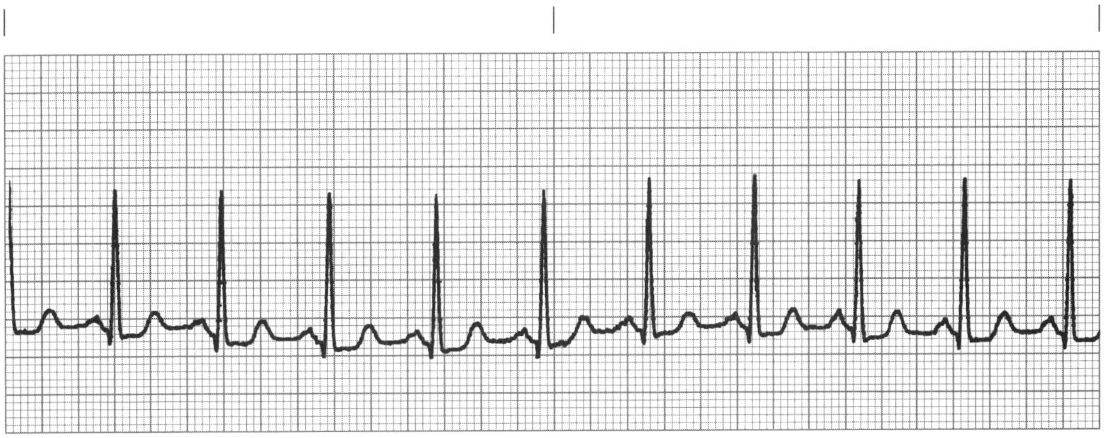

Regularity: _____ Rate: _____ P-Waves: _____
PRI: _____ QRS: _____ Interp: _____

Medical Emergencies

Rhythm 12

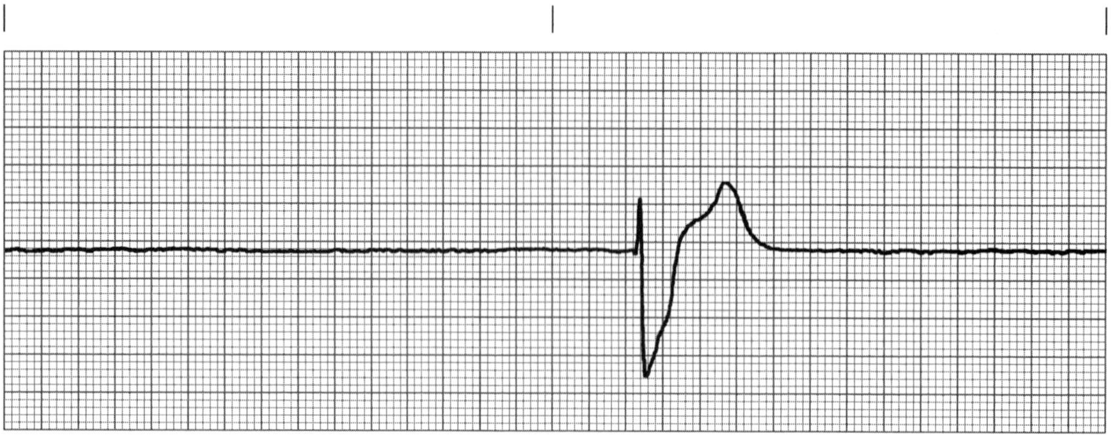

Regularity: _____ Rate: _____ P-Waves: _____
PRI: _____ QRS: _____ Interp: _____

Rhythm 13

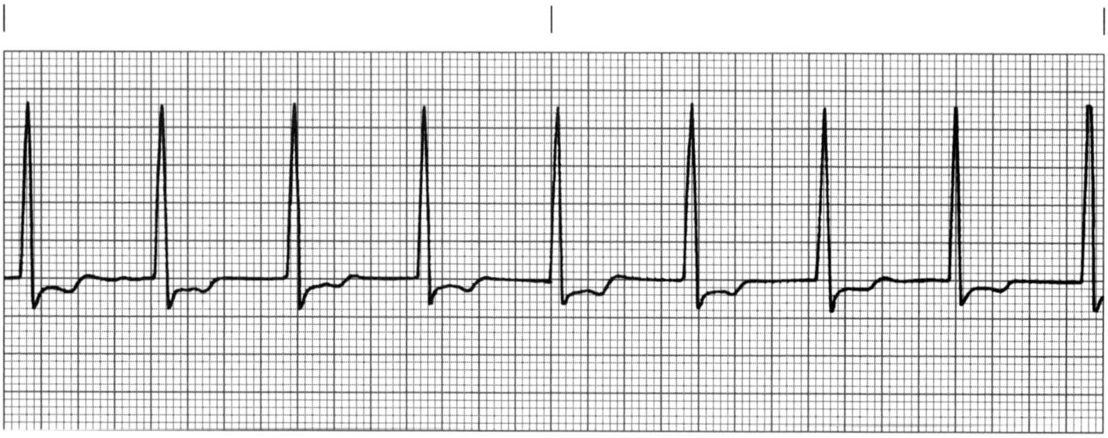

Regularity: _____ Rate: _____ P-Waves: _____
PRI: _____ QRS: _____ Interp: _____

Rhythm 14

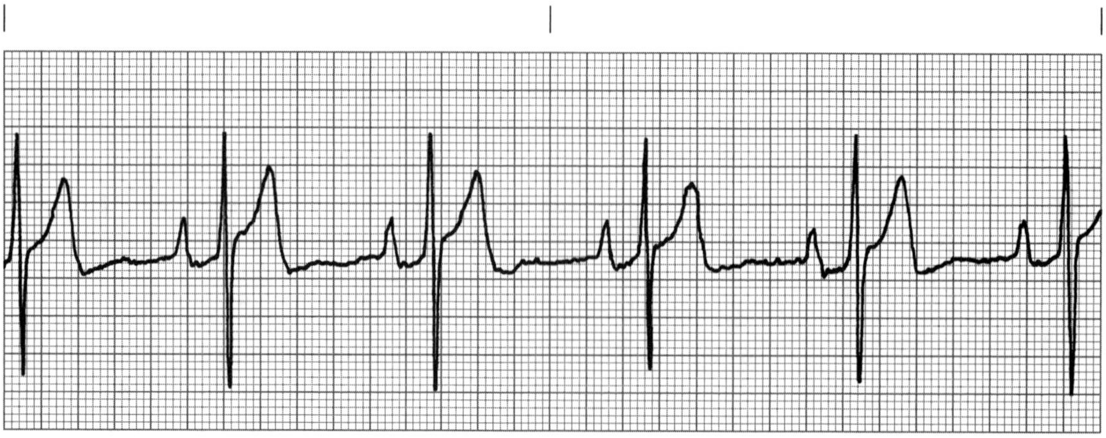

Regularity: _____ Rate: _____ P-Waves: _____
PRI: _____ QRS: _____ Interp: _____

Rhythm 15

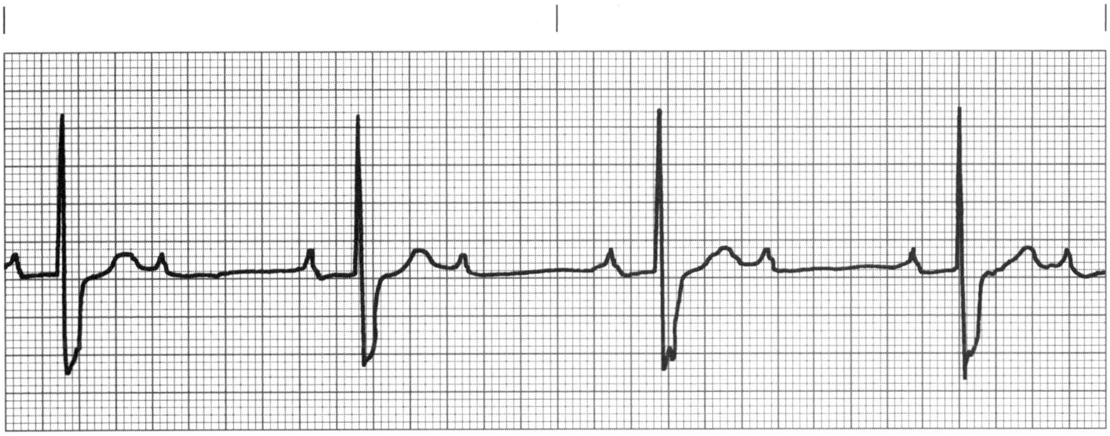

Regularity: _____ Rate: _____ P-Waves: _____
PRI: _____ QRS: _____ Interp: _____

Rhythm 16

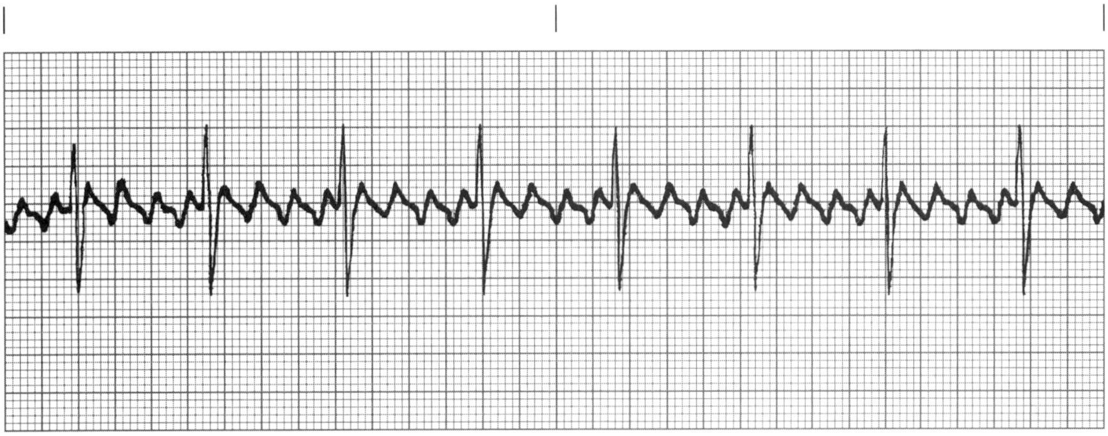

Regularity: _____ Rate: _____ P-Waves: _____
PRI: _____ QRS: _____ Interp: _____

Rhythm 17

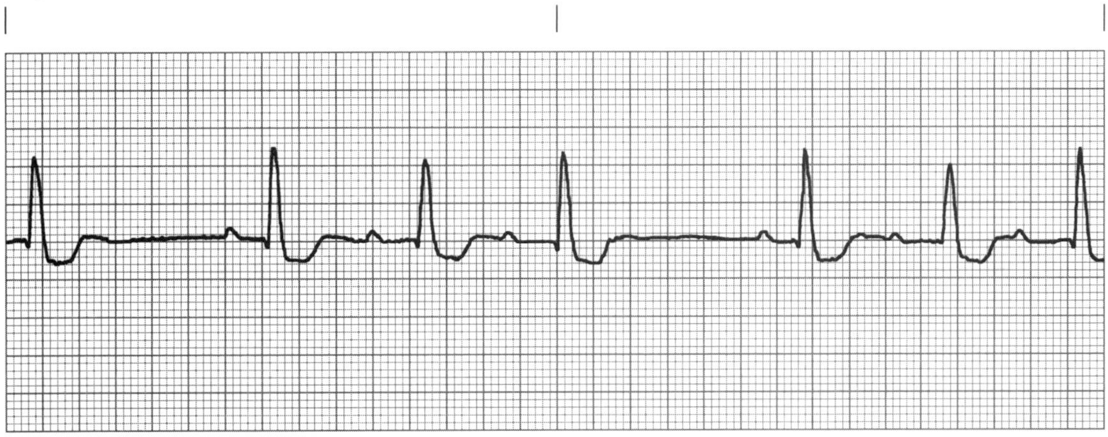

Regularity: _____ Rate: _____ P-Waves: _____
PRI: _____ QRS: _____ Interp: _____

Medical Emergencies

Rhythm 18

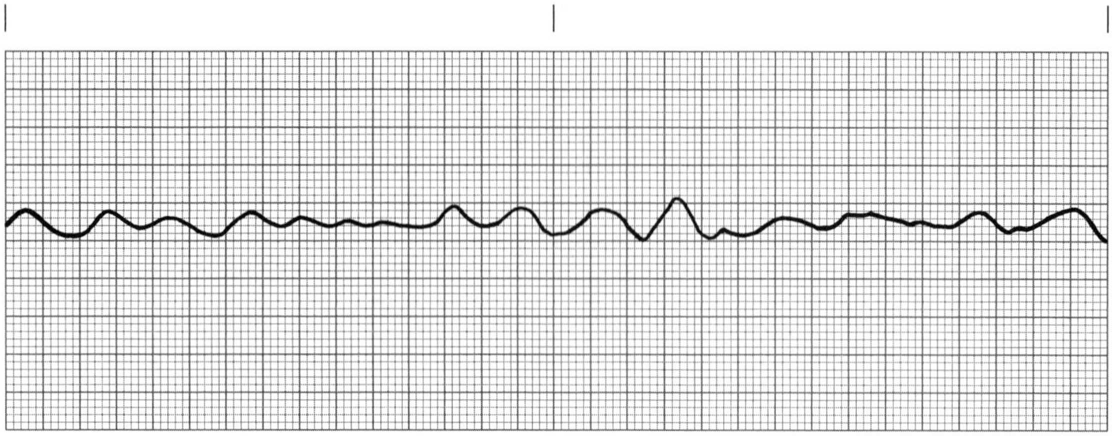

Regularity: _____ Rate: _____ P-Waves: _____
PRI: _____ QRS: _____ Interp: _____

Rhythm 19

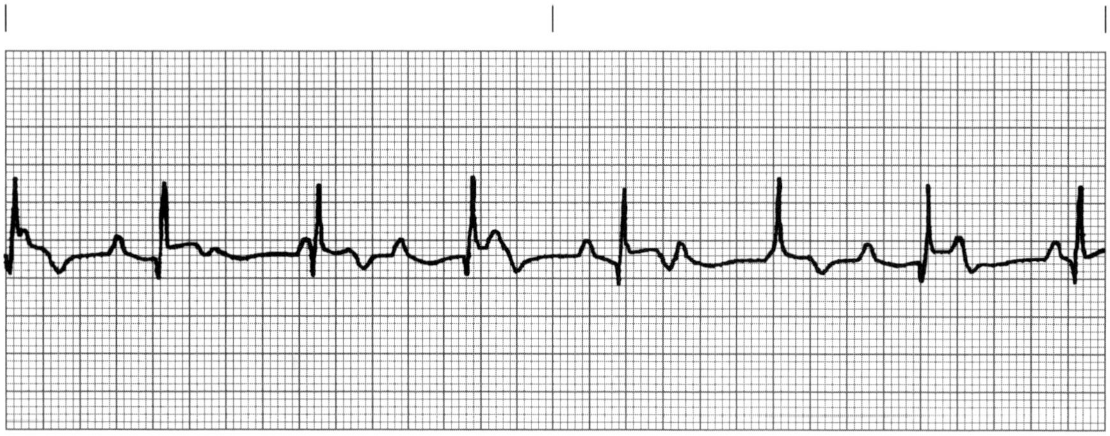

Regularity: _____ Rate: _____ P-Waves: _____
PRI: _____ QRS: _____ Interp: _____

Rhythm 20

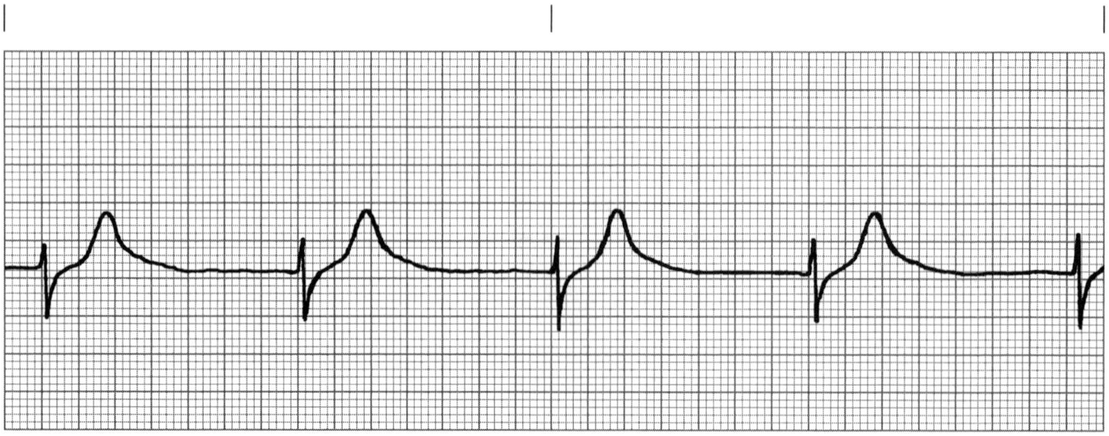

Regularity: _____ Rate: _____ P-Waves: _____
PRI: _____ QRS: _____ Interp: _____

Rhythm 21

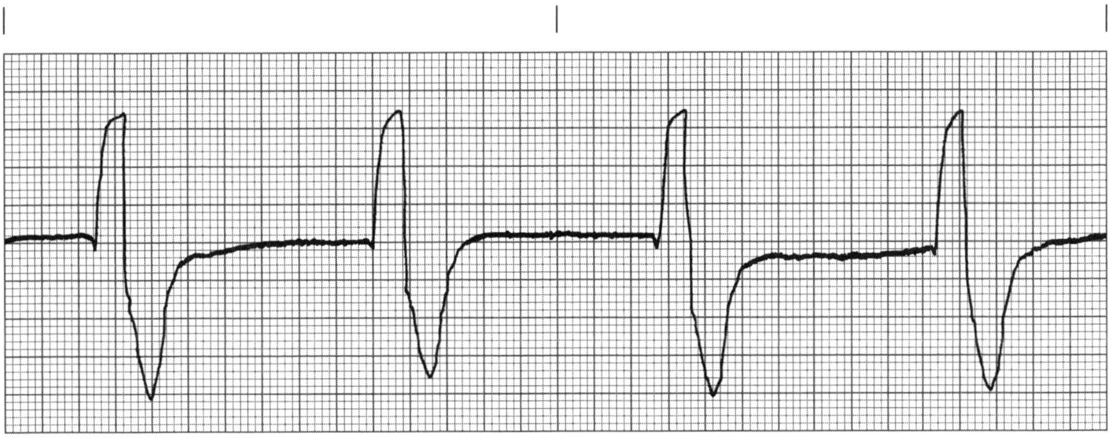

Regularity: _____ Rate: _____ P-Waves: _____
PRI: _____ QRS: _____ Interp: _____

Rhythm 22

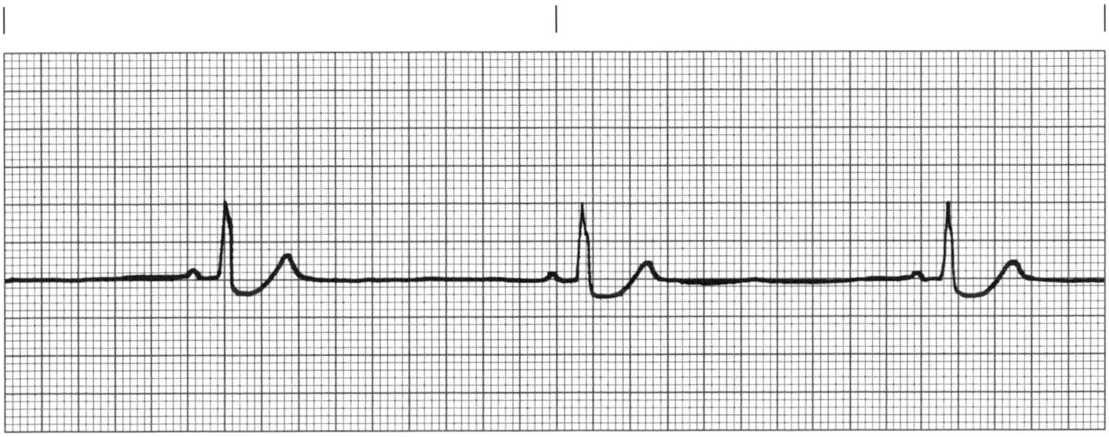

Regularity: _____ Rate: _____ P-Waves: _____
PRI: _____ QRS: _____ Interp: _____

Rhythm 23

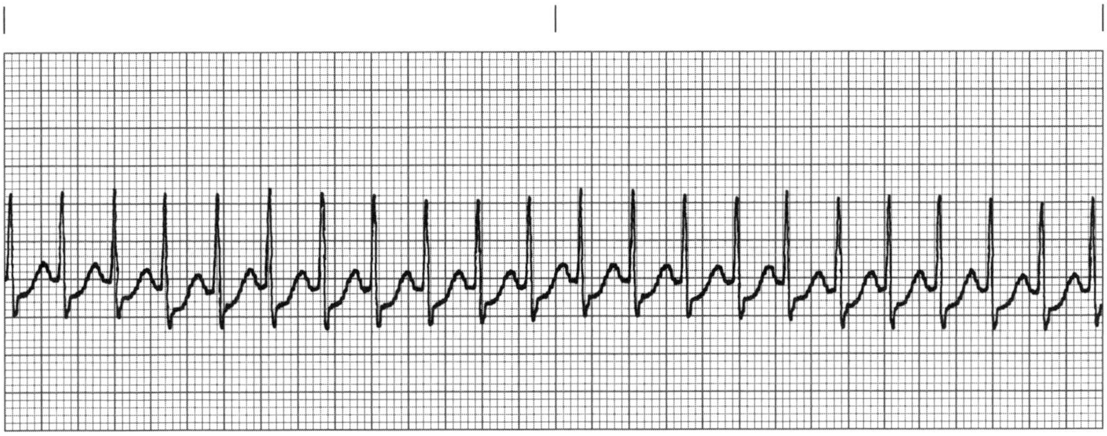

Regularity: _____ Rate: _____ P-Waves: _____
PRI: _____ QRS: _____ Interp: _____

Rhythm 24

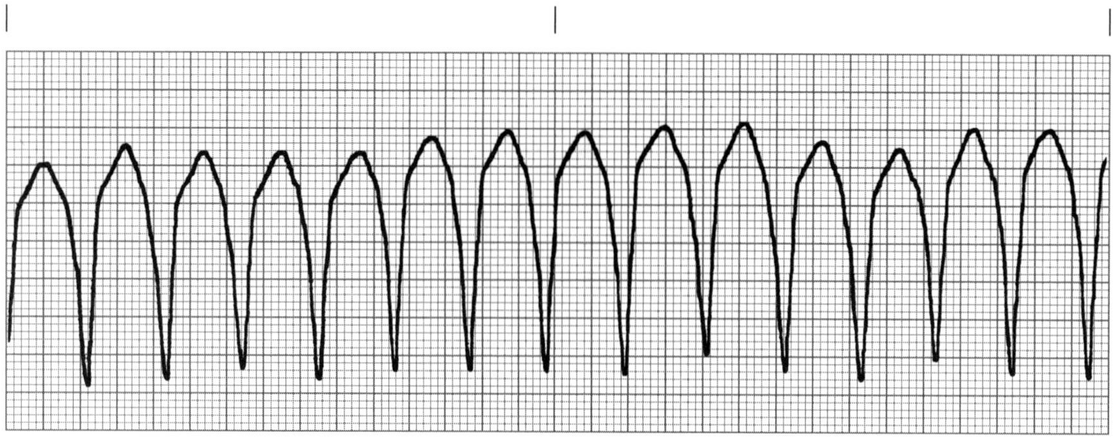

Regularity: _____ Rate: _____ P-waves: _____
PRI: _____ QRS: _____ Interp: _____

Rhythm 25

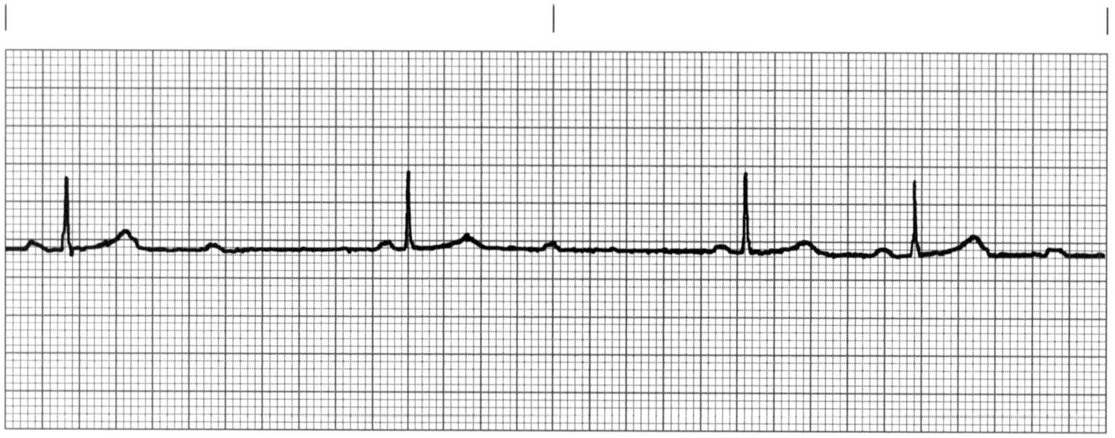

Regularity: _____ Rate: _____ P-Waves: _____
PRI: _____ QRS: _____ Interp: _____

Rhythm 26

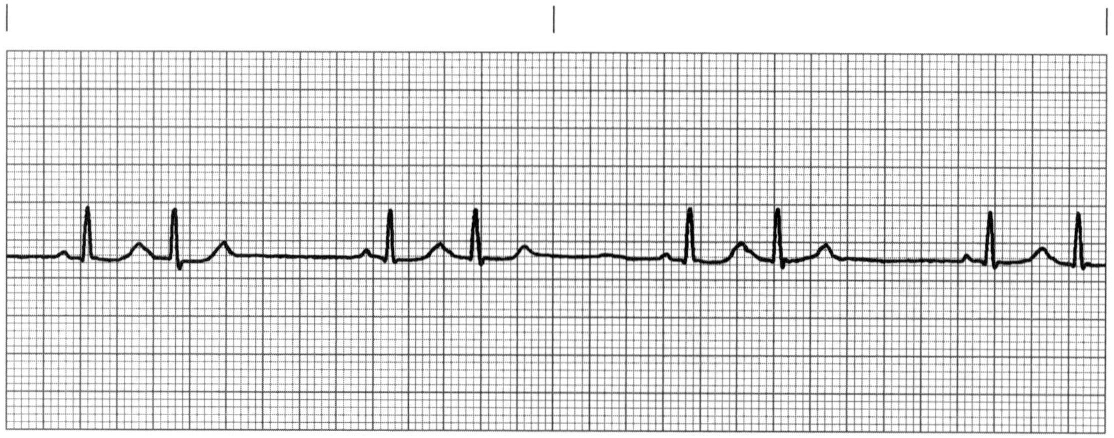

Regularity: _____ Rate: _____ P-Waves: _____
PRI: _____ QRS: _____ Interp: _____

Rhythm 27

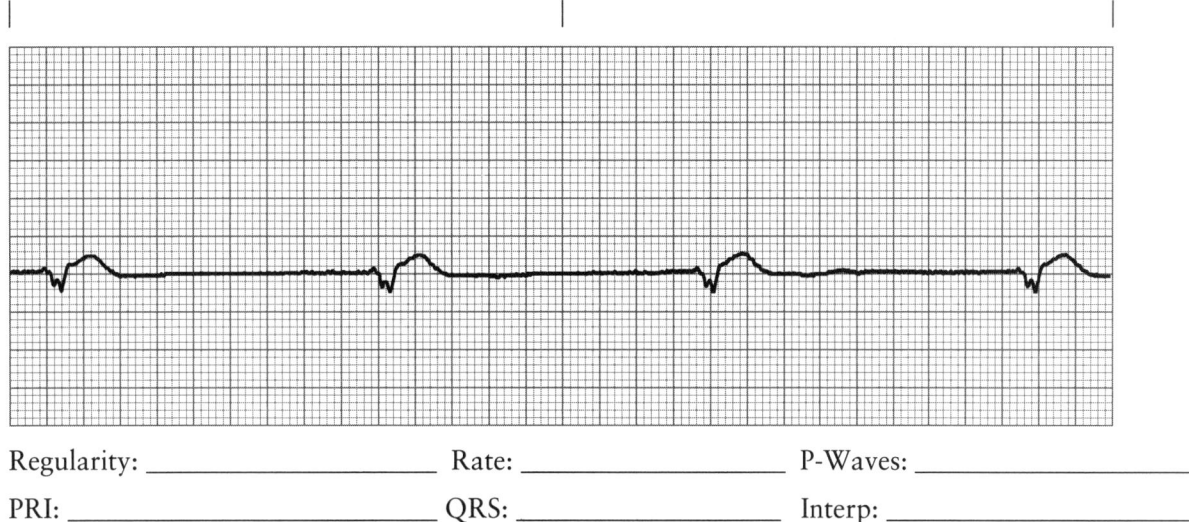

Regularity: _____ Rate: _____ P-Waves: _____
PRI: _____ QRS: _____ Interp: _____

Part 2: Assessment and Management of the Cardiovascular Patient

Review of Chapter Objectives

After reading this part of the chapter, you should be able to:

1. **Identify and describe the components of the focused history as it relates to the patient with cardiovascular compromise.** pp. 1187–1191

   The focused history for cardiac situations uses the same format you learned for pulmonology, the SAMPLE format: Signs/Symptoms, Allergies, Medications, Past medical history, Last oral intake, and Events preceding the incident.

   - **Signs/Symptoms.** The most common symptoms of cardiac disease/compromise include chest pain or discomfort, dyspnea, cough, syncope, and palpitations.

     Use the OPQRST format (also something you encountered with pulmonology) to assess chest pain or discomfort: Onset of pain, Provocation/Palliation of pain, Quality of pain, Region where felt/Radiation, Severity, and Timing (duration). (See also objective 15 for full detail.) Questions concerning dyspnea are similar: You want to know how long it has lasted and whether it is continuous or intermittent. Was onset rapid or gradual? Does anything specific either worsen or palliate the dyspnea, and is it exertional or not? Last, be sure to see if orthopnea exists: Does sitting upright give any relief? Questions about cough center on whether it is chronic or acute and whether it suggests congestive heart failure (dry or productive, presence of any wheezing with cough, and so on).

     In addition, observe and question for these possible signs/symptoms: level of consciousness, diaphoresis, restlessness/anxiety, feeling of impending doom, nausea/vomiting, fatigue, palpitations, edema of extremities or positional (sacral), headache, syncope, behavioral change, facial expression, limitation of activity, signs of recent trauma. Many signs/symptoms of cardiovascular disease and compromise can be subtle or change (either rapidly or gradually) over time.

   - **Allergies.** Check for allergies to medication (prescription and over-the-counter) or X-ray contrast dyes. Try to distinguish between details suggestive of side effect (such as GI upset) and those of allergy (rash, hives, anaphylactic shock).

- **Medications.** Check both for current medications (again, prescription and over-the-counter) and recent medication changes. If there has been a recent change, ask why. Look for the use of cardiovascular drugs such as nitroglycerin, propranolol or other beta-blockers, digitalis (digoxin, Lanoxin), diuretics (Lasix, Dyazide), antihypertensives (Capoten, Prinivil, Vasotec), antidysrhythmics (Quinaglute, Mexitil, Tambocor), lipid-lowering agents (Mevacor, Lopid), and erectile dysfunction medications (Viagra, Levitra, Cialis). If possible, check directly (by inspecting the med tray, if there is one) or indirectly (by history) about drug compliance and bring containers to the hospital with you.
- **Past medical history.** Ask directed questions about history of heart disease, MI, stroke, high blood pressure, as well as why suggestive drugs are taken. Specific problems you should inquire about include history of rheumatic heart disease (valvular problems), previous cardiac surgery, congenital cardiac anomalies, pericarditis or other inflammatory cardiac disease, or congestive heart failure (CHF). Relevant problems of other organ systems include pulmonary disease/COPD, diabetes mellitus, renal disease, hypertension, atherosclerosis. Also ask whether there is any family history of illness/death (particularly early deaths before age 50) from cardiovascular disease or other relevant disorders. Last, be sure to ask whether patient smokes or smoked tobacco and whether he/she knows his/her cholesterol level.
- **Last oral intake.** Valuable as a screening question for anyone with a possible surgical condition, this also gives you the chance to ask about most recent caffeine or tobacco use, as well as whether there was a recent fatty meal. (For some patients, this may help steer you to gallbladder disorders.)
- **Events preceding incident.** Ask what the patient was doing just before onset of symptoms. Was there emotional stress or physical exertion? Was there sexual activity? If the patient is male, does he take Viagra? It is often uncomfortable to take a sexual history, but sometimes the information gained is lifesaving, and you can explain to the patient the possible importance of the answer.

2. Identify and describe the details of inspection, auscultation, and palpation specific to the cardiovascular system. pp. 1191–1194

Always do visual inspection first. (1) Look for tracheal position. If it isn't in its normal midline position but is toward one side, there may be a pneumothorax. (2) Check neck veins for signs of jugular distention (have the patient elevated about 45° and with head turned to the side). Jugular venous distention (JVD) is evidence of back pressure from causes such as heart (pump) failure or cardiac tamponade. (3) Thorax and chest movement while breathing should be observed with proper exposure so you can see chest shape (barrel chests may indicate COPD) and effort during respiration, such as retractions of the soft tissues between the ribs. Accessory muscles are used when breathing is difficult and may include those of the neck, back, and abdomen. Always look for surgical scars; a scar over the sternum may indicate prior cardiac surgery. (4) Evaluate the epigastrium while the chest wall is exposed, looking for distention and visible pulsations. Pulsations may signal an aortic aneurysm dissection or rupture. (5) Position-dependent edema may be found in the ankles or sacral area, depending on whether the patient has been sitting or lying in bed. Pitting edema (a depression that persists after you stop applying firm pressure) is significant. (6) Skin changes associated with cardiovascular disease include pallor and diaphoresis (indicating increased sympathetic tone and peripheral vasoconstriction) or a mottled appearance (often an indicator of chronic cardiac failure). (7) Subtle changes associated with cardiovascular disease include not only surgical scars but subcutaneous batteries for a pacemaker or nitroglycerin skin patches.

Auscultation includes listening to the lungs, to the heart, and over the carotid arteries. (1) Assess the lung fields for equality and for sounds such as crackles, rhonchi (whistling or snoring-like sounds), or wheezes, which may signal pulmonary edema or primary pulmonary disease. Note that patients with pulmonary edema may have foamy, blood-tinged sputum evident at the mouth and nose. In advanced cases, you may even hear a gurgling-like sound as the patient breathes. (2) It is difficult to auscultate the heart well in the field because of the number and intensity of background noises. Ideally, you want to listen for heart sounds at four classic sites: aortic, pulmonic, mitral (left AV valve), and tricuspid (right AV valve). The point on the chest wall where heartbeat is loudest or is best felt is called the point of maximum impulse (PMI). (3) Auscultation over the carotid arteries may reveal bruits, murmur sounds due to turbulent flow. A bruit over any artery indicates partial obstruction due to atherosclerosis. Never attempt carotid sinus massage in a patient with a bruit because you might dislodge atherosclerotic material that could lodge in a cerebral artery causing a stroke or other mishap.

Palpation should cover three areas: peripheral pulse, thorax, and epigastrium. (1) Determine rate and regularity of the pulse as well as equality. A pulse deficit (intensity less than expected) may indicate underlying peripheral vascular disease and should be reported to medical direction. (2) Thoracic palpation is extremely important and may reveal crepitus, akin to "bubble wrap" crackling under your fingers, which suggests subcutaneous emphysema. Check for tenderness or possible rib fracture. Remember that at least 15 percent of MI patients have some associated chest wall tenderness. (3) Abdominal exam may reveal distention or pulsations.

3. **Identify and define the heart sounds and relate them to hemodynamic events in the cardiac cycle.** pp. 1192–1193

   Everyone is familiar with the lub-dub of normal heart sounds. The first component, called S_1, is produced by the closing of the AV valves during ventricular systole (at the beginning of the ventricular contraction that expels blood into the aorta and pulmonary artery). The second heart sound (S_2) is produced by the closure of the aortic and pulmonary valves as the ventricles begin to relax and the heart fills with blood again (at early diastole).

4. **Describe the differences between normal and abnormal heart sounds.** pp. 1192–1193

   Any extra heart sounds (beyond S_1 and S_2) are abnormal. The sound termed S_3 is associated with congestive heart failure, and it has a cadence like that of the word Kentucky; when it is present, it follows S_2. The fourth heart sound, S_4, appears just before S_1 when it is present, and it is associated with increased effort of atrial contraction. Its cadence resembles that of Tennessee.

5. **Define pulse deficit, pulsus paradoxus, and pulsus alternans.** pp. 1194, 1222

   A pulse deficit is the less intense of two peripheral pulses that you would expect to be equal, for instance, the right and left carotid or right or left radial pulses. The pulse with the deficit often reflects an artery that is partially blocked by atherosclerosis. Pulsus paradoxus is related to a change in blood pressure with respiration. Specifically, pulsus paradoxus exists when systolic blood pressure decreases by more than 10 mmHg with inspiration, and it is due to compression of either the great vessels or the ventricles. Pulsus alternans exists when the pulse alternates between weak and strong intensity over time. In such cases, pulses may be felt as thready or weak on examination.

6. **Identify the normal characteristics of the point of maximum impulse (PMI).** p. 1193

   The point on the chest wall where heartbeat is loudest on auscultation is usually the point where palpation finds the strongest impulse of the beating heart. This location is called the point of maximum impulse (PMI). You can find additional information about the PMI and cardiac examination in Division 2.

7. **Based on field impressions, identify the need for rapid intervention for the patient in cardiovascular compromise.** pp. 1186–1194

   As with any other patient, your first responsibilities are to check airway, breathing, circulation, and the possibility of shock. Only after you have managed life-threatening problems (and if new, life-threatening problems don't develop) can you communicate with and support the patient and family. Note that interventions in the field beyond the absolutely essential are generally limited to administration of analgesia or nitrates for chest pain, treatment of pulmonary edema, and administration of appropriate analgesia for peripheral vascular emergencies. Do be sure, however, to look for the obvious and subtle signs of cardiovascular disease during the focused history and physical. The discovery of an abdominal pulsation that might signal aortic aneurysm dissection or rupture in a patient with some signs of early shock changes the dynamic for intervention and transportation greatly.

8. Describe the incidence, morbidity, and mortality associated with myocardial conduction defects. p. 1216

Remember that dysrhythmias arising from coronary heart disease, or CHD (often part of myocardial ischemia or infarction), cause many of the sudden deaths associated with CHD, and these deaths are too numerous. About 225,000 Americans have CHD-induced deaths before they can reach a hospital; this amounts to roughly one death per minute. Dysrhythmias are the most common complication of MI and the most common cause of death from an MI. Life-threatening dysrhythmias can develop very early in the course of myocardial ischemia and can cause sudden death (immediate or within one hour of onset of symptoms).

Conduction abnormalities also arise directly from disease or from drug effects or electrolyte abnormalities. Among the forms of AV block, third-degree block is the most serious: In this type, none of the impulses originating in the atria reach the ventricles. Ventricular rate and rhythm are dependent on development of a ventricular escape rhythm. This can lead to morbidity through symptomatic bradycardia and heart failure. In some situations, cardiac arrest and death may result. Bundle branch block can result from age-related deterioration, MI, or transient causes such as drugs and electrolyte abnormalities. Part of your concern with cases of left bundle branch block should lie in the fact that nothing else can be determined from the ECG regarding possible ischemic change. Thus, a patient with left bundle branch block can have a significant MI and ECG changes will not be seen; this can increase the morbidity or mortality from the MI.

9. Identify the clinical indications, components, and the function of transcutaneous and permanent artificial cardiac pacing. pp. 1179, 1182–1183, 1206, 1207–1208

Permanent artificial pacemakers are generally inserted into patients who have chronic high-grade AV block or sick sinus syndrome or who have had episodes of severe symptomatic bradycardia in the past. The pacemaker (the pulse generator) is implanted near the heart, and its discharge lead is inserted into either the right ventricle or right atrium and ventricle, depending on whether it is a ventricular-type pacemaker or a dual-chambered pacemaker (see Figure 28-45). The battery packs are usually palpable in their subcutaneous position (often in the shoulder or axillary region). Permanent pacemakers are of two functional types: Either they can pace continuously or they can pace when the heart's natural rate falls below a preset number of beats per minute. (The two types are called fixed-rate and demand pacemakers.) In all cases, the pacemaker should enable the patient to have a heart rate and rhythm that supports adequate cardiac output.

Transcutaneous cardiac pacing (TCP) allows electrical pacing of the heart through the skin via specially designed thoracic electrodes. You will need to have one of the newer cardiac monitor/defibrillators with an appropriate built-in pacing device. TCP may be highly beneficial for patients with symptomatic bradycardia such as high-degree AV block, atrial fibrillation with slow ventricular response, or other significant bradycardias and asystole. You can use TCP if pharmacological intervention fails and if the patient is hypotensive or hypoperfusing to try to establish a rate and rhythm compatible with adequate cardiac output. You can also use TCP to provide overdrive pacing to suppress recurrent tachycardia or in torsade de pointes, a specific form of ventricular tachycardia.

10. Explain what each setting and indicator on a transcutaneous pacing system represents and how the settings may be adjusted. pp. 1207–1208

One system setting is for heart rate: The range available is typically 60 to 80 bpm, and you will consult with medical direction about setting the appropriate rate. The output setting (in amps) should initially be set to 0 and then gradually increased until you see the pacemaker spike on ECG that shows ventricular capture. Maintenance rate and output are arranged with medical direction. With a patient in asystole, output is generally begun at the maximum setting, with output gradually lowered if ventricular capture occurs.

11. Describe the techniques of applying a transcutaneous pacing system. pp. 1206, 1207

There are eleven steps involved in applying and monitoring TCP. (1) Establish IV access and ECG monitoring and administer oxygen. (2) Place the patient in a supine position. (3) Confirm symptomatic bradycardia (the usual indication) and medical direction's order for TCP. (4) Apply the pacing electrodes according to the manufacturer's directions. Be sure they adhere well to the skin. (5) Connect the electrodes. (6) Set desired heart rate on the pacemaker. (7) Turn output setting to 0. (8) Turn on pacer. (9) Slowly increase output until you see ECG spikes indicating ventricular capture. (10) Check the patient's pulse and blood pressure and adjust rate and amperage (output) per instructions from medical direction. (11) Monitor patient response to treatment.

12. Describe the characteristics of an implanted pacemaking system.   pp. 1179, 1181–1182

See the first part of objective 9 on permanent pacemakers.

13. Describe the epidemiology, morbidity, mortality, and pathophysiology of angina pectoris.   pp. 1211–1212

Angina pectoris, or pain in the chest, occurs when the myocardial demand for oxygen exceeds the available supply through the coronary arteries. Myocardial ischemia causes the chest pain. Usually, reduced blood flow through the coronary arteries is correlated with permanent partial obstruction by atherosclerotic lesions. Angina can also result from spasm of the coronary arteries (arterial vasospasm), temporarily reducing the diameter of the lumen and blood flow. About two-thirds of patients with vasospastic angina (commonly called Prinzmetal's angina) have atherosclerosis involving the coronaries. Epidemiologically, though, this still means roughly one-third of patients with Prinzmetal's angina do not have significant coronary atherosclerosis and thus may not fit the risk factor profile for atherosclerosis.

The epidemiology, morbidity, and mortality of cardiovascular disease, including coronary heart disease (CHD, disease of the coronary arteries), are covered in depth in objectives 1 and 3 of Part 1 of this chapter.

14. Describe the assessment and management of a patient with angina pectoris.   pp. 1213–1214

During assessment, remember that weak or absent peripheral pulses (especially when symmetric or global) may signal impending shock, which requires immediate intervention. Pallor and cyanosis of the skin or cold extremities also suggest shock. Because angina is a progressive disorder, a history of angina does not mean that the current episode is "safe." If it is important enough to activate EMS, it is important enough for your full attention and the suspicion of serious underlying problems such as acute MI. Listen to the history of the current event: The chief complaint is usually sudden onset chest pain. Pain may radiate or be localized to the chest. Angina usually lasts 3 to 5 minutes, although it may last as long as 15 minutes, and it is generally relieved by rest and/or nitroglycerin. Prinzmetal angina is often accompanied by S-T segment elevation on ECG, which may indicate myocardial tissue ischemia. Breathing may or may not be labored, but you should check for lung sounds after ensuring the airway is patent. Listen for congestion, especially at the bases. Although the anginal patient's rate and rhythm may be altered, they may be normal, and peripheral pulses should be equal and normal. Typically, blood pressure rises during the anginal episode and normalizes afterward. Ask the patient for his/her baseline BP, as hypertension may be present. If it is possible without prolonging the time on scene, get an ECG tracing. A 12-lead ECG provides more information and should be done if possible.

Management includes placing the patient at physical and emotional rest to decrease myocardial oxygen demand: Give oxygen, generally at high-flow rate. Establish IV access on scene or en route to the hospital. Conduct the ECG; do not, however, delay transport to perform it. You can give nitroglycerin sublingually as a tablet or spray. If symptoms persist after 1 to 2 doses, raise your suspicion for a more serious condition such as acute MI. Nifedipine and other calcium channel blockers can also be used for relief of anginal pain: Morphine may be used for nonresponsive chest pain.

Patients with an initial episode of angina or an episode that does not respond to medication are usually admitted for observation. Immediate transport is indicated if relief does not come after oxygen and nitrates. The absence of relief may signal the beginning of infarction, and in this case reperfusion is crucial. Hypotension may occur, especially if nitroglycerin has been given. It indicates transport as well because it can lead to or worsen hypoperfusion of myocardial tissue.

S-T segment changes, particularly elevation, also indicate the need for rapid, efficient transport: Transport should be WITHOUT lights or siren, if possible, in order to minimize patient anxiety.

If the patient refuses transport, be sure you clearly explain that immediate evaluation is vital because of the potential for problems such as MI. If you can't reverse the patient's decision, be sure the patient reads and signs the refusal and understands the potential risks. Ask that they contact their cardiologist or other physician for follow-up as soon as possible.

15. **Identify what is meant by the OPQRST of chest pain assessment.** pp. 1187–1188

Use the OPQRST format (also something you encountered with pulmonology) to assess chest pain or discomfort: Onset of pain, Provocation/Palliation of pain, Quality of pain, Region where felt/Radiation, Severity, and Timing (duration). Questions about onset include when pain began and what was happening at the time. Ask a patient who has had prior episodes of chest pain to compare this one with prior episodes. If it is described as similar to pain that signaled a prior heart attack, you can strongly assume the pain is cardiac in origin. Questions on provocation and palliation of pain also may point to angina or toward another cause. In particular, ask about any relationship to exertion of any type or palliation with rest. If there have been multiple episodes, ask whether it takes less to trigger an episode now than in the past. Ask a general question about the quality of the pain and let the patient describe it. Common words include sharp, tearing, pressured, or heavy. Radiation of chest pain may occur to arm(s), neck, jaw, and/or back. Again, ask if this pattern fits earlier episodes. Ask the patient to evaluate the severity of the pain on a scale of 1 to 10 (be sure you use the same scale that will be used at the hospital in order to standardize response significance): You can ask the same question later to assess efficacy of therapy. Timing questions get information on how long the pain has lasted (write down the time the patient first noted pain as this may affect decisions later regarding possible fibrinolytic therapy) as well as whether pain has been constant or intermittent or has changed with time (Better? Worse?).

16. **List other clinical conditions that may mimic signs and symptoms of coronary artery disease and angina pectoris.** p. 1212

Causes of chest pain fall into four categories: cardiovascular, respiratory, gastrointestinal, and musculoskeletal. You'll note that the causes range from the troublesome but benign (dyspepsia, or heartburn) to the life threatening (aortic dissection). Cardiovascular causes include coronary artery disease and angina, but also pericarditis and dissection of the thoracic aorta. Respiratory causes include pulmonary embolism, pneumothorax, pneumonia, and pleurisy (pleural inflammation). GI causes are diverse: cholecystitis (gallbladder origin), pancreatitis, hiatal hernia, esophageal disease, gastroesophageal reflux (GERD), peptic ulcer disease, and dyspepsia. Musculoskeletal causes include chest wall syndrome, costochondritis, acromioclavicular disease, herpes zoster (shingles), chest wall trauma, and chest wall tumors. You should always be prepared to treat patients with chest pain as if they may have cardiac ischemia or another major disease process. Only after you have excluded these possibilities should you consider the less critical causes.

17. **Identify the ECG findings in patients with angina pectoris.** p. 1213

An ECG should be done on scene; if that would delay transport, it may be done en route. If possible, get a 12-lead ECG because it provides more information. Typical findings in patients with angina include S-T depression and/or T wave inversion. After relief of pain, ECG usually returns to baseline. The most common finding in angina is S-T depression, although Prinzmetal patients typically show S-T elevation. Note that S-T segment changes are not specific, and dysrhythmias and ectopy may not be seen either. Be sure to transmit the ECG to medical direction and discuss as necessary.

18. **Based on the pathophysiology and clinical evaluation of the patient with chest pain, list the anticipated clinical problems according to their life-threatening potential.** p. 1212

Because angina, whether typical (obstructive) or vasospastic (namely, Prinzmetal's angina), reflects myocardial ischemia, progression to myocardial infarction is always possible. ECG monitoring may pick up signs of ischemia or infarction, as well as related cardiac problems such as dysrhythmia and ectopy, all of which can rapidly develop into life-threatening conditions. Aortic dissection is a life-threatening emergency, as can be pericarditis if pressure on the heart decreases cardiac output to the point of hypoperfusion of the heart (causing angina) or other vital organs such as the brain. Pulmonary embolism may also present as a life-threatening emergency if the embolus is very large or affects flow into both lungs. Pneumothorax and pneumonia are always serious, but they may also be life threatening in a patient with previously compromised cardiopulmonary function. Pleurisy, suspected cholecystitis or pancreatitis, and esophageal disease and peptic ulcer disease are also serious. If any of the GI conditions involve hemorrhage, the patient's condition may become unstable, especially if cardiopulmonary compromise exists. Always carry a degree of suspicion of impending or possible shock. Other causes, including the musculoskeletal causes as well as GI problems such as hiatal hernia, merit medical workup, but these patients are unlikely to be unstable on scene or during transport. In some cases, such as known GERD, dyspepsia, or costochondritis, a patient with no other signs of a serious condition and no change in condition while you are on scene may refuse transport. You should always advocate follow-up as quickly as possible with the personal physician because the complaint was severe enough to warrant the call to EMS.

19. **Describe the epidemiology, morbidity, mortality, and pathophysiology of myocardial infarction.** pp. 1214–1215

Each year about 466,000 Americans die from coronary heart disease (CHD), and myocardial infarction (MI) is the usual direct cause of death. In addition, an American suffers a nonfatal MI every 29 seconds. Myocardial infarction, the death of myocardial tissue, is the result of prolonged oxygen deprivation or when myocardial oxygen demand exceeds oxygen supply for an extended period. MI is most often associated with atherosclerotic heart disease (ASHD, which is the same as atherosclerotic coronary heart disease). The precipitating event is often development of a thrombus in a partially occluded artery, with the thrombus completely occluding the vessel. Other pathophysiologic bases for MI include coronary artery spasm, microemboli as can be seen with cocaine use, acute volume overload, hypotension (causing myocardial hypoperfusion), or acute respiratory failure (leading to acute hypoxia). Trauma can also cause MI, often by loosening atherosclerotic plaque in the coronary artery, blocking it.

The region of the heart affected and the size of the eventual infarcted area depend on the coronary artery involved and the specific site of the obstruction. Most infarctions involve the left ventricle. Obstruction of the left coronary artery or its branches may result in infarction of the anterior or lateral ventricle or the interventricular septum. Right coronary artery occlusions tend to result in infarction of the inferior or posterior wall of the left ventricle or infarction of the right ventricle.

The pathophysiologic progression of events starts with ischemia, followed by cell death. The infarcted tissue becomes necrotic and eventually forms scar tissue, if the affected individual survives. Ischemic tissue at the periphery of the infarct will survive but may become the origin of dysrhythmias. Dysrhythmias are the most common complication of MI and the most common cause of death from an MI.

Infarction of myocardium can cause congestive heart failure. Heart failure implies that the heart is working poorly but adequately. If the heart cannot meet body oxygen demand, cardiogenic shock results. Last, if the damaged portion of the ventricular wall is too weakened, it may form a ventricular aneurysm and rupture, causing death.

Based on pathophysiology, the basic strategies of intervention are pain relief and reperfusion. For reperfusion to be effective, rapid, safe transport is essential.

20. **List the mechanisms by which a myocardial infarction may be produced from traumatic and nontraumatic events.** p. 1214

See objective 19.

21. **Identify the primary hemodynamic changes produced in myocardial infarction.** pp. 1214–1215

In order for myocardial tissue to become ischemic, there is either hypoperfusion or low blood oxygen. Hypoperfusion is the typical cause of ischemia and eventual infarction. If the affected myocardium includes conductive tissue, dysrhythmias such as ventricular tachycardia or ventricular fibrillation may result. Even if rhythm is preserved, it is possible that infarction can cause pump failure of either the right or left ventricle or both, resulting in heart failure. If the pump failure is severe, cardiogenic shock develops.

22. **List and describe the assessment parameters to be evaluated in a patient with a suspected myocardial infarction.** pp. 1215–1216

Initial size-up, inspection, and vital signs may reveal a lot. Is breathing labored? Is the patient diaphoretic and pale? Are there other signs of shock? Remember that blood pressure usually elevates during an episode of ischemia and then returns to normal. Hypotension more likely suggests cardiac compromise and possible shock. Peripheral pulses should be regular and equal. Irregularities may suggest dysrhythmia.

As you move through the OPQRST mnemonic, look for these signs of MI: sudden onset chest pain that proves to be severe, constant, and unrelenting over a period longer than 30 minutes. Pain may radiate to the arms (usually the left), neck, back, or into the epigastrium. Myocardial ischemia can easily produce pain in the 8–10 range and the pain may be associated with nausea and vomiting. Unlike the situation with angina, neither rest nor nitroglycerin will palliate MI pain. Remember that patients with diabetes mellitus may NOT have this picture even when an MI is in evolution. These patients may minimize the severity of their discomfort or simply complain of feeling unwell. Typically, these patients do not have nausea and vomiting. MIs typically evolve over 48 to 72 hours, and so the pain seen at 24 to 48 hours may be very different than if you had seen the patient in the first 12 to 24 hours after onset of discomfort.

Emotion may suggest MI. Patients with severe chest pain often are very frightened and complain of a sense of doom or fear of death. Denial of emotional upset or severity of pain does not mean a benign episode. Denial may hide severe fear or pain.

Auscultation of the lung fields may show clear fields or congestion in the bases. Other physical findings typical of MI include pallor and diaphoresis, coldness in the extremities, and possible change in body temperature. Heart rate and rhythm may be irregular or not. Blood pressure may be baseline, high, or low.

The ECG should be checked first for underlying rhythm and any sign of dysrhythmia. If you have a 12-lead ECG, look at the S-T segment and QRS complex. Check S-T segment for height, depth, and overall contour. Note any depression or elevation. A pathological Q wave (one deeper than 5 mm and wider than 0.04 sec) can indicate infarcted tissue or extensive transient ischemia. Anticipate dysrhythmias.

Next, assess whether the patient is a likely candidate for rapid transport and reperfusion therapy with fibrinolytic agents. The time window for fibrinolytic therapy to be effective is generally considered to be the first 6 hours from onset of symptoms. Consult medical direction. Note that some patients will have contraindications to fibrinolytic therapy, including bleeding or clotting disorders, possible blood in the stool, uncontrolled hypertension, recent trauma, recent hemorrhagic stroke, or recent surgery. Generally, signs of acute injury or pathological Q waves indicate transport for reperfusion if you are within the 6-hour window. If you are uncertain whether the patient meets criteria for reperfusion therapy, assume that he/she does. Be sure to relay information to medical direction including time of pain onset, any S-T segment change (particularly elevation), and location of ischemia or infarct according to a 12-lead ECG.

23. **Identify the anticipated clinical presentation of a patient with a suspected acute myocardial infarction.** pp. 1215–1216

See objective 22.

24. **Differentiate the characteristics of the pain/discomfort occurring in angina pectoris and acute myocardial infarction.** p. 1215

Typical picture of angina: The chief complaint is usually sudden onset chest pain. Pain may radiate or be localized to the chest. Angina usually lasts 3 to 5 minutes, although it may last as long as 15 minutes, and it is generally relieved by rest and/or nitroglycerin. Breathing may or may not be labored, but you should check for lung sounds after ensuring airway is patent.

Typical picture of MI: There is a sudden onset chest pain that proves to be severe, constant, and unrelenting over a period longer than 30 minutes. Pain may radiate to the arms (usually the left), neck, back, or into the epigastrium. An MI can produce pain in the 8–10 range and the pain may be associated with nausea and vomiting. Unlike the situation with angina, neither rest nor nitroglycerin will palliate MI pain. Blood pressure may be high, low, or baseline, but it is unlikely to change solely with decrease in pain.

25. **Identify the ECG changes characteristically seen during evolution of an acute myocardial infarction.** p. 1216

See objective 22.

26. **Identify the most common complications of an acute myocardial infarction.** pp. 1214–1216

Dysrhythmias are the most common complication and one of the most common causes of death associated with MI. Congestive heart failure, or even overt cardiogenic shock, can also occur with an MI, especially when the infarcted area is very large or represents tissue loss on top of previous losses from prior MIs. Rupture of ventricular aneurysms, weakened areas of a ventricular wall due to MI, is another complication and cause of sudden death.

27. **List the characteristics of a patient eligible for fibrinolytic therapy.** pp. 1218–1220

The most essential element of eligibility is time from onset of symptoms, as a duration beyond 6 hours from onset is generally correlated with poor success of fibrinolytic therapy. In addition, patients who have contraindications to fibrinolytic therapy include persons with bleeding or clotting disorders, possible blood in the stool (GI bleeding), uncontrolled hypertension, recent trauma, recent surgery, or recent hemorrhagic stroke.

28. **Describe the "window of opportunity" as it pertains to reperfusion of a myocardial injury or infarction.** p. 1218

Reperfusion therapy with a fibrinolytic agent is most likely to be successful from the onset of symptoms to 6 hours later. Sometimes the window is expanded slightly for a younger patient or one with serious complications.

29. **Based on the pathophysiology and clinical evaluation of the patient with a suspected acute myocardial infarction, list the anticipated clinical problems according to their life-threatening potential.** pp. 1214–1220

Dysrhythmias are the most common complication and one of the most common causes of death associated with myocardial infarction. Cardiogenic shock results from loss of cardiac function such that the minimal oxygen needs of the body are not met. A lesser loss of cardiac function can result in congestive heart failure. An uncommon complication that can result in death is rupture of a ventricular aneurysm.

30. **Specify the measures that may be taken to prevent or minimize complications in the patient suspected of myocardial infarction.** pp. 1216–1220

Act expediently and calmly and keep the patient in as much physical and emotional rest as possible. Provide supplemental oxygen to decrease myocardial oxygen demand and increase available oxygen. Always have good IV access (possibly more than one IV line). Be sure to ask about medication allergies (especially to any that may have been used previously in a cardiac setting) before the patient or family may become unable to give you this information. Transport as rapidly as possible with no lights or sirens if possible. Delay in transport, however, is preferable to a patient's refusal to leave the scene.

31. Describe the most commonly used cardiac drugs in terms of therapeutic effect and dosages, routes of administration, side effects, and toxic effects. pp. 1199, 1200, 1218; see Chapter 6

The classes of drugs you are most likely to use in the setting of an MI are antidysrhythmics, sympathomimetics, and drugs specific for use in the setting of ischemia (including the fibrinolytics), along with less frequently used prehospital medications.

Antidysrhythmics
Antidysrhythmics control or suppress dysrhythmias. Among the most commonly used are atropine, lidocaine, procainamide, bretylium, adenosine, amiodarone, and verapamil.

- Atropine sulfate is a parasympatholytic agent (one that decreases parasympathetic effect by acting as an anticholinergic) used to treat symptomatic bradycardias, especially those arising in the atria, and is sometimes used as part of a treatment regimen for asystole. Dose is 0.5–1.0 mg IV for bradycardia and 1.0 mg for asystole, repeated every 3 to 5 minutes as needed until a total dose of 0.04 mg/kg is reached. Endotracheal (ET) doses are 2.0–2.5 times the IV doses. Side effects include blurred vision, dilated pupils, dry mouth, tachycardia, and drowsiness. It has no contraindications in the EMS setting.
- Lidocaine is a first-line antidysrhythmic used to treat and prevent life-threatening ventricular dysrhythmias such as ventricular tachycardia. It suppresses abnormal irritability in the ventricles while having little effect on normal myocardial tissue. Dose is 1.0–1.5 mg/kg slow IV push (50 mg/min) for ectopy, or normal IV push in cardiac arrest. An IV drip is prepared by mixing 1 gram into 250 cc D_5W or saline. Typical maintenance dose is 2–4 mg/minute. Maximum bolus dose is 300 mg. The drug can be given IV bolus, IV drip, or through an ET tube. Side effects include drowsiness, seizures, confusion, bradycardia, heart blocks, and nausea and vomiting. Lidocaine is contraindicated by the presence of second- or third-degree AV block.
- Procainamide is a second-line antidysrhythmic to lidocaine, and it is used for ventricular dysrhythmias refractory to lidocaine or for patients who are allergic to lidocaine. It is administered by slow IV bolus or IV drip. IV bolus is 100 mg given over 5 minutes, with a maximum dose of 17 mg/kg. Discontinue when the dysrhythmia is suppressed, hypotension ensues, the QRS complex widens 50 percent, or the maximum dose is given. Drip rate is the same as for lidocaine. Side effects and contraindications are the same as for lidocaine.
- Bretylium is a second-line antidysrhythmic used to treat life-threatening ventricular dysrhythmias, especially ventricular fibrillation. Although its mechanism of action is poorly understood, bretylium apparently raises the ventricular fibrillation threshold. Bretylium is administered by IV bolus and IV drip. Dose is 5 mg/kg IV push with drip rate of 1–2 mg/min. A subsequent dose of 10 mg/kg is repeated if the dysrhythmia persists. Maximum dose is 30 mg/kg. Side effects include hypo- or hypertension, dizziness, syncope, seizures, and nausea and vomiting. Bretylium is now being used less frequently because of development of other agents.
- Adenosine is used to manage supraventricular tachydysrhythmias. It is a naturally occurring nucleoside that acts on the AV node to slow conduction and inhibit reentry pathways. It is given by IV rapid bolus through a venous site as close to the heart as possible. Flush the line with saline immediately after giving adenosine to ensure drug delivery. Initial dose is 6 mg (rapid push) followed by a 15–30 cc saline flush. If the tachydysrhythmia is not eliminated, a second dose of 12 mg and, if needed, a third dose of 12 mg may be given. Maximum dose is 30 mg. Side effects include apprehension, burning sensation, heavy sensation in the arms, hypotension, chest pressure, diaphoresis, numbness or tingling, dyspnea, tightness in the throat and/or groin pressure, headache, and nausea and vomiting. Adenosine is contraindicated in the presence of second- or third-degree AV block or in sick sinus syndrome unless a pacemaker is present.
- Amiodarone (Cordarone) is an antidysrhythmic used in management of recurring ventricular fibrillation and hemodynamically unstable ventricular tachycardia (nonperfusing tachycardia). Amiodarone is also being used more frequently in the prehospital setting of cardiac arrest. Although it is a second-line drug in the United States, it is a first-line agent in several Commonwealth countries. Dosage is 150–300 mg by slow IV infusion. Side effects include hypotension (the most common), bradycardia, and AV blocks. It is contraindicated in cardiogenic shock, marked sinus bradycardia, and second- or third-degree AV block.

- Verapamil is a calcium channel blocker that slows heart rate in symptomatic atrial tachycardias. It is used to terminate paroxysmal supraventricular tachycardia as well as to control the rapid ventricular response often seen with atrial flutter or fibrillation. It is administered by slow IV bolus with a maximum dose of 30 mg.

Sympathomimetic agents

Sympathomimetic agents are similar to the naturally occurring hormones epinephrine and norepinephrine, and they mimic sympathetic nervous system stimulation on either alpha or beta adrenergic receptors. Alpha receptor stimulation causes peripheral vasoconstriction and beta receptor stimulation increases heart rate and cardiac contractility, causes bronchodilation, and peripheral vasodilation. Stimulation of dopaminergic receptors in the renal and mesenteric vascular beds causes dilation. Commonly used sympathomimetic agents include epinephrine, norepinephrine, isoproterenol, dopamine, and dobutamine.

- Epinephrine, which acts on alpha and beta receptors, is the mainstay of cardiac arrest resuscitation. It is used with ventricular fibrillation, asystole, and pulseless electrical activity. It is also sometimes used for bradycardia refractory to atropine. It is given as IV bolus, subcutaneously, and via ET tube. Dose is 1 mg of 1:10,000 solution given every 3 to 5 minutes.
- Norepinephrine has alpha agonist properties greater than those of epinephrine. It acts on beta receptors to a lesser degree. It is used occasionally in hemodynamically significant hypotension and cardiogenic shock, although dopamine is the first-line agent for these conditions. Norepinephrine may be effective if total peripheral resistance is low, such as in neurogenic shock. It is administered by IV infusion via drip by placing 4 mg into 1000 cc of D_5W (ONLY) to give a concentration of 4 mcg/cc. Initial loading dose is 8–12 mcg/min to give blood pressure of 80–100 mmHg systolic. Maintenance dose is 2–4 mcg/min. Side effects include anxiety, trembling, headache, dizziness, and nausea and vomiting. It can also cause bradycardia. DO NOT use norepinephrine in patients with hypotension from hypovolemia.
- Isoproterenol is rarely used with the advent of TCP, but it is a potent beta agonist that increases heart rate and cardiac contractility. It is used in bradycardia refractory to atropine and to manage asystole. Isoproterenol is given via IV infusion. Add 1 mg to 250 cc D_5W or saline to give 4 mcg/cc. The drip rate is 2–20 mcg/min. Common procedure is to start with a low dose and titrate upward until a satisfactory rate is achieved. TCP is preferred to use of isoproterenol.
- Dopamine (Intropin) is a vasopressor that increases cardiac output. It stimulates both alpha and beta receptors. It has the advantage over other drugs of preserving renal perfusion at recommended doses. Dose is given via IV drip by mixing 800 mg into 500 cc D_5W or saline to give a concentration of 1600 mcg/cc (400 mg into 250 cc also works). Dopamine's effects are dose-related: At 1–2 mcg/kg/min, renal artery dilation occurs; at 2–10 mcg/kg/min, beta receptors are primarily stimulated; at 10–15 mcg/kg/min, both beta and alpha receptors are stimulated; and at 15–20 mcg/kg/min, alpha receptors are primarily stimulated. Side effects include nervousness, headache, dysrhythmias, palpitations, chest pain, dyspnea, and nausea and vomiting. Note: Dopamine is contraindicated for hypovolemic shock until fluid resuscitation has been completed.
- Dobutamine (Dobutrex), like dopamine, increases cardiac output and increases stroke volume. It has little effect on heart rate and is occasionally used in isolated left heart failure until medications such as digitalis can take effect. Dobutamine is given by IV infusion by mixing 250 mg into 250 cc D_5W or saline to give a concentration of 1000 mcg/cc. Dose is 2–10 mcg/kg/min titrated to effect. Its side effects are the same as dopamine's. Do not use dobutamine as the sole agent in hypovolemic shock unless fluid resuscitation is complete. Dopamine is preferred over dobutamine to increase cardiac output in cardiogenic shock.

Drugs used for myocardial ischemia

Drugs used to treat myocardial ischemia and relieve its pain include oxygen, nitrous oxide, nitroglycerin, morphine, and nalbuphine.

- Oxygen is important because it increases the blood's oxygen content and aids oxygenation of peripheral and cardiac tissues. It is indicated in any situation where hypoxia or ischemia is possible.

- Nitrous oxide (Nitronox) is purely an analgesic with no significant hemodynamic effects. However, delivery in fixed combination with 50 percent oxygen can increase myocardial oxygen supply. Nitrous oxide is self-administered by inhalation via a modified demand valve to the desired effect. Its effects subside within 2 to 5 minutes. Side effects include CNS depression and potential respiratory depression. Do not give nitrous oxide to patients who cannot comprehend verbal instructions or who are intoxicated with alcohol or other drugs.
- Nitroglycerin is an organic nitrate that dilates peripheral arteries and veins, reducing preload and afterload and myocardial oxygen demand. It may cause some coronary artery dilation, thus increasing blood flow through the collateral circulation. Nitroglycerin use often helps to distinguish the pain of angina from that of an MI. Nitroglycerin does not relieve the pain of an MI, but it should be given before morphine because it works in conjunction with morphine in an MI. Dosage is one tablet sublingually repeated every 5 minutes up to a total of three tablets. Monitor blood pressure before each dose. Its side effects include headache, dizziness, weakness, hypotension, and tachycardia. Note that nitroglycerin loses potency as soon as the bottle is opened to the air. Always use the nitroglycerin you bring with you and check the date before administration.
- Morphine sulfate is a narcotic drug that is important in managing MI. It reduces myocardial oxygen demand by reducing both preload and afterload. It also acts directly on the CNS to relieve pain, and it reduces sympathetic discharge, which can further decrease myocardial oxygen demand. Dosage is in 1–2 mg increments via slow IV push, titrated to pain relief. Monitor blood pressure before each dose. Side effects include nausea and vomiting, abdominal cramping, respiratory depression, hypotension, and potential altered mental status. Toxic effects are apnea and severe hypotension. Check for drug allergy before administration.
- Nalbuphine (Nubain) is used in some EMS systems instead of morphine. Nalbuphine is an analgesic, but it lacks the desirable hemodynamic effects of morphine. Dose is 10–20 mg IV, IM, or subcutaneously. Side effects include sedation, clammy skin, dizziness, dry mouth, hypotension, hypertension, and nausea and vomiting. It is contraindicated in patients who have taken depressants or alcohol.
- Fentanyl is a synthetic opiate analgesic that is shorter acting and more potent. It has fewer side effects than morphine sulfate due to its short action. Onset is immediate with peak effects occurring within 3 to 5 minutes. The adult dose is from 25–50 mcg.

Fibrinolytic agents

The use of fibrinolytic agents as a definitive treatment for myocardial ischemia is one of the most important recent advances in medicine. In some instances, fibrinolytic therapy may even have benefit in the field, and this is especially true in areas with a long transit time to a definitive care facility. Fibrinolytic agents are generally very expensive, and their use requires a 12-lead ECG. Alteplase (tPA, Activase) and reteplase (Retavase) are fibrinolytic agents. Although aspirin is not a fibrinolytic agent, it merits discussion in this section.

- Aspirin is important in treatment of cardiac ischemia because it inhibits platelet aggregation and thus is effective in treating coronary ischemia and stroke secondary to thrombus development. The standard dosage is 325 mg by mouth, although some physicians prefer smaller doses. Baby aspirin may be useful because it can be chewed, thus more quickly reaching a therapeutic blood level. Its most common side effect is GI upset, although bleeding can be a problem in certain patients.
- Alteplase (Activase, tPA). Alteplase, or tPA (tissue plasminogen activator) is a potent fibrinolytic agent that is manufactured through recombinant technology, which means it is the same as the biological compound. This minimizes chances of allergic reaction. TPA is effective if given within 6 hours of onset of coronary ischemia. It is given as a bolus dose followed by infusion. The typical dose is 100 mg given over 1.5 to 2 hours. Complications of tPA include hemorrhage, which can be fatal. Also, when reperfusion occurs, potentially life-threatening dysrhythmias can develop.
- Reteplase (Retavase) is another human plasminogen activator. It functions in a manner similar to tPA and has the same basic side effects and complications. It is administered as a single 10-unit bolus by IV push over 2 minutes. A second 10-unit bolus is given 30 minutes afterward. This dosing regimen makes reteplase attractive for prehospital care.

- Tenectplase (TNKase) is a newer generation fibrinolytic that is more fibrin specific and with a longer half-life than tPA. The typical dose is 30–50 mg IV bolus over 5 seconds.

Other prehospital drugs

Less frequently used agents you may administer in the prehospital setting include furosemide, diazepam, promethazine, and sodium nitroprusside.

- Furosemide (Lasix) is a potent loop diuretic that also relaxes the venous system with effects seen within 5 minutes. Its diuretic effect decreases intravascular fluid volume. Dose is 40 mg slow IV push (40 mg/min). If the patient takes furosemide or another diuretic, you may need to double the dosage. Side effects include hypotension, ECG changes, chest pain, dry mouth, hypokalemia, hypochloremia, hyponatremia, and hyperglycemia. Furosemide should only be used in life-threatening emergencies during pregnancy because it can cause fetal abnormalities.
- Diazepam (Valium) is not an analgesic but rather an anti-anxiety drug, and it may be given to patients who are extremely apprehensive or agitated. Dose is 2–5 mg IV or deep IM.
- Promethazine (Phenergan) has sedative, antihistamine, antiemetic, and anticholinergic properties. It also potentiates narcotics, making it useful in the MI setting by reducing the nausea associated with morphine while enhancing its effects. Dosage is 12.5–25.0 mg given slow IV push or deep IM (25.0 mg/min). Its side effects are drowsiness, sedation, blurred vision, tachycardia, bradycardia, and dizziness. Promethazine is contraindicated in unresponsive patients or those taking large doses of depressants. Extrapyramidal symptoms (namely, dystonia) have been reported with promethazine.
- Sodium nitroprusside (Nipride) is a potent arterial and venous vasodilator, making it popular for use in hypertensive crisis. It is given as an IV infusion, which makes administration more controlled and the patient's response more predictable.
- Vasopressin is the naturally occurring antidiuretic hormone and at high doses has sympathomimetic effects. It appears to increase coronary, cerebral, and other vital organ perfusion during cardiac arrest.

Drugs infrequently used in the prehospital setting

Lastly, certain medications commonly associated with in-hospital use or long-term patient use are included in this discussion. You are most likely to use these often if you work in an emergency department. Drugs in this group include digitalis, beta-blockers, calcium channel blockers, and alkalinizing agents.

- Digitalis (digoxin, Lanoxin) is a cardiac glycoside that increases cardiac contractility and cardiac output. It slows impulse conduction through the AV node and decreases the ventricular response to certain supraventricular dysrhythmias such as atrial flutter or fibrillation and paroxysmal supraventricular tachycardia. It is also used long term to treat heart failure. The dose is 8–12 mcg/kg slow IV push over 15 to 20 minutes. If possible, obtain the patient's digitalis level beforehand (if the patient is on digoxin) before administering any cardiac glycoside. Most patients taking digitalis will remain therapeutic at 10–15 mcg/kg over a 24-hour period. Giving digitalis to patients who already take a cardiac glycoside involves complicated calculations, which makes it impractical for prehospital use in most settings. Its side effects include fatigue, muscle weakness, agitation, hallucinations, headache, malaise, dizziness, vertigo, stupor, blurred vision and yellow-green halo vision, photophobia, diplopia, and nausea and vomiting. Digitalis toxicity, which is not uncommon in some patients, can cause almost any dysrhythmia, including some of the same dysrhythmias it is used to treat, and these will often be refractory to traditional antidysrhythmic drugs. Digitalis is contraindicated in any digitalis-induced toxicity, ventricular fibrillation, or ventricular tachycardia not caused by CHF.
- Beta-blockers are frequently used to control dysrhythmias, hypertension, and angina. Many beta-blockers such as propranolol (Inderal) are nonselective; other beta-blockers such as metoprolol are selective for either B_1 or B_2 receptors. Beta-blockers may precipitate CHF, heart block, or asthma in patients predisposed to them. The beta-blocker labetalol (Trandate, Normodyne) effectively decreases blood pressure. It is given by IV bolus and infusion. The IV

bolus is 20 mg over 20 minutes and may be repeated at 40–80 mg over 10 minutes. Maximum bolus is 300 mg. Drip is established by mixing 200 mg into 160 cc D$_5$W, and the drip dose is 2 cc/min.

- Calcium channel blockers are a relatively new class of antihypertensive medications that include verapamil (Isoptin, Calan), diltiazem (Cardizem), and nifedipine (Procardia). Nifedipine is now being used in addition to nitroglycerin to treat angina. Like nitroglycerin, it is a vasodilator but with a different mechanism. It is given orally. Calcium channel blockers are being used increasingly for angina, dysrhythmias, and other cardiovascular problems.

- Alkalinizing agents such as sodium bicarbonate are used late in the management of cardiac arrest, if at all. Occasionally, metabolic acidosis from another disorder may cause pulseless electrical activity, asystole, ventricular tachycardia, or ventricular fibrillation. In these cases, sodium bicarbonate may aid in converting to a perfusing rhythm. Adequate CPR, prompt defibrillation, and appropriate drug administration should always precede the use of bicarbonate. Sodium bicarbonate has few side effects and no contraindications in the emergency setting. Dose is initially 1 mEq/kg followed by 0.5 mEq/kg every 10 minutes. When possible, doses should be based on arterial blood gas (ABG) results.

32. Describe the epidemiology, morbidity, mortality, and physiology associated with heart failure. pp. 1220–1221

Heart failure is the clinical syndrome in which the heart's pumping capacity is compromised so that cardiac output cannot meet the body's needs. Heart failure can be typed as right ventricle or left ventricle failure or bilateral heart failure. Left ventricular failure occurs when the left ventricle's ability to pump fails, causing back pressure of blood into the pulmonary circulation, which results in pulmonary edema. Right ventricular failure is due to loss of pumping ability in the right ventricle, resulting in back pressure of blood into the systemic venous circulation causing venous congestion. The most common cause of right heart failure is preexistent left heart failure. Other causes of right ventricular failure include systemic hypertension, pulmonary hypertension due to COPD, or cor pulmonale. All of these causes relate to an initial increase in the pressure in the pulmonary arteries, which then results in right ventricular enlargement, and, if untreated, right ventricular failure. Pulmonary embolism causes right ventricular failure if the clot is large enough to block a major pulmonary vessel.

33. Identify the factors that may precipitate or aggravate heart failure. pp. 1220–1221

There are many causes of heart failure, including valve disorders and coronary or myocardial disease. Dysrhythmias may aggravate heart failure by further decreasing cardiac output, decreasing myocardial perfusion, or both. Other factors that can contribute to heart failure include excess fluid or salt intake, fever (sepsis), hypertension, pulmonary embolism, or excessive alcohol or drug use. Failure can manifest with exertion in a patient who has an underlying disease or who has progressive cardiac disease. Specific causes of left heart failure include MI, valvular disease, chronic hypertension, and dysrhythmias. Because MI is a common cause of left ventricular failure, suspect that all patients with pulmonary edema may have had an MI. Causes of right ventricular failure include initial MI of the left ventricle, systemic hypertension, pulmonary hypertension due to COPD, and cor pulmonale. Another major cause of right ventricular failure is pulmonary embolism.

34. Define acute pulmonary edema and describe its relationship to left ventricular failure. pp. 1220–1221

As the left ventricle's pumping ability falls, it cannot pump out all of the blood delivered to it from the lungs. Consequently, left atrial pressure rises and is transmitted to the pulmonary veins and the pulmonary capillary beds. When pulmonary capillary pressure increases sufficiently, blood plasma is forced into the alveoli and interstitial spaces; this is pulmonary edema (swelling of the lungs). Progressive fluid accumulation in the alveoli decreases the lungs' oxygenation capacity and can cause hypoxia that can be fatal.

35. Differentiate between early and late signs and symptoms of left ventricular failure and those of right ventricular failure. pp. 1220–1221

For left ventricular failure, the cardinal symptom is dyspnea due to pulmonary edema. Signs include cyanosis; tachycardia; noisy, labored breathing; crackles; cough; blood-tinged, frothy sputum; and a gallop rhythm of the heart. The major signs of right ventricular failure: neck veins engorged and pulsating, edema of body and extremities, engorged liver and spleen, abdominal distention with ascites (fluid), as well as tachycardia.

Congestive heart failure (CHF) is a general term for ventricular failure (left, right, or both) that causes excess fluid to accumulate in body tissues (hence, congestion). The excess fluid manifests as edema, which may be pulmonary, peripheral, sacral, or within the abdomen as ascites. You may find it in the acute setting of MI, pulmonary edema, or pulmonary hypertension. In the chronic setting, it can reflect cardiac enlargement.

36. Define and explain the clinical significance of paroxysmal nocturnal dyspnea, pulmonary edema, and dependent edema. pp. 1221–1222

Paroxysmal nocturnal dyspnea (PND) is an episode of waking during the night due to shortness of breath, and it reflects the presence of pulmonary edema. If these episodes become more frequent (more nights or more times/night), it suggests worsening of the underlying pathophysiologic process. Pulmonary edema reflects backup of fluid into the pulmonary alveoli and interstitium, but it does not necessarily imply etiology. Left ventricular failure, however, is probably the best known and most common cause, and you should look for other signs of congestive heart failure in a patient who presents with signs of pulmonary edema. If pulmonary edema seems to be very acute in onset, look for precipitating causes, such as cardiac dysrhythmia or acute MI. Dependent edema represents edema in the gravity-dependent portions of the body. For a bedridden patient, this often manifests as sacral edema. Sometimes edema will be so severe it will eliminate your ability to find a pulse in the affected area (such as a pedal pulse). If edema is severe enough to be pitting edema (a situation in which you press firmly into the affected tissue, lift the finger, and find that the depression caused by your finger persists), you can make a semi-quantitative evaluation by scoring as 0 to 4+.

37. List the interventions prescribed for the patient in acute congestive heart failure. pp. 1223–1224

Manage a patient with severe CHF by assessing in an ongoing manner for life-threatening symptoms and intervene promptly while readying the patient for rapid transport. Do not allow the patient to exert in any way, including standing up. Positioning in a seated position with feet dangling promotes venous pooling and, consequently, reduced preload. Administer high-flow oxygen. If necessary, provide positive-pressure ventilations with either a demand valve or a bag-valve-mask device. Establish an IV line at a keep-vein-open rate or place a saline or heparin lock. Place ECG electrodes. If the patient is extremely diaphoretic, apply tincture of Benzoin first so electrodes will be tightly adherent to skin. Record a baseline ECG and continue monitoring.

Medication use will be according to your local protocols or the order of medical direction. Always remember to ask about drug allergies or reactions to any medication.

Transport as a nonemergency unless clinical conditions say otherwise. Indications for emergency transport include hypertension or hypotension, severe respiratory distress or pending respiratory failure, or life-threatening dysrhythmias. If you feel nonemergency transport will compromise the patient's condition, use lights and siren.

38. Describe the most commonly used pharmacological agents in the management of congestive heart failure in terms of therapeutic effect, dosages, routes of administration, side effects, and toxic effects. pp. 1999, 1200, 1223; see Chapter 6

The drugs most likely to be used in the setting of left ventricular failure and pulmonary edema include morphine sulfate, nitroglycerin, furosemide (Lasix), dopamine (Intropin), dobutamine (Dobutrex), promethazine (Phenergan), and nitrous oxide (Nitronox). Dosages and other information on these medications are given in objective 31.

39. Define and describe the incidence, mortality, morbidity, pathophysiology, assessment, and management of the following cardiac related problems:

Cardiac tamponade   pp. 1224–1225

Cardiac tamponade exists when an accumulation of material (air, pus, serum, blood, or a combination) inside the pericardium places pressure on the heart such that diastolic filling is impaired and stroke volume falls. Tamponade may evolve gradually; common progressive causes include pericarditis and benign or malignant neoplasms. Rare medical causes of tamponade include hypothyroidism and renal disease. Acute onset tends to occur when the cause is trauma or MI. Specific traumatic causes include CPR and penetrating and nonpenetrating chest trauma. Regardless of cause and regardless of gradual or acute onset, cardiac tamponade can lead to death.

During the initial patient assessment, you may suspect cardiac tamponade. If so, limit history taking to questions that might reveal a precipitating cause. Use the OPQRST mnemonic to get information about the patient's symptoms: The most frequent chief complaints in tamponade are chest pain or dyspnea, and pain may be either dull or sharp. On physical exam, cardiac tamponade often presents with a characteristic picture: dyspnea and orthopnea, with clear lung sounds. Typically, peripheral pulses are rapid and weak. In the early stage, venous pressure is often elevated and you may see jugular vein distention. Blood pressure often reveals a decrease in systolic pressure, pulsus paradoxus, and narrowing pulse pressures. Heart sounds may be normal early in tamponade, but they are more likely (especially later) to become muffled or faint because of the presence of the tamponade-producing material in the pericardial sac.

Use of the ECG, whether single monitor lead or 12-lead, is not a diagnostic tool, but it may support your clinical suspicions. ECG findings are generally inconclusive; however, ectopy is usually a late sign due to irritation of the heart's epicardial tissue by the pericardial effusion. QRS and T wave voltages are low, and nonspecific T wave changes occur. S-T segments may elevate. Electrical alternans (weak voltage alternating with normal voltage) may appear in the P, QRS, T, or S-T segments.

Management is primarily supportive except when shock or low perfusion is detected. Maintain airway and deliver high-flow oxygen. If clinically indicated, use endotracheal intubation and maintain circulation with IV support, medications, or CPR. Again, before giving any medication ask about allergies. Medications frequently used in the setting of cardiac tamponade include morphine sulfate, nitrous oxide, furosemide, dopamine, and dobutamine. Rapid transport is indicated.

Hypertensive emergency   pp. 1225–1226

Hypertensive emergency occurs when there is a life-threatening elevation of blood pressure. This develops in about 1 percent of patients with hypertension. Clinically, the emergency is usually characterized by a rapid increase in diastolic pressure (generally, to greater than 130 mmHg) accompanied by restlessness and confusion, blurred vision, and nausea and vomiting. It often occurs with hypertensive encephalopathy, a consequence of severe hypertension marked by severe headache, vomiting, visual changes including transient blindness, paralysis, seizures, and stupor or coma. With modern medications, hypertensive encephalopathy has become rare, although it is still seen in the hospital setting. Both ischemic and hemorrhagic strokes are more common results of severe hypertension and can have devastating consequences. Hypertensive emergency can also cause left ventricular failure and pulmonary edema.

The major causes of hypertensive emergency include noncompliance with antihypertensive drugs or other prescribed medications and lack of treatment for hypertension. Risk factors include age (older age) and race (hypertension is more common in blacks, and morbidity and mortality appear to be higher, too). Among pregnant women, one cause of hypertension is preeclampsia (also called toxemia of pregnancy), which can appear at any point after the 20th week of pregnancy.

Assessment findings on physical exam of a patient with hypertensive emergency commonly include a chief complaint of headache accompanied by any of the following: nausea, vomiting, blurred vision, shortness of breath, epistaxis, and dizziness (vertigo). The patient may be semiconscious or unconscious and seizing. In toxemia of pregnancy, the woman usually has edema of hands or face. Photosensitivity and headache are common complaints in this group. Determine whether there is a documented history of hypertension and to what degree prescribed medications have been taken. Find out whether the patient may have borrowed someone else's medications or taken herbal or over-the-counter drugs. Skin may be pale or flushed, normal, cool, or warm. Look for edema. The patient may confirm PND, orthopnea, vertigo, epistaxis, tinnitus, or visual acuities. Look for possible motor or sensory deficits in parts of the body or on one side. ECG findings are generally inconclusive unless there is an underlying cardiac condition such as angina or MI. If left ventricular failure is present, pulmonary edema may be present. Otherwise, lungs are generally clear. The pulse is strong and may feel bounding. Hypertension is present with systolic pressure greater than 160 mmHg and/or diastolic pressure greater than 90 mmHg. Signs or symptoms of hypertensive encephalopathy in the presence of measured hypertension should be considered a hypertensive emergency.

Management centers on positioning for comfort and watching for possible airway compromise if vomiting or stroke occurs. Give oxygen and decide upon transport based on clinical presentation. Attempt supportive IV therapy on scene or en route. Place pregnant patients on their left sides and transport as smoothly and quietly as possible.

Medications that may be used in the prehospital setting have notably changed recently; know your local protocol. Medications often used include morphine, furosemide, nitroglycerin, sodium nitroprusside, and labetalol (Trandate, Normodyne).

Cardiogenic shock pp. 1226–1229

Cardiogenic shock is the extreme state of heart failure: Cardiac output is so low it cannot sustain minimal physiologic activity. Clinically, you will see it after existing dysrhythmias, hypovolemia, or altered vascular tone have been corrected, leaving only the possibility of endogenous pump failure. This failure of the heart and overwhelming of any compensatory mechanisms usually happens after an extensive MI, often involving more than 40 percent of the left ventricle, or with diffuse ischemia. Note that cardiogenic shock can occur at any age, but it is most often seen as an end-stage event in geriatric patients with underlying disease. Mortality rate is high for elderly patients following massive MI or septic shock because end-organ damage is so severe that life cannot be sustained.

Numerous mechanisms can lead to cardiogenic shock, and onset may be gradual or acute. Among mechanical causes are tension pneumothorax and cardiac tamponade. Interference with ventricular emptying or afterload (such as pulmonary embolism and prosthetic or natural valve dysfunction) can also cause shock. Impairment in cardiac contractility is also a general cause: examples include MI, myocarditis, and recreational drug use. Trauma is another general cause, either primarily through cardiac damage or secondarily through hypovolemia. Finally, shock can develop secondarily to underlying conditions such as neurologic, GI, renal, or metabolic disorders.

Assessment findings depend on whether the patient is in an early phase of shock or a most advanced state. Look for evidence of a possible contributing cause such as hypovolemia, sepsis, or trauma. Among direct cardiac causes, you will most often see cardiogenic shock in the setting of MI if the MI affects the anterior wall or 40 percent or more of the left ventricle. Information about the patient's medications may give clues about preexisting pump compromise. Inquire about the degree of compliance with medication regiments and ask about borrowed or over-the-counter drugs, which might have unpredictable interaction effects.

The altered mental status associated with advancing shock may begin as restlessness and progress through confusion to loss of consciousness. Airway findings include dyspnea, productive cough, or labored breathing. Tachypnea is often present due to pulmonary edema. Also common is a history of paroxysmal nocturnal dyspnea. Typical ECG findings include tachycardia and atrial dysrhythmias such as atrial tachycardia. Ectopy is also common.

MI often precedes cardiogenic shock; symptoms will be compatible with those expected with MI. Expect hypotension to develop as shock progresses. Systolic pressure will often fall to less than 80 mmHg. Try to correct any discovered dysrhythmias.

Management of cardiogenic shock begins by placing the patient in a position of comfort. With pulmonary edema, this may be sitting upright. Treatment consists mostly of caring for underlying conditions (such as MI or CHF) and supportive care. Remember to treat heart rate and rhythm and transport rapidly. Medications that may be used in this setting include the vasopressors dopamine, dobutamine, and norepinephrine. Other medications include morphine, promethazine, nitroglycerin, nitrous oxide, furosemide, digitalis, and sodium bicarbonate.

Cardiac arrest
pp. 1229–1233

Cardiac arrest and sudden death account for 60 percent of all deaths from coronary heart disease. Cardiac arrest is defined as the absence of ventricular contractions that immediately results in systemic circulatory failure. Sudden death is any death that occurs within one hour of the onset of symptoms. At autopsy, signs of MI are not present, and authorities generally believe lethal dysrhythmia secondary to severe atherosclerosis is the most common cause of death. The risk factors for sudden death are similar to those for ASHD and CHD. Other causes of sudden death include drowning, acid–base imbalance, electrocution, drug intoxication, electrolyte imbalance, hypoxia, hypothermia, pulmonary embolism, stroke, hyperkalemia, trauma, and end-stage renal disease.

Assessment for cardiac arrest shows an unresponsive, apneic, pulseless individual. After initiating CPR, place ECG leads and initiate monitoring. Dysrhythmias you may find include ventricular tachycardia or fibrillation, asystole, or PEA. If you find asystole, confirm it in two or more leads. Question bystanders with the goal of finding some specific, prognostic information: Did anyone witness the arrest? If CPR was begun before you arrived, try to learn as precisely as possible the length of time between arrest and initiation of effective CPR. Often, the emergency room physician will also want to know total down time from the beginning of the arrest until arrival at the emergency department. Also, try to get a list of the patient's medications as well as a past history.

Management starts with simultaneous efforts on the ABCs. Ventilate with a bag-valve-mask using 100 percent oxygen. Intubate or insert an airway as quickly as possible. If ECG changes indicate defibrillation or synchronized cardioversion, perform it in conjunction with CPR, stopping CPR only long enough to apply the pads or paddles and deliver the shock. If the patient has an internal pacemaker or defibrillator, be sure not to defibrillate over the device.

After starting CPR and advanced airway management, get IV access with a venous site as close to the heart as possible (for instance, the antecubital area in the arm or the external jugular vein). Follow IV medications with a 30 to 45 second flush to ensure complete delivery. After each flush, set the line to a keep-vein-open rate. Agents used with cardiac arrest include amiodarone, atropine, lidocaine, procainamide, bretylium, epinephrine, norepinephrine, dopamine, dolbutamine, and vasopressin.

If blood pressure and pulse return, be aware that the blood pressure itself may be low, normal, or high because of the drugs administered. Pulse may return with a bradycardic, normal, or tachycardic rate. Ventricular ectopy is the most serious concern. If the patient presented in ventricular tachycardia or ventricular fibrillation or if ectopy is seen postarrest, use an antidysrhythmic such as lidocaine.

Transport should be done as safely and smoothly as possible and with lights and siren.

40. Identify the limiting factor of pericardial anatomy that determines intrapericardiac pressure. p. 1224

The limitation is in the volume of material that can be held in the pericardial sac without exerting undue pressure on the heart. The normal volume is about 25 cc in an adult. As this volume is exceeded, pressure is exerted on the heart, and it can eventually reach the point of significantly limiting the extent to which the heart can fill during diastole or contract to expel blood during systole. This is cardiac tamponade.

41. Describe how to determine if pulsus paradoxus, pulsus alternans, or electrical alternans is present. pp. 1222, 1224

Pulsus paradoxus is determined by measuring blood pressure during respirations. A systolic pressure that falls more than 10 mmHg during inspiration is pulsus paradoxus. Pulsus alternans is an alternation between weak and strong peripheral pulses; this is determined by palpation of the pulse. Electrical alternans is determined by ECG analysis: It consists of an alternating pattern of normal and very low voltage.

42. Explain the essential pathophysiological defect of hypertension in terms of Starling's law of the heart. pp. 1221, 1226

Starling's law states that the greater the stretch on myocardial muscle (the preload), the greater will be the force of contraction. This is true until the muscle is overstretched, at which point contraction becomes weaker. Afterload also affects stroke volume. An increase in afterload (peripheral vascular resistance) is an increase in the pressure against which the ventricle must pump, and thus increased afterload decreases stroke volume. Hypertension, or high blood pressure, is a state in which afterload is chronically increased, and thus this represents a chronic stressor on the ventricular myocardium.

43. Rank the clinical problems of patients in hypertensive emergencies according to their sense of urgency. pp. 1225–1226

Hypertensive emergency in the general sense is a state in which diastolic blood pressure has risen to dangerous levels (greater than 130 mmHg), mandating a lowering of blood pressure within one hour to minimize or avoid risk for end-organ changes such as hypertensive encephalopathy, renal failure, or blindness. Hypertensive encephalopathy is a life-threatening situation in which stroke, coma, left ventricular failure, or pulmonary edema may occur. A hypertensive emergency in a pregnant patient with preeclampsia poses a high risk of the obstetric complication of abruption of the placenta or progression to eclampsia, with its seizures and risk of death for the woman and unborn fetus.

44. Identify the drugs of choice for hypertensive emergencies, cardiogenic shock, and cardiac arrest, including their indications, contraindications, side effects, route of administration, and dosages. pp. 1999, 1200, 1226, 1227–1229, 1230; see Chapter 6

- **Hypertensive emergencies.** Drugs include morphine sulfate, furosemide, nitroglycerin, sodium nitroprusside, and labetalol.
- **Cardiogenic shock.** Drugs include dopamine, dobutamine, norepinephrine, morphine sulfate, promethazine, nitroglycerin, nitrous oxide, furosemide, digitalis, and sodium bicarbonate.
- **Cardiac arrest.** Drugs include atropine, lidocaine, procainamide, bretylium, epinephrine, norepinephrine, isoproterenol, dopamine, dobutamine, and sodium bicarbonate.

General descriptions, specific doses, contraindications, and side effects of these medications are given in objective 31. Two medications not covered in detail in objective 31 are discussed below.

Labetalol (Trandate, Normodyne). The IV bolus is 20 mg over 20 minutes, and it may be repeated at 40–80 mg over 10 minutes. Maximum bolus is 300 mg. Drip is established by mixing 200 mg into 160 mL D_5W, and the drip dose is 2 cc/min.

Sodium bicarbonate. Sodium bicarbonate is used late in the management of cardiac arrest, if at all. Occasionally, metabolic acidosis from another disorder may cause pulseless electrical activity, asystole, ventricular tachycardia, or ventricular fibrillation. In these cases, sodium bicarbonate may aid in converting to a perfusing rhythm. Adequate CPR, prompt defibrillation, and appropriate drug administration should always precede the use of bicarbonate. Sodium bicarbonate has few side effects and no contraindications in the emergency setting. Dose is initially 1 mEq/kg followed by 0.5 mEq/kg every 10 minutes. When possible, doses should be based on arterial blood gas (ABG) results.

45. Describe the major systemic effects of reduced tissue perfusion caused by cardiogenic shock. pp. 1226–1227

A chief effect is CNS compromise, which may manifest early as restlessness or agitation and later as confusion or unconsciousness. Impaired renal function due to poor perfusion may be seen as oliguria or anuria. The decrease in blood flow to the extremities as blood is shunted to core organs is seen as cold, clammy, pale skin.

46. **Explain the primary mechanisms by which the heart may compensate for a diminished cardiac output and describe their efficiency in cardiogenic shock.** pp. 1226–1227

The three basic mechanisms that increase cardiac output are increase in contractility, increase in preload, or decreasing peripheral resistance. Increased myocardial contractile force will help to increase stroke volume. Increased preload increases the stretch on the myocardium, and, within limits (this is Starling's law), this results in increased contraction force and increased stroke volume. Last, decreasing peripheral resistance (afterload) decreases the force that the ventricles must exert in order to expel blood into the aorta and pulmonary arteries.

47. **Identify the clinical criteria and progressive stages of cardiogenic shock.** pp. 1226–1227

See objective 39.

48. **Describe the dysrhythmias seen in cardiac arrest.** p. 1229

The dysrhythmias seen most frequently in cardiac arrest are ventricular tachycardia, ventricular fibrillation, asystole, and pulseless electrical activity (PEA). Asystole should always be confirmed in two more ECG leads.

49. **Explain how to confirm asystole using the 3-lead ECG.** p. 1229

An ECG tracing of asystole is shown in Part 1 of this chapter. On each lead, you should see an absence of all cardiac electrical activity: There will be no discernible components of the ECG sequence (no P waves, QRS complexes, or T waves).

50. **Define the terms *defibrillation* and *synchronized cardioversion*.** pp. 1199, 1204

Defibrillation is the process of passing an electrical current through a fibrillating heart in order to depolarize all cells and allow them to repolarize uniformly, thus restoring an organized cardiac rhythm. Synchronized cardioversion is a controlled form of defibrillation for patients who have some organized cardiac activity with a pulse. A synchronizing circuit interprets the QRS cycle and delivers an electrical discharge during the R wave of the QRS complex, reducing the likelihood of delivering the cardioversion during the vulnerable period of the QRS cycle and reducing the likelihood of triggering ventricular fibrillation. Indications for synchronized cardioversion include perfusing ventricular tachycardia, paroxysmal supraventricular tachycardia, rapid atrial fibrillation, and 2:1 atrial flutter.

51. **Specify the methods of supporting the patient with a suspected ineffective implanted defibrillation device.** p. 1201

When external defibrillation is required, be sure that you do not place paddles over the generator of an implanted automatic defibrillator or pacemaker, because this can damage or disable the implanted device.

52. **Describe resuscitation and identify circumstances and situations where resuscitation efforts would not be initiated.** pp. 1229–1233

Objective 39 covers initial resuscitation procedures as well as care after return of spontaneous pulse. In some situations, the patient will not survive despite resuscitation efforts, and in these cases resuscitation is contraindicated and should not be begun: These settings are rigor mortis, fixed dependent lividity (pooling of blood in gravity-dependent fashion), decapitation, and incineration. Less obvious but equally important settings include those where there is a valid advance directive to withhold resuscitation.

53. **Identify communication and documentation protocols with medical direction and law enforcement used for termination of resuscitation efforts.** pp. 1232–1233

In some settings, resuscitation will begin but criteria for termination of resuscitation may exist. These include (1) age 18 years or older; (2) arrest that is presumed cardiac in origin and not associated with a treatable cause such as hypothermia, overdose, or hypovolemia; (3) successful and maintained endotracheal intubation; (4) ACLS standards having been applied throughout the arrest; (5) on-scene efforts having been sustained for 25 minutes or the patient remaining in asystole through four rounds of ALS drugs; (6) patient rhythm that is asystolic or agonal when the decision to terminate is made and persistence of this rhythm until resuscitation is actually terminated, and (7) victims of blunt trauma who presented in asystole or developed asystole on scene.

You should be equally familiar with criteria that exclude termination of resuscitation: (1) age under 18 years, (2) cause that might benefit from in-hospital treatment, (3) persistent or recurring ventricular tachycardia or fibrillation, (4) transient return of a pulse, (5) signs of neurologic viability, (6) arrest witnessed by EMS personnel, (7) and family or other responsible party opposed to termination.

Review local protocols and contact medical direction before attempting to terminate resuscitation. The medical director or other physician may use the following information: (1) medical condition of the patient, (2) known etiologic factors, (3) therapy rendered, (4) family's presence and appraisal of the situation, (5) communication of any resistance or uncertainty on the part of the family, and (6) maintenance of continued documentation including ECG.

Law enforcement regulations will require that all local, state, and federal laws pertaining to death be followed. The officer may also be required to assign the patient to the medical examiner if he/she does not have a physician. Check with your local law enforcement agencies to determine their protocols.

54. Describe the incidence, morbidity, mortality, pathophysiology, assessment, and management of vascular disorders including occlusive disease, phlebitis, aortic aneurysm, and peripheral artery occlusion. pp. 1233–1237

Conditions discussed in the chapter as peripheral vascular emergencies include atherosclerosis (which is an occlusive disease), aneurysm, acute arterial occlusion, and deep venous thrombosis.

- Atherosclerosis is the progressive degenerative disease affecting medium and large arteries that underlies many cardiovascular emergencies. It is the cause of coronary artery disease and can affect the carotid, aortic, and cerebral arteries, among others. In atherosclerosis, fats are deposited under the inner layer of the artery, causing injury that subsequently damages the middle, muscle-containing tissue layer as well. Progression occurs as calcium is deposited in the fatty material, forming plaques. Small hemorrhages typically occur around atherosclerotic plaques, further damaging the artery. As the disease progresses, the luminal diameter narrows and blood flow may be impaired to the distal tissues. Eventually, the artery may become totally blocked. If tearing occurs in the arterial wall, the vessel may become dilated and frail; this constitutes an atherosclerotic aneurysm. Arteriosclerosis is the related process in which disruption of tissue layers destroys the elasticity of the vessel and contributes to hypertension. You are already familiar with some of the clinical states due to atherosclerosis and arteriosclerosis: angina, MI, carotid bruits, and stroke.
- Aneurysms are dilatations of vessels. There are actually several types of aneurysms, including atherosclerotic, dissecting, infectious, congenital, and traumatic. Most aneurysms are due to atherosclerotic damage and occur in the aorta, the largest artery in the body and the one with the highest blood pressure. Infectious aneurysms are usually syphilitic in nature and are now rare. Congenital aneurysms can occur with several disease states including Marfan's syndrome, a genetic disorder of connective tissue. Aortic aneurysms are not uncommon in individuals with Marfan's syndrome because the aortic wall is relatively weak from birth.
- Aneurysms form in the aorta when blood infiltrates the wall through a tear in its innermost layer. An abdominal aortic aneurysm secondary to atherosclerosis is a fairly common finding in persons aged 60 to 70 years and ten times as common in men than in women. Signs and symptoms of an abdominal aneurysm include abdominal, back, or flank pain, hypotension, and an urge to defecate caused by retroperitoneal leakage of blood. Degenerative changes in the smooth muscle and elastic tissue of the aorta cause most dissecting aortic aneurysms. The original tear often results from cystic medial necrosis, a degeneration of connective tissue associated with hypertension and, to some extent, aging. Hypertension is clearly a risk factor; it is present in 75 to 85 percent of cases. It occurs most frequently in

those older than 40 to 50 years, although it can occur in younger individuals, especially pregnant women. There can also be a hereditary factor. A dissecting aortic aneurysm is one where a rapid inrushing of blood into the wall causes the layers of the wall to separate and eventually rupture. A dissecting aortic aneurysm is extremely painful, and this is one reason you gently search for pulsating masses during the focused abdominal exam of a patient with back, chest, or abdominal pain.

- Acute arterial occlusion is the sudden blockage of an artery due to trauma, thrombosis, embolus, tumor, or idiopathic means. Emboli are probably most common. They can arise within a chamber of the heart (mural emboli), from a thrombus in the left ventricle, from an atrial thrombus secondary to atrial fibrillation, or from a thrombus caused by abdominal aortic atherosclerosis. Arterial occlusions (from emboli leaving the aorta) most commonly involve vessels in the abdomen or extremities. Emboli leaving the heart via the left ventricle can cause embolic strokes, and emboli leaving the right ventricle (perhaps secondary to atrial fibrillation) can cause pulmonary embolisms.

- Deep venous thrombosis is a blood clot in a vein, usually one in the thigh or calf of the leg. Predisposing factors include recent history of trauma, inactivity, pregnancy, or varicose veins. The patient often complains of gradually increasing pain and tenderness; the affected leg and foot are typically swollen because of occluded venous drainage. Skin may be warm and red. Gentle palpation of the calf and thigh will reveal tenderness, and you may be able to palpate cordlike clotted veins.

- Assessment of peripheral vascular disorders starts with the ABCs. Breathing is usually unaffected except in the case of pulmonary emboli. If you find decompensated shock, the cause is most likely to be aneurysm, arterial occlusion, or pulmonary embolus. Circulation is typically compromised distal to the occlusion. Check circulation for the five Ps: pallor, pain, pulselessness, paralysis, and paresthesias. Also check the skin for mottling distal to the affected area. Use the OPQRST acronym to learn more about the patient's pain or other complaint. Find out if this is a new event or a recurrence.

- On physical exam, alteration in breathing and heart rate and rhythm are most common, with pulmonary embolus and aortic aneurysm the two conditions most likely to be life threatening. Unequal bilateral blood pressures may indicate a high thoracic aortic aneurysm that affects flow to one arm. Peripheral pulses may be normal, diminished, or absent, dependent on the site of obstruction. Bruits may be audible over a carotid artery partially occluded by atherosclerotic material. ECG findings generally do not contribute to diagnosis or treatment. However, if you find ectopy or dysrhythmias, treat them.

- Management of the patient with a peripheral vascular emergency is largely supportive. Place the patient in a position of comfort. Give oxygen by nonrebreather mask if you suspect pulmonary embolus, aortic aneurysm, or acute arterial occlusion or if either hypotension or a hypoperfusion state exists. Ask about drug allergies before giving any medication. Agents you may use in this setting include nitrous oxide and morphine. Transport as soon as possible. Indications for rapid transport with lights and siren include any situation in which medications do not relieve symptoms or in which you suspect pulmonary embolism, aortic aneurysm, or arterial occlusion. Also consider hypotension or hypoperfusion to be an emergency meriting rapid transport.

55. Identify the clinical significance of claudication and presence of arterial bruits in a patient with peripheral vascular disorders. pp. 1233–1237

Claudication is severe pain in a calf muscle due to inadequate blood supply. It typically occurs with exertion and subsides with rest. It is, in many respects, a peripheral parallel to cardiac angina. Arterial bruits are another sign of partial arterial blockage, usually due to atherosclerosis. Bruits are soft sounds heard over an artery (often the carotids) and represent the turbulent blood flow due to partial obstruction.

56. Describe the clinical significance of unequal arterial blood pressure readings in the arms. p. 1236

Unequal bilateral blood pressures may indicate an aneurysm high in the thoracic aorta; this is due to unequal flow to the left and right extremities.

57. Recognize and describe the signs and symptoms of dissecting thoracic or abdominal aneurysm. pp. 1233–1234

Pain and evolution of shock (including alterations in heart rate and rhythm) are the most common symptom and sign of a dissecting aortic aneurysm. Abdominal aneurysms often present initially with abdominal, back, or flank pain accompanied by development of hypotension. The patient may complain of an urge to defecate if blood leaks into the retroperitoneal space. Thoracic aneurysms also present with pain; look for unequal bilateral blood pressures in the arms as evidence of the dissecting aneurysm.

58. Differentiate between signs and symptoms of cardiac tamponade, hypertensive emergencies, cardiogenic shock, and cardiac arrest. pp. 1224–1229

Cardiac tamponade typically presents as dyspnea and chest pain, the latter of which may be either dull or sharp. Onset may be sudden or gradual. Classical physical findings include orthopnea, pulsus paradoxus, and narrowing pulse pressures. (In addition, you may see elevated venous pressures in the early phase represented by jugular venous distention.) The ECG is not a diagnostic tool, but you may well see diminished voltages and electrical alternans.

Hypertensive emergencies often show signs of hypertensive encephalopathy: confusion, headache, vomiting, visual changes, or seizures. The extreme hypertension found on blood pressure measurement (diastolic greater than 130 mmHg) is diagnostic.

Cardiogenic shock presents with the signs typical of shock: tachycardia, hypotension, poor peripheral perfusion. History may reveal evidence of chronic heart disease (medications, surgical scars, PND, or current medication regimen) or an acute event such as an MI as clues to the cardiac origin of shock. The usual heart rhythm is sinus tachycardia, but dysrhythmias are not uncommon. Peripheral edema may be so severe that pulses are not palpable.

Cardiac arrest presents with a completely unresponsive patient with no spontaneous breathing or pulse. ECG may show asystole or PEA or may show a dysrhythmia such as ventricular tachycardia or ventricular fibrillation.

59. Utilize the results of the patient history, assessment findings, and ECG analysis to differentiate between, and provide treatment for, patients with the following conditions: pp. 1186–1237

- **Cardiovascular disease.** Objectives 54–57 all deal with elements of peripheral vascular disease. Assessment findings are specific to the region of the vascular system affected by occlusion. Central findings such as tachypnea and change in heart rate or rhythm suggest pulmonary embolism or aortic aneurysm. Care is largely supportive unless a life-threatening problem (such as hypotension or dysrhythmia) develops.
- **Chest pain.** Chest pain can have a cardiac (pericarditis, angina, or MI) or vascular (aortic aneurysm) origin, or it can reflect problems of the respiratory system, GI tract, or musculoskeletal system (see objective 15). Look for pain on exertion that is relieved by rest and/or nitroglycerin as a sign of possible angina and pain that is unremitting for an MI. With both you may well see ECG changes including sinus tachycardia, S-T segment depression or elevation, ectopy, or dysrhythmias.
- **In need of a pacemaker.** A patient with a history of high-degree AV block or symptomatic bradycardia or atrial fibrillation has inadequate cardiac output for body needs during the periods of those dysrhythmias. If medications don't convert the dysrhythmia to a rhythm compatible with adequate cardiac output, a pacemaker should be considered. Other patients may have recurrent episodes of life-threatening dysrhythmias such as ventricular tachycardia or ventricular fibrillation, and they may also need a pacemaker.
- **Angina pectoris.** The typical presentation for angina is pain lasting from 3 to 5 minutes, or perhaps as long as 15 minutes, that is relieved by rest and/or nitroglycerin. Prinzmetal's (vasospastic) angina most often occurs at rest or without a known trigger but has similar duration. Prinzmetal's angina is often accompanied by S-T segment elevation on ECG. A patient with fixed (obstructive) angina may show S-T depression and/or T wave inversion on 12-lead ECG. Relief of pain is generally associated with resolution of ECG disturbances.

- **A suspected myocardial infarction.** The patient with an acute MI has chest pain that is severe, constant, and lasts longer than 30 minutes. Neither rest nor nitroglycerin relieves the pain, and the patient may be fearful or feel a sense of doom. On ECG, check the S-T segment for depression, which suggests ischemia, or elevation, which suggests tissue injury. A pathological Q wave (deeper than 5 mm and longer than 0.04 sec) can indicate either widespread transient ischemia or infarcted tissue. Ectopy and dysrhythmia can appear without warning.
- **Heart failure.** Heart failure, inadequacy of pumping ability to meet the body's oxygen demand, can be left-sided, right-sided, or both. Left-sided ventricular failure typically presents with dyspnea and the following additional signs: cyanosis, tachycardia, noisy, labored breathing, crackles, cough, blood-tinged, often frothy sputum, and galloping heart sounds. Decreased lung sounds on exam reflect pulmonary edema. Right-sided ventricular failure typically presents with tachycardia, jugular venous distention, edema of body and extremities, engorged (palpable) liver and spleen, and abdominal distention due to ascites fluid. History will usually reflect past cardiac disease or pulmonary disease (COPD). Paroxysmal nocturnal dyspnea suggests left heart failure.
- **Cardiac tamponade.** Cardiac tamponade may be gradual or acute in onset depending on the origin of the material filling the pericardium and exerting pressure on the heart. Assessment typically finds dyspnea and orthopnea and pulsus paradoxus. ECG is not considered diagnostic, but you may see decreased voltage and electrical alternans in these patients.
- **A hypertensive emergency.** The patient with a hypertensive emergency will have extreme hypertension (diastolic greater than 130 mmHg) and usually will show some signs of hypertensive encephalopathy such as headache, visual change, nausea and vomiting, restlessness, or seizures or coma.
- **Cardiogenic shock.** Cardiogenic shock represents shock of cardiac origin: Exam will show characteristic signs of shock (hyperperfusion to extremities, hypotension, tachycardia) but history and exam will rule out extracardiac causes such as hypovolemia or sepsis. ECG may reveal an underlying acute event such as MI.
- **Cardiac arrest.** Patients in cardiac arrest are unresponsive, apneic, and pulseless. ECG may show asystole, PEA, or ventricular tachycardia or ventricular fibrillation. Confirm arrest in two or more ECG leads before beginning management.

60. **Based on the pathophysiology and clinical evaluation of the patient with chest pain, characterize the clinical problems according to their life-threatening potential.** p. 1212

Among cardiac causes, ischemia and MI are life threatening. Pericarditis becomes immediately life threatening if tamponade develops. Among vascular causes, dissection of the thoracic aorta is also immediately life threatening. Most of the respiratory causes are slightly less urgent (such as pneumonia and pleurisy), although both pulmonary embolism and pneumothorax can be immediately life threatening, especially in an individual with preexisting respiratory or cardiovascular compromise. The GI causes of chest pain most likely to prove truly urgent are those associated with GI hemorrhage: These may include esophageal disease and peptic ulcer disease. Cholecystitis and pancreatitis are serious medical emergencies, but they are generally slightly less urgent than cases involving active hemorrhage. Hiatal hernia, GERD, and dyspepsia require medical care but are relatively unlikely to require urgent care. Most musculoskeletal causes are not urgent and do not have immediate life-threatening potential, although chest trauma may involve injury to the respiratory and/or cardiovascular systems.

61. **Given several preprogrammed patients with cardiac complaints, provide the appropriate assessment, treatment, and transport.** pp. 1186–1237

During your training as an EMT-Paramedic you will participate in many classroom sessions involving simulated patients. You will also spend some time in the emergency departments of local hospitals as well as in advanced-level ambulances gaining clinical experience. During these times, use your knowledge of cardiac disease to help you assess and care for the simulated or real patients you attend.

Content Self-Evaluation

MULTIPLE CHOICE

_____ 1. Chest pain is the most common chief complaint among patients with cardiac disease, but not all patients with cardiac disease will have chest pain.
   A. True
   B. False

_____ 2. Which element of the OPQRST acronym represents those activities that either increase or decrease the severity of a symptom or complaint?
   A. "O"
   B. "P"
   C. "Q"
   D. "R"
   E. "S"

_____ 3. Which patient might you expect not to have chest pain while experiencing an MI?
   A. the young male
   B. the middle-aged female
   C. the athlete
   D. the diabetic
   E. the patient with no recent exertion

_____ 4. A family cardiac history is significant unless the family member had heart problems before the age of 40.
   A. True
   B. False

_____ 5. Auscultation of the carotid artery reveals a murmur. This finding is:
   A. normal.
   B. suggestive of the need for carotid massage.
   C. called a bruit.
   D. indicative of hypertension.
   E. a contraindication for thrombolytic therapy.

_____ 6. Which of the following is likely to cause a poor ECG signal?
   A. excessive body hair
   B. dried conductive gel
   C. poor electrode placement
   D. diaphoresis
   E. all of the above

_____ 7. Atropine, lidocaine, and adenosine are in which group of drugs?
   A. sympathomimetics
   B. sympatholytics
   C. fibrinolytics
   D. antidysrhythmics
   E. drugs used for myocardial ischemia and its pain

_____ 8. Dopamine, dobutamine, and epinephrine are in which group of drugs?
   A. sympatholytics
   B. drugs used for myocardial ischemia and its pain
   C. antidysrhythmics
   D. parasympathomimetics
   E. sympathomimetics

_____ 9. Nitrous oxide, nitroglycerin, fentanyl, and morphine are in which group of drugs?
   A. sympathomimetics
   B. drugs used for myocardial
   C. antidysrhythmics
   D. antiatherosclerotics ischemia and its pain
   E. sympatholytics

_____ 10. A potent loop diuretic used to relax the venous system and decrease intravascular fluid volume is:
   A. promethazine.
   B. alteplase.
   C. furosemide.
   D. sodium nitroprusside.
   E. isoproterenol.

_____ 11. Digitalis (digoxin) has all the following effects EXCEPT it:
   A. increases the force of cardiac contraction.
   B. suppresses atrial ectopy as an antidysrhythmic.
   C. increases cardiac output.
   D. decreases ventricular response to certain supraventricular dysrhythmias.
   E. decreases conduction through the AV node.

_____ 12. The alkalizing agents such as sodium bicarbonate are first line drugs in the treatment of asystole.
   A. True
   B. False

_____ 13. Repeated countershocks decrease the transthoracic resistance and allow the delivery of more energy to the heart.
   A. True
   B. False

_____ 14. Indications for synchronized cardioversion in an unstable patient include all of the following EXCEPT:
   A. rapid atrial fibrillation.
   B. nonperfusing ventricular tachycardia.
   C. paroxysmal supraventricular tachycardia.
   D. perfusing ventricular tachycardia.
   E. 2:1 atrial flutter.

_____ 15. When using the transthoracic pacer, you should set the rate at:
   A. between 60 and 80.
   B. between 40 and 60.
   C. between 80 and 100.
   D. never lower than 75.
   E. the patient's current heart rate.

_____ 16. To assure the defibrillator delivers the electrical energy at the right time during the heart's electrical sequence you must be sure the defibrillator is in the synchronized cardioversion mode and:
   A. the patient is premedicated.
   B. the energy is set to 100 joules.
   C. there is R wave capture.
   D. the defibrillator is fully energized.
   E. all of the above

_____ 17. If initial carotid massage does not slow the heart rate, massage both arteries simultaneously.
   A. True
   B. False

_____ 18. Potentially urgent noncardiac causes of chest pain include all of the following EXCEPT:
   A. stroke.
   B. peptic ulcer disease.
   C. pneumothorax.
   D. pulmonary embolism.
   E. esophageal disease.

_____ 19. The type of myocardial infarction where the injury affects the full thickness of the myocardium is termed:
   A. a non-Q wave infarction.
   B. angina.
   C. angina pectoris.
   D. a transmural infarction.
   E. a subendocardial infarction.

_____ 20. The greatest threat to the patient's life caused by the myocardial infarction is:
A. hypoxia.
B. dysrhythmias.
C. cardiac enzyme release.
D. pulmonary emboli.
E. nerve injury.

_____ 21. Always consider the possibility of cardiac tamponade when you encounter a patient:
A. with a chest wall tumor.
B. with muffled or distant heart and lung sounds.
C. with a gallop rhythm (S_1, S_2, S_3, S_4 heart sounds).
D. who has just entered ventricular fibrillation.
E. who received CPR and later deteriorated.

_____ 22. Causes of cardiogenic shock include all of the following EXCEPT:
A. subendocardial MI.
B. tension pneumothorax.
C. pulmonary embolism.
D. diffuse myocardial ischemia.
E. prosthetic valve malfunction.

_____ 23. Return of spontaneous circulation occurs when resuscitation results in resumption of a pulse; spontaneous breathing may or may not return.
A. True
B. False

_____ 24. Which of the following is NOT a criteria for termination of resuscitation efforts?
A. Successful and maintained endotracheal intubation.
B. Patient remains in asystole after four rounds of ALS drugs.
C. On-scene ALS efforts have been sustained for 25 minutes.
D. Arrest is associated with blunt trauma, hypothermia, or drug overdose.
E. ACLS standards have been applied throughout the arrest.

_____ 25. Which of the following is not a sign or symptom of abdominal aortic aneurysm?
A. hypotension
B. back pain
C. blood in the urine
D. urge to defecate
E. abdominal pain

MATCHING

Write the letter of the definition in the space provided next to the term to which it applies.

_____ 26. orthopnea

_____ 27. bruit

_____ 28. paroxysmal nocturnal dyspnea

_____ 29. pulsus paradoxus

_____ 30. pulsus alternans

_____ 31. intermittent claudication

_____ 32. thrombophlebitis

A. inflammation and clots within a vein

B. relief of dyspnea on sitting upright

C. alternation of weak and strong pulse over time

D. pain in the calf muscles secondary to local ischemia

E. episodes of being awakened at night by shortness of breath

F. murmur heard over an artery due to turbulent blood flow

G. drop of more than 10 mmHg in systolic BP with inspiration

Write the letter of the clinical setting in the space provided next to the procedure that should be carried out in that setting.

_____ 33. defibrillation

_____ 34. transcutaneous cardiac pacing

_____ 35. precordial thump

_____ 36. synchronized cardioversion

_____ 37. carotid sinus massage

A. effort made immediately after onset of ventricular fibrillation or pulseless ventricular tachycardia that may cause conversion to organized rhythm

B. passage of electrical current through the heart during a specific part of the cardiac cycle to terminate certain dysrhythmias

C. manipulation of an arterial baroreceptor in an effort to increase parasympathetic tone

D. electrical pacing of the heart with use of special skin electrodes

E. passage of electrical current through a fibrillating heart to depolarize a critical mass of myocardium, resulting in conversion to an organized rhythm

Write the letter of the cardiac condition in the space provided next to the ECG finding that would suggest it.

_____ 38. pathological Q wave

_____ 39. S-T segment elevation

_____ 40. T wave inversion

_____ 41. S-T segment depression

A. infarcted tissue or extensive transient ischemia

B. myocardial ischemia

C. myocardial injury

D. old infarcted tissue that has formed a scar

Write the letter of the probable diagnosis in the space provided next to the appropriate description of the condition. A letter response may be used more than once or not at all.

A. pulmonary edema
B. heart failure
C. acute MI
D. left ventricular failure
E. right ventricular failure
F. cardiac arrest
G. cardiac tamponade
H. hypertensive encephalopathy

_____ 42. constant chest pain that is not relieved by rest or nitroglycerin and lasts longer than 30 minutes

_____ 43. progressive fluid accumulation in the lungs

_____ 44. syndrome in which the heart's pumping ability does not meet body needs

_____ 45. unresponsiveness with apnea and pulselessness

_____ 46. jugular venous distention, engorged liver, edema, tachycardia

_____ 47. pulsus paradoxus and electrical alternans

_____ 48. dyspnea, orthopnea, decreased systolic BP with narrowing pulse pressures

_____ 49. severe headache, visual disturbance, seizures, stupor, diagnostic vital signs

Chapter 29

Neurology

Review of Chapter Objectives

After reading this chapter, you should be able to:

1. **Describe the incidence, morbidity, and mortality of neurological emergencies.**   p. 1244

   Diseases and conditions of the nervous system affect millions of Americans: You will see neurological emergencies in the field, and you will also see patients who present with another complaint but who have coexisting neurological conditions. Epilepsy affects about 2.5 million persons, who may present with a neurological emergency or have another condition complicated by their seizure disorder. Strokes are medical emergencies, and they affect about 500,000 people annually, of whom about 150,000 die. Strokes are also a frequent source of considerable morbidity. Recent studies have shown that early recognition and intervention in certain strokes due to thromboembolism may decrease their morbidity and mortality. Neoplasms affecting the CNS occur in about 40,000 persons annually; morbidity and mortality depend on variables including tumor type and location. The miscellaneous group termed the degenerative disorders account for considerable morbidity for many Americans, and they often account for premature death, as well. Multiple sclerosis affects about 300,000 to 400,000 Americans, and typical first presentation is at the age range of 20 to 40 years. Parkinson's disease affects more than 500,000 Americans, who are typically 60 years or older.

   Other neurological conditions are extremely common and of variable cause and rate of morbidity/mortality. For instance, nearly half of all Americans will have a syncopal episode (that is, faint) in their lifetime, and syncope accounts for roughly 3 percent of all emergency department visits. Headaches of various causes are extremely common, with nearly 45 million persons affected by chronic headaches. Low back pain can be either acute or chronic, and roughly 60 to 90 percent of Americans will experience some type of lower back pain in their lifetimes.

2. **Identify the risk factors most predisposing to diseases of the nervous system.**   pp. 1258–1259, 1263–1264, 1267, 1268, 1276

   Risk factors differ for the various types of neurological conditions. Strokes are vascular in nature (hemorrhagic or occlusive), and the major risk factors for stroke reflect this: atherosclerosis, heart disease, diabetes, abnormal blood lipid levels, hypertension, sickle cell disease, use of oral contraceptives, and the cardiac dysrhythmia atrial fibrillation. Some chronic conditions such as epilepsy reflect different causes and thus have different risk factors. Epilepsy can develop in patients who have had head trauma, brain tumors, or certain vascular disorders such as stroke. Most cases are considered idiopathic, which means the cause is unknown. Syncope is similar in having very different causes. Syncopal episodes can be due to cardiovascular (such as dysrhythmias or mechanical problems) origin or noncardiovascular (metabolic, neurologic, or psychiatric) origin; indeed, many episodes are considered idiopathic even after workup. Headaches tend to be classified as vascular (such as migraine), tension, or organic (the last including headaches due to tumor, infection,

©2007 Pearson Education, Inc.
Essentials of Paramedic Care, 2nd ed.

or other conditions). Some of the risk factors for low back pain may be gender-related. Symptoms in women over age 60 years, for example, often reflect postmenopausal osteoporosis. Occupations involving exposure to vibrations from vehicles or machinery or jobs requiring repetitious lifting also are associated with risk for low back pain. Other causes include compression or trauma to the sciatic nerve or its roots, as can happen with a herniated intervertebral disk. Most cases, though, are also idiopathic.

3. **Discuss the anatomy and physiology of the nervous system.** (see Chapter 3)

The nervous system is the body's chief control for virtually every major function. It is divided physically into the central nervous system (CNS) and peripheral nervous system (PNS). The CNS consists of the brain and spinal cord. If the body were visualized as a computer, the CNS would be the central processing unit. Both very basic functions, such as continuance of heartbeat and respiration, and complex functions, such as listening to Mozart and anticipating a musical passage you particularly like, are controlled by cells in the brain. Messages within the CNS, as well as those that connect it with the rest of the body, travel as nerve impulses. The complex network of nerves outside the CNS makes up the peripheral nervous system. The messages that carry information regarding critical body functions such as respiration pass through a part of the PNS called the autonomic nervous system; these functions do not require any conscious effort to maintain them. In contrast, messages that involve voluntary, or conscious, actions and thoughts travel through the other part of the PNS, the somatic nervous system. Both the autonomic and somatic nervous systems have two parallel tracks: one of nerves that carry messages to the brain, and a second that carries messages from the brain. In terms of the computer analogy, the PNS carries the various input and output messages that run between the brain and spinal cord and the rest of the body. The autonomic nervous system is also structurally and functionally broken into two parts: the sympathetic and parasympathetic nervous systems. These two parts work together to make sure the net balance of stimulatory and inhibitory messages from the brain keep body functions such as blood pressure within normal limits.

The basic structural and functional unit is the neuron, or nerve cell. Nerve cells have a body that contains the essential cell machinery of nucleus, mitochondria, and so forth. Nerve processes (usually there are many) that are capable of receiving impulses from other neurons or body cells are called dendrites. An impulse that is picked up by a dendrite travels toward the cell body. Another process, the axon, carries the impulse away from the cell body. Axons may have multiple tips, which means the neuron has the capacity to send the impulse onward to more than one other nerve or other cell. Dendrites associated with neurons of the major senses organs (such as the eye or ear) convert an environmental stimulus into a nerve impulse that can be forwarded via the axon to other nerves, and eventually the brain. Dendrites associated with neurons that monitor internal conditions such as PaO_2 also convert that information into an impulse and send it to the brain. Eventually all such information is analyzed by neurons in the brain and response impulses travel back through the PNS. These impulses eventually affect a motor neuron, causing a muscle cell to contract, or affect another type of cell such as one in a gland. Messages cannot pass directly from an axon to a dendrite because there is a tiny physical gap, called a synapse, between each pair of neurons. As the wave of electrical depolarization (due to ion fluxes of potassium rapidly leaving the neuron and sodium rapidly entering) reaches the axon tip, it causes a chemical called a neurotransmitter to be released into the synapse. (There are multiple neurotransmitters within the body. Either acetylcholine or norepinephrine is found in the neurons of the PNS. Neurotransmitters within the CNS include dopamine and serotonin.) When the neurotransmitter crosses the synapse and is taken up by the dendrite on the other side, a wave of depolarization is started in that dendrite and the nerve impulse is then carried toward the cell body.

Most of the CNS is protected by the bones of the cranium and spine. The spinal column is made up of 33 vertebrae running from the neck to the junction with the pelvis. There is also an inner shock-absorbing, cushioning protection system. The cells of the brain and spinal cord are bathed in cerebrospinal fluid, and there are three layers of protective membranes between the neural surface and the outer protective bone. These meninges are called the dura mater, arachnoid membrane, and pia mater (in outer-to-inner sequence).

As you look at a human brain, it has six obvious structural regions: the cerebrum, the diencephalon, the mesencephalon (or midbrain), the pons, the medulla oblongata, and the cerebellum.

Sometimes, the terminology is simplified as follows: the forebrain (cerebrum and diencephalon), the midbrain, and the hindbrain (the brainstem—pons, medulla oblongata—and the cerebellum). The largest part of the brain, with its characteristic folded outer surfaces, is the cerebrum. The cerebrum has left and right sides, or hemispheres, which are connected physically and functionally by tissue called the corpus callosum. The cerebrum is responsible for intelligence, learning, memory, and language, as well as analysis and response to sensory and motor activities. The diencephalon is covered by the cerebrum, and it is made up of a number of vital structures: the thalamus, hypothalamus, and the limbic system. This primal part of the brain is responsible for many involuntary functions such as temperature regulation, sleep, water balance, stress response, and emotion. It also has an important role in regulating the autonomic nervous system. The brainstem consists of the mesencephalon, pons, and medulla oblongata. The mesencephalon is located between the diencephalon and the pons, and it plays a role in motor coordination. It is the major region controlling eye movement. The pons is a major connection point between the upper portions of the brain and the medulla and cerebellum. The medulla oblongata itself marks the division between the brain and the spinal cord. The major centers for control of respiration, cardiac activity, and vasomotor activity are located here. The cerebellum is located in the posterior fossa of the cranium, and it also has two hemispheres, which are closely coordinated to the brainstem and higher centers. The cerebellum coordinates fine motor movement, posture, equilibrium, and muscle tone.

The hemispheres of the cerebrum do not contain identical centers. Rather, the functional responsibilities of the cerebrum have been mapped as a whole. Important centers with clinical implications for you in cases such as stroke or trauma include the following: (1) speech, which is located in the temporal lobe; (2) vision, which is located in the occipital lobe; (3) personality, which is located in the frontal lobes; (4) sensory, which is located in the parietal lobes; and (5) motor, which is located in the frontal lobes. As noted previously, balance and coordination are located in the cerebellum. A last important center is called the reticular activating system (RAS), which operates in the lateral portion of the medulla, pons, and especially the mesencephalon. The RAS sends impulses to and receives messages from the cerebral cortex (the outer portion of the cerebrum). This diffuse system of interlaced cells is responsible for maintaining consciousness and the ability to respond to external stimuli.

The brain receives about 20 percent of the body's total blood flow per minute. Vascular supply to the brain is provided by two systems, a physical arrangement that provides secondary supply if one system is occluded or severed. The anterior system is the carotid, and the posterior system is the vertebrobasilar. They join at the circle of Willis before entering the structures of the brain itself. Venous drainage is via the venous sinuses and the internal jugular veins. As previously noted, there is also cerebrospinal fluid (CSF) bathing the tissues of the brain and spinal cord. Most of the intracranial CSF is found in the ventricles.

The spinal cord is 17 to 18 inches long on average in adults. It leaves the brain at the medulla and passes through an opening in the skull called the foramen magnum to enter the spinal canal. The spinal cord, which ends near the level of the first lumbar vertebra (the reason why spinal taps are done below that level), conducts impulses to and from the peripheral nervous system and locally for motor reflexes. Thirty-one pairs of nerves exit the spinal cord between adjacent vertebrae. The dorsal nerve roots carry afferent fibers, ones carrying impulses to the brain. The ventral roots carry efferent fibers, which carry impulses from the brain to the periphery. Each nerve root has a corresponding area of skin called a dermatome, to which it supplies sensation. In the field, you may be able to correlate sensory deficits to the level of a spinal cord problem. The reason why our protective motor reflexes are so fast and effective lies in the fact that the afferent and efferent impulses are coordinated in the spinal cord—they do not travel the whole way to the brain before coming back. However, because they are mediated in the spinal cord, they lack fine motor control.

The peripheral nervous system (PNS) contains 12 pairs of cranial nerves, which extend directly from the lower surface of the brain and exit through small holes in the skull, and the peripheral nerves, which exit from the spinal cord as noted previously. The nerves of the PNS control both voluntary and involuntary activities. The cranial nerves supply nervous control for the head, neck, and certain thoracic and abdominal organs. The peripheral nerves can be divided into four classes: (1) somatic sensory, afferent nerves that carry impulses concerned with touch, pressure, pain, temperature, and position; (2) somatic motor, efferent nerves that carry impulses to the skeletal (voluntary) muscles; (3) visceral (autonomic) sensory, afferent nerves that carry impulses of sensation from the visceral organs (examples being fullness in the bladder or distension of the rectum); and (4) visceral (autonomic) motor, efferent nerves that serve the involuntary cardiac muscle and the smooth muscle of the viscera and the glands.

The involuntary division of the PNS is called the autonomic nervous system, and it has two components: the sympathetic nervous system and the parasympathetic nervous system. The sympathetic system is associated with the primitive "fight-or-flight" response to sensory stimuli. Its major nerve roots are located near the thoracic and lumbar part of the spinal cord. Stimulation causes increased heart rate and blood pressure, pupillary dilation, rise in blood sugar, as well as bronchodilation, all responses that ready the body for stress. The neurotransmitters norepinephrine and epinephrine mediate its actions, and sympathetic activity is also closely correlated to activity in the adrenal gland medulla, tissue that is of nervous system origin and that also relies on norepinephrine and epinephrine. The parasympathetic nervous system is responsible for controlling vegetative functions such as normal heart rate and blood pressure. It is associated with the cranial nerves and the sacral plexus of nerves, and it is mediated by the neurotransmitter acetylcholine. When stimulated, it causes a decrease in heart rate, an increase in digestive activity, pupillary constriction, and a reduction in blood sugar.

4. **Define and discuss the epidemiology (including the morbidity/mortality and preventative strategies), pathophysiology, assessment findings, and management for the following neurologic problems:**

   a. **Coma and altered mental status**   pp. 1256–1257

   Altered mental status is extremely common, as you'll understand when you consider the wide variety of causes. Morbidity and mortality are often correlated to cause. Vigilant assessment and management on your part will optimize your patient's chances, regardless of causes. An alteration in mental status is the hallmark sign of CNS injury or illness; as such, any alteration, be it subtle or as florid as coma, requires evaluation. In coma, the patient cannot be aroused by even powerful external stimuli such as pain. The two mechanisms generally capable of causing altered mental status are structural lesions (such as tumor, trauma, degenerative disease, or another process that destroys or encroaches on the substance of the brain) and toxic-metabolic states (such as the presence of toxins including ammonia or the absence of vital substances such as oxygen, glucose, or thiamine). Causes of toxic-metabolic disturbances include anoxia, diabetic ketoacidosis, hepatic failure, hypoglycemia, renal failure, thiamine deficiency, and toxic exposure (for instance, cyanide). Some of the most common causes you'll see for altered mental status (meaning they can cause a structural lesion or a toxic-metabolic state) are the following: (1) drugs, including depressants such as alcohol, hallucinogens, and narcotics; (2) cardiovascular, including anaphylaxis, cardiac arrest, stroke, dysrhythmias, hypertensive encephalopathy, and shock; (3) respiratory, including chronic obstructive pulmonary disease (COPD), inhalation of a toxic gas such as carbon monoxide, and hypoxia; and (4) infectious, such as AIDS, encephalitis, and meningitis.

   During history taking and assessment, remember the mnemonic AEIOU-TIPS, and look for signs of these common causes: A (acidosis or alcohol), E (epilepsy), I (infection), O (overdose), U (uremia, or kidney failure), T (trauma, tumor, or toxin), I (insulin, either hypoglycemia or ketoacidosis), P (psychosis or poison), S (stroke, seizure). During physical assessment, use the AVPU method for determining level of consciousness. Unresponsive patients require especially vigilant monitoring and protection of the airway. Remember that in some cases you will not be able to determine the cause of the problem in the prehospital setting.

   Management begins with the ABCs. The initial priority is the airway; be sure to immobilize the C-spine in cases of suspected head or neck injury. Then attend to breathing, administering supplemental oxygen, and assisting ventilations if needed. An unresponsive patient requires an airway adjunct. As an evaluation of circulation, check heart rate and rhythm and blood pressure. Then perform the following steps:
   - IV of normal saline or lactated Ringer's solution at a keep-vein-open rate; alternatively place a heparin lock.
   - Determine blood glucose level with reagent strip or glucometer. If serum glucose is low, give 50 percent dextrose to mediate the hypoglycemia. Even if the patient is an

uncontrolled diabetic, any transient hyperglycemia will do limited harm at most in the short prehospital period. In many cases of hypoglycemia, dextrose can be lifesaving, and you may see an immediate response. Glucose may also be lifesaving for the alcoholic patient with hypoglycemia.
- Administer naloxone if there is suspicion of narcotic overdose. (See Chapter 34, "Toxicology and Substance Abuse," for details.)
- If there is suspicion of alcoholism, consider use of 100 mg thiamine (Vitamin B1).

In chronic alcoholism, intake, absorption, and use of thiamine is impaired. Among these patients, you may see Wernicke's syndrome, a condition marked by loss of memory and disorientation that is associated with a diet deficient in thiamine. Of even greater concern is Korsakoff's psychosis, marked by memory disorder, because it may be irreversible. Thus, the administration of thiamine as per local protocols and the judgment of medical direction may be important.

If increased intracranial pressure is possible, as in a closed head injury, ventilate the patient at 12 breaths per minute. The decrease in carbon dioxide causes cerebral vasoconstriction and reduces brain swelling. DO NOT hyperventilate, as this can decrease CO_2 to dangerously low levels. Medical direction may order use of mannitol (Osmotrol) to cause a diuresis that may shift fluid from the intravascular space through the kidneys.

b. Seizures pp. 1264–1267

A seizure is a temporary alteration in behavior due to a massive discharge of one or more groups of neurons in the brain. Seizures can be induced in anyone under certain stressful conditions such as hypoxia or rapidly decreasing blood glucose. Febrile seizures often occur in young children with a sudden increase in body temperature. Structural diseases of the brain such as tumors, head trauma, toxic eclampsia, and vascular disorders can also cause a seizure. Recurrent seizures without such a known cause are termed epilepsy. Epilepsy affects about 2.5 million persons, who may present with a neurological emergency or have another condition complicated by their seizure disorder. Most cases of epilepsy are idiopathic, that is, without known cause, whereas others arise secondary to damage from strokes, head trauma, tumor surgery or radiation, and so on.

Assessment begins with history according to the patient or bystanders, as well as physical impression. Remember that many people think the only kind of seizure is a "grand mal," so a bystander who does not know the patient may suggest he is on drugs, or that he fainted, or give other information that is misleading. In addition, other medical conditions can present similarly to a seizure: Examples are migraine headaches, cardiac dysrhythmias, hypoglycemia, or orthostatic hypotension. Hyperventilation, as well as a number of CNS conditions, can cause stiffness in the extremities. Decerebrate movements can be caused by increased intracranial pressure. Thus, there is often more potential harm than good in administering an anticonvulsant.

The patient history should include an attempt to ascertain the following information: (1) history of seizures, and, if so, particulars of type, nature, and frequency; (2) recent history of head trauma; (3) possibility of alcohol or other drug use; (4) recent history of fever, headache, or stiff neck; (5) history of diabetes, heart disease, or stroke; and (6) current medications. During physical exam, look for evidence of head injury or injury to the tongue and for evidence of alcohol or drug abuse. Be sure to document any dysrhythmias.

Active management may not be needed for many types of seizures, including short generalized tonic-clonic seizures that have ended before you arrive. Management for most generalized seizures in process is supportive: Manage the airway, make sure the patient does not injure himor herself, and monitor for possible hyper- or hypothermia, depending on environmental conditions. General procedures include the following: (1) assurance of scene safety; (2) maintenance of airway (DO NOT force objects between the patient's teeth or push objects into the mouth that may initiate vomiting); (3) administration of high-flow oxygen; (4) establishment of IV access, running normal saline or lactated Ringer's solution at keep-vein-open rate; (5) determination of blood glucose level, with 50 percent glucose given in hypoglycemia; (6) physical protection of patient from surroundings; (7) maintenance of temperature; (8) postictal positioning on left side with suction if required; (9) monitoring of cardiac rhythm; (10) consideration of an anticonvulsant if seizure is prolonged (greater than 5 minutes); and (11) transport the patient in supine or lateral recumbent position in quiet, reassuring atmosphere.

Status epilepticus, two or more generalized seizures without intervening return of consciousness, can be a life-threatening emergency. The most common cause in adults with epilepsy is failure to comply with medication regimen. Status is a major emergency because it involves a prolonged period of apnea with the possibility of CNS hypoxia. The most valuable intervention is to protect the airway and to deliver 100 percent oxygen, preferably by BVM device. After airway and breathing have been addressed, start an IV with normal saline at keep-vein-open rate, monitor cardiac rhythm, give 25 g of 50 percent dextrose IV push if hypoglycemia is present, give 5–10 mg diazepam IV push for an adult, and continue to monitor airway. Note that some patients will require large doses of diazepam, and this may cause respiratory depression. Depression, if significant, can be reversed with flumazenil, although this may also result in the return of seizures.

c. Syncope   pp. 1267–1268

Syncope, or fainting, is characterized by a sudden, temporary loss of consciousness caused by insufficient blood flow to the brain, with recovery almost immediate upon supine positioning. Syncope is very common, accounting for roughly 3 percent of all emergency department visits. It can occur at any age. Symptoms may include prior feelings of dizziness or light-headedness or there may be no warning at all. By definition, if return of consciousness does not occur within a few moments, the event is NOT syncope; it is something more serious. (Review Table 29-2, text page 1261, for help in distinguishing between syncope and seizure.)

There are three pathophysiologic mechanisms for syncope: cardiovascular, noncardiovascular, and idiopathic. Cardiovascular causes include dysrhythmias or mechanical problems such as an abnormally functioning heart valve. Noncardiovascular causes include metabolic, neurological, or psychiatric conditions. For instance, hypoglycemia, a transient ischemic attack (TIA), or an anxiety attack may all precipitate syncope. Idiopathic, as always, means there is no known cause even after careful evaluation. Management begins with an attempt to find and treat the underlying cause. If no cause is established, the patient should be transported to an appropriate emergency department for evaluation. Field management is somewhat similar to that for seizure: assure scene safety, maintain open airway, administer high-flow oxygen and assist ventilations as needed, check circulatory status (heart rate and rhythm, blood pressure), check and continue monitoring mental status, start IV with normal saline or lactated Ringer's at keep-vein-open rate, determine blood glucose level, monitor cardiac rhythm, and transport in a reassuring environment.

d. Headache   pp. 1268–1270

Headaches, either acute or chronic, are a tremendously common complaint: You've probably had problems with a headache at least once. Nearly 45 million Americans suffer from chronic headaches. There are three general categories of headache: vascular, tension, and organic. Headaches of vascular origin include migraines and cluster headaches. Migraines occur more commonly in women, whereas cluster headaches occur more commonly in men. Migraines are typically characterized by intense, throbbing pain, sensitivity to light or sound, nausea, vomiting, and sweating. Migraines may last from several minutes to several days. They typically present as one-sided headaches and they may be preceded by an aura. Cluster headaches usually occur as a series of one-sided headaches that are sudden in onset, intense, and continue for roughly 15 minutes to 4 hours. Symptoms may include nasal congestion, drooping eyelid, and an irritated eye. Tension headaches account for a significant percentage of headaches. Most personnel in emergency medicine have, or will have, a tension headache. Some people experience them on a daily basis. These persons may wake with a headache that worsens over the course of the day. The typical tension headache has a dull, achy pain that feels as if forceful pressure is being applied to the neck or head. The last class of headache, organic headaches, is less common. They occur in association with tumor, infection, or other diseases of the brain, eye, or other body system.

Because headaches can herald serious illness or precede a catastrophic event such as a ruptured aneurysm, it is always important to keep these possible underlying causes in mind when you speak with a patient complaining of headache. A continuous throbbing headache, particularly if over the occiput, accompanied by fever, confusion, and stiffness of the neck is classic for meningitis. Sudden onset pain, often described as "the worst pain of my life," or changes in pain pattern should all be considered possible signs of conditions as grave as intracranial hemorrhage. In general, any headache of acute onset or of changing pattern demands immediate attention on your part.

A complete and thorough history is important in evaluating the patient with headache. Questions that may evoke valuable information include the following: What were you doing when the pain started? Does anything make the pain worse (such as light, sound, or movement)? What is the quality of the pain, throbbing, crushing, tension? Does pain radiate to the neck, arm, back, or jaw? What is the severity of the pain on a scale of 1 to 10 and has severity changed? How long has the headache been present (is it acute or chronic)? You will see that the same line of questioning about pain is used in other settings, too, as with patients who complain of abdominal pain (Chapter 32, "Gastroenterology").

Management is supportive and generally includes the following: (1) assurance of scene safety; (2) protection of airway; (3) placement of patient in position of comfort (often accomplished by patients themselves); (4) high-flow oxygen with ventilation assistance as needed; (5) IV with normal saline or lactated Ringer's at keep-vein-open rate, determination of blood glucose, monitoring of cardiac rhythm; (6) transport with reassurance in an environment that is calm and quiet; and (7) consideration of use of antiemetics or analgesics. Antiemetics that might be helpful for migraine include prochlorperazine (Compazine) and abortive agents such as sumatriptan (Imitrix).

e. Neoplasms pp. 1270–1272

Neoplasm is a general term for "new growth," and it is used to describe tumors that arise after birth. Neoplasms of the CNS affect about 40,000 Americans per year. These neoplasms can be divided into benign and malignant tumors based on several characteristics. The cells of a benign tumor generally resemble normal cells, grow relatively slowly, and tend to remain confined to one location. In contrast, malignant tumors of the CNS often have cells that are primitive in appearance and don't resemble normal cells, grow quickly, and may invade adjacent healthy tissue or spread within the CNS. Both kinds of CNS tumors can be dangerous because any tumor growth can place pressure on other tissues and impair their function and because the pressure cannot be relieved by expansion of the cranial space. In adults, the cranium is rigid and fixed. Pressure exerted by a tumor causes increased intracranial pressure. There are numerous types of brain tumors, and the cause is unknown for most of them.

CNS tumors present with many signs and symptoms dependent on the size, type, and location of the tumor. It isn't your role in the field to diagnose new tumors; rather, you are more likely to have patients with previously diagnosed tumors or patients who present with problems that may reflect a CNS tumor. Common complaints among persons with undiagnosed brain tumors include the following: headache (often severe and recurrent), new onset seizures, nausea and vomiting, behavioral or cognitive changes, weakness or paralysis of one or more limbs or one side of the face, change in sensation in one or more limbs or one side of the face, new onset uncoordination, difficulty walking or unsteady gait, dizziness, and double vision. Be alert for any of these signs and be sure to obtain a thorough history. In addition to the SAMPLE questions, ask the following: (1) What is the state of your general health? (2) Have you had any seizure activity, headache, or nosebleed? (3) Have you ever had surgery for removal of a brain tumor, chemotherapy, radiation therapy, holistic therapy, or any form of experimental treatment?

Management is largely supportive, with the goal of reducing anxiety and palliating symptoms. The general steps of field management have much in common with those for seizures and headaches. Assure scene safety, and protect the airway. Position the patient for comfort, generally with head elevated. Use high-flow oxygen and assist ventilations as needed. Start an IV with normal saline or lactated Ringer's at keep-vein-open rate or use a saline or heparin lock. Monitor cardiac rhythm and consider narcotic analgesia if approved by medical direction. Consider diazepam if seizures are present. Medical direction may recommend either antiinflammatory medication (dexamethasone) and/or diuretics. Last, transport in a calm, quiet environment while reassuring the patient.

f. Abscess p. 1272

A brain abscess is a pocket of pus localized to one area of the brain. They are uncommon, accounting for 2 percent of intracranial masses. Signs and symptoms are similar to those of a neoplasm and include headache, lethargy, hemiparesis (weakness on one side of the body), seizures, rigidity of the neck, nausea, and vomiting. Fever is frequently present, suggesting an infectious cause. Your field management is supportive and similar to that for neoplasm or meningitis.

g. Stroke
pp. 1257–1263

Stroke is a general term for injury or death of brain tissue, usually due to interruption of blood flow to that region of the cerebrum. The term "brain attack" is being used more frequently because of some similarities between stroke and heart attack, the latter also being due to oxygen deprivation. You should also realize that there are more treatment similarities to heart attacks. Strokes due to thromboembolic causes may be aborted or minimized with use of fibrinolytic agents now used with heart attack (such as tissue plasminogen activator, tPA). The importance to you is that prompt recognition and transport of stroke patients is greater than ever. Stroke patients who may be candidates for fibrinolytic therapy must receive definitive treatment within 3 hours of onset.

Strokes are the third most common cause of death and a frequent cause of considerable disability among middle-aged and elderly persons. Major risk factors include atherosclerosis, heart disease, hypertension, diabetes, abnormal blood lipid levels, use of oral contraceptives, and sickle cell disease. Strokes can be caused either by occlusion of an artery or by hemorrhage. Both interrupt blood flow to distal tissues. An occlusive stroke is caused by blockage of the artery, resulting in ischemia to brain tissue that may progress to infarction if oxygen deprivation continues long enough. Infarcted brain tissue swells, further damaging nearby tissue that might have only a marginal blood supply itself. If swelling is sufficiently severe, herniation (protrusion of tissue through the foramen magnum, the opening at the base of the skull through which the spinal cord emerges from the cranium) can occur. Occlusive strokes are either thrombotic or embolic in origin.

Thrombotic strokes are due to a thrombus, or blood clot, that forms in and then obstructs a cerebral artery. Thrombosis is often related to atherosclerotic change in the artery. Unsurprisingly, the signs and symptoms of a thrombotic stroke are often gradual in onset. The stroke often occurs at night and is characterized by the patient waking with altered mental status and/or loss of speech, sensation, or motor function. An embolic stroke is caused by a solid, liquid, or gaseous mass that is carried to the site of obstruction from a remote site. The most common brain emboli are blood clots that often arise from diseased blood vessels in the neck (namely, the carotid artery) or from abnormal cardiac contraction. Atrial fibrillation often results in atrial dilation, a precursor to clot formation. Other types of emobli include air, tumor tissue, and fat. Typically, embolic strokes present with sudden onset of severe headaches. Hemorrhagic strokes are due to bleeding within brain tissue, and they can be categorized as intracerebral or subarachnoid (see Figure 29-7, text page 1260). They are discussed in detail below under intracranial hemorrhage.

Prompt and proper assessment of a stroke in progress is very important. Signs and symptoms will depend on the type of stroke and the area of the brain affected by it. Onset of symptoms may be acute, and the patient may be unconscious. You may observe stertorous breathing due to paralysis of part of the soft palate. Respiratory expirations may be puffs of air out of the cheeks and mouth. The patient's pupils may be unequal. If so, the larger pupil will be on the side of the hemorrhage. Paralysis, when present, usually involves one side of the face, one arm, or one leg. Speech disturbances may be noted, and the patient's skin may be cool and clammy.

In list form, common signs and symptoms of stroke include the following: one-sided facial drooping, headache, confusion and agitation, dysphasia (difficulty in speech), aphasia (inability to speak), dysarthria (impairment of tongue and muscles making speech difficult), vision problems such as blindness in one eye or double vision, hemiparesis (one-sided weakness), hemiplegia (one-sided paralysis), paresthesias, inability to recognize by touch, gait disturbances or uncoordinated motor movements, dizziness, incontinence, or coma.

Management of stroke emphasizes early recognition; supportive measures; prompt, rapid transport; and notification of the emergency department (see algorithm in Figure 29-8, text page 1263). Remember that aggressive airway management is vital in these patients. Other field measures include the following: (1) assurance of scene safety, including body substance isolation; (2) airway management including suction as needed; (3) ventilation assistance as needed: If the patient is apneic or breathing is inadequate, provide positive-pressure ventilation at 20/minute. Hyperventilation eliminates excessive CO_2 levels. Avoid hyperventilation because excessively low CO_2 levels can cause profound cerebral vasoconstriction. If breathing is adequate, give oxygen via nonrebreather mask at 15 L/minute; (4) complete a detailed patient history; (5) keep patient supine or in recovery position. If the patient has congestive heart failure, place patient in semi-upright position as needed. If patient has altered mental status and you suspect potential for airway compromise, keep him or her in left lateral recumbent, or recovery position; (6) determine blood glucose level: if hypoglycemia is present, consider 50 percent dextrose by IV push; (7) start an IV of normal saline or lactated Ringer's at a keep-vein-open rate or place a saline or heparin lock (avoiding dextrose solutions, which may increase intracranial pressure due to osmotic effect); (8) monitor cardiac rhythm; (9) protect paralyzed extremities; (10) reassure patient and explain all procedures as the patient may be able to understand even if he or she cannot respond; and (11) transport without excessive movement or noise.

h. Intracranial hemorrhage   pp. 1259–1263

Hemorrhagic strokes are due to blood within brain tissue, and they can be categorized as intracerebral or subarachnoid. These intracranial hemorrhages often occur with sudden onset of a severe headache. Most intracranial hemorrhages occur in a hypertensive patient when a small vessel deep within brain tissue ruptures. Subarachnoid hemorrhages most commonly result from either congenital blood vessel anomalies or from head trauma. Congenital anomalies include aneurysms and arteriovenous malformations. Aneurysms tend to be on the brain's surface and may either hemorrhage into brain tissue or into the subarachnoid space. Hemorrhage within brain tissue may tear and separate normal brain tissue. Release of blood into the ventricles containing CSF may paralyze vital centers. If blood impairs drainage of CSF, the resultant increase in intracranial pressure may cause herniation of brain tissue.

i. Transient ischemic attack   pp. 1260–1261

A transient ischemic attack (TIA) is a temporary manifestation of the signs and/or symptoms of stroke that is due to temporary interference with blood supply to the affected part of the brain. These symptoms may persist for a few minutes or for hours, but they almost always resolve within 24 hours. After the attack (because it reflects ischemia, not infarction), there is no evidence of brain or neurological damage. The most common cause is carotid artery disease (provoking an embolic event). Other causes can be small emboli of different origin, decreased cardiac output, hypotension, overmedication with antihypertensive medications, or cerebrovascular spasm. Part of the importance of recognizing TIAs is that they may be the precursor to a stroke. One third of TIA patients suffer a stroke soon afterward. A TIA is typically sudden in onset, with specific signs and symptoms depending on the part of the brain involved.

In the prehospital setting, it is virtually impossible to distinguish a TIA from a stroke. While taking the history, try to get the following information: previous neurological symptoms, if any; initial symptoms and their progression; changes in mental status; precipitating factors, if any; dizziness; palpitations; history of hypertension, cardiac disease, sickle cell disease, or previous TIA or stroke. Because TIAs and strokes are generally indistinguishable in the field, the management is the same. (See Stroke above.)

j. Degenerative neurological diseases   pp. 1272–1275

The term "degenerative neurological disease" characterizes diseases that selectively affect one or more functional systems of the CNS. Generally, they produce symmetrical and progressive involvement of the CNS, affect similar areas of the brain, and produce similar clinical signs and symptoms. Examples discussed in the text include Alzheimer's disease, muscular dystrophy, multiple sclerosis, dystonias, Parkinson's disease, central pain syndrome, Bell's palsy, amyotrophic lateral sclerosis, myoclonus, spina bifida, and poliomyelitis. Alzheimer's disease is perhaps the most important of the degenerative disorders because of its frequency and its devastating nature. It is the most common cause of dementia in the elderly. Alzheimer's results from neuronal cell death and disappearance in the cerebral cortex, causing marked atrophy of the brain. Initially, patients have problems with short-term memory, and this usually progresses to problems with thought and intellect. Patients also develop a shuffling gait and have stiffness of body muscles. As the disease progresses, the patient develops aphasia and psychiatric problems. In its final stages, the patient may become virtually decorticate, losing all ability to think, speak, and move. Muscular dystrophy (MD) actually refers to a group of genetic diseases characterized by progressive muscle weakness and degeneration of skeletal muscle fibers. The heart and other involuntary muscles are affected in some types of MD. The most common form is Duchenne's MD. Some forms begin in childhood whereas others do not appear until midlife. Prognosis depends on the type and individual progression of the disorder. Multiple sclerosis (MS) is another common and potentially devastating degenerative disorder. It involves inflammation of certain nerve cells followed by demyelination (loss of the fatty insulation surrounding nerve fibers in the CNS). Prevalence in the United States is approximately 300,000–400,000 persons. Most are women who first developed symptoms between ages 20 and 40 years. The pathophysiology of MS involves autoimmune attack against myelin. Signs and symptoms include weakness of one or more limbs, sensory loss, paresthesias, and changes in vision. Symptoms may wax and wane over years, and they may range from mild to severe. Severe cases leave the patient so debilitated she may not be able to care for herself.

The dystonias are characterized by muscle contractions that cause twisting, repetitive movements, abnormal postures, or freezing in the middle of an action. Early symptoms include deterioration in handwriting, foot cramps, or tendency of one foot to drag after walking or running. In some cases, symptoms become more noticeable and widespread over time. In other individuals, there is little or no progression over time. Parkinson's disease is a motor system disorder also called a "shaking palsy." Parkinson's is characterized chemically by a deficiency of dopamine in the CNS, and treatment is generally aimed at increasing levels in the brain. Parkinson's is common, and you will see it. Roughly 500,000 Americans are affected, and more than 50,000 new cases are reported annually. It affects men and women equally and has an average age at onset of 60 years. It usually does not develop in persons under 40. Parkinson's is chronic and progressive, and its signs fall into four categories: tremor (which usually begins in the hand and may progress to involve the arm, a foot, or the jaw), rigidity (resistance to movement among muscles in opposing pairs), bradykinesia (slowing or loss of normal, spontaneous movement), and postural instability (with development of a forward or backward lean, stooped posture, or tendency to fall easily).

Central pain syndrome results from damage or injury to the brain, brainstem, or spinal cord, and it is marked by intense, steady pain that may be described as burning, aching, tingling, or "pins and needles." It occurs in patients who, at some point in the past, have had strokes, multiple sclerosis, limb amputation, or spinal cord injury. Pain medications generally do not provide relief, and patients often rely on sedatives or other means of keeping the CNS free from stress. One example is trigeminal neuralgia, which is caused by abnormal impulse conduction along the trigeminal nerve (cranial nerve V). It often has brief episodes of intense facial pain. The fear of a possible attack may be debilitating. Medications including carbamazepine (Tegretol) may be helpful, and surgery may be indicated for select cases.

Bell's palsy is the most common form of facial paralysis, affecting roughly 40,000 Americans yearly. It results from inflammation of the facial nerve (cranial nerve VII) and is marked by one-sided facial paralysis, inability to close the eye on the affected side, pain, tearing of that eye, drooling, hypersensitivity to sound, and impaired taste. Multiple causes exist, among them head trauma, herpes simplex virus, and Lyme disease. Treatment is usually aimed at protecting the eye. Corticosteroids may be used for inflammation when pain is severe. Most patients recover within 3 months. Amyotrophic lateral sclerosis (ALS, or Lou Gehrig's disease), affects 20,000 Americans with roughly 5,000 new cases reported each year. ALS involves progressive degeneration of the nerve cells that control voluntary movement. It is marked by weakness, loss of motor control, difficulty speaking, and cramping. Eventually a weakened diaphragm and intercostal muscles lead to breathing problems. There is currently no effective therapy and no cure, and prognosis continues to be poor, with death within 3 to 5 years of diagnosis (often as a result of pulmonary infection). Myoclonus refers to temporary involuntary twitching or spasm of a muscle or muscle group. It is generally considered not a disorder, but a symptom. It occurs with a variety of disorders including multiple sclerosis, Parkinson's, and Alzheimer's. Pathologic myoclonus may limit a person's ability to eat, walk, and talk. Treatment consists of medication that reduces symptoms, often antiepileptic drugs such as clonazepam, phenytoin, and sodium valproate.

Spina bifida (SB) is a congenital neural defect due to failure of one or more fetal vertebrae to close properly during development, leaving a portion of the spinal cord unprotected. Long-term effects include impairment in physical mobility, and most individuals have some form of learning disability. The three most common types are myelomeningocele, the most severe form, in which the spinal cord and meninges protrude from the opening in the spine, meningocele, in which the meninges only protrude through the spinal opening, and SB occulta, the mildest form, in which one or more vertebrae are malformed and covered only by a layer of skin. Treatment includes surgery, medication, and physiotherapy appropriate for the extent of deformity. Poliomyelitis (polio) is an infectious disease that sometimes results in permanent paralysis.

The acute disease is marked by fatigue, headache, fever, vomiting, stiffness of the neck, and pain in the hands and feet. New cases in the United States are rare due to routine childhood vaccination. However, thousands of pre-vaccine polio survivors are alive today and you may see them as patients. Many of these individuals require supportive care.

Assessment of any of the degenerative disorders requires your personal impressions and history taking to determine the chief complaint. The patient may be having a flare-up of a problem or they may have an unrelated complaint. In all cases, make your assessment, intervene for any life-threatening problems, and learn exactly what prompted a call for EMS. Management relies on treating the chief complaint. You don't want to overlook the underlying condition, but you also don't want it to get in the way of recognizing and treating a more immediately serious problem. While providing care, you should keep in mind these general aspects of patients who have a disorder in this group: Mobility may be affected, and the patient may need assistance to move. Communication may be difficult. Take the time to ensure open communication with patient, family, caregivers, or bystanders. Respiratory compromise may be a concern, particularly in exacerbations of ALS or some other conditions. Any breathing problem is a priority. Last, recognize the anxiety attendant with these disorders. Approach the patient and family with compassion. The following specific guidelines may be useful for a number of patients: Determine blood glucose; this may help you detect whether altered mental status is due to hypoglycemia. Establish an IV with normal saline or lactated Ringer's at a keep-vein-open rate. Monitor cardiac rhythm during transport.

5. Describe and differentiate the major types of seizures. pp. 1264–1265

Seizures can be clinically grouped as generalized or partial on a pathophysiologic basis. Generalized seizures begin with an electrical discharge in a small part of the brain but the abnormal activity spreads to involve the entire cerebral cortex. In contrast, partial seizures may remain confined to a small area, causing localized malfunction, or they may spread and become secondarily generalized seizures.

Generalized seizures include tonic-clonic (also commonly called grand mal) and absence seizures. A tonic-clonic seizure is a generalized motor seizure that produces a temporary loss of consciousness. Usually, it includes a tonic phase (in which muscle tone is increased) and a clonic phase (in which muscles in the extremities jerk rhythmically). In some cases, temporary paralysis of the intercostal muscles causes an interruption in breathing and cyanosis may become evident. When respirations resume, you may see copious amounts of frothy oral secretions. Incontinence is also common during a seizure, and you may note agitation or confusion, drowsiness, or even coma following a seizure, depending on the norm for that patient. Absence seizures present very differently. They are characterized by a sudden onset of a brief (typically 10- to 30-second) loss of consciousness or awareness. Loss of consciousness may be so brief that the casual observer misses it altogether. These idiopathic seizures of childhood rarely occur after age 20 years. Note that absence seizures may not respond to your normal treatment modalities.

Pseudoseizures, also called hysterical seizures, are not true electrical seizures. Rather, they represent psychiatric phenomena. The patient typically presents with sharp, bizarre movements that may be interrupted with a terse command such as "Stop it!"

Partial seizures may be either simple or complex. Simple seizures involve local motor, sensory, or autonomic dysfunction in one area of the body; there is no loss of consciousness. You should remember, however, that they may spread in area of involvement and progress to a generalized, tonic-clonic seizure. Complex seizures, which usually originate in the temporal lobe, are often characterized by an aura and focal findings such as alterations in mental status or mood. Patients in the midst of such a seizure may appear intoxicated or mentally unstable: They may be confused, stagger, have purposeless movements, or show sudden personality changes. These seizures typically last 1 to 2 minutes, and the patient will slowly come back to baseline after that period.

6. Describe the phases of a generalized seizure. pp. 1264–1265

Although patients are individuals with their own seizure patterns, many tonic-clonic seizures progress through seven phases: (1) aura, a subjective sensation that serves as a warning to those patients who experience it; (2) loss of consciousness, during the aura sensation, if there is one; (3) tonic phase; (4) hypertonic phase, during which you will see extreme muscular rigidity, including hyperextension of the back; (5) clonic phase of muscle spasms (often including the jaw) marked by rhythmic movements; (6) post-seizure, during which the patient is in a coma; and (7) postictal, during which the patient awakens.

7. **Define the following:**

   The degenerative neurological diseases are discussed in some detail in objective 4j, and you may wish to check that section for review on any or all of these disorders.

   a. Muscular dystrophy p. 1272

   Muscular dystrophy (MD) is actually a group of genetic diseases characterized by progressive muscle weakness and degeneration of the skeletal or voluntary muscle fibers.

   b. Multiple sclerosis pp. 1272–1273

   Multiple sclerosis (MS) is a disease that involves inflammation of certain nerve cells followed by demyelination; the destruction of the insulating myelin sheath is due to autoimmune activity.

   c. Dystonia p. 1273

   The dystonias are a group of disorders characterized by muscle contractions that cause twisting and repetitive movements, abnormal posturing, or freezing in the middle of an action.

   d. Parkinson's disease p. 1273

   Parkinson's disease is a chronic and progressive disorder of the motor system within the CNS and is characterized by tremor, rigidity, bradykinesia, and postural instability.

   e. Trigeminal neuralgia pp. 1273–1274

   Trigeminal neuralgia is due to abnormal conduction of impulses along the trigeminal nerve (cranial nerve V). The condition is an example of a central pain syndrome.

   f. Bell's palsy p. 1274

   Bell's palsy, the most common form of facial paralysis, is a one-sided phenomenon with unknown cause, marked by inability to close the eye, pain, tearing of the eye, drooling, hypersensitivity to sound, and impairment of taste.

   g. Amyotrophic lateral sclerosis p. 1274

   Amyotrophic lateral sclerosis (ALS), or Lou Gehrig's disease, is a progressive degenerative condition of specific nerve cells that control voluntary movement; it is marked by weakness, loss of motor control, difficulty speaking, and cramping.

   h. Peripheral neuropathy pp. 1246–1247

   Peripheral neuropathy is not considered a degenerative neurological condition; rather, it is a descriptive term that includes any malfunction or damage of the peripheral nerves. Results may include muscle weakness, loss of sensation, impaired reflexes, and malfunction of internal organs. Diabetes is one of the major causes of peripheral neuropathy involving multiple nerves (also called a polyneuropathy).

   i. Myoclonus p. 1274

   Myoclonus is a temporary, involuntary twitching or spasm of a muscle or group of muscles. It is actually a symptom rather than a disorder. A very benign example of myoclonus is hiccups. Pathological myoclonus may be part of disorders including Alzheimer's, Parkinson's, and multiple sclerosis.

   j. Spina bifida p. 1274

   Spina bifida (SB) is a congenital neural defect that results from failure of one or more vertebrae to close properly during fetal development. The defect may range from the asymptomatic (vertebral malformation covered by skin) to the severe (protrusion of spinal cord and meninges through an opening in the spine).

   k. Poliomyelitis p. 1274

   Poliomyelitis (polio) is a viral infectious disease characterized by inflammation of the CNS, which sometimes results in permanent paralysis.

8. **Define and discuss the pathophysiology, assessment findings, and management for nontraumatic spinal injury, including:**

   a. Low back pain pp. 1275–1276

   Low back pain, defined as pain felt between the lower rib cage and the gluteal muscles, often radiating to the thighs, is an extremely common complaint but only occasionally the reason for an EMS call. Men and women are equally affected, but you should keep in mind that back pain in women over 60 years may represent the first sign of osteoporosis, an important medical condition. Vertebral fractures from causes other than osteoporosis are also possible causes. Other causes of low back pain include sciatica, which is reflected as severe pain along the path of the sciatic nerve down the back of the thigh and inner leg. Sciatica may be due to compression or trauma to the sciatic nerve or its roots, perhaps from a herniated intervertebral disk or an osteoarthritic lumbosacral vertebral bone. Sciatica may also be due to inflammation of the nerve secondary to metabolic, toxic, or infectious causes. Pain at the level of L-3, L-4, L-5, and S-1 may be due to inflammation of interspinous bursae. External to the spine are other causes of low back pain: inflammation or sprain of muscles and ligaments that attach to the spine. Most low back pain, though, is found to be idiopathic.

Assessment of back pain is based on chief complaint, history, and physical exam. When the complaint is low back pain, a precise diagnosis is likely to be difficult. Preliminary diagnosis may focus on occupational risk from repetitive lifting or exposure to machinery vibrations. Listen for clues in the history about the nature and timing of the pain and whether the current complaint is acute pain or exacerbation of a chronic condition. Your priorities in the field are to determine whether pain is due to a life-threatening or non-life-threatening condition. Note: The presence of any identifiable neurological deficit may point to a serious underlying cause, as may a gradual onset of pain consistent with degenerative disk disease or tumor growth. The location of the injury may be revealed on exam by a limited range of motion in the lumbar spine, point tenderness on palpation, alterations in sensation, pain, and temperature at a localized point, or pain or paresthesia below a point of injury. Always keep in mind that you are unlikely to be able to determine the cause of the pain in the field. Your primary goal is to look for signs of life-threatening problems and to gather historical and exam information that will be useful to the receiving physician. You will also need to decide, perhaps after consultation with medical direction, whether immobilization (and, if so, to what degree) is necessary during transport.

If there are no clear life-threatening problems requiring intervention, management is primarily aimed at minimizing pain and immobilizing as per local protocol. If there is no historical reason to suspect injury in the past or an underlying condition such as osteoporosis (which makes patients vulnerable to pathologic fracture), C-spine immobilization may still be recommended as a comfort measure during transport. Also remember that some patients will require parenteral analgesia and diazepam before they can lie on a stretcher. Consult medical direction if you feel your patient might fit into this category. Last, remember to provide ongoing assessment en route with special attention to the ABCs, vitals, and the possible presence or development of motor or sensory deficits that might indicate a critical condition capable of compromising ventilatory efforts.

b. Herniated intervertebral disk   p. 1276

Intervertebral disks may rupture due to injury or due to degeneration associated with aging. Degenerative disk disease is most common in patients over 50 years of age. A herniated disk occurs when the gelatinous center of the disk extrudes through a tear in the tough outer capsule, and the resulting pain is due to pressure on the spinal cord or to muscle spasm at the site. The disks themselves are not innervated. Non-injury-related herniation may also be caused by improper lifting. Men aged 30 to 50 years are more prone to herniated disks than are women. Herniation is most common at levels L-4, L-5, and S-1, but it also may occur at C-5, C-6, and C-7. Assessment and management are discussed under low back pain in objective 8a.

c. Spinal cord tumors   p. 1276

A cyst or tumor along the spine or intruding into the spinal canal may cause pain by pressing on the spinal cord, causing degenerative changes in bone, or interrupting blood supply. The specific manifestations depend on location and type of tumor or cyst. Assessment and management are discussed under low back pain in objective 8a.

9. Differentiate between neurologic emergencies based on assessment findings.   pp. 1247–1277

Because many signs and symptoms of neurologic dysfunction are subtle, you should use the observations made during scene size-up and formation of general impressions to look for evidence suggesting focus on the neurological system. Environmental clues may include medical equipment, medication bottles, Medic-Alert identification, alcohol bottles, and so on. Note, for instance, if the patient is conscious, and, if so, is he confused or lucid? Are his posture and gait normal? Speech can give many clues, particularly if either the patient or a bystander can tell you if the speech you hear is normal for the patient. Skin color, temperature, and moisture are valuable, as is any evidence of facial drooping or muscle spasm. Mental status can then be quickly ascertained through the AVPU method. Assessment of higher cerebral functioning includes assessment of emotional status. Try to evaluate the patient's affect, thought patterns, perceptions, judgments, and memory and attention. ANY alteration from the patient's normal mental status or mood is considered significant and warrants further assessment. After that level of assessment is done, evaluate for the ABCs, including respiration pattern, effort of breathing, heart rate, rhythm, and ECG pattern. An unresponsive patient can be evaluated further with use of the Glasgow Coma Scale (GCS). Be aware that a midlevel GCS score (such as 5, 6, or 7) that drops on reevaluation has grim implications.

Scene size-up and initial history will usually make clear whether trauma is involved or not. Regardless of whether trauma is a factor, try to get information on the presence or severity of medical conditions that are risk factors for neurologic conditions, hypertension, heart disease, diabetes, atherosclerosis, as well as any chronic neurologic conditions such as epilepsy. In addition, history should try to establish whether current complaint is acute, an exacerbation of a chronic problem, or a chronic state.

Physical exam of a patient with a neurologic emergency includes the standard head-to-toe exam as well as a more detailed neurological evaluation. Look closely at the patient's face. The ability to smile, frown, or wrinkle the forehead gives information about the status of the facial nerve. Although slight pupillary asymmetry is normal, abnormal pupils can be an early indicator of increasing intracranial pressure. If both pupils are dilated and don't react to light, suspect brainstem injury or serious anoxia. If the pupils are dilated but still react, injury may be reversible. Most of all, remember that any patient with altered mental status and a unilaterally dilated pupil is in the "immediate transport" category. When you check the pupils, look for contact lenses. If present, they should be removed, placed in their container or saline solution, and transported with the patient.

Respiratory derangements are common with CNS illness or injury. Five abnormal breathing patterns may be commonly observed in this setting: Cheyne-Stokes respiration is a pattern marked by apnea lasting 10 to 60 seconds followed by gradually increasing depth and frequency of respiration. It can be seen with brain damage due to trauma or cerebral hemorrhage and with chronic hypoxia. Kussmaul's respirations are deep, rapid breaths caused by severe metabolic or CNS problems. Central neurogenic hyperventilation is caused by a lesion in the CNS and is marked by rapid, deep, noisy respirations. Ataxic respirations are poor breaths due to CNS damage causing ineffective thoracic muscular coordination. Apneustic respiration is breathing marked by prolonged inspiration unrelieved by expiration attempts and it is due to damage in the upper pons. Always remember that CO_2 has a critical effect on cerebral vessels: Increased levels cause vascular dilation, whereas low levels cause vasoconstriction. This is the basis for controlled hyperventilation in settings where some degree of vasoconstriction might minimize brain swelling.

Cardiovascular status is always important. Even if a primary cardiovascular problem is not present, CNS events are likely to cause changes to the cardiovascular system. In particular, assess heart rate, ECG rhythm, bruits over the carotid arteries, and possible presence of jugular venous distension, a sign of ineffective cardiac pumping. You should be aware that vital signs and changes in them are crucial in following the course of a neurological emergency. Note Cushing's reflex, a grouping of four characteristics in vital signs that signals increased intracranial pressure: increased blood pressure, decreased pulse rate, decreased respirations, and increased temperature. The earliest signs are the decrease in pulse rate and an increase in blood pressure and temperature.

The exam for neurologic system status is covered in detail on text pages 1251–1253. Note that the components of the exam include sensorimotor evaluation (if posture is abnormal, consider whether it might be decorticate or decerebrate in nature), motor system status, and cranial nerve status.

Last, be particularly aware with elderly patients and with patients with a chronic neurological condition (such as the degenerative disorders) that it is vital to know the patient's baseline values in all areas before you can put your current findings into the context of acute changes or not. Interviewing family members or caregivers may be very helpful.

10. **Given several preprogrammed nontraumatic neurological emergency patients, provide the appropriate assessment, management, and transport.** pp. 1244–1277

The priorities for someone who is unconscious or clearly in urgent distress with neurologic difficulties are the same as for a patient who is affected by a potentially life-threatening emergency of another origin: Ensure adequate airway, breathing (ventilation), and circulation. This is particularly important for someone whose emergency may be originating in, or affecting, the CNS: The brain requires a constant supply of oxygen, glucose, and vitamins. After 10 to 20 seconds without blood flow, unconsciousness will occur. Significant deprivation of oxygen (anoxia) or glucose (hypoglycemia) can cause seizures or coma. You should always give high-flow oxygen to a patient with a neurologic emergency and give glucose to any one found to be hypoglycemic.

Neurologic injuries and illnesses usually require treatment as soon as possible to prevent progressive damage. In the case of thromboembolic stroke, this may be particularly true because therapies are coming into use that can minimize the region of brain tissue infarcted in the stroke or even prevent the progression of tissue ischemia to tissue infarction. Patients who show altered mental status and/or any clear neurologic impairment (pupillary dilation, especially unilateral, facial drooping, slurred speech, abnormal posturing—if these appear to be new or progressing findings) that may suggest TIA or stroke need immediate intervention and transport. Management of seizures and syncope often mandates prompt intervention and care, as well.

You will see many calls for complaints such as low back pain and headache. These conditions may be relatively minor or the signal of a serious underlying disorder. History suggesting new onset, severe pain, or clearly progressive pain indicates the need for aggressive assessment and management, whereas other patients with chronic pain of either origin also require full assessment but may need only supportive care.

Patients with known CNS neoplasms or degenerative neurological conditions may present with a complaint related to their underlying disease or a problem of completely different origin. Be aware that these persons are always more vulnerable to oxygen or glucose deprivation from another source (for example, cardiac disease or diabetes, respectively); in addition, remember that some patients will have airways vulnerable to compromise secondary to muscle paralysis or other neurologic causes.

Content Self-Evaluation

MULTIPLE CHOICE

_____ 1. The two mechanisms that generally cause altered mental status are:
  A. occlusive and hemorrhagic strokes.
  B. systemic diseases and drugs or toxic agents.
  C. structural lesions and toxic-metabolic states.
  D. head trauma and CNS disease.
  E. toxic-metabolic states and brain tumors.

_____ 2. Peripheral neuropathy can affect muscle activity, sensation, and reflexes, but not internal organ function.
  A. True
  B. False

_____ 3. If the patient is able to smile, frown, and wrinkle forehead muscles, which cranial nerve is intact?
  A. I   D. XI
  B. V   E. XII
  C. VII

4. The Glasgow Coma Scale assesses eye opening, verbal response, and motor response. Which correlation of score and likely outcome is incorrect?
   A. score of 3 or 4, 10 percent favorable outcome
   B. score of 8 or higher, 94 percent favorable outcome
   C. score of 5–7 that increases to 8 or higher, 80 percent favorable outcome
   D. score of 5–7, 50 percent favorable outcome in adults and 90 percent in children
   E. score of 5–7 that decreases by one point, 10 percent favorable outcome

5. Two interventions that may be indicated in treatment of a patient with altered mental status, a low blood glucose level, and suspected alcoholism are:
   A. 50 percent dextrose and naloxone
   B. 50 percent dextrose and mannitol (Osmotrol)
   C. 50 percent dextrose and thiamine
   D. thiamine and mannitol (Osmotrol)
   E. thiamine and hyperventilation

6. A condition characterized by a loss of memory and disorientation and often associated with chronic alcoholism and a diet deficient in thiamine is:
   A. Korsakoff's psychosis.
   B. Wernicke's syndrome.
   C. Lein's psychosis.
   D. Esselstyne's syndrome.
   E. Makynen seizure.

7. The type of stroke caused by a ruptured cerebral artery is a(n) _____ stroke.
   A. occlusive
   B. embolic
   C. thrombotic
   D. hemorrhagic
   E. aneural

8. If a stroke patient is apneic or breathing inadequately, controlled positive-pressure hyperventilation may be beneficial because it:
   A. causes cerebral vasoconstriction, decreasing cerebral swelling.
   B. causes a reflex increase in respiration rate.
   C. eliminates excess CO_2 levels.
   D. increases CO_2 levels toward normal range.
   E. increases the ability of brain cells to take up any available oxygen.

9. Among the many types of epileptic seizures, the most likely to require intervention on your part are:
   A. absence seizures.
   B. tonic-clonic seizures.
   C. petit mal seizures.
   D. simple partial seizures.
   E. complex partial seizures.

10. The phase of a seizure in which a patient experiences alternating contraction and relaxation of the muscles is the _____ phase.
    A. tonic
    B. clonic
    C. aural
    D. hypertonic
    E. postical

11. All of the following are characteristics of a complex partial seizure EXCEPT:
    A. auditory hallucinations.
    B. a sense of deja vu.
    C. localized tonic-clonic movement of one extremity.
    D. unusual odors.
    E. strange tastes.

_____ 12. If a patient with suspected syncope does not regain consciousness within a few moments, the event is NOT syncope, but something more serious.
   A. True
   B. False

_____ 13. The two most common causes of headache are:
   A. vascular and organic.
   B. vascular and neurogenic.
   C. tension and vascular.
   D. tension and organic.
   E. tension and neurogenic.

_____ 14. A disease that is chronic and is characterized by progressive motor disorder with tremor, rigidity, bradykinesia, and postural instability is:
   A. Alzheimer's.
   B. Reed-Sternberg's.
   C. Parkinson's.
   D. Lou Gehrig's.
   E. Bell's palsy.

_____ 15. Which one of the following is NOT a degenerative neurological disorder?
   A. multiple sclerosis (MS)
   B. Parkinson's disease
   C. Bell's palsy
   D. muscular dystrophy
   E. vertebral disk disease

Matching

Write the two letters giving the cause and description of the abnormal breathing pattern in the space provided next to the name of the pattern.

_____ 16. Cheyne-Stokes respiration

_____ 17. central neurogenic hyperventilation

_____ 18. Kussmaul's respiration

_____ 19. ataxic respirations

_____ 20. apneustic respirations

A. rapid, deep respirations

B. brain damage due to trauma or cerebral hemorrhage and with chronic hypoxia

C. ineffective thoracic muscular coordination due to CNS damage

D. severe metabolic or CNS conditions

E. rapid, deep, noisy respirations involving hyperventilation

F. prolonged inspiration unrelieved by expiration attempts

G. brief period of apnea followed by increasing depth and frequency of respirations

H. lesion in the CNS

I. poor respirations

J. pattern due to damage in the upper part of the pons

Write the two letters giving the major cause and characteristic of presentation in the space provided next to the type of stroke to which they apply. A letter may be used more than once.

_____ 21. thrombotic stroke

_____ 22. intracerebral hemorrhage

_____ 23. embolic stroke

_____ 24. subarachnoid hemorrhage

A. gradual development of signs/symptoms, often first noticed on waking during night
B. congenital blood vessel abnormalities or head trauma
C. sudden onset of severe headache
D. blood clot that forms in an area of a cerebral artery narrowed by atherosclerosis
E. rupture of a small blood vessel within brain tissue
F. lodging of a blood clot, air bubble, tumor tissue, or fat in an artery that is far from its site of origin

Endocrinology

Review of Chapter Objectives

After reading this chapter, you should be able to:

1. **Describe the incidence, morbidity, and mortality of endocrinologic emergencies.** pp. 1282, 1284–1285, 1289

   Many people have endocrine disorders that involve excessive or deficient hormone production or function. The incidence of such disorders is widely variable. Some disorders are readily controlled by hormone replacement therapy; others are more complex and thus more difficult to manage. The most common of all of the endocrine disorders is diabetes mellitus, affecting at least 8 million Americans.

2. **Identify the risk factors that predispose a person to endocrinologic disease.** pp. 1284–1285, 1289, 1292

   Diabetes mellitus is the most commonly encountered endocrine disorder. Among the predisposing factors that have been identified for this condition are heredity, viral infection, autoimmune antibodies, and obesity.

   Heredity is thought to be the key factor in the predisposition for Graves' disease, although autoimmune antibodies are known to trigger the excess production of thyroid hormone. Severe physiologic stress has been found to be a common triggering factor for thyrotoxicosis (thyroid storm). On the other hand, hypothyroidism or myxedema may be either congenital or acquired.

   The risk of adrenal gland disorders is increased by the administration of glucocorticoids or may be a consequence of abnormalities of the anterior pituitary gland or the adrenal cortex. Approximately half of all adrenal gland disorders are due to autoimmune disorders or may be aggravated by acute physiologic stress.

3. **Discuss the anatomy and physiology of the endocrine system.** (see Chapter 3)

   There are eight major structures associated with the endocrine system located throughout the body: the hypothalamus, pituitary gland, thyroid gland, parathyroid glands, thymus, pancreas, adrenal glands, and gonads. The pineal gland is also part of the endocrine system.

   The hypothalamus, located deep within the cerebrum of the brain, is the junction between the endocrine system and the central nervous system. About the size of a pea, the pituitary gland is located adjacent to the hypothalamus within the cerebrum. The pineal gland is also located adjacent to the hypothalamus. The double-lobed thyroid gland is located in the neck anterior to and just below the cartilage of the larynx. The parathyroid glands are very small and are found on the posterior lateral surface of the thyroid gland. The thymus is located in the mediastinum just behind the sternum. The pancreas is located in the upper abdomen behind the stomach and between the duodenum and the spleen. The adrenal glands are somewhat triangular in shape and are located on the superior surface of the kidneys. Gonads can be found in the lower pelvis in women, with each ovary resembling an almond in size and shape. In men, the gonads are located in the scrotum.

The endocrine system is closely linked to the nervous system and plays a critical role in our ability to maintain life by regulating many bodily functions through chemical substances called hormones. The endocrine system is made up of ductless glands, which manufacture and secrete hormones that act in adjacent tissues or travel via the bloodstream to target organs or other endocrine glands to produce specific or generalized effects. Hormones regulate metabolic activity, growth and development, as well as mediate chemical reactions, maintain homeostatic balance, and initiate our adaptive response to stress.

4. **Discuss the pathophysiology, assessment findings, need for rapid intervention and transport, and management of endocrinologic emergencies.** pp. 1282–1293

As you review the anatomy and physiology of the endocrine system, it is clearly evident that the endocrine system is closely linked to the nervous system and controls a variety of physiologic processes that are essential for survival. The causes of endocrine disorders are variable and include heredity, congenital anomalies, viral infection, and autoimmune disease processes. The most commonly encountered endocrine emergencies in the prehospital setting are related to diabetes mellitus and disorders of the thyroid or adrenal glands. You should review the sections of the text that clarify the differences in clinical presentation, assessment, and management of these disorders.

5. **Describe osmotic diuresis and its relationship to diabetes mellitus.** p. 1284

Osmosis is the tendency for water molecules to migrate across a semipermeable membrane so that the concentrations of particles approach equivalence on both sides. When blood glucose levels rise above 180 mg/dL, no more glucose can be reabsorbed through the renal tubules and glucose begins to be lost (or "spill") into the urine. This causes the osmotic pressure, or concentration of particulates, to rise inside the kidney tubule to a level higher than that of the blood. Water follows glucose into the urine to cause a marked water loss termed osmotic diuresis that is the basis for the polyuria (excessive urination) associated with untreated diabetes.

6. **Describe the pathophysiology of adult and juvenile onset diabetes mellitus.** pp. 1284–1285

Juvenile onset or Type I diabetes mellitus is a serious disease characterized by very low production of insulin by the beta cells of the pancreas. In many cases, there is no insulin being produced. It is called juvenile onset diabetes because of the average age of the patient at the time of diagnosis. Type I diabetes is also known as insulin-dependent diabetes because patients require regular injections of insulin to control their disease. Heredity appears to be an important factor in determining which people will develop Type I diabetes. The cause of Type I diabetes is not clear. Other factors attributed to triggering juvenile onset diabetes are viral infection, an autoimmune response, or genetically determined premature deterioration of beta cells. The immediate cause of Type I diabetes is the destruction of pancreatic beta cells.

Type II diabetes mellitus, also known as non-insulin-dependent diabetes, is responsible for almost 90 percent of all cases of diabetes. Type II diabetes usually begins in later life and is often associated with obesity, so it is known as adult onset diabetes. Type II diabetes is associated with a moderate decline in insulin production accompanied by a marked decrease in the utilization of the insulin within the body. The cause is not clearly understood, although obesity is believed to play a role in its development. Increased weight, along with the increased size of fat cells, causes a relative deficiency in the number of insulin receptors, thus making the fat cells less responsive to insulin. Type II diabetes is usually managed through a combination of diet, exercise, and the administration of medications to reduce either blood glucose or enhance the efficiency of insulin. Occasionally insulin administration is required.

7. **Differentiate between the pathophysiology of normal glucose metabolism and diabetic glucose metabolism.** pp. 1282–1284

Metabolism, which means "to change," is a term used to refer to all of the chemical and energy transformations within the body. Two kinds of change take place in the cell. One kind builds complex molecules from simple ones (anabolism), such as the synthesis of glycogen from glucose. The other kind breaks down complex molecules into simpler ones (catabolism), such as occurs with the breakdown of glucose into carbon dioxide, water, and energy (in the form of ATP). When materials are abundant after meals and the glucose is high, insulin enables cells to use glucose directly and to store energy as glycogen, protein, and fat. Insulin stimulates glucose pathways. In contrast, glucagon, the dominant hormone during periods of low blood glucose, stimulates catabolic pathways to produce usable energy from the body's stores.

The rate at which glucose can enter the cell is dependent upon insulin levels. Insulin combines with insulin receptors on the surface of the cell membrane, allowing glucose to enter the cell by increasing the permeability of the cell membrane. The rate at which glucose can be transported into the cells can be accelerated tenfold by insulin.

Sometimes the body cannot use glucose as its primary energy source, as is the case in patients with diabetes mellitus. Without insulin, the amount of glucose that can be transported into the cells is far too small to meet the body's energy demands. Without insulin, the glucose remains in the bloodstream, resulting in hyperglycemia. Carbohydrate depletion is also seen in other conditions, such as a high-fat, low-carbohydrate diet or starvation (which can be associated with some eating disorders). Under these conditions, the body slowly switches from glucose to fat as the primary energy source. Adipose cells break down fats into their component free fatty acids, and the blood concentration of these acids rises considerably.

Most of the fatty acids are used directly by the body's cells as an energy source. The liver takes in some, where the catabolism of fatty acids produces acetoacetic acid. When more acetoacetic acid is released by the liver than can be effectively utilized by body cells, it accumulates in the bloodstream along with two other closely related substances, acetone and β-hydroxybutyric acid. The three substances are collectively called ketone bodies. Their presence in excessive quantities is called ketosis.

8. Describe the mechanism of ketone body formation and its relationship to ketoacidosis. pp. 1283, 1285–1287

When the body's carbohydrate stores begin to become depleted, small amounts of glucose can be formed by the breakdown of protein and fat through the process of gluconeogenesis. The byproducts of amino acid breakdown include carbon dioxide and water and the formation of urea. The breakdown of fat results in the formation of carbon dioxide, water, and ketone bodies.

The normal blood ketone level in humans is low because ketones are usually metabolized as rapidly as they are formed. If there are low levels of glucose stored in the cells, the ability of the body to oxidize the ketones is soon exceeded and ketones begin to build up in the bloodstream, resulting in a condition known as ketosis. This results in an increased amount of acid in the body fluids. The resulting metabolic acidosis is often severe and can be fatal.

9. Discuss the physiology of the excretion of potassium and ketone bodies by the kidneys. p. 1284

Whenever the flow rate of fluid inside the tubules of the kidney rises, as in osmotic diuresis, an increase in excretion of potassium occurs. This leads to the potential for significant hypokalemia and its effects, such as potentially life-threatening cardiac dysrhythmias. In ketotic states, ketone bodies are excreted through respiration and will also spill into the urine.

10. Describe the relationship of insulin to serum glucose levels. pp. 1282–1288

Insulin is a glucagon antagonist and lowers the blood glucose level by promoting energy storage. Insulin increases the rate at which various body cells take up glucose by changing the permeability of the cell membranes. These changes also make the cell more permeable to potassium, magnesium, and phosphate ions, as well as many amino acids. Because the liver rapidly breaks down insulin, the hormone must be secreted constantly.

Homeostasis of blood glucose is remarkably effective. In nondiabetics, when blood glucose is high, as after a meal, the beta cells of the pancreas release insulin. Insulin enables cells to use glucose directly as well as to store energy as glycogen, protein, and fat. If you were to draw a venous blood sample to measure fasting blood glucose levels, you'd find the level in healthy individuals is usually between 80–90 mg glucose/dL blood. In the first 60 to 90 minutes after a meal the level will increase to approximately 120–140 mg/dL before dropping off to near-fasting levels as insulin is released to move the glucose from the bloodstream into the cells. Conversely, when blood glucose levels are low, the alpha cells of the pancreas release glucagon to raise the blood glucose level.

11. **Describe the effects of decreased levels of insulin on the body.** pp. 1284–1288

Insulin deficiency contributes to the development of hyperglycemia. Without insulin to facilitate the movement of large glucose molecules across cell membranes, the blood glucose level rises even as the intracellular level of glucose plummets. At the same time, the alpha cells of the pancreas release glucagon to increase blood glucose by stimulating the breakdown of glycogen, as well as stimulating the breakdown of body proteins and fats with subsequent chemical conversion to glucose (gluconeogenesis).

12. **Describe the effects of increased serum glucose levels on the body.** p. 1288

With a rise in blood glucose levels, as is the case in Type I diabetes, the body's cells cannot take up circulating glucose. Glucose then spills into urine, leading to a large water loss, via osmotic diuresis, and significant dehydration. This can lead to significant loss of potassium and hypokalemia.

13. **Discuss the pathophysiology, assessment findings, and management of the following endocrine emergencies:**

   a. **Nonketotic hyperosmolar coma** pp. 1285–1286, 1287–1288

   This condition is a complication of Type II diabetes due to inadequate insulin activity and is marked by high blood glucose, marked dehydration, and decreased mental function.

   Development of the coma is slower than with ketoacidosis. Early signs include increased urination and thirst. Later signs may include orthostatic hypotension, dry skin, and tachycardia.

   This condition is difficult to distinguish from ketoacidosis in the field. Field management focuses on maintaining ABCs and fluid resuscitation.

   b. **Diabetic ketoacidosis** pp. 1285–1287

   Diabetic ketoacidosis is a serious, potentially life-threatening complication of diabetes mellitus. It occurs when profound insulin deficiency is coupled with increased glucagon activity.

   The onset is slow, lasting from 12 to 24 hours. In its early stages, the signs and symptoms include increased thirst, excessive hunger, urination, and malaise. Increased urination results from the osmotic diuresis accompanying glucose spillage into the urine. Intensified thirst is caused by the body's attempt to replace the fluids lost by increased urination. Nausea, vomiting, marked dehydration, tachycardia, and weakness characterize diabetic ketoacidosis. The skin is usually warm and dry. Coma is not uncommon. The breath may have a sweet or acetone-like character due to the increased ketones in the blood. Very deep, rapid respirations, called Kussmaul's respirations, also occur. Kussmaul's respirations represent the body's attempt to compensate for the metabolic acidosis produced by the ketones and organic acids present in the blood. It may be complicated by several electrolyte imbalances. The most significant is decreased potassium. Decreased potassium (hypokalemia) can lead to serious dysrhythmias or even death.

   The approach used with the patient suffering from diabetic ketoacidosis is essentially the same as with any unconscious patient. You should first complete your initial assessment of airway, breathing, and circulation. You will then complete your focused history and physical exam. Pay particular attention to the presence of a Medic-Alert bracelet and/or insulin in the refrigerator. Also, obtain a history from bystanders. The fruity odor of ketones occasionally can be detected on the breath. If possible, complete the rapid test for blood glucose.

   It is not uncommon for patients in ketoacidosis to have blood glucose levels well in excess of 300 mg/dL. The field management of such cases is focused on maintenance of ABCs and fluid resuscitation to counteract the patient's dehydration. Treatment should include drawing a red top tube (or the tube specified by local protocols) of blood. Following this, you should administer one to two liters of normal saline per protocol. If transport time is lengthy, the medical direction physician may request intravenous or subcutaneous administration of regular insulin.

If the blood glucose level cannot be quickly determined, draw a red top tube of blood for analysis and start an IV of normal saline. Following this, administer 50 mL (25 g) of 50 percent dextrose solution. This additional glucose load will not adversely affect the ketoacidotic patient because it is negligible compared to the total quantity present in the body. If the patient is alcoholic, consider administering 100 mg of thiamine. Transportation to an appropriate facility should be expedited.

c. Hypoglycemia   p. 1288

Hypoglycemia, or low blood glucose, is a potentially life-threatening medical emergency. Sometimes called insulin shock, it can occur if a patient accidentally or intentionally injects too much insulin, eats an inadequate amount of food after taking insulin, or has overexercised and burned up all available glucose. Untreated, the insulin will cause the blood glucose to drop to a very low level. The longer the period of hypoglycemia persists, the greater the risk that the brain cells will be permanently damaged or even killed.

The signs and symptoms of hypoglycemia are many and varied. An abnormal mental status is the most important and often the earliest sign. In the earliest stages of hypoglycemia, the patient may appear restless or impatient or complain of hunger. As the blood sugar falls lower, he or she may display inappropriate anger or display a variety of bizarre behaviors. Physical signs may include diaphoresis and tachycardia. If the blood sugar falls to a critically low level, the patient may sustain a hypoglycemic seizure or become comatose. In contrast to diabetic ketoacidosis, hypoglycemia can develop quickly. When encountering a patient behaving bizarrely, you should always consider hypoglycemia.

In suspected cases of hypoglycemia, perform the initial assessment quickly. Inspect the patient for a Medic-Alert bracelet. If possible, determine the blood glucose level. If the blood glucose level is noted to be less than 60 mg/dL, draw a red top tube of blood and start an IV of normal saline. Next, administer 50–100 mL (25–50 g) of 50 percent dextrose intravenously. If the patient is conscious and able to swallow, complete glucose administration with orange juice, sodas, or commercially available glucose pastes.

If the blood glucose cannot be obtained and if the patient is unconscious, you should start an IV of normal saline and administer 50–100 mL (25–50 g) of 50 percent dextrose. Expedite transport to the nearest medical facility. If you suspect alcoholism, administer 100 mg of thiamine prior to the administration of dextrose.

d. Hyperglycemia   pp. 1287–1288

Diabetes mellitus results from either inadequate amounts of circulating insulin or inadequate utilization of insulin. This means that there is an excess of blood glucose while there is an intracellular deficit. In diabetes, glucose builds up in the bloodstream, especially after meals. The blood glucose level rises higher and returns to normal more slowly in the diabetic than in the non-diabetic. An oral glucose tolerance test uses this phenomenon in the diagnosis of diabetes. The diabetic's inadequate insulin level and impaired glucose tolerance are partly due to the decreased entry of glucose into the cells, thus leaving more glucose in the bloodstream.

The second cause of hyperglycemia in the diabetic results from difficulties with the function of the liver. When blood glucose levels are high, insulin secretion is normally increased and the breakdown of glycogen is decreased. In the diabetic, however, insulin secretion is decreased, and the alpha cells secrete glucagon to stimulate glycogenolysis by the liver, thus raising the blood glucose level.

In Type I diabetes the decreased insulin secretion is accompanied by a steady accumulation of glucose in the blood. Hyperglycemia acts like an osmotic diuretic and glucose "spills over" into the urine (glycosuria) pulling large amounts of water with it (polyuria). The body's attempt to dilute the concentration of glucose in the bloodstream results in intracellular dehydration and stimulates thirst (polydipsia). As the cells become glucose-depleted, they begin to use proteins and fats as an energy source resulting in weight loss and the formation of harmful by-products, such as ketones and organic-free fatty acids. The body's response to this state of cellular starvation is to trigger hunger in the patient (polyphagia). If the acids and ketones continue to collect in the blood, severe metabolic acidosis occurs and coma ensues, resulting in serious brain damage or death.

Type II diabetes does not usually result in diabetic ketoacidosis. It can, however, develop into a life-threatening emergency termed hyperglycemic hyperosmolar nonketotic (HHNK) coma. In Type II diabetes, when blood glucose levels exceed 600 mg/dL, the high osmolality of the blood causes an osmotic diuresis and marked dehydration of body cells. However, sufficient insulin is produced to prevent the manufacture of ketones and the complications of metabolic acidosis. In this respect, the condition differs from diabetic ketoacidosis.

e. Thyrotoxicosis   pp. 1289–1290

Thyrotoxic crisis, more commonly known as "thyroid storm," is a life-threatening medical emergency, which can be fatal within as little as 48 hours if not treated. It is usually associated with severe physiologic (trauma, infection, uncontrolled diabetes mellitus, and so on) or psychological stress. You will also encounter thyroid storm from an accidental or intentional overdose of thyroid hormone. Many patients with thyrotoxicosis have underlying Graves' disease (hyperthyroidism).

The signs and symptoms associated with thyroid storm reflect the patient's profound hypermetabolic state and increased adrenergic response. The patient may be hyperthermic (with temperatures as high as 105°) and tachycardic (especially common are atrial tachydysrhythmias), with a high pulse pressure and dyspnea. Mental status changes range from agitation and restlessness to delirium and coma. Nausea, vomiting, and diarrhea are also often present. Death often follows heart failure and profound cardiovascular collapse.

Field management is focused on supportive care with oxygenation, ventilatory assistance, fluid resuscitation, and cardiac monitoring, along with expedited transport to definitive care to block the high circulating levels of thyroid hormones.

f. Myxedema   pp. 1290–1291

Inadequate levels of the thyroid hormones in adults produce hypothyroidism or myxedema, which results in a generalized decrease in metabolism. While it may occur in males or females of any age, it is most commonly seen among middle-aged females or as a consequence when surgery or radiation is used to treat hyperthyroidism.

This disorder tends to have a gradual onset, and the initial signs and symptoms tend to be quite subtle and include hoarse voice and slow speech, facial bloating, weakness, cold intolerance, lethargy, and fatigue as well as altered mental states, particularly depression. Additionally, the skin and hair are quite dry and coarse in texture. Patients with hypothyroidism are treated with replacement thyroid hormone, usually synthetic T_4 agents such as levothyroxine (Synthroid).

Rarely do these patients require emergency treatment for their hypothyroidism unless it progresses to myxedema coma; however, you will encounter many patients who take thyroid replacement hormones.

Myxedema coma, a life-threatening complication of hypothyroidism, is not uncommon in colder climates but is unusual in warm ones. It is most often seen in older patients who have pulmonary or vascular disease. Other contributing factors include a history of thyroid disease, exposure to cold, infection, trauma, or drugs that suppress the central nervous system such as sedatives and hypnotics. The mortality rate associated with myxedema coma is high.

Myxedema coma usually has a gradual onset, with lethargy and depression that progresses to coma. Other signs and symptoms include extreme hypothermia (temperatures as low as 75°F are not uncommon), low amplitude bradycardia, carbon dioxide retention, and profound respiratory depression.

Emergency management of myxedema coma is focused on maintenance of the ABCs and, as always, careful monitoring of the patient's cardiac and oxygenation status; most patients will require intubation and ventilatory assistance. Active rewarming is contraindicated due to the risk of cardiac dysrhythmias and the potential to cause vasodilatation, which may contribute to cardiovascular collapse. Although it is appropriate to initiate intravenous access, care must be taken to limit fluids since fluid and electrolyte imbalance is common. Follow local protocols or contact medical direction for specific orders based on your patient's presentation.

g. Cushing's syndrome   pp. 1291–1292

Chronic high levels of glucocorticoids result in the development of Cushing's syndrome or hyperadrenalism. Cushing's syndrome may occur as a result of long-term glucocorticoid (steroid) therapy, or by abnormalities of the adrenal glands, or by a pituitary tumor triggering excessive secretion of adrenocorticotropic hormone (ACTH), which stimulates the adrenals to produce excessive amounts of glucocorticoids.

Presenting signs and symptoms include: weight gain, particularly through the trunk of the body, face, and neck, with a typical "moon-faced" appearance and often a "buffalo hump" due to the fat deposits in these areas; skin changes, such as the thinning of the skin to an almost transparent appearance, a tendency to bruise easily, delayed healing from even minor wounds, and the development of facial hair among women; increased vascular sensitivity; hypertension; mood swings and memory impairment or decreased ability to concentrate.

Treatment involves removing the cause, such as the surgical removal of a tumor, or adjusting the dosage of glucocorticoids. While it is unlikely that you would encounter a patient with an acute hyperadrenal crisis, you are very likely to encounter patients who exhibit signs and symptoms of Cushing's syndrome. These patients have a higher incidence of cardiovascular disease, hypertension, and stroke than the general population and are prone to infection. When performing your assessment, be alert for the signs mentioned above, which are associated with high glucocorticoid levels. Pay particular attention to skin preparation when starting intravenous lines, due to the fragility of these patients' skin and their susceptibility to infection. Your observations noted in your patient care report and relayed to the receiving hospital staff may contribute to the early diagnosis and treatment of this disorder, especially in those patients who do not have a primary care provider whom they see on a regular basis.

h. Adrenal insufficiency, or Addison's disease   pp. 1292–1293

Most commonly, adrenal insufficiency, or Addison's disease, is an idiopathic autoimmune disorder causing atrophy of the adrenal glands and resulting in the inadequate production of the adrenal hormones, such as cortisol, aldosterone, and androgens. Other causes include pituitary or hypothalamic dysfunction, adrenal hemorrhage, infections, such as tuberculosis, acquired immunodeficiency syndrome (AIDS), or sudden cessation of long-term or high-dose therapy with synthetic glucocorticoids.

Chronic adrenal insufficiency is characterized by progressive weakness, fatigue, decreased appetite, and weight loss. Hyperpigmentation of the skin and mucous membranes is one of the earliest signs. The hyperpigmentation tends to be most significant in sun-exposed areas, joints, and pressure points. Patients with Addison's disease are prone to hypotension, hypoglycemia, hyponatremia, and hyperkalemia. About half of the patients will have gastrointestinal problems such as nausea, vomiting, or diarrhea, which will exacerbate the electrolyte imbalances and increase the potential for cardiac dysrhythmias.

Acute adrenal insufficiency, known as Addisonian crisis, is a life-threatening medical emergency characterized by profound hypotension and shock, which can be rapidly fatal. It is most commonly seen in those patients with Addison's disease who've been exposed to stress such as acute infection, trauma, dehydration, or emotional duress. It has been suggested that adrenal insufficiency should be considered in any patient with unexplained cardiovascular collapse. Vomiting and diarrhea tend to increase the volume depletion and subsequent hypotension. It is not uncommon for patients to report abdominal pain, which tends to mimic an acute abdomen. Fever, weakness, and confusion are also common.

Lifelong replacement hormone therapy and careful monitoring of electrolyte levels are used to treat chronic adrenal insufficiency. Most of this is provided by the primary care physician. Patient education is critical to maintenance of well-being. All patients with Addison's disease are advised to wear a Medic-Alert tag in addition to carrying an identification card detailing their current medication regimen and physician's phone number.

Emergency management is focused on maintenance of the ABCs and, as always, careful monitoring of the patient's cardiac and oxygenation status as well as blood glucose level. Hypoglycemia poses its own threat to the patient's well-being, so blood glucose levels should be assessed and 25–50 g of 50 percent dextrose should be administered to patients with levels less than 50 mg/dL or those with altered mental status. Obtaining a baseline 12-lead EKG is important due to the potential for dysrhythmias related to electrolyte imbalance. Fluid resuscitation should be aggressive. Follow your local protocol or contact medical direction for specific orders based on your patient's presentation. Immediate transport to an appropriate facility is imperative since definitive treatment includes the administration of glucocorticoids and/or mineralocorticoids in conjunction with correcting other electrolyte or hormonal abnormalities.

14. **Describe the actions of epinephrine as it relates to the pathophysiology of hypoglycemia.** p. 1288

Hypoglycemia, or low blood sugar, reflects high insulin and low glucose levels. Regardless of the cause, when insulin levels are high, glucagon may be ineffective in raising blood glucose levels. In prolonged fasts, almost half the glucose normally produced through gluconeogenesis is of renal origin. This activity is stimulated by epinephrine.

15. **Describe the compensatory mechanisms utilized by the body to promote homeostasis when hypoglycemia is present.** pp. 1282, 1288

When blood glucose levels fall, the alpha cells of the pancreas secrete glucagon. Glucagon stimulates the breakdown of glycogen into glucose for release into the bloodstream. This process, called glycogenolysis, takes place throughout the body but occurs primarily in the liver. In addition to stimulating the breakdown of glycogen, glucagon also stimulates the breakdown of proteins and fats with subsequent conversion to glucose. This process of producing sugar from nonsugar sources is called gluconeogenesis. Both of these processes contribute to the maintenance of homeostasis by raising blood glucose levels.

16. **Differentiate among different endocrine emergencies based on assessment and history.** pp. 1282–1293

As you proceed through your course, you will encounter a variety of real and simulated patients with endocrinologic disorders and emergencies. Use the information provided in this chapter of your text, as well as the application of this information as demonstrated by your instructors, preceptors, and mentors to enhance your own ability to differentiate endocrinologic emergencies.

17. **Given several scenarios involving endocrine emergency patients, provide the appropriate assessment, management, and transportation.** pp. 1281–1293

Throughout your classroom, clinical, and field training, you will encounter a variety of real and simulated patients with endocrinologic emergencies. Use the information provided in this chapter of your text, as well as the application of this information as demonstrated by your instructors, preceptors, and mentors to enhance your ability to assess, manage, and transport patients with endocrinologic emergencies.

Content Self-Evaluation

MULTIPLE CHOICE

_____ 1. Which of the following is an exocrine gland?
   A. pineal
   B. thymus
   C. salivary
   D. parathyroid
   E. adrenal

_____ 2. The term describing the sum of cellular processes that produce energy and molecules needed for growth and repair is:
   A. anabolism.
   B. catabolism.
   C. metabolism.
   D. homeostasis.
   E. physiology.

_____ 3. Insulin's primary function is to:
   A. metabolize glucose at the cellular level.
   B. free glucose from muscle storage sites.
   C. promote cell uptake of glucose.
   D. store glucose at the cellular level.
   E. enhance the function of glucagon.

_____ 4. Diabetes mellitus is caused by the inadequate production or activity of:
   A. polypeptide.
   B. glucagon.
   C. somatostatin.
   D. cortisol.
   E. insulin.

_____ 5. Osmotic diuresis, a characteristic of untreated diabetes, contributes to the development of:
   A. polydipsia and polyphagia.
   B. polydipsia and polyuria.
   C. polyuria and polyphagia.
   D. polyuria.
   E. polyphagia.

_____ 6. All of the following are signs and symptoms of diabetic ketoacidosis EXCEPT:
   A. abdominal pain.
   B. deep rapid respirations.
   C. decreased mental function.
   D. cold, clammy skin.
   E. tachycardia.

_____ 7. Diabetic ketoacidosis, characterized by high blood glucose and metabolic acidosis, occurs as a result of all of the following EXCEPT:
   A. profound insulin deficiency.
   B. decreased glucagon activity.
   C. cessation of insulin injections.
   D. physiologic stress.
   E. overexertion.

_____ 8. Kussmaul's respirations are a primary compensatory mechanism for reducing acidosis in the patient with diabetic ketoacidosis.
   A. True
   B. False

_____ 9. Which of the following signs or symptoms will be present in the patient experiencing diabetic ketoacidosis?
   A. acetone breath odor
   B. apathy
   C. diplopia
   D. drooling
   E. diaphoresis

_____ 10. Kussmaul's respirations are seen in which of the following conditions?
   A. diabetic ketoacidosis
   B. hyperglycemic hyperosmolar nonketotic coma
   C. hypoglycemia
   D. insulin shock
   E. thyrotoxicosis

_____ 11. The most important sign or symptom associated with hypoglycemia is:
   A. tachycardia.
   B. cool, clammy skin.
   C. altered mental status.
   D. polydipsia.
   E. polyphagia.

_____ 12. Hyperglycemic hyperosmolar nonketotic acidosis differs from diabetic ketoacidosis because significant production of ketone bodies is prevented by the action of:
   A. polypeptide.
   B. glucagon.
   C. somatostatin.
   D. cortisol.
   E. insulin.

_____ 13. Even in the absence of a blood glucose level, altered mental status in a known diabetic should always be treated with 50 percent dextrose.
   A. True
   B. False

_____ 14. All of the following are signs and symptoms associated with thyrotoxic crisis EXCEPT:
   A. high fever.
   B. bradycardia.
   C. hypotension.
   D. delirium.
   E. vomiting.

_____ 15. Potential triggers for myxedema coma include all of the following EXCEPT:
   A. excessive thyroid medication.
   B. infection.
   C. trauma.
   D. cold environment.
   E. CNS depressants.

_____ 16. Signs and symptoms associated with myxedema coma include all of the following EXCEPT:
   A. hypothermia.
   B. decreased mental status.
   C. low amplitude bradycardia.
   D. CO_2 retention.
   E. seizures.

_____ 17. Which disorder exhibits prominent weight gain in the trunk, face, and neck, with accumulation of fat on the upper back and easily bruised, translucent skin?
   A. Addison's disease
   B. Cushing's syndrome
   C. Graves' disease
   D. myxedema
   E. "thyroid storm"

_____ 18. Long-term exposure to excess glucocorticoids or abnormalities to either the adrenal cortex or pituitary gland may cause hyperadrenalism.
   A. True
   B. False

_____ 19. Addison's disease is characterized by high corticosteroid activity that causes major disturbances in water and electrolyte balance.
   A. True
   B. False

_____ 20. Which disorder exhibits progressive weakness, fatigue, decreased appetite, and weight loss?
   A. Addison's disease
   B. Cushing's syndrome
   C. Graves' disease
   D. myxedema
   E. "thyroid storm"

Allergies and Anaphylaxis

Review of Chapter Objectives

After reading this chapter, you should be able to:

1. **Describe the incidence, morbidity, and mortality of anaphylaxis.** p. 1296

   Anaphylaxis results from an exposure to a particular substance that sets off a chain of biochemical events that can ultimately lead to shock and death. While the exact incidence is unknown, an estimated 400 to 800 deaths annually in the United States are attributed to anaphylaxis. Two of the most common fatal causes of anaphylaxis are attributed to injected penicillin and stings from bees and wasps (Hymenoptera). Between 100 and 500 deaths per year are attributed to penicillin, while 25 to 40 persons die each year from Hymenoptera stings. Overall, the incidence of anaphylaxis seems to be declining due to better recognition and treatment, particularly the availability of numerous potent antihistamines.

2. **Identify the risk factors most predisposing to anaphylaxis.** p. 1296

   Anaphylaxis is the fastest and most severe form of immediate hypersensitivity reaction. Some persons have an allergic tendency. This allergic tendency is genetically passed from parent to child and is characterized by the presence of large quantities of IgE antibodies.

3. **Discuss the anatomy and physiology of the organs and structures related to anaphylaxis.** pp. 1296–1298

   The immune system is a complex system responsible for combating infection. Components of the immune system can be found in the blood, the bone marrow, and the lymphatic system. The immune response is a complex cascade of events that occurs following activation by an invading substance.

   Following exposure to a particular antigen, large quantities of IgE antibodies are released. These antibodies attach to the membranes of basophils and mast cells, causing them to release histamine, heparin, and other chemicals into the surrounding tissue. The release of these chemical mediators causes a response in the cardiovascular, respiratory, and gastrointestinal systems as well as in the skin.

4. **Discuss the pathophysiology of allergy and anaphylaxis.** pp. 1296–1299

   The signs and symptoms associated with allergy and anaphylaxis are due to the physiologic changes triggered by the chemical mediators of the immune response that are released from the basophils and mast cells. Histamine is the primary mediator of all allergic reactions. It is a potent substance that causes bronchoconstriction, vasodilation and increased vascular permeability, and increased intestinal motility. Other chemical substances are also released that have effects similar to or synergistic with histamine, such as SRS-A (slow-reacting substance of anaphylaxis), which results in an asthma-like attack or asphyxia.

5. **Describe the common routes of substance entry into the body.** p. 1298

Allergens can enter the body through various routes including oral ingestion, inhalation, topically, and through injection or envenomation. The vast majority of anaphylactic reactions result from injection or envenomation.

6. **Define allergic reaction, anaphylaxis, antigen, antibody, and natural and acquired immunity.** pp. 1296–1299

An allergic reaction is an exaggerated immune response to a foreign protein or other substance, while anaphylaxis is an unusual or exaggerated allergic reaction to a foreign protein or other substance.

An antigen is any substance that is capable, under appropriate conditions, of inducing a specific immune response. An antibody is a member of a unique class of chemicals that are manufactured by specialized cells of the immune system. The antibody is the principal agent of a chemical attack on an invading substance. Following exposure to an antigen, antibodies are released from cells of the immune system. The antibodies attach themselves to the invading substance so it can be removed from the body by other cells of the immune system.

Natural immunity refers to the immunity that is present at birth; also called innate immunity, it is genetically determined. Acquired immunity is immunity that develops over time and results from exposure to an antigen.

7. **List common antigens most frequently associated with anaphylaxis.** p. 1297

Any substance that is capable, under appropriate conditions, of inducing a specific immune response is known as an antigen. Most antigens are proteins. The following agents are among those that commonly trigger anaphylaxis: antibiotics, foods, or insect stings. Refer to Table 31-1 on text page 1297 for a more complete list.

8. **Discuss human antibody formation.** pp. 1296–1298

Antibodies are a unique class of chemicals that are manufactured by specialized cells of the immune system, called B cells. Another name for antibodies is immunoglobulins (Igs), and there are five different classes: IgA, IgD, IgE, IgG, and IgM. Following exposure to an antigen, antibodies are released from cells of the immune system. The antibodies attach themselves to the invading substance to facilitate removal of the substance from the body by other cells of the immune system. This response is known as humoral immunity.

If the body has never been exposed to a particular antigen, the response of the immune system is different than if it has been previously exposed. The initial response to an antigen is called the primary response. Following exposure to a new antigen, several days pass before both the cellular and humoral components of the immune system respond. Generalized antibodies (IgG and IgM) are released first.

Simultaneously other components of the immune system begin to develop antibodies specific to the new antigen. The cells also develop a memory of the particular antigen and, if there is a subsequent exposure to this same substance, the immune system response is much faster. This is known as the secondary response. As part of this secondary response, antibodies specific for the offending antigen are released. Antigen-specific antibodies are much more effective in facilitating removal of the offending antigen than the generalized antibodies released during the primary response.

9. **Describe the physical manifestations of anaphylaxis.** pp. 1299–1301, 1303

The signs and symptoms of anaphylaxis begin within 30 to 60 seconds following exposure for the vast majority of patients. The more rapid the onset, the more severe the patient presentation.

Respiratory manifestations of anaphylaxis include laryngeal edema and bronchoconstriction. Cardiovascular symptoms include tachycardia plus massive vasodilation resulting in profound hypotension. The combination of respiratory and cardiovascular signs will lead to a rapid deterioration of the patient's mental status. Generalized flushing and urticaria are common, as is angioedema about the head, face, and neck. Nausea, vomiting, and diarrhea may accompany hypermotility of the gastrointestinal tract.

10. Identify and differentiate between the signs and symptoms of an allergic reaction and anaphylaxis. p. 1303

Allergic reactions can range from a mild skin rash to a severe life-threatening multisystem response. Allergic reaction, also known as hypersensitivity, takes two forms, delayed or immediate. Delayed hypersensitivity is the result of cellular immunity and does not involve antibodies. It may occur hours to days after exposure and is very common. Delayed hypersensitivity usually presents as a skin rash and is often due to exposure to certain drugs and chemicals, for instance, poison ivy. Other signs and symptoms may include mild bronchoconstriction, mild intestinal cramps, or diarrhea, while the patient's mental status and vital signs will remain normal.

Immediate hypersensitivity is antibody-mediated immunity and often has a genetic link. The range of clinical presentation is widely variable. Examples of these reactions include hay fever, drug and food allergies, eczema, and asthma. Allergens can enter the body by various routes, but as a rule, those that enter by injection tend to have more rapid and more severe effects. Immediate hypersensitivities may be merely annoying, like the itching eyes and runny nose of hay fever, or may pose a real and immediate life threat, as seen in the anaphylactic reaction described in this chapter.

The signs and symptoms of anaphylaxis begin within seconds following exposure. The more rapid the onset of symptoms, the more severe the patient presentation. Respiratory manifestations of anaphylaxis include laryngeal edema and bronchoconstriction. Cardiovascular symptoms include tachycardia plus massive vasodilation resulting in profound hypotension. A rapid deterioration of the patient's mental status accompanies the cardiovascular collapse. Generalized flushing and urticaria are common, as is angioedema about the head, face, and neck. Nausea, vomiting, and diarrhea may accompany hypermotility of the gastrointestinal tract. Refer to Table 31-2 on text page 1303 for a comparison of signs and symptoms of mild allergic reactions and severe allergic reactions or anaphylaxis.

11. Explain the various treatment and pharmacological interventions used in the management of allergic reactions and anaphylaxis. pp. 1301–1303

The first priority in the management of allergic reactions and anaphylaxis is to establish and maintain the patient's airway. Administer oxygen immediately along with ventilatory support as needed. You should be prepared to intubate, recognizing that laryngeal edema may change the size and appearance of the airway.

Establish vascular access as soon as possible and be prepared to run crystalloid solutions wide open if the patient is hypotensive.

Epinephrine is the drug of choice for severe allergic reaction and anaphylaxis. In mild to moderate cases, administer 0.3–0.5 mg of 1:1,000 epinephrine subcutaneously; while in severe reactions and anaphylaxis, administer 0.3–0.5 mg of intravenous 1:10,000 epinephrine. Remember that the effects of epinephrine wear off quickly, so be prepared to repeat boluses in 3 to 5 minutes. It may be necessary to establish a continuous epinephrine infusion.

Antihistamines, such as diphenhydramine, are widely used for the management of allergic reactions due to their ability to block histamine receptors. The usual dosage is 25–50 mg given either intravenously or intramuscularly. It may also be helpful to administer beta agonist agents via handheld nebulizer to help reverse bronchospasm. Adult patients should receive 0.5 mL of albuterol in 3 mL of normal saline.

As is always the case, your management approach should always be dictated by local protocols. Other medications that may be used to manage severe anaphylaxis include corticosteroids, such as SoluMedrol, to suppress the inflammatory response or vasopressors, such as dopamine, to enhance cardiac output. You'll recall that adequate fluid resuscitation prior to initiating vasopressor therapy is important.

12. Correlate abnormal findings in assessment with the clinical significance in the patient with an allergic reaction or anaphylaxis. pp. 1299–1301, 1303

The central physiological action in severe allergic reaction and anaphylaxis is the massive release of histamine and other chemical mediators of the immune system. The resultant bronchospasm, airway edema, peripheral vasodilation, and increased capillary permeability can take a patient from his or her usual state of health to the brink of death in mere seconds. This chemically caused transformation is readily evident in the patient's clinical presentation: air hunger, dyspnea, angioedema, tachycardia, and hypotension. Your timely intervention is imperative to your patient's survival.

13. Given several preprogrammed and moulaged patients, provide the appropriate assessment, care, and transport for the allergic reaction and anaphylaxis patient. pp. 1296–1303

Throughout your classroom, clinical, and field training, you will encounter a variety of real and simulated patients with allergic reactions or anaphylaxis emergencies. Use the information provided in this chapter of your text, as well as the application of this information as demonstrated by your instructors, preceptors, and mentors to enhance your ability to assess, manage, and transport these patients.

Content Self-Evaluation

MULTIPLE CHOICE

_____ 1. The type of immunity resulting from a direct attack of a foreign substance by specialized cells of the immune system is known as:
  A. humoral.
  B. cellular.
  C. natural.
  D. acquired.
  E. genetic.

_____ 2. The unique class of chemicals that are manufactured by specialized cells of the immune system to attack invading foreign proteins is:
  A. allergens.
  B. antigens.
  C. toxins.
  D. antibodies.
  E. pathogens.

_____ 3. Any substance that is capable, under appropriate conditions, of inducing a specific immune response is a(n):
  A. immunoglobulin.
  B. antigen.
  C. toxin.
  D. antibody.
  E. pathogen.

_____ 4. The type of immunity that is present at birth and has no relation to a previous exposure to a particular antigen is:
  A. humoral.
  B. cellular.
  C. natural.
  D. acquired.
  E. genetic.

_____ 5. The type of immunity that develops over time as a result of exposure to an antigen is:
  A. humoral.
  B. cellular.
  C. natural.
  D. acquired.
  E. genetic.

_____ 6. An allergic reaction is best defined as an exaggerated, sometimes potentially life-threatening response by the immune system to a foreign substance.
   A. True
   B. False

_____ 7. All of the following are common allergens EXCEPT:
   A. insect stings.
   B. drugs.
   C. antibodies.
   D. seafood.
   E. radiology contrast materials.

_____ 8. The vast majority of anaphylactic reactions occur as a result of:
   A. inhalation.
   B. ingestion.
   C. injection.
   D. topical exposure.
   E. genetics.

_____ 9. The antibody most commonly associated with hypersensitivity reactions is:
   A. IgA.
   B. IgD.
   C. IgE.
   D. IgG.
   E. IgM.

_____ 10. The primary chemical mediator of an allergic reaction is:
   A. heparin.
   B. histamine.
   C. SRS-A.
   D. basophil.
   E. the mast cell.

_____ 11. All of the following are physiologic effects associated with the release of the chemical mediators of anaphylaxis EXCEPT:
   A. bronchodilation.
   B. vasodilation.
   C. increased intestinal motility.
   D. increased vascular permeability.
   E. secretion of gastric acids.

_____ 12. Urticaria, a wheal and flare reaction characterized by red raised bumps that appear on the skin, is due to:
   A. bronchodilation.
   B. vasodilation.
   C. increased intestinal motility.
   D. decreased vascular permeability.
   E. secretion of gastric acids.

_____ 13. The first line parenteral drug for the management of anaphylaxis is:
   A. oxygen.
   B. diphenhydramine.
   C. epinephrine.
   D. methylprednisolone.
   E. albuterol.

_____ 14. The first priority when responding to a patient with an anaphylactic reaction is to:
   A. protect the airway.
   B. administer diphenhydramine.
   C. stabilize the cervical spine.
   D. ensure scene safety.
   E. establish vascular access.

_____ 15. Hypotension that is seen in severe anaphylaxis is due to:
   A. internal hemorrhage.
   B. inadequate oxygenation.
   C. bradycardia.
   D. vasodilation.
   E. gastrointestinal hypermotility.

Chapter 32

Gastroenterology

Review of Chapter Objectives

After reading this chapter, you should be able to:

1. **Describe the incidence, morbidity, and mortality of gastrointestinal emergencies.** p. 1307

   Gastrointestinal (GI) emergencies account for over 500,000 emergency visits and hospitalizations annually. Of that total, more than 300,000 are due to GI bleeding. These numbers are expected to increase over time due to the aging American population and the trend of delaying treatment until over-the-counter medications no longer control symptoms. You will see GI emergencies in your practice, and it is likely that a large proportion will involve older persons. The number of patients over age 60 years in this patient population has risen from roughly 3 percent to over 45 percent in only a few years.

2. **Identify the risk factors most predisposing to gastrointestinal emergencies.** p. 1307

   Many of the most common risk factors are self-induced by patients. They include excessive alcohol and tobacco consumption, stress, ingestion of caustic substances, and poor bowel habits. Because of the various risk factors and possible causes of GI emergencies, it is particularly important that you know how to complete a thorough focused history and examination before making a field diagnosis and how to assess the seriousness of the emergency and possible prevention strategies to minimize organ damage.

3. **Discuss the anatomy and physiology of the gastrointestinal system.** (see Chapter 3)

   The GI tract is a long tube that extends from the mouth to the anus and is divided structurally and functionally into different parts. In general, the GI system is divided into the upper and lower GI tracts. The upper GI tract includes the mouth, esophagus, stomach, and duodenum, whereas the lower GI tract includes the remainder of the small intestine and the large intestine, rectum, and anus. In the upper GI tract, food is ingested and preliminary physical and chemical digestion is begun. In the lower GI tract, digestion of food is completed, nutrients are absorbed into the body, and remaining fiber, intestinal bacteria, and other materials are eliminated through the anus as feces. In addition, three additional organs—the liver, gallbladder, and pancreas—are intimately associated with the GI system both structurally (through connections with the duodenum) and functionally. The vermiform appendix, a blind sac found at the junction of the small and large intestines, does not have any apparent physiologic role in GI function but is important to you because of the inflammatory condition called appendicitis, which you will see in patients in the field.

4. **Discuss the pathophysiology of abdominal inflammation and its relationship to acute pain.** pp. 1307–1308

   Sudden onset, or acute, pain can be caused by a variety of mechanisms, one of which is inflammation. Inflammation of hollow organs such as the appendix or gallbladder produces pain that is

©2007 Pearson Education, Inc.
Essentials of Paramedic Care, 2nd ed.

characteristically poorly localized and crampy in nature (visceral pain). When inflammation is widespread within the abdomen, as happens after an inflamed appendix ruptures, inflammation of the peritoneal membrane (peritonitis) results in pain that is usually localized and sharp in nature (somatic pain). It is important for you to become familiar with the different types of pain because they often represent progressive stages in an inflammatory condition—for example, appendiceal pain that changes from visceral to somatic pain over time.

5. **Define somatic, visceral, and referred pain as they relate to gastroenterology.** p. 1308

Somatic pain is characteristically sharp and localized, and it originates in the peritoneal membrane or within elements of the wall of the abdominal cavity, such as skeletal muscle. Bacterial irritation, which is common after perforation of the gut or rupture of the appendix or gallbladder, causes somatic pain where the degree of extension of irritation through the abdominal cavity is often paralleled in the physical extent of the abdomen in which pain is perceived. Visceral pain is typically crampy and vague in character and poorly localized; it is commonly due to inflammation, distention, or ischemia in the walls of the GI tract (which is hollow) or in the capsule of a solid organ such as the liver. Referred pain is not a type of pain; rather, it is the term applied to any pain that is felt in a site other than the site of origin. Appendicitis is often first felt as periumbilical pain.

6. **Differentiate between hemorrhagic and nonhemorrhagic abdominal pain.** p. 1310

Recall that many GI emergencies are hemorrhagic. If hemorrhage results from perforation or rupture of an organ, pain will often be sudden in onset, somatic in nature, and extend in location as blood spreads through the abdominal cavity. Hemorrhage within the GI tract may initially produce visceral pain that is more characteristic of a nonhemorrhagic process such as inflammation or ischemia. Hemorrhage that is extensive enough to cause abdominal distention implies serious volume loss and will also be reflected in altered vital signs. Finally, pain from a dissecting aortic aneurysm (a grave, non-GI surgical emergency) is often felt between the shoulder blades.

7. **Discuss the signs and symptoms and differentiate between local, general, and peritoneal inflammation relative to acute abdominal pain.** p. 1308

Local inflammation within the GI tract often produces visceral pain associated with sympathetic nervous system stimulation (which typically results in nausea, vomiting, diaphoresis, and tachycardia). General inflammation within the abdomen often includes bacterial or chemical irritation of the peritoneum (the origins of peritonitis) and is thus associated with increasingly widespread somatic pain. Peritonitis (inflammation of the peritoneum) often represents the end stage of a generalized inflammatory or hemorrhagic process; as such, it is often associated with the most significant physical signs including altered vitals or overt shock. Because pain associated with peritonitis is often very severe, it is typical to find the patient lying with knees to chest as this position minimizes stretch of the already inflamed peritoneum.

8. **Describe the questioning technique and specific questions when gathering a focused history in a patient with abdominal pain.** pp. 1309–1310

Questioning is done with the SAMPLE technique (Symptoms, Allergies, Medication, Past medical history, Last oral intake, and Events leading to the current complaint). Specific questions about the present illness typically use the OPQRST-ASPN mnemonic to gather information about the abdominal pain:

- Onset of pain (sudden or slow)
- Provocation or palliation of pain in terms of position or activity such as walking
- Quality (or nature) of the pain
- Region where pain is felt, along with any radiation of pain (For instance, radiation of pain among different locations implies similar neural pathways as referred pain and may give clues to origin of problem.)
- Severity of pain at the moment and over time

- Time over which pain has been felt (Note that any patient with pain lasting over 6 hours is considered a surgical emergency and requires transport to an appropriate facility for evaluation.)
- Associated Symptoms, such as vomiting (if yes, ask about appearance of vomitus), change in bowel habits (if "diarrheal," inquire whether stool may suggest hemorrhage via foul-smelling, tarry appearance or obvious blood), or lost appetite
- Pertinent Negatives such as absence of change in GI tract function associated with positives such as pelvic pain, change in urinary habits, or positive cardiovascular history (Remember that diaphragmatic irritation with pain felt in neck or shoulder may reflect inferior myocardial infarction.)

9. **Describe the technique for performing a comprehensive physical examination on a patient complaining of abdominal pain.** p. 1310

Always start with the least invasive step, visual inspection. This includes checking the patient's appearance and positioning as well as visually inspecting the abdomen for signs of distention or discoloration. Be sure to get a complete set of baseline vital signs early in the process. Changes in vitals along with alterations in mental status may indicate early shock due to hemorrhage or other processes. Auscultation and percussion often do NOT provide useful information in the field; however, if you do auscultate, be sure to do so before palpating in order to avoid perturbation in abdominal sounds. Palpation with gentle pressure should start in the LEAST affected area and move toward the point of greatest pain. Remember to immediately stop palpation if you feel any pulsation. Further palpation may cause rupture of the affected blood vessel or organ.

10. **Discuss the pathophysiology, assessment findings, and management of the following gastroenterological problems:**

Upper gastrointestinal bleeding pp. 1311–1312

The six most common causes of hemorrhage in the upper GI tract are (in descending order) peptic ulcer disease, gastritis, variceal rupture, Mallory-Weiss syndrome (esophageal laceration, generally secondary to vomiting), esophagitis, and duodenitis. Note that ulcers and gastritis account for 75 percent of cases (with 50 percent due to ulcers). Irritation and erosion of the GI lining is the most common pathophysiologic basis for bleeding, and involvement of the stomach lining underlies 75 percent of upper GI bleeds. Because most such cases involve chronic, low-level hemorrhage, many patients can be cared for on an outpatient basis. However, brisk upper GI bleeds may be life threatening. Assessment findings that can help to distinguish the severity of the bleed include presence and severity of hematemesis (vomiting of blood) and/or melena (passage of partially digested blood represented as dark, tarry stools). Look for subtle signs of shock and manage accordingly. Besides shock, another potentially grave complication of some bleeds is airway compromise due to aspiration of vomitus (when vomiting is present). Be sure to support the airway, and beware of vomiting in patients who are lying in a supine position. A patient with pain characteristic of peritonitis, especially with discoloration or bulging of the abdomen, may have a life-threatening blood loss. General management centers on airway, oxygenation, and circulatory status. Position to minimize risk of aspiration, provide high-flow oxygen, and start two large-bore IV lines (one with blood tubing and one for volume replacement with normal saline). Base fluid resuscitation on patient condition and response to treatment.

Lower gastrointestinal bleeding pp. 1317–1318

Hemorrhage from the lower GI tract is most commonly associated with chronic medical conditions and the anatomic changes of advancing age. Typical causes include diverticulosis, colorectal lesions, and inflammatory bowel disease. Remember that lower GI bleeds rarely result in the massive hemorrhage that can be associated with esophageal or stomach pathology. Assessment should establish whether the problem is new in onset or chronic (be sure to look for scars from previous surgical procedures). Questions about stool or inspection of stool may show melena, which usually indicates a slow lower GI bleed, or bright red blood, which indicates severe hemorrhage with rapid passage through the intestines or a source in the distal colon. Distal GI causes include hemorrhoids and rectal fissures. Be sure to assess for abdominal signs such as discoloration or bulging and maintain ongoing check for signs of early shock. General management centers on the patient's physiologic status. Watch airway and oxygenation closely, and use oxygen if necessary. Establish IV access and fluid resuscitation based on patient's findings or shift in findings over time. If there are any signs of significant blood loss, be sure one IV line is capable of use for blood transfusion.

Acute gastroenteritis   pp. 1314–1315

Acute gastroenteritis involves inflammation of the stomach and intestines associated with sudden onset vomiting, diarrhea, or both. It is very common; the underlying inflammation causes erosion of the mucosal and submucosal layers of the GI tract with blood loss and damage to the intestinal villi. Triggers can include alcohol or tobacco use, use of nonsteroidal antiinflammatory agents, stress, and GI or systemic infection. The most common and striking finding is copious volumes of watery diarrhea secondary to damage to the intestinal lining. Diarrhea may contain blood. In general, patients are often febrile and suffering from general malaise as well as nausea and vomiting. Watch for any signs of early shock such as altered mental status, development of pale, clammy skin, or changes in vitals. Abdominal tenderness is common; distention is uncommon unless significant amounts of gas are in the intestines. In cases of severe dehydration, watch for problems such as cardiac dysrhythmia secondary to electrolyte disturbance. Management is supportive and palliative, with any needed support for airway (position to minimize odds of aspiration), oxygenation, or circulation. Fluid resuscitation via oral or IV route may be indicated. Be sure you take appropriate precautions during patient care to prevent spread of any possible infectious disease.

Colitis   p. 1318

Colitis is a general term for inflammation of the large intestine. Ulcerative colitis, which you may see in the field, is an inflammatory bowel disease that frequently affects relatively young people (with average age of 20 to 40 years at onset). Mild disease may only affect the distal colon, and it may present in the field with bloody diarrhea and discomfort. More severe disease may affect the entire colon, and this may present with severe, bloody diarrhea, electrolyte disturbances, or even hypovolemic shock. Management is tied to the patient's condition and includes appropriate support of oxygenation and circulation. If the patient has bouts of nausea and vomiting, beware of possible aspiration and airway compromise. Any patient who presents with a lower GI bleed or colicky, visceral-type pain should be transported for diagnostic evaluation.

Gastroenteritis   pp. 1314–1315

Gastroenteritis, inflammation of the stomach and intestines, is characterized by longer-term changes in the mucosa, thus distinguishing it from acute gastroenteritis. Gastroenteritis is usually due to microbial infection, with viral infection most common. However, patients with bacterial infection are usually the sickest. Common findings are fever, nausea, vomiting, diarrhea, lethargy, and, in the most severe cases, shock. Infection with *H. pylori* (the most common infectious cause in the United States) commonly presents with heartburn, abdominal pain, and the presence of gastric ulcers. Management includes appropriate infection precautions and patient care centered on monitoring of ABCs and transport. When outbreaks are associated with natural disaster or other possible contamination of water supply, be sure to protect yourself by use of proper sanitation and protection of water and food supplies.

Diverticulitis   pp. 1319–1320

Diverticulitis represents inflammation secondary to infection of diverticula, the outpouchings of intestinal mucosa and submucosa common in older Americans. Diverticulitis frequently starts with occlusion of a diverticulum by fecal material followed by bacterial infection. Complications include colonic hemorrhage or perforation. Common presenting signs of diverticulitis include low-grade fever, nausea and vomiting, and point tenderness on palpation. Because roughly 95 percent of cases involve the sigmoid colon, another name for this condition is "left-sided appendicitis." Management is supportive, with attention to the ABCs. Signs of shock suggest significant hemorrhage.

Appendicitis   pp. 1322–1323

Appendicitis is inflammation of the vermiform appendix. You will encounter acute appendicitis in the field, most commonly in older children and young adults. Untreated appendicitis can result in rupture with subsequent peritonitis. The pathophysiology has parallels to that of diverticulitis: The appendix becomes obstructed with fecal material, and the resultant inflammation and infection cause the characteristic discomfort, which may present initially as periumbilical, visceral pain, but later becomes the well-known somatic, right lower quadrant pain. Somatic pain or signs of peritonitis suggest significant inflammation with ischemia or infarction of the appendix or appendiceal rupture, respectively. Other findings such as fever, anorexia, and nausea or vomiting relate to the stage of appendiceal inflammation. Exam findings range from vague abdominal discomfort on palpation (in early cases) to clear peritonitis. Management during transport centers on positioning for comfort, managing airway to avoid aspiration, and establishing IV access. Monitor as you would for bowel obstruction and be aware of any early signs of shock.

Ulcer disease   pp. 1315–1317
Peptic ulcers, created secondary to mucosal erosion by gastric acid, can occur anywhere in the GI tract and are particularly common in the duodenum and stomach. You will see ulcer cases and GI problems complicated by the presence of peptic ulcers. Pathophysiology includes genetic predisposition (seen as positive family history) as well as risk factors such as stress, use of nonsteroidal antiinflammatory drugs, acid-stimulating products such as alcohol and nicotine, and chronic infection with *H. pylori*. The common mechanism is a breach of the mucous layer that protects the mucosa from the acid secreted in the stomach. Findings can vary widely. Chronic pain is typically worse when the stomach is empty and is relieved by eating or drinking coating liquids such as milk. Acute pain, particularly when somatic in character, may suggest rupture of the ulcer with hemorrhage into the abdomen. Bleeds manifest similarly to other upper GI hemorrhages and are handled similarly. In severely ill patients, appearance suggests severity of distress (such as lying still with knees drawn to chest), and there are often signs of shock. Management depends on physiologic status and involves monitoring of ABCs with appropriate intervention for possible or overt shock.

Bowel obstruction   pp. 1320–1322
Bowel obstruction involves partial or complete blockage of a portion of the small or large intestine. Rapid diagnosis and treatment are essential to avoid complications such as bowel infarction. The four most common causes are hernias, intussusception, volvulus, and adhesions. The most common site is the small intestine due to smaller diameter and greater length and motility of intestinal loops. Chronic obstruction is often due to a progressive process such as tumor growth or adhesions. Acute obstruction may be due to ingestion of a foreign body or incarceration and strangulation of a hernia or loop of intussuscepted bowel. Findings suggestive of obstruction include pain (which is often diffuse and visceral in nature) and vomiting. The character of the vomitus (for example, feces-like material) may suggest the approximate site of the obstruction. Significant ischemia or infarction is suggested by findings of early or overt shock. Visual inspection may reveal distention, peritonitis, or free air within the abdomen. Ask about scars that indicate prior surgery and look for discoloration that may indicate the presence of free blood in the abdominal cavity. Palpation may be useful in localizing discomfort but beware of any but light pressure because heavier pressure may cause rupture of the obstructed segment. Treatment depends on the patient's physiologic status, with attention and support of the ABCs. Remember to place one IV line capable of blood transfusion if there are any indications of significant hemorrhage.

Crohn's disease   pp. 1318–1319
Crohn's disease, like ulcerative colitis, is an inflammatory bowel disease. However, the pathologic inflammation can occur anywhere in the GI tract from the mouth to the rectum. After inflammation damages the mucosa and submucosa, granulomas form that further damage the wall of the GI tract. Patients with Crohn's frequently have narrowing of damaged segments, occasionally to the point of complete obstruction. Other findings include diarrhea and intestinal or perianal abscesses or fistulas. Because of the variety of sites involved in different patients, as well as the variety of complications due to progressive damage, prehospital diagnosis is nearly impossible. You should remember that an acute flare-up of symptoms accompanied by absence of bowel sounds suggests intestinal obstruction, which is a surgical emergency. Because significant hemorrhage is unusual, however, hypovolemic shock is infrequent among these patients. Prehospital management is largely palliative, with specific monitoring and support of the ABCs. Evidence of obstruction or shock calls for high-flow oxygen and circulatory support including IV access and fluid resuscitation.

Pancreatitis   p. 1324
Pancreatitis is inflammation of the pancreas. The four main pathologic types are metabolic, mechanical, vascular, and infectious. Metabolic causes (specifically alcoholism) account for over 80 percent of cases. Alcohol causes deposition of platelet plugs in the acini. As flow of digestive

secretions from the pancreas is impaired, digestive enzymes become activated while within the pancreas, damaging pancreatic tissue. Progression of this chronic damage can lead to hemorrhage, which presents as sudden onset nausea, vomiting, and severe pain that is in the left upper quadrant and may radiate to the back or the epigastric region. Mechanical pancreatitis is due to gallstones or elevated serum lipids. As digestive secretions accumulate behind the obstruction, pancreatic tissue damage occurs, edema develops, and blood flow is secondarily impaired, causing further damage due to ischemia. Mechanical pancreatitis is often acute in onset. Vascular causes of pancreatitis include thromboembolism and ischemia secondary to shock. Findings of mild pancreatitis include visceral pain, often epigastric in location, abdominal distension, nausea and vomiting, and elevated blood amylase and lipase. Findings in severe pancreatitis include refractory hypotensive shock, blood loss, and respiratory failure. As with other conditions involving hemorrhage, management of severe pancreatitis centers on support of ABCs including use of high-flow oxygen and appropriate IV access.

Esophageal varices pp. 1313–1314

A varix is a swollen vein, and esophageal varices (plural) are usually due to hypertension in the portal system. Varices are subject to rupture and hemorrhage, and mortality in these cases exceeds 35 percent. The most common cause is liver damage secondary to alcohol consumption (via cirrhosis of the liver and portal hypertension). The other common cause is ingestion of caustic substances, which damage the esophagus directly and eventually cause rupture of an esophageal vein. Initial presentation of rupture features painless bleeding with evolution of signs of hemodynamic instability. Hematemesis can be both forceful and large in volume. Clotting time increases as high portal pressure backs up blood into the spleen, destroying platelets. Because tamponade isn't possible in the prehospital setting, management centers on rapid transport with care focusing on aggressive airway management (including orotracheal intubation if needed), use of high-flow oxygen, and IV fluid resuscitation.

Hemorrhoids p. 1320

Hemorrhoids are small masses of swollen veins in the rectum or anus (internal and external hemorrhoids, respectively). Most are of unknown origin and occur in midlife, although some result from recognizable causes such as pregnancy or portal hypertension. In addition, external hemorrhoids can be caused by heavy lifting with straining. Although hemorrhoids frequently bleed during defecation, particularly in the setting of constipation, significant hemorrhage is rare. The typical cause for your call will be distress over the presence of bright red blood with defecation. The physical findings are usually benign, with hemodynamic stability and absence of signs of shock (skin is warm and dry, tachycardia is consistent with anxiety). Emotional assurance and monitoring for continued physiologic stability (due to possibility that bleeding is the first sign of a lower GI bleed) is usually sufficient during transport. Either signs of significant bleeding or bleeding hemorrhoids in an alcoholic patient warrant closer monitoring and transport for immediate care.

Cholecystitis pp. 1323–1324

Roughly 90 percent of cases of cholecystitis, inflammation of the gallbladder, are due to gallstones. Cholecystitis caused by stones can be acute or chronic. In both cases, the basic pathophysiology involves obstruction of the flow of bile by gallstones, with resultant inflammation of the gallbladder. Bacterial infection can also cause chronic cholecystitis. An acute attack is characterized by right upper quadrant pain, often with referred pain in the right shoulder. The right subcostal region may be tender due to muscle spasm. Sympathetic nervous stimulation may cause pale, cool, clammy skin. Prehospital care centers on palliation of distress and monitoring of ABCs with use of oxygen if needed and with establishment of IV access.

Acute hepatitis pp. 1324–1325

Acute hepatitis, inflammation of the liver, can result from any injury to liver cells associated with an infectious or inflammatory process. Viral hepatitis is most common, and alcoholic hepatitis secondary to cirrhosis is also common. Symptoms range from mild manifestations to overt liver failure and death, and mortality is high due to the wide range of potential causes. You will find that presentation often parallels severity of hepatitis: Common complaints include right upper quadrant tenderness not relieved by eating or antacids and development of clay-colored stools (this secondary to decreased bile production). If bilirubin retention exists, scleral icterus and jaundice may be present. Palpation may reveal liver enlargement, and fever may be due to infection or tissue necrosis. Presence of cool, clammy, diaphoretic skin suggests hemorrhage of a hepatic lesion. Secure ABCs and establish IV access. Be particularly careful in consideration of use of any pharmacologic agent because liver failure may impair drug metabolism. Never forget to use personal protective equipment and to use body substance isolation precautions.

11. **Differentiate between gastrointestinal emergencies based on assessment findings.** pp. 1308–1310

Assessment includes initial size-up, SAMPLE focused history with attention to current complaint, personal medical and family history, and physical examination. History of present illness will reveal whether condition is acute, chronic, or an acute flare-up of a chronic problem. The relation of pain (if any) with last oral intake may suggest ulcers (in which eating typically relieves pain) or, in contrast, cholecystitis (where pain may worsen after eating, particularly a fatty meal). The presence of chest pain rather than abdominal pain (or in addition to abdominal pain) may mean a condition has generated referred pain: Examples include gastroesophageal reflux (heartburn), gastric or duodenal ulcers, or cholecystitis. A change in nature of pain from visceral to somatic may infer a progression of abdominal pathology. Always remember before starting the physical exam that the majority of GI emergencies entail bleeding from the upper or lower GI tract: Watch for signs of hemorrhage in vitals (and changes in vitals) and on visual inspection of the abdomen, as well as examination of any vomitus or stool.

12. **Given several preprogrammed patients with abdominal pain and symptoms, provide the appropriate assessment, treatment, and transport.** pp. 1307–1325

Care of any hemorrhagic case entails close monitoring of ABCs with attention to airway (minimizing risk of aspiration of any vomitus), breathing (high-flow oxygen is often indicated), and circulation (establishment of one or two IV lines with ability for blood transfusion where appropriate, and fluid resuscitation as needed). Although there are some conditions such as Crohn's disease in which bleeding rarely leads to hypovolemic shock, you should always be prepared to treat shock. Cases that seem to represent progressive, nonhemorrhagic conditions such as appendicitis, cholecystitis, or diverticulitis should also be monitored for stability and signs of acute events such as rupture or hemorrhage. Last, be aware that GI emergencies often present in older patients with coexisting morbid conditions and monitor cardiopulmonary status and other organ function carefully. Take close note of conditions such as alcoholism, consider GI problems associated with them (such as hepatitis, pancreatitis, or esophageal varices), and adjust assessment and treatment accordingly.

Content Self-Evaluation

MULTIPLE CHOICE

_____ 1. Which of the following statements about gastrointestinal (GI) emergencies is NOT true?
   A. GI emergencies account for about 5 percent of all annual visits to the emergency department.
   B. The majority of GI emergencies entail GI hemorrhage.
   C. The number of GI emergencies is expected to rise, in part due to aging of the population.
   D. The risk factors for GI emergencies are well known, and most (such as familial predisposition to GI conditions) are out of control of the patient.
   E. The number of GI emergencies is expected to rise, in part due to delays in seeking treatment by patients who treat themselves as long as symptoms allow.

_____ 2. Risk factors for GI disease include excessive use of alcohol and tobacco, stress, ingestion of caustic substances, and poor bowel habits.
   A. True
   B. False

_____ 3. All of the following statements about physical examination of the abdomen are true EXCEPT:
   A. visual inspection should always be done first.
   B. palpation should always precede auscultation.
   C. of auscultation, percussion, palpation, and visual inspection, palpation may be most likely to produce a lot of useful information.
   D. discoloration of the skin (specifically, ecchymosis) may indicate where hemorrhage has occurred into the abdominal cavity.
   E. abdominal distension may be an ominous sign, suggesting either free air in the abdomen or loss of a large amount of circulating volume.

_____ 4. Three organs intimately associated with the GI tract are the:
   A. teeth, tongue, and epiglottis.
   B. appendix, gallbladder, and parotid gland.
   C. cystic duct, the bile duct, and the common bile duct.
   D. appendix, the rectum, and the anus.
   E. liver, pancreas, and gallbladder.

_____ 5. The chief function of the upper GI tract is digestion, whereas the chief functions of the lower GI tract are absorption of nutrients and excretion of wastes.
   A. True
   B. False

_____ 6. Major causes of upper GI hemorrhage include all of the following EXCEPT:
   A. gastritis.   D. peptic ulcers.
   B. rupture of an esophageal varix.   E. Mallory-Weiss syndrome.
   C. gastroenteritis.

_____ 7. Severe, potentially life-threatening upper GI hemorrhage is common with:
   A. variceal and hemorrhoidal rupture and bleeding.
   B. peptic ulcer disease and Crohn's disease.
   C. esophageal varices and hepatic cirrhosis.
   D. esophageal varix rupture and esophageal Mallory-Weiss tears.
   E. eroded gastric ulcers and eroded ulcerative colitis lesions.

_____ 8. Blood is indicated by melena, stool containing small or large amounts of bright red blood, and hematochezia, dark, tarry, foul-smelling stool.
   A. True
   B. False

_____ 9. A common difference between acute gastroenteritis and gastroenteritis is that gastroenteritis is more likely to be caused by microbial infection.
   A. True
   B. False

_____ 10. Conditions that routinely call for the paramedic to take infectious precautions include:
   A. hepatitis and cirrhosis.
   B. peptic ulcer disease and gastroenteritis.
   C. cholecystitis and pancreatitis.
   D. gastroenteritis and appendicitis.
   E. hepatitis and gastroenteritis.

_____ 11. Patients with peptic ulcer disease typically have worsening of pain after eating, whereas patients with cholecystitis typically have relief of pain after eating.
   A. True
   B. False

_____ 12. Any patient who presents with lower GI bleeding or colicky abdominal pain should be transported to the emergency department for evaluation.
   A. True
   B. False

_____ 13. Conditions that typically have lesions in the rectum and anus include:
   A. diverticulosis and hemorrhoids.
   B. ulcerative colitis and Crohn's disease.
   C. ulcerative colitis and hemorrhoids.
   D. volvulus and intussusception.
   E. hernias and hemorrhoids.

_____ 14. Among the most common causes of bowel obstruction are:
   A. intestinal tumors, volvulus, and hernias.
   B. intussusception, volvulus, and hemorrhoids.
   C. adhesions, hernias, and intestinal tumors.
   D. hernias, volvulus, and adhesions.
   E. appendicitis, volvulus, and diverticulitis.

_____ 15. Acute pancreatitis is most commonly caused by:
   A. excessive use of alcohol and tobacco.
   B. gallstones and excessive use of alcohol.
   C. infectious GI disease and gallstones.
   D. drug toxicity and excessive use of alcohol.
   E. vascular disease causing ischemia and gallstones causing obstruction of the pancreatic duct.

MATCHING

Write the letter of the type of pain in the space provided next to the appropriate description of the pain.

A. somatic   D. radiated

B. peritonitis   E. referred

C. visceral

_____ 16. pain originating in the walls of hollow organs that is typically produced by the processes of inflammation, distension, or ischemia

_____ 17. pain perceived in a location other than the one from which it originates

_____ 18. pain frequently characterized by the patient as sharp and well localized

_____ 19. condition caused by presence of free blood or GI contents within the abdominal cavity, which is typically perceived by the patient as somatic pain that is eased in a knee-chest position

_____ 20. pain frequently originating in the capsules of solid organs and typically perceived by the patient as sharp or tearing in character

_____ 21. pain between the shoulder blades that may be produced by a dissecting abdominal aorta

_____ 22. pain that an appendicitis patient may perceive when the inflamed appendix ruptures

_____ 23. pain that seems to the patient to move from one location to another

Urology and Nephrology

Review of Chapter Objectives

After reading this chapter, you should be able to:

1. **Describe the incidence, morbidity, mortality, and risk factors predisposing to urologic and nephrologic emergencies.** pp. 1329–1330, 1335, 1331–1339, 1343–1344, 1345–1346

   Renal (kidney) and urologic (urinary tract) disorders are very common, affecting about 20 million Americans, so you will definitely see emergencies related to these disorders in the field. The seriousness of these disorders is demonstrated by two statistics: Roughly 250,000 Americans have the most severe form of long-term kidney failure (end-stage failure) and require either dialysis or transplantation to live. More than 50,000 Americans die annually from some form of kidney disease. Some emergencies are not necessarily life threatening but are very painful to experience and common in the population: Over 500,000 persons are treated annually for kidney stones. Persons most at risk for severe kidney problems include older patients, persons with diabetes mellitus, persons with chronic hypertension, and individuals with more than one risk factor. The two risk factors most significant for end-stage renal failure are hypertension and diabetes, which account for more than half of all cases. The risk factors for kidney stones are very different. Some kinds of stones follow a familial pattern, suggesting genetic predisposition. Other risk factors include physical immobilization, use of certain medications (anesthetics, opiates, and psychotropic drugs), and metabolic disorders such as gout. Finally, urinary tract infection, which accounts for over 6 million office visits yearly, has identified risk factors: female gender, paraplegic persons and others (notably some persons with diabetes) with nerve disruption to the bladder, pregnancy, and regular use of instrumentation such as catheters.

2. **Discuss the anatomy and physiology of the organs and structures related to the urinary system.** (see Chapter 3)

   The two major organs of the urinary system are the kidneys and the urinary bladder. Two major structures are the ureters and the urethra. The kidney is the critical organ of the urinary system: The kidneys perform the vital functions of the urinary system, which include:

   - Maintenance of blood volume with proper balance of water, electrolytes, and pH
   - Retention of key substances such as glucose and removal of toxic wastes such as urea
   - Major role in regulation of arterial blood pressure
   - Control of the development of red blood cells

   The first two roles are achieved through the production of urine in the kidneys. The kidneys' role in regulation of blood pressure is achieved in part through control of the body's fluid volume.

©2007 Pearson Education, Inc.
Essentials of Paramedic Care, 2nd ed.

In addition, they produce an enzyme called renin, which acts to activate a hormone (chemical messenger) called angiotensin, which is part of a hormonal pathway that acts to retain water in the body (increase blood pressure).

The structural and functional unit within the kidney is the nephron, and each kidney contains about 1 million nephrons, establishing the functional reserve that most people take for granted. Blood is filtered into the first part of the nephron, the glomerulus, and then moves through a length of specialized tubule. As the fluid moves through the parts of the tubule, movement of water and some materials out of the tubule and into the blood occurs (reabsorption), as does movement of some materials out of blood and into the tubule (secretion). The kidneys can maintain an exquisitely fine control over the relative activity of reabsorption and secretion for virtually every substance that is filtered into the glomerulus. The ability of the kidney to retain glucose, excrete wastes such as urea, and thus perform all of its vital roles is extraordinary, and life depends upon it. When kidney function is too low or nonexistent, an individual will die unless the function is replaced through artificial dialysis or through kidney transplantation. The final role of the kidney, control over development of red blood cells, is achieved through production and release of a hormone called erythropoietin, which stimulates red blood cell synthesis in the bone marrow.

Each ureter runs from a kidney to the bladder, and urine moves out of the kidney through them to reach the bladder. Because ureters are very small in internal diameter, they can become blocked by internal objects such as kidney stones. The bladder is a muscular sac that expands to hold urine. During urination, stored urine is eliminated from the bladder (and the body) through the tube called the urethra.

In women, the structures of the urinary system and the reproductive system are completely separate. In men, however, reproductive fluid (semen) is also eliminated from the body through the urethra. Thus, consideration of symptoms of urinary tract trouble in men is sometimes more complex than consideration of the same problem in women. For instance, infection in a man's urethra can come directly through sexual activity.

The genitourinary systems of men include some specifically reproductive organs and structures: the testes (the primary male reproductive organs, which produce testosterone and sperm cells) and tubing called the epididymis and vas deferens, through which sperm cells leave the testes and move toward the urethra. Sperm leaves the vas deferens to enter the urethra as it passes through the substance of the other male reproductive organ, the prostate gland, which produces fluid that mixes with sperm to produce semen, the male reproductive fluid. The prostate will be important to you in field work because it surrounds the first part of the male urethra. Prostate enlargement, which occurs routinely with age, can compress the urethra to the point of closure. This can result in retention of urine and a medical emergency call.

3. Define referred pain and visceral pain as they relate to urology. p. 1331

Visceral pain and referred pain have the same underlying pathophysiology as they do in the setting of GI emergencies. In the setting of urology, visceral pain usually arises in the walls of hollow structures such as the ureters, bladder, and urethra or the male vas deferens or epididymis. Visceral pain is characteristically described as aching or crampy and feels deeply internal within the body and poorly localized. Visceral pain can mark the first presentation of both kidney stones and urinary tract infection (although both are better known for somatic pain patterns that arise later). Referred pain, which is felt in a location other than the one of origin, has some notable urologic examples. Pyelonephritis, inflammation within the kidney, is often referred to the neck or shoulder.

4. Describe the questioning technique and specific questions the paramedic should use when gathering a focused history in a patient with abdominal pain. pp. 1332–1333

Recall Chapter 32, "Gastroenterology," where you learned about the focused history relating to abdominal pain that might be GI in origin. The technique is similar when the GI system is not the focus of attention. For instance, initial questioning still follows the OPQRST format (shown below with some specific questions in parentheses):

- Onset of pain (Sudden or slow? Activity at the time?)
- Provocation or palliation of pain (Pain on urination, inability to void or void normally, and palliation with walking all may suggest urinary tract origin.)

- Quality of the pain (Visceral pain is common with urinary emergencies; a change to somatic pain, particularly flank pain, may suggest ureteral obstruction by a stone.)
- Region where pain is felt, along with any radiation of pain (Listen for suggestions of referred/radiated pain; in postpubertal women, be sure to get menstrual history and follow-up comments suggesting OB/GYN problems.)
- Severity of pain currently and over time (Most urinary conditions don't cause the abrupt switch to somatic pain—with increase in severity—seen with a ruptured appendix, for instance.)
- Time over which pain has been felt (Note that any patient with pain lasting over 6 hours is considered a surgical emergency and requires transport to an appropriate facility for evaluation.) When in doubt, consider the case a potential surgical emergency and treat/transport as such.

Additional questions center on:

- Previous history of similar event (Note that kidney stones and infections may be recurrent problems; family history may also be helpful.)
- Nausea/vomiting (Because nausea and vomiting can be caused purely by autonomic nervous system discharge, this is not necessarily a sign localizing to GI system; nausea and vomiting is common with severe pain associated with kidney stones.)
- Changes in bowel habits (Diarrhea may suggest a GI condition; constipation may be less helpful as a clue to the origin of a problem.)
- Weight loss (Loss over hours to days suggests dehydration, whereas longer-term loss suggests chronic illness or GI dysfunction.)
- Last oral intake, include beverages (Learning this is necessary for possible surgical cases; timing of a meal may also suggest acute onset problem or aggravation of an existing one.)
- Chest pain (Consider MI but also consider referred pain; note that diabetic persons may not have typical pain pattern during MI due to neuropathy.)

5. Describe the technique for performing a comprehensive physical examination of a patient complaining of abdominal pain. pp. 1333–1334

The physical exam includes overall impressions as well as examination of the abdomen. Elements include both patient appearance and posture/activity. Walking often suggests urinary origin: Walking that relieves pain may suggest a kidney stone, and walking hunched up in a febrile person complaining of back pain may suggest kidney infection. Additionally, altered level of consciousness in the absence of fever may suggest hemorrhage and evolution of hypovolemic shock. Hemorrhage should lead you to consider GI or reproductive (OB) emergencies. Patients undergoing dialysis may have chronic changes in mental status during dialysis; try to discern whether the level you see is the norm for that person or represents an acute or subacute change. Also consider the apparent state of the patient's health and his or her personal appearance, which can often give leads to a chronic condition or one of acute onset. Skin color and appearance can suggest chronic anemia (pale, cool, dry skin), shock (pale, clammy skin), or fever (dry, flushed).

Examination of the abdomen was covered in Chapter 32. Percussion may be very useful in the setting of urology. Pain on percussion of the flanks may suggest kidney inflammation and infection, and pain on percussion of the pelvic rim may suggest problems in the bladder. Remember that pregnancy may also be found during physical examination as you palpate above the pelvic rim. A ruptured ectopic pregnancy may be suggested by lower quadrant pain that increases with palpation and evidence of hemorrhage. In older men, palpation above the pelvic rim may reveal the enlarged, fluctuant mass of an obstructed bladder due to prostatic hypertrophy. In all men, exam includes examination of the scrotum and penis. Urethral discharge may suggest infection. Scrotal masses may be painful (such as infectious epididymitis) or nonpainful (testicular cancer, which is most common in young men, or a varicocele). Ask questions about acute or longer-term presence of any mass. For men with an apparently obstructed bladder, find out when they last urinated and whether there had been any change in pattern.

Generally, nephrologic and urologic emergencies don't produce acute abnormalities on exam, unlike GI emergencies. However, pain from an inflamed or infected kidney may be felt in the flank, and pelvic pain may suggest bladder origin or a reproductive problem in either a man or woman. Always consider possible miscarriage from either an ectopic pregnancy or an intrauterine one in girls and women of childbearing age.

6. Define acute renal failure. p. 1335

Acute renal failure is defined as a sudden (over a period of a day or days) drop in urine output to less than 400–500 mL per day. Low urine output is oliguria, whereas no urine output is anuria.

7. Discuss the pathophysiology of acute renal failure. pp. 1335–1337

There are three types of acute renal failure (ARF) based on pathophysiology: prerenal, renal, and postrenal. You may see all three types in the field. Remember that acute renal failure may be reversible if recognized and treated early enough.

- Prerenal ARF is due to insufficient blood flow to the kidneys. This type accounts for 40 to 80 percent of cases, and it is the most likely to be reversible if perfusion is restored. Common causes in the field include cardiac failure (often an MI), hemorrhage, dehydration, shock, and sepsis, as well as anomalies of a renal artery or vein.
- Renal ARF is due to a pathologic process within the kidney tissue itself. The three general causes are damage to small vessels and/or glomeruli, tubular cell damage, and interstitial damage. In each type, nephron function is lost.
- Postrenal ARF is due to obstruction at some point distal to the kidneys: both ureters, the bladder outlet, or the urethra. Postrenal ARF may be reversible if the obstruction is identified and removed before permanent kidney damage occurs.

8. Recognize the signs and symptoms related to acute renal failure. pp. 1337–1338

Timing of voiding difficulty can provide vital information: A normal history with sudden onset inability to void may suggest distal obstruction, whereas feeling ill over a number of days with some decrease in voiding may suggest chronic renal problems with an acute aggravation: Ask for renal history. Some triggers of acute renal failure may be obvious: dehydration secondary to diarrhea, hemorrhage, shock, sepsis. Visual inspection may reveal cool, pale, moist skin (which suggests shunting of blood to core, including kidneys, if shock is absent) and edema in hands, feet, or face. Physical findings may reveal the trigger for the failure: A distended, discolored abdomen may suggest severe intraabdominal hemorrhage with hypoperfusion to kidneys.

9. Describe the management of acute renal failure. p. 1338

Because acute renal failure can cause life-threatening metabolic complications (consider the key role of the kidneys in regulation of fluid volume, electrolytes, and pH), provide close monitoring and support of the ABCs. High-flow oxygen should be used, and patient positioning and IV fluid resuscitation are important. In general, you want to protect fluid volume and cardiovascular function to minimize damage due to renal hypoperfusion and eliminate or reduce exposure to any potentially nephrotoxic drug.

Drug information may be available from medical direction; likewise, specific advice for care of dialysis patients may also be obtained before or during transit.

10. Integrate pathophysiological principles and assessment findings to formulate a field impression and implement a treatment plan for the patient with acute renal failure. pp. 1335–1338

If onset is acute and without evidence of distal obstruction, prerenal ARF may be suggested. Be sure to treat any identifiable potential trigger condition and aggressively protect fluid volume and oxygenation. Always remember that prerenal ARF may be reversible if you act quickly and correctly; this is still true in patients with chronic renal failure. Quick action may also preserve remaining function if renal causes are suspected. Renal causes may require the hospital setting for definitive treatment, but the treatment staples are the same as for prerenal. If history or exam suggests postrenal obstruction, be sure to get as much information as possible for use by hospital staff. For instance, known cancer in the abdomen or pelvis may suggest bilateral ureteral obstruction. Advanced age in men may suggest acute renal retention secondary to prostate enlargement, and history in boys or men of recent sexual activity, recreational drugs, or parties may suggest the possible presence of a foreign body in the urethra.

11. Define chronic renal failure. pp. 1338–1339

Chronic renal failure is inadequate kidney function due to the permanent loss of nephrons (usually representing a loss of at least 70 to 80 percent of total nephrons). When metabolic instability sets in (around 80 percent loss), the condition is termed end-stage renal failure, and either dialysis or kidney transplantation is required to survive.

12. Discuss the pathophysiology of chronic renal failure. pp. 1339–1340

The three processes that can underlie chronic renal failure are the same as those producing acute renal failure: damage to small blood vessels or glomeruli, tubular cell injury, and damage to interstitial tissue. In each case, surviving nephrons adapt by structural changes that increase function, but these changes damage the nephrons themselves over time, leading to greater loss of nephron numbers. Common causes of damage to blood vessels and glomeruli include systemic hypertension, atherosclerosis, diabetes, and systemic lupus erythematosus, an autoimmune disease. Causes of tubular cell injury include nephrotoxic drugs and heavy metals and distal obstruction with backup of urine into the kidney. Finally, interstitial damage can be caused by infections including pyelonephritis and tuberculosis.

13. Recognize the signs and symptoms related to chronic renal failure. pp. 1340–1341

All of the kidney's major functions are deranged or lost in chronic renal failure. The general syndrome of signs and symptoms associated with chronic failure is termed uremia or uremic syndrome, so-called for the characteristic buildup of the waste urea. Clinical elements of uremia are found in Table 33-3 on text page 1340. They include peripheral and pulmonary edema, hypertension, hyperkalemia and acidosis, congestive heart failure and accelerated atherosclerosis, headache, impaired mental status, seizures, muscle irritability, anorexia/nausea/vomiting, ulcers and GI bleeding, glucose intolerance due to cellular resistance to insulin, jaundice, uremic frost, pruritus, easy bleeding, chronic anemia, and vulnerability to infection. In addition, children and young adults may show poor growth and development, including delayed sexual maturation.

14. Describe the management of chronic renal failure. pp. 1341–1343

Long-term management will focus on dialysis (either hemodialysis or peritoneal dialysis, dependent on individual circumstances) or transplantation.

15. Integrate pathophysiological principles and assessment findings to formulate a field impression and implement a treatment plan for the patient with chronic renal failure. pp. 1339–1343

Immediate management is similar to that for acute renal failure. Focus on close monitoring and support of the ABCs with high-flow oxygen, positioning to support blood flow to internal organs and brain, and administration of IV fluid if hypovolemia is suggested. Chief prevention strategies are protection of fluid volume and cardiovascular function with correction of major electrolyte disturbances as merited by individual findings and the philosophy of erring on the side of conservative treatment. Close monitoring of the ECG may give you time to adjust and respond to cardiac problems caused by fluid overload or electrolyte disturbances. Life-threatening conditions should always be treated and lesser conditions or complications noted for consideration by the receiving staff. Where possible, be sure your impressions clearly note which conditions have been chronic (or the norm) for the patient and which findings represent acute changes. As indicated and allowed by medical direction, fluid lavage may be considered for patients who use peritoneal dialysis.

16. Define renal dialysis. pp. 1342–1343

Renal dialysis is artificial replacement of some of the kidneys' vital functions. Two different technologies, hemodialysis and peritoneal dialysis, are widely used. Both rely on the physiologic principles of osmosis and equalization of osmolarity across a semipermeable membrane. As blood flows over such a membrane, many critical substances such as urea and sodium, potassium, and hydrogen ions move from blood into the hypo-osmolar solution, the dialysate, thus reducing the concentrations in blood. The overall effect is to lessen or eliminate temporarily volume overload and toxically high blood concentrations of electrolytes, urea, and other substances.

In hemodialysis, the patient's blood is passed through a machine containing a semipermeable membrane. Vascular access is established through a permanent anastamosis of an artery and vein in the forearm. If such a fistula is not possible, an indwelling catheter may be placed in the internal jugular vein. In peritoneal dialysis, the peritoneal membrane is used as the semipermeable membrane and dialysate solution is introduced into, and then removed from, the abdominal cavity via an indwelling catheter.

17. **Discuss the common complications of renal dialysis.** pp. 1342–1343

Complications common to both forms of dialysis include physiologically destabilizing shifts in blood volume and composition and blood pressure during and shortly after dialysis. Other complications common to both forms include shortness of breath or dizziness and neurologic abnormalities ranging from headache to seizure or coma. Hypotension may represent dehydration, hemorrhage, or infection. Shortness of breath or chest pain may reflect cardiac dysrhythmias, ischemia, or even MI. In many cases the neurologic abnormalities represent shifts in the chemical milieu of the brain. Seizures are usually responsive to benzodiazepines.

Complications specific to hemodialysis include bleeding at the needle puncture site, local infection, and stenosis or obstruction of the internal fistula. Under normal flow conditions, you will hear or feel a bruit or thrill. Leading complications requiring hospitalization include thrombosis, infection, and development of an aneurysm. The latter are particularly common in patients in whom artificial graft material was used to construct the fistula. The most common complications in patients undergoing peritoneal dialysis include infection in the catheter or tunnel containing the catheter, or in the peritoneum itself. Because the incidence of peritonitis is roughly one episode per year, you may find the signs of peritonitis in this patient group.

18. **Define renal calculi.** pp. 1343–1344

Renal calculi (calculus, singular) are crystal aggregations in the kidney's urine collecting system. The same condition is referred to as nephrolithiasis. Although overall morbidity and mortality are low, brief hospitalizations are common for patients because of the severity of the pain as stones move through the renal pelvis, ureter, bladder, and urethra.

19. **Discuss the pathophysiology of renal calculi.** p. 1344

Some kinds of stones form as part of a systemic metabolic disorder such as gout (excess uric acid) or primary hyperparathyroidism (excess calcium). Most stones, however, form due to a more general imbalance between the amount of water flowing through the kidney tubing and the mineral ions, uric acid, and other relatively insoluble substances that are dissolved in that water. Trigger events for stone formation include change in diet, activity, or climate, all of which can alter water conservation or the amount of one or more such substances in the blood and, thus, the filtrate. Calcium stones are the most common and are most frequently seen in men aged 20 to 30 years. This type of stone is likely to recur and is likely to be found in a family history. Struvite stones are also common; their formation is often related to chronic urinary tract infection or frequent bladder catheterization. Perhaps because of the tie to infection, these stones are more common in women. Struvite stones can grow to fill the renal pelvis; in such cases, they present a "staghorn" appearance on X-rays. The less common stones are made of uric acid or cystine. Uric acid stones can occur in the presence of gout (about 50 percent of cases); they are also more common men and tend to occur in families. Cystine stones are the least common, and they are associated with excess cystine in filtrate. There is probably at least a partial genetic predisposition, and they are known to occur in families.

20. **Recognize the signs and symptoms related to renal calculi.** p. 1345

The assessment almost always focuses on pain as the chief complaint; the pain associated with kidney stones is generally conceded to be among the most severe known, ranking up there with labor pain. Typical history is a vague onset of discomfort in the flank progressing within an hour or so to an extremely sharp pain that may remain in the flank or radiate downward toward the pelvis or scrotum in men. Migrating pain suggests that the stone is in the lowest third of the involved ureter. Stones that lodge low in the ureter or within the bladder wall characteristically cause bladder symptoms such as frequency, urgency, and painful urination. In women these symptoms may make it difficult to distinguish stones from an infection. Physical exam will almost always reveal someone in considerable distress, often agitated and walking restlessly. High blood pressure and tachycardia may correlate with the degree of pain. Skin is typically cool, clammy, and pale due to autonomic discharge. Abdominal exam may be difficult to perform or assess given patient restlessness and muscle guarding secondary to pain.

21. Describe the management of renal calculi. p. 1345

Management, as always, begins with the ABCs. Position for comfort, but be ready for vomiting, particularly if pain is severe or last oral intake recent. IV access may be needed for analgesic administration (if needed and appropriate per local protocol) or fluid to promote urine formation and movement of the stone through the urinary tract.

22. Integrate pathophysiological principles and assessment findings to formulate a field impression and implement a treatment plan for the patient with renal calculi. pp. 1343–1345

The common pathophysiology for all types of stones rests on an imbalance of water and relatively insoluble substances in the kidney filtrate. The type and size of stone, as well as current site in the urinary tract, may be discerned from personal and family history, as well as physical examination. Assessment for treatment (prior to and during transport) focuses on nature, site, and severity of pain. A urine sample may reveal blood in the presence of any type of stone. A urine sample may be particularly valuable from a woman patient because of inclusion of infection in the differential diagnosis, especially when bladder symptoms are present. Because passage of the stone is the ultimate goal, IV fluid may be beneficial as soon as it can be started as it promotes urine formation. Analgesia may be necessary, dependent on the individual patient and local protocol.

23. Define urinary tract infection. pp. 1345–1346

Infection of the urinary tract implies infection in the urethra, bladder, or kidney, or the prostate gland in men. Urinary tract infections (UTI) are extremely common, accounting for about 6 million office visits per year, and you will see them in the field.

24. Discuss the pathophysiology of urinary tract infection. pp. 1346–1347

Because bacteria usually enter via the urethra, infections are more common in women (who have a much shorter urethra), paraplegic patients or others who require catheterization, and diabetic persons who have neuropathy involving the bladder. UTIs are generally divided into those affecting the lower urinary tract (namely, urethritis, cystitis, and prostatitis) and those of the upper urinary tract (pyelonephritis). Lower UTIs are much more common because of bacterial entrance via the urethra and NOT commonly via the bloodstream. Sexually active females may be at higher risk due to indirect factors (use of contraceptives vaginally and unintentional introduction of enteric flora into the urethra), and direct sexual transmission of infection can occur in males. Pyelonephritis usually occurs due to an infection that ascends through the urinary tract. The infectious inflammation can affect the interstitium, nephrons, or both. Incidence is highest during pregnancy and among the sexually active, paralleling the epidemiology of lower UTIs. Intrarenal abscesses can result, and rupture with spillage of contents into adjacent perirenal fat can cause formation of a perinephric abscess. Note that the likely pathogens are distinctly different in community-acquired and nosocomial infections.

25. Recognize the signs and symptoms related to urinary tract infection. p. 1347

The typical triad of a lower UTI consists of painful urination, frequent urge to urinate, and difficulty in beginning and continuing flow. Pain frequently is visceral in character before voiding, progresses to severe, burning pain during and after urination, and then receding to visceral pain again. Many women will have a past medical history of such episodes, which may or may not have been diagnosed and treated. Vitals generally reflect those of someone in pain, with slight tachycardia and an increase in blood pressure. Exam will probably show tenderness over the pubis and cool, clammy skin. Patients with pyelonephritis typically have a fever and feel more generally ill. Their pain is typically in the flank or lower back with occasional reference to the neck or shoulder. Pain tends to be somewhat more somatic in character: moderately severe or severe and constant. The triad of lower urinary tract symptoms may or may not be present. (If not, ask whether they have been present recently.) The exam of a patient with pyelonephritis will be more striking, with a restless and ill appearance; warm, dry skin if fever is present; and possible tenderness over the flank. Lloyd's sign, tenderness on percussion of the lower back at the costovertebral angle, indicates pyelonephritis.

26. Describe the management of a urinary tract infection. p. 1347

Management centers on monitoring and support of the ABCs. Positioning may help the patient with severe pain; be prepared in case the patient vomits. Analgesics are usually unnecessary; severely painful cases of pyelonephritis may be the exception. As with renal stones, hydration to increase and dilute urine flow is generally helpful. Use of IV fluid eliminates the risk of vomiting and satisfies treatment guidelines for possible surgical cases.

27. Integrate pathophysiological principles and assessment findings to formulate a field impression and implement a treatment plan for the patient with a urinary tract infection. pp. 1345–1347

Lower UTIs typically arise from infection that has entered via the urethra and has damaged tissue in the lower urinary tract. Hydration increases urine formation and promotes a more dilute urine (in a patient with normal renal function), and so it may help ease the symptoms of urgency, frequency, and pain in the patient with a lower UTI. Lack of systemic signs indicates that normal monitoring of ABCs is probably sufficient before and during transport. Patients with pyelonephritis (upper UTI) are more likely to show fever and other signs of systemic infection. IV hydration is also indicated for the same reasons and because IV access may be needed if physiologic instability develops or the patient is deemed later to be a surgical case. Transport for diagnosis and definitive treatment (appropriate antibiotic therapy) provides the link to long-term care.

28. Apply epidemiology to develop prevention strategies for urologic and nephrologic emergencies. p. 1330

Urinary tract infections, which include genitourinary infections in men, are the most typical urologic emergency. IV hydration promotes formation of a dilute urine that will help to eliminate bacteria within the urinary tract and decrease the triad of symptoms typically associated with lower UTIs: pain, frequency, and urgency. In elderly men, pain or poor urination may frequently be due to obstruction by an enlarged prostate: In these cases, the enlarged bladder will be felt on exam. Hydration is also useful for patients with pyelonephritis. ABCs should always be supported. Because UTIs, particularly lower UTIs, are more common among diabetic patients with neuropathy, it is also wise to assess diabetic status for signs of instability while monitoring ABCs as in all other patients. Remember to relay all relevant information on fetal age, presence of any complications, and so on, in pregnant women presenting with UTIs to the receiving facility so they can arrange appropriate OB support.

Prevention strategies are probably most critical for the nephrologic emergencies directly involving kidney function (acute and chronic renal failure) and indirectly involving function (renal calculi with possible obstruction of the distal urinary tract). Prevention strategies in patients with acute renal failure (ARF), particularly cases that may be prerenal in origin, center on protection of fluid volume (usually through IV fluid) and support of cardiovascular function. Close monitoring of the ABCs is critical because of the possibility of metabolic derangements secondary to renal failure. Although reversibility is less likely with renal and postrenal ARF, the same strategies are important. Avoidance of nephrotoxic drugs is important, as is alleviation of postrenal obstruction as soon as possible.

29. Integrate pathophysiological principles to the assessment of a patient with abdominal pain. pp. 1331–1334

Abdominal pain is questioned in similar ways whether or not the system of origin (GI, urinary tract, reproductive) is suspected from the initial size-up or complaint. The distinction of visceral and somatic pain may be useful in discerning cause, as is any referred pain pattern. For instance, most urologic/nephrologic emergencies typically feature visceral pain. However, renal stones are notorious for severe, somatic pain when they lodge somewhere in the distal urinary tract. Although the presence of nausea and vomiting is generally not helpful (if not due to GI disturbance, it is frequently due to autonomic discharge), presence of diarrhea suggests GI origin. Similarly, pain associated with urination suggests urinary tract origin.

30. **Synthesize assessment findings and patient history information to accurately differentiate between pain of a urologic or nephrologic emergency and that of another origin.** pp. 1331–1334

As noted in Chapter 32, many GI emergencies feature hemorrhage, and discernment through vital signs and physical exam of likely hemorrhage is an important first step in looking for system of origin. Examination of vomitus or diarrhea is also helpful. Gross examination of urine may not be helpful; however, gross blood is consistent with kidney stone in an otherwise appropriate presentation, and cloudiness of urine may represent the large numbers of white cells that may be present in pyelonephritis. Remember the typical pain patterns: GI emergencies often start with visceral pain (frequently located higher than in urinary tract conditions) and progress to somatic pain if an inflamed or damaged structure ruptures; postrupture peritonitis is not unusual. In contrast, most urologic/nephrologic emergencies feature visceral pain felt in the pelvis or male scrotum. Somatic-like pain felt in the flank, shoulder, or neck may suggest a kidney stone. Tenderness in the lower back at the costovertebral angle may suggest pyelonephritis, particularly if systemic signs of infection are present. If the urinary system appears likely, be sure to address the issue of renal function. Prevention strategies to prevent further loss of nephrons are vital to implement expediently.

31. **Develop, execute, and evaluate a treatment plan based on the field impression made in the assessment.** pp. 1324–1347

Because acute renal failure can cause life-threatening metabolic complications (consider the key role of the kidneys in regulation of fluid volume, electrolytes, and pH), close monitoring and support of the ABCs are essential. High-flow oxygen should be used, and positioning and IV fluid resuscitation are important. In general, you want to protect fluid volume and cardiovascular function to minimize damage due to renal hypoperfusion and eliminate or reduce exposure to any potentially nephrotoxic drug. The same applies to an acute problem in a patient with chronic renal failure. It is always important to prevent nephron loss, even in patients who already have compromise. In patients with renal calculi, it is important to promote urine formation and flow in an effort to move the stone through the distal urinary tract. In urinary tract infections (either lower or upper), IV hydration may promote formation of dilute urine that will flush some microbes from the urinary tract and relieve some of the pain, frequency, and urgency that might be present. Monitoring of the ABCs and support of any acute complications is always mandated.

Content Self-Evaluation

MULTIPLE CHOICE

_____ 1. The major functions of the urinary system include all EXCEPT:
   A. maintenance of blood volume.
   B. control of development of white blood cells.
   C. regulation of arterial blood pressure.
   D. maintenance of the balance of electrolytes and blood pH.
   E. removal of many toxic wastes from the blood.

_____ 2. From which of these diseases do more than 250,000 Americans suffer?
   A. colitis
   B. diabetes
   C. end-stage renal failure
   D. pancreatitis
   E. prostatic hypertrophy

_____ 3. Pain arising in hollow organs such as the ureter and bladder is known as:
   A. parietal pain.
   B. referred pain.
   C. somatic pain.
   D. visceral pain.
   E. parenteral pain.

_____ 4. Pain that occurs when afferent nerve fibers carrying the pain message merge with other pain-carrying fibers at the spinal cord junction is called:
   A. parietal pain.
   B. referred pain.
   C. somatic pain.
   D. visceral pain.
   E. parenteral pain.

_____ 5. Typical questions to ask when obtaining a focused history related to abdominal pain include all of the following EXCEPT:
   A. previous history of similar event.
   B. sudden or gradual unintended weight loss.
   C. presence of chest pain.
   D. last oral intake.
   E. last date of sexual activity, if sexually active.

_____ 6. Indications that a woman's abdominal pain might be of obstetric (pregnancy-related) origin include all of the following EXCEPT:
   A. known pregnancy or last menstrual period not in immediate past.
   B. frequency and urgency of urination.
   C. indications of intraabdominal hemorrhage.
   D. presence of blood in the vagina and on the vulva.
   E. palpation of the uterus above the pelvic rim.

_____ 7. Lloyd's sign, which is an indication of pyelonephritis, is associated with:
   A. pain on percussion of the costovertebral angle.
   B. pain on palpation of the anterior costal margin.
   C. periumbilical tenderness.
   D. rebound pain at the level of the umbilicus.
   E. pain on inhalation.

_____ 8. Patients most at risk for kidney disorders are the elderly, persons with diabetes mellitus, hypertension, or both, and patients with more than one risk factor.
   A. True
   B. False

_____ 9. Oliguria is defined as low urine output (roughly 400–500 mL daily or less), whereas anuria is complete absence of urine output.
   A. True
   B. False

_____ 10. In its earliest phase, postrenal ARF is reversible.
   A. True
   B. False

_____ 11. The two factors responsible for more than half of all cases of end-stage renal failure are:
   A. damage due to nephrotoxic drugs and other substances and hypertension.
   B. pyelonephritis and diabetes mellitus.
   C. diabetes mellitus and hypertension.
   D. infections and glomerulonephritis.
   E. atherosclerosis and hypertension.

_____ 12. Common elements of uremic syndrome include all of the following EXCEPT:
   A. peptic ulcer.
   B. hyperkalemia and metabolic acidosis.
   C. easy bleeding and bruising.
   D. hypoglycemia.
   E. chronic anemia.

_____ 13. Always be alert for development of physiologic instability in patients with chronic renal failure, regardless of initial presentation.
   A. True
   B. False

_____ 14. All of the following may be complications related to hemodialysis or peritoneal dialysis EXCEPT:
   A. chest pain.
   B. dyspnea.
   C. hypertension.
   D. seizure.
   E. infection.

_____ 15. All of the following statements about kidney stones are true EXCEPT:
   A. Renal calculi and nephrolithiasis are synonymous terms for kidney stones.
   B. Brief hospitalization for kidney stones is common because of the severity of pain while a stone is being passed.
   C. Immobilization and use of opiates and psychotropic drugs are risk factors for stones.
   D. Calcium and uric acid stones tend to run in families, suggesting a genetic link.
   E. Calcium stones are associated with chronic urinary tract infection or frequent bladder catheterization.

_____ 16. Which of the following types of renal calculi is found more often in women than in men?
   A. calcium stones
   B. cystine stones
   C. struvite stones
   D. uric acid stones
   E. oxalate stones

_____ 17. Male patients with kidney stones rarely have referred pain in the testicle on the affected side.
   A. True
   B. False

_____ 18. Risk factors for urinary tract infection include all of the following EXCEPT:
   A. female gender.
   B. pregnancy.
   C. advanced age.
   D. persons requiring routine bladder catheterization.
   E. persons with conditions causing urinary stasis.

_____ 19. The pathophysiology of urinary tract infections is due primarily to:
   A. bacterial infections.
   B. decreases in sexual intercourse.
   C. sexually transmitted disease infections.
   D. urinary tract lesions.
   E. viral infections.

_____ 20. Prostatis is the inflammation of the prostate gland.
   A. True
   B. False

Chapter 34

Toxicology and Substance Abuse

Review of Chapter Objectives

After reading this chapter, you should be able to:

1. **Describe the incidence, morbidity, and mortality of toxic and drug abuse emergencies.**　　p. 1351

   Toxicological emergencies are defined as those relating to exposure to a toxin, which is a chemical substance that causes adverse effects within the exposed individual. The term *toxin* includes drugs and poisons. Over the years, both the number and severity of toxicological emergencies has increased, so this is an area with which you must become familiar and must take steps to remain current in your knowledge. The estimated number of poisonings is over 4 million per year (and the term *poisonings* excludes drug overdoses). Roughly 10 percent of all EMS calls involve toxic exposures. About 70 percent of all accidental poisonings involve children under the age of 6 years; however, these poisonings tend to be relatively mild, accounting for only 5 percent of fatalities. Adult poisonings and drug overdoses are less frequent but they account for over 90 percent of hospital admissions for toxic exposures and 95 percent of the fatalities in this category.

2. **Identify the risk factors most predisposing to toxic emergencies.**　　p. 1351

   Age is an important risk factor: About 70 percent of all accidental poisonings involve children under the age of 6 years. A child who has had an accidental ingestion has a 25 percent chance of another, similar ingestion within one year. Intentional exposure as a form of drug experimentation or suicide is common in older children and young adults. Although adult poisonings and overdoses are less frequent, they account for 90 percent of hospital admissions for exposure to a toxic substance and 95 percent of fatalities. Among adults, most poisonings and drug overdoses are intentional. For instance, 80 percent of all attempted suicides involve a drug overdose. Interpersonal violence is a second risk factor: Poisoning in an older child can be the result of an intentional act by a parent or caregiver. Third, specific settings and situations make accidental poisoning more likely: Exposure in an industrial workplace or on a farm is increasingly common. Finally, use of medications is itself a risk factor. Most often, accidental exposures among older children and adults represent hypersensitivity reactions or dosage errors when taking prescribed medications.

3. **Discuss the anatomy and physiology of the organs and structures related to toxic emergencies.**　　pp. 1352–1353

   Agents that are ingested through the mouth are exposed to the teeth, tongue, and mucous membranes of the mouth, as well as the throat and esophagus, before entering the stomach. As with intentionally ingested foods, agents remain in the stomach for a period of time before they pass into the small intestine (length of time depends on the amount of stomach contents, whether contents are liquid or solid, and so on). Most absorption into the bloodstream takes place during passage of the agent through the small intestine.

Agents that are inhaled pass through the nose (possibly also the mouth), pharynx, trachea, and other increasingly small airways before reaching the alveoli of the lungs. Absorption is largely at the distal end of the respiratory tree, the alveolar-capillary interface, which is the normal site for gas exchange (typically oxygen and carbon dioxide). Because the epithelial lining of the airways is relatively delicate, local effects can occur through tissue irritation in these medial structures.

With surface absorption, the agent must pass through the skin or mucous membranes to which it has been applied in order to enter the body and cause local or systemic effects (the latter if agent is absorbed into bloodstream).

In cases of injection, the needle passes through the skin and subcutaneous tissues to reach a vein. The amount and depth of skin and subcutaneous tissue varies widely on different body sites. Typically, skin is thin and there is little subcutaneous tissue at sites with easy venous access such as the forearms and hands, as well as the comparable sites on the lower extremities. Be aware that drug addicts who have sclerosed readily available veins may have the ability to inject substances successfully into very small and usually inaccessible vessels.

4. Describe the routes of entry of toxic substances into the body. pp. 1352–1353

There are four routes of entry into the body: ingestion, inhalation, surface absorption, and injection. Ingestion via the mouth is the most common route of entry for toxic exposure. Inhalation of a poison into the lungs results in rapid absorption from the alveolar air into the blood. Causative agents are in the form of gases, vapors, fumes, or aerosols. Surface absorption applies to cases in which entry is through the skin or mucous membranes. Injection applies when the toxic agent is injected under the skin, into muscle, or directly into the bloodstream.

5. Discuss the role of poison control centers in the United States. p. 1351

Poison control centers assist in the treatment of poison victims and provide information on new products and new treatment recommendations. They are usually based in major medical centers serving large populations, and many have computer systems that allow staff to rapidly and accurately access information. Centers are available to you 24 hours a day, 7 days a week: Take the time to memorize the telephone number of the center serving your area. Your center can help you determine the potential toxicity for your patient when you give them the following information: type of agent, amount and time of exposure, and physical condition of the patient. With this information, you may be able to start the current, definitive treatment in the field. The center can notify the receiving facility before you get the patient there.

6. Discuss the pathophysiology, assessment findings, need for rapid intervention and transport, and management of toxic emergencies. pp. 1350–1386

- **Pathophysiology:** With each route of entry, there is a general pattern of possible toxic effects depending on the type and amount of agent involved: Immediate effects involve the tissues exposed to the toxic agent during entry. Delayed, systemic effects are related to absorption into the bloodstream and circulation throughout the body. In ingestion, corrosive agents can cause immediate injury through burns of the lips, oral mucous membranes, tongue, throat, and esophagus. Delayed effects can arise from absorption via the small intestine into the blood with effects on distant organs and tissues. In inhalation, immediate injury can occur from irritation of the airways resulting in extensive edema and damaged tissue. Delayed, systemic effects occur when the agent travels through the bloodstream and interacts with distant organs and tissues. In surface absorption, immediate injury can occur in the involved skin or mucous membranes. Delayed effects again relate to absorption into the bloodstream. With injection, immediate injury is seen as irritation at the injection site, usually visible as red, irritated, edematous skin. Delayed, systemic effects are again due to distribution throughout the body via the bloodstream.

- **Assessment:** Certain basic principles of assessment apply to most toxicological emergencies. For instance, maintain a high index of suspicion that a poisoning or drug overdose may have occurred. During scene size-up, look for potential dangers to yourself and other rescuers, such as a threat of violence from suicidal patients and the threat of accidental injection from used needles that may be hidden on the patient's person or at the scene. In cases with chemicals and hazardous materials, it is crucial that you use the proper clothing and equipment. Be sure that such articles are distributed to team members who have been trained in their use.

  Assessment of the patient begins with a history if the patient appears to be able to give one. Critical questions include what kind of toxin the patient was exposed to and when exposure occurred (so you have clues for likelihood of immediate or delayed effects or both). Physical involves a rapid head-to-toe exam with full vital signs.

- **Time needs:** In accordance with your local protocols, relay information to Poison Control. Generally speaking, you never want to delay initiation of supportive or definitive care or transport because of delays in sending information to, or receiving information from, Poison Control. Time is of the essence, literally. Ongoing assessment is particularly important for this group of patients because they can deteriorate rapidly. Repeat initial assessment and vitals every 5 minutes for critical or unstable patients and every 15 minutes for stable patients. Specific assessment findings are given for each type of agent.

- **General management:** The preliminary steps of management include securing rescuer safety and removing the patient from any toxic environment. Support ABCs as you would with any other patient, keeping in mind that damage may have occurred to the mouth, pharynx, and/or airway in inhalation injury, and to the mouth and pharynx in ingestion incidents. The direct access to the cardiovascular system that occurs with injection cases may also complicate support of the ABCs.

The first management step specific to toxicological emergencies is decontamination, that is, minimization of toxicity by reducing the amount of toxin absorbed into the body. Decontamination involves three steps: The first is reduction of intake of toxin (steps will be route-specific, such as removal from fume-filled atmosphere in inhalation, removal of clothes and cleansing of skin in surface absorption, removal of stinger in injection, and so on).

The second step is reduction of absorption after toxin is in the body, and this usually applies to ingestion incidents. The most common method entails use of activated charcoal to bind molecules of the toxin to it and prevent absorption into the bloodstream. Gastric lavage (stomach pumping) is of limited use as a step to reduce absorption. Lavage must be done within about one hour of exposure to be effective, and its possible complications (aspiration and perforation) are significant. Lavage is uncommon except in specific circumstances, for example, when the toxin doesn't bind to activated charcoal or when the toxin has no antidote. The third step in decontamination is enhanced elimination of toxin from the body. Cathartics enhance gastric mobility and thus may shorten the time the toxin is in the GI tract. Know the limitations in use of cathartics in your area, especially among pediatric patients, in whom they can induce severe electrolyte disturbances. Whole bowel irrigation with use of a gastric tube seems to be effective and carries few potential complications; however, its use is limited to only a few centers.

The third management step specific to toxicological emergencies is use of an antidote, a substance that neutralizes the specific toxin and counteracts its effects in the body. As you can see in Table 34-1 on text page 1355, there are not many antidotes, and few are 100 percent effective. Your best guide is to be thoroughly knowledgeable with your local protocols, the directions given by the Poison Control Center, and by counsel given by medical direction.

7. **List the most common poisonings, pathophysiology, assessment findings, and management of poisoning by ingestion, inhalation, absorption, injection, and overdose.** pp. 1352–1386

Ingestion is the most common route of poisoning that you will see. Frequently ingested poisons include household products, petroleum-based agents such as gasoline and paint, cleaning agents such as alkalis and soaps, cosmetics, drugs (prescription, nonprescription, and illicit), plants, and foods. Some poisons can remain in the stomach for several hours, which may permit removal of the poison from the stomach and the body before systemic absorption can occur via passage through the small intestine. In at least one case, ingestion of aspirin, removal from the stomach is difficult because the ingested tablets bind together to form one large bolus. Useful questions for historical assessment include: (1) What did you ingest? (Obtain samples or containers whenever possible.) (2) When did you ingest the substance? (3) How much did you ingest? (4) Did you drink any alcohol? (5) Have you attempted to treat yourself? (including induction of vomiting) (6) Have you been under mental health care, and, if so, why? (The answer may indicate potential for suicide.) (7) What is your weight? A physical assessment exam is especially important because a history may be unavailable or unreliable. Your exam should provide physical evidence of intoxication and discover comorbid conditions that may affect treatment or response. Pay particular attention to skin, eyes, mouth, chest, circulation status, and abdomen (review text page 1356). Be aware that a patient may have ingested multiple substances. Management centers on prevention of aspiration, intubation where necessary (RSI may be required to avoid patient's clamping down on tube), use of high-flow oxygen, and IV access for volume replacement and possible IV drug administration. Remember that it is always important to have ongoing cardiac monitoring and reassessment of vital signs.

Toxic inhalations can be self-induced or due to accidental exposure. Commonly inhaled poisons include toxic gases, carbon monoxide, ammonia, chlorine, freon, toxic vapors, fumes, or aerosols (from products such as paint and other hydrocarbons, glue, and so on), carbon tetrachloride, methyl chloride, tear gas, mustard gas, amyl nitrite, butyl nitrite, and nitrous oxide. Inhaled toxins primarily cause direct injury in the respiratory system, and these problems may be most severe in patients who inhaled a chemical or propellant concentrated in either a paper or plastic bag.

Given the pathophysiology of inhaled toxins, you should look for signs/symptoms related to three major systems: the central nervous system (dizziness, headache, confusion, hallucinations, seizures, or coma), the respiratory system (tachypnea, cough, hoarseness, stridor, dyspnea, retractions, wheezing, chest pain or tightness, crackles or rhonchi), and the heart (dysrhythmias). Management starts with protecting yourself from any toxins in the atmosphere and removal of the patient from the injurious environment. Follow these guidelines: Wear protective clothing, use appropriate respiratory protection, and remove the patient's contaminated clothing. Then you can perform the initial assessment, history, and physical examination focusing on the central nervous system, as well as the respiratory and cardiac systems. Support ABCs as you would with any other patient, keeping in mind that damage may have occurred to the mouth, pharynx, and/or airway as a direct, immediate injury. Contact medical direction and your Poison Control Center according to your particular protocols.

For surface absorption, the most common contacts are with poisonous plants such as poison ivy, poison sumac, and poison oak. Many toxic chemicals can be absorbed through the skin. Organophosphates, which are used as pesticides, are easily absorbed through the skin and mucous membranes, as is cyanide. The signs and symptoms vary widely depending on the toxin involved. Whenever you suspect surface absorption, take the following general steps: (1) wear protective clothing; (2) use appropriate respiratory protection; (3) remove the patient's contaminated clothing; (4) perform initial assessment, history, and physical exam; (5) initiate supportive measures; and (6) contact Poison Control Center and medical direction.

Female insects in the class Hymenoptera (honeybees, hornets, yellow jackets, wasps, and fire ants) are common causes of injection injury. In addition, spiders, ticks, snakes, and certain marine animals are known causes of toxic exposure by injection. In addition to intentional injections, most poisonings by injection involve bites and stings from insects and animals. Be alert for the possibility of allergic reactions or anaphylaxis. Over time, beware of delayed systemic reactions. General principles of field management include the following: (1) protection of all rescue personnel because the culprit organism may still be in the area; (2) removal of the patient from danger of repeated injection (particularly in the case of yellow jackets, wasps, or hornets); (3) whenever possible and safe, obtain the injury-causing organism and bring it to the emergency department; (4) perform initial assessment and rapid physical exam; (5) prevent or delay further absorption of the poison; (6) initiate supportive measures as needed; (7) watch for anaphylaxis; (8) transport as rapidly as possible; and (9) contact Poison Control Center and medical direction per protocols.

8. **Define the following terms:**

   a. **Substance or drug abuse** p. 1380

   Substance or drug abuse is use of a pharmacological product for purposes other than medically defined reasons.

b. Substance or drug dependence   **p. 1380**

Substance or drug dependence is the same thing as addiction: Physiological dependence exists if discontinuance of the drug would cause adverse physical reactions. Psychological dependence exists if discontinuance of the drug would cause the presence or increase in tension or emotional stress.

c. Tolerance   **p. 1380**

Tolerance is a phenomenon associated with continued use of a drug; it implies that the user must take increasingly large doses of the drug in order to achieve the same effect.

d. Withdrawal   **p. 1380**

Withdrawal refers to alcohol or drug discontinuance in which the patient's body reacts severely when deprived of the abused substance.

e. Addiction   **p. 1380**

Addiction is the same thing as dependence: Addiction can have a physiological or psychological component or both.

9. List the most commonly abused drugs (both by chemical name and by street names).   **pp. 1381, 1382–1383**

The most commonly abused drugs include: (1) alcohol in its fermented and distilled forms; (2) barbiturates such as phenobarbital and thiopental; (3) cocaine (both crack and rock forms); (4) narcotics/opiates such as heroin, codeine, meperidine, morphine, hydromorphone, pentazocine, methadone, Darvon, and Darvocet; (5) marijuana and hashish (also called grass or weed on the street); (6) amphetamines such as Benzedrine, Dexedrine, and Ritalin (called speed on the street); (7) hallucinogens including LSD, STP, mescaline, psilocybin, and PCP (also called angel dust); (8) sedatives from different chemical families such as Seconal, Valium, Librium, Xanax, Halcion, Restoril, Dalmane, and phenobarbital; and (9) the benzodiazepines, Valium, Librium, Xanax, Halcion, Restoril, Dalmane, Centrax, Ativan, and Serax.

10. Describe the pathophysiology, assessment findings, and management of commonly used drugs.   **pp. 1380–1386**

In addition to the specific drugs discussed in objective 11, it is notable that many groups of drugs produce definable toxic syndromes. Knowledge of these syndromes is useful because it helps you cluster information for compounds that produce similar clinical pictures. (1) Anticholinergic toxidrome is caused by belladonna alkaloids, atropine, scopolamine, synthetic anticholinergics, and incidental anticholinergics such as antihistamines, tricyclic antidepressants, and phenothiazines. Signs and symptoms include dry skin/mucous membranes, blurred near vision, fixed dilated pupils, tachycardia, hyperthermia and flushing, lethargy, and CNS signs, respiratory failure, and cardiovascular collapse. Management is as described for the tricyclics in objective 11. (2) Narcotic toxidrome is due to illicit drugs such as heroin and opium, prescription narcotics such as meperidine and methadone, and combination medications including narcotic agents such as hydromorphone, diphenoxylate (Lomotil), and oxycodone. Assessment findings include CNS depression, pinpoint pupils, slowed respirations, hypotension, and positive response to naloxone. Note that pupils may be dilated and excitement may predominate the clinical picture. Management is described in objective 11. (3) The sympathomimetic toxidrome is caused by aminophylline, amphetamines, caffeine, cocaine, ephedrine, dopamine, methylphenidate (Ritalin), and phencyclidine. Features include CNS excitation, hypertension, seizures, and tachycardia (hypotension with caffeine). Management is discussed in objective 11.

11. List the clinical uses, street names, pharmacology, assessment findings, and management for patients who have taken the following drugs or been exposed to the following substances:

a. Cocaine   **pp. 1361, 1381, 1382**

Cocaine has sympathomimetic effects, and assessment findings include CNS excitation, dilated pupils, hyperactivity, hypertension, seizures, tachycardia, and hypotension if taken with caffeine. Benzodiazepines may be required for seizures or diazepam 5–10 mg can be given as a seizure precaution; beta-blockers are contraindicated because their unopposed alpha receptor stimulation can cause cardiac ischemia, increased hypertension, and hyperthermia. General measures include ABCs, respiratory support and oxygenation, ECG monitoring, IV access, and treatment of any life-threatening dysrhythmia.

  b. **Marijuana and cannabis compounds**   **p. 1383**

Marijuana and related compounds can be smoked (inhaled) or taken orally, and pertinent signs and symptoms include euphoria, dry mouth, dilated pupils, and altered sensation. Management centers on ABCs, reassurance and speaking in a quiet voice, and ECG monitoring if indicated.

  c. **Amphetamines and amphetamine-like drugs**   **pp. 1381, 1383**

Amphetamines are CNS stimulants that can be taken orally or injected. Assessment findings include exhilaration, hyperactivity, dilated pupils, hypertension, psychosis, tremors, and seizures. Management centers on ABCs, oxygenation and ECG monitoring, IV access, treatment of any life-threatening dysrhythmia, and diazepam 5–10 mg as a seizure precaution. Diazepam and haloperidol in combination may be useful in controlling hyperactivity.

  d. **Barbiturates**   **pp. 1381, 1382**

The barbiturates, which are CNS depressants, can be taken orally or injected. Signs and symptoms include lethargy, emotional lability, incoordination, slurred speech, nystagmus, coma, hypotension, and respiratory depression. Management focuses on ABCs and respiratory support with oxygenation, IV access, ECG monitoring, and contact with Poison Control. Alkalinization of urine and diuresis may improve elimination of barbiturates from the body.

  e. **Sedative-hypnotics**   **p. 1383**

Sedative-hypnotics are generally taken orally, and they are also CNS depressants. Assessment findings include altered mental status, hypotension, slurred speech, respiratory depression, shock, bradycardia, and seizures. Management centers on ABCs with respiratory support and oxygenation, IV access, ECG monitoring, and possible use of naloxone dependent on agent taken and advice of medical direction.

  f. **Cyanide**   **pp. 1359, 1362**

Cyanide can enter the body by different routes dependent on the product in which it is found. It is present in household items such as rodenticides and silver polish, as well as in foods such as fruit pits and seeds. It can be liberated into inhalable form through burning of nitrogen-containing products such as plastics, silks, or synthetic carpets. Cyanide also forms in patients on long-term therapy with nitroprusside. Regardless of entry, cyanide acts extremely quickly as a cellular asphyxiant, inhibiting the vital process of cellular respiration. Signs and symptoms include a burning sensation in mouth and throat, headache, confusion, combative behavior, hypertension, and tachycardia, followed by hypotension and further dysrhythmias, seizures and coma, and pulmonary edema. Management relies on removal from the source, immediate supportive measures, and treatment with a cyanide antidote kit containing amyl nitrite ampules, a sodium nitrite, and a sodium thiosulfate solution. Adding nitrites to blood converts some hemoglobin to methemoglobin, which binds cyanide, removing it from its free form in the blood. Thiosulfate binds with cyanide to form a soluble nontoxic compound. Note: Cyanide is rapidly toxic, so it is crucial you be familiar with a cyanide antidote kit if your unit carries one.

  g. **Narcotics/opiates**   **pp. 1361, 1381, 1382**

The narcotics can be taken orally or by injection. Pertinent assessment findings include CNS depression, constricted pupils, respiratory depression, hypotension, bradycardia, pulmonary edema, and coma. General management centers on ABCs with respiratory support and oxygenation, IV access, and ECG monitoring. You may use the antidote naloxone, which can be titrated to relieve symptoms of toxicity without provoking withdrawal symptoms in addicts. General instructions involve use of 1–2 mg naloxone IV or endotracheally per medical direction until respiration improves. Larger doses (2–5 mg) may be required in the management of Darvon overdose and alcoholic coma.

  h. **Cardiac medications**   **p. 1363**

The number of available cardiac medications grows continually, and many classes exist, including antidysrhythmics, beta-blockers, calcium channel blockers, glycosides, ACE inhibitors, and so forth. General pharmacology includes regulation of heart function by reducing heart rate, suppressing automaticity, reducing vascular tone, or some combination of these. Although overdose can be intentional, it often is due to an error in dosage. At the level of overdose, signs and symptoms include (1) nausea and vomiting; (2) headache, dizziness, and confusion; (3) profound hypotension; (4) cardiac dysrhythmias (usually bradycardic); (5) cardiac conduction blocks; and (6) bronchospasm and pulmonary edema (especially with beta-blockers). Management centers on initiating standard toxicological emergency assessment and treatment immediately. Severe bradycardia may not respond well to atropine, so you should have an external pacing device at hand. Some cardiac medications have antidotes; these include calcium for calcium channel blockers, glucagon for beta-blockers, and digoxin-specific Fab (Digibind) for digoxin. Contact medical direction before giving any of these antidotes.

i. **Caustics** pp. 1363–1364

Caustic substances can either be acids or alkalis, and such substances are common at home and in the industrial workplace. Strong caustics can cause severe burns at the site of contact; if ingested, they can cause tissue destruction at the lips, mouth, esophagus, and more distal regions of the GI tract. Strong acids by definition have a pH less than 2; they are found in plumbing solutions and bathroom cleaners. Contact usually produces immediate, severe pain due to tissue coagulation and necrosis. Often this type of burn produces an eschar over the site, which may act as a shield to protect deeper tissues from damage. Because the substance is in the stomach much longer than the esophagus, the stomach is the more likely to sustain damage. Immediate or delayed hemorrhage is possible, as is perforation. Absorption of acids into the bloodstream produces acidemia, which needs to be managed along with the local, direct effects. Strong alkaline agents by definition have a pH greater than 12.5; they are present in solid or liquid form in household products such as drain cleaners. These agents cause local injury through liquefaction necrosis. Because of a delay in pain sensation, these agents are often present longer at the site of contact, allowing for greater tissue damage and deeper tissue injury. Solid products can stick to the oropharynx or esophagus, causing bleeding, perforation, and inflammation of central chest structures. Liquid alkalis are more likely to injure the stomach because, like the liquid strong acids, they pass quickly through the esophagus. Within 1 to 2 days of exposure to a strong alkali, complete loss of mucosal tissue can occur, followed either by gradual healing or further bleeding, necrosis, and stricture formation. Assessment findings include facial burns; pain in the lips, tongue, throat, and/or gums; drooling and trouble swallowing; hoarseness, stridor, or shortness of breath; and shock from bleeding and vomiting. Both assessment and initiation of management must be rapid and aggressive to avoid significant morbidity and mortality. As with other toxicological situations, protect yourself and initiate standard toxicological assessment and treatment: Pay particular attention to the airway. Injury to the oropharynx and/or larynx may make airway control and ventilation very difficult and may go so far as to require cricothyrotomy. Because caustic substances do not adhere to activated charcoal, there is no indication for it. It is controversial whether ingestion of milk or water acts effectively to coat the stomach lining or dilute the caustic. It is clear that rapid transport is essential. Hydrofluoric acid, which is used to clean glass in laboratory settings and in etching glass in artwork, is a specific example of a strong acid that can be lethal in even small exposure doses. Management specific to this agent is immersion of the exposed limb in iced water with magnesium sulfate, calcium salts, or benzethonium chloride.

j. **Common household substances** pp. 1363–1364

Many of these substances contain caustic agents (either strong acids or strong alkalis) as major ingredients; see objective i for details.

k. **Drugs abused for sexual purposes/sexual gratification** p. 1381

This group includes a number of miscellaneous agents that are used to stimulate and enhance sexual experience but do not have medically approved indications for such use. MDMA, popularly known as Ecstasy, is an example. Ecstasy is a modified form of methamphetamine and has similar, although milder, effects. Look for its use on college campuses and in nightclub settings. Initial signs and symptoms of use include anxiety, tachycardia, nausea, and hypertension, followed by relaxation, euphoria, and feelings of enhanced emotional insight. Studies indicate prolonged use may cause brain damage. Cases that can lead to death have the following assessment findings: confusion, agitation, tremor, high temperature, and diarrhea. No specific treatment exists, so supportive measures should be taken. Flunitrazepam, or Rohypnol, is illegal in the United States but has been used as a "date rape drug" when slipped into a woman's drink. The drug is a strong benzodiazepine that causes sedation and amnesia. When this drug is suspected, treat as for other benzodiazepines but remember to look for consequences of sexual assault and be sure to treat them as well.

l. Carbon monoxide   **pp. 1359, 1361, 1362–1363**

Carbon monoxide is a tasteless, odorless gas that is often created by incomplete combustion. Because of its chemical structure, it has an affinity for hemoglobin over 200 times greater than that of oxygen. Once carbon monoxide has bound to hemoglobin, it is very difficult to displace and it causes an effective hypoxia. Because of the variability of signs and symptoms (depending on dose and duration of exposure), many people ignore poisoning until toxic levels are in the blood. Early symptoms resemble those of the flu. Combining likely causes of carbon monoxide generation with early symptoms raises this red flag: Beware carbon monoxide poisoning in multiple patients living together in a poorly heated and ventilated space who have "flu-like" symptoms. Specific signs and symptoms include headache, nausea and vomiting, confusion or other manifestation of altered mental status, and tachypnea. Because of the difficulty of displacing carbon monoxide from hemoglobin, definitive treatment may require use of a hyperbaric chamber (in which oxygen is present at greater than atmospheric pressure). In the field, take these steps: Ensure safety of rescuing personnel, remove the patient(s) from contaminated area, begin immediate ventilation of affected area, and initiate supportive measures including high-flow oxygen via nonrebreather device (this last care step is critical).

m. Alcohols   **pp. 1361, 1381, 1382, 1383–1386**

Ethyl alcohol is the form of alcohol in beverages, and it is the single most common substance of abuse among Americans. Alcoholism, dependence on alcohol, progresses in much the same way as drug dependence discussed earlier in the chapter. The early symptoms of alcohol use, especially at low doses, include loss of inhibitions and emotionally excitatory effects, which can cause some of the aberrant behaviors associated with alcohol intoxication. Once ingested, alcohol is completely absorbed from the stomach and intestinal tract within approximately 30 to 120 minutes. After absorption, it is widely distributed in blood to all body tissues, and concentrations of alcohol in the brain rapidly approach the level in the blood. Alcohol's major physiologic effects are as a CNS depressant: Toxicity can include stupor, coma, and death. Because the liver is the major site of detoxification within the body, compromise of liver function increases the course and severity of alcohol intoxication. Another significant health effect is peripheral vasodilation, which results in flushing of the skin and a feeling of warmth. In cold conditions, this can increase loss of body heat and help to produce hypothermia. Alcohol-related diuresis is due to inhibition of vasopressin, a hormone responsible for homeostasis of water balance. The dry mouth associated with hangovers may in part be due to the alcohol-induced dehydration. Methanol, wood alcohol, is so toxic it is not safe for human consumption. However, methanol toxicity can occur either as an accident or because an alcoholic individual could not obtain ethyl alcohol. Methanol causes visual disturbances, abdominal pain, and nausea and vomiting even at low doses. Occasionally, methanol toxic patients complain of headache or dizziness or present with seizures and obtundation. Ethylene glycol, a related compound, can also be involved in toxic emergencies. It produces similar symptoms, but its CNS effects, including hallucinations, coma, and seizures, present at even earlier stages.

Assessment findings in an individual with chronic alcoholism include poor nutrition, alcoholic hepatitis, liver cirrhosis with subsequent esophageal varices, loss of sensation in hands and feet, loss of cerebellar function shown as poor balance and coordination, pancreatitis, upper GI hemorrhage (which is often fatal), hypoglycemia, subdural hematoma secondary to falls, and rib and extremity fractures, also secondary to falls. When you are in the field, keep in mind that conditions such as a subdural hematoma, sepsis, and diabetic ketoacidosis can, along with other conditions, mimic alcohol intoxication. For instance, the breath odor of ketoacidosis can resemble that of alcohol.

Abrupt discontinuance of alcohol by a dependent individual may provoke a withdrawal syndrome that can prove to be potentially lethal. Withdrawal symptoms can occur several hours after sudden abstinence and last up to 5 to 7 days. Common signs and symptoms include a coarse tremor of hands, tongue, and eyelids; nausea and vomiting; general weakness; increased sympathetic tone; tachycardia; sweating; hypertension; orthostatic hypotension; anxiety, irritability or depressed mood; and poor sleep. Seizures may occur, as can delirium tremens

(DTs). DTs usually develop on the second or third day of withdrawal and are characterized by a decreased level of consciousness associated with hallucinations and misinterpretation of nearby events. Both seizures and delirium tremens are ominous signs.

Alcohol intoxication, whether acute or chronic, should not be underestimated as a toxic emergency. In cases of suspected alcohol abuse, manage as follows: (1) Establish and maintain the airway, (2) determine if other drugs or substances are involved, (3) start an IV with lactated Ringer's solution or normal saline, (4) use a Chemstrip and give 25 g $D_{50}W$ if the patient is hypoglycemic, (5) administer 100 mg thiamine IV or IM, (6) maintain a sympathetic and supportive attitude with the patient, and (7) transport to emergency department for further care. Note: Medical direction may suggest diazepam in severe cases of seizure or hallucination.

n. **Hydrocarbons** p. 1365

Numerous household substances contain hydrocarbons, organic compounds composed primarily of carbon and hydrogen. Hydrocarbons include kerosene, naphtha, turpentine, mineral oil, chloroform, toluene, and benzene, and they are found in lighter fluid, paint, glue, lubricants, solvents, and aerosol propellants. Exposure can be via ingestion, inhalation, or surface absorption. Signs and symptoms of hydrocarbon exposure vary according to agent, dose, and route of exposure, but common problems include burns due to local contact, respiratory signs (wheezing, dyspnea, hypoxia, or pneumonitis from aspiration or inhalation), CNS signs (headache, dizziness, slurred speech, ataxia, and obtundation), foot and wrist drop with numbness and tingling, and cardiac dysrhythmias. Research has shown that fewer than 1 percent of hydrocarbon poisonings require physician care. In cases where you know the agent in question and in which the patient is asymptomatic, medical direction may permit the patient to stay at home. On the other hand, hydrocarbon poisonings can be very serious. If the patient is symptomatic, does not know the causative agent, or has taken a specific agent (such as halogenated or aromatic hydrocarbon compounds) that requires GI decontamination, standard toxicological emergency procedures and prompt transport are indicated.

o. **Psychiatric medications** pp. 1365–1367

The tricyclic antidepressants were standard therapy for depression for years, despite concerns that their generally narrow therapeutic window made accidental toxic-level exposure, as well as intentional overdose, potentially common. Despite the introduction of newer, safer antidepressants, a number of tricyclics are still in use for depression, as well as chronic pain syndromes and migraine prophylaxis. Agents still in use include amitriptyline (Elavil), amoxapine, clomipramine, doxepin, imipramine, and nortriptyline. Signs and symptoms on assessment include dry mouth, blurred vision, urinary retention, and constipation. Late into overdose, you may find confusion and hallucinations, hyperthermia, respiratory depression, seizures, tachycardia and hypotension, and cardiac dysrhythmias (such as heart block, wide QRS complex, and torsade de pointes.) In addition to standard toxicological procedures, cardiac monitoring is critical because dysrhythmias are the most common cause of death. If you suspect a mixed overdose with a benzodiazepine, DO NOT use Flumazenil because it might precipitate a seizure. If significant cardiac toxicity is evident, sodium bicarbonate may be used as an additional therapy; contact medical direction as needed.

p. **Newer antidepressants and serotonin syndromes** pp. 1366–1367

In the recent past, a number of new antidepressants that are not related to the tricyclics have been introduced. Because of their high safety profile in both therapeutic and overdose amounts, these drugs have virtually replaced the tricyclics in clinical practice. This group includes trazodone (Desyrel), bupropion (Wellbutrin), and the large group of drugs known as selective serotonin reuptake inhibitors (SSRIs). Drugs in this group include Prozac, Luvox, Paxil, and Zoloft. Their pharmacology, as indicated by group name, centers on prevention of reuptake of serotonin from neural synapses in the brain, theoretically raising the amount of serotonin available to modulate brain function. The usual signs and symptoms in overdose cases are generally mild, including drowsiness, tremor, nausea and vomiting, and sinus tachycardia. Occasionally trazodone and bupropion cause CNS depression and seizures, but deaths are rare, and they have been reported in situations with mixed overdoses and multiple ingestions. You should know that the SSRIs have been associated with serotonin syndrome, a constellation of signs/symptoms correlated with increased serotonin level and triggered by increasing the dose of SSRI or adding a second drug such as a narcotic or another antidepressant. Serotonin syndrome is marked by the following: (1) agitation, anxiety, confusion, and insomnia; (2) headache, drowsiness, and coma; (3) nausea, salivation, diarrhea, and abdominal cramps; (4) cutaneous piloerection and flushed skin; (5) hyperthermia and tachycardia; and (6) rigidity, shivering, incoordination, and myoclonic jerks. Because of the lower morbidity and mortality in these drugs compared with overdoses with the older antidepressants, standard toxicological emergency procedures suffice. The patient should discontinue all serotonergic drugs and you should institute supportive measures. Benzodiazepines or beta-blockers are occasionally used to improve patient comfort, but they are rarely given in the field.

q. Lithium p. 1367

Lithium is the most effective drug used in the treatment of bipolar disorder (a psychiatric disorder also known as manic depression). Pharmacology is unclear. However, it is known that lithium has a narrow therapeutic index, making toxicity relatively common during normal use and in overdose situations. Assessment findings of toxicity include thirst and dry mouth, tremor, muscle twitching, increased reflexes, confusion, stupor, seizures, coma, nausea, vomiting, diarrhea, and bradycardia and dysrhythmias. Lithium overdose should be treated primarily with supportive measures. Use standard toxicological procedures but remember that activated charcoal does not bind lithium and should not be used. Alkalinization of the urine with sodium bicarbonate and diuresis with mannitol may increase elimination of lithium, but severe toxicity requires hemodialysis.

r. MAO inhibitors p. 1366

Monoamine oxidase inhibitors (MAO inhibitors) have been used historically as psychiatric agents, primarily as antidepressants. Recently they have found limited use as treatment for obsessive-compulsive disorder. These drugs have always had relatively limited usage for several reasons: They have a narrow therapeutic index, multiple drug interactions, potentially serious interactions with foods rich in tyramine (for instance, red wine and cheese), and high morbidity and mortality in overdose incidents. The pharmacology of MAO inhibitors directly affects CNS neurotransmitters: The drugs inhibit the breakdown of norepinephrine and dopamine while increasing the molecular components necessary to produce more. Remember that overdose with this group of drugs is very serious, even though symptoms may not appear for up to 6 hours. Assessment findings include headache, agitation, restlessness, tremor, nausea, palpitations, tachycardia, severe hypertension, hyperthermia, and eventually bradycardia, hypotension, coma, and death. Newer MAO inhibitors have been introduced into the marketplace; they appear to be less toxic and avoid the food interactions that involved the older generation of MAO inhibitors. They are reversible in effect; however, overdose outcome data are not yet available for these drugs. Management includes reversal if the drug is in the newer class of reversible MAO inhibitors, prompt institution of standard toxicological procedures, and, if needed, symptomatic support for seizures and hyperthermia with use of benzodiazepines. If a vasopressor is needed, use norepinephrine.

s. Nonprescription pain medications: (1) nonsteroidal antiinflammatory agents; (2) salicylates; (3) acetaminophen pp. 1368–1369

1. Nonsteroidal antiinflammatory agents (called NSAIDs) are a large, commonly used group of drugs such as naproxen sodium, indomethacin, ibuprofen, and ketorolac (Toradol). Overdose is common, and assessment findings include headache, ringing in the ears (tinnitus), nausea, vomiting, abdominal pain, swelling of the extremities, mild drowsiness, dyspnea, wheezing, pulmonary edema, and rash and itching. There is no specific antidote for NSAID toxicity, so use general overdose procedures including supportive care and transport to the emergency department for evaluation and any necessary symptomatic treatment.

2. Salicylates are some of the most common over-the-counter drugs taken and among the most common taken in overdose. They include aspirin, oil of wintergreen, and some prescription combination medications. About 300 mg/kg aspirin can cause toxicity. In these amounts, the salicylate inhibits normal energy production and acid buffering in the body, resulting in metabolic acidosis that further injures other organ systems. Assessment findings include tachypnea, hyperthermia, confusion, lethargy and coma, cardiac failure and dysrhythmias, abdominal pain and vomiting, and noncardiogenic (inflammatory) pulmonary edema and adult respiratory distress syndrome. The findings of chronic overdose

are somewhat less severe and tend not to include abdominal complaints. It is thus difficult to distinguish chronic overdose from early acute overdose or acute overdose that has progressed past the initial abdominal irritation stage. In all cases, management of salicylate poisoning should be treated with use of standard toxicological emergency procedures. Activated charcoal definitely reduces drug absorption and should be used. If possible, learn the time of ingestion because blood levels measured at the right interval can be indicative of the expected degree of injury. Most symptomatic patients require generous IV fluids and may need urine alkalinization with sodium bicarbonate. Severe cases may require dialysis.

3. Acetaminophen (paracetamol, Tylenol) has few side effects in normal dosage, and it is one of the most commonly used drugs in America for fever/pain. It is also a common ingredient in combination medications and is found in some prescription combination medications. In large doses, acetaminophen can be very dangerous: A dose of 150 mg/kg is considered toxic and may result in death secondary to liver damage. A highly reactive metabolite is responsible for most adverse effects, but this is avoided in most cases by detoxification. When large amounts enter the body in overdose, this detoxification system is overloaded and gradually depleted, leaving the metabolite in the circulation to cause liver necrosis. It is important for you to learn and remember that the signs and symptoms of toxicity appear in four stages: Stage 1—0.5 to 24 hours after ingestion, marked by nausea, vomiting, weakness, and fatigue; Stage 2—24 to 48 hours, marked by abdominal pain, decreased urine, and elevated liver enzymes; Stage 3—72 to 96 hours, marked by liver function disruption; and Stage 4—4 to 14 days, marked by gradual recovery or progressive liver failure. Field management relies on standard toxicological procedures. Again, it is important to find time of ingestion because this may allow blood levels to be drawn at a time appropriate to predict potential injury. An antidote (N-acetylcysteine, or NAC, Mucomyst) is available and highly effective. However, NAC is usually given based on clinical and lab studies and in the hospital setting.

t. **Theophylline** p. 1369

Theophylline is a member of the group of drugs called xanthines. It is generally used by patients with asthma or COPD because it has moderate bronchodilation and mild antiinflammatory effects. It has a narrow therapeutic index and high toxicity, so it has been used less frequently recently. Thus, it is not a factor as often as it once was in overdose injuries. Assessment findings include agitation, tremors, seizures, cardiac dysrhythmias, and nausea and vomiting. Theophylline can cause significant morbidity and mortality. In an overdose setting, you must start toxicological emergency procedures immediately. Theophylline is on a short list of drugs that have significant entero-hepatic circulation. Thus, activated charcoal in multiple doses over time will continuously remove more and more theophylline from the body. Dysrhythmias should be treated according to ACLS procedures.

u. **Metals** pp. 1361, 1369–1370

With the exception of iron, heavy metal overdose is rare. Metals that can cause toxicity include lead, arsenic, and mercury, all of which affect numerous enzyme systems in the body and thus cause a variety of symptoms. Some also have direct local effects when ingested and they accumulate in various organs.

- **Iron:** The body needs only small daily amounts of iron; excess amounts are easily obtained through nonprescription supplements and multivitamins. Children have the tendency to overdose on iron by taking too many candy-flavored chewable vitamins containing iron. Symptoms occur when more than 20 mg/kg of elemental iron are ingested. Excess iron causes GI injury and possible hemorrhagic shock, especially if it forms concretions (lumps formed when tablets fuse together). Patients with significant iron ingestions may have visible tablets or concretions in the stomach or small intestine on X-ray. Other signs and symptoms include vomiting (often hematemesis) and diarrhea, abdominal pain, shock, liver failure, metabolic acidosis with tachypnea, and eventual bowel scarring and possible obstruction. It is essential to start standard toxicological procedures promptly. Because iron inhibits GI motility, tablets remain in the stomach for a long time and may possibly be easier to remove via gastric lavage (especially if concretions are not present). Because activated charcoal does not bind metals, it should not be used for iron overdose or for any other metal overdose. Deferoxamine, a

chelating agent, may be used in iron overdose as an antidote because it binds iron such that less enters cells to cause damage.
- **Lead and mercury:** Both metals are found in varying amounts in the environment. Lead was often used in glazes and paints before its toxic potential was realized. Mercury is a contaminant from industrial processing and is also found in some thermometers and temperature-control switches in homes. Both acute and chronic overdose are possible with both metals. Signs and symptoms of heavy metal toxicity include headache, irritability, confusion, coma, memory disturbance, tremor, weakness, agitation, and abdominal pain. Chronic poisoning can result in permanent neurological injury, which makes it crucial that heavy metal levels be monitored in the environment of a patient with toxicity. You need to remember the signs and symptoms of heavy metal poisoning and promptly institute standard procedures. Although activated charcoal is not helpful, various chelating agents (such as DMSA, BAL, and CDE) are available and may be used in definitive management in the hospital.

v. **Plants and mushrooms** pp. 1371–1372

Plants, trees, and mushrooms are common contributors to accidental toxic ingestions. You should know that many decorative home plants can present a toxic danger to children. Most poison control centers distribute pamphlets that list relevant household plants. In nature, it is impossible to identify all toxic plants and mushrooms. A general approach for you to take is to obtain a sample of the offending plant if possible, trying to find a complete leaf, stem, or flower. Mushrooms are very difficult to identify from small pieces. Because many ornamental plants contain irritating material, be sure to examine the patient's mouth and throat for redness, blistering, or edema. Identify other findings during the focused physical exam. Mushroom poisonings generally involve a mistake in identification of edible mushrooms or accidental ingestion by children. Mushrooms in the class *Amanita* account for over 90 percent of deaths; they produce a poison that is extremely toxic to the liver and carry a mortality rate of about 50 percent. Signs and symptoms of poisonous plant ingestion include excessive salivation, lacrimation, diaphoresis, abdominal cramps, nausea, vomiting, and diarrhea, as well as decreasing levels of consciousness, eventually progressing to coma. Contact Poison Control if at all possible for guidance on management. If contact isn't possible, follow the procedures outlined under food poisoning (text pages 1370–1371).

12. **Discuss common causative agents or offending organisms, pharmacology, assessment findings, and management for a patient with food poisoning, a bite, or a sting.** pp. 1370–1371, 1373–1380

Food poisoning can be due to a variety of causes including bacteria, viruses, and bacterial-associated chemical toxins. All notoriously produce varying degrees of gastrointestinal distress. Bacterial food poisonings range in severity. Bacterial exotoxins (secreted by bacteria) and enterotoxins (exotoxins associated with GI diseases) cause nausea, vomiting, diarrhea, and abdominal pain. Food contaminated with the bacteria *Shigella*, *Salmonella*, or *E. coli* can produce more severe reactions, often leading to electrolyte imbalance and hypovolemia. The world's most toxic poison is produced by *Clostridium botulinum*, and exposure presents as severe respiratory distress or even arrest. Fortunately, botulism rarely occurs except in cases of improper food storage procedures such as canning. A variety of seafood poisonings result from toxins produced by dinoflagellate-contaminated shellfish such as clams, mussels, oysters, and scallops. This exposure syndrome is called paralytic shellfish poisoning and can lead to respiratory arrest in addition to the GI symptoms. Toxicological emergencies can also arise from toxins found within commonly eaten fish. Bony fish poisoning (Ciguatera poisoning) is most frequent in fish caught in the Pacific Ocean or along the tropical reefs of Florida and the West Indies. Ciguatera may have an incubation period of 2 to 6 hours before producing myalgia and paresthesia. Scombroid (histamine) poisoning results from bacterial contamination of mackerel, tuna, bonitos, and albacore. Both Ciguatera and scombroid poisoning cause the standard GI symptoms; scombroid poisoning also produces immediate facial flushing due to histamine-induced vasodilation.

Except for botulism, food poisoning is rarely life threatening and treatment is largely supportive. In cases of suspected food poisoning, contact Poison Control and medical direction, and take the following steps: (1) perform necessary assessment; (2) collect samples of suspected food source; and (3) support ABCs with airway maintenance, high-flow oxygen, intubation or assisted ventilation as needed, and establish IV access. In addition, consider administration of antihistamines (especially in seafood poisonings) and antiemetics.

Spider and snake bites can be common and significant toxicological emergencies in certain parts of the country. The brown recluse spider lives in southern and midwestern states. It is found in large numbers in Tennessee, Arkansas, Oklahoma, and Texas. It has also been reported in Hawaii and California. The brown recluse is about 15 mm in length; generally lives in dark, dry locations; and can often be found in or around a house. The bites themselves are usually painless, and bites often occur at night while the victim is asleep. The initial, local reaction occurs within minutes and consists of a small erythematous macule surrounded by a white ring. Over the next 8 hours or so localized pain, redness, and swelling develop. Tissue necrosis develops over days to weeks. Other symptoms include fever, chills, nausea, vomiting, joint pain, and in severe cases, bleeding disorders (namely, disseminated intravascular coagulation, DIC). Treatment is largely supportive, and there is no antivenin. Antihistamines may reduce systemic reactions and surgical excision may be required for necrotic tissue. Black widow spiders live in all parts of the continental United States and are often found in woodpiles or brush. The female spider bites, and the venom is very potent, causing excessive neurotransmitter release at the synaptic junctions. Immediate, local reaction includes pain, redness, and swelling. Progressive muscle spasms of all large muscles can develop and are usually associated with severe pain. Other systemic symptoms are nausea, vomiting, sweating, seizures, paralysis, and decreased level of consciousness. Field treatment is largely supportive, with reassurance an important factor. IV muscle relaxants may be needed for severe spasms. If medical direction orders it, you may use diazepam or calcium gluconate. Calcium chloride is ineffective and should not be used. Because hypertensive crisis is possible, monitor BP carefully. Transport as rapidly as possible so antivenin can be given in the hospital.

There are several thousand snake bites annually in the United States, but few deaths. The assessment findings depend on the snake, location of the bite, and the type and amount of venom injected. Two families of poisonous snakes are native to the United States: the pit vipers (cottonmouths, rattlesnakes, and copperheads) and the coral snake, a distant relative of the cobra. Pit viper venom contains hydrolytic enzymes capable of destroying most tissue components. They can produce hemolysis, destroy other tissue elements, and may affect the clotting ability of the blood. They produce tissue infarction and necrosis, especially at the site of the bite. A severe pit viper bite can produce death within 30 minutes. However, most fatalities occur from 6 to 30 hours after the bite, with 90 percent within the first 48 hours. Assessment findings for pit viper bites include fang marks (often little more than a scratch or abrasion); swelling and pain at wound site; continued oozing from wound; weakness, dizziness, or faintness; sweating and/or chills; thirst; nausea and vomiting; diarrhea; tachycardia and hypotension; bloody urine and GI hemorrhage (these are late); ecchymosis; necrosis; shallow respirations progressing to respiratory failure; and numbness and tingling around face and head. The first goal in treatment is to slow absorption of venom; remember that about 25 percent of bites are dry; that is, no venom is injected. Antivenin is available but should only be considered for severe cases as evidence by marked systemic signs and symptoms. Routine treatment involves keeping the patient supine, immobilizing the affected limb with a splint, maintaining the extremity in a neutral position without any constricting bands, and giving supportive care with high-flow oxygen, IV with crystalloid fluid, and rapid transport. Note: DO NOT apply ice, cold pack, or freon spray to wound; DO NOT apply an arterial tourniquet; and DO NOT apply electrical stimulation from any source in an attempt to retard or reverse venom spread. Coral snakes, which are small and with small fangs, are primarily found in the southwest. A mnemonic that you should remember is "Red touch yellow, kill a fellow; red touch black, venom lack." This indicates the stripe pattern of the coral snake: red-yellow-black-yellow-red. Coral snake venom contains some of the same enzymes as pit viper venom, but it additionally has a neurotoxin that will result in respiratory and skeletal muscle paralysis. Assessment findings include the following (noting that there may be no local or systemic effects for as long as 12 to 24 hours): localized numbness, weakness, and drowsiness; ataxia; slurred speech and excessive salivation; paralysis of tongue and larynx producing difficulty in swallowing and breathing; drooping of eyelids; double vision; dilated pupils; abdominal pain, nausea, and vomiting; loss of consciousness;

seizures; respiratory failure; and hypotension. Treatment includes the following steps: (1) Wash the wound with lots of water, (2) apply a compression bandage and keep extremity at the level of the heart, (3) immobilize the limb with a splint, (4) start an IV with crystalloid fluid, and (5) transport to the emergency department for antivenin. Note: DO NOT apply ice, cold pack, or freon spray to the wound; DO NOT incise the wound; and DO NOT apply electrical stimulation from any device in an attempt to retard or reverse venom spread.

Stings (injection injuries) can come from insects and marine animals. Many people die from allergic reactions to insect stings, particularly wasps, bees, hornets, and fire ants. Only the common honeybee leaves a stinger. Wasps, hornets, yellow jackets, and fire ants sting repeatedly until removed from contact. Assessment findings include localized pain, redness, swelling, and a skin wheal. Idiosyncratic reactions are not considered allergic if they respond well to antihistamines. Signs and symptoms of an allergic reaction include localized pain, swelling, redness, and skin wheal, itching or flushing of skin or rash, tachycardia, hypotension, bronchospasm, or laryngeal edema, facial edema, and uvular swelling. General management includes washing of the sting area; gentle removal of stinger, if present (scrape, do not squeeze); application of cool compresses; and observation for allergic reaction or anaphylactic shock. Marine animal injection injuries are a threat in some coastal areas, especially in warmer, tropical waters. Toxin injection can be from jellyfish or coral stings or from punctures by the bony spines of animals such as sea urchins and stingrays. All marine venoms contain substances that produce pain that is disproportionate to the size of the injury. These toxins are unstable and heat sensitive, and heat will relieve the pain and inactivate the venom. Signs and symptoms of marine animal injection include intense local pain and swelling, weakness, nausea and vomiting, dyspnea, tachycardia, and hypotension or shock (in severe cases). In any case of suspected injection, treat by establishing and maintaining airway, application of a constriction bandage between the wound and the heart no tighter than a watchband (to occlude lymphatic flow only), application of heat or hot water, and inactivation or removal or any stingers. Because both fresh and salt water contain considerable bacterial and viral pollution, you should always be alert to possible secondary infection of a wound. In cases of marine-acquired infections, be sure to consider *Vibrio* species.

13. **Given several scenarios of poisoning or overdose, provide the appropriate assessment, treatment, and transport.** pp. 1350–1386

Remember that the basic assessment of a patient with a toxicological emergency includes careful scene size-up, protection of rescue personnel, and rapid response to any needs to support the ABCs. Treatment includes decontamination and use of antidotes, where available. Rapid transport is standard. Detailed specifics for many drugs, toxic substances, and animal bites and stings are given in other objectives for this chapter.

Content Self-Evaluation

MULTIPLE CHOICE

1. Which of the following statements about the epidemiology of toxicological emergencies is NOT true?
    A. The frequency of toxicological emergencies continues to increase both in number and severity.
    B. About 70 percent of accidental poisonings occur among children aged 6 years or younger.
    C. Toxicological emergencies account for about 1 percent of emergency department visits and EMS responses.
    D. More serious poisonings, especially in older children, may represent intentional poisoning by a parent or caregiver.
    E. Adult poisonings and overdoses account for 95 percent of the fatalities in this category.

_____ 2. Immediate effects of toxic ingestion are often localized to the site of entry, whereas delayed effects are often systemic in nature.
   A. True
   B. False

_____ 3. Many inhalation exposures are accidental, and leading agents include the following:
   A. carbon dioxide, carbon tetrachloride, and ammonia.
   B. toxic vapors, plants, and chlorine.
   C. carbon monoxide, nitrous oxide, and petroleum-based products such as gasoline.
   D. carbon monoxide, ammonia, and toxic vapors.
   E. chlorine, cleaners (soaps and alkalis), and carbon monoxide.

_____ 4. All of the following are guidelines to follow in cases of toxicological emergencies EXCEPT:
   A. maintaining a high index of suspicion for possible poisonings.
   B. recording everything you see or smell at the scene that might help determine cause.
   C. taking appropriate measures to protect all rescue personnel and any bystanders.
   D. centering general management on support of ABCs, decontamination of the patient, and use of an antidote, if there is one.
   E. removing the patient from a toxic environment as promptly as possible.

_____ 5. Never delay supportive measures or transport due to a delay in contacting the Poison Control Center.
   A. True
   B. False

_____ 6. The most common route of entry for toxic substances is:
   A. inhalation.   D. injection.
   B. ingestion.   E. adsorption.
   C. surface absorption.

_____ 7. The three principles of decontamination are:
   A. removal of patient from toxic environment, reduction in intake of toxin, and increase in elimination of toxin from body.
   B. removal of patient from toxic environment, removal of patient's clothing and washing of patient's body, and increase in elimination of toxin from body.
   C. removal of patient from toxic environment, reduction in intake of toxin, and use of antidote, if one.
   D. removal of patient's clothing and washing of body, reduction in intake of toxin, and reduction in absorption of toxin already in body.
   E. reduction in intake of toxin into the body, reduction of absorption of toxin already in the body, and increase in elimination of toxin from the body.

_____ 8. The most widely used means of reducing absorption of toxins in the body is:
   A. gastric lavage (stomach pumping).   D. whole bowel irrigation.
   B. activated charcoal.   E. chelating agents.
   C. syrup of ipecac.

_____ 9. Do not involve law enforcement in a possible suicide case until it is clear that suicide was intended.
   A. True
   B. False

_____ 10. Flumazenil is an antidote for which of the following ingested substances?
   A. arsenic   D. ethylene glycol
   B. benzodiazepines   E. methyl alcohol
   C. cyanide

_____ 11. Which of the following is not a question commonly asked of a poisoning patient during the focused history?
   A. How much of the agent(s) did you ingest?
   B. How long ago did you ingest the agent(s)?
   C. Were any people with you when you ingested the agent(s)?
   D. What is your weight?
   E. Have you attempted to treat yourself in any way?

_____ 12. The physical exam is crucial in toxicological emergencies, and it has two purposes: (1) documenting physical evidence of intoxication and (2) detecting any underlying illness or condition that might affect either patient's symptoms or outcome of exposure.
   A. True
   B. False

_____ 13. All of the following statements are correct when treating ingestion emergencies EXCEPT:
   A. Maintaining the ABCs is the top priority along with monitoring of all vitals.
   B. Prevention of aspiration is a major objective, and intubation may be necessary.
   C. An IV at keep-vein-open rate is recommended for all potentially dangerous ingestion incidents.
   D. Induce vomiting unless it is against local protocol or you are told not to do so by Poison Control.
   E. Follow general treatment guidelines with decontamination procedures.

_____ 14. The first priorities, in proper order, with surface-absorption exposures are to remove the patient from the toxic environment, perform the initial assessment, and then ensure your safety.
   A. True
   B. False

_____ 15. All of the following are respiratory signs or symptoms of a toxic inhalation exposure EXCEPT:
   A. bradycardia.   D. tachypnea.
   B. chest tightness.   E. dizziness.
   C. cough.

_____ 16. The typical signs and symptoms of carbon monoxide poisoning include:
   A. a burning sensation in mouth and throat, headache, and confusion.
   B. headache, seizure or coma, and tachypnea.
   C. tachypnea, pulmonary edema, and a burning sensation in mouth and throat.
   D. tachypnea, tachycardia, headache, and confusion.
   E. headache, nausea and vomiting, and confusion or other altered mental status.

_____ 17. The narcotic toxidrome is characterized by CNS depression, whereas the sympathomimetic toxidrome is characterized by CNS excitation.
   A. True
   B. False

_____ 18. Response to poisoning with one of the cardiac medications often involves bradycardia, which may require use of:
   A. atropine.   D. digoxin.
   B. an external pacing device. E. calcium.
   C. a beta-blocker.

_____ 19. Common assessment findings for ingestion of a caustic include all of the following EXCEPT:
   A. chest and abdominal pain.   D. hoarseness and/or stridor.
   B. drooling and trouble swallowing. E. pain in the lips, tongue, throat, or gums.
   C. facial burns.

_____ 20. A patient has spilled a large quantity of an unknown acid on his skin. Treatment should consist of:
   A. contacting Poison Control for instructions.
   B. covering the area with activated charcoal.
   C. diluting the acid with bicarbonate.
   D. irrigation with copious amounts of water.
   E. irrigation with copious amounts of milk.

_____ 21. Ingestion of alkalis usually results in:
   A. immediate and intense pain.
   B. bradycardia.
   C. local burns to the mouth and throat.
   D. ulceration and perforation of the stomach lining.
   E. liquefaction necrosis.

_____ 22. Drugs with narrow therapeutic indexes are more likely to be involved in accidental toxicological emergencies. Two such drugs are:
   A. lithium and the selective serotonin reuptake inhibitors (SSRIs).
   B. tricyclic antidepressants and salicylates.
   C. tricyclic antidepressants and lithium.
   D. tricyclic antidepressants and SSRIs.
   E. salicylates and lithium.

_____ 23. It is particularly important to know the time of ingestion when a blood test (timed properly) can predict degree of damage. Two drugs to which this statement especially applies are:
   A. acetaminophen and tricyclics.
   B. SSRIs and tricyclics.
   C. acetaminophen and nonsteroidal antiinflammatory drugs.
   D. salicylates and nonsteroidal antiinflammatory drugs.
   E. salicylates and acetaminophen.

_____ 24. If you suspect mixed ingestion with tricyclics and benzodiazepines, do NOT use Flumazenil because it may precipitate seizures.
   A. True
   B. False

_____ 25. Serotonin syndrome includes all of the following signs and symptoms EXCEPT:
   A. nausea, diarrhea, and abdominal cramps.
   B. hypotension.
   C. agitation and confusion.
   D. hyperthermia.
   E. rigidity, incoordination, and myoclonic jerks.

_____ 26. Chelating agents are often useful in cases of toxicity due to:
   A. lithium.   D. heavy metals.
   B. theophylline.   E. salicylates.
   C. some cardiac medications.

_____ 27. All of the following statements are true about MAO inhibitors EXCEPT:
   A. Overdose cases may be very serious, even though initial signs/symptoms may appear hours after ingestion.
   B. MAO inhibitors have been used to treat depression and obsessive-compulsive disorder.
   C. MAO inhibitors as a group have a narrow therapeutic index.
   D. MAO inhibitors may interact negatively with foods containing tyramine, such as cheese and wine.
   E. In overdose, death usually follows the eventual signs of tachycardia, hypertension, and coma.

_____ 28. In cases of suspected food poisoning or poisoning involving plants and mushrooms, it is important to bring samples along with the patient if possible.
A. True
B. False

_____ 29. In cases involving bites or stings, fatalities are most likely among patients who have an allergic reaction or anaphylaxis to insect stings.
A. True
B. False

_____ 30. In common toxic drug ingestions, the use of benzodiazepines is frequently recommended with:
A. alcohol, narcotics, and barbiturates.
B. alcohol, hallucinogens, and barbiturates.
C. cocaine, amphetamines, and hallucinogens.
D. cocaine, alcohol, and amphetamines.
E. cocaine, amphetamines, and barbiturates.

_____ 31. Alcohol is a(n):
A. depressant.
B. narcotic.
C. opiate.
D. stimulant.
E. oxidant.

_____ 32. Signs and symptoms associated with amphetamine usage include all of the following EXCEPT:
A. constricted pupils.
B. exhilaration.
C. hypertension.
D. psychosis.
E. tremors.

_____ 33. Altered mental status and slurred speech are signs/symptoms of Xanax overdose.
A. True
B. False

_____ 34. Which of the following statements about delirium tremens is NOT true?
A. They usually develop 2 to 3 days after withdrawal of alcohol.
B. They can occur in individuals who have experienced recent binge drinking.
C. DTs are marked by a decreased level of consciousness with hallucinations.
D. Seizures and delirium tremens are ominous signs.
E. DTs are associated with a significant mortality rate.

MATCHING

Write the letter of the definition in the space provided next to the term to which it applies.

_____ 35. injection

_____ 36. tolerance

_____ 37. toxin

_____ 38. inhalation

_____ 39. poisoning

_____ 40. substance abuse

_____ 41. therapeutic index (or window)

_____ 42. ingestion

_____ 43. delirium tremens (DTs)

_____ 44. enterotoxin

_____ 45. decontamination

_____ 46. surface absorption

_____ 47. overdose

_____ 48. toxidrome

_____ 49. withdrawal

_____ 50. addiction

A. an exposure to a nonpharmacological toxic substance

B. entry of a substance into the body via a break in the skin

C. result of drug discontinuance in which body reacts severely to absence of drug

D. group of clinical signs and symptoms consistently associated with exposure to a particular type of toxin

E. dependence on a drug—physiological, psychological, or both

F. potentially lethal syndrome found when alcohol withdrawn from chronic abusers

G. dosage range between effective and toxic dosages

H. need to progressively increase dosage to achieve same effect

I. process of minimizing toxicity by reducing amount of toxin absorbed into the body

J. entry of a substance into the body via the skin or mucous membranes

K. exposure to an amount of pharmacological substance greater than normally tolerated

L. bacterial exotoxin that produces GI symptoms and diseases such as food poisoning

M. entry of a substance into the body via the respiratory tract

N. any chemical that causes adverse effects on an organism exposed to it

O. use of pharmacological product for purposes other than those medically defined for it

P. entry of a substance into the body via the GI tract

Chapter 35

Hematology

Review of Chapter Objectives

After reading this chapter, you should be able to:

1. **Identify the anatomy and physiology of the hematopoietic system.** (see Chapter 3)

   The components of the hematopoietic system include the blood, bone marrow, liver, spleen, and kidneys. The process of hematopoiesis forms the cellular components of blood. In the fetus, this first takes place outside the bone marrow in the liver, spleen, lymph nodes, and thymus. By the fourth month of gestation, the bone marrow begins to produce blood cells. After birth and across the span of life, bone marrow continues to fulfill this critical function barring the development of some pathological process.

   In hematopoiesis, the stem cell reproduces to maintain a constant population of cells. Some stem cells further differentiate into myeloid multipotent stem cells that, in turn, differentiate into unipotent progenitors, which ultimately mature into the formed elements of blood: red blood cells (RBCs), white blood cells (WBCs), and platelets. Pluripotent stem cells may also differentiate into common lymphoid stem cells, ultimately becoming lymphocytes. Erythropoietin, the hormone responsible for red blood cell production, is produced by the kidneys and, to a lesser extent, the liver. The liver also removes toxins from the blood and produces many of the clotting factors and proteins in plasma. The spleen plays an important role in the immune system with its cells that scavenge abnormal blood cells and bacteria.

2. **Discuss the following:** (see Chapter 3)

   Plasma
   Plasma is a thick, pale yellow fluid consisting predominately of water, electrolytes, and proteins. It also contains some fats, carbohydrates, and chemical messengers. Plasma is the medium that carries the formed elements of the blood cells.

   Red blood cells (erythrocytes)
   Erythropoiesis—the process of RBC production—is triggered by the secretion of erythropoietin. The secretion occurs whenever the kidney's renal cells sense hypoxia. Erythropoietin, in turn, causes the bone marrow to produce more red blood cells, which increases the oxygen-carrying capacity of the blood.

   Red blood cells have a life span of about 4 months, although hemorrhage, hemolysis (RBC destruction), or sequestration by the liver or spleen may significantly reduce this time. The spleen and liver contain macrophages (a specialized type of scavenger white blood cell) that can remove damaged or abnormal cells from circulation.

   Hemoglobin
   Hemoglobin is an iron compound found in the red blood cells. It has a great affinity for oxygen and helps transport oxygen from the pulmonary capillaries to the tissues. One gram of hemoglobin can carry 1.34 milliliters of oxygen.

Hematocrit

Hematocrit is the packed cell volume of red blood cells per unit of blood. This measurement is obtained by spinning a blood sample in a centrifuge to separate the cellular elements from the plasma. Red cells—the heaviest component of the blood (due to the hemoglobin's iron)—settles to the bottom of the tube. The white blood cells form the next layer, while plasma floats on top. The height of the RBCs is divided by the total height of the tube's contents (cellular components + plasma) and is reported as a percentage. The normal range is from 40 to 52 percent, although women tend to have slightly lower levels than men.

White blood cells (leukocytes)

White blood cells originate in the bone marrow from undifferentiated stem cells. The process by which the stem cells differentiate into the various immature forms of white blood cells—known as blasts—is known as leukopoiesis. The three main blasts include granulocytes, monocytes, and lymphocytes. While leukocytes provide protection from foreign invasion, each type of white blood cell has its own unique function. Healthy people have between 5,000 and 9,000 white blood cells per milliliter of blood. The presence of illness, however, can cause that number to rise to more than 16,000.

Granulocytic white blood cells include three types—eosinophils, neutrophils, and basophils. Basophils act as storage sites for the body's histamine. When stimulated, the basophils degranulate and release the histamine, typically in an allergic reaction. Eosinophils can inactivate the chemical mediators of an acute allergic reaction, thus modulating the anaphylactic response. The main purpose of neutrophils is to fight infection.

Monocytes, the second main grouping of white blood cells, serve as "trash collectors." They move throughout the body engulfing both foreign invaders and dead neutrophils. Some monocytes remain in circulation, while others migrate to other sites to further mature into macrophages. Monocytes and macrophages also secrete growth factors to stimulate the formation of red blood cells and granulocytes. Some macrophages become fixed within tissues of the liver, spleen, lungs, and lymphatic system, becoming part of the reticuloendothelial system. Here they have the capability of stimulating lymphocyte production in an immune response.

Lymphocytes, the third main grouping of white blood cells, circulate in the blood. They are also found in the lymph fluid and nodes, bone marrow, spleen, liver, lungs, skin, and intestine. These highly specialized cells contain surface receptor sites specific to a single antigen and initiate an immune response in order to rid the body of infectious agents.

Platelets, clotting, and fibrinolysis

Platelets, or thrombocytes, function to form a plug at an initial bleeding site and to secrete several factors important to clotting. Normally, platelets number between 150,000 and 450,000 per milliliter. They are derived from megakaryocytes that come from an undifferentiated stem cell in the bone marrow. They can survive from 7 to 10 days, after which they are removed from circulation by the spleen.

Damage to cells or to the tunica intima (innermost lining of the blood vessels) triggers clotting, or the "coagulation cascade." Cascading can be activated by either an intrinsic pathway (trauma to blood cells from turbulence) or an extrinsic pathway (damage to vessels).

Following the intrinsic pathway, platelets release substances that lead to the formation of prothrombin activator. In the presence of calcium, the prothrombin converts to thrombin, which in turn converts fibrinogen to stable fibrin. The fibrin traps blood cells and more platelets to form a clot.

Following the extrinsic pathway, smooth muscle fibers in the tunica media (middle lining of the blood vessels) contract. The resulting vasoconstriction reduces the size of the injury, which reduces blood flow through the area. This action limits blood loss and allows platelet aggregation (formation of a platelet plug) and the subsequent conversion of the prothrombin activator.

Clotting factors or proteins are primarily produced in the liver and circulate in an inactive state. Prothrombin and fibrinogen are the best known of these factors. Damaged cells send out a chemical message that activates a specific clotting factor. This activates each protein in a sequence geared toward stable clot formation.

An enzyme on the surface of the platelet membrane makes it sticky. This stickiness allows platelet aggregation to occur.

Fibrinolysis, the process through which plasmin dismantles a blood clot, does not signal the end of the coagulation cascade. Once a fibrin clot is formed, it releases a chemical called plasminogen, which is subsequently converted to plasmin. Plasmin begins dismantling or lysing a clot, which may take hours or days. This allows the scarring process to take place.

Hemostasis
Hemostasis involves three mechanisms to prevent or control blood loss: (1) vascular spasms that reduce the size of a vascular tear, (2) platelet plugs (an aggregate of platelets that adheres to collagen), and (3) the formation of stable fibrin clots (coagulation).

3. **Identify the following:** (see Chapter 4)

Inflammatory process
The inflammatory process is a nonspecific defense mechanism that wards off damage caused by some microorganism or trauma. The process helps localize damage, while simultaneously destroying the source and facilitating repair. The process may be triggered by various agents—infectious, chemical, or immunologic—or by trauma. Following local tissue injury, chemical messengers are released. These chemicals attract white blood cells, increase capillary permeability, and cause vasodilatation, which in turn produces the redness, swelling, warmth, and pain associated with inflammation.

Systemic inflammation is another type of inflammatory process. It occurs as a result of bacterial infection. Fever, which commonly accompanies systemic inflammation, is thought to occur in response to the chemical mediators released by macrophages seeking to rid the body of an infectious agent. These same mediators act on the brain, triggering sympathetic nervous system stimulation and causing heat conservation, vasoconstriction, and fever.

Cellular and humoral immunity
Lymphocytes, the primary cells of the immune system, include two types—T cells and B cells. T cells, which mature in the thymus, are responsible for handling mediated or cellular immunity. In humoral immunity, B cells produce antibodies to combat infection. Cellular immunity is responsible for antigen-triggered release of effector cells. This type of immunity causes the following: (1) delayed hypersensitivity reactions, (2) transplant rejection, and (3) defense against intracellular organisms. Humoral immunity occurs when an antigen triggers the development and release of specific antibodies necessary for the body's defense.

Alterations in immunologic response
A variety of factors—drugs, diseases, genetic conditions, and infection—can trigger alterations in the body's immunologic response. Genetics and viral infection, for example, can cause the immune system to develop antibodies against the body's own tissues, which leads to a variety of localized or systemic diseases. Immunosuppressive drugs, like those used to prevent transplant rejection, and cancer chemotherapy agents (as well as cancer itself) can also cause alterations, the most significant of which is a reduced ability to fight infections. Alterations in immunity may also be acquired through infection with the human immunodeficiency virus (HIV), which has an affinity for T lymphocytes, rendering the body at great risk of opportunistic infections.

Regardless of the cause, alterations in immunologic response and the resultant risk of infection make it imperative for the EMS provider to protect the patient from disease-causing agents. You must practice good hand-washing techniques, BSI, correct IV procedures, and proper wound care.

4. **Identify blood groups.** pp. 1390–1391

The presence of certain antigens (proteins) on the surface of a donor's red blood cells allows the patient's body to recognize it as "self" or "not self." Following a transfusion, antibodies in the patient's own blood attack any foreign antigens that may be present in the transfused blood, causing a reaction. The presence or absence of such antigens and antibodies provides us with the blood typing system used today—a system designed to prevent reactions to transfusions.

To see how this system works, consider these cases. Someone with A antigen on his or her red blood cells would have anti-B antibodies. This person is said to have type A blood. Conversely, someone with B antigens would have anti-A antibodies, resulting in type B blood. Other people have both A and B antigens, but neither anti-A or anti-B antibodies. Their blood type is AB. With regard to transfusions, these individuals are known as universal recipients because they lack any antibodies to attack foreign blood cells. Yet other people have neither A nor B antigens, but have both anti-A and anti-B antibodies. Their blood type is O. Individuals with type O blood are called universal donors because their blood has no antigens to trigger a reaction.

In addition to the presence of A and B antigens, blood typing must take into account another factor—the Rh antigen found on red blood cells. People with the Rh factor are said to be Rh positive; people without it are said to be Rh negative. When identifying an individual on the basis of blood type, all of these elements are taken into account. For example, one person may be O positive, while another might be AB negative.

5. List erythrocyte disorders. pp. 1397–1399

Erythrocyte disorders include anemia, sickle cell disease, and polycythemia. Of the three, anemia is the most common disorder. It is typically classified as a hematocrit (red blood cell count) of less than 37 percent in women and 40 percent in men. The reduction may be due to blood loss, the destruction of red blood cells (hemolytic anemia), or diseases that limit the production of red blood cells. Anemia is not a disease, but the sign of an underlying problem.

Sickle cell anemia is an inherited disorder of red blood cell production, so named because the red blood cells become sickle-shaped when oxygen levels are low. The cells are less flexible and increase the viscosity of the blood, which in turn leads to vasooclussive crisis and multiple organ damage. The C-shaped cells survive for only a short time, typically 10 to 20 days.

Polycythemia is an abnormally high hematocrit due to excess production of red blood cells. It is rare and most frequently occurs in persons over 50 years of age. The increased hematocrit predisposes the patient to thrombosis and platelet dysfunction.

6. List leukocyte disorders. pp. 1399–1401

Disorders or problems of the white blood cells (leukocytes) have a significant impact on the body's defense system. These problems include leukopenia (too few white blood cells) or leukocytosis (too many white blood cells). A variation of leukopenia is neutropenia in which there are too few neutrophils; this is potentially dangerous, as the absolute count for neutrophils is an excellent indicator of the immune system's status. Improper white cell formation may also cause disorders such as leukemia (cancer of the hematopoietic cells) or lymphoma (cancer of the lymphatic system).

7. List platelet and clotting disorders. pp. 1401–1402

The common platelet disorders include thrombocytosis, thrombocytopenia, hemophilia, and von Willebrand's disease. Thrombocytosis is an increase in the production and number of platelets secondary to other disorders and usually leaves the patient asymptomatic.

Thrombocytopenia is an abnormal decrease in the number of platelets. It is due to decreased platelet production, sequestration of platelets in the spleen, destruction of platelets, or any combination of the three. Acute idiopathic thrombocytopenia purpura (ITP) results from destruction of platelets by the immune system. It is most commonly seen in children following a viral infection or in adult women with autoimmune disease.

Hemophilia is a blood disorder in which one of the proteins necessary for blood clotting is missing or defective. When a person with hemophilia is injured, the bleeding will take longer to stop because the body cannot form stable fibrin clots. Prolonged hemorrhage may result, even from what might otherwise be a minor wound.

Von Willebrand's disease is a condition in which the vWF component of factor VIII is deficient. This factor is necessary for normal platelet adhesion—an essential part of the clotting process. The disease is not associated with the deep muscle or joint bleeding of hemophilia, nor is it usually as serious, although nosebleeds, excessive menstruation, and gastrointestinal bleeds can occur.

8. Describe how acquired factor deficiencies may occur. pp. 1401–1402

People who lack clotting factors can have bleeding disorders, which can occur as a result of genetics or medications. Some medications such as aspirin, dipyridamole (Persantine), and ticlopidine (Ticlid) decrease the stickiness of platelets by altering the surface enzyme that allows platelet aggregation. Others such as heparin and warfarin (Coumadin) cause changes within the clotting cascade to prevent clot formation. Heparin, working together with antithrombin III (a naturally occurring thrombin inactivator), inactivates thrombin to prevent formation of the fibrin clot. Coumadin blocks the activity of vitamin K, which is necessary to generate the activated forms of clotting factors II, VII, IX, and X, thus effectively interrupting the clotting cascade.

9. Identify the components of the physical assessment as they relate to the hematology system. pp. 1392–1396

Many times hematological disorders are discovered and diagnosed when the patient seeks assistance for another medical condition, as the signs and symptoms associated with hematological problems may be quite varied. Patients with infection, white blood cell abnormalities (immunocompromised and prone to infection), or transfusion reactions may present with febrile symptoms. Acute hemodynamic compromise can be found in patients with anemia secondary to acute blood loss, coagulation disorders, or autoimmune disease. Confirmation of hematological disorders is usually dependent on laboratory analysis, but a complete history will go a long way toward developing an accurate diagnosis.

Additional specific considerations include mental status, dizziness, vertigo, or syncope, all of which may be indicative of anemia. Visual problems should alert you to the possibility of autoimmune disorders or sickle cell disease.

Skin color may be another indicator of hematological problems. Jaundice may indicate liver disease or hemolysis of red blood cells, while polycythemia is often associated with a florid (reddish) appearance, as pallor is with anemia. Observe for petechiae or purpura and bruising. Itching is commonly associated with hematological problems because of an excess of bilirubin resulting from liver disease or a breakdown of hemoglobin. Many patients report itching over a bruise. Look for evidence of prolonged bleeding, such as multiple bandages over a relatively minor wound.

Palpate the lymph nodes of the neck, clavicle, axilla, and groin. Enlarged lymph nodes are commonly seen in conjunction with hematopoietic disorders.

Gastrointestinal effects may be quite varied. Patients with clotting disorders may report epistaxis, bleeding gums, or melena. Many patients with clotting disorders report atraumatic bleeding of the gums. Ulcerations of the gums and oral mucosa as well as thrush (viral infection of the mouth) are often seen with immunocompromised patients. Abdominal pain is often seen in patients with hematological disorders. You may also be able to discern hepatic or splenic enlargement on your abdominal exam.

You should always ask about joint pain and examine the major joints closely in any patient who you suspect may have hematological problems. Minor trauma can cause significant hemarthrosis in patients with clotting disorders such as hemophilia. Many patients with autoimmune disorders frequently complain of arthralgia (joint pain) in all of their major joints.

You may see a variety of cardiorespiratory presentations that are linked to hematological disorders. Signs of hypoxia, such as tachypnea, tachycardia, and even chest pain, may be indicative of anemia. Occasionally, patients with bleeding disorders may develop hemoptysis. As always, you should be alert to signs and symptoms of shock and be prepared to initiate prompt therapy.

Genitourinary signs and symptoms associated with hematological problems may include hematuria, bleeding into the scrotal sac, excessive menstrual bleeding, and infection. Sickle cell disease is the most common cause for priapism seen in the emergency setting. Recognize that a detailed physical exam of the genitourinary system is not appropriate in the prehospital setting.

10. Describe the pathology and clinical manifestations and prognosis associated with:

Anemia pp. 1397–1398

The most common disease associated with red blood cells is defined as a hematocrit of less than 37 percent in women and less than 40 percent in men. The majority of patients remain asymptomatic until their hematocrit drops below 30 percent. Anemia is either due to a reduction in the total number of RBCs or quality of hemoglobin. It may also be due to acute or chronic blood loss. Anemia is a sign of an underlying disease process that is either destroying RBCs and hemoglobin or decreasing their production. Anemias may be hereditary or acquired.

The signs and symptoms associated with anemia are related to the associated hypoxia that results from the decrease in RBCs or hemoglobin. Depending on the rapidity of onset, signs and symptoms may be subtle or dramatic, determined to some degree by the patient's age and underlying state of health. Signs and symptoms may include fatigue, dizziness, headache, pallor, and tachycardia, or dyspnea with exertion. If the anemia develops rapidly, it may overwhelm the body's compensatory mechanisms, in which case you may observe postural or frank hypotension, tachycardia, peripheral vasoconstriction, and decreased mental status.

Anemia may be self-limited or can be a lifelong illness requiring transfusions on a recurring and periodic basis. Confirmation of the illness and determination of its cause will be predictive of its prognosis.

Leukemia   p. 1400

Cancers of the hematopoietic cells occur when the precursors of white blood cells in the bone marrow begin to replicate abnormally. Initially, the proliferation of WBCs is confined to the bone marrow but then spreads to the peripheral circulation. Leukemia is classified by the type of cell involved and may be either acute or chronic. Examples include acute or chronic lymphocytic leukemia, acute or chronic myelogenous leukemia, or hairy cell leukemia. Although leukemias may occur across the life span, some are more commonly associated with specific age groups. For instance, acute lymphocytic leukemia (ALL) is seen predominately in children and young adults, while chronic lymphocytic leukemia (CLL) is most common in the sixth and seventh decades of life.

The signs and symptoms of leukemia are variable, although anemia and thrombocytopenia (decreased number of platelets) are common. These patients often appear acutely ill, complain of fatigue, and are febrile due to secondary infection. Lymph nodes will be enlarged. The history often includes weight loss and anorexia, as well as a feeling of abdominal fullness or pain that occurs as a result of liver and spleen enlargement.

The management of leukemia is a marvel of modern medicine as treatments such as chemotherapy, radiation therapy, and bone marrow transplantation have resulted in cures of specific types. Where ALL was once a virtual death sentence, now more than 50 percent of the pediatric patients live a normal life with the disease cured or in remission.

Lymphomas   pp. 1400–1401

Lymphomas are cancers of the lymphatic system. Malignant lymphoma is classified by the cell type involved, which indicates the stem cell from which the malignancy arises. The cancer may be either Hodgkin's or non-Hodgkin's lymphoma. In the United States, approximately 40,000 people are diagnosed with non-Hodgkin's lymphoma each year, while 7,500 are diagnosed with Hodgkin's lymphoma.

The most common presenting sign of non-Hodgkin's lymphoma is painless swelling of the lymph nodes, while those with Hodgkin's lymphoma typically have no related symptoms. Some patients report fever, night sweats, anorexia, weight loss, and pruritis.

The long-term survival rate is much better with Hodgkin's lymphoma. Many people with this disease who were treated with radiation, chemotherapy, or both are considered cured.

Polycythemia   p. 1399

Polycythemia is an abnormally high hematocrit due to excess production of red blood cells. A relatively rare disorder, it typically occurs in people over the age of 50. It can also develop secondary to dehydration. The increased red blood cell load increases the patient's risk of thrombosis, which causes most polycythemia-related deaths.

The signs and symptoms of polycythemia vary. The primary finding is a hematocrit of 50 percent or greater, which is usually accompanied by an increased number of white blood cells and platelets. The large number of RBCs may cause platelet dysfunction resulting in bleeding abnormalities such as epistaxis, spontaneous bruising, and gastrointestinal bleeding. Other complaints may include headache, dizziness, blurred vision, and itching. Severe cases can result in congestive heart failure.

Disseminated intravascular coagulopathy   p. 1402

Disseminated intravascular coagulopathy (DIC), also called consumption coagulopathy, is a disorder of coagulation caused by the systemic activation of the coagulation cascade. Normally, inhibitory mechanisms localize coagulation to the affected area through a combination of rapid blood flow and absorption of the fibrin clot. In DIC, circulating thrombin cleaves to fibrinogen, forming fibrin clots throughout the circulation. This condition results in widespread thrombosis and, occasionally, end-organ ischemia.

Bleeding, the most frequent sign of DIC, occurs due to the reduced fibrinogen level, consumption of coagulation factors, and thrombocytopenia. It most commonly results from sepsis, hypotension, obstetrical complications, severe tissue injury, brain injury, cancer, and major hemolytic transfusion reactions. The patient may exhibit a purpuric rash, often over the chest and abdomen. The disease is quite grave and has a poor prognosis.

Hemophilia   pp. 1401–1402

Hemophilia is a disorder in which one of the proteins necessary for blood clotting is missing or defective. A deficiency of factor VIII is called hemophilia A, which is the most common inherited disorder of hemostasis. The severity of the disease is related to the amount of available circulating factor VIII, and patients are classified as mild, moderate, or severe on that basis. A deficiency of factor IX is known as hemophilia B or Christmas disease, which is more rare but also more severe than hemophilia A.

Hemophilia is a sex-linked inherited bleeding disorder. The gene with the defective encoding is carried on the X chromosome; this means that if the mother is a carrier, her son will inherit this disorder. Conversely, female offspring who inherit the defective gene from their mother will be carriers, but will not exhibit the clotting defect. In order for a female to exhibit the defect, she must inherit the defect from both parents, that is, a mother who is a carrier and a father who has hemophilia. Hemophilia A affects 1 in 10,000 males.

The signs and symptoms of hemophilia include prolonged bleeding, numerous bruises, deep muscle bleeding characterized as pain or a "pulled muscle," and bleeding in the joints known as hemarthrosis.

Sickle cell disease   pp. 1398–1399

This disease is an inherited disorder of RBC production that causes hemoglobin to be produced in a "C" or sickle shape during low oxygen states. These patients also have hemolytic anemia as a result of destruction of abnormal red blood cells. The average life span of sickled cells is about one sixth that of a normal red cell—approximately 10 to 20 days versus 120 days. Additionally, the sickled shape increases the blood's viscosity, leading to sludging and obstruction of capillaries and small vessels. Blockage of blood flow to various tissues and organs is common usually following periods of stress. The process, called a vasoocclusive crisis, is characteristic of the disease and over time leads to organ damage, particularly in the cardiovascular, renal, and neurologic systems.

Sickle cell disease primarily affects African Americans, although other ethnic groups may also be affected, such as Puerto Ricans and people of Spanish, French, Italian, Greek, or Turkish ancestry. If both parents carry the sickle cell gene, the chances are 1 in 4 that their child will have normal hemoglobin.

Patients will develop three types of problems. Vasoocclusive crisis causes severe abdominal and joint pain, priapism, and renal or cerebrovascular infarcts. Hematological crises present with a drop in hemoglobin, sequestration of RBCs in the spleen, and problems with bone marrow function. Infectious crises mark the third type of problem as the patients are functionally immunosuppressed and the loss of splenic function makes them vulnerable to infection. Infections become increasingly common and often are the cause of death.

Multiple myeloma   pp. 1402–1403

Multiple myeloma is a cancerous disorder of plasma cells, the type of B cell responsible for producing immunoglobulins (antibodies). Rarely seen in patients under the age of 40, approximately 14,000 new cases are diagnosed each year.

Usually, multiple myeloma begins with a change or mutation in a plasma cell in the bone marrow. These cancerous cells crowd out the normal healthy cells and lead to a reduction in blood cell production. The patient then becomes anemic and prone to infection. The first sign is often a pain in the back or ribs as the diseased marrow weakens the bones and as a result, pathological fractures may occur. The resulting anemia leads to fatigue, and reduced platelet production places the patient at risk of bleeding. Calcium levels rise as a result of the bone destruction, and this often leads to renal failure.

11. **Given several preprogrammed patients with hematological problems, provide the appropriate assessment, management, and transport.**   pp. 1390–1403

Throughout your classroom, clinical, and field training, you will encounter a variety of real and simulated patients with hematological problems. Use the information provided in this chapter of your text, as well as the application of this information as demonstrated by your instructors, preceptors, and mentors to enhance your ability to assess, manage, and transport these patients.

Content Self-Evaluation

MULTIPLE CHOICE

_____ 1. The surface protein on a blood cell that allows blood to be typed is known as a(n):
   A. antibody.
   B. antigen.
   C. thrombocyte.
   D. granulocyte.
   E. monocyte.

_____ 2. The rarest blood type in the United States is:
   A. A.
   B. AB.
   C. B.
   D. O.
   E. none of the above

_____ 3. The blood type known as a universal donor is:
   A. A.
   B. AB.
   C. B.
   D. O.
   E. none of the above

_____ 4. The process of red blood cell destruction is known as:
   A. sequestration.
   B. fibrinolysis.
   C. hemolysis.
   D. hematopoiesis.
   E. phagocytosis.

_____ 5. Tiny red dots found on the skin that may be indicative of hematological disorders are called:
   A. purpura.
   B. jaundice.
   C. ecchymosis.
   D. petechiae.
   E. bruises.

_____ 6. An excess of bilirubin, either from liver disease or the breakdown of hemoglobin, can cause:
   A. gingivitis.
   B. generalized sepsis.
   C. arthralgia.
   D. priapism.
   E. pruritis.

_____ 7. Often, one of the earliest indications of hematological problems is:
   A. gingivitis.
   B. generalized sepsis.
   C. arthralgia.
   D. priapism.
   E. pruritis.

_____ 8. Which disease may result in slower blood clotting?
   A. AIDS
   B. cholecystitis
   C. cirrhosis
   D. pancreatitis
   E. malaria

_____ 9. The condition in which patients with hemophilia develop swollen, discolored, and painful joints with minimal trauma is:
   A. leukotaxis.
   B. dysthralgia.
   C. ecchymotic arthralgia.
   D. hemarthrosis.
   E. arthralgia.

_____ 10. A deficiency of _____ is linked to anemia.
   A. calcium
   B. copper
   C. iron
   D. potassium
   E. magnesium

_____ 11. A hematocrit of 50 percent or greater is the principal finding in:
   A. anemia.
   B. leukopenia.
   C. polycythemia.
   D. thrombocytopenia.
   E. non-Hodgkin's lymphoma.

_____ 12. Painless swelling of lymph nodes is the most common presenting sign of:
   A. anemia.
   B. leukopenia.
   A. polycythemia.
   D. thrombocytopenia.
   E. non-Hodgkin's lymphoma.

_____ 13. An abnormal decrease in the number of platelets, which can be induced by many drugs, is:
   A. anemia.
   B. leukopenia.
   E. polycythemia.
   D. thrombocytopenia.
   E. non-Hodgkin's lymphoma.

_____ 14. Patients with hemophilia A are deficient in blood clotting factor:
   A. VII.
   B. VIII.
   C. IX.
   D. X.
   E. XII.

_____ 15. The disease referred to as consumption coagulopathy is often caused by any of the following EXCEPT:
   A. hemolytic transfusion reactions.
   B. hypertension.
   C. obstetrical complications.
   D. sepsis.
   E. hypotension.

Chapter 36
Environmental Emergencies

Review of Chapter Objectives

After reading this chapter, you should be able to:

1. **Define "environmental emergency."** p. 1407

   An environmental emergency is a medical condition caused by or exacerbated by environmental factors such as weather, terrain, atmospheric pressure, or other local factors.

2. **Describe the incidence, morbidity, and mortality associated with environmental emergencies.** p. 1423

   The types of environmental emergencies most associated with any EMS provider's service are specific to that region: mountainous, coastal, desert, and so forth. In general, though, environmental emergencies are very common, and most paramedics will see such emergencies in their practice. It is vital that paramedics learn which types of emergencies are most likely to occur in their locales and that they know the special rescue techniques and resources needed and available for such emergencies.

   Specifics on morbidity and mortality: About 4,500 persons die annually from drowning in the United States, making drowning the third most common cause of accidental death across age groups. Approximately 40 percent of these deaths are among children under age 5 years. There is a second peak among teenagers and a third among the elderly (the last due to bathtub incidents). Many more people each year sustain serious injury from near-drowning. Roughly 85 percent of near-drowning victims are male, and two thirds of them do not know how to swim. Commonly, these situations are associated with freshwater settings, especially swimming pools.

3. **Identify risk factors most predisposing to environmental emergencies.** p. 1407

   General risk factors that place an individual at greater risk for an environmental emergency include age (very young and very old), poor general health, fatigue, predisposing medical conditions, and certain prescription or over-the-counter medications. Among drowning and near-drowning cases, alcohol use by an adult victim or the supervising adult is common.

4. **Identify environmental factors that may cause illness or exacerbate a preexisting illness or complicate treatment or transport decisions.** p. 1407

   Environments with certain characteristics are more likely to have emergencies: For instance, deserts may have tremendous variation in temperature between the hottest part of the day and overnight.

©2007 Pearson Education, Inc.
Essentials of Paramedic Care, 2nd ed.

Other such factors include current season, local weather patterns, atmospheric (high altitude) or hydrostatic (underwater) pressure, and the type of terrain. Rough or isolated terrain may significantly increase time for EMS response and for transport to the appropriate treating facility.

5. Define "homeostasis" and relate the concept to environmental influences. p. 1407

Homeostasis is the body's ability to maintain a steady and normal internal environment despite changing external conditions. In this chapter, external conditions that are explored in the context of environmental emergency are (1) extremes in temperature, (2) drowning (freshwater or saltwater), and (3) atmospheric (high altitude) or hydrostatic (underwater diving) pressure.

6. Identify normal, critically high, and critically low body temperatures. pp. 1408–1410

In the core of the body, temperature usually varies within 1° of 98.6°F (37°C). Heat exhaustion occurs at core temperatures above 100°F (37.8°C), and heatstroke can occur at 105°F (40.6°C) and higher. In contrast, mild hypothermia is associated with core temperatures of roughly 90–95°F (32–35°C). Severe hypothermia develops when core temperature drops below 90°F (32°C). The upper and lower core body temperatures compatible with survival are roughly 114°F and 86°F, respectively.

7. Describe several methods of temperature monitoring. p. 1409

Core body temperature can be monitored with a tympanic or rectal thermometer. Peripheral body temperature, which is usually a little bit lower, can be measured with use of an oral thermometer or a thermometer placed under the armpit (an axillary temperature). Approximate peripheral temperature or change in peripheral temperature can often be discerned by touch.

8. Describe human thermal regulation, including system components, substances used, and wastes generated. pp. 1407–1411, 1416

The human body does not generate "cold," it generates heat, and this process is called thermogenesis. There are three types of thermogenesis: The most basic and vital type is thermoregulatory thermogenesis, in which the nervous system and endocrine system work together to control the rate of cellular metabolism, which directly changes the rate of internal heat production. In work-induced thermogenesis, heat is produced through the work of skeletal muscles during exercise. In a cool or cold environment, muscles will produce some additional heat through shivering. The last type of heat generation is diet-induced thermogenesis, and it reflects the heat generated by cells as they process food and nutrients and eventually metabolize the breakdown products.

The body's thermal regulation is achieved through coordination of the nervous and endocrine systems. This is intuitively logical because these two systems are the control systems for all major body functions. Cells in the hypothalamus, a structure at the base of the brain, have the ability to act as a thermostat. As nerve cells, they sense the temperature of the core blood passing by them and they can receive messages from temperature sensors located in other parts of the body. Additional sensor cells for core temperature are located in the spinal cord, abdomen, and around the great veins in the chest. Peripheral sensors are in the skin and subcutaneous tissue.

On a cool day, peripheral temperature may drop. When the hypothalamic cells get the message, the cells act as endocrine cells, producing and secreting a hormone into the blood that acts to increase work-induced thermogenesis. Heat is produced through shivering. Also piloerection, or "goose bumps," the standing of small hairs, results in decreased air flow over the skin surface. If the environment is so cold that both peripheral and core temperature drop, the hypothalamic cells secrete hormones that increase heat production through all three means: thermoregulatory, work-induced, and diet-induced thermogenesis. (In the last, body cells burn fats and thus produce more heat.) In addition, core temperature, which is critical for survival, is maintained in part by reducing blood flow (and thus heat) to the most peripheral tissues, the skin and subcutaneous tissues. In contrast, when the thermostat cells sense peripheral temperature is too high (as when you exercise vigorously), they stop releasing the hormone that stimulates thermogenesis. Not only is heat production slowed, but mechanisms to dissipate heat into the external environment are also activated.

These include dilation of blood vessels in the skin and subcutaneous tissue (why people flush in the heat) and sweating.

This method of control, in which the production of a substance (in this case, heat) is turned off by the presence of that substance, is called negative feedback. Heat feeds back on the thermostat cells to turn off production of more heat. Think about the thermostat and furnace in a house. They work in a very similar fashion.

Thermogenesis consumes nutrient fuel for cells—fats, proteins, and carbohydrates—and it results in waste products such as carbon dioxide and water (from cellular respiration and fat breakdown) and urea (from protein breakdown). Extensive skeletal muscle use may also result in lactic acid accumulation. Heat dissipation through sweating consumes water, urea, and salts that are lost onto the skin surface.

9. List the common forms of heat and cold disorders. pp. 1411–1423

The common heat disorders are variants of hyperthermia, elevated core body temperature: In terms of increasing severity, these conditions are heat (muscle) cramps, heat exhaustion, and heatstroke. Cold disorders are frostbite, trench foot, and hypothermia.

10. List the common predisposing factors and preventive measures associated with heat and cold disorders. pp. 1411–1412, 1416–1417

Important predisposing factors for hyperthermia include age, general health, and medications. Both the very young and the very old have less responsive heat-regulating systems and can tolerate less variation in their core body temperature. Persons who have diabetes with autonomic neuropathy are at higher risk for hyperthermia because damage to the autonomic nervous system may interfere with proper messaging to the CNS about temperature and may interfere with the heat-dissipating processes of vasodilation and sweating. Several groups of medications can affect body temperature. Diuretics predispose to dehydration, which impairs ability to sweat. Beta-blockers interfere with vasodilation, impair ability to increase heart rate in response to volume loss, and may interfere with temperature messages to the CNS. Psychotropics and antihistamines interfere with thermoregulation within the CNS. Additional factors include acclimatization to local conditions, length and intensity of heat exposure, and environmental factors such as humidity and wind. Preventive measures for heat disorders include three major elements. First, maintenance of adequate fluid intake is vital, and remember that thirst alone is an inadequate indicator for dehydration. Second, you should allow yourself time for acclimatization to the hot environment, which results in more perspiration with lower salt concentration, thus conserving body-fluid volume. Last, it is important to limit exposure to hot environments.

Important predisposing factors for hypothermia are the same: age, general health, and medications. Both the very young and the very old have less responsive heat-generating systems to combat cold exposure and cannot tolerate cold environments. The elderly may become hypothermic in environments that are only somewhat cool to others. Persons with inadequately treated hypothyroidism have suppressed metabolisms, which prevents proper responsiveness to cold. In addition, malnutrition, hypoglycemia, Parkinson's disease, fatigue, and other medical conditions can interfere with the body's ability to combat cold exposure. Drugs that interfere with heat-generating mechanisms include narcotics, alcohol, phenothiazines, barbiturates, antiseizure medications, antihistamines and other allergy medications, antipsychotics, sedatives, antidepressants, and various analgesics such as aspirin, acetaminophen, and NSAIDs. Additional factors include prolonged or intense exposure, which directly affects both morbidity and mortality, and coexisting weather conditions (such as high humidity, brisk winds, or accompanying rain, all of which magnify the effect of cold). Preventive measures can decrease the morbidity of cold-related injury, and these include dressing warmly; being rested, which maximizes the ability of the heat-generating mechanisms to replenish energy reserves; appropriate eating at proper intervals to support metabolism; and limitation of exposure to cold environments.

11. Define heat illness, hypothermia, frostbite, near-drowning, decompression illness, and altitude illness. pp. 1411, 1416, 1422, 1423, 1428, 1433

- Heat illness is increased core body temperature (CBT) due to inadequate thermolysis (heat dissipation).

- Hypothermia is a state of low body temperature, particularly low core body temperature.
- Frostbite is environmentally induced freezing of body tissues causing destruction of cells.
- Near-drowning is an incident of potentially fatal submersion in liquid that did not result in death or in which death occurred more than 24 hours after submersion.
- Decompression illness is the development of nitrogen bubbles within body tissues due to a rapid reduction of air pressure when a diver returns to the surface; this is commonly called "the bends."
- High altitude illness is caused by a decrease in ambient pressure causing a low-oxygen environment and resultant hypoxia.

12. Describe the pathophysiology, signs and symptoms, and predisposing factors, preventive actions, and treatment for heat cramps, heat exhaustion, heatstroke, and fever. pp. 1411–1416

Heat cramps are caused by overexertion and dehydration in a hot environment. They occur when the temperature- and exercise-induced sweating (which consumes water and electrolytes including sodium) depletes the body of so much water and electrolytes that the actively exercising skeletal muscle fibers cramp. Signs and symptoms include cramping in fingers, arms, legs, or abdominal muscles. Patients are generally mentally alert with a feeling of weakness, but they may be dizzy or faint. Vital signs are stable, although temperature may be normal or slightly elevated. Skin is likely to be moist and warm. Note that heat cramps may be painful but they are NOT considered to be an actual heat illness. The general predisposing factors and preventive measures for all heat-related disorders are discussed with objective 10. Treatment for heat cramps is usually easily accomplished. First, remove the patient from the hot environment to a cooler one such as a shady area or an air-conditioned ambulance. For severe cramps, you can administer an oral saline solution (approximately 4 tsp salt/gallon water) or a sports electrolyte drink. Do NOT use salt tablets, which are not absorbed readily and can irritate the stomach, causing ulceration or hypernatremia. If the patient cannot take liquids readily, an IV of normal saline may be needed. Palliative care may include muscle massage or moist towels over patient's head and the cramping muscles.

Heat exhaustion, which is considered a mild heat illness, is an acute reaction to heat exposure, and it is the most common heat-related illness seen by EMS providers. The loss of water and electrolytes (notably sodium) from working in a hot environment, combined with general vasodilation as a heat-dissipating mechanism, leads to a decreased circulating blood volume, venous pooling, and reduced cardiac output. The presenting symptoms are due to dehydration and sodium loss secondary to sweating. Because the symptoms are not unique to heat exhaustion, diagnosis requires presentation in the appropriate environmental setting. Remember that untreated heat exhaustion can progress to heatstroke. The signs and symptoms of heat exhaustion include increased body temperature (over 100°F, 37.8°C); cool, clammy skin with heavy perspiration; rapid, shallow breathing; and a weak pulse. Signs of active thermolysis may include diarrhea and muscle cramps. The patient will feel weak and, in some cases, may lose consciousness. There also may be CNS symptoms such as headache, anxiety, paresthesia, and impaired judgment or even psychosis. The general predisposing factors and preventive measures for all heat-related disorders are discussed with objective 10. Treatment includes removal of the patient from the hot environment and placement in a supine position. For severe cramps, you can administer an oral saline solution (approximately 4 tsp salt/gallon water) or a sports electrolyte drink. Do NOT use salt tablets, as discussed above. If the patient cannot take liquids readily, an IV of normal saline may be needed. Remove some clothing and fan the patient to increase heat dissipation. Be careful not to cool the patient to the point of chilling him or her. Stop fanning if shivering develops, and consider covering the patient lightly. If shock is suspected, treat accordingly. If symptoms do not resolve, consider the possibility of increased core body temperature and evolution of heatstroke.

Heatstroke is a true environmental emergency, one in which the body's hypothalamic temperature regulation is lost and there is uncompensated hyperthermia resulting in cell death and damage to the brain, liver, and kidneys. Generally, heatstroke is characterized by body temperature above 105°F (40.6°C), CNS disturbances, and (usually) cessation of perspiration. It is thought that sweating stops either because of destruction of sweat glands or because of sensory overload resulting in their temporary dysfunction. Patients may present with signs and symptoms including cessation of sweating, hot skin that is either moist or dry (depending on whether sweat has dried), very high core temperatures, deep respirations that become shallow and rapid respirations that may later slow, a rapid, full pulse that may slow later, hypotension with low or absent diastolic reading, confusion or disorientation or unconsciousness, and possible seizures. Field management centers on immediate cooling of the patient's body and replacement of fluids. First, remove the patient from the environment; if this is not done, other measures will be only minimally useful. Initiate rapid active body cooling to a target temperature of 102°F (39°C). This can be accomplished en route to the hospital. Remove the patient's clothing and cover with sheets soaked in tepid water. If necessary, either fanning or misting may be used. Be sure you avoid overcooling because this can trigger reflex hypothermia. Tepid water avoids the risk of producing reflex peripheral vasoconstriction and shivering that can be produced by exposure to cold water. In addition, use high-flow oxygen and assist respirations if they are shallow. Use pulse oximetry if available. Administer fluid therapy orally (if possible) or IV. In many cases, orally will suffice. Remember in this setting that electrolyte replacement is not nearly as necessary as water/volume replacement. If IVs are needed, start one or two and make the initial infusion with the line(s) wide open. Be sure to monitor the ECG because dysrhythmias can develop at any time. Avoid vasopressors and anticholinergic drugs because they may inhibit sweating and can contribute to development of a hyperthermic state in high-humidity, high-temperature environments. Lastly, monitor body temperature for trends toward target temperature or for other shift. If you work in a hot climate, try to make sure your thermometers measure above 106°F and below 95°F.

Fever (or pyrexia) is defined simply as elevation of body temperature above the normal for the individual. The body develops fever when pathogens cause infection, in turn stimulating productions of pyrogens, substances produced either by the pathogen or by cells involved in an inflammatory or immune response to the pathogen. Pyrogens produce fever by resetting the hypothalamic thermostat to a high level. The increase in temperature is largely due to increased metabolic activity. When production of pyrogen stops (or pathogen attack stops), the thermostat resets to normal and fever ends. Although fever typically presents in a setting of infectious disease, it may be difficult to distinguish from heatstroke, particularly if there is no history available and CNS signs are apparent. If you are unsure of diagnosis, treat for heatstroke. Treatment for fever should be undertaken when the patient is uncomfortable or when a child has a history of febrile seizures. Remove extra layers of clothing or bedclothes to allow body cooling. Consider use of an antipyretic agent such as acetaminophen or ibuprofen. Acetaminophen is available in rectal suppository form if vomiting is a concern. Note that sponge baths and cool-water immersion should not be used because they can cause a rapid drop in temperature with reflex shivering and increase in body temperature.

13. **Describe the contribution of dehydration to the development of heat disorders.** p. 1415

Dehydration often accompanies heat disorders because it inhibits vasodilation and heat dissipation (thermolysis). Dehydration leads to orthostatic hypotension and the following symptoms: nausea, vomiting, abdominal distress, vision disturbances, decreased urine output, poor skin turgor, and signs of hypovolemic shock. These may present along with the signs and symptoms of heatstroke. When assessment suggests dehydration, rehydration is critical. IV fluids may be needed, especially when the patient has altered mental status or is nauseated. An adult with moderate to severe dehydration may require 2 to 3 liters of IV fluids or more.

14. **Describe the differences between classical and exertional heatstroke.** p. 1414

Heatstroke is often divided into two types: classic and exertional. In classic heatstroke, the patient probably has chronic disorders, and increased core body temperature is due to deficient thermoregulatory function. Predisposing conditions include age, diabetes, and other medical conditions. In classic heatstroke, hot, red, dry skin is common. In contrast, exertional heatstroke often occurs in persons in good general health, and the increased core body temperature is due to overwhelming heat stress. Contextually, there is excessive ambient temperature, excessive exertion, prolonged exposure, and poor acclimatization. In exertional heatstroke, skin may well be moist from prior sweat. If heatstroke is tied to exertion, you may find severe metabolic acidosis caused by lactic acid accumulation. Hyperkalemia may also develop due to release of potassium from injured muscle cells, renal failure, or metabolic acidosis.

15. Identify the fundamental thermoregulatory difference between fever and heatstroke. p. 1415

The fundamental difference is that the trigger for temperature disruption is endogenous (internal) in fever and exogenous (external) in heatstroke. In fever, the hypothalamic thermostat is actually reset to a high level by pyrogens, substances associated with infection and the body's responses to it. The thermostat resets to the normal level when pyrogens disappear from the body. In heatstroke, exposure to high ambient temperatures depletes the body of the materials necessary for compensation (such as water and electrolytes for perspiration) and then causes the hypothalamic thermoregulatory processes to be lost. The ensuing uncompensated hyperthermia, with very high core body temperatures, begins the process of organ damage (if untreated) with potential for death.

16. Discuss the role of fluid therapy in the treatment of heat disorders. pp. 1412, 1413, 1414

Objective 13 discusses the role of dehydration in heat disorders. Because dehydration plays an increasingly significant role in heat cramps, heat exhaustion, and heatstroke, rehydration becomes increasingly pivotal to treatment success. Remember in milder forms of heat disorders, such as heat cramps, that the patient's perception of thirst is a poor indication of the degree of dehydration present. Fluid, whether it is administered orally or IV, is important in restoring the body's thermolytic abilities. In heat exhaustion and heatstroke, replacement of fluid (often by IV due to patient nausea, inability to swallow, or inability to take in fluids orally fast enough to be successful) is critical. Remember that an adult with moderate to severe dehydration can require 2 or 3 liters or more of replacement fluid.

17. Describe the pathophysiology, predisposing factors, signs, symptoms, and management of the following:

a. hypothermia pp. 1416–1422

Hypothermia is defined as a state of low core body temperature, which can be due to inadequate heat generation, excessive cold stress, or a combination of both. Hypothermia can be discussed in several contexts. First, it can be mild (core temperature greater than 90°F or 32°C) or severe (core temperature less than 90°F). In both forms signs and symptoms of hypothermia are present. Onset of symptoms can be acute (falling through ice into a lake), subacute (hikers trapped on a mountain during a winter snowstorm), or chronic (homeless individuals living outdoors during the winter). In many cases of acute and subacute hypothermia, the individual may not have any underlying predisposing factors for hypothermia: The pathophysiology of hypothermia rests on exposure to unsurvivable cold (as in the example of falling in the lake) or extended exposure to very cold conditions (the hiking example). In both settings, the body's ability for thermogenesis is simply overwhelmed. In other cases, an individual with impaired capacity for compensation is exposed to normal or cool conditions and develops hypothermia when a healthy individual would not or develops hypothermia before a healthy person would do so. Medical conditions that predispose to hypothermia include inadequately treated hypothyroidism, which depresses the body's metabolic rate; brain tumors or head trauma, which may impair hypothalamic function; as well as myocardial infarction, diabetes, hypoglycemia, drugs, poor nutrition, sepsis, or very young or old age.

Signs and symptoms of hypothermia are given in Table 36-2 (text page 1418). Your assessment of an individual with mild hypothermia will likely reveal lethargy; shivering; lack of coordination; pale, cold, dry skin; and an early rise in blood pressure, heart rate, and respiratory rates. In severe hypothermia, you may find no shivering, loss of voluntary muscle control, hypotension, and an unpredictable pulse and respiration. On the ECG, you may find dysrhythmias. The most common presenting dysrhythmia is atrial fibrillation. With progressive cooling of the body core, a variety of dysrhythmias may appear, with eventual bradycardia or asystole. Note: The severely hypothermic patient requires assessment of pulse and respirations for at least 30 seconds every 1 to 2 minutes. Management includes: (1) removal of wet garments; (2) protection against further heat loss and wind chill (calling for passive external warming with blankets, moisture barriers, etc.); (3) maintenance of patient in horizontal position; (4) avoidance of rough handling, which can trigger dysrhythmias; (5) monitoring of core temperature; and (6) monitoring of cardiac rhythm. Persons with mild hypothermia may be rewarmed with active external techniques such as warmed blankets or heat packs. In contrast, active rewarming of the severely hypothermic patient is best carried out in the hospital because of the possibility of complications such as ventricular fibrillation. If transport to the hospital will require more than 15 minutes, you may need to begin active rewarming in the field. Beware of rewarming shock and cold diuresis, both of which are discussed on text page 1421. As a final aid in putting the pieces of hypothermia care together, review the algorithm on text page 1420.

b. superficial and deep frostbite pp. 1422–1423

Frostbite is an environmentally induced freezing of body tissues. As tissues freeze due to the excessive cold, ice crystals form within cells and water is drawn from cells into the extracellular space. As the ice crystals expand, cells are destroyed. Damage to blood vessels from ice crystal formation causes loss of vascular integrity, which results in further tissue swelling and loss of distal blood flow. Peripheral tissues are more exposed to cold and thus more likely to be involved in frostbite. Thus, frostbite is largely seen in the extremities and in areas of the head and face. Predisposing factors are the same as those for hypothermia, and they are discussed with objective 10. The role of predisposing factors is often straightforward in terms of pathophysiology. A patient with diabetes, for instance, may have impaired peripheral circulation, and this relatively low flow of warm blood may make the extremities more vulnerable to frostbite. Two types of frostbite are defined based on the extent of tissue freezing: superficial and deep frostbite. Superficial frostbite (also called frostnip) involves some freezing of epidermal tissue, resulting in initial redness followed by blanching and diminished sensation. Deep frostbite involves both the epidermal and subcutaneous layers; there is a white, hardened appearance. Sensation is lost. Subfreezing temperatures are necessary for frostbite (otherwise, cellular water wouldn't freeze) but are not necessary for hypothermia. You will find that many patients with frostbite also do have hypothermia. You will also find that there is tremendous variation in presentation of frostbite. Some patients will feel little pain at the outset, whereas others will complain of bitter pain. Physical exam is a better indicator of the extent of frostbite. In superficial frostbite, there will be some degree of compliance felt beneath the frozen layer upon palpation; in deep frostbite, the frozen part will be hard and noncompliant. Treatment involves the following steps. First, do not thaw the affected area if there is any possibility of refreezing and do not massage the frozen area or rub with snow. Both may result in more extensive damage. Do administer analgesia prior to thawing, and do transport to the hospital for rewarming by immersion. If transport will be delayed, thaw the frozen part in a 102–104°F water bath. Water will need to be changed frequently as it cools. Do cover the thawed part with loosely applied, dry, sterile dressings and elevate and immobilize the thawed part. Do not puncture or drain blisters, and do not rewarm frozen feet if they are required for walking out of a hazardous situation.

c. near-drowning pp. 1423–1426

Near-drowning is defined as submersion that is survived for at least 24 hours. The pathophysiology parallels that of drowning. Following submersion, a conscious person will have complete apnea for up to 3 minutes as an involuntary reflex as he struggles to keep his head above water, and during this period blood is shunted to the heart and brain. During apnea, $PaCO_2$ will rise to greater than 50 mmHg while PaO_2 falls to less than 50 mmHg. The hypoxic stimulus eventually overrides the sedative effects of the hypercarbia, resulting in CNS stimulation. While conscious, the panicky victim typically swallows a lot of water, stimulating severe laryngospasm and bronchospasm. Especially in near-drowning victims, this effect prevents significant influx of water into the lungs (and is thus termed a dry drowning or near-drowning). Another effect of laryngospasm is worsening hypoxia, which causes a deepening coma. Morbidity or delayed mortality in near-drowning is primarily due to asphyxia from airway obstruction secondary to water in the airways (if a wet event) or laryngospasm and bronchospasm (if a dry near-drowning). Water in the lungs of a near-drowning survivor may cause lower-airway disease. A number of factors affect survival, and these include the cleanliness of the water, the duration of submersion, and the age and general health of the victim. Children have a longer survival time and a greater probability of successful resuscitation. Most significant is water temperature. In general, the colder the water, the greater the chance for survival. Usually, you expect brain death after 4 to 6 minutes without oxygen. However, some patients in cold water (below 68°F) may be resuscitated after 30 minutes or more in cardiac arrest. A possible physiologic factor in this phenomenon is the mammalian diving reflex. When a person dives into cold water, the submersion of the face inhibits breathing, drops heart rate, and causes vasoconstriction in tissues relatively resistant to asphyxia even as blood flow to the heart and brain continue. The colder the water, the greater the shunting of blood to brain and heart. This is the origin of the saying "the cold water drowning victim is not dead until he is warm and dead."

Field treatment for near-drownings in either saltwater or freshwater is similar: The first goal is to correct the profound hypoxia. Treatment includes the following steps: Remove the patient from the water. If possible, initiate ventilation while the victim is still in the water. Note that both steps require a trained, equipped rescue swimmer. Suspect head and neck injury if there was a fall or a dive involved; rapidly place victim on long backboard and use C-spine precautions. Then, protect from heat loss by removing wet clothing, laying the patient on a warm surface, and covering the body to the extent possible. The remaining steps are familiar to all resuscitations: Examine for airway patency, breathing, and pulse. If needed, begin CPR and defibrillation. Manage the airway as needed with suctioning and airway adjuncts. Administer 100 percent oxygen. Use respiratory rewarming, if available and if transport time will exceed 15 minutes. Establish an IV of lactated Ringer's or normal saline for venous access and run at 75 mL/hr. Follow ACLS protocols if the patient is normothermic. If hypothermic, the patient should be treated for hypothermia as discussed in the text. Note: Resuscitation is NOT indicated if immersion is known to have been extremely prolonged (unless hypothermia IS present) or if there is evidence of decomposition. All near-drowning victims should be admitted for observation for possible late complications including adult respiratory distress syndrome (ARDS).

d. decompression illness   pp. 1428, 1429–1431

Decompression illness, or the bends, is due to nitrogen bubbles coming out of solution in the blood and tissues, causing increased pressure on various body structures and occluding circulation in small blood vessels. This occurs in joints, tendons, the spinal cord, skin, brain, and inner ear. The trigger is a rapid ascent after exposure to a depth of 33 feet or more for a time sufficient to allow body tissues to become saturated with nitrogen. Predisposing factors for the individual include older age, obesity, fatigue, alcohol consumption before or after dive, and a history of medical problems. General factors are cold water diving, diving in rough water, strenuous diving conditions, history of previous decompression incident, overstaying time at a given dive depth, diving at 80 feet or more, too rapid an ascent, heavy exercise before or after dive, flying after diving (within 24 hours), or driving to high altitude after dive. Signs and symptoms include joint and abdominal pain, fatigue, paresthesia, and CNS disturbances. If the nitrogen bubbles occlude blood flow such that areas of local ischemia develop, tissue damage may occur.

Patients with decompression illness usually seek treatment within 12 hours of ascent, but some may not seek help until 24 hours afterward. Early oxygen therapy may reduce symptoms substantially, and divers who are given high-concentration oxygen have a significantly better treatment outcome. Prehospital management includes a number of steps. First, assess ABCs and administer CPR, if needed. Administer oxygen at 100 percent concentration with a nonrebreather mask. Intubate if the patient is unconscious. Keep the patient in a supine position and protect him or her from excessive heat or cold, wetness, or noxious fumes. If the patient is conscious and alert, give nonalcoholic liquids such as fruit juice or oral balanced salt solutions. Evaluate and stabilize the patient at the nearest emergency department prior to transfer to a recompression chamber for definitive therapy. Begin IV fluid replacement with electrolyte solutions if the patient is unconscious or seriously injured, otherwise use lactated Ringer's solution. DO NOT use 5 percent dextrose in water. If there is evidence of CNS involvement, give dexamethasone, heparin, or diazepam as instructed by medical direction. If air evacuation is used, cabin pressure must be maintained at sea level to avoid worsening of the illness. Be sure to send the diving equipment for examination, if possible.

e. diving emergency   pp. 1427–1433

The underlying physiology of diving emergencies is based on dissolution of gases in water, specifically, oxygen, carbon dioxide, nitrogen, and other gases dissolved in a diver's blood and body tissues. Pressure increases during descent, causing more gas to dissolve. During ascent, decreasing pressure allows gases to come out of solution, and they are eliminated gradually through respiration. If ascent is too rapid, however, dissolved gases, primarily nitrogen, come out of solution and expand in volume quickly, forming bubbles in the blood, brain, spinal cord, inner ear, muscles, and joints. Scuba diving injuries are due to barotrauma (changes in pressure), pulmonary overpressure, arterial gas embolism, decompression illness, cold, panic, or a combination. Accidents generally occur at one of four phases of the dive: on the surface, during descent, at the bottom, or during ascent. Risk factors at the surface include presence of lines or kelp in which a diver can become entangled, cold water, which might induce shivering or even blackout, and boats or other large objects in the area. Barotrauma during descent is a factor in emergencies occurring during that period. If the diver cannot equilibrate the pressure between the nasopharynx and middle ear, he or she can experience severe pain, ringing in the ears, dizziness, and hearing loss, any of which can cause disorientation or panic, leading to an emergency. A similar problem of disequilibration can occur in the sinuses, producing frontal headache or pain below the eyes. Emergencies at the bottom often involve nitrogen narcosis, a state of stupor commonly called "rapture of the deep." Other emergencies occur when a diver begins to run out of oxygen and panics. Injury during ascent can involve barotrauma or decompression illness. The most serious form of barotrauma is pulmonary overpressure, a condition in which expansion of air within the alveoli is greater than the tissue can handle and rupture of alveoli occur. If this occurs, the lung sustains structural damage and air entering the circulatory system can cause an arterial gas embolism. Pneumomediastinum (air in the mediastinum) and pneumothorax can also occur.

In a diving emergency, gather all evidence of air embolism and decompression illness together. Specific questions center on the timing and nature of the phases of the dive, as well as the diver's experience and state of equipment. Signs and symptoms of pulmonary overpressure include substernal chest pain, respiratory distress, and diminished breath sounds. Treatment is the same as for pneumothorax of any other origin (see Chapter 27, "Pulmonology"). The signs and symptoms of arterial gas embolism (AGE) begin within 2 to 10 minutes of ascent with a rapid, dramatic onset of sharp tearing pain and other symptoms related to the specific organ system affected by lack of blood flow. The most common presentation resembles that of a stroke, with confusion, vertigo, visual disturbances, and loss of consciousness. Presentation may include hemiplegia as well as cardiopulmonary collapse. The key to diagnosis is the history of the dive. Treatment after assessment of ABCs includes use of 100 percent oxygen via nonrebreather mask, placement of patient in supine position, frequent monitoring of vitals, IV fluids at a keep-vein-open rate, and use of a corticosteroid if ordered by medical direction. Transport to a recompression chamber as rapidly as possible under conditions that keep air pressure at that of sea level. Pneumomediastinum produces substernal chest pain, irregular pulse, abnormal heart sounds, reduced blood pressure and narrow pulse pressure, and change in voice. Cyanosis may or may not be present. Field management includes use of high-concentration oxygen via nonrebreather mask, IV with lactated Ringer's or normal saline per medical direction, and transport to an emergency department. Nitrogen narcosis causes the same concerns regarding mental and physical function as present with any other type of intoxication, with the addition of a person's functioning underwater during a dive. Altered level of consciousness and impaired judgment are key in assessment. Treatment involves return to shallow depth as this produces self-resolution.

Less frequent diving problems include oxygen toxicity due to prolonged exposure to high partial pressures of oxygen, hyperventilation, and hypercapnia due to inadequate clearance of carbon dioxide through the breathing equipment. Oxygen toxicity can lead to lung damage or even seizures. Hyperventilation due to excitement or panic may lead to muscle cramps or even decreased level of consciousness. Hypercapnia may also lead to unconsciousness. Finally, poorly prepared air tanks may be contaminated with other gases, which can increase the risk of hypoxia, narcosis, and accidental injury.

f. altitude illness pp. 1433–1436

In contrast to diving emergencies, high altitude illnesses are due to decreased ambient pressure creating a low-oxygen environment. As barometric pressure decreases at higher altitudes, lower oxygen availability can both trigger related disorders and aggravate existing medical conditions such as angina, congestive heart failure, COPD, and hypertension. Even in very healthy individuals, rapid ascent to high altitudes without time for acclimatization can cause illness. It is difficult to predict who will be affected by altitude illness: The predictor is hypoxic ventilatory response. There are two medications that may act to prevent altitude illness: acetazolamide and nifedipine. High altitude illness begins to be manifest at approximately 8,000 ft (2,400 m) above sea level. Aspen, Colorado is located at 2,438 m, and it has 26 percent less oxygen per volume of air than at sea level. The range considered high altitude is 4,900–11,500 ft. Here, the hypoxic environment causes decreased exercise tolerance, although without major disruption of normal oxygen transport in the blood. The range for very high altitude is 11,500–18,000 ft, and this causes extreme hypoxia during exercise or sleep. Extreme altitude (greater than 18,000 ft) will cause severe illness in virtually everyone. Some signs and symptoms of altitude illness include malaise, anorexia, headache, sleep disturbance, and respiratory distress that worsens with exertion. Specific disorders include acute mountain sickness, high altitude pulmonary edema, and high altitude cerebral edema.

Acute mountain sickness (AMS) usually manifests in an unacclimatized person who ascends rapidly to an altitude of 2,000 m (6,600 ft) or higher. Signs and symptoms include lightheadedness, breathlessness, weakness, headache, and nausea and vomiting. More serious signs can develop, especially if the person continues to ascend: weakness to the point of requiring assistance to dress and eat, severe vomiting, decreased urine output, shortness of breath, and altered level of consciousness. Mild AMS is self-limiting and often improves in 1 to 2 days if no further ascent occurs. Treatment for AMS consists of halting ascent or possibly lowering altitude, use of acetazolamide and antinauseants as needed. Supplemental oxygen will relieve symptoms but is typically used only in severe cases. Definitive treatment for all high altitude illnesses is descent.

High altitude pulmonary edema (HAPE) results from increased pulmonary pressure and hypertension caused by changed blood flow in higher altitude. Children are most susceptible, and men are more susceptible than women. Initial symptoms include dry cough, mild shortness of breath on exertion, and slight crackles in the lungs. Symptoms of progression include severe dyspnea and cyanosis, coughing productive of frothy sputum, and weakness that may progress to coma and death. In its early stages, HAPE is completely reversed by descent and use of oxygen. If immediate descent is not possible, oxygen can completely reverse HAPE but requires 36 to 72 hours to do so. Such a supply is rarely available to mountain climbers. An alternative is a portable hyperbaric bag, the use of which simulates a descent of roughly 5,000 ft. Acetazolamide may decrease symptoms. Other medications such as morphine, nifedipine, and furosemide may be useful but carry risk for complications such as hypotension and dehydration.

The exact cause of high altitude cerebral edema (HACE) is unknown. It usually presents as deteriorating neurological status in a patient with AMS or HAPE. The increased fluid in the brain tissue causes increased intracranial pressure. Symptoms include altered mental status, ataxia, decreased level of consciousness, and coma. If descent isn't possible, oxygen and steroids and a hyperbaric bag may help.

If coma develops, it may persist for days after descent to sea level, but it usually resolves, although it may leave residual disability.

18. Identify differences between mild, severe, chronic, and acute hypothermia. p. 1417

As discussed with objective 17a, mild hypothermia is defined by a core temperature greater than 90°F (32°C) in the presence of signs/symptoms of hypothermia, whereas severe hypothermia is defined as core temperature less than 90°F in the presence of signs/symptoms of hypothermia. Acute hypothermia involves sudden exposure to a cold environment as can happen when someone falls through the ice on a frozen lake. Chronic hypothermia may occur in predisposed persons in ambient temperatures inadequately cold to produce hypothermia in a healthy, appropriately dressed individual. In the United States, look for it among homeless persons who have endured frequent and prolonged cold stress outdoors.

19. Discuss the impact of severe hypothermia on standard BCLS and ACLS algorithms and transport considerations. pp. 1419–1422

Severe hypothermia (core temperature less than 86°F or 30°C) mandates a switch from passive rewarming and some degree of active external rewarming to active internal rewarming, which may include use of warm IV fluids; warm, humid oxygen; peritoneal lavage; extracorporeal rewarming; and esophageal rewarming tubes. If pulse or breathing is absent, severe hypothermia mandates continuance of CPR but withholding of IV fluids and limitation of electrical conversion to three times maximum. There are also specific considerations for resuscitation when core temperature is 86°F or less (discussed on text pages 1419–1422). Drug metabolism in the severely hypothermic patient is significantly decreased, and levels may accumulate that will become toxic when the patient is rewarmed. In addition, it may not be possible to electrically defibrillate a heart that is at a temperature less than 86°F.

20. Differentiate between freshwater and saltwater immersion as they relate to near-drowning. p. 1424

There are differences between freshwater and saltwater near-drowning because of the difference in the salt content of the water. You should know, however, that although the pathophysiology is different, there is no difference in the end result or in field management. In freshwater settings, a massive amount of hypotonic water diffuses across the alveolar/capillary interface, resulting in hemodilution, an expansion in blood plasma volume with relative reduction in erythrocyte concentration. Hemodilution produces a thickening of the alveolar walls with inflammatory cells, hemorrhagic pneumonitis, and destruction of surfactant. Surfactant is the lipid substance secreted by lung cells that regulates surface tension on the fluid lining the alveoli, helping to keep them open. Loss of surfactant leads to fluid buildup in the small airways with atelectasis. Because some blood flowing through the lungs is now not oxygenated, hypoxemia results. Saltwater settings are different because the ambient water is hypertonic to that in the body. Thus, water is drawn from the bloodstream into the alveoli, producing pulmonary edema and profound shunting. Hypoxemia again results. In addition, saltwater near-drownings feature respiratory and metabolic acidosis due to retention of carbon dioxide and the development of anaerobic metabolism.

21. Discuss the incidence of "wet" versus "dry" drownings and the differences in their management. p. 1424

While conscious, the panicky victim typically swallows a lot of water into the stomach, stimulating severe laryngospasm and bronchospasm. Especially in near-drowning victims, this effect prevents significant influx of water into the lungs (and is thus termed a dry drowning or dry near-drowning). Another effect of laryngospasm is worsening hypoxia, which causes a deepening coma. Morbidity or delayed mortality in near-drowning is primarily due to asphyxia from airway obstruction secondary to water in the airways (if a wet event) or laryngospasm and bronchospasm (if a dry near-drowning). Water in the lungs of a near-drowning survivor may cause lower-airway disease. Dry drownings occur in about 10 percent of drowning victims, which means wet drownings are by far more common.

22. Discuss the complications and protective role of hypothermia in the context of near-drowning. pp. 1423, 1424

In general, the colder the water, the greater the patient's chance for survival. Usually, you expect brain death after 4 to 6 minutes without oxygen. However, some patients in cold water (below 68°F) may be resuscitated after 30 minutes or more in cardiac arrest. A possible physiologic factor in this phenomenon is the mammalian diving reflex. When a person dives into cold water, the submersion of the face inhibits breathing, drops heart rate, and causes vasoconstriction in tissues relatively resistant to asphyxia even as blood flow to the heart and brain continues. The colder the water, the greater the shunting of blood to brain and heart. This is the origin of the saying "the cold water drowning victim is not dead until he is warm and dead."

23. Define self-contained underwater breathing apparatus (scuba). p. 1426

Scuba is the commonly known abbreviation for self-contained underwater breathing apparatus, a portable system that contains compressed air that is delivered to a diver so he or she can breathe underwater.

24. Describe the laws of gases and relate them to diving emergencies and altitude illness.   pp. 1426–1427

Three laws pertaining to the behavior of gases under different physical conditions relate to environmental emergencies.

- Boyle's law states that a volume of gas is inversely proportional to its pressure when temperature remains constant. As you increase pressure (as happens during a dive), gas is compressed into increasingly smaller volumes. One liter of air at the surface fills 500 mL at 33 feet of water depth, and the same one liter fills only 250 mL at 66 feet. As a diver ascends, pressure decreases toward that at the surface and the gas present in tissues and in the blood expands to occupy ever greater volumes. The reason controlled ascent is so important is that the sudden dissolution of gas into bubble form associated with rapid ascent causes occlusion of small blood vessels, the disorder known as decompression illness. With increasing altitudes, the gas molecules in air expand to occupy an increasingly larger volume, and thus a lungful of air contains even less gas (including oxygen), and hypoxemia and tissue hypoxia can result.
- Dalton's law states that the total pressure of a mixture of gases (such as air) is equal to the sum of the partial pressures of each individual gas. Air is roughly 78 percent nitrogen, 21 percent oxygen, and 1 percent carbon dioxide and other trace gases. As altitude changes (upward or downward), those proportions remain the same. The fraction of oxygen in air does not change.
- Henry's law states that the amount of a gas dissolved in a given volume of fluid is proportional to the pressure of the gas above it. This law is most relevant to diving. As a person descends to greater depths, oxygen is increasingly used up in cellular metabolism, whereas nitrogen, which is inert, does not change in quantity. Instead, it dissolves into body water. As the person ascends, those gases (particularly nitrogen, because it is present in the greatest amount) come out of the blood and tissues and form bubbles. The correct rate of ascent allows the gas to form bubbles at a rate for which the body can compensate.

25. Differentiate between the various diving emergencies.   pp. 1427–1428

See the discussion with objective 17e. Briefly, one disorder, nitrogen narcosis, is unrelated to change in pressure (barotrauma). Instead, it reflects the sedative and intoxicating effect of nitrogen on the CNS. Disorders related to barotrauma include decompression illness during rapid ascent, in which nitrogen bubbles forming in blood and other body fluids cause severe pain and the possibility of areas of ischemia secondary to occlusion of small blood vessels by bubbles. Lung overinflation associated with rapid ascent can cause pulmonary overpressure accidents, in which air expansion can rupture alveoli, resulting in hemorrhage and reduced oxygen and carbon dioxide transport, as well as complications due to air leakage.

26. Identify the various conditions that may result from pulmonary overpressure accidents.   pp. 1428, 1431

Lung overinflation associated with rapid ascent can cause pulmonary overpressure accidents, in which air expansion can rupture alveoli, resulting in hemorrhage and reduced oxygen and carbon dioxide transport, as well as air leakage into the mediastinum, a condition termed pneumomediastinum. Another condition associated with pulmonary overpressure is arterial gas embolism (AGE), in which a large bubble of free air can enter the circulation, travel through the left side of the heart, and eventually lodge at some point in the systemic circulation, setting up the possibility of cardiac, pulmonary, or cerebral compromise.

27. Describe the function of the Divers Alert Network (DAN) and how its members may aid in the management of diving-related illnesses.   p. 1433

The Divers Alert Network (DAN) serves as a nonprofit consultant for diving-related health concerns, and it can be contacted through Duke University Medical Center in North Carolina. There are both emergency (919-684-8111) and nonemergency (919-684-2948) telephone numbers.

28. **Describe the specific function and benefit of hyperbaric oxygen therapy for the management of diving accidents.** pp. 1429–1430

Decompression illness may require recompression, which can be accomplished by placing the patient in a hyperbaric oxygen chamber (a chamber in which pressure of oxygen is maintained at greater-than-atmospheric levels). In this setting, nitrogen redissolves, relieving the illness. Controlled decompression then allows the nitrogen to come out of solution and be eliminated without forming bubbles. Arterial gas embolism also requires prompt treatment in a recompression chamber so the air embolism can dissolve, relieving the ischemia associated with its occlusion of a blood vessel. These are the only diving-related conditions for which hyperbaric oxygen is standard. In some cases, it may also be required for patients with pulmonary overpressure.

29. **Define acute mountain sickness (AMS), high altitude pulmonary edema (HAPE), and high altitude cerebral edema (HACE).** pp. 1434–1436

- Acute mountain sickness (AMS) represents sudden-onset hypoxia in a person unacclimatized to their current altitude. Signs and symptoms are generally mild and the illness often resolves spontaneously within 1 to 2 days of living at the higher altitude. AMS usually develops after a rapid ascent to an altitude of 2,000 m (6,600 ft) or higher.
- High altitude pulmonary edema (HAPE) is a more serious condition caused by increased pulmonary pressure and hypertension due to altitude-induced changes in blood flow. Either immediate descent or 36 to 72 hours of supplemental oxygen usually relieves the condition.
- High altitude cerebral edema (HACE) reflects increased intracranial pressure due to increased fluid in the brain. The pathophysiologic mechanism is unclear. Even with proper treatment, residual disability may result if coma developed before definitive treatment (descent, oxygen, steroids) could improve the patient's condition.

30. **Discuss the symptomatic variations presented in progressive altitude illnesses.** pp. 1434–1436

The symptoms associated with AMS are so mild that the patient may never request treatment, and they resemble those associated with severe overexertion (in both cases because the root cause is insufficient oxygen and stressed body systems). In HAPE, symptoms of similar severity (cough, shortness of breath on exertion) progress to those of a clearly serious illness: dyspnea, possibly with cyanosis, and coughing productive of frothy sputum. Weakness can progress to coma. The presentation of HACE may follow presentation of AMS or HAPE. The presentation of HACE itself reflects the progressive neurologic deterioration associated with increased intracranial pressure: altered mental status and decreasing level of consciousness, ataxia, and coma.

31. **Discuss the pharmacology appropriate for the treatment of altitude illnesses.** pp. 1435–1436

If AMS requires medication, treatment usually consists of acetazolamide and antinauseants such as prochlorperazine. Supplemental oxygen will relieve symptoms but is usually reserved for severe cases. HAPE in its early stages can be treated with rapid descent and supplemental oxygen. If descent is not an option, oxygen in combination with a portable hyperbaric bag is useful; pharmacological adjuncts include acetazolamide, morphine, nifedipine, and furosemide. Acetazolamide carries the least risk for complications. HACE is treated with descent, oxygen with a hyperbaric bag, and steroids to reduce intracranial swelling.

32. **Given several preprogrammed simulated environmental emergency patients, provide the appropriate assessment, management, and transportation.** pp. 1407–1436

Attention to the ABCs is always important, and this doesn't change with environmental emergencies. The need to move the patient from the harmful environment to one conducive to recovery is special, although not unique (as with inhalation toxicological emergencies). Among the heat disorders, heatstroke is the most serious, and rapid transport is always required.

Hypothermia always requires transport to a hospital setting. The urgency in rewarming varies with the degree of hypothermia, as do some potential complications on rewarming such as cardiac dysrhythmias. Superficial and deep frostbite differ in the depth of tissue affected by freezing; care while en route to the hospital is similar. Early recognition is important to the EMS provider, but prevention is the most important of all steps.

Near-drownings require immediate care and rapid transport to the hospital. Although more than 90 percent of near-drowning patients survive without sequelae, ARDS can occur as a potentially deadly late complication. Emergencies related to air pressure (diving and altitude) can vary in severity and setting, but immediate care and removal to an appropriate environment as soon as possible are key to treatment. Again, these emergencies are better prevented than treated. Knowing what resources are available in the area is important to treating any of these types of emergencies.

Content Self-Evaluation

MULTIPLE CHOICE

_____ 1. General risk factors that predispose a person to developing an environmental illness include all of the following EXCEPT:
   A. predisposing medical conditions such as diabetes.
   B. fatigue.
   C. high levels of fluid intake.
   D. use of certain over-the-counter or prescription medications.
   E. age: either very young or old persons.

_____ 2. Homeostasis is the body's ability to maintain a steady, normal internal environment in the face of changing external conditions.
   A. True
   B. False

_____ 3. Which process is NOT one that results in body heat loss into the environment?
   A. evaporation   D. radiation
   B. convection   E. diffusion
   C. respiration

_____ 4. Which group of medications does NOT predispose a person to hyperthermia?
   A. psychotropics   D. beta-blockers
   B. antiepileptics   E. antihistamines
   C. diuretics

_____ 5. Thirst is an adequate indicator of dehydration.
   A. True
   B. False

_____ 6. Dehydration is often intimately associated with heat disorders because it inhibits peripheral vasodilation and limits sweating.
   A. True
   B. False

_____ 7. In situations where it is unclear whether the diagnosis is fever or heatstroke, always treat for both conditions.
   A. True
   B. False

518 ESSENTIALS OF PARAMEDIC CARE

_____ 8. Medical conditions that may predispose to hypothermia include all of the following EXCEPT:
   A. hypothyroidism.
   B. malnutrition.
   C. Parkinson's disease.
   D. thin body build.
   E. hypoglycemia.

_____ 9. Rewarming is not the mirror image of the cooling process.
   A. True
   B. False

_____ 10. Which is NOT appropriate as a rewarming measure for mild to moderate hypothermia?
   A. warmed blankets
   B. warmed IV fluids
   C. peritoneal lavage
   D. heat packs
   E. heat lamp

_____ 11. Management guidelines for frostbite include all of the following negatives EXCEPT:
   A. do not thaw affected area if possibility of refreezing exists.
   B. do not massage the frozen area or rub with snow.
   C. do not puncture or drain any blisters.
   D. do not warm frozen feet if patient will need to walk out of hostile environment.
   E. do not give analgesia prior to thawing.

_____ 12. The physiology of freshwater and saltwater drownings differs, and these differences contribute to differences in prognosis and field management.
   A. True
   B. False

_____ 13. Resuscitation of a drowning victim is not indicated when:
   A. respirations have ceased.
   B. cardiac asystole exists.
   C. the patient has been pulled from freezing water and is very cold himself.
   D. immersion is known to have been extremely long.
   E. head or neck injury due to trauma is evident.

_____ 14. Which gas law is most applicable to decompression illness?
   A. Boyle's law
   B. Dalton's law
   C. Henry's law
   D. Ohm's law
   E. Venturi's law

_____ 15. Which of the following might be administered IV to a near-drowning patient?
   A. plasmanate
   B. dextran
   C. lactated Ringer's
   D. D_5W
   E. hetastarch

_____ 16. One of the most severe complications of near-downing is:
   A. "the squeeze."
   B. ARDS.
   C. DAN.
   D. barotrauma.
   E. pneumomediastinum.

_____ 17. The condition whose chief signs and symptoms include altered levels of consciousness and impaired judgment is:
   A. AGE.
   B. "the squeeze."
   C. "the bends."
   D. pneumomediastinum.
   E. nitrogen narcosis.

_____ 18. The condition whose signs and symptoms include substernal chest pain, irregular pulse, abnormal heart sounds, reduced blood pressure and narrow pulse pressure, and a change in voice is:
   A. AGE.
   B. "the squeeze."
   C. "the bends."
   D. pneumomediastinum.
   E. nitrogen narcosis.

_____ 19. The condition whose signs and symptoms include altered mental status, ataxia, decreased level of consciousness, and coma is:
   A. AGE.
   B. DAN.
   C. HACE.
   D. HAPE.
   E. AMS.

_____ 20. A condition induced by reduced atmospheric pressure and related to changes in pulmonary blood flow is:
   A. AGE.
   B. DAN.
   C. HACE.
   D. HAPE.
   E. AMS.

MATCHING

Write the letter of the clinical characteristics in the space provided next to the appropriate disorder.

_____ 21. heat exhaustion

_____ 22. deep frostbite

_____ 23. high altitude cerebral edema

_____ 24. severe hypothermia

_____ 25. acute mountain sickness (early phase)

_____ 26. pulmonary overpressure

_____ 27. nitrogen narcosis

_____ 28. mild hypothermia

_____ 29. decompression illness

_____ 30. high altitude pulmonary edema

A. moderately decreased core temperature, shivering, lethargy, early rise in heart and respiratory rates

B. dry cough and dyspnea progressing to cough productive of frothy sputum and severe dyspnea

C. severe pain and CNS disturbances that develop during a rapid ascent from a dive to depth below 40 feet

D. environmentally induced freezing of skin and subcutaneous tissues with hardness on palpation, no sensation

E. altered mental status and decreasing level of consciousness, ataxia

F. substernal chest pain that develops during ascent, often from shallow depths, associated with respiratory distress and diminished breath sounds

G. lightheadedness, shortness of breath, nausea after rapid ascent to altitude of 6,600 feet or more

H. stuporous state that develops during deep dives rather than during descent or ascent

I. somewhat increased core temperature, rapid, shallow respirations, weak pulses

J. severely decreased core temperature, no shivering, hypotension, dysrhythmias, undetectable pulse and respirations

Chapter 37

Infectious Disease

Review of Chapter Objectives

After reading this chapter, you should be able to:

1. **Describe the specific anatomy and physiology pertinent to infectious and communicable diseases.** pp. 1443–1446; also see Chapter 4

   The body's first line of defense against many infectious agents is the skin. Additionally, components of the respiratory system also assist in this endeavor by creating turbulent airflow, while nasal hairs trap pathogens and mucus in the lower airways also traps and kills pathogens. Cilia in the airways move the mucus to the mouth and nose for expulsion. Other bacteria are removed from the body via feces and urine. However, there are three body systems that specifically protect against disease; these are the immune system, the complement system, and the lymphatic system.

   The immune system fights disease by protecting the body from foreign invaders in a mechanism initiated by the inflammatory response and involving white blood cells. There are two types of immune system response: cell-mediated immunity that employs T lymphocytes and humoral immunity that depends on the B lymphocytes to form antibodies. The complement system recognizes surface proteins, providing alternative pathways to combat infection. The lymphatic system is a secondary circulatory system that collects overflow fluid from tissue spaces and filters it before returning it to the circulatory system. The spleen is an essential organ of the lymphatic system whose white pulp generates antibodies and produces B and T lymphocytes, while the red pulp removes unwanted particulate matter, such as old or damaged red blood cells.

2. **Define specific terminology identified with infectious/communicable diseases.** pp. 1441–1482

   Infectious diseases are illnesses caused by infestations of biological organisms, such as bacteria, viruses, fungi, protozoans, or helminths. Microorganisms that normally reside in our bodies without causing disease are referred to as normal flora and protect us from pathogens (disease-causing organisms). Opportunistic pathogens are ordinarily nonharmful bacteria that cause disease only under unusual circumstances, such as a weakened immune system.

3. **Discuss public health principles relevant to infectious/communicable diseases.** pp. 1441–1442

   The task of public health epidemiologists is to study how infectious diseases affect populations, as well as to predict and describe how disease moves from individuals to populations and determine what the impact of the disease is on the population. Paramedics must evaluate the host (patient), what they believe to be the infectious agent, and the environment. Based on that assessment, they may opt to use more aggressive personal protective equipment. They must also consider the patient, those in the patient's environment, and the environment where the patient is being transported all to be at risk for infection.

4. **Identify public health agencies involved in the prevention and management of disease outbreaks.** p. 1442

Local agencies including hospitals, fire departments, and EMS agencies cooperate with state and local health departments to monitor and report the incidence and prevalence of disease. Additionally, there are numerous federal agencies involved in tracking the morbidity and mortality of infectious disease, as well as setting standards for workplace disease prevention and control standards. These include: the U.S. Department of Health and Human Services (DHHS) Centers for Disease Control and Prevention (CDC), the National Institute for Occupational Safety and Health (NIOSH), and the U.S. Department of Labor's Occupational Safety and Health Administration (OSHA).

5. **List and describe the steps of an infectious process.** pp. 1446–1449

The elements of disease transmission include the interactions of host, infectious agent, and environment. Infectious agents invade hosts by either direct or indirect transmission, and may be bloodborne, airborne, or transmitted by fecal-oral route. Factors that affect the likelihood that an exposed individual will become infected and then actually develop disease include correct mode of entry, virulence (strength), number of organisms transmitted, and host resistance.

6. **Discuss the risks associated with infection.** pp. 1441, 1446–1449

Infection is the presence of an agent within the host, without necessarily causing disease. Not all exposures result in transmission of microorganisms, nor are all infectious agents communicable. Risk of infection is considered theoretical if transmission is acknowledged to be possible but has not actually been reported. It is considered measurable if factors in the infectious agent's transmission and associated risks have been identified from reported data. Generally, the risk of disease transmission increases if a patient has open wounds, increased secretions, active coughing, or any ongoing invasive treatment where exposure to an infectious body fluid is likely.

7. **List and describe the stages of infectious diseases.** pp. 1446–1449

Exposure to an infectious agent may result in contamination or penetration. Penetration implies that infection has occurred, but infection should never be equated with disease. Once infected, the host goes through a latent period when he cannot transmit an infectious agent to someone else. This is followed by the communicable period when the host may exhibit signs of clinical disease and can transmit the infectious agent to another host. The time between exposure and the appearance of symptoms is known as the incubation period, which may range from a few days to months or years.

Most viruses and bacteria have antigens that stimulate the body to produce antibodies. The presence of these antibodies in the blood indicates exposure to the particular disease that they fight. This process is known as seroconversion. The window phase refers to the time between exposure and seroconversion. The disease period is the duration from the onset of signs and symptoms of disease until the resolution of symptoms or death.

8. **List and describe infectious agents, including bacteria, viruses, fungi, protozoans, and helminths (worms).** pp. 1443–1446

- Bacteria: microscopic single-celled organisms (1–20 micrometers in length) that can be differentiated by their reaction to a chemical staining process; classified by type as spheres (cocci), rods, spirals.
- Viruses: disease-causing organisms that are much smaller than bacteria and are only visible with an electron microscope; obligate intracellular parasites, they can grow and reproduce only within a host cell.
- Fungi: plantlike microorganisms, most of which are not pathogenic.
- Protozoans: single-celled parasitic organisms with flexible membranes and ability to move; rarely a cause of disease in humans, but commonly considered opportunistic pathogens in those patients with compromised immune function.

- Helminths (worms): parasitic organisms that live in or on another organism and are common causes of disease where sanitation is poor; various forms include pinworms, hookworms, trichinella.

9. Describe characteristics of the immune system. (see Chapters 4 and 31)

The immune system is the body's mechanism for defending against foreign invaders. The various cells involved in the immune response are sometimes collectively referred to as the reticuloendothelial system (RES) because their locations are so widely scattered throughout the body. *Reticulo* means network and *endothelial* refers to certain cells that line blood vessels, the heart, and various body cavities. Key to the immune system's response is the ability to differentiate "self" from "nonself." Once an invader is recognized as "nonself," a series of actions is initiated to eradicate the foreign material; this process is known as the inflammatory response. This response involves selected leukocytes (white blood cells) that attack the infectious agent in a process called phagocytosis. Neutrophils act first and then 12 to 24 hours later are followed by macrophages. The macrophages release chemotactic factors, which trigger additional immune system responses.

The complement system provides an alternative pathway to deal with foreign invaders more quickly than is accomplished through cell-mediated or humoral immunity. This system of at least 20 proteins works with antibody formation and the inflammatory reaction to combat infection by starting a cascade of biochemical events triggered by tissue injury.

10. Describe the processes of the immune system defenses, including humoral and cell-mediated immunity. (see Chapters 4 and 31)

There are two types of immune system response: cell-mediated immunity, which generates various forms of T lymphocytes that react against specific antigens, and humoral-mediated immunity, which results from antibodies (immunoglobulins) formed from mature B lymphocytes in the lymph nodes and bone marrow. Humoral immunity is responsible for the immune system properties of memory and specificity. Other classes of white blood cells, monocytes, eosinophils, basophils, and natural killer (NK) cells also participate in the general immune response. There are five classes of human antibodies: IgG—major class of immunoglobulin in the immune response; it crosses the placental barrier and thus plays an important role in producing immunity prior to birth; IgM—formed early in most immune responses; IgA—primary immunoglobulin in exocrine secretions; IgD—acts as an antigen receptor and is present on the surface of B lymphocytes; IgE—attaches itself to mast cells in the respiratory and intestinal tracts, playing a critical role in allergic reactions.

11. In specific diseases, identify and discuss the issues of personal isolation. pp. 1449–1484

Understanding the mechanism for disease transmission, as well as the relationship between infectious agent, host, and environment, will allow the EMS provider to make appropriate decisions regarding personal protection against disease. To supplement the body's natural defenses against disease, EMS providers must protect themselves against infectious exposures. Prevention is the most effective approach to infectious disease. All body fluids are possibly infectious, and universal precautions should be followed at all times.

12. Describe and discuss the rationale for the various types of personal protection equipment. pp. 1449–1453

Personal protective equipment provides an additional barrier to exposure, thus minimizing the risk of infection from bloodborne and airborne organisms. Isolating all body substances and avoiding contact with them further reduces risk of exposure. Using disposable items for patient care also decreases risk, as does exercising caution around "sharps." Thorough and vigorous hand washing also goes a long way to reduce inadvertent contamination. Dispose of biohazard wastes as proscribed by local laws and regulations. Decontaminate and disinfect infected equipment according to local SOPs and protocols.

13. Discuss what constitutes a significant exposure to an infectious agent. pp. 1453–1454

All exposures to blood, blood products, or any potentially infectious material should be immediately reported to the designated infectious disease control officer (IDCO). The nature of the exposure is assessed based on route (percutaneous, mucosal, or cutaneous), dose, and nature of the infectious agent. For instance, in the case of HIV, the highest risk exposure involves percutaneous exposure with a large volume of blood, a high antibody titer against a retrovirus in the source patient, deep percutaneous injury, or actual intramuscular injection.

14. Describe the assessment of a patient suspected of, or identified as having, an infectious/communicable disease. pp. 1454–1455

When assessing any patient, you should maintain a high index of suspicion that an infectious agent may be involved. Evaluate every environment for its suitability to transmit infectious agents and always maintain appropriate BSI.

Be alert to clues about the potential for infectious disease based on the patient's past medical history and medication use, as well as his or her chief complaint and the history of present illness. Look for general indicators of infection, such as unusual skin signs or rashes, fever, weakness, profuse sweating, malaise, or dehydration. Follow the standard format for assessing medical patients.

15. Discuss the proper disposal of contaminated supplies such as sharps, gauze, sponges, and tourniquets. pp. 1451–1452

Any patient care supplies (gauze, sponges, and tourniquets) that have been contaminated by blood or body fluids should be disposed of as biohazard waste in leakproof biohazard bags and in accordance with local protocol. Dispose of all contaminated sharps in properly labeled puncture-resistant containers.

16. Discuss disinfection of patient care equipment and areas where patient care occurred. pp. 1452–1453

Decontaminate infected equipment according to local protocols in the appropriate designated area. The decontamination process begins with the removal of surface dirt and debris using soap and water, then disinfect as appropriate, and finally sterilize if required. There are four levels of decontamination:

- low-level disinfection—appropriate for routine cleaning and removing visible body fluids
- intermediate-level disinfection—appropriate for cleaning equipment that has been in contact with intact skin
- high-level disinfection—required for all reusable devices that have come in contact with mucous membranes
- sterilization—required for all contaminated invasive instruments

17. Discuss the seroconversion rate after direct significant HIV exposure. pp. 1448–1449

HIV is detected through the presence of antibodies specific to HIV. When a person develops antibodies after exposure to a disease, his previously negative test will be positive indicating that seroconversion has taken place. The estimated probability of a health care worker becoming infected by a work-related exposure to virus-containing blood is 0.2 to 0.44 percent.

18. Discuss the causative agent, body systems affected and potential secondary complications, routes of transmission, susceptibility and resistance, signs and symptoms, patient management and protective measures, and immunization for each of the following:

- **HIV (Human immunodeficiency virus)** pp. 1447, 1451, 1556–1558
  —HIV is a retrovirus with affinity for human T lymphocytes with the CD4 marker.
  —Transmitted via blood, blood products, and body fluids, HIV enters the body through breaks in the skin, mucous membranes, eyes, or by placental transmission (13–30 percent transmission rate).

- —Destruction of the immune system leads to the development of opportunistic infections and cancers.
  - —There is no vaccine or cure, although postexposure prophylaxis with triple therapy (two reverse transcriptase inhibitors and one protease inhibitor) may be helpful.
  - —Practice BSI for all potential blood-body fluid exposures during patient care activities.
- **Hepatitis A** pp. 1447, 1459
  - —Hepatitis A virus (HAV) is transmitted by fecal–oral route. It has an incubation period of 3 to 5 weeks, with greatest probability of transmission in the latter half of that period.
  - —The disease causes inflammation of the liver (also known as viral or infectious hepatitis) evidenced by general malaise, fever, anorexia, nausea and vomiting, and possibly jaundice, although many infections are asymptomatic.
  - —Vaccines (Havrix and Vaqta) provide effective active immunization.
  - —EMS workers should employ universal precautions against bloodborne or fecal–oral transmission.
- **Hepatitis B** pp. 1447, 1459–1460
  - —Hepatitis B virus (HBV) is transmitted by direct contact with contaminated blood or body fluids and is very highly infectious. There is a 1.9 to 40 percent transmission rate via cutaneous exposure and a rate of 5 to 35 percent via needle stick. The HBV incubation period is 8 to 24 weeks.
  - —HBV causes inflammation of the liver (also known as serum hepatitis) evidenced by general malaise, fever, anorexia, nausea and vomiting, and possibly jaundice, cirrhosis, and malignancies. Some 60 to 80 percent of infections, however, are asymptomatic.
  - —Vaccines (Recombivax HB, Engerix B) provide effective immunization after completion of series of three IM injections and follow-up antibody screening.
  - —Employ universal precautions against bloodborne transmission.
- **Hepatitis C** pp. 1447, 1460
  - —Hepatitis C virus (HCV) is transmitted by direct contact with contaminated blood or body fluids.
  - —A majority of patients have chronic hepatitis C, which has the ability to cause active disease years later.
  - —HCV often causes liver fibrosis, which progresses over the years to cirrhosis.
  - —Effective vaccines do not yet exist, although there has been some success in treating disease with alpha interferon, often in combination with ribavirin.
  - —Employ universal precautions against bloodborne transmission.
- **Hepatitis D** p. 1460
  - —Hepatitis D virus (HDV) seems only to coexist with hepatitis B.
  - —HDV virus is transmitted by direct contact with contaminated blood or body fluids.
  - —HDV causes inflammation of the liver evidenced by general malaise, fever, anorexia, nausea and vomiting, and possibly jaundice, cirrhosis, and malignancies.
  - —Immunization against HBV confers immunity to HDV.
  - —Employ universal precautions against bloodborne transmission.
- **Hepatitis E** pp. 1460–1461
  - —Hepatitis E virus is transmitted, like hepatitis A, by the fecal–oral route; it is more commonly associated with contaminated drinking water.
  - —Hepatitis E causes inflammation of the liver evidenced by general malaise, fever, anorexia, nausea, and vomiting. It occurs primarily in young adults, with highest rates among pregnant women.
  - —Employ universal precautions against fecal–oral transmission.
- **Tuberculosis (TB)** pp. 1461–1463
  - —The causative bacteria of the disease is *Mycobacterium tuberculosis*.
  - —TB is commonly transmitted through airborne droplets but may also be contracted by direct inoculation through mucous membranes and broken skin or by drinking contaminated milk.
  - —The communicability of TB is variable, with an incubation period of 4 to 12 weeks, although disease usually develops from 6 to 12 months after infection.
  - —TB primarily affects the respiratory system, including a highly contagious form in the larynx, and may spread to other organ systems causing extrapulmonary TB.

—No vaccine exists, although postexposure prophylaxis is helpful.
—Protect against disease transmission by practicing universal precautions, plus donning an N95 (or HEPA) respirator, as well as employing appropriate respiratory precautions while performing CPR or intubation; masking the patient will also reduce exposure to droplet nuclei.

- **Meningococcal meningitis**   pp. 1466–1468
  —The causative organism for meningococcal meningitis is *Neisseria meningitidis*.
  —The infection asymptomatically colonizes in the upper respiratory tract of healthy individuals and then is transmitted by respiratory droplets.
  —Presentation includes fever, chills, headache, nuchal rigidity with flexion, arthralgia, lethargy, malaise, altered mental status, vomiting and seizures; characteristic petechiae rash common in pediatric cases.
  —The incubation period is from 2 to 4 days, but potentially as long as 10 days.
  —Meningococcal vaccines are available against some of the serotypes but are not routinely recommended for immunization of health care workers; postexposure drug prophylaxis is effective.
  —Practice universal precautions and use masks on self and patient.

- **Pneumonia**   pp. 1447, 1463–1464
  —Pneumonia's causative organism may be bacterial, viral, or fungal, although the most common pathogen is *Streptococcus pneumoniae*.
  —It is transmitted by airborne droplet inhalation.
  —Acute lung infection is characterized by fever, chills, dyspnea, productive cough, pleuritic chest pain, and adventitious lung sounds indicative of consolidation.
  —An effective vaccine exists for at risk populations: children under 2 years of age, adults over age 65, and anyone without a spleen. Routine vaccination of EMS personnel is not required.
  —Use of respiratory precautions is advised.

- **Severe Acute Respiratory Syndrome (SARS)***   pp. 1464–1465
  —SARS is caused by a coldlike virus.
  —It is transmitted by respiratory droplets deposited on the membranes of the mouth, nose, and eyes.
  —The incubation period is 2 to 7 days but may extend to 10 to 14 days. The patient should be considered contagious as long as he displays symptoms.
  —Signs and symptoms include those of severe respiratory distress (altered mental status, one-to-two-word dyspnea, cough, cyanosis, and hypoxia) as well as rhinorrhea, chills, myalgias, headache, and diarrhea.
  —SARS patients are treated like any patient with pneumonia and severe respiratory illness.

- **Tetanus**   pp. 1476–1477
  —*Clostridium tetani* bacillus is the causative organism.
  —Tetanus is transmitted by exposure to *C. tetani* spores, which are present in the soil, street dust, and feces. The condition is often associated with puncture wounds, deep lacerations, or injections.
  —Localized symptoms include rigidity of muscles in close proximity to wound. Generalized symptoms include pain and stiffness of the jaw that may progress to cause muscle spasm and rigidity of the entire body; respiratory arrest may result.
  —The incubation period is variable (usually 3 to 21 days, or 1 to 3 months); shorter periods are linked to more severe illness.
  —Universal precautions should afford sufficient protection, although respiratory protection and goggles are advised for intubation.
  —Vaccinations usually begin in childhood (DTP or diphtheria-tetanus toxoid, pertussis) and every 10 years thereafter; postexposure prophylaxis is often recommended.

- **Rabies**   pp. 1475–1476
  —The causative organism is the rabies virus, a member of the Rhabdovirus family and *Lyssavirus* genus, which affects the nervous system.
  —Rabies is transmitted in the saliva of an infected animal by bites, through an opening in the skin, or by direct contact with a mucous membrane. Once it enters the body, it then travels

Note: This objective is in addition to the listed DOT objectives.

along motor and sensory fibers to the spinal ganglia corresponding to the site of invasion and then to the brain, creating an encephalomyelitis that is almost always fatal.
—Rabies is characterized by a nonspecific prodrome that typically lasts 1 to 4 days (malaise, fever, chills, sore throat, myalgia, anorexia, nausea, vomiting, and diarrhea); this is followed by the encephalitic phase that begins with periods of excessive motor activity, followed by confusion, hallucinations, tetany, and seizures. Focal paralysis appears and if untreated causes death within 2 to 6 days. Attempts to drink water may produce laryngospasm, causing profuse drooling associated with hydrophobia.
—BSI precautions are appropriate and the use of masks may be prudent.
—Several options for rabies immunization are available and are recommended for animal care workers. Postexposure prophylaxis should be discussed on a case-by-case basis with a physician.

- **Hantavirus** p. 1473
  —This family of viruses is carried by rodents such as the deer mouse.
  —Transmission is primarily by inhalation of aerosols caused by the stirring up of the dried urine, saliva, and fecal droppings of these rodents. Contamination of food and autoinoculation after handling objects tainted by rodent droppings may also cause transmission.
  —Hantavirus causes hantavirus pulmonary syndrome (HPS) whose signs and symptoms include fatigue, fever, muscle aches, headaches, nausea, vomiting and diarrhea, and—after 4 to 10 days—pulmonary edema occurs. Hemodynamic compromise occurs approximately 5 days after onset.
  —There is no vaccine available.
  —Wear masks when in dusty, unoccupied buildings for extended periods of time.

- **Chickenpox** pp. 1465–1466
  —Chickenpox is caused by the varicella zoster virus (VZV) in the herpes virus family.
  —It is transmitted by airborne droplet inhalation plus direct contact with weeping lesions or contaminated linens.
  —Respiratory symptoms include malaise and low-grade fever, followed by a rash that starts on the face and trunk and progresses to the rest of the body including the mucous membranes. The fluid-filled vesicles that form the rash rupture, leaving small ulcers that scab over within a week.
  —The incubation period is from 10 to 21 days.
  —An effective vaccine exists (Varivax) and is required in some states for admission to elementary school or day care; it is also recommended for susceptible health care workers.
  —Employ universal precautions and place masks on patients. Extensive decontamination of the ambulance and any equipment used for a patient with chickenpox is strongly recommended.

- **Mumps** pp. 1447, 1469
  —The mumps virus is a member of the genus *Paramyxovirus*.
  —It is transmitted through respiratory droplets and direct contact with saliva of infected patients.
  —The infection is characterized by painful enlargement of the salivary glands. It presents as a feverish cold followed by swelling and stiffening of the parotid salivary gland in front of the ear, often bilaterally.
  —The incubation period is 12 to 25 days.
  —A mumps live-virus vaccine is available and should be administered with measles and rubella (MMR) to all children over 1 year of age.
  —Standard BSI precautions are advised; EMS personnel should not work without an established MMR immunity.

- **Rubella** p. 1470
  —The carrier is the rubella virus of the genus *Rubivirus*.
  —It is transmitted by inhalation of infective droplets.
  —Rubella is generally milder than measles. It is characterized by a low-grade fever and sore throat, and accompanied by a fine, pink rash on the face, trunk, and extremities that lasts about 3 days.
  —The incubation period is 12 to 19 days.

- —Immunization should be combined with mumps and measles (MMR) and, due to its devastating effects in a developing fetus, every woman should be immunized prior to becoming pregnant.
- —Standard BSI precautions are advised; EMS personnel should not work without an established MMR immunity.

- **Measles** pp. 1447, 1469–1470
  - —The carrier is the measles virus of the genus *Morbilli*.
  - —It is transmitted by droplet inhalation and direct contact.
  - —Known also as rubeola or hard measles, it is characterized by fever, conjunctivitis, malaise, cough, and nasopharyngeal congestion. Koplik's spots (bluish-white specks with a red halo approximately 1 mm in diameter) appear on the oral mucosa, followed within 24 to 48 hours by a maculopapular rash lasting about 6 days, moving from head to toe.
  - —The incubation period is 7 to 14 days.
  - —Immunization is 97 to 99 percent effective and is usually administered in conjunction with mumps and rubella (MMR).
  - —Standard BSI precautions are advised, along with vigilant hand washing and masks; EMS personnel should not work without an established MMR immunity.

- **Pertussis (whooping cough)** pp. 1470–1471
  - —Pertussis is caused by the bacterium *Bordetella pertussis*.
  - —It is transmitted via respiratory secretions or in an aerosolized form and is highly contagious.
  - —The disease has a three-phase clinical presentation. The catarrhal phase of 1 to 2 weeks resembles a common cold and fever. In the paroxysmal phase of 1 month or longer, fever subsides and the patient develops a mild cough that quickly becomes severe and violent. Rapid consecutive coughs are accompanied by deep high-pitched inspiration, and coughing produces copious thick mucus and may lead to increased intracranial pressure and, potentially, intracerebral hemorrhage. Finally, in the convalescent phase, the frequency and severity of the coughs decrease, and the patient is no longer contagious.
  - —The incubation period is 6 to 20 days.
  - —Mask the patient and observe standard BSI precautions, including postexposure hand washing. Booster doses of DTP (diphtheria-tetanus toxoid, pertussis) should be considered.

- **Influenza** pp. 1447, 1468–1469
  - —Influenza is caused by viruses designated types A, B, C.
  - —It is transmitted by airborne droplet inhalation, direct contact, or autoinoculation.
  - —The disease is characterized by sudden onset of chills, fever (usually of 3 to 5 days duration), malaise, muscle aches, nasal discharge, and cough that may be severe and of long duration.
  - —The incubation period is from 1 to 3 days.
  - —Immunization is available and recommended for the elderly, those who live in institutional settings, military recruits, and health care workers.
  - —Antiviral agents such as amantadine are available but are only effective against type A.
  - —Universal BSI precautions and good hand washing are recommended.

- **Mononucleosis** p. 1471
  - —The causative organism of mononucleosis is Epstein-Barr virus (EBV).
  - —It is transmitted by direct oropharyngeal contact with an infected person.
  - —Clinical presentation includes fatigue, fever, sore throat, oral discharges, and tender, enlarged lymph nodes. Splenomegaly is not uncommon.
  - —The incubation period is 4 to 6 weeks.
  - —No vaccine is available.
  - —Observe universal BSI precautions, and good hand washing practices are recommended.

- **Herpes Simplex 1 and 2** pp. 1447, 1471–1472, 1480
  - —There are two forms of herpes simplex, herpes simplex virus type 1 (HSV-1) and herpes simplex virus type 2 (HSV-2).
  - —HSV-1 is transmitted in the saliva of carriers.
  - —HSV-1 affects the oropharynx, face, lips, skin, fingers, and toes, although it can cause meningoencephalitis in newborns and aseptic meningitis in adults. Following an incubation period of 2 to 12 days, fluid-filled vesicles form that soon deteriorate to small ulcers. Lesions may be

accompanied by fever, malaise, and dehydration. Lesions usually disappear in 2 to 3 weeks but may recur throughout the patient's life.
— HSV-2 is sexually transmitted, although it may be transmitted during childbirth as the infant moves through the birth canal.
— Presentation of HSV-2 includes vesicular lesions on the genitals, rectum, anus, perineum, or mouth depending on the type of sexual activity. Females may be asymptomatic. Fever and enlarged lymph nodes often accompany initial infection. Lesions last up to several weeks and may recur throughout the patient's lifetime.
— Immunization is not available for either form.
— Universal precautions are absolutely essential, along with good hand washing.

- **Syphilis** pp. 1447, 1478–1479
  — Syphilis is caused by the spirochete *Treponema pallidum*.
  — It is transmitted by direct contact with exudates from other syphilitic lesions of the skin and mucous membranes, semen, blood, saliva, and vaginal discharges.
  — The disease has four stages: primary syphilis—painless lesion forms 3 to 6 weeks after exposure; secondary syphilis—bacteremic stage occurs 5 to 6 weeks after lesion heals; maculopapular rash on hands and feet, condyloma latum (painless wartlike lesions on warm, moist skin areas that are very infectious); latent stage—symptoms abate for months to years; tertiary syphilis—wide variety of presentations (cardiovascular, neurologic).
  — The incubation period is 3 weeks.
  — No immunization is available.
  — Universal precautions are absolutely essential along with use of good hand washing practices.

- **Gonorrhea** pp. 1447, 1448
  — Gonorrhea is caused by a gram-negative bacterium, *Neisseria gonorrhoeae*.
  — It is transmitted by direct contact with exudates of mucous membranes, primarily from direct sexual contact.
  — Presentation varies: in men, it most commonly causes dysuria and purulent discharge, then epididymitis; in women, there is commonly no pain or discharge unless it develops into pelvic inflammatory disease.
  — The incubation period is 10 to 14 days.
  — Universal precautions are absolutely essential along with use of good hand washing practices.

- **Chlamydia** p. 1480
  — Chlamydia is caused by a genus of intracellular parasites most like gram-negative bacteria, *Chlamydia trachomatis*.
  — It is transmitted by sexual activity and by hand-to-hand transfer of eye secretions; it often coexists with gonorrhea.
  — Presentation varies with symptoms in a manner similar to gonorrhea, but less severe: in men, it most commonly causes dysuria and purulent discharge, then epididymitis; women may have no pain or discharge unless it develops into pelvic inflammatory disease.
  — The incubation period is 10 to 14 days.
  — Universal precautions are absolutely essential along with use of good hand washing practices.

- **Scabies** p. 1482
  — Scabies is caused by infestation of a mite, *Sarcoptes scabiei*.
  — The condition is contracted by exposure through close personal contact, from hand holding to sexual contact. Mites remain viable on clothing or bedding for up to 48 hours.
  — Upon attaching to a new host, the female burrows into the epidermis to lay eggs within 2½ minutes. Larvae hatch shortly and are full-grown adults in 10 to 20 days. Primary symptom of the condition is intense itching.
  — The incubation period is 2 to 6 weeks after infestation. It remains communicable until all mites and eggs are destroyed.
  — No immunization is available.
  — Bag and remove all linens immediately. Decontaminate stretcher and patient compartment as for lice. Remove and decontaminate any clothing that may have contacted the patient.

- **Lice (Pediculosis)**   **pp. 1481–1482**
  - There are three varieties of infestation: *Pediculus humanus var. capitis* (head lice), *Pediculus humanus var. corporis* (body lice), and *Pthirus pubis* (pubic lice or crabs).
  - Lice are transmitted by direct contact, which may or may not be associated with sexual activity.
  - Eggs hatch within 7 to 10 days.
  - Infestation results in parasitic infection of the skin of the scalp, trunk, or pubic area, which is primarily characterized by intense itching. Red macules, papules, and urticaria commonly appear on the shoulders, buttocks, abdomen, or genital areas.
  - No immunization is available.
  - Spray the ambulance interior close to the cot and the area by the patient's head with an insecticide, preferably one containing permethrin. Wipe and clean all surfaces to remove insecticide residues.
- **Lyme disease**   **pp. 1447, 1477–1478**
  - Lyme disease is caused by the tick-borne spirochete *Borrelia burgdorferi*.
  - It is transmitted by the bite of an infected tick.
  - A flat, painless red lesion may appear at the bite site (and may appear to resemble a bull's eye). This may be accompanied by malaise, headache, and muscle aches; then the spirochete spreads to the skin, nervous system, heart, and joints. Meningitis, cardiac conduction defects, and arthritis are common. Recurrence can appear months to years after initial exposure.
  - The incubation period ranges from 3 to 32 days.
  - Immunization is available (LYMErix) as a series of three vaccinations.
  - Employ universal precautions. Also, when responding in wooded areas, check for ticks, and spray the ambulance compartment with an arthropod-effective insecticide.
- **Gastroenteritis**   **pp. 1473–1474**
  - Causative organisms for the condition may be viruses, bacteria, and parasites.
  - It is highly contagious via the fecal–oral route, including the ingestion of contaminated food or water.
  - Prolonged vomiting and diarrhea may cause dehydration and electrolyte disturbances.
  - No immunization is available.
  - Follow universal precautions and use aggressive hand washing.

19. **Discuss other infectious agents known to cause meningitis including streptococcus pneumonia, haemophilus influenza type B, and various varieties of viruses.**   **pp. 1466–1468**

Meningitis is often caused by other infectious agents, particularly *Streptococcus pneumoniae* and *Haemophilus influenzae type B*. Streptococcus is the most common cause of adult pneumonia and the leading cause of otitis media in children. Vaccines have proven to be very effective, especially in children. *Haemophilus* was once the leading cause of meningitis in children from 6 months to 3 years of age but the development of a vaccine in the early 1980s has virtually eliminated its incidence. While a variety of viruses have also been known to cause meningitis, in otherwise healthy individuals viral meningitis is a self-limited disease that lasts 7 to 10 days.

20. **Identify common pediatric viral diseases.**   **pp. 1465–1466, 1469–1471, 1472**

The most common cause of viral illness in children is respiratory syncytial virus (RSV), most commonly causing pneumonia and bronchiolitis in infants and young children. Croup and pharyngitis have also been attributed to viruses, such as the parainfluenza virus and rhinovirus. All of these are transmitted by direct inhalation of infected droplets or through exposed mucosal surfaces, as well as autoinoculation from unwashed hands after handling contaminated surfaces.

21. **Discuss the characteristics of and organisms associated with febrile and afebrile diseases including bronchiolitis, bronchitis, laryngitis, croup, epiglottitis, and the common cold.**   **pp. 1468–1473**

The common cold (viral rhinitis) is caused by any of the more than 100 serotypes of rhinovirus. Transmission is caused by direct inhalation of infected droplets or through exposed mucosal surfaces, as well as autoinoculation from unwashed hands after handling contaminated surfaces. The incubation period is from 12 hours to 5 days, with an average of 48 hours. Generally, it is a mild illness characterized by nasal congestion, rhinitis, and cough.

Bronchiolitis, bronchitis, laryngitis, croup, and epiglottitis may have bacterial or viral origins, although epiglottitis is most commonly due to *Haemophilus influenzae, Streptococcus pneumoniae,* or *Staphylococcus aureus,* while croup is usually viral.

All of these are transmitted by direct inhalation of infected droplets or through exposed mucosal surfaces, as well as autoinoculation from unwashed hands after handling contaminated surfaces.

22. Articulate the pathophysiological principles of an infectious process given a case study of a patient with an infectious/communicable disease. pp. 1441–1484

As already discussed, the interactions between a host, an infectious agent, and the environment are the elements of disease transmission. Recognizing that infectious agents invade hosts through either direct or indirect transmission, you should generally be able to determine which is applicable given the patient presentation. Your role as an EMS provider is to interrupt disease transmission while providing safe and effective care for your patient, based on your recognition of signs and symptoms and your knowledge of the physiologic priorities for emergency care.

23. Given several preprogrammed infectious disease patients, provide the appropriate body substance isolation procedure, assessment, management, and transport. pp. 1441–1484

Throughout your training, you will encounter a variety of real and simulated patients with a variety of infectious diseases. Use the information provided in your text as well as the application of this information as demonstrated by your instructors, preceptors, and mentors to enhance your ability to assess, manage, and transport these patients. Remember that prevention is the best approach and, for that reason, you should presume that every patient is potentially infectious and take appropriate precautions to minimize your exposure. Your own personal accountability in the area of infection control is equally important. Do not go to work if you have any signs or symptoms of illness, keep your immunizations up to date, and always practice effective hand washing.

Content Self-Evaluation

MULTIPLE CHOICE

_____ 1. Microscopic single-celled organisms that can be differentiated by their reaction to a chemical staining process are called:
- A. helminths.
- B. bacteria.
- C. viruses.
- D. fungi.
- E. protozoans.

_____ 2. Single-celled parasitic organisms that are a common cause of opportunistic infection are called:
- A. helminths.
- B. bacteria.
- C. viruses.
- D. fungi.
- E. protozoans.

_____ 3. All microorganisms that reside in our bodies are pathogenic.
- A. True
- B. False

_____ 4. Visible only by electron microscope, obligate intracellular parasites that resist antibiotic treatment are called:
   A. helminths.
   B. bacteria.
   C. viruses.
   D. fungi.
   E. protozoans.

_____ 5. All of the following are airborne diseases EXCEPT:
   A. meningitis.
   B. tuberculosis.
   C. measles.
   D. syphilis.
   E. influenza.

_____ 6. The presence of an infectious agent within the host, without necessarily causing disease, is referred to as:
   A. infection.
   B. contamination.
   C. communicable.
   D. exposure.
   E. virulence.

_____ 7. All of the following are factors that affect disease transmission EXCEPT:
   A. mode of entry.
   B. virulence.
   C. dose of organism.
   D. host resistance.
   E. type of organism.

_____ 8. Surface proteins on viruses and bacteria that stimulate the production of antibodies are called:
   A. pathogens.
   B. prokaryotes.
   C. antigens.
   D. prions.
   E. eukaryotes.

_____ 9. The creation of antibodies following an exposure to a disease is called:
   A. incubation.
   B. seroconversion.
   C. latency.
   D. infection.
   E. contamination.

_____ 10. Sterilization is the recommended level of decontamination for all equipment used by EMS personnel.
   A. True
   B. False

_____ 11. At the scene of a motor vehicle accident, all of the following are appropriate infection control measures EXCEPT:
   A. wearing gloves and changing them between patients.
   B. using protective eyewear or face shields to limit splash exposures.
   C. recapping needles to reduce risk of needlestick to others.
   D. decontaminating all reusable equipment.
   E. putting all contaminated dressings in a leakproof biohazard bag.

_____ 12. Risk factors for developing infectious disease include:
   A. immunosuppression.
   B. diabetes.
   C. artificial heart valves.
   D. alcoholism.
   E. all of the above

_____ 13. Which of these infectious diseases poses the greatest risk to EMS personnel as a result of work-related exposures?
   A. AIDS
   B. tuberculosis
   C. hepatitis A
   D. hepatitis B
   E. hantavirus

_____ 14. The most significant problem associated with HIV is:
   A. opportunistic infection.   D. blindness.
   B. hemorrhage.   E. splenomegaly.
   C. dementia.

_____ 15. The most common form of hepatitis transmitted by the fecal–oral route is:
   A. hepatitis A.   D. hepatitis D.
   B. hepatitis B.   E. hepatitis E.
   C. hepatitis C.

_____ 16. Primarily a respiratory disorder, the most common preventable adult infectious disease in the world is:
   A. hepatitis A.   D. pneumonia.
   B. tuberculosis. E. influenza.
   C. HIV.

_____ 17. Your 60-year-old patient reports an acute onset of high fever, chills, dyspnea, pleuritic chest pain, and a productive cough. You suspect:
   A. hantavirus.   D. pneumonia.
   B. tuberculosis. E. influenza.
   C. HIV.

_____ 18. Your patient has a low-grade fever and malaise and is covered from head to toe with fluid-filled vesicles and small ulcers. You suspect:
   A. measles.   D. meningitis.
   B. rubella.   E. scabies.
   C. chickenpox.

_____ 19. Your patient reports an acute onset of high fever, stiff neck, and severe headache. You suspect:
   A. measles.   D. meningitis.
   B. rubella.   E. scabies.
   C. chickenpox.

_____ 20. All of the following are viral infections that may be contracted in the EMS setting EXCEPT:
   A. measles.   D. meningitis.
   B. rubella.   E. scabies.
   C. chickenpox.

_____ 21. The most important personal precaution against disease transmission is:
   A. effective hand washing.
   B. up-to-date immunizations.
   C. postexposure prophylaxis.
   D. disinfection of equipment.
   E. compliance with infection control policies.

_____ 22. Your partner reports a sudden onset of fever, chills, malaise, muscle aches, nasal discharge, and a cough. You suspect:
   A. hantavirus.   D. pneumonia.
   B. tuberculosis. E. influenza.
   C. HIV.

_____ 23. All of the following are causative organisms for food poisoning EXCEPT:
   A. *Escherichia coli.*   D. *Salmonella.*
   B. *Haemophilus influenzae.* E. *Shigella.*
   C. *Campylobacter.*

_____ 24. The clinical presentation of encephalitis often mimics that of meningitis.
　　　　A. True
　　　　B. False

_____ 25. All of the following are sexually transmitted diseases EXCEPT:
　　　　A. HSV-2.　　　　　　　　D. HPV.
　　　　B. chlamydia.　　　　　　 E. gonorrhea.
　　　　C. HAV.

Psychiatric and Behavioral Disorders

Review of Chapter Objectives

After reading this chapter, you should be able to:

1. **Define behavior and distinguish among normal behavior, abnormal behavior, and the behavioral emergency.** pp. 1487–1488

   Behavior is a person's observable conduct and activity, while a behavioral emergency is a situation in which a patient's behavior becomes so unusual, bizarre, or threatening that it alarms the patient or another person and requires the intervention of EMS and/or mental health personnel. The differentiation between "normal" and "abnormal" behavior is largely subjective and widely variable based on culture, ethnic group, socioeconomic class, environment, and personal interpretation and opinion.

2. **Discuss the prevalence of behavioral and psychiatric disorders.** pp. 1487–1488

   It is estimated that 20 percent of the population has some type of mental health problem and that as many as 1 in 7 will require treatment for an emotional disturbance.

3. **Discuss the pathophysiology of behavioral and psychiatric disorders.** pp. 1488–1489

   The general causes of behavioral and psychiatric disorders are biological (organic), psychosocial, and sociocultural. Biological (organic) causes are related to disease processes or structural changes in the brain. Psychosocial causes are related to the patient's personality, dynamics of unresolved conflict, or crisis management methods. Sociocultural causes are related to the patient's actions and interactions within society. It should be noted that many psychiatric disorders are due to altered brain chemistry.

4. **Discuss the factors that may alter the behavioral or emotional status of an ill or injured individual.** pp. 1488–1489

   Remember that you cannot be sure that a patient is suffering from a purely psychological condition until you have completely ruled out medical conditions, such as hypoglycemia, traumatic injury, and substance abuse. Failure to comply with the prescribed medication regimen may cause exacerbation of a patient's psychiatric condition and lead to the development of a behavioral emergency. Societal events (rape, assault, and acts of violence) may contribute to alterations in someone's emotional status, as can interpersonal events, such as death of a loved one or loss of a relationship.

©2007 Pearson Education, Inc.
Essentials of Paramedic Care, 2nd ed.

5. **Describe the medical legal considerations for management of emotionally disturbed patients.** p. 1504

The laws of consent specify that any competent person has the right to refuse to consent to treatment. Further, no competent person may be transported against his/her will. Any person who is in imminent danger of harming him-/herself or others is not considered competent to refuse treatment and transport. Most states have laws that allow persons fitting this criterion to be transported against their will to a hospital or approved psychiatric facility for evaluation.

6. **Describe the overt behaviors associated with behavioral and psychiatric disorders.** pp. 1492–1502

Overt behaviors that may be associated with behavioral emergencies include hand gestures (clenched fists, wringing hands, and so on) or postures (cowering, visible tension, and so on) that you may observe in your patient. The patient may display strange or threatening facial expressions. The patient's speech may reveal disorientation, fixations, unrealistic judgments, or unusual thought processes. Other behaviors you may observe include pacing, picking at one's skin, or appearing to pull things from the air. There are many different kinds of such overt behaviors, and they can differ or overlap depending on the specific disorder.

7. **Define the following terms:**

- **Affect** p. 1490
  Visible indicators of mood or the impression that someone else may have about one's mood based on one's appearance. For instance, a person with a flat affect gives the appearance of being disinterested and is often lacking facial expression.
- **Anger** p. 1495
  This can be described as feelings of hostility or rage to compensate for an underlying feeling of anxiety.
- **Anxiety** p. 1494
  This is a state of uneasiness, discomfort, apprehension, and restlessness.
- **Confusion** p. 1490
  This is a state of being unclear or unable to make a decision easily.
- **Depression** p. 1495
  This is a profound sadness or feeling of melancholy.
- **Fear** p. 1490
  Fear is a feeling of alarm and discontent in the expectation of danger.
- **Mental status** p. 1490
  This is defined as the state of the patient's cerebral functioning.
- **Open-ended question** p. 1490
  This is the type of question that cannot be answered by "yes" or "no" and requires a longer response from the person being questioned.
- **Posture** p. 1489
  This term refers to the position, attitude, or bearing of the body.

8. **Describe verbal techniques useful in managing the emotionally disturbed patient.** pp. 1490–1491

The key to dealing with the emotionally disturbed patient is to listen carefully. Place yourself at the patient's level, but keep a safe and proper distance, not invading the patient's personal space. Ask open-ended questions that require your patient to respond in detail. Be comfortable with silence and take whatever time is necessary to get the whole story of the situation. Do not lie to or make fun of the patient. Be nonjudgmental.

9. **List the appropriate measures to ensure the safety of the paramedic, the patient, and others.** pp. 1489, 1504

As with any call, determining scene safety is critical. Many behavioral emergencies, for which you are dispatched, will also warrant mutual response by law enforcement personnel. Gain control of the scene. Remove anyone who agitates the patient or adds confusion to the scene. Examine the environment for signs of violence and potential weapons. Approach every situation cautiously and when feasible observe the patient from a distance first before approaching. Avoid invading the patient's personal space. Watch for signs of aggression. If a patient becomes violent, use of restraint may become necessary; in such cases, carefully follow your service's protocols for such circumstances and be sure to document your actions thoroughly.

10. **Describe the circumstances when relatives, bystanders, and others should be removed from the scene.** p. 1490

It is important to gain control of the scene as quickly as possible. Remove anyone who agitates the patient or adds to the confusion on the scene. Generally, it is a good idea to limit the number of people around the patient. You may even find it necessary to totally clear the room or to move the patient to a quiet area.

11. **Describe techniques to systematically gather information from the disturbed patient.** pp. 1490–1491, 1503–1504

Your interpersonal skills are crucial to your success as an EMS professional but never more so than when you are caring for a patient who is having a behavioral emergency. Limit environmental distractions at the scene. Introduce yourself and note how the patient responds to you, altering your approach if the patient becomes agitated. Establish eye contact. Place yourself at the patient's level. Listen carefully. Take your time. Do not physically threaten the patient. Ask open-ended questions. Be truthful with the patient and never play along with hallucinations or delusions. Focus your questioning and assessment on the immediate problem.

12. **Identify techniques for physical assessment in a patient with behavioral problems.** pp. 1489–1491, 1502–1507

All of the interpersonal skills discussed above that allow you to effectively interview patients will need to be incorporated into your physical assessment activities. Generally, the examination of a behavioral emergency patient is largely conversational. If you need to perform hands-on assessment activities, defer their completion until you have had the opportunity to establish rapport and, even then, do not make any sudden moves that may startle the patient. If a patient is restrained, be sure to monitor him or her frequently and carefully to ensure that the airway is patent and that he or she is not experiencing positional asphyxia.

13. **List situations in which you are expected to transport a patient forcibly and against his will.** p. 1504

Any person who is in imminent danger of harming him-/herself or others is not considered competent to refuse treatment and transport. Patients who are suicidal or homicidal meet this criterion. Most states have laws that allow persons fitting this criterion to be transported against their will for evaluation. The authority to make this decision varies from state to state. Other situations are not so clear-cut and require you to use clinical judgment and follow your service's protocols.

14. **Describe restraint methods necessary in managing the emotionally disturbed patient.** pp. 1504–1507

The primary objective is to restrict the patient's movement to prevent him from harming himself or others. Your own agency's rules will dictate the appropriate technique and method for restraint. The following rules always apply: use minimum necessary force; use appropriate devices; remember that restraint is not punitive; and carefully monitor anyone who is restrained. Before initiating any restraint activities, make sure that you have sufficient help, as this minimizes the potential for injury to the patient or yourself.

15. List the risk factors and behaviors that indicate a patient is at risk for suicide. p. 1501

All of the following are considered to be risk factors for suicide: previously attempted suicide, depression, age (15 to 24 years of age or over 40), substance abuse, social isolation, major separation trauma, major physical stresses, loss of independence, suicide of a parent. Also significant is having possession of a mechanism for suicide and having a specific plan and/or expressing it.

16. Use the assessment and patient history to differentiate between the various behavioral and psychiatric disorders. pp. 1489–1502

Most psychiatric disorders have two diagnostic elements: symptoms of the disease/disorder and indications that the disease/disorder has impaired major life functions or interfered with the activities of daily living. It is not the role of EMS personnel to diagnose behavioral disorders, as this can be a difficult task even for skilled mental health professionals. The overview of psychiatric disorders is intended to increase your general understanding of behavioral problems.

The most helpful thing you can do is to perform a mental status exam (MSE) as part of your routine assessment. The elements of an MSE include: general appearance, behavioral observations, orientation, memory, sensorium, perceptual processes, mood and affect, intelligence, thought processes, insight, judgment, and psychomotor ability.

17. Given several preprogrammed behavioral emergency patients, provide the appropriate scene size-up, initial assessment, focused assessment, and detailed assessment, then provide the appropriate care and patient transport. pp. 1487–1507

Throughout your training, you will encounter a variety of real and simulated patients with behavioral or psychiatric emergencies. Use the information in the text, as well as the application of this information as demonstrated by your instructors, preceptors, and mentors to enhance your ability to assess, manage, and transport patients with behavioral emergencies. Every emergency call has an element of behavioral emergency in it; your patience and professionalism will help minimize the emotional component for everyone involved.

Content Self-Evaluation

MULTIPLE CHOICE

_____ 1. Organic causes for behavioral emergencies include all of the following EXCEPT:
   A. tumor.
   B. depression.
   C. substance abuse.
   D. infection.
   E. hypoglycemia.

_____ 2. It is always safe to assume that a patient exhibiting bizarre behavior is suffering from a psychological problem or disease.
   A. True
   B. False

_____ 3. The term that describes the state of a patient's cerebral functioning is:
   A. affect.
   B. mood.
   C. mental status.
   D. orientation.
   E. sensorium.

_____ 4. The best approach for gaining information from a behavioral emergency patient is to:
   A. ask questions requiring yes or no answers.
   B. talk loudly to establish control.
   C. ask open-ended questions.
   D. physically restrain the patient before questioning.
   E. move quickly to expedite transport and then question.

_____ 5. The structured exam designed to quickly evaluate a patient's level of mental functioning is the:
   A. neurologic exam.
   B. mental status exam.
   C. psychiatric evaluation.
   D. Glasgow Coma Score.
   E. stroke assessment scale.

_____ 6. The most likely way to provoke violence or aggression in a behavioral emergency patient is to:
   A. listen carefully to his responses.
   B. appear patient and unhurried.
   C. ask open-ended questions.
   D. invade his personal space.
   E. avoid rapid or sudden movements.

_____ 7. Panic attack, phobias, and posttraumatic stress syndrome are classified as:
   A. types of schizophrenia.
   B. personality disorders.
   C. variants of depression.
   D. bipolar disorders.
   E. anxiety disorders.

_____ 8. The most prevalent form of psychiatric problem is:
   A. schizophrenia.
   B. personality disorder.
   C. depression.
   D. bipolar disorder.
   E. anxiety disorder.

_____ 9. Profound sadness, diminished ability to concentrate, and feelings of worthlessness are commonly associated with:
   A. schizophrenia.
   B. personality disorders.
   C. depression.
   D. bipolar disorders.
   E. anxiety disorders.

_____ 10. Medications commonly used in the management of schizophrenia are:
   A. antipsychotics.
   B. sedatives.
   C. antihistamines.
   D. antipsychotics and sedatives.
   E. sedatives and antihistamines.

_____ 11. Common causes of dementia include all of the following EXCEPT:
   A. Alzheimer's disease.
   B. head trauma.
   C. cardiac seizure.
   D. Parkinson's disease.
   E. AIDS.

_____ 12. Hallucinations, delusions, and disorganized thought, speech, and behavior are commonly associated with:
   A. schizophrenia.
   B. personality disorders.
   C. depression.
   D. bipolar disorders.
   E. anxiety disorders.

_____ 13. The compelling desire to use a substance, inability to reduce use of a substance, and repeated unsuccessful efforts to quit using that substance are indicators of:
   A. psychological dependence.
   B. physical dependence.
   C. substance tolerance.
   D. factitious disorder.
   E. somatoform disorder.

_____ 14. In general, which of the following restraints should the paramedic not use when physically restraining an agitated patient?
   A. sheets
   B. plastic ties
   C. wristlets
   D. chest Posey
   E. all of the above

_____ 15. When a pediatric or geriatric patient is experiencing a behavioral emergency, the paramedic should always consider using chemical restraints.
   A. True
   B. False

MATCHING

Write the letter of the word or phrase in the space provided next to its definition.

A. delirium
B. dementia
C. schizophrenia
D. delusions
E. hallucinations
F. catatonia
G. paranoid
H. bipolar disorder
I. personality disorder
J. depersonalization

_____ 16. Feeling detached from oneself

_____ 17. Condition characterized by relatively rapid onset of widespread disorganized thought

_____ 18. Fixed false beliefs

_____ 19. Condition that results in persistently maladaptive behavior

_____ 20. Sensory perceptions with no basis in reality

_____ 21. Condition characterized by one or more manic episodes, with or without subsequent or alternating periods of depression

_____ 22. Condition characterized by immobility, rigidity, and stupor

_____ 23. Common disorder involving significant behavioral changes and disorganized thought

_____ 24. Preoccupation with feelings of persecution

_____ 25. Condition involving gradual development of memory impairment and cognitive disturbance

Chapter 39

Gynecology

Review of Chapter Objectives

After reading this chapter, you should be able to:

1. **Review the anatomic structures and physiology of the female reproductive system.** (see Chapter 3)

   The most important female reproductive structures are located within the pelvic cavity. Essential to reproduction, these structures include the ovaries, fallopian tubes, uterus, and vagina. The external genitalia have accessory functions, in that they protect body openings and play an important role in sexual functioning.

2. **Identify the normal events of the menstrual cycle.** (see Chapter 3)

   A monthly hormonal cycle prepares the uterus to receive a fertilized egg. The first 2 weeks of the cycle (known as the proliferative phase) are dominated by estrogen causing the uterine lining to thicken. In response to a surge of luteinizing hormone, ovulation takes place and an egg is released from the ovary. The secretory phase is the stage of the menstrual cycle immediately surrounding ovulation. If the egg is not fertilized, the woman's estrogen level drops sharply while the progesterone level dominates. Uterine vascularity increases in anticipation of implantation. If fertilization does not occur, estrogen and progesterone levels fall, triggering vascular changes leaving the endometrium ischemic. The ischemic endometrium is shed during the menstrual phase (menstruation), along with a discharge of blood, mucus, and cellular debris. Menstrual flow usually lasts 3 to 5 days, with an average blood loss of 50 mL.

3. **Describe how to assess a patient with a gynecological complaint.** pp. 1510–1511

   The most common gynecological complaints are abdominal pain and vaginal bleeding. Complete your initial assessment in the usual manner and then proceed with a focused history and physical exam. Specific questions will need to be asked that are pertinent to reproductive function and dysfunction. If pertinent, be sure to gather information about her obstetrical history, including pregnancies and deliveries. It is important to document the date of the patient's last menstrual period (LMP). You should also ask what form of birth control, if any, she uses and, if pertinent, whether she uses it regularly. Pay particular attention to the physical exam, which will be limited to assessment of the abdomen and potentially (in the presence of serious bleeding) inspection of the patient's perineum. Gently auscultate and palpate the abdomen. Be sure to note the color, character, and volume of any blood lost. An internal vaginal exam should never be performed in the prehospital setting.

©2007 Pearson Education, Inc.
Essentials of Paramedic Care, 2nd ed.

541

4. Explain how to recognize a gynecological emergency. pp. 1510–1511

As with any emergency situation, vital signs are useful clues as to your patient's status as well as its severity. Be alert for early signs of shock or a positive tilt test, both of which point to significant blood loss. If possible, estimate blood loss. The use of two sanitary pads per hour is considered significant bleeding.

5. Describe the general care for any patient experiencing a gynecological emergency. pp. 1512, 1514, 1515

Management of gynecological emergencies is focused on supportive care. Rely on your initial assessment guidance in your decision making about oxygen therapy, ventilatory support, and vascular access. In the presence of shock, follow your local protocols for fluid resuscitation and use of the PASG. In cases of heavy bleeding, do not pack dressings in the vagina. Continue to monitor the patient's status and bleeding en route to definitive care. Equally important is the psychological support that you give your patient. Protect her modesty and privacy.

6. Describe the pathophysiology, assessment, and management of the following gynecological emergencies.

   a. Pelvic inflammatory disease pp. 1512–1513

   Pelvic inflammatory disease (PID), the most common cause of nontraumatic abdominal pain in women in the childbearing years, is an infection of the female reproductive tract that is most commonly caused by gonorrhea or chlamydia. Predisposing factors include: multiple sexual partners, prior history of PID, recent gynecological procedure, or an IUD. The patient will look acutely ill and will often present with diffuse lower abdominal pain, and may also have fever, chills, nausea, vomiting, and possibly a foul-smelling vaginal discharge. The patient may also walk with a shuffling gait due to pain. Blood pressure may be normal, and fever may or may not be present. Palpation of the lower abdomen usually elicits moderate to severe pain. The primary management in the field is supportive care and a position of comfort during transport. If the patient appears septic, then administer oxygen and initiate IV therapy.

   b. Ruptured ovarian cyst p. 1513

   Cysts are fluid-filled pockets, and, when they develop in the ovary, they can rupture and be a source of abdominal pain. The rupture spills a small amount of blood into the abdomen, irritating the peritoneum and causing abdominal pain and rebound tenderness. Usually the patient complains of moderate to severe unilateral abdominal pain that may radiate to the back; it may be associated with vaginal bleeding. The patient may also report pain during intercourse or a delayed menstrual period. The primary management in the field is supportive care and a position of comfort during transport.

   c. Cystitis p. 1513

   A bacterial infection of the urinary bladder (cystitis) is a common cause of abdominal pain that may be accompanied by urinary frequency, dysuria, and a low-grade fever. The pain is generally located just above the symphysis pubis unless the infection has spread to the kidneys, in which case there is likely to be flank pain as well. The primary management in the field is supportive care and a position of comfort during transport.

   d. Mittelschmerz p. 1513

   Mid-cycle abdominal pain may accompany ovulation. The unilateral lower quadrant pain is usually self-limited and may be accompanied by mid-cycle spotting. Treatment is symptomatic.

   e. Endometritis p. 1513

   Endometritis, an infection of the uterine lining, is an occasional complication of miscarriage, childbirth, or gynecologic procedures. Commonly reported signs and symptoms include mild to severe lower abdominal pain, a bloody and foul-smelling discharge, and fever that may mimic PID. The primary management in the field is supportive care and a position of comfort during transport. If the patient appears septic, then administer oxygen and initiate IV therapy.

   f. Endometriosis pp. 1513–1514

   Endometriosis is a condition in which endometrial tissue is found outside the uterus. Most commonly, it is found in the abdomen and pelvis. Regardless of the site, the tissue responds to the hormones of the menstrual cycle, thus bleeding in a cyclic manner. The condition is most common in women between 30 and 40 and is rare in postmenopausal women. The patient complains of dull, cramping pelvic pain, usually related to menstruation. The primary management in the field is supportive care and a position of comfort during transport.

- g. **Ectopic pregnancy** p. 1514

   Ectopic pregnancy is the implantation of a fetus outside of the uterus, most commonly in the fallopian tubes. Patients usually report severe unilateral abdominal pain that may radiate to the shoulder on the affected side, a late or missed menstrual period, and sometimes vaginal bleeding. As the fetus develops, the tube can rupture, triggering a massive, life-threatening hemorrhage. Absorb the bleeding but do not pack the vagina. Ectopic pregnancy is a surgical emergency, and the primary management in the field is supportive care and a position of comfort during transport, as well as oxygen administration and IV therapy for fluid resuscitation.

- h. **Vaginal hemorrhage** p. 1514

   Nontraumatic vaginal hemorrhage is rarely encountered in the prehospital setting unless it is severe. Do not presume that such bleeding is due to normal menstrual flow. Most commonly, it is due to a spontaneous abortion (miscarriage) and is associated with cramping abdominal pain and the passage of clots and tissue. Other possible causes include cancerous lesions, PID, or the onset of labor. Absorb bleeding but do not pack the vagina. The primary management in the field is supportive care and a position of comfort for the patient, as well as oxygen administration and IV therapy for fluid resuscitation. If the bleeding is due to miscarriage, this will likely be a significant emotional event for your patient, so your kind and considerate care is important.

   Traumatic vaginal bleeding may result from sexual assault, blunt-force injuries to the lower abdomen, seat-belt injuries, objects inserted into the vagina, self-attempts at abortion, and lacerations following childbirth. Bleeding in such cases should be managed by direct pressure over a laceration or a cold pack applied to a hematoma. Never pack the vagina. Provide expedited transport to the hospital, with oxygen administration and IV access as necessary.

7. **Describe the assessment, care, and emotional support of the sexual assault patient.** pp. 1515–1516

   Sexual assault victims are unique patients with unique needs. The psychological care of these patients is as important, if not more so, than the physical care they may need. Confine your questions to the physical injuries that the patient may have received. Unless your patient is unconscious, do not touch the patient, even to take vital signs, without her permission. Explain what's going to be done before initiating any treatment. Avoid touching the patient other than to take vital signs or to examine other physical injuries. Do not examine the external genitalia of the sexual assault victim unless there is life-threatening hemorrhage. Consider the patient to be a crime scene and protect that scene; handle clothing as little as possible, collect all bloody articles as potential evidence, do not allow the patient to change clothes or bathe and do not clean wounds if possible. Be sure to document the treatment of the sexual assault victim carefully, thoroughly, and objectively.

8. **Given several preprogrammed gynecological patients, provide the appropriate assessment, management, and transportation.** pp. 1510–1516

   Throughout your classroom, clinical, and field training, you will encounter a variety of real and simulated gynecologic patients. Use the information provided in this chapter of your text, as well as the application of this information as demonstrated by your instructors, preceptors, and mentors to enhance your ability to assess, manage, and transport these patients. Keep in mind that gynecological emergencies are likely to be very stressful situations for your patients, and they will appreciate your gentle, considerate care and professionalism.

Content Self-Evaluation

MULTIPLE CHOICE

_____ 1. Painful discomfort during menstrual periods is known as:
   A. menarche.
   B. dyspareunia.
   C. cystitis.
   D. dysmenorrhea.
   E. pelvic inflammatory disease.

_____ 2. The term used to describe the number of times a woman has been pregnant is parity.
   A. True
   B. False

_____ 3. Which of the following questions is LEAST likely to get an accurate response from a female who is complaining of abdominal pain?
   A. Are you currently menstruating?
   B. Are you sexually active?
   C. Could you be pregnant?
   D. Have you ever experienced this pain before when menstruating?
   E. Have you experienced dizziness?

_____ 4. The term used to describe the number of deliveries a woman has had is:
   A. gravida.
   B. gravity.
   C. parity.
   D. parita.
   E. completa.

_____ 5. A palpable abdominal mass found midway between the symphysis pubis and the umbilicus in the lower abdomen of a 25-year-old woman is most likely to be a(n):
   A. tumor.
   B. intrauterine pregnancy of 5 months gestation.
   C. intrauterine pregnancy of 4 months gestation.
   D. intrauterine pregnancy of 3 months gestation.
   E. ovarian cyst.

_____ 6. Pelvic inflammatory disease is most often caused by:
   A. gonorrhea and chlamydia.
   B. streptococcus and staphylococcus.
   C. gonorrhea and HIV.
   D. chlamydia and streptococcus.
   E. HIV and staphylococcus.

_____ 7. Mid-cycle abdominal pain associated with ovulation is known as:
   A. endometriosis.
   B. PID.
   C. a miscarriage.
   D. cystitis.
   E. mittelschmerz.

_____ 8. Endometriosis is an infection of the uterine lining.
   A. True
   B. False

_____ 9. The most effective means to control non-traumatic vaginal hemorrhage is to apply direct pressure to the perineum.
   A. True
   B. False

_____ 10. All of the following signs and symptoms are associated with endometritis EXCEPT:
   A. history of gynecologic procedure.
   B. severe abdominal pain.
   C. fever.
   D. bradycardia.
   E. bloody, foul-smelling discharge.

_____ 11. All of the following signs and symptoms are associated with a ruptured ovarian cyst EXCEPT:
   A. dyspareunia.
   B. severe abdominal pain.
   C. fever.
   D. delayed menstrual period.
   E. irregular bleeding.

_____ 12. If a female patient presents with severe unilateral abdominal pain that radiates to the shoulder on one side, a missed menstrual period, and vaginal bleeding, you should suspect:
   A. mittelschmerz.
   B. ectopic pregnancy.
   C. PID.
   D. endometriosis.
   E. cystitis.

_____ 13. A female reports that during intercourse she felt a sudden and sharp tearing sensation. She is now bleeding from the external genitalia, although the bleeding is minimal. Management should include:
   A. asking the woman to hold a dressing over the area.
   B. establishing an IV and beginning fluid resuscitation regardless of blood loss.
   C. packing the vagina with sterile dressings.
   D. palpating the interior of the vagina to determine the extent of bleeding.
   E. securing a hot pack over the vaginal opening with tape.

_____ 14. The prehospital priorities for care of the sexual assault victim include all of the following EXCEPT:
   A. examining for perineal tears.
   B. determining if life-threatening injuries exist.
   C. providing emotional support.
   D. preserving evidence.
   E. protecting patient's privacy.

_____ 15. The BEST management for a victim of a sexual assault is:
   A. aggressive questioning and internal examination.
   B. discouraging the patient from dressing since this may taint evidence.
   C. examining the genitalia.
   D. psychological and emotional support.
   E. prompt summoning of law enforcement officials.

Chapter 40

Obstetrics

Review of Chapter Objectives

After reading this chapter, you should be able to:

1. **Describe the anatomic structures and physiology of the reproductive system during pregnancy.** pp. 1519–1522

   The primary "organ of pregnancy" is the placenta, which arises from the site on the uterine wall where the blastocyst (fertilized egg) implants itself. This temporary, blood-rich structure serves as a lifeline for the developing fetus via the umbilical cord. Its functions include the transfer of heat while exchanging oxygen and carbon dioxide, delivering nutrients, and removing waste. The placenta also serves as an endocrine gland throughout the pregnancy, secreting hormones necessary for fetal survival as well as the estrogen and progesterone required to maintain the pregnancy. The placenta is also a protective barrier against harmful substances that might cross the placental barrier to the fetus.

   The fetus develops within the amniotic sac, a thin-walled membranous covering containing amniotic fluid that surrounds and protects the fetus during intrauterine life.

2. **Identify the normal events of pregnancy.** pp. 1522–1525

   Fetal development begins at the moment of conception (fertilization). Normally, the duration of pregnancy is 40 weeks after the date of the mother's last menstrual period or 280 days. This is comparable to 10 lunar months or 9 calendar months. This time period is divided into trimesters, each of 3 calendar months' duration.

   Implantation of the fertilized egg into the uterine wall occurs during the preembryonic stage that lasts approximately 14 days. The embryonic stage begins at day 15 and ends at approximately 8 weeks, by which time all of the body systems have been formed. It is midway through this stage that the fetal heart begins to beat. The period from 8 weeks' gestation until delivery is known as the fetal stage. The gender of the infant can usually be determined by 16 weeks, and by the 20th week, fetal heart tones are audible by stethoscope. The mother usually feels fetal movement (quickening) by the 24th week. By the 38th week, the baby is considered to be full term.

3. **Describe how to assess an obstetrical patient.** pp. 1525–1527

   The initial assessment for an obstetric patient is the same as for any other patient. Utilization of the SAMPLE history will allow you to obtain specific information about the pregnancy. Ask about gravidity, parity, length of gestation, and EDC (estimated date of confinement or due date). You should also obtain information about past OB/GYN history (e.g., C-section) or complications as well as prenatal care. Determine current medications and any drug allergies as well. It is important to obtain the past medical history because pregnancy may aggravate preexisting medical problems or trigger new ones such as gestational diabetes. It is possible to estimate the due date by

©2007 Pearson Education, Inc.
Essentials of Paramedic Care, 2nd ed.

measuring fundal height above the symphysis pubis. Continue the physical exam, which is essentially the same for any patient, while being mindful of the need for modesty and privacy.

4. Identify the stages of labor and the paramedic's role in each stage. pp. 1537–1539

Labor is the physiologic and mechanical process by which the baby, placenta, and amniotic sac are expelled through the birth canal. The three stages of labor are dilatation, expulsion, and placental. The first stage (dilatation stage) begins with the onset of true labor and ends with the complete dilatation and effacement of the cervix. The second stage (expulsion stage) begins with the complete dilatation of the cervix and ends with the delivery of the baby. The third and final stage of labor (placental stage) begins immediately after the birth of the baby and ends with the delivery of the placenta. The role of the paramedic during labor is to assist in the delivery and to recognize and treat life-threatening problems for the mother or baby.

5. Differentiate between normal and abnormal delivery. pp. 1544–1549

Normally, most infants present from the birth canal in a headfirst, face-down position (vertex presentation), which allows the infant to be delivered vaginally. Abnormal delivery situations generally preclude vaginal delivery and are likely to require caesarean section, so transport must be expedited. These situations include breech presentation (buttocks present first), prolapsed cord (umbilical cord protrudes from the birth canal), limb presentation (baby's arm or leg protrudes from the birth canal) or occiput posterior presentation (baby's brow is facing forward).

6. Identify and describe complications associated with pregnancy and delivery. pp. 1527–1537, 1549–1550

Medical complications of pregnancy include ectopic pregnancy, bleeding problems, supine hypotensive syndrome, gestational diabetes, and hypertensive disorders. Ectopic pregnancy refers to the implantation of the fertilized egg outside of the uterus. Abdominal pain and evidence of intraabdominal and/or vaginal bleeding usually herald this event. Bleeding is generally differentiated as painful or painless. Vaginal bleeding, accompanied by cramping abdominal pain, prior to the 20th week of gestation is almost always associated with a spontaneous abortion. Painless bleeding is most commonly associated with placenta previa where, due to abnormal implantation of the placenta on the uterine wall, labor is accompanied by bleeding. Painful bleeding is the hallmark of abruptio placenta or the premature separation of the placenta from the uterine wall. It poses an immediate life threat to mother and child.

Supine hypotensive syndrome occurs most commonly in the third trimester as a result of compression of the inferior vena cava by the gravid uterus. Insulin resistance and decreased glucose tolerance characterize gestational diabetes, occurring in the last 20 weeks of pregnancy. Hypertensive disorders of pregnancy (formerly called toxemia) include preeclampsia or eclampsia and chronic and transient hypertension. Major motor seizures are the hallmark of eclampsia, which is the most serious of the hypertensive disorders, posing a life threat to the mother and child.

Some complications associated with delivery are discussed in objective 5. Other problems can occur after delivery. One of these is postpartum hemorrhage, which is the loss of 500 cc or more of blood immediately following delivery. A common cause of the condition is lack of uterine muscle tone, and it occurs most frequently in the multigravida, with multiple births, and with the births of large infants. Uterine rupture is another complication of delivery. It can result from blunt abdominal trauma, prolonged uterine contractions, or a surgically scarred uterus. Uterine rupture presents with a patient in excruciating abdominal pain and often in shock. Uterine inversion occurs when the uterus turns inside out after delivery and extends through the cervix. Blood loss from 800 to 1,800 cc occurs, and the patient often experiences profound shock. Pulmonary embolism can also occur after pregnancy as a result of venous thromboembolism. It often presents with sudden dyspnea accompanied by sharp chest pain and a sense of impending doom.

7. Identify predelivery emergencies. pp. 1527–1537

Recognition of a predelivery emergency is based on information obtained from the focused history and physical exam that relates to the reported abnormality, such as pain, discomfort, or bleeding.

While any of the complications listed above has potential to be an emergency, the most likely are abruptio placenta and eclampsia, both of which pose potential life threats to mother and child and require prompt and appropriate intervention.

8. State indications of an imminent delivery. pp. 1538–1539

Increasing frequency and duration of contractions and the sensation of needing to move one's bowels (urge to push) are all signs of impending delivery. However, crowning is the definitive sign that birth is imminent.

9. Identify the contents of an obstetrical kit and explain the use of each item. pp. 1539–1542

Commercially prepared OB kits are available from a variety of sources and contain the following items for use in the event of a field delivery: toweling or drape material, bulb syringe, two plastic umbilical clamps, and scissors. The toweling is used for draping the patient to minimize contamination of the baby during the birth. A bulb syringe is necessary for suctioning the baby's mouth and nose, while the cord clamps and scissors are used when separating the infant from its mother by clamping and cutting the umbilical cord.

10. Differentiate the management of a patient with predelivery emergencies from a normal delivery. p. 1527

Management of predelivery emergencies requires that the paramedic correctly recognize their presence based on information obtained from the focused history and physical exam and then expedite transport while anticipating the development of shock and maintaining adequate oxygenation, fluid resuscitation as necessary, and, if appropriate, pharmacological intervention. Most of the time, the mother will be transported in the left lateral recumbent position.

11. State the steps in the predelivery preparation of the mother. pp. 1538–1539

The first priority is to provide the mother with privacy. Then, time permitting, administer oxygen via a nasal cannula and establish vascular access. Position the mother on her back with knees and hips flexed and buttocks slightly elevated, or the mother may prefer squatting or to be in a semi-Fowler's position with knees and hips flexed. Drape the mother's perineum to minimize contamination of the infant during delivery.

12. Establish the relationship between body substance isolation and childbirth. p. 1539

Normally, preparation for childbirth in the prehospital setting would entail thoroughly washing hands and forearms before donning a gown, in addition to sterile gloves and goggles. Body substance isolation for childbirth generally includes draping the mother to minimize contamination of the baby during delivery.

13. State the steps to assist in the delivery of a newborn. pp. 1539–1542

Key EMS actions during a routine (normal) delivery are primarily supportive, but you should remain vigilant to signs of impending problems. Providing gentle support to the perineum as the delivery progresses decreases the likelihood of an explosive delivery causing vaginal tears and the potential for neonatal head trauma. While supporting the head, gently slide your finger along the head and neck to ensure that the cord is not wrapped around the baby's head and neck. As the head emerges from the vaginal opening, suction the airway (mouth first, then nose) to ensure that the airway is clear prior to the neonate taking his first breath. It may be necessary to tear the amniotic sac to release the amniotic fluid and permit the baby to breathe.

Gently guide the baby's head downward to allow delivery of the upper shoulder. Do not pull! Then gently guide the baby's body upward to allow delivery of the lower shoulder. Once the shoulders are delivered, the rest of the body will be quickly delivered. Keep the baby at the level of the mother's hips until the cord has been clamped and cut. Once the body has fully emerged from the birth canal, the baby should again be suctioned until the airway is clear. After clamping the umbilical cord at 10 cm and 15 cm from the baby and cutting in between, carefully dry the baby and wrap in a warming blanket to prevent hypothermia.

14. Describe how to care for the newborn.   pp. 1542–1544

The essential emergency care of the newborn includes the establishment and maintenance of adequate airway and breathing status and the prevention of heat loss. Support the infant's head and torso, using both hands. Maintain warmth, repeat suctioning of the mouth and nose as needed until the airway is clear, and then assess using the APGAR score. Do not delay resuscitation or transport to perform APGAR scoring.

15. Describe how and when to cut the umbilical cord.   p. 1542

Once the baby's body has been delivered, suction the airway until clear while keeping the baby at the level of the mother's hips until the cord has been clamped and cut. Do not "milk" the cord. Supporting the baby's body, place the first umbilical clamp approximately 10 cm from the baby and the second clamp at 15 cm and carefully cut in between.

16. Discuss the steps in the delivery of the placenta.   pp. 1541, 1542

Following delivery of the baby, the vaginal opening will continue to ooze blood. Do not pull on the umbilical cord! Eventually, the cord will appear to lengthen indicating separation of the placenta from the uterine wall. Once the placenta is expelled through the vaginal opening, it should be placed in a biohazard bag and be transported to the hospital for examination.

17. Describe the management of the mother postdelivery.   pp. 1542, 1549–1550

The mother should receive fundal massage to control postpartum bleeding and the perineum should be inspected for tears. Continuously monitor vital signs. If not accomplished prior to delivery, vascular access should be established should fluid resuscitation become necessary.

18. Summarize neonatal resuscitation procedures.   pp. 1543–1544

If the infant's respirations are below 30 per minute and tactile stimulation does not increase the rate to a normal range (30–60), immediately assist ventilations using a pediatric bag-valve mask with high-flow oxygen. If the heart rate is below 80 and does not increase in response to ventilations, initiate chest compressions. Transport to a facility with neonatal intensive care capabilities.

19. Describe the procedures for handling abnormal deliveries, complications of pregnancy, and maternal complications of labor.   pp. 1527–1537, 1544–1550

Management of abnormal deliveries or complications of pregnancy and labor require that the paramedic correctly recognize the problem and expedite transport while anticipating the development of shock and maintaining adequate oxygenation, fluid resuscitation as necessary and, if appropriate, pharmacological intervention. Most of the time, the mother will be transported in the left lateral recumbent position. When the baby's position (breech presentation, prolapsed cord, or limb presentation) dictates, the mother should be placed on oxygen and then assisted in assuming the knee-chest position. Additionally, in the management of prolapsed cord, two gloved fingers should be placed inside the vagina to prevent the baby's weight from compressing the cord and inhibiting oxygen delivery to the baby.

20. Describe special considerations when meconium is present in amniotic fluid or during delivery.   p. 1549

The presence of meconium (fetal fecal matter) in the amniotic fluid is indicative of a fetal hypoxic incident. The thicker and darker the color of the meconium staining in the amniotic fluid, the higher the risk of fetal morbidity. Once the head has emerged from the birth canal, suction the mouth and nose thoroughly while still on the perineum. However, if the meconium is thick, visualize the glottis and use an endotracheal tube to suction the hypopharynx and trachea until clear. Failure to suction will cause the meconium to be pushed further down the trachea and into the lungs.

21. Describe special considerations of a premature baby. pp. 1536–1537

Premature infants are ill suited for extrauterine life, particularly with regard to their pulmonary function. All of the concerns about caring for a neonate are exaggerated when the neonate is less than 38 weeks' gestation. Of greatest concern are airway maintenance, maintaining body temperature, ventilatory support, and oxygen delivery. These critically ill neonates should be taken immediately to a facility with neonatal intensive care capabilities.

22. Given several simulated delivery situations, provide the appropriate assessment, management, and transport for the mother and child. pp. 1519–1550

Throughout your training, you will encounter a variety of real and simulated obstetric patients. Use the information provided in this chapter, as well as the application of this information as demonstrated by your instructors, preceptors, and mentors to enhance your ability to assess, manage, and transport these patients. Keep in mind that this is likely to be a stressful situation for your patient, and she will appreciate your kind, considerate care and professionalism.

Content Self-Evaluation

MULTIPLE CHOICE

_____ 1. Thickening of the uterine lining in anticipation of implantation of the fertilized egg is stimulated by:
   A. estrogen.
   B. progesterone.
   C. follicle-stimulating hormone.
   D. luteinizing hormone.
   E. oxytocin.

_____ 2. All of the following are placental functions EXCEPT:
   A. acting as the "organ of pregnancy."
   B. production of hormones.
   C. serving as a protective barrier.
   D. providing fertilization.
   E. providing a means of heat transfer.

_____ 3. The normal duration of pregnancy is:
   A. 40 weeks.
   B. 280 days.
   C. 10 lunar months.
   D. 9 calendar months.
   E. all of the above

_____ 4. Blood volume increases by what percentage during pregnancy?
   A. 10 percent
   B. 25 percent
   C. 30 percent
   D. 45 percent
   E. 60 percent

_____ 5. The fetus receives its blood from the placenta by means of the:
   A. umbilical vein.
   B. umbilical artery.
   C. inferior vena cava.
   D. superior vena cava.
   E. aorta.

_____ 6. Fetal circulation changes to normal circulation with the:
   A. onset of labor.
   B. expulsion from the birth canal.
   C. baby's first breath.
   D. clamping of the umbilical cord.
   E. dilation and effacement of the cervix.

_____ 7. When performing a focused history on a pregnant patient, which of the following questions would be appropriate?
A. Are you experiencing any pain or discomfort?
B. Have you had any vaginal discharge or bleeding?
C. When is your due date?
D. Have you ever been pregnant before?
E. all of the above

_____ 8. All of the following are common signs or symptoms of a predelivery emergency EXCEPT:
A. abdominal pain or trauma.
B. vaginal bleeding or discharge.
C. painful deformed extremities.
D. altered mental status or seizures.
E. hypertension or hypotension.

_____ 9. All of the following are causes of bleeding during pregnancy EXCEPT:
A. abortion.
B. ovarian cyst.
C. ectopic pregnancy.
D. placenta previa.
E. abruptio placenta.

_____ 10. Treatment of a female patient who is 16 weeks pregnant, is complaining of cramping abdominal pain, and has bright red vaginal bleeding should include all of the following EXCEPT:
A. packing the vagina to control bleeding.
B. treating for shock if indicated.
C. maintaining oxygenation.
D. providing emotional support.
E. saving any tissue and clots for evaluation.

_____ 11. You suspect the patient in the situation described in question 10 is having a(n):
A. abortion.
B. ovarian cyst.
C. ectopic pregnancy.
D. placenta previa.
E. abruptio placenta.

_____ 12. Pelvic inflammatory disease, endometriosis, and tubal ligation are predisposing factors for:
A. abortion.
B. ovarian cyst.
C. ectopic pregnancy.
D. placenta previa.
E. abruptio placenta.

_____ 13. You find that your patient is 36 weeks pregnant, has an altered mental status, and is reported to have had a major motor seizure, which you suspect is due to:
A. placenta previa.
B. eclampsia.
C. epilepsy.
D. abruptio placenta.
E. supine hypotensive syndrome.

_____ 14. Care of the patient in question 13 should include all of the following EXCEPT:
A. administering high-flow oxygen via a nonrebreather mask.
B. protecting the patient from injury if seizures recur.
C. minimizing noise and light to prevent seizure activity.
D. administering magnesium sulfate per protocol.
E. transporting on right side to protect airway.

_____ 15. All of the following are signs and symptoms of an imminent delivery EXCEPT:
A. the presence of crowning.
B. contractions occurring every 1 to 2 minutes.
C. passage of "bloody show."
D. sensation of an urge for bowel movement.
E. rupture of membranes.

_____ 16. The stage of labor that begins with complete cervical dilatation and ends with the delivery of the fetus is called the dilatation stage.
   A. True
   B. False

_____ 17. Your patient has just delivered a healthy baby boy. Following the delivery of the placenta, her vaginal bleeding seems to increase. Which of the following best describes what you should do to provide emergency care for this patient?
   A. Massage the uterus and position your patient on her right side.
   B. Administer oxygen and firmly massage the uterus.
   C. Massage the uterus and pack the vagina to control bleeding
   D. Administer oxygen and pack the vagina with sanitary napkins.
   E. Provide fluid resuscitation and position patient on her right side.

_____ 18. Meconium-stained amniotic fluid should first be managed by:
   A. immediate transport to the hospital for physician evaluation.
   B. administration of oxygen to the mother to resolve fetal distress.
   C. suctioning of the mouth and nose before the infant takes his first breath.
   D. stimulation of the infant to encourage coughing to clear meconium from airway.
   E. expediting completion of delivery to decrease fetal distress.

_____ 19. Management of a limb presentation should include all of the following EXCEPT:
   A. administration of high-flow oxygen to the mother.
   B. immediate transport to the hospital.
   C. attempting to push the limb back into the vagina.
   D. positioning the mother with her head down and pelvis elevated.
   E. providing reassurance to the mother.

_____ 20. The administration of an IV fluid bolus to control premature labor is based on increasing intravascular volume and thus causing inhibition of:
   A. antidiuretic hormone.   D. luteinizing hormone.
   B. progesterone.   E. follicle-stimulating hormone.
   C. estrogen.

_____ 21. Elements of the APGAR assessment include appearance, pulse, grimace, activity, and respirations.
   A. True
   B. False

_____ 22. Acrocyanosis in the neonate is always a sign of inadequate oxygenation.
   A. True
   B. False

_____ 23. You have just assisted with the delivery of a baby girl. She has shallow, gasping respirations and a heart rate that is less than 100 beats per minute. Which of the following best describes your emergency care for this patient?
   A. administering "blow-by" oxygen and monitoring her pulse for 60 seconds
   B. assisting ventilations with a BVM and reassessing in 30 seconds
   C. administering high-flow oxygen with a nonrebreather mask
   D. assisting ventilations with a BVM and beginning chest compressions
   E. continuing to monitor and expedite transport

_____ 24. Shoulder dystocia is commonly associated with diabetic or obese mothers and:
   A. prematurity.   D. hormonal deficits.
   B. hormonal excesses.   E. fetal distress.
   C. postterm pregnancy.

_____ 25. If the uterus protrudes from the vaginal opening following the delivery of the placenta, you should:
   A. wrap it tightly in dry towels.
   B. wrap it in dextrose-soaked dressings.
   C. make no more than three attempts to replace it.
   D. make no more than one attempt to replace it.
   E. cover it with plastic wrap.

MATCHING

Write the letter of the definition in the space provided next to the term it describes.

_____ 26. amniotic sac

_____ 27. ovulation

_____ 28. fetus

_____ 29. placenta

_____ 30. umbilical cord

_____ 31. effacement

_____ 32. Braxton-Hicks contractions

_____ 33. parity

_____ 34. tocolysis

_____ 35. puerperium

A. Unborn infant from the third month of pregnancy to birth
B. Fetal lifeline, a placental extension through which the child is nourished
C. Organ of pregnancy for the exchange of oxygen and waste products
D. Transparent membrane forming the sac, which holds the fetus
E. Release of an egg from the ovary
F. The time period surrounding the birth of the fetus
G. Thinning and shortening of the cervix during labor
H. Number of pregnancies carried to term
I. Process of stopping labor
J. Painless, irregular uterine contractions

Essentials of Paramedic Care

Division 5

Special Considerations/Operations

Chapter 41

Neonatology

Review of Chapter Objectives

With each chapter of the Workbook, we identify the objectives and the important elements of the text content. You should review these items and refer to the pages listed if any points are not clear.

After reading this chapter, you should be able to:

1. **Define newborn and neonate.** p. 1555

   A newborn is a baby in the first few hours of its life, also called a newly born infant. A neonate is a baby less than one month old.

2. **Identify important antepartum factors that can affect childbirth.** p. 1556

   Antepartum factors are those that occur before the onset of labor. Examples of important antepartum factors that can adversely affect childbirth include multiple gestation, inadequate prenatal care, a mother who is younger than 16 years of age or older than 35, a history of perinatal morbidity or mortality, postterm gestation, drugs or medications, and a mother with a history of toxemia, hypertension, or diabetes.

3. **Identify important intrapartum factors that can determine high-risk newborn patients.** p. 1556

   Intrapartum factors are those that occur during childbirth. Examples of intrapartum factors that can help determine high-risk newborn patients include a mother with premature labor, meconium-stained amniotic fluid, rupture of membranes more than 24 hours prior to delivery, use of narcotics within 4 hours of delivery, an abnormal presentation, prolonged labor or precipitous delivery, and a prolapsed cord or bleeding.

4. **Identify the factors that lead to premature birth and low-birth-weight newborns.** pp. 1556, 1573, 1576–1577

   A premature or low-birth-weight newborn is an infant born prior to 37 weeks of gestation or with a birth weight ranging from 0.6 to 2.2 kg (1 pound, 5 ounces, to 4 pounds, 13 ounces). Factors that lead to premature birth or low-birth-weight newborns include, among others, maternal narcotic use or trauma. For a full list of factors, see Chapter 40, "Obstetrics," in Division 4.

5. **Distinguish between primary and secondary apnea.** p. 1557

   When an infant is born, it may experience hypoxia. This is usually relieved by the initial gasps for air. If this asphyxia continues, respiratory movement may cease altogether. The infant may then enter a period of apnea known as primary apnea. In most cases, simple stimulation and exposure to oxygen will reverse bradycardia and assist in the development of pulmonary perfusion. With ongoing asphyxia, the infant will enter a period known as secondary apnea. Always assume that apnea in the newborn is secondary apnea and rapidly treat it with ventilatory assistance.

6. Discuss pulmonary perfusion and asphyxia.   **p. 1557**

With the first breaths, the lungs rapidly fill with air, which displaces the remaining fetal fluid. The pulmonary arterioles and capillaries open, decreasing pulmonary vascular resistance. The blood is now diverted from the ductus arteriosus to the pulmonary circulation. However, if hypoxia or severe acidosis occurs, the pulmonary vascular bed may constrict and the ductus may reopen. This will retrigger fetal circulation with its attendant shunting, ongoing hypoxia, and ultimately asphyxia (if the situation is not managed quickly and correctly).

7. Identify the primary signs utilized for evaluating a newborn during resuscitation.   **pp. 1559–1560**

The newborn should be assessed immediately after birth. The primary signs used for evaluating a newborn during resuscitation include respiratory rate, heart rate, and skin color. The newborn's respiratory rate should average 40 to 60 breaths per minute. The normal heart rate is between 150 and 180 beats per minute at birth, slowing to 130 to 140 beats per minute thereafter. A pulse less than 100 beats per minute indicates distress and requires emergency intervention. Some cyanosis of the extremities is common immediately after birth. However, if the newborn is cyanotic in the central part of the body or if peripheral cyanosis persists, the newborn must be treated with 100 percent oxygen.

8. Identify the appropriate use of the APGAR scale.   **pp. 1559–1560**

The APGAR scale—designed for use at 1 and 5 minutes after birth—helps distinguish between newborns who need only routine care and those who need greater assistance. The system also predicts long-term survival. A severely distressed newborn (one with an APGAR score of less than 4) requires immediate resuscitation.

9. Calculate the APGAR score given various newborn situations.   **pp. 1559–1560; also see Chapter 40**

To calculate the APGAR score, a value of 0, 1, or 2 is given for each of the following categories: pulse rate (heart rate), grimace (irritability), activity (muscle tone), and respiratory rate.

10. Formulate an appropriate treatment plan for providing initial care to a newborn.   **pp. 1560–1563**

Treatment of the newborn begins by preparing the environment and assembling the equipment needed for delivery and immediate care of the newborn. The initial care of the newborn follows the same priorities as for all patients. Complete the initial assessment first. Correct any problems detected in the initial assessment before proceeding to the next step. The majority of term newborns require no resuscitation beyond suctioning of the airway, mild stimulation, and maintenance of body temperature by drying and warming with blankets.

11. Describe the indications, equipment needed, application, and evaluation of the following management techniques for the newborn in distress:

    a. Blow-by oxygen   **pp. 1565, 1567**

    Blow-by oxygen—the process of blowing oxygen across a newborn's face—is applied if central cyanosis is present or if the adequacy of ventilations is uncertain. If possible, the oxygen should be warmed and humidified.

    b. Ventilatory assistance   **pp. 1565, 1567–1568**

    Positive-pressure ventilation should be applied to a newborn if any of the following conditions exist: heart rate less than 100 beats per minute, apnea, or persistence of central cyanosis after administration of supplemental oxygen. A bag-valve-mask unit is the device of choice. A self-inflating bag of appropriate size should be used (450 mL is optimal). If prolonged ventilation is required, it may be necessary to disable the pop-off valve.

   c. Endotracheal intubation   **pp. 1564, 1566–1567, 1568**

This technique involves placement of an endotracheal (ET) tube into the trachea of a newborn, usually for suctioning meconium. Endotracheal intubation requires appropriately sized tubes without cuffs and a laryngoscope. After suctioning, a fresh tube should be inserted for mechanical ventilation. (See Procedure 41-2 for more details.) Endotracheal intubation should be carried out in the following situations: The bag-valve mask does not work, tracheal suctioning is needed, prolonged ventilation will be required, a diaphragmatic hernia is suspected, or an inadequate respiratory effort is found.

   d. Orogastric tube   **p. 1570**

An orogastric, or nasogastric, tube is used to relieve significant gastric distention, most often caused by a leak around an uncuffed endotracheal tube. The tube should be inserted through the nose or mouth, then through the esophagus into the stomach. An endotracheal tube should be in place to avoid misplacing the gastric tube into the trachea. Make sure the newborn is well oxygenated and that the tube is correctly measured (from the tip of the newborn's nose, around the ear, to the xiphoid process). Lubricate the end of the tube before inserting and then check placement by injecting 10 cc of air into the tube and auscultating a bubbling sound (or sound of rushing air) over the epigastrium.

   e. Chest compressions   **pp. 1570, 1571**

Chest compressions should be applied to newborns with heart rates of less than 60 beats per minute or with heart rates between 60 and 80 beats per minute that do not increase with 30 seconds of positive-pressure ventilation and supplemental oxygen. Begin chest compressions by encircling the newborn's chest, placing both thumbs on the lower one third of the sternum. Compress the sternum 1.5 to 2.0 cm (½ to ¾ inch) at a rate of 120 times per minute. Maintain a ratio of 3 compressions to 1 ventilation. Reassess the newborn after 20 cycles of compressions (1-minute intervals). Discontinue compressions if the spontaneous heart rate exceeds 80 beats per minute.

   f. Vascular access   **pp. 1570, 1571**

Vascular access—a method for administering fluids and drugs—should be considered if ventilation and oxygenation fail to correct cardiopulmonary arrests or in cases of persistent bradycardia, hypovolemia, respiratory depression secondary to narcotics, and metabolic acidosis. Vascular access can most readily be managed by using the umbilical vein. The umbilical cord contains three vessels—two arteries and one vein, with the vein being the largest of the three. Equipment for venous access includes a scalpel blade, a 5 French umbilical catheter, a three-way stopcock, umbilical tape, and saline. Be sure to save enough of the umbilical stump (cut to 1 cm above the abdomen) in case neonatal personnel have to place additional lines. Also, if the catheter is inserted too far, it may become wedged against the liver, and it will not function.

12. Discuss the routes of medication administration for a newborn.   **pp. 1570, 1571, 1572**

Medications for the newborn may be administered by peripheral vein cannulation, intraosseous cannulation, umbilical vein cannulation, and endotracheal tube.

13. Discuss the signs of hypovolemia in a newborn.   **p. 1578**

Hypovolemia is the leading cause of shock in the newborn. It may result from dehydration, hemorrhage, or third-spacing of fluids, with dehydration being by far the most common cause. Signs of hypovolemia include pale color, cool skin, diminished peripheral pulses, delayed capillary refill (despite a normal ambient temperature), mental status changes, and diminished urination (oliguria).

14. Discuss the initial steps in resuscitation of a newborn.   **pp. 1564–1573**

Resuscitation of the newborn follows an inverted pyramid. In chronological order, initial steps include drying, warming, positioning, suctioning, and tactical stimulation; administration of supplemental oxygen; bag-valve ventilation; and chest compressions. If these steps fail, advanced measures include intubation and administration of medications.

15. Discuss the effects of maternal narcotic usage on the newborn. p. 1573

Maternal narcotic use has been shown to produce low-birth-weight infants. Such infants may demonstrate withdrawal symptoms—tremors, startles, and decreased alertness. They also face a serious risk of respiratory depression at birth.

16. Determine the appropriate treatment for the newborn with narcotic depression. p. 1573

Naloxone, which is extremely safe even at high doses, is the treatment of choice for respiratory depression secondary to maternal narcotic use within four hours of delivery. Ventilatory support must be provided prior to administration of naloxone. Due to the long duration of the narcotic, which may exceed the duration of the naloxone, repeat administration will be needed. Keep in mind, however, that the naloxone may induce a withdrawal reaction in an infant born to a narcotic-addicted mother. Medical direction may advise that naloxone NOT be administered if the mother is drug addicted, recommending prolonged ventilatory support instead.

17. Discuss appropriate transport guidelines for a newborn. p. 1573

Paramedics are frequently called upon to transport a high-risk newborn from a facility where stabilization has occurred to a neonatal intensive care unit. During transport you will help maintain the newborn's body temperature, control oxygen administration, and maintain ventilatory support. Often, a transport isolette with its own heat, light, and oxygen source is available. If a self-contained isolette is not available for transport, you might wrap the newborn in several blankets, keep the infant's head covered, and place hot-water bottles containing water heated to no more than 40°C (104°F) near, but not touching, the newborn. DO NOT use chemical packs to keep the newborn warm.

18. Determine appropriate receiving facilities for low- and high-risk newborns. p. 1573

Low-risk newborns need to be taken to a hospital with an obstetrical unit, whereas high-risk newborns are often taken directly or transferred to a facility with a neonatal intensive care unit (NICU).

19. Describe the epidemiology, including the incidence, morbidity/mortality, risk factors and prevention strategies, pathophysiology, assessment findings, and management for the following neonatal problems:

a. Meconium aspiration pp. 1574–1575

Meconium-stained amniotic fluid occurs in approximately 10 to 15 percent of deliveries, mostly in postterm or small-for-gestational-age newborns. Meconium aspiration accounts for a significant proportion of neonatal deaths. Fetal distress and hypoxia can cause meconium to be passed into the amniotic fluid. Either in utero or more often with the first breath, thick meconium is aspirated into the lungs, resulting in small airway obstruction and aspiration pneumonia. The infant may have respiratory distress within the first hours, or even the first minutes, of life as evidenced by tachypnea, retraction, grunting, and cyanosis in severely affected newborns. The partial obstruction of some airways may lead to a pneumothorax.

An infant born through thin meconium may not require treatment, but depressed infants born through thick, particulate (pea-soup) meconium-stained fluid should be intubated immediately, prior to the first ventilation. Before stimulating such infants to breathe, apply suction with a meconium aspirator attached to an endotracheal tube. Connect to suction at 100 cc/H$_2$O or less to remove meconium from the airway. Withdraw the ET tube as suction is applied. It may be necessary to repeat this procedure to clear the airway. The patient should then be taken to a facility that can manage a high-risk neonate.

b. Apnea p. 1575

This condition is a common finding in the preterm infant or infants weighing under 1,500 grams (3 pounds, 5 ounces), infants exposed to drugs, or infants born after prolonged or difficult labor and delivery. Typically, the infant fails to breathe spontaneously after stimulation, or the infant experiences respiratory pauses of greater than 20 seconds. Apnea can be due to hypoxia, hypothermia, narcotic or central nervous system depressants, weakness of the respiratory muscles, septicemia, metabolic disorders, or central nervous system disorders.

Management begins with tactile stimulation, followed by bag-valve-mask ventilation, with the pop-off valve disabled. If the infant does not breathe on its own, or if the heart rate is below 60 with adequate ventilation and chest compressions, perform tracheal intubation with direct visualization. Gain circulatory access, and monitor the heart rate continuously. If the apnea is due to a narcotic administered within the past 4 hours, consider naloxone. Remember, however, that the use of a narcotic antagonist is generally contraindicated if the mother is a drug abuser. Throughout the treatment, keep the infant warm to prevent hypothermia.

c. Diaphragmatic hernia pp. 1575–1576

This is a rare condition seen in approximately 1 out of every 2,200 live births. The defect is caused by the failure of the pleuroperitoneal canal to close completely. The survival rate for newborns who require mechanical ventilation in the first 18 to 24 hours is approximately 50 percent, and it approaches 100 percent if there is no distress in the first 24 hours of life.

Protrusion of abdominal viscera through the hernia into the thoracic cavity occurs in varying degrees. Assessment findings may include little to severe distress present from birth; dyspnea and cyanosis unresponsive to ventilations; small, flat (scaphoid) abdomen; bowel sounds in the chest; and heart sounds displaced to the right. If you suspect a diaphragmatic hernia, position the infant with its head and thorax higher than the abdomen and feet. This will help to displace the abdominal organs downward. Place a nasogastric or orogastric tube and apply low, intermittent suctioning. DO NOT use bag-valve-mask ventilation, which can worsen the condition by causing gastric distension. If necessary, cautiously administer positive-pressure ventilation through an endotracheal tube. A diaphragmatic hernia usually requires surgical repair, which should be explained to the parents along with the need for quick transport.

d. Bradycardia p. 1576

Bradycardia is most commonly caused by hypoxia in newborns. However, the bradycardia may also be due to several other factors, including increased intracranial pressure, hypothyroidism, or acidosis. In cases of hypoxia, the infant experiences minimal risk if the hypoxia is corrected quickly. In providing treatment, follow the procedures in the inverted pyramid. Resist the inclination to treat the bradycardia with pharmacological measures alone. Keep the newborn warm and transport to the nearest facility.

e. Prematurity pp. 1576–1577

A premature newborn is an infant born prior to 38 weeks of gestation or with weight ranging from 0.6 to 2.2 kg (1 pound, 5 ounces, to 4 pounds, 13 ounces.) Mortality decreases weekly with gestation beyond the onset of fetal viability. Premature newborns are at greater risk of respiratory suppression, head or brain injury caused by hypoxemia, changes in blood pressure, intraventricular hemorrhage, and fluctuations in serum osmolarity. They are also more susceptible to hypothermia than full-term newborns. The degree of immaturity determines the physical characteristics of a premature newborn. Premature newborns often appear to have a larger head relative to body size. They may have large trunks and short extremities, transparent skin, and few wrinkles.

Prematurity should not be a factor in short-term treatment. Resuscitation should be attempted if there is any sign of life, and the measures of resuscitation should be the same as those for newborns of normal weight and maturity. Maintain a patent airway and avoid potential aspiration of gastric contents.

f. Respiratory distress/cyanosis pp. 1577–1578

Prematurity is the single most common factor causing respiratory distress and cyanosis in the newborn. The problem occurs most frequently in infants less than 1,200 grams (2 pounds, 10 ounces) and 30 weeks of gestation. Premature infants have an immature central respiratory control center and are easily affected by environmental or metabolic changes. There are many factors contributing to respiratory distress, including lung or heart disease, central nervous system disorders, meconium aspiration, metabolic problems, obstruction of the nasal passages, shock and sepsis, and diaphragmatic hernia. Expect the following assessment findings: tachypnea, paradoxical breathing, intercostal retractions, nasal flaring, and expiratory grunt.

In providing treatment, follow the inverted pyramid, paying particular attention to airway and ventilation. Suction as needed and provide a high concentration of oxygen. If prolonged ventilation will be required, consider placing an ET tube. Perform chest compressions, if indicated. Consider dextrose ($D_{10}W$ or $D_{25}W$) if the newborn is hypoglycemic. Maintain body temperature and transport to the most appropriate facility.

g. Seizures   pp. 1578–1579

Neonatal seizures differ from seizures in a child or an adult, because generalized tonic-clonic convulsions rarely occur in the first month of life. Types of seizures in the neonate include:

- **Subtle seizures**—consist of chewing motions and excessive salivation, blinking, sucking, swimming movements of the arms, pedaling movements of the legs, apnea, and color changes.
- **Tonic seizures**—characterized by rigid posturing of the extremities and trunk; sometimes associated with fixed deviation of the eyes.
- **Focal clonic seizures**—consist of rhythmic twitching of muscle groups in the extremities and face.
- **Multifocal seizures**—exhibit signs similar to focal clonic seizures except multiple muscle groups are involved and clonic activity randomly migrates.
- **Myoclonic seizures**—characterized by brief focal or generalized jerks of the extremities or parts of the body that tend to involve distal muscle groups.

The causes of neonatal seizures include sepsis, fever, hypoglycemia, hypoxic ischemic encephalopathy, metabolic disturbances, meningitis, development abnormalities, or drug withdrawal. Assessment findings of seizures include decreased level of consciousness and seizure activity as already described. Treatment focuses on airway management, oxygen saturation, and administration of an anticonvulsant. You might administer a benzodiazepine (usually lorazepam) for status epilepticus or dextrose ($D_{10}W$ or $D_{25}W$) for hypoglycemia.

h. Fever   p. 1579

Neonates do not develop fever as easily as older children. Therefore, any fever in a neonate requires extensive evaluation because it is more likely to be caused by a life-threatening condition such as pneumonia, sepsis, or meningitis. In fact, fever may be the only sign of meningitis in a neonate. Because of their immature development, they do not exhibit the classic symptoms such as a stiff neck. Assessment findings of a fever include changes in mental status (irritability or somnolence), decreased feeding, skin warm to the touch, and rashes or petechia. Term infants may form beads of sweat on their brow, but not on the rest of their body. Premature infants, on the other hand, will have no visible sweat at all.

Treatment of the neonate with a fever will, for the most part, be limited to ensuring a patent airway and adequate ventilation. Do not use cold packs, as they may drop the temperature too quickly and cause seizures. If the newborn becomes bradycardic, provide chest compressions.

i. Hypothermia   pp. 1579–1580

Hypothermia presents a common and life-threatening condition for newborns. The high body surface to body volume relationship in newborns makes them extremely sensitive to environmental temperatures, especially right after delivery when they are wet. In treating hypothermia—a body temperature below 35°C (95°F)—try to control the loss of heat through evaporation, conduction, convection, and radiation. Also remember that hypothermia can be an indicator of sepsis in the newborn. Regardless of the cause, the increase in the metabolic demands can produce a variety of related conditions including metabolic acidosis, pulmonary hypertension, and hypoxemia.

In assessing hypothermic newborns, remember that they do not shiver. Instead, expect the following findings: pale color, skin cool to the touch (especially in the extremities), acrocyanosis, respiratory distress, possible apnea, bradycardia, central cyanosis, initial irritability, and lethargy in later stages. Management focuses on ensuring adequate ventilations and oxygenation. Chest compressions may be necessary with bradycardia.

j. Hypoglycemia   p. 1580

Newborns are the only age group that can develop severe hypoglycemia and not have diabetes mellitus. Hypoglycemia is more common in premature or small-for-gestational-age infants, the smaller twin, and newborns of diabetic mothers, as these infants have decreased glucose utilization. Hypoglycemia may be due to a number of factors, including inadequate glucose intake or increased glucose utilization, stress (which can cause blood sugar to fall to a critical level), respiratory illnesses, hypothermia, toxemia, CNS hemorrhage, asphyxia, meningitis, and sepsis. Infants receiving glucose infusions can develop hypoglycemia if the infusion is suddenly stopped.

Infants with hypoglycemia may be asymptomatic, or they may exhibit symptoms such as apnea, color changes, respiratory distress, lethargy, seizures, acidosis, and poor myocardial contractility. Assessment findings may include twitching or seizures, limpness, lethargy, eye-rolling, high-pitched cry, apnea, irregular respirations, and possible cyanosis. Treatment begins with management of airway and ventilations. Administer chest compressions, if needed. With medical direction, administer dextrose ($D_{10}W$ or $D_{25}W$). Remember—persistent hypoglycemia is a serious condition and can have catastrophic effects on the brain.

k. Vomiting pp. 1580–1581

Vomiting in a neonate may result from a variety of causes and rarely presents as an isolated symptom. Vomiting—the forceful ejection of stomach contents—rarely occurs during the first weeks of life and may be confused with regurgitation or "spitting up." Causes of vomiting include a tracheoesophageal fistula, an upper gastrointestinal obstruction, increased intracranial pressure, or an infection. Vomiting containing dark blood signals a life-threatening illness. Keep in mind, however, that vomiting of mucus—which may occasionally be streaked with blood—in the first few hours after birth is not uncommon.

Assessment findings may include distended stomach, signs of infection, increased ICP, or drug withdrawal. Because vomitus can be aspirated, management considerations focus on ensuring a patent airway to prevent aspiration. If you detect respiratory difficulty, suction or clear the vomitus from the airway and oxygenate as needed. Fluid administration may be necessary to prevent dehydration. Remember that, as with older patients, vagal stimulation may cause bradycardia in the neonate.

l. Diarrhea p. 1581

Diarrhea can cause severe dehydration and electrolyte imbalances in the neonate. Normally five to six stools per day can be expected, especially in breast-fed infants. Causes of diarrhea in a neonate include bacterial or viral infection, gastroenteritis, lactose intolerance, phototherapy, neonatal abstinence syndrome (NAS), thyrotoxicosis, and cystic fibrosis. In managing an infant with diarrhea, remember BSI precautions. Management consists of maintenance of airway and ventilations, adequate oxygenation, and chest compressions, if indicated. With medical direction, fluid therapy might be administered to prevent or treat dehydration.

m. Common birth injuries pp. 1581–1582

A birth injury occurs in an estimated 2 to 7 of every 1,000 live births in the United States. About 5 to 8 of every 100,000 infants die of birth trauma and 25 of every 100,000 die of anoxic injuries. These injuries account for 2 to 3 percent of infant deaths. Risk factors for birth injury include prematurity, postmaturity, cephalopelvic disproportion, prolonged labor, breech presentation, explosive delivery, and a diabetic mother.

Birth injuries can take various forms. Cranial injuries may include molding of the head and overriding of the parietal bones, erythema, abrasions, ecchymosis, subcutaneous fat necrosis, subconjunctival and retinal hemorrhage, subperiosteal hemorrhage, and fracture of the skull. Often the infant will develop a large scalp hematoma, called a caput succedaneum, during the birth process, but this condition will usually resolve over a week's time. Other birth injuries include peripheral nerve injury, injury to the liver, rupture of the spleen, adrenal hemorrhage, fractures of the clavicle or extremities, and hypoxia-ischemia.

Assessment findings may include diffuse (sometimes ecchymotic) edematous swelling of soft tissues around the scalp, paralysis below the level of the spinal cord injury, paralysis of the upper arm with or without paralysis of the forearm, diaphragmatic paralysis, movement on only one side of the face when crying, inability to move the arm freely on the side of the fractured clavicle, lack of spontaneous movement of the affected extremity, hypoxia, and shock. Management of a newborn who has suffered a birth injury is specific to injury but always centers on protection of the airway, provision of adequate ventilation, and chest compressions, if necessary.

n. Cardiac arrest p. 1582

The incidence of neonatal cardiac arrest is related primarily to hypoxia. The condition can be caused by primary or secondary apnea, bradycardia, persistent fetal circulation, or pulmonary hypertension. Unless appropriate interventions are initiated immediately, the outcome is poor.

Risk factors for cardiac arrest in newborns include bradycardia, intrauterine asphyxia, prematurity, drugs administered to or taken by the mother, congenital neuromuscular diseases, congenital malformations, and intrapartum hypoxemia. Assessment findings may include peripheral cyanosis, inadequate respiratory effort, and ineffective or absent heart rate. In managing the neonatal cardiac arrest, follow the inverted pyramid for resuscitation and administer drugs or fluids according to medical direction.

o. **Post-arrest management** p. 1582

Post-arrest management involves maintenance of the infant's body temperature, prompt transport to the appropriate facility, and delicate handling of the parents or caregivers.

20. **Given several neonatal emergencies, provide the appropriate procedures for assessment, management, and transport.** pp. 1555–1582

During your classroom, clinical, and field training, you will assess and develop a management plan for the real and simulated patients you attend. Use the information presented in this chapter, the information on neonatal emergencies in the field provided by your instructors, and the guidance given by your clinical and field preceptors to develop the skills needed to assess, manage, and transport the newborn and neonate patient. Continue to refine these skills once your training ends and you begin your career as a paramedic.

Content Self-Evaluation

MULTIPLE CHOICE

_____ 1. Examples of antepartum factors indicating possible complications in newborns would include multiple gestation and:
   A. premature labor.
   B. inadequate prenatal care.
   C. abnormal presentation.
   D. prolapsed cord.
   E. prolonged labor.

_____ 2. Examples of intrapartum factors indicating possible complications in newborns would include the use of narcotics within 4 hours of delivery and:
   A. meconium-stained amniotic fluid.
   B. postterm gestation.
   C. a mother under 16 years old.
   D. toxemia or diabetes.
   E. a mother over 35 years old.

_____ 3. When the fetus is in the uterus, the respiratory system is:
   A. working at a very rapid speed.
   B. working at a very slow speed.
   C. essentially nonfunctional.
   D. essentially functional.
   E. flushed with meconium.

_____ 4. Factors that stimulate the baby's first breath include:
   A. mild acidosis.
   B. hypoxia.
   C. hypothermia.
   D. initiation of stretch reflexes in the lungs.
   E. all of the above

_____ 5. Persistent fetal circulation is a condition in which the:
   A. ductus arteriosus remains closed.
   B. ductus arteriosus reopens.
   C. pulmonary vascular bed dilates.
   D. both A and C
   E. both B and C

_____ 6. Always assume that apnea in the newborn is secondary apnea and rapidly treat it with ventilatory assistance.
   A. True
   B. False

_____ 7. Most of the fetal development that could lead to congenital problems occurs during the:
   A. first trimester.
   B. second trimester.
   C. third trimester.
   D. onset of labor.
   E. intrapartum period.

_____ 8. Some infants are born with a defect in their spinal cord. In some cases, the spinal cord and associated structures may be exposed. This abnormality is called diaphragmatic hernia.
   A. True
   B. False

_____ 9. A congenital hernia of the umbilicus found in the neonate is called a(n):
   A. choanal atresia.
   B. Pierre Robin Syndrome.
   C. spina bifida.
   D. meningomyelocele.
   E. omphalocele.

_____ 10. A congenital condition characterized by a small jaw combined with a cleft palate, downward displacement of the tongue, and an absent gag reflex is called a(n):
   A. cleft lip.
   B. omphalocele.
   C. cleft palate.
   D. Pierre Robin Syndrome.
   E. choanal atresia.

_____ 11. The APGAR score should be assigned at 1 and 10 minutes after the infant's birth.
   A. True
   B. False

_____ 12. The G in APGAR stands for:
   A. gravida.
   B. gestation.
   C. grimace.
   D. gray tone.
   E. none of the above

_____ 13. A dark green material found in the intestine of the full-term newborn is called:
   A. bile.
   B. meconium.
   C. mucus.
   D. vomitus.
   E. hyperbilirubinemia.

_____ 14. Loss of heat by the newborn can occur through:
   A. evaporation.
   B. convection.
   C. conduction.
   D. radiation.
   E. all of the above

_____ 15. Immediately after birth, the newborn's core temperature is expected to drop 4° or more from its birth temperature.
   A. True
   B. False

_____ 16. Prior to cutting the umbilical cord, it should not be "milked" as this can cause:
   A. polycythemia.
   B. anemia.
   C. hyperbilirubinemia.
   D. hemophilia.
   E. both A and C

_____ 17. An increase in the level of bilirubin in the blood can cause:
   A. jaundice.
   B. pallor.
   C. cyanosis.
   D. flushing.
   E. anemia.

_____ 18. The most important indicator of neonatal distress is the fetal respiratory rate.
   A. True
   B. False

_____ 19. EMS units should contain all of the following equipment in their neonatal resuscitation kit EXCEPT a(n):
   A. meconium aspirator.
   B. laryngoscope with size 3 and 4 blades.
   C. device to secure the endotracheal tube.
   D. umbilical catheter and 10 mL syringe.
   E. DeLee suction trap.

_____ 20. Following the inverted pyramid of neonatal resuscitation, which would be done first?
   A. intubation
   B. bag-valve-mask ventilations
   C. chest compressions
   D. drying and warming
   E. administration of medications

_____ 21. In distressed newborns, monitor the heart rate with external electronic monitors.
   A. True
   B. False

_____ 22. The danger of deep suctioning a newborn is that it can cause a(n):
   A. vagal response.   D. allergic reaction.
   B. increased heart rate.   E. tachypnea.
   C. decreased respiratory rate.

_____ 23. Suctioning of a newborn should last no longer than 10 seconds.
   A. True
   B. False

_____ 24. Normal newborn respirations are approximately _____ times a minute.
   A. 10–30   D. 40–70
   B. 20–50   E. 60–90
   C. 30–60

_____ 25. Insertion of an endotracheal tube is recommended when prolonged ventilation of a newborn will be required.
   A. True
   B. False

_____ 26. Initiate chest compressions in the newborn with which of the following?
   A. heart rate greater than 100
   B. heart rate less than 60
   C. no respirations
   D. heart rate between 60 and 80 that does not improve
   E. both B and D

_____ 27. The proper sized catheter to cannulate the umbilical vein is:
   A. 14 ga.
   B. 22 ga.
   C. 10 Fr.
   D. 5 Fr.
   E. 2 Fr.

_____ 28. Naloxone may induce withdrawal in the newborn of a mother who is drug addicted.
   A. True
   B. False

_____ 29. Remove the endotracheal tube as you suction the neonate with possible meconium aspiration.
   A. True
   B. False

_____ 30. Which of the following is NOT a causative factor for apnea?
   A. CNS depressants
   B. caffeine
   C. septicemia
   D. metabolic disorders
   E. weak respiratory muscles

_____ 31. The most common cause of bradycardia in the newborn is:
   A. increasing intracranial pressure.
   B. narcotic overdose.
   C. cerebral palsy.
   D. hypoxia.
   E. congenital cardiac problems.

_____ 32. Which of the following is a reason premature infants lose heat more readily?
   A. decreased subcutaneous fat
   B. increased surface area to weight ratio
   C. immature temperature control mechanisms
   D. cannot shiver and generate heat
   E. all of the above

_____ 33. The initial bolus of fluid for the dehydrated neonate is:
   A. 10 mL/kg.
   B. 20 mL/kg.
   C. 40 mL/kg.
   D. 60 mL/kg.
   E. none of the above

_____ 34. Hypothermia is a common and life-threatening condition in neonates.
   A. True
   B. False

_____ 35. Hypoglycemia is only associated with severe diabetes mellitus in the newborn.
   A. True
   B. False

Chapter 42 Pediatrics

Review of Chapter Objectives

After reading this chapter, you should be able to:

1. **Discuss the paramedic's role in the reduction of infant and childhood morbidity and mortality from acute illness and injury.** pp. 1587–1589

   When considering the reduction of pediatric morbidity and mortality, your role as a paramedic centers around two key concepts. First, you must realize that pediatric injuries have become a major health concern. Second, you should remember that children are at a higher risk of injury than adults and that they are more likely to be adversely affected by the injuries that they suffer.

   In addition to pediatric injuries, paramedics are often responsible for treating the ill child. There are many aspects of disease and disease processes that are unique to children. It is important that the paramedic be familiar with these, as early intervention is often the key to reduced morbidity and mortality.

2. **Identify methods/mechanisms that prevent injuries to infants and children.** pp. 1588–1589

   As a paramedic, you can help reduce the rate of injury by taking advantage of opportunities to share "teaching points" in your daily life, both personally and professionally. Take part in, or offer to organize, school or community programs in injury prevention or health care. Engage student interest in the EMS profession by volunteering to speak at "career days," emphasizing those aspects of your job that relate to young people. Use nonurgent ambulance calls as a chance to educate family members or caregivers on the importance of "childproofing" a home or neighborhood. Work with appropriate agencies in initiating or conducting safety inspections, block watches, and more.

3. **Describe Emergency Medical Services for Children (EMSC) and how it can affect patient outcome.** p. 1588

   Emergency Medical Services for Children (EMSC) is a federally funded program aimed at improving the health of pediatric patients who suffer life-threatening illnesses and injuries. EMSC falls under the management of the Maternal and Child Health Bureau, which is an agency of the U.S. Department of Health and Human Services. As part of a nationally coordinated effort, the EMSC program has identified a number of pediatric health care concerns, including: community education, data collection, quality improvement, injury prevention, access, prehospital care, emergency care, definitive care, finance, rehabilitation, a systems approach to pediatric care, and ongoing health care from birth to young adulthood.

4. Identify the common family responses to acute illness and injury of an infant or child. p. 1590

As you might expect, the reaction of parents or caregivers to a pediatric emergency will vary. Initial responses by parents or caregivers might include shock, grief, denial, anger, guilt, fear, or complete loss of control. Their behavior may change during the course of the emergency.

5. Describe techniques for successful interaction with families of acutely ill or injured infants and children. p. 1590

Communication is the key to successful interaction with families of acutely ill or injured pediatric patients. Preferably only one paramedic will speak with adults at the scene. This will avoid any chance of conflicting information and allow a second paramedic to focus on the child. If parents or caregivers sense your confidence and professionalism, they will regain control and trust your suggestions for care. As with the child, most parents and caregivers feel overwhelmed by fear.

If conditions permit, you should allow one of the parents or caregivers to remain with the child at all times. Some family members may be extremely emotional in emergency situations. The child will react more positively to a family member who appears calm and reassuring. If a parent or caregiver is "out of control," have another person take him or her away from the immediate area to settle down. Maintain a reasonable level of suspicion if a child shows a pattern of injuries, some old and some new. In such cases, the parent or caregiver may try to cover up what may be an abusive situation. They may also try to block examination and treatment.

6. Identify key anatomical, physiological, growth, and developmental characteristics of infants and children and their implications. pp. 1590–1593

Children are broken into age groups because they differ in terms of anatomical, physiological, growth, and developmental characteristics. The following are some of the differences:

Newborns (first hours after birth). The term *newborn* refers to a baby in the first hours of extrauterine life. These patients are assessed using the APGAR scoring system, which was described in Chapters 40 and 41. Resuscitation of the newborn generally follows the inverted pyramid and the guidelines established in the Neonatal Advanced Life Support (NALS) curriculum.

Neonates (ages birth to 1 month). The neonate typically loses up to 10 percent of its birth weight as it adjusts to extrauterine life. This lost weight, however, is ordinarily recovered within 10 days. Gestational age affects early growth. Children born at term (40 weeks) should follow accepted developmental guidelines. Infants born prematurely will not be as developed, either neurologically or physically, as their term counterparts.

The neonatal stage of development centers on reflexes. The neonate's personality also begins to form. Obviously, the history must be obtained from the parents or caregivers. However, it is also important to observe the child. Common illnesses in this age group include jaundice, vomiting, and respiratory distress. The approach to this age group should include several factors. First, the child should always be kept warm. Observe skin color, tone, and respiratory activity. The absence of tears when crying may indicate dehydration. The lungs should be auscultated early during this exam, while the infant is quiet.

Infants (ages 1 to 5 months). Infants should have doubled their birth weight by 5 to 6 months of age and can follow the movement of others with their eyes. Muscle control develops in a cephalocaudal ("head-to-tail") progression, with control spreading from the trunk toward the extremities. Although the infant's personality continues to form, it still centers strongly on the parents or caregivers. Concentrate on keeping these patients warm and comfortable, allowing them to remain in the parent's or caregiver's lap, if possible. A pacifier or bottle can be used to help keep the baby quiet during the examination.

Infants (ages 6 to 12 months). Patients in this age group are active and enjoy exploring the world with their mouths. In this stage of development, the risk of foreign body airway obstruction (FBAO) becomes a serious concern. Infants who are 6 months and older have more fully formed personalities and express themselves more readily than younger babies. They have a considerable anxiety toward strangers. They don't like lying on their backs, and they tend to cling to their mother, though the father "will do." Common illnesses and accidents include febrile seizures, vomiting, diarrhea, dehydration, bronchiolitis, car accidents, croup, child abuse, poisonings, falls, airway obstructions, and meningitis. These children should be examined while sitting in the lap of the parent or caregiver. The exam should progress in a toe-to-head order, since starting at the face may upset the child. If time and conditions permit, allow the child to become familiar with you before beginning the examination.

Toddlers (ages 1 to 3 years). Great strides in gross motor development occur during this stage. Children tend to run underneath or stand on almost anything. As they grow older, toddlers become braver and more curious or stubborn. They begin to stray away from the parents or caregivers more frequently. Yet these remain the only people who can comfort them quickly, and most children will cling to a parent or caregiver if frightened. At ages 1 to 3, language development begins. Although the majority of the history comes from interaction with the parent or caregiver, it is possible to ask the toddler simple questions.

Accidents of all types are the leading cause of injury deaths in pediatric patients ages 1 to 15. Common accidents in this age group include motor vehicle collisions, homicides, burn injuries, drownings, and pedestrian accidents. Common illnesses and injuries in the toddler age group include vomiting, diarrhea, febrile seizures, poisonings, falls, child abuse, croup, and meningitis. Keep in mind that FBAO is still a high risk for toddlers.

Be cautious when treating toddlers. Approach toddlers slowly and try to gain their confidence. Conduct the exam in a toe-to-head order. The child may be difficult to examine and may resist being touched. Be sure to tell the child if something will hurt. If at all possible, avoid procedures on the dominant arm/hand, which the child will try to pull away.

Preschoolers (ages 3 to 5 years). Children in this age group show a tremendous increase in fine and gross motor development. Language skills increase greatly. However, if frightened, these children often refuse to speak. They usually have vivid imaginations and may see monsters as part of their world. Preschoolers may have tempers and will express them. During this stage of development, children fear mutilation and may feel threatened by treatment. Avoid frightening or misleading comments. When evaluating a child in this age group, question the child first, keeping in mind that imagination may interfere with the facts. The child often has a distorted sense of time, and thus you must rely on the parents or caregivers to fill in the gaps. Common illnesses and accidents in this age group include croup, asthma, poisonings, auto accidents, burns, child abuse, ingestion of foreign bodies, drownings, epiglottitis, febrile seizures, and meningitis.

Start the examination with the chest and evaluate the head last. Do not lie or try to trick the patient. Avoid baby talk. If time and situation permit, give the preschooler health care choices.

School-age children (ages 6 to 12 years). School-age children are active and carefree. Growth spurts sometimes lead to clumsiness. The personality continues to develop, and these children are proud and protective of their parents and caregivers. Common illnesses and injuries for this age group include drownings, auto accidents, bicycle accidents, falls, fractures, sports injuries, child abuse, and burns.

When examining school-age children, give them responsibility for providing the history. However, remember that children may be reluctant to provide information if they sustained an injury while doing something forbidden. The parents or caregivers can fill in the pertinent details. During assessment, respect the modesty of school-age children. Also, remember to be honest and tell the child what is wrong.

Adolescents (ages 13 to 18). Adolescence covers the period from the end of childhood to the start of adulthood (age 18). It begins with puberty, roughly at age 13 for males and 11 for females. Puberty is highly child specific and can begin at various ages. Adolescents vary significantly in their development. Those over age 15 are physically nearer to adults in terms of their vital signs but emotionally may still be children. Regardless of physical maturity, remember that teenagers as a group are "body conscious." The slightest possibility of a lasting scar may be a tremendous issue to the adolescent patient. Common illnesses and injuries in this age group include mononucleosis, asthma, auto collisions, sports injuries, drug and alcohol problems, suicide gestures, and sexual abuse. Remember that pregnancy is also possible in female adolescents.

In examining an adolescent patient, it may be wise to conduct the interview away from the parents or caregivers. If you must perform a detailed physical exam, respect the teenager's sense of privacy. If the patient exhibits modesty or bodily shame, have a paramedic of the same sex as the teenager conduct the exam. Although patients in this age group are not legally adults, keep in mind that most of them see themselves as grown up and will take offense at the use of the word *child*.

7. **Outline differences in adult and childhood anatomy, physiology, and "normal" age-group-related vital signs.** pp. 1593–1597

   Anatomical or physiological differences in infants and children as compared with adults include:

   - A proportionally larger tongue
   - Smaller airway structures
   - Abundant secretions
   - Deciduous (baby) teeth
   - Flatter nose and face
   - Head heavier relative to body and less-developed neck structures and muscles
   - Fontanelle and open sutures (soft spots) palpable on top of a young infant's head
   - Thinner, softer brain tissue
   - Head larger in proportion to the body
   - Shorter, narrower, more elastic (flexible) trachea
   - Shorter neck
   - Abdominal breathers with a faster respiratory rate
   - In the case of newborns, breathe primarily through the nose (obligate nose breathers)
   - Larger body surface relative to their body mass
   - Softer bones
   - More exposed spleen and liver
   - More easily dehydrated
   - Less blood and in greater danger of developing severe shock or bleeding to death from a relatively minor wound
   - Immature temperature control mechanism (unstable in babies)

   Age-related differences in vital signs include:

   - Pulse rates (average) by age group:
     - Newborn: 100–180
     - Infant 0 to 5 months: 100–160
     - Infant 6 to 12 months: 100–160
     - Toddler 1 to 3 years: 80–110
     - Preschooler 3 to 5 years: 80–110
     - School-age child 6 to 10 years: 65–110
     - Early adolescent 11 to 14 years: 60–90
   - Respiratory rates (average) by age group:
     - Newborn: 30–60
     - Infant 0 to 5 months: 30–60
     - Infant 6 to 12 months: 30–60
     - Preschooler 3 to 5 years: 22–34
     - School-age child 6 to 10 years: 18–30
     - Early adolescent 11 to 14 years: 12–26
   - Blood pressure (average/mmHg at rest) by age group:

Age Group	Systolic Approx. 90 plus 2/3 age	Diastolic Approx. 2/3 systolic
Preschooler 3 to 5 years:	average 98 (78–116)	average 65
School-age child 6 to 10 years:	average 105 (80–122)	average 69
Early adolescent 11 to 14 years:	average 114 (88–140)	average 76

8. Describe techniques for successful assessment and treatment of infants and children. pp. 1597–1623

Many of the components of the initial patient assessment can be done during a visual examination of the scene ("assessment from the doorway"). Whenever possible, involve the parent or caregiver in efforts to calm or comfort the child. Depending on the situation, you may decide to allow the parent or caregiver to remain with the child during treatment and transport. The developmental stage of the patient and the coping skills of the parents or guardians will be key factors in making this decision.

When interacting with parents or other responsible adults, pay attention to the way in which parents or caregivers interact with the child. Are the interactions appropriate to the emergency? Are family members concerned? Are they angry? Are they overly emotional or entirely indifferent?

From the time of dispatch, you will continually acquire information relative to the patient's condition. As with all patients, personal safety must be your first priority. In treating pediatric patients, follow the same guidelines in approaching the scene as you would with any other patient. Observe for potentially hazardous situations, and make sure you take appropriate BSI precautions. Remember that infants and young children are at especially high risk for infection.

9. Discuss the appropriate equipment used to obtain pediatric vital signs. p. 1605

Remember that poorly taken vital signs are of less value than no vital signs at all. Therefore, you must have the correct equipment to obtain pediatric vital signs. Items include appropriate-sized BP cuffs, a pediatric stethoscope, and so on. Modern noninvasive monitoring devices all have their application to emergency care. These devices may include pulse oximeter, automated blood pressure devices, self-registering thermometers, and ECGs. However, these devices may frighten a child. Before applying any monitoring device, explain what you are going to do and then demonstrate the device.

10. Determine appropriate airway adjuncts, ventilation devices, and endotracheal intubation equipment; their proper use; and complications of use for infants and children. pp. 1606–1617

As a general rule, use airway adjuncts in pediatric patients only if prolonged artificial ventilations are required. There are two reasons for this. First, infants and children often improve quickly through the administration of 100 percent oxygen. Second, airway adjuncts may create greater complications in children than in adults.

Keeping this in mind, be sure to have available the appropriate-sized airway adjuncts for each pediatric age group. Basic equipment includes oral and nasal airways, a pediatric BVM, smaller-sized suction catheters, smaller-sized masks for the BVM, age-appropriate nasogastric tubes, and a pediatric laryngoscope, blades, and ET tubes. It is also a good idea to carry a Braslow® tape, which, after measuring the child's height, displays the appropriate sizes of tubes.

The biggest complication of airway management for the pediatric patient is the possibility of overinflation, which allows air to gather in the stomach. Gastric distention can cause pressure on the diaphragm, making full expansion of the lungs difficult. For specific techniques in airway management in the pediatric patient, review the steps and scan sheets in the textbook, especially those dealing with advanced airway and ventilatory management.

11. List the indications and methods of gastric decompression for infants and children. pp. 1617–1619

If gastric distention is present in a pediatric patient, you may consider placing a nasogastric tube (NG tube). In infants and children, gastric distention may result from overly aggressive artificial ventilations or from air swallowing. Placement of an NG tube will allow you to decompress the stomach and the proximal bowel of air. An NG tube can also be used to empty the stomach of blood or other substances. Indications for use of nasogastric intubation include an inability to achieve adequate tidal volumes during ventilation due to gastric distention and the presence of gastric distention in an unresponsive patient.

As with nasopharyngeal airways, an NG tube is contraindicated in pediatric patients who have sustained head or facial trauma. Because the NG tube might migrate into the cranial sinuses, consider the use of an orogastric tube instead. Other contraindications include possible soft-tissue damage in the nose and inducement of vomiting.

In determining the correct length of NG tube, measure the tube from the top of the nose, over the ear, to the tip of the xiphoid process. To insert an NG tube, you should:

- Oxygenate and continue to ventilate, if possible.
- Measure the NG tube from the tip of the nose, over the ear, to the tip of the xiphoid process.
- Lubricate the end of the tube. Then pass it gently downward along the nasal floor to the stomach.
- Auscultate over the epigastrium to confirm correct placement. Listen for bubbling while injecting 10–20 cc of air into the tube.
- Use suction to aspirate stomach contents.
- Secure the tube in place.

12. Define pediatric respiratory distress, failure, and arrest. pp. 1624–1626

The severity of respiratory compromise can be quickly classified into the following categories:

Respiratory distress. The mildest form of respiratory impairment is classified as respiratory distress. The most noticeable finding is the increased work of breathing. The signs and symptoms of respiratory distress include a normal mental status deteriorating to irritability or anxiety, tachypnea, retractions, nasal flaring (in infants), good muscle tone, head bobbing, grunting, and cyanosis that improves with supplemental oxygen. If not corrected immediately, respiratory distress will lead to respiratory failure.

Respiratory failure. Respiratory failure occurs when the respiratory system is not able to meet the demands of the body for oxygen intake and for carbon dioxide removal. It is characterized by inadequate ventilation and oxygenation. During respiratory failure, the carbon dioxide level begins to rise as the body is not able to remove it. This ultimately leads to respiratory acidosis. The signs and symptoms of respiratory failure include irritability or anxiety deteriorating to lethargy, marked tachypnea later deteriorating to bradypnea, marked retractions later deteriorating to agonal respirations, poor muscle tone, marked tachycardia later deteriorating to bradycardia, and central cyanosis. Respiratory failure is a very ominous sign. If immediate intervention is not provided, the child will deteriorate to full respiratory arrest.

Respiratory arrest. The end result of respiratory impairment, if untreated, is respiratory arrest. The cessation of breathing typically follows a period of bradypnea and agonal respirations. The signs and symptoms of respiratory arrest include unresponsiveness deteriorating to coma, bradypnea deteriorating to apnea, absent chest wall movement, bradycardia deteriorating to asystole, and profound cyanosis. Respiratory arrest will quickly deteriorate to full cardiopulmonary arrest if appropriate interventions are not made. The child's chances of survival markedly decrease when cardiopulmonary arrest occurs.

13. Differentiate between upper airway obstruction and lower airway disease. pp. 1626–1632

Obstruction of the upper airway can be caused by many factors and may be partial or complete. Obstruction can result from inflamed or swollen tissues, which may be caused by infection or by aspirating a foreign body. Two medical conditions that can lead to upper airway obstruction in pediatric patients include croup and epiglottitis. Appropriate care depends on prompt and immediate identification of the disorder and its severity.

Suspect lower airway distress when the following conditions exist: an absence of stridor, presence of wheezing during exhalation, and increased work of breathing. Common causes of lower airway disease include respiratory diseases such as asthma, bronchiolitis, and pneumonia. Although infrequent, you may also encounter cases of foreign body lower airway aspiration, especially in toddlers and preschoolers.

14. Describe the general approach to the treatment of children with respiratory distress, failure, or arrest from upper airway obstruction or lower airway disease. pp. 1626–1632

The general approach to the child with respiratory distress or failure from an upper or lower airway problem is to assess the child in the least stressful way possible and to administer oxygen. If the child has a complete upper airway obstruction, the appropriate FBAO maneuvers will need to be quickly done. If the child is in respiratory arrest, begin BVM resuscitation and consider the need for ET tube insertion. An NG tube may be useful to minimize gastric distention. If the child is in respiratory failure, assisted ventilations should also be considered.

In cases of upper airway obstruction, keep this precaution in mind: Because it is difficult to distinguish croup from epiglottitis in the prehospital setting, never examine the oropharynx. If epiglottitis is present, examination of the oropharynx may result in laryngospasm and complete airway obstruction. In fact, if the patient is maintaining his or her airway, do not put anything into the child's mouth, including a thermometer. In the case of foreign body aspiration, do not attempt to look into the child's mouth if the obstruction is partial. Instead make the child comfortable and administer humidified oxygen. If the obstruction is complete, clear the airway with accepted basic life support techniques. However, DO NOT perform blind finger sweeps, as this can push a foreign body deeper into the airway.

When treating lower airway diseases, the primary goal is to support ventilations through the use of supplemental, humidified oxygen and appropriate pharmacological therapy such as bronchodilator medications (asthma and bronchiolitis). If prolonged ventilation will be required, perform endotracheal intubation.

15. Discuss the common causes and relative severity of hypoperfusion in infants and children. pp. 1632–1636

The second major cause of pediatric cardiopulmonary arrest—after respiratory impairment—is shock. Shock can most simply be defined as inadequate perfusion of the tissues with oxygen and other essential nutrients and inadequate removal of metabolic waste products.

When compared with the incidence of shock in adults, shock is an unusual occurrence in children because their blood vessels constrict so efficiently. However, when the blood pressure does drop, it drops so far and so fast that the child may quickly develop cardiopulmonary arrest. A number of factors place infants and young children at risk for shock. Newborns and neonates will develop shock as a result of a loss of body heat. Other causes include dehydration (from vomiting and/or diarrhea), infection (particularly septicemia), trauma, and blood loss. Less common causes of shock in infants and children include allergic reactions, poisoning, and cardiac events.

As in adults, the severity of shock in a pediatric patient is classified as compensated shock, decompensated shock, and irreversible shock. It can also be categorized as cardiogenic or noncardiogenic. Cardiogenic shock results from an inability of the heart to maintain an adequate cardiac output to the circulatory tissues. Cardiogenic shock in a pediatric patient is ominous and often fatal. Noncardiogenic shock—types of shock that result from causes other than inadequate cardiac output—is more frequently encountered in pediatric patients, because they have a much lower incidence of cardiac problems that adults. Causes of noncardiogenic shock may include hemorrhage, abdominal trauma, systemic bacterial infection, spinal cord injury, and others.

16. Identify the major classifications of pediatric cardiac rhythms. pp. 1637–1640

Dysrhythmias in children are uncommon. When dysrhythmias occur, bradydysrhythmias are the most common. Supraventricular tachydysrhythmias are very uncommon. Dysrhythmias can cause pump failure, ultimately leading to cardiogenic shock. Children have a very limited capacity to increase stroke volume. The primary mechanism through which they increase cardiac output is through changes in the heart rate. The treatment of dysrhythmias is specific for the dysrhythmia in question.

17. Discuss the primary etiologies of cardiopulmonary arrest in infants and children. pp. 1624–1625, 1632

The primary causes of cardiopulmonary arrest in infants and children include untreated respiratory failure, immaturity of the cardiac conductive system, bradycardia, hypoxia, vagal stimulation (rare), drug overdose, drowning, multiple system trauma, electrocution, pericardial tamponade, tension pneumothorax, acidosis, hypothermia, hypoglycemia, and FBAO.

18. Discuss age-appropriate sites, equipment, techniques, and complications of vascular access for infants and children. pp. 1619–1620

Intravenous techniques for children are basically the same as for adults. (See Chapter 7, "Medication Administration.") However, additional veins may be accessed in an infant. These include veins of the neck and scalp, as well as of the arms, hands, and feet. The external jugular vein, however, should only be used in life-threatening situations.

The use of intraosseous (IO) infusion has become popular in the pediatric patient. This is especially true when large volumes of fluid must be administered, as occurs in hypovolemic shock, and when other means of venous access are unavailable. The indications for IO include the existence of shock or cardiac arrest, an unresponsive patient, or an unsuccessful attempt at a peripheral IV insertion. The contraindications for IO infusion include the presence of a fracture in the bone chosen for infusion and a fracture of the pelvis or extremity fracture in the bone proximal to the chosen site.

In performing IO perfusion, you can use a standard 16- or 18-gauge needle (either hypodermic or spinal). However, an intraosseous needle is preferred and significantly better. Basic steps are as follows: Prep the anterior surface of the leg below the knee with antiseptic solution (povidone iodine), and insert the needle in twisting fashion 1–3 centimeters below the tuberosity. Insertion should be slightly inferior in direction (to avoid the growth plate) and perpendicular to the skin. Signs of correct placement of the needle into the marrow cavity include a lack of resistance as the needle passes through the bony cortex, the ability of the needle to stand upright without support, the ability to aspirate bone marrow into a syringe, or free flow of the infusion without infiltration into the subcutaneous tissues.

19. Describe the primary etiologies of altered level of consciousness in infants and children. pp. 1623–1647, 1653–1654, 1663

The primary causes of an altered level of consciousness in infants and children include infection (fever), traumatic brain injury, respiratory failure (hypoxia), hypoperfusion, and dysrhythmias. Although metabolic causes such as seizures and hypoglycemia are fairly uncommon, they can and do produce altered levels of consciousness in children. Shunt failures may also present as altered mental status.

20. Identify common lethal mechanisms of injury in infants and children. pp. 1649–1651

The most common pediatric mechanisms of injury (MOI) include falls, motor vehicle crashes, car versus pedestrian collisions, drownings and near-drownings, penetrating injuries, burns, and physical abuse.

21. Discuss anatomical features of children that predispose or protect them from certain injuries. pp. 1654–1655

Head. Small children have larger heads in proportion to the rest of their bodies. For this reason, when they fall or are thrown through the air, they often land head first, predisposing them to serious head injury. The larger relative mass of the head and lack of neck muscle strength also provide increased momentum in acceleration-deceleration injuries and a greater stress on the cervical spine. Because the skull is softer and more compliant in infants and young children than in adults, brain injuries occur more readily.

Chest and abdomen. Infants and young children lack the rigid rib cages of adults. Therefore, they suffer fewer rib fractures and more intrathoracic injuries. Remember that chest injuries are the second most common cause of pediatric trauma death. Because of the compliance of the chest wall, severe intrathoracic injury can be present without signs of external injury. Likewise, their relatively underdeveloped abdominal musculature affords minimal protection to the viscera, particularly the spleen.

Extremities. Because children have more flexible bones than adults, they tend to have incomplete fractures such as bend fractures, buckle fractures, and greenstick fractures. Therefore, you should treat "sprains" and "strains" as fractures and immobilize accordingly. In younger children, the bone growth plates have not yet closed. Some growth plate fractures can lead to permanent disability if not managed correctly.

Body surface. There are three distinguishing features of the pediatric patient's skin and BSA. First, the skin of an infant or child is thinner than that of an adult. Second, infants and children generally have less subcutaneous fat. Finally, they have a larger body-surface-area-to-weight ratio. As a result of these features, children risk greater injury from extremes in temperature or thermal exposure. They lose fluids and heat more quickly than adults and have a greater likelihood of dehydration and hypothermia. They also burn more easily and deeper than adults, which explains why burns are one of the leading causes of death among pediatric trauma patients.

22. **Describe aspects of infant and child airway management that are affected by potential cervical spine injury.** pp. 1651–1653

An infant's open airway is in the neutral or extended position but not in the hyperextended position. This needs to be kept in mind when positioning the infant who may have sustained a neck injury where there can be little to no movement of the neck for fear of worsening the potential neck injury. Children under the age of 6 usually have large heads in proportion to the rest of their bodies. Therefore, it is often necessary to pad behind the shoulders when a cervical collar is applied as a part of the spinal immobilization. Keep infants, toddlers, and preschoolers with the cervical spine in a neutral in-line position by placing padding from the shoulders to the hips.

Always make sure that you use appropriate-sized pediatric immobilization equipment. These supplies may include rigid cervical collars, towel or blanket rolls, foam head blocks, commercial pediatric immobilization devices, vest-type or short wooden backboards, and long boards with the appropriate padding.

23. **Identify infant and child trauma patients who require spinal immobilization.** pp. 1621, 1623

Children are not small adults. Although spinal injuries are not as common as in adults, they do occur, especially because of a child's disproportionately larger and heavier head. Any time an infant or child sustains a significant head injury, assume that a neck injury may be present. Children can suffer a spinal cord injury with no noticeable damage to the vertebral column as seen on cervical spine X-rays. Thus, negative cervical spine X-rays do not necessarily assure that a spinal cord injury does not exist. As a result, children should remain immobilized until a spinal cord injury has been ruled out by hospital personnel.

Remember that many children, especially those under age 5, will protest or fight restraints. Try to minimize the emotional stress by having a parent or caregiver stand near or touch the child.

24. **Discuss fluid management and shock treatment for infant and child trauma patients.** pp. 1632–1636, 1653

Fluid management and shock treatment for pediatric trauma patients should include administration of supplemental oxygen and establishment of intravenous access. However, DO NOT delay transport to gain venous access. Management of the airway and breathing takes priority over management of circulation, as circulatory compromise is less common in children than in adults.

When obtaining vascular access, remember the following:

- If possible, insert a large-bore catheter into a peripheral vein.
- Reassess the patient's vital signs and give additional boluses of 20 mL/kg—up to 100 mL/kg if there is no improvement.

- Once venous access is obtained, administer an initial fluid bolus of 20 mL/kg of lactated Ringer's or normal saline.
- Reassess the patient's vital signs and re-bolus with another 80–100 mL/kg if there is no improvement.
- If improvement does not occur after the second bolus, there is likely to be a significant blood loss that may require surgical intervention. Rapid transport is essential.

25. Determine when pain management and sedation are appropriate for infants and children. p. 1653

Many pediatric injuries are painful and analgesics are indicated. These include burns, long-bone fractures, dislocations, and others. Unless there is a contraindication, pediatric patients should receive analgesics. Commonly used analgesics include meperidine, morphine, and fentanyl. It is best to avoid using synthetic analgesics (e.g., butorphanol [Stadol], nalbuphine [Nubain]), as their effects on children are unpredictable. Also, certain pediatric emergencies may benefit from sedation. These include such problems as penetrating eye injuries, prolonged rescue from entrapment in machinery, cardioversion, and other painful procedures. Always consult medical direction if you feel pediatric analgesia or sedation may be required.

26. Define child abuse, child neglect, and sudden infant death syndrome (SIDS). pp. 1656–1661

Child abuse is the intentional effort by a parent or caregiver to harm a child physically, psychologically, or sexually. Abuse can also take the form of child neglect (either physical or emotional), in which the physical, mental, and/or emotional well-being of the child is ignored.

Sudden infant death syndrome (SIDS) is defined as the sudden death of an infant during the first year of life from an illness of unknown etiology, with peak incidence occurring at 2 to 4 months.

27. Discuss the parent/caregiver responses to the death of an infant or child. p. 1657

The responses of the parent or caregiver to the death of a child include the normal grief reactions. Initially, there may be shock, disbelief, and denial. Other times, the parents or caregivers may express anger, rage, hostility, blame, or guilt. Often, there is a feeling or inadequacy as well as helplessness, confusion, and fear. The grief process is likely to last for years, as in the case of a SIDS death.

28. Define children with special health care needs and technology-assisted children. pp. 1661–1664

In recent years medical technology has lowered infant mortality rates and allowed a greater number of children with special needs to live at home. Some of these infants and children include:

- Premature babies
- Infants and children with lung disease, heart disease, or neurological disorders
- Infants and children with chronic diseases, such as cystic fibrosis, asthma, childhood cancers, cerebral palsy, and others
- Infants and children with altered functions from birth (e.g., spina bifida, congenital birth defects, and cerebral palsy)

On some calls, you may be asked to treat technology-assisted children who depend, in varying degrees, upon special equipment. Commonly found devices include tracheostomy tubes, apnea monitors, home artificial ventilators, central intravenous lines, gastric feeding tubes, gastrostomy tubes, and shunts. (For more on these devices, see Chapter 46, "Acute Interventions for the Chronic-Care Patient.")

29. Discuss basic cardiac life support (CPR) guidelines for infants and children. pp. 1599–1602, 1606–1611

The CPR guidelines for infants and children are periodically revised. The Brady website at: www.bradybooks.com will provide the most up-to-date information on these standards.

30. Integrate advanced life support skills with basic cardiac life support for infants and children. pp. 1611–1621, 1637–1640

This is a skills objective that should be practiced in the classroom lab setting. You should work through simulated "mega-codes" that involve both BLS and ALS responders administering all the appropriate treatments as specified in their regional protocols and the American Heart Association's PALS algorithms.

31. Discuss the indications, dosage, route of administration, and special considerations for medication administration in infants and children. pp. 1620–1622

When administering medications to any patient of any age, the paramedic needs to know the indications, contraindications, correct dose, correct route of administration, and any expected side effects of the medication. Specifically, when administering the medications to infants and children, be very careful and accurate with the dose. Most medication doses are weight specific, so it will be necessary to have a rough idea of the weight of the patient or to use some other tool such as the Braslow tape.

The objectives of medication therapy in pediatric patients include:

- Correction of hypoxemia
- Increased perfusion pressure during chest compressions
- Stimulation of spontaneous or more forceful cardiac contractions
- Acceleration of the heart rate
- Correction of metabolic acidosis
- Management of pain (see objective 25)
- Treatment of seizures (see objective 33)

In administering medications to pediatric patients, consult with medical direction.

32. Discuss appropriate transport guidelines for low- and high-risk infants and children. p. 1623

In managing a pediatric patient, never delay transport to perform a procedure that can be done en route to the hospital. After deciding upon necessary interventions—first BLS, then ALS—determine the appropriate receiving facility. In reaching your decision, consider three factors: time of transport, specialized facilities, and specialized personnel. If you live in an area with specialized prehospital crews such as Critical Care Crews and Neonatal Nurses, their availability should weigh in your decision. Consider whether the patient would benefit by transfer to one of these crews. (For more on transport guides for low- and high-risk infants, see Chapter 41, "Neonatology.")

33. Describe the epidemiology, including the incidence, morbidity/mortality, risk factors, prevention strategies, pathophysiology, assessment, and treatment of infants and children with:

a. Respiratory distress/failure pp. 1624–1632

Respiratory emergencies constitute the most common reason EMS is called to care for a pediatric patient. Respiratory illnesses can cause respiratory compromise due to their effect on the alveolar/capillary interface. Some illnesses are quite minor, causing only minor symptoms, while others can be rapidly fatal. Your approach to the child with a respiratory emergency will depend upon the severity of respiratory compromise (see objectives 12 and 13). If the child is alert and talking, then you can take a more relaxed approach. However, if the child is ill-appearing and exhibiting marked respiratory difficulty, then you have to immediately intervene to prevent respiratory arrest and possible cardiopulmonary arrest.

Pediatric patients with late respiratory failure or respiratory arrest require aggressive treatment. This includes:
- Establishment of an airway
- Administration of high-flow supplemental oxygen

- Mechanical ventilation with a bag-valve-mask device attached to a reservoir delivering 100 percent oxygen
- Endotracheal intubation if mechanical ventilation does not rapidly improve the patient's condition
- Consideration of gastric decompression with an orogastric or nasogastric tube if abdominal distension is impeding ventilation
- Consideration of needle decompression of the chest if a tension pneumothorax is suspected
- Consideration of cricothyrotomy if complete obstruction is present and the airway cannot be obtained by any other method
- Obtain venous access, and transport to a facility equipped to handle critically ill children

b. Hypoperfusion pp. 1632–1636

As noted, shock is the second major cause of pediatric cardiopulmonary arrest. For an overview of the causes and degrees of severity of hypoperfusion in infants and children, see objective 15.

The definitive care of shock takes place in the emergency department of a hospital. Because shock is a life-threatening condition in pediatric patients, it is important to recognize early signs and symptoms—or even the possibility of shock in a situation where the signs and symptoms may not have yet developed. In a situation in which you suspect a possibility of shock, provide oxygen to boost tissue perfusion and transport as quickly as possible. Also, keep the patient in a supine position and take steps to protect the child from hypothermia and agitation that might worsen the condition. In some cases (compensated shock), fluid therapy as ordered by medical direction can buy time until the patient arrives at an appropriate treatment center. (See objective 24 for more on fluid therapy and shock management.)

c. Cardiac dysrhythmias pp. 1637–1640

Dysrhythmias in children are uncommon. When dysrhythmias occur, bradydysrhythmias are the most common. Supraventricular tachydysrhythmias are very uncommon. Dysrhythmias can cause pump failure, ultimately leading to cardiogenic shock. Children have a very limited capacity to increase stroke volume. The primary mechanism through which they increase cardiac output is through changes in the heart rate. The treatment of dysrhythmias is specific for the dysrhythmia in question.

d. Neurologic emergencies pp. 1640, 1642–1643

Neurologic emergencies in childhood are fairly uncommon. However, seizures can and do occur. In fact, they are a frequent reason for summoning EMS. In addition to seizures, meningitis tends to show up more often in children than in adults. Although your chances of encountering either of these two diseases are small, both are life-threatening and should be promptly identified and treated.

Seizures. The etiology for seizures is often unknown. However, several risk factors have been identified. They include fever, hypoxia, infections, idiopathic epilepsy (epilepsy of unknown origin), electrolyte disturbances, head trauma, hypoglycemia, toxic ingestions or exposure, tumor, or CNS malformations. Management of pediatric seizure is essentially the same as for the seizing adult. Place patients on the floor or on the bed. Be sure to lay them on their side, away from furniture. Do not restrain patients, but take steps to protect them from injury. Maintain the airway, but do not force anything, such as a bite stick, between the teeth. Administer supplemental oxygen. Then take and record all vital signs. If the patient is febrile, remove excess layers of clothing, while avoiding extreme cooling. If status epilepticus is present, institute the following steps:

- Start an IV of normal saline or lactated Ringer's and perform a glucometer evaluation.
- Administer diazepam as follows:
  —Children 1 month to 5 years: 0.2–0.5 mg slow IV push every 2 to 5 minutes up to a maximum of 2.5 milligrams.
  —Children 5 years and older: 1 mg slow IV push every 2 to 5 minutes to a maximum of 5 milligrams.
- Contact medical direction for additional dosing. Diazepam can be administered rectally if an IV cannot be established.
- If the seizure appears to be due to a fever and a long transport time is anticipated, medical direction may request the administration of acetaminophen to lower the fever. Acetaminophen is supplied as an elixir or as suppositories. The dose should be 15 mg/kg body weight.

Meningitis. Meningitis is an infection of the meninges, the lining of the brain and spinal cord. Meningitis can result from either a virus or a bacteria. These infections can be rapidly fatal if they are not promptly recognized and treated appropriately. Prehospital care of the pediatric patient with meningitis is supportive. Rapidly complete the initial assessment and transport the child to the emergency department. If shock is present, treat the child with IV fluids (20 mL/kg) and oxygen.

e. Trauma   pp. 1648–1651

Trauma is the number one cause of death in infants and children. Most pediatric injuries result from blunt trauma. As noted in objective 21, children have thinner and more pliable body walls that allow forces to be more readily transmitted to body contents, increasing the possibility of injury to internal tissues and organs. If you serve in an urban area, you can expect to see a higher incidence of penetrating trauma, mostly intentional and mostly from gunfire or knife wounds. There is also a significant incidence of penetrating trauma outside the cities (mostly unintentional) from hunting and agricultural accidents.

Although pediatric patients can be injured in the same way as adults, children tend to be more susceptible to certain types of injuries than grownups. Falls, for example, are the single most common cause of injury in children. Other mechanisms of injury include motor vehicle collisions, car versus pedestrian collisions, drownings and near-drownings, penetrating injuries, burns, and physical abuse.

The treatment of trauma is injury specific. It involves management of the ABCs, management of the injury (e.g., spinal immobilization, splinting of fractures, control of bleeding), and treatment for possible shock.

f. Abuse and neglect   pp. 1657–1661

Child abuse is the second leading cause of death in infants less than 6 months of age. An estimated 2,000 to 5,000 children die each year as a result of abuse or neglect. There are several characteristics common among abused children. Often the child is seen as "special" and different from others. Premature infants and twins stand a higher risk of abuse than other children. Many abused children are less than 5 years of age. Physically and mentally handicapped children as well as those with special needs are at greater risk. So are uncommunicative children. Boys are more often abused than girls. A child who is not what the parents wanted (e.g., the "wrong" gender) is at increased risk of abuse, too.

Signs of abuse or neglect can be startling. As a guide, the following findings should trigger a high index of suspicion:

- Any obvious or suspected fractures in a child under 2 years of age
- Injuries in various stages of healing, especially burns and bruises
- More injuries than usually seen in children of the same age or size
- Injuries scattered on many areas of the body
- Bruises or burns in patterns that suggest intentional infliction
- Increased intracranial pressure in an infant
- Suspected intraabdominal trauma in a young child
- Any injury that does not fit with the description of the cause given

Information in the medical history may also raise the index of suspicion. Examples include:

- A history that does not match the nature or severity of the injury
- Vague parental accounts or accounts that change during the interview
- Accusations that the child injured himself or herself intentionally
- Delay in seeking help
- Child dressed inappropriately for the situation
- Revealing comment by bystanders, especially siblings

Suspect child neglect if you spot any of the following conditions:

- Extreme malnutrition
- Multiple insect bites

- Long-standing skin infections
- Extreme lack of cleanliness
- Verbal or social skills far below those you would expect for a child of similar age and background
- Lack of appropriate medical care

In cases of child abuse or neglect, the goals of management include appropriate treatment of injuries, protection of the child from further abuse, and notification of proper authorities.

g. Special health care needs, including technology-assisted children   pp. 1661–1664

For most of human history, infants and children with devastating congenital conditions or diseases died or remained confined to a hospital. In recent decades, however, medical technology has lowered infant mortality rates and allowed a greater number of children with special needs to live at home. For examples of children with special needs and some of the technological devices used to assist them, see objective 28.

In treating pediatric patients with special needs, remember that they require the same assessment as other patients. (Recall that in the initial assessment, "disability" refers to a patient's neurological status—not to the child's special need.) Keep in mind that the child's special need is often an ongoing process, which may make the parent or caregiver an excellent source of information. In most cases, you should concentrate on the acute problem—the reason for the call. In managing patients with special needs, try to keep several thoughts in mind.

- Avoid using the term *disability* (in reference to the child's special need). Instead, think of the patient's many abilities.
- Never assume that the patient cannot understand what you are saying.
- Involve the parents, caregivers, or the patient, if appropriate, in treatment. They manage the illness or congenital condition on a daily basis.
- Treat the patient with a special need with the same respect as any other patient.

h. SIDS   pp. 1656–1657

The incidence of SIDS in the United States is approximately 2 deaths per 1,000 births. It is the leading cause of death between 2 weeks and 1 year of age, with peak incidence occurring at 2 to 4 months. SIDS occurs most frequently in the fall and winter months. It tends to be more common in males than in females. It is more prevalent in premature and low-birth-weight infants, in infants of young mothers, and in infants whose mothers did not receive prenatal care. Infants of mothers who used cocaine, methadone, or heroin during pregnancy are at greater risk. Occasionally, a mild upper respiratory infection will be reported prior to the death. SIDS is not caused by external suffocation from blankets or pillows. Neither is it related to allergies to cow's milk or regurgitation and aspiration of stomach contents. It is not thought to be hereditary.

Current theories vary about the etiology of SIDS. Some authorities feel it may result from an immature respiratory center in the brain that leads the child to simply stop breathing. Others think there may be an airway obstruction in the posterior pharynx as a result of pharyngeal relaxation during sleep, a hypermobile mandible, or an enlarged tongue. Studies strongly link SIDS to a prone sleeping position. Soft bedding, waterbed mattresses, smoking in the home, and/or an overheated environment are other potential associations. A small percentage of SIDS may be abuse related.

Unless the infant is obviously dead, undertake active and aggressive care of the infant to assure the family or caregivers that everything possible is being done. A first responder or other personnel should be assigned to assist the parents or caregivers and to explain the procedure. At all points, use the baby's name.

34. Given several preprogrammed simulated pediatric patients, provide the appropriate assessment, treatment, and transport.   pp. 1587–1664

During your classroom, clinical, and field training, you will be presented with real and simulated pediatric patients and assess and treat them. Use the information provided in this chapter and the information and skills you gain from your instructors and clinical and field preceptors to develop your skill on caring for these patients. Continue to refine newly learned skills once your training ends and you begin your paramedic career.

Content Self-Evaluation

MULTIPLE CHOICE

_____ 1. The leading cause of death in pediatric patiens in the United States is:
   A. AIDS.
   B. asthma.
   C. trauma.
   D. neglect.
   E. cardiac arrest.

_____ 2. Factors that account for high rates of pediatric injury include all of the following EXCEPT:
   A. weather.
   B. geography.
   C. dangers in the home.
   D. HMOs.
   E. motor vehicle accidents.

_____ 3. The federally funded program aimed at improving the health of pediatric patients who suffer from life-threatening illnesses and injuries is called:
   A. EMSC.
   B. PBTLS.
   C. PALS.
   D. APLS.
   E. TRIPP.

_____ 4. The most common response of children to illness or injury is:
   A. denial.
   B. fear.
   C. excitement.
   D. indifference.
   E. grief.

_____ 5. Treatment of a pediatric patient begins with:
   A. obtaining vital signs.
   B. placement of an ET tube.
   C. administration of oxygen.
   D. focused head-to-toe exam.
   E. communications and psychological support.

_____ 6. While caring for the pediatric patient, whenever possible, the paramedic should:
   A. avoid discussing painful procedures.
   B. administer high-flow oxygen.
   C. allow a parent or caregiver to stay with the child.
   D. use correct medical and anatomical terms.
   E. stand in an authoritative posture.

_____ 7. The term *neonate* describes a baby that is:
   A. newly born.
   B. 10 days or less in age.
   C. up to 1 month in age.
   D. 1 to 5 months in age.
   E. 6 months or more in age.

_____ 8. The age group for which foreign body airway obstruction (FBAO) becomes a concern is:
   A. infants ages 1 to 5 months.
   B. infants ages 6 to 12 months.
   C. toddlers.
   D. preschoolers.
   E. school-age children.

_____ 9. An infant's airway differs from that of an adult in all of the following ways EXCEPT that it:
   A. is narrower at all levels.
   B. has a softer and more flexible trachea.
   C. is less likely to be blocked by secretions.
   D. has a greater likelihood of soft-tissue injury.
   E. is more prone to obstruction by the tongue.

_____ 10. In comparing pediatric heart and respiratory rates with those of an adult, infants and young children have:
   A. about the same heart and respiratory rates as an adult.
   B. slower heart rates and slower respiratory rates.
   C. slower heart rates and faster respiratory rates.
   D. faster heart rates and slower respiratory rates.
   E. faster heart rates and faster respiratory rates.

_____ 11. Unlike an adult, the trachea of a child can collapse if the neck and head are hyperextended because:
   A. the trachea is softer and more flexible.
   B. a child's tongue takes up more space proportionately.
   C. the cricoid rings are firmer.
   D. a child's larynx is higher.
   E. the airway is wider at all levels.

_____ 12. The two abdominal organs that are most likely to suffer traumatic injury in a pediatric patient are the:
   A. kidney and gallbladder.
   B. liver and spleen.
   C. stomach and small intestine.
   D. colon and appendix.
   E. bladder and pancreas.

_____ 13. A child's larger body-surface-area-to-weight ratio causes a pediatric patient to be:
   A. resilient to temperature changes.
   B. prone to hypothermia.
   C. difficult to assess.
   D. prone to excess subcutaneous fat.
   E. less likely to lose fluids quickly.

_____ 14. Although infants and children have a circulating blood volume proportionately larger than adults, their absolute blood volume is:
   A. about the same.
   B. smaller.
   C. even larger.
   D. rate dependent.
   E. variable.

_____ 15. The pediatric assessment triangle focuses on airway, breathing, and circulation.
   A. True
   B. False

_____ 16. In an infant or small child, tachypnea, an abnormally rapid rate of breathing, may indicate:
   A. fear.
   B. pain.
   C. inadequate oxygenation.
   D. exposure to cold.
   E. all of the above

_____ 17. A respiratory rate of 18 to 30 breaths per minute would be considered normal for a(n):
   A. newborn.
   B. 6-month-old infant.
   C. toddler.
   D. preschooler.
   E. school-age child.

_____ 18. Which of the following approaches is the correct method for conducting the physical examination of an infant or a very young child?
   A. toe-to-head
   B. head-to-chest
   C. head-to-toe
   D. chest-to-head
   E. both A and B

_____ 19. To obtain the blood pressure of a pediatric patient, the cuff should be _____ the width of the patient's arm.
   A. one fourth
   B. one third
   C. one half
   D. two thirds
   E. three fourths

584 ESSENTIALS OF PARAMEDIC CARE

_____ 20. Poorly taken vital signs are of less value than no vital signs at all.
   A. True
   B. False

_____ 21. Medication administration in the pediatric patient is modified to the patient's:
   A. age.
   B. height.
   C. weight.
   D. level of distress.
   E. level of consciousness.

_____ 22. The hallmark of pediatric management is:
   A. frequent pulse checks.
   B. prompt transport.
   C. administration of fluids.
   D. adequate oxygenation.
   E. diagnosis of medical conditions.

_____ 23. As a rule, an oropharyngeal airway should only be used on pediatric patients who:
   A. have sustained head or facial trauma.
   B. are known to suffer from seizures.
   C. show signs of cardiac arrest.
   D. exhibit a vagal response.
   E. lack a gag reflex.

_____ 24. The only indication for cricothyrotomy in the pediatric patient is:
   A. a foreign body airway obstruction.
   B. desire to suction the airway.
   C. failure to obtain an airway by any other method.
   D. desire to ventilate by a BVM.
   E. both A and C

_____ 25. An indication for performing endotracheal intubation in a pediatric patient includes:
   A. need to gain access for suctioning.
   B. necessity of providing a route for drug administration.
   C. need for prolonged artificial ventilations.
   D. failure to provide adequate ventilations with a BVM.
   E. all of the above

_____ 26. The optimal positioning of the head for pediatric intubation in the absence of a spinal injury is:
   A. neutral.
   B. hyperextended.
   C. sniffing.
   D. head-tilt.
   E. spine.

_____ 27. If gastric distention is present in a pediatric patient, a paramedic might consider placing a(n):
   A. oropharyngeal airway.
   B. nasopharyngeal airway.
   C. needle cricothyrotomy.
   D. nasogastric tube.
   E. endotracheal tube.

_____ 28. In obtaining vascular access in a pediatric patient, the external jugular vein should only be used in life-threatening situations.
   A. True
   B. False

_____ 29. The indications for use of intraosseous infusion include all of the following EXCEPT:
   A. a patient less than 6 years old.
   B. existence of shock or cardiac arrest.
   C. presence of a facture in the pelvis.
   D. an unresponsive patient.
   E. failure to place a peripheral IV.

_____ 30. You are more likely to use electrical therapy on pediatric patients than adult patients.
   A. True
   B. False

_____ 31. All of the following are symptoms of epiglottitis EXCEPT:
   A. a rapid onset.
   B. occasional stridor.
   C. a barking cough.
   D. drooling.
   E. a fever of approximately 102–104°F.

_____ 32. In treating a patient with epiglottitis, a paramedic should:
   A. take blood pressure readings regularly.
   B. attempt to visualize the oropharynx.
   C. take the child's temperature orally.
   D. place the child in a supine position.
   E. none of the above

_____ 33. Common causes of lower airway distress include all of the following EXCEPT:
   A. pneumonia.
   B. asthma.
   C. croup.
   D. bronchiolitis.
   E. status asthmaticus.

_____ 34. When a child experiences a severe asthma attack without wheezing, this is:
   A. an ominous sign.
   B. because of a lack of expectorant.
   C. a sign of improvement.
   D. because of an inability to cough.
   E. common, and should not alarm the paramedic.

_____ 35. All of the following are signs and symptoms of shock in a child EXCEPT:
   A. pale, cool, clammy skin.
   B. impaired mental status.
   C. absence of tears when crying.
   D. increased urination.
   E. a rapid respiratory rate.

_____ 36. Cardiogenic shock is more frequently encountered in prehospital pediatric care than noncardiogenic shock.
   A. True
   B. False

_____ 37. When dysrhythmias do occur in children, the most common form is a(n):
   A. bradydysrhythmia.
   B. supraventricular tachydysrhythmia.
   C. ventricular tachydysrhythmia.
   D. asystole.
   E. ventricular fibrillation.

_____ 38. A pediatric patient is seen by a paramedic for a seizure. Assessment and history reveal that the child has a fever of 101°F, was very sleepy and irritable before the seizure, and has had no similar episodes. The child complained of a stiff neck and headache earlier in the day. You suspect that the episode may have been caused by:
   A. febrile convulsions.
   B. meningitis.
   C. hypoglycemia.
   D. hypoxia.
   E. hyperglycemia.

_____ 39. Whenever a glucometer reading reveals a blood sugar of less than 70 mg/dL, a paramedic might suspect:
   A. hypoxia.
   B. hyperglycemia.
   C. hypoglycemia.
   D. ketoacidosis.
   E. dehydration.

_____ 40. The single most common cause of trauma-related injuries in children is:
   A. motor vehicle collisions.
   B. burns.
   C. falls.
   D. physical abuse.
   E. drownings.

_____ 41. Appropriate-sized pediatric immobilization equipment includes all of the following EXCEPT:
   A. towel or blanket roll.
   B. vest-type device (KED).
   C. sandbag.
   D. straps and cravats.
   E. padding.

_____ 42. All of the following are true statements about SIDS EXCEPT that it:
   A. occurs most frequently in the fall and winter.
   B. is not caused by external suffocation by blankets.
   C. tends to be more common in females than in males.
   D. is not thought to be hereditary.
   E. is possibly linked to a prone sleeping position.

_____ 43. Child abuse can take the form of:
   A. psychological abuse.
   B. physical abuse.
   C. sexual abuse.
   D. neglect.
   E. all of the above

_____ 44. In cases of suspected child abuse, management goals include all of the following EXCEPT:
   A. protection of the child from further injury.
   B. notification of proper authorities.
   C. appropriate treatment of injuries.
   D. cross-examination of the parents or caregivers.
   E. documentation of all findings and statements.

_____ 45. A surgical connection that runs from the brain to the abdomen in a pediatric patient is called a(n):
   A. central IV.
   B. tracheostomy.
   C. shunt.
   D. inner cannula.
   E. epigastric tube.

Chapter 43

Geriatric Emergencies

Review of Chapter Objectives

After reading this chapter, you should be able to:

1. **Discuss the demographics demonstrating the increasing size of the elderly population in the United States.** pp. 1669–1670

   Between 1960 and 1990, the number of elderly people in the United States nearly doubled. By late 1998, the total reached more than 34 million, with nearly 400,000 people age 95 and older. As the 2000s opened, demographers talked about the "graying of America," a process in which the number of elderly is pushing up the average age of the U.S. population as a whole. In 2030, when the post–World War II baby boomers enter their 80s, more than 70 million people will be age 65 or older. By 2040, the elderly will represent roughly 20 percent of the population. In other words, one in five Americans will be age 65 or older.

2. **Assess the various living environments of elderly patients.** pp. 1670–1671

   The elderly live in both independent and dependent living environments. Many continue to live alone or with their partner until well into their 80s or 90s. The "oldest" old are the most likely to live alone, and, in fact, nearly half of those age 85 and older live by themselves. The great majority of these people—an estimated 78 percent—are women. This is because married men tend to die before their wives, and widowed men tend to remarry more often than widowed women. Elderly persons living alone represent one of the most impoverished and vulnerable parts of society.

   Usually the elderly own their own homes or apartments. In addition to these traditional residences, they may choose among a variety of options for assisted living. Among the elderly who receive help, more than 43 percent rely on paid assistance. Another 54 percent use unpaid assistance, and 3 percent use both types of help. Those elderly who turn to dependent care arrangements select live-in nursing, life-care communities, congregate care, or personal-care homes. Approximately 5 percent of the elderly live in nursing homes.

3. **Discuss society's view of aging and the social, financial, and ethical issues facing the elderly.** pp. 1669–1671

   After years of working and/or raising a family, an elderly person must not only find new roles to fulfill but, in many cases, must overcome the societal label of "old person." A lot of elderly people disprove ageism—and all the stereotypes it engenders—by living happy, productive, and active lives. Others, however, feel a sense of social isolation or uselessness. Physical and financial difficulties reinforce these feelings and help create an emotional context in which illnesses can occur.

©2007 Pearson Education, Inc.
Essentials of Paramedic Care, 2nd ed.

589

Successful medical treatment of elderly patients involves an understanding of the broader social content in which they live.

As a group, most elderly people worry about income, aggravated by fixed retirement payments or loss of benefits when a partner dies. Tight finances and limited mobility may prevent an independent elderly person from maintaining adequate nutrition and safety. As a result, elderly patients may be at increased risk of accidental hypothermia, carbon monoxide poisoning, or fires. They may also reduce their medications, or "half dose," to save money.

In the course of caring for elderly patients, ethical concerns frequently arise. You may be confronted with multiple decision makers, particularly in dependent living environments. You may also have a question about the patient's competency to give informed consent or refusal of treatment. Finally, you may be faced with advanced directives, such as "living wills" and Do Not Resuscitate (DNR) orders.

*Supplemental objective: Describe the resources available to assist the elderly, and create strategies to refer at-risk patients to appropriate community services. pp. 1669–1671

In treating the elderly, remember that the best intervention is prevention. The goal of any health care service, including EMS, should be to help keep people from becoming sick or injured in the first place. As a paramedic, you can reduce morbidity among the elderly by taking part in community education programs and by cooperating with agencies or organizations that support the elderly. The specific resources may differ from community to community, but some possibilities include senior centers, Meals on Wheels, religious organizations with programs for the elderly, governmental agencies, or national and state associations such as the AARP, the Alzheimer's Association, or the Association for Senior Citizens.

Many EMS agencies have developed a means for referring elderly patients to appropriate follow-up services. Consider preparing a checklist with descriptions of services in your area as well as the names of contact people and their phone numbers. The checklists can be given to elderly patients as needed.

4. Discuss common emotional and psychological reactions to aging, including causes and manifestations. pp. 1669–1671

When behavioral or psychological problems develop later in life, they are often dismissed as normal age-related changes. This attitude denies an elderly person the opportunity to correct a treatable condition and/or overlooks an underlying physical disorder. Studies have shown that the elderly retain their basic personalities and their adaptive cognitive abilities. Intellectual decline and regressive behavior are not normal age-related changes and could in fact have a physiological cause, such as head trauma.

It is important to keep in mind the emotionally stressful situations facing many elderly people such as isolation, loneliness, loss of independence, loss of strength, fear of the future, and more. The elderly are at risk for alcoholism as well as facing a higher incidence of secondary depression as a result of neuroleptic medications such as Haldol or Thorazine.

The emotional well-being of the elderly impacts upon their overall physical health. Therefore, it is important that you note evidence of altered behavior in any elderly patient that you assess and examine. Also, keep in mind that many emotional conditions, such as depression, are normal reactions to stressful situations and can be resolved with appropriate counseling and treatment. Finally, remember that medical disorders in the elderly often present as functional impairment and should be treated as an early warning of a possibly undetected medical problem.

5. Apply the pathophysiology of multisystem failure to the assessment and management of medical conditions in the elderly patient. p. 1672

The body becomes less efficient with age, increasing the likelihood of malfunction. The body of an elderly patient is susceptible to all the disorders of young people, but its maintenance, defense, and repair processes are weaker. As a result, the elderly often suffer from more than one illness or disease at a time. On average, six medical disorders may coexist in an elderly person and perhaps even more in the old-old. Furthermore, disease in one organ system may result in the deterioration of other systems, compounding existing acute and/or chronic conditions.

Because of concomitant diseases (comorbidity) in the elderly, complaints may not be specific to any one disorder. Common complaints of the elderly include fatigue and weakness, dizziness/vertigo/syncope, falls, headaches, insomnia, dysphagia, loss of appetite, inability to void, and/or constipation/diarrhea.

Elderly patients often accept medical problems as a part of aging and fail to monitor changes in their condition. In some cases, such as a silent myocardial infarction, pain may be diminished or absent. In others, a complaint may seem trivial, such as constipation.

Although many medical problems in the young and middle-aged populations present with a standard set of signs and symptoms, the changes involved in aging lead to different presentations. In pneumonia, for example, some classic symptoms such as fever, chest pain, and a cough may be diminished or absent.

6. **Compare the pharmacokinetics of an elderly patient to that of a young patient, including drug distribution, metabolism, and excretion.** pp. 1672–1673

In general, a person's sensitivity to drugs increases with age. When compared with younger patients, the elderly experience more adverse drug reactions, more drug-drug interactions, and more drug-disease interactions. Because of age-related pharmacokinetic changes such as a loss of body fluids and atrophy of organs, drugs concentrate more readily in the plasma and tissues of elderly patients. As a result, drug dosages often must be adjusted to prevent toxicity. Additionally, due to differences in the GI tract, medications are metabolized and excreted at a slower rate in the elderly patient.

7. **Discuss the impact of polypharmacy, dosing errors, increased drug sensitivity, and medication noncompliance on assessment and management of the elderly patient.** pp. 1672–1673

If medications are not correctly monitored, polypharmacy can cause a number of problems among the elderly. In taking a medical history of an elderly patient, remember to ask questions to determine if the patient is taking a prescribed medication as directed. Noncompliance with drug therapy, usually underadherence, is common among the elderly. Up to 40 percent do not take medications as prescribed. Of these individuals, 35 percent experience some type of medical problem.

Factors that can decrease compliance in the elderly include limited income, memory loss (due to decreased or diseased neural activity), limited mobility, sensory impairment (cannot hear/read/understand directions), multiple or complicated drug therapies, fear of toxicity, childproof containers (especially difficult for arthritic patients), and lengthy drug therapy plans.

8. **Discuss the use and effects of commonly prescribed drugs for the elderly patient.** pp. 1672–1673, 1703–1705

Functional changes in the kidneys, liver, and gastrointestinal system slow the absorption and elimination of many medications in the elderly. In addition, the various compensatory mechanisms that help buffer against medication side effects are less effective in the elderly than in younger patients.

Approximately 30 percent of all hospital admissions are related to drug-induced illness. About 50 percent of all drug-related deaths occur in people over the age of 60. Accidental overdoses may occur more frequently in the aged due to confusion, vision impairment, self-selection of medications, forgetfulness, and concurrent drug use. Intentional drug overdose also occurs in attempts at self-destruction. Another complicating factor is the abuse of alcohol among the elderly.

9. **Discuss the problem of mobility in the elderly, and develop strategies to prevent falls.** p. 1673

Regular exercise and a good diet are two of the most effective prevention measures for ensuring mobility among the elderly. Some elderly may suffer from a severe medical problem, such as crippling arthritis. They may fear for their personal safety, either from accidental injury or intentional injury, such as robbery. Certain medications also may increase their lethargy. Whatever the cause, a lack of mobility can have detrimental physical and emotional effects. Some of these include poor nutrition, difficulty with elimination, poor skin integrity, a greater predisposition for falls, loss of independence and/or confidence, depression from "feeling old," and isolation.

Falls present an especially serious problem for the elderly. Fall-related injuries represent the leading cause of accidental death among the elderly and the seventh highest cause of death overall. As a result, the paramedic should consider strategies for making a home safe for the elderly and point these out to the elderly patient or family of the elderly patient, whichever may be appropriate. Examples of hazards that can easily be corrected include torn or slippery rugs, chairs without armrests, chairs with low backs, chairs with wheels, obstructing furniture, slippery bathtubs, dim lighting, high cabinet shelves, missing handrails on stairways, and high steps on stairways.

10. Discuss age-related changes in sensations in the elderly, and describe the implications of these changes for communication and patient assessment. pp. 1673, 1675–1678

Most elderly patients suffer from some form of age-related sensory changes. Normal physiological changes may include impaired vision or blindness, impaired or loss of hearing, an altered sense of taste or smell, and/or a lower sensitivity to pain or touch. Any of these conditions can affect your ability to communicate with the patient. In general, be prepared to spend more time obtaining histories from elderly patients.

11. Discuss the problems with continence and elimination in the elderly patient, and develop communication strategies to provide psychological support. pp. 1674–1675

The elderly often find it embarrassing to talk about problems with continence and elimination. They may feel stigmatized, isolated, and/or helpless. When confronted with these problems, DO NOT make a big deal out of them. Respect the patient's dignity, and assure the person that, in many cases, the problem is treatable.

Remember, too, that problems with continence and elimination are not necessarily caused by aging. They may be the result of drug therapy or medical conditions such as diabetes. As a result, in assessing a patient with incontinence or constipation, inquire about their medications and any chronic medical disorders. Also keep in mind the variety of other conditions that can result from problems with continence or elimination. In the case of incontinence, for example, a patient may experience rashes, skin infections, skin breakdown (ulcers), urinary tract infections, sepsis, and falls or fractures (caused by a frequent need to eliminate). In elderly people with cerebrovascular disease or impaired baroreceptor reflexes, efforts to force a bowel movement can lead to a transient ischemic attack (TIA) or syncope.

12. Discuss factors that may complicate the assessment of the elderly patient. pp. 1673, 1675–1679

In assessing an elderly patient, keep in mind the variety of causes of functional impairment. If identified early, an environmental or disease-related condition can often be reversed. Your success depends upon a thorough understanding of age-related changes and the implications of these changes for patient assessment and management. You will need to recall at all times the complications that can arise from comorbidity (having more than one disease at a time) and polypharmacy (concurrent use of a number of drugs).

Communications challenges may also complicate the assessment. Patients may be blind, have speech difficulties, or have some kind of hearing loss that can make assessment more difficult. They also often have a lower sensitivity to pain or touch.

In general, assessment of the elderly patient follows the same basic approach used with any other patient. However, you should keep in mind these points:

- Set a context for illness, taking into account the patient's living situation, level of activity, network of social support, level of dependence, medication history (both prescriptive and nonprescriptive), and sleep patterns.

- Pay close attention to an elderly person's nutrition, noting conditions that may complicate or discourage eating.
- Keep in mind that elderly patients may minimize or fail to report important symptoms. Therefore, try to distinguish the patient's chief complaint from the patient's primary problem.
- Because of presence of multiple chronic diseases, treat the patient on a "threat-to-life" basis.
- Recall at all times that alterations in the temperature-regulating mechanism can result in a lack of fever, or a minimal fever, even in the presence of a severe infection.
- When confronted with a confused patient, try to determine whether the patient's mental status represents a significant change from normal for them. DO NOT assume that a confused, disoriented patient is "just senile," thus failing to assess for a serious underlying problem.
- Remember that some patients are often easily fatigued and cannot tolerate a long physical examination. Also, because of problems with temperature regulation, the patient may be wearing several layers of clothing.
- Be aware that the elderly patient may minimize or deny symptoms because of a fear of institutionalization or a loss of self-sufficiency.
- Try to distinguish signs of chronic disease from acute problems. For example:
  —Peripheral pulses may be difficult to evaluate because of peripheral vascular disease and arthritis.
  —The elderly may have nonpathological crackles (rales) upon lung auscultation.
  —The elderly often exhibit an increase in mouth breathing and a loss of skin elasticity, which may be confused with dehydration.
  —Dependent edema may be caused by inactivity, not congestive heart failure.

13. Discuss the principles that should be employed when assessing and communicating with the elderly. pp. 1673, 1676–1678

To improve your skill at assessing and communicating with the elderly, keep in mind these principles.

- Always introduce yourself.
- Speak slowly, distinctly, and respectfully.
- Speak to the patient first, rather than to family members, caregivers, or bystanders.
- Speak face to face, at eye level with eye contact.
- Locate the patient's hearing aid or eyeglasses, if needed.
- DO NOT shout at the patient. This will not help if the patient is deaf, and it may distort sounds for the patient who has some level of hearing.
- Write notes, if necessary.
- Allow the patient to put on the stethoscope, while you speak into it like a microphone.
- Turn on the room lights.
- If a patient has forgotten to put in dentures, politely ask the person to do so.
- Display verbal and nonverbal signs of concern and empathy.
- Remain polite at all times.
- Preserve the person's dignity.
- Always explain what you are doing and why.
- Use your power of observation to recognize anxiety—tempo of speech, eye contact, tone of voice—during the telling of the history.

14. Compare the assessment of a young patient with that of an elderly patient. pp. 1675–1685

The assessment of the older person differs from that of a younger person in a number of ways. The elderly often have complicated medical histories that entail numerous chronic conditions. They also usually take multiple medications (both prescribed and nonprescribed), which in turn may produce a variety of physical and/or psychological side effects. As stated in previous objectives, remain sensitive to the special fears of an elderly patient, particularly the fear of increased dependency, and unique stresses of that age group, such as loss of long-term partners or friends. Allow for the extra time necessitated by communication challenges. DO NOT rush the elderly patient through an assessment unless it is absolutely necessary because of a life-threatening condition.

15. Discuss common complaints of elderly patients.   **pp. 1672, 1685–1713**

Common complaints of elderly patients include fatigue and weakness, dizziness, vertigo or syncope, falls, headaches, insomnia, dysphagia, loss of appetite, inability to void, and constipation or diarrhea. Many of these complaints in and of themselves would not be too serious. However, given the context of complicated medical histories of the elderly, each of these complaints are important and should be followed up and taken very seriously.

16. Discuss the normal and abnormal changes of age in relation to the:

a. Pulmonary system   **pp. 1680–1681**

The effects of aging on the respiratory system begin as early as age 30. Without regular exercise and/or training, the lungs start to lose their ability to defend themselves and to carry out their prime function of ventilation. Age-related changes in the respiratory system include decreased chest wall compliance, loss of lung elasticity, increased air trapping due to collapse of the smaller airways, and reduced strength and endurance of the respiratory muscles. In addition, there is a decrease in an effective cough reflex and the activity of the cilia. The decline of these two defense mechanisms leave the lungs more susceptible to recurring infection. Other factors that may affect pulmonary function in the elderly are kyphosis (exaggeration of the normal posterior curvature of the spine), chronic exposure to pollutants, and long-term cigarette smoking.

b. Cardiovascular system   **pp. 1681–1682**

A number of variables unrelated to aging influence cardiovascular functions—diet, smoking and alcohol use, education, socioeconomic status, and even personality traits. Of particular importance is the level of physical activity.

This said, the cardiovascular system still experiences, in varying degrees, age-related deterioration. Changes include a loss of elasticity and hardening of the arteries, an increase in the size and bulk of the left ventricle (hypertrophy), development of fibrosis (formation of fiber-like connective/scar tissue), and changes in the rate, rhythm, and overall efficiency of the heart.

c. Nervous system   **pp. 1681, 1682–1683**

Unlike cells in other organ systems, cells in the central nervous system cannot reproduce. The brain can lose as much as 45 percent of its cells in certain areas of the cortex. Overall, there is an average 10 percent reduction in brain weight from age 20 to age 90. Keep in mind, however, that reductions in brain weight and ventricular size are not well correlated with intelligence, and elderly people may still be capable of highly creative and productive thought. In addition to shrinkage of brain tissue, the elderly may experience some memory loss, clinical depression, altered mental status, and impaired balance. Keep in mind that these changes vary greatly and may not be seen in all elderly patients, even at the close of very long lives.

d. Endocrine system   **pp. 1681, 1683**

The elderly experience a variety of age-related hormonal changes. Women, for example, experience menopause, the result of reductions in estrogen production. Men also experience a decline in levels of testosterone. In addition, the elderly commonly experience a decline in insulin sensitivity and/or an increase in insulin resistance. Finally, thyroid disorders, especially hypothyroidism and thyroid nodules, increase with age as well.

e. Gastrointestinal system   **pp. 1681, 1683–1684**

Age affects the gastrointestinal system in various ways. The volume of saliva may decrease by as much as 33 percent, leading to complaints of dry mouth, nutritional deficiencies, and a predisposition to choking. Gastric secretions may decrease to as little as 20 percent of the quantity present in younger people. Esophageal and intestinal motility also decrease, making swallowing more difficult and delaying digestive processes. The production of hydrochloric acid also declines, further disrupting digestion and, in some adults, contributing to nutritional anemia. Gums atrophy and the number of taste buds decrease, reducing even further the desire to eat.

Other conditions may also develop. Hiatal hernias are not age-related per se, but can have serious consequences for the elderly. The hernias may incarcerate, strangulate, or, in the most severe cases, result in massive GI hemorrhage. A diminished liver function, which is associated with aging, can delay or impede detoxification. It also can reduce the production of clotting proteins, which in turn leads to bleeding abnormalities.

f. Thermoregulatory system   pp. 1681, 1684

As people age, the thermoregulatory system becomes altered or impaired. Aging seems to reduce the effectiveness of sweating in cooling the body. Older people tend to sweat at higher core temperatures and have less sweat output per gland than younger people. As people age, they also experience deterioration of the autonomic nervous system, including a decrease in shivering and lower resting peripheral blood flow. In addition, the elderly may have a diminished perception of the cold. Drugs and disease can further alter an elderly patient's response to temperature extremes, resulting in hyperthermia or accidental hypothermia.

g. Integumentary system   pp. 1681, 1684

As people age, the skin loses collagen, a connective tissue that gives elasticity and support to the skin. Without this support, the skin is subject to a great number of injuries from bumping or tearing. In addition, the skin thins as people age. Because cells reproduce more slowly, older patients often suffer more severe skin injuries than younger patients and healing takes a longer time. As a rule, the elderly are at a higher risk of secondary infections, skin tumors, drug-induced eruptions, and fungal or viral infections. Decades of exposure to the sun also makes the elderly vulnerable to melanoma and other sun-related carcinomas.

h. Musculoskeletal system   pp. 1681, 1684

An aging person may lose as much as 2 to 3 inches of height from narrowing of the intervertebral disks and osteoporosis (softening of bone tissue due to the loss of essential minerals). This is especially evident in the vertebral bodies, thus causing a change in posture. The posture of the aged individual often reveals an increase in the curvature of the thoracic spine (kyphosis) and slight flexion of the knee and hip joints. The demineralization of bone makes the elderly patient much more susceptible to hip and other fractures.

In addition to skeletal changes, a decrease in skeletal muscle weight commonly occurs with age—especially with sedentary individuals. To compensate, elderly women develop a narrow, short gait, while older men develop a wide gait. These changes make the elderly more susceptible to falls.

17. Describe the incidence, morbidity/mortality, risk factors, prevention strategies, pathophysiology, assessment, need for intervention and transport, and management for elderly medical patients with:

a. Pneumonia, chronic obstructive disease, and pulmonary embolism   pp. 1686–1689

Pneumonia. Pneumonia is an infection of the lung usually caused by a bacterium or virus. Aspiration pneumonia is also common in the elderly due to difficulty in swallowing.

Pneumonia is the fourth leading cause of death in people age 65 and older. Its incidence increases with age at a rate of 10 percent for each decade beyond age 20. It is found in 60 percent of autopsies performed on the elderly. Reasons for the high incidence of pneumonia among the elderly include decreased immune response, reduced pulmonary function, increased colonization of the pharynx by gram-negative bacteria, abnormal or ineffective cough reflex, and decreased effectiveness of mucociliary cells of the upper respiratory system. The elderly who are at the greatest risk for contracting pneumonia are frail adults and those with multiple chronic diseases or compromised immunity.

Common signs and symptoms of pneumonia include increasing dyspnea, congestion, fever, chills, tachypnea, sputum production, and altered mental status. Occasionally, abdominal pain may be the only symptom.

Prevention strategies include prophylactic treatment with antibiotics. Efforts should also be taken to reduce exposure to infectious patients and to promote patient mobility. Once a person has contracted the disease, treatment includes management of all life threats, maintenance of adequate oxygenation, and transport to the hospital for diagnosis and further management.

Chronic obstructive pulmonary disease (COPD). COPD is really a collection of diseases characterized by chronic airflow obstruction with reversible and/or irreversible components. Although each COPD has its own distinct features, elderly patients commonly have two or more types at the same time. COPD usually refers to some combination of emphysema, chronic bronchitis, and, to a lesser degree, asthma. Pneumonia, as well as other respiratory disorders, can further complicate chronic obstructive pulmonary disease in the elderly.

In the United States, COPD is among the 10 leading causes of death. Its prevalence has been increasing over the past 20 years due to factors such as genetic predisposition, exposure to environmental pollutants, existence of a childhood respiratory disease, and cigarette smoking (a contributing factor in up to 80 percent of all COPD cases).

The physiology of COPD varies but may include inflammation of the air passages with increased mucus production or actual destruction of the alveoli. Usual signs and symptoms include a cough, increased sputum production, dyspnea, accessory muscle use, pursed-lip breathing, tripod positioning, exercise intolerance, wheezing, pleuritic chest pain, and tachypnea.

The most effective prevention involves elimination of tobacco products and reduced exposure to cigarette smoke. Once the disease is present, appropriate self-care measures include exercise, avoidance of infections, appropriate use of medications, avoidance of unnecessary stress, and, when necessary, calling EMS. When confronted with an elderly patient with COPD, treatment is essentially the same as for all age groups: supplemental oxygen and possibly drug therapy, usually for reducing dyspnea.

Pulmonary embolism (PE). Pulmonary embolism should always be considered as a possible cause of respiratory distress in the elderly. Although statistics for the elderly are unavailable, approximately 650,000 cases occur annually in the United States. Of this number, a pulmonary embolism is the primary cause of death in 100,000 people. Nearly 11 percent of PE deaths take place in the first hour, and another 38 percent in the second hour.

Blood clots are the most frequent cause of a PE. However, the condition may also be caused by fat, air, bone marrow, tumor cells, or foreign bodies. Risk factors for developing pulmonary embolism include deep venous thrombosis; prolonged immobility (common among the elderly); malignancy (tumors); paralysis; fractures of the pelvis, hip, or leg; obesity; trauma to the leg vessels; major surgery; presence of a venous catheter; use of estrogen (in women); and atrial fibrillation.

Definitive diagnosis of a pulmonary embolism takes place in a hospital setting. However, the condition should be suspected in a patient with the acute onset of dyspnea. Often, it is accompanied by pleuritic chest pain and right heart failure. If the PE is massive, you can expect severe dyspnea, cardiac dysrhythmias, and ultimately cardiovascular collapse.

The goals of field treatment are to manage and minimize complications of the condition. General treatment considerations include delivery of high-flow oxygen via mask, maintaining oxygen levels above an SaO_2 of 90 percent. Establishment of an IV for possible administration of medications, upon advice from medical direction, is appropriate. However, vigorous fluid therapy should be avoided, if possible. Rapid transport is essential. Position the patient in an upright position and avoid lifting the patient by the legs or knees, which may dislodge thrombi in the lower extremities. During transport, monitor changes in skin color, pulse oximetry, and breathing rate and rhythm.

b. Myocardial infarction, heart failure, dysrhythmias, aneurysm, and hypertension pp. 1689–1692

The leading cause of death in the elderly is cardiovascular disease. Assessment and treatment of cardiovascular disease in the elderly patient is often complicated by non-age-related factors and disease processes in other organ systems. Commonly found cardiovascular disorders in the elderly include the following. (Additional disorders, including syncope, can be found in the text.)

Myocardial infarction (MI). Myocardial infarction involves actual death of muscle tissue due to partial or complete occlusion of one or more of the coronary arteries. The greatest number of patients hospitalized for acute MI are older than age 65. The elderly patient with MI is less likely to present with classic symptoms, such as chest pain, than a younger counterpart. Atypical presentations that may be seen in the elderly include the absence of pain, exercise intolerance, confusion/dizziness, syncope, dyspnea (common in patients over age 85), neck or dental pain, epigastric pain, and fatigue/weakness.

The mortality rate associated with myocardial infarction doubles after age 70. Elderly patients are more likely to suffer silent myocardial infarction. They also tend to have larger myocardial infarctions. The majority of the deaths that occur in the first few hours after a myocardial infarction are due to dysrhythmias such as ventricular fibrillation.

Field management is the same as that listed for angina, except that the nitro often does not work and morphine may be necessary if the patient's BP tolerates it. It may also be necessary to manage dysrhythmias and hypotension with medications. These patients need to be quickly evaluated and transported to a facility that can administer clot busters or provide emergency cardiac catheterization and angioplasty, if necessary.

Heart failure. Heart failure takes place when the cardiac output cannot meet the body's metabolic demands. The incidence rises exponentially after age 60 and is the most common diagnosis in hospitalized patients over the age of 65. The causes of heart failure fall in one of four categories—impairment to flow, inadequate cardiac filling, volume overload, and myocardial failure. Factors that place the elderly at risk for heart failure include prolonged myocardial contractions, noncompliance with drug therapy, anemia, ischemia, thermoregulatory disorders, hypoxia, infection, and use of nonsteroidal antiinflammatory drugs.

Signs and symptoms of heart failure vary. In most patients, regardless of age, some form of edema exists. Assessment findings for the elderly may include musculoskeletal injury, fatigue (left failure), two-pillow orthopnea, dyspnea on exertion, dry hacking cough progressing to a productive cough, dependent edema (right failure), nocturia, anorexia, hepatomegaly (enlarged liver), and ascites.

Nonpharmacologic management of heart failure includes modifications in diet, exercise, and reduction in weight, if necessary. Pharmacologic management may include treatment with diuretics, vasodilators, antihypertensive agents, or inotropic agents. Check to see if the patient is already on any of these medications and if the patient is compliant with scheduled doses.

Dysrhythmias. Many cardiac dysrhythmias develop with age, but atrial fibrillation is the most common dysrhythmia encountered. Dysrhythmias occur primarily as a result of the degeneration of the patient's conductive system. Anything that decreases myocardial blood flow can produce a dysrhythmia. They may also be caused by electrolyte abnormalities.

To complicate matters further, the elderly do not tolerate extremes in heart rate as well as a younger person would. In addition, dysrhythmias can lead to falls due to cerebral hypoperfusion. They can also result in congestive heart failure (CHF) or a transient ischemic attack (TIA).

Treatment considerations depend upon the type of dysrhythmia. Patients may already have a pacemaker in place. In such cases, keep in mind that pacemakers have a low but significant rate of complications such as a failed battery, fibrosis around the catheter site, lead fracture, or electrode dislodgment. In a number of situations, drug therapy is indicated. Whenever you discover a dysrhythmia, remember that an abnormal or disordered heart rhythm may be the only clinical finding in an elderly patient suffering acute myocardial infarction.

Aneurysms. An aneurysm, or rupture of the vessel, often results from aortic dissection—a degeneration of the wall of the aorta, either in the thoracic or abdominal cavity. Approximately 80 percent of thoracic aneurysms are due to atherosclerosis combined with hypertension. The remaining cases occur secondary to other factors, including Marfan's syndrome or blunt trauma to the chest. Patients with dissections will often present with tearing chest pain radiating through to the back or, if a rupture/aneurysm occurs, cardiac arrest.

The distal portion of the aorta is the most common site for an abdominal aneurysm. Approximately one in 250 people over age 50 dies from a ruptured abdominal aneurysm. Patients may present with tearing abdominal pain or unexplained low back pain. Pulses in the legs are diminished or absent and the lower extremities feel cold to the touch. There may be sensory abnormalities such as numbness, tingling, or pain in the legs. The patient may fall when attempting to stand.

Treatment of the aneurysm depends upon the size, location, and severity of the condition. In the case of thoracic aortic dissection, continuous IV infusion and/or administration of drug therapy to lower the arterial pressure and to diminish the velocity of left ventricle contraction may be indicated. Rapid transport is essential, especially for the older patient who most commonly requires care and observation in an intensive care unit.

Hypertension. Because hypertension is not widely seen in less-developed nations, experts believe that the condition is not a normal age-related change. Today more than 50 percent of Americans over age 65 have clinically diagnosed hypertension—defined as blood pressure greater than 140/90 mmHg. Prolonged elevated blood pressure will eventually damage the heart, brain, or kidneys. As a result of hypertension, elderly patients are at a greater risk for heart failure, stroke, blindness, renal failure, coronary heart disease, and peripheral vascular disease. In men with blood pressure greater than 160/95 mmHg, the risk of mortality nearly doubles.

Hypertension increases with atherosclerosis, which is more common in the elderly than other age groups. Other contributing factors include obesity and diabetes. The condition is often a "silent" disease because it produces no clinically obvious signs or symptoms. It may be associated with nonspecific complaints such as headache, tinnitus, epistaxis (nosebleed), slow tremors, and nausea or vomiting.

Hypertension can be prevented or controlled through diet, exercise, cessation of smoking, and compliance with medications. Management of the condition depends upon its severity and the existence of other conditions. For example, hypertension is often treated with beta-blockers—medications that are contraindicated in patients with chronic obstructive lung disease, asthma, or heart block greater than first degree. Diuretics, another common drug used for treating hypertension, should be prescribed with care for patients on digitalis. Keep in mind that centrally acting agents are more likely to produce negative side effects in the elderly. Unlike younger patients, the elderly may experience depression, forgetfulness, sleep problems, or vivid dreams and/or hallucinations.

c. **Cerebral vascular disease, delirium, dementia, Alzheimer's disease, and Parkinson's disease** pp. 1693–1696

Cerebral vascular disease (CVA). Cerebral vascular disease (stroke/brain attack) is the third leading cause of death in the United States. Annually, about 500,000 people suffer strokes and about 150,000 die. Incidence of stroke and the likelihood of dying from a stroke increases with age. Occlusive stroke is statistically more common in the elderly and relatively uncommon in younger individuals. Older patients are at higher risk of stroke because of atherosclerosis, hypertension, immobility, limb paralysis, congestive heart failure, and atrial fibrillation. Transient ischemic attacks (TIAs) are also more common in older patients, more than one third of whom will develop a major permanent stroke.

Strokes fall into one of two categories. Brain ischemia—injury to brain tissue caused by an inadequate supply of oxygen and nutrients—accounts for about 80 percent of all strokes. Brain hemorrhage, the second major category, may be either subarachnoid hemorrhage or intracerebral hemorrhage. Because of the various kinds of strokes, signs and symptoms can present in many ways—altered mental status, coma, paralysis, slurred speech, a change in mood, and seizures. Stroke should be highly suspected in any elderly patient with a sudden change in mental status.

Keep two things in mind when treating stroke. One, complete the Glasgow Coma Scale for later comparison at the ED. Second, transport the patient as rapidly as possible. In the case of stroke, "time is brain tissue." By far the most preferred treatment is prevention. Preventive strategies include control of hypertension, treatment of cardiac disorders, treatment of blood disorders, cessation of smoking, cessation of recreational drugs, moderate use of alcohol, regular exercise, and good eating habits.

Delirium, dementia, and Alzheimer's disease. Approximately 15 percent of all Americans over the age of 65 have some degree of dementia or delirium. Dementia is chronic global mental impairment, often progressive or irreversible. The best-known form of dementia is Alzheimer's disease, a condition that affects an estimated 4 million Americans. Delirium is a global mental impairment of sudden onset and self-limited duration.

Possible causes of delirium include subdural hematoma, tumors and other mass lesions, drug-induced changes or alcohol intoxication, CNS infections, electrolyte abnormalities, cardiac failure, fever, metabolic disorders (including hypoglycemia), chronic endocrine abnormalities (including hypothyroidism and hyperthyroidism), and postconcussion syndrome. Common signs and symptoms include acute onset of anxiety, an inability to focus, disordered thinking, irritability, inappropriate behavior, fearfulness, excessive energy, or psychotic behavior such as hallucinations or paranoia. Aphasic or speaking errors and/or prominent slurring may be present.

Dementia is more prevalent in the elderly than delirium. Over 50 percent of all nursing home patients have dementia. The mental deterioration is often called "organic brain syndrome," "senile dementia," or "senility." Causes of dementia include small strokes, atherosclerosis, age-related neurological changes, neurological diseases, certain hereditary diseases, and Alzheimer's disease. Signs and symptoms include progressive disorientation, shortened attention span, aphasia or nonsense talking, and hallucinations.

Alzheimer's disease, a particular type of dementia, is a chronic degenerative disorder that attacks the brain and results in impaired memory, thinking, and behavior. It goes through stages, each with different signs and symptoms, the culmination of which is death.

Parkinson's disease. Parkinson's disease is a degenerative disorder involving changes in muscle response, including tremors, loss of facial expressions, and gait disturbances. It usually appears in people over the age of 50 and peaks at age 70. The disease affects one million Americans, with 50,000 new cases each year. The causes include viral encephalitis, atherosclerosis of cerebral vessels, reaction to certain drugs or toxins (antipsychotics or carbon monoxide), metabolic disorders (anoxia), tumors, head trauma, and degenerative disorders (Shy-Drager syndrome).

There is no known cure for Parkinson's disease. In calls involving a Parkinson's patient, observe for conditions that may have involved the EMS system, such as a fall or the inability to move. Manage treatable conditions and transport as needed.

d. Diabetes and thyroid diseases   pp. 1696–1697

Diabetes. An estimated 20 percent of older adults have diabetes mellitus, primarily Type II diabetes. Almost 40 percent have some type of glucose intolerance. Reasons the elderly develop this disorder include poor diet, decreased physical activity, loss of lean body mass, impaired insulin production, and resistance by body cells to the actions of insulin. The condition may present, in the early stages, with vague symptoms as fatigue or weakness. Allowed to progress, diabetes can result in neuropathy and visual impairment.

Elderly patients on insulin risk hypoglycemia, especially if they accidentally take too much insulin or do not eat enough food following injection. The lack of good nutrition can be particularly troublesome to elderly diabetic patients. They often find it difficult to prepare meals, fail to enjoy food because of diminished taste, have trouble chewing food, or are unable to purchase adequate and/or enough food because of limited income.

Many diabetics use self-monitoring devices to monitor their glucose levels. Self-treatment involves diet, exercise, and the use of sulfonylurea agents and/or insulin. In EMS calls involving diabetic or hypoglycemic elderly patients, follow care steps similar to those taken with younger patients. However, remember that diabetes places the elderly at increased risk of other complications, including atherosclerosis, delayed healing, retinopathy (disorders of the retina), altered renal function, and severe peripheral vascular disease, leading to foot ulcers and even amputations. In the case of hypoglycemia, DO NOT rule out alcohol as a complicating factor.

Thyroid diseases. With normal aging, the thyroid gland undergoes moderate atrophy and changes in hormone production. An estimated 2 to 5 percent of the people over 65 experience hypothyroidism, a condition resulting from inadequate levels of thyroid hormones. It affects women in greater numbers than men, and the prevalence rises with age.

Less than 33 percent of the elderly present with typical signs and symptoms of hypothyroidism. When they do, their complaints are often attributed to aging. Common nonspecific complaints in the elderly include mental confusion, anorexia, falls, incontinence, decreased mobility, and muscle or joint pain. Treatment involves thyroid hormone replacement.

Hyperthyroidism is less common among the elderly but may result from medication errors such as an overdose of thyroid hormone replacement. The typical symptom of heat intolerance is often present. Otherwise, hyperthyroidism presents atypically in the elderly with nonspecific features or complaints such as atrial fibrillation, failure to thrive (weight loss and apathy combined), abdominal distress, diarrhea, exhaustion, and depression.

Diagnosis and treatment of thyroid disorders does not take place in the field. Elderly patients with known thyroid problems should be encouraged to go to the hospital for medical evaluation.

e. Gastrointestinal problems, GI hemorrhage, and bowel obstruction   pp. 1697–1699

Gastrointestinal problems. Gastrointestinal emergencies are common among the elderly. The most frequent emergency is GI bleeding. However, older people will also describe a variety of other gastrointestinal complaints—nausea, poor appetite, diarrhea, and constipation, to name a few. Remember that like other presenting complaints in the elderly, these conditions may be symptomatic of a more serious disease.

Prompt management of a GI emergency is essential for old and young alike. However, keep in mind that older patients are more intolerant of hypotension and anoxia than younger patients. The elderly also face a significant risk of hemorrhage and shock. Treatment of GI emergencies in the elderly includes airway management, support of breathing and circulation, high-flow oxygen therapy, IV fluid replacement with a crystalloid solution, PASG placement (if indicated), and, above all else, rapid transport.

GI hemorrhage. Gastrointestinal hemorrhage falls into two general categories: upper GI bleed and lower GI bleed. Upper GI bleeds include peptic ulcer disease, gastritis, esophageal varices, and Mallory-Weiss tears. Lower GI bleeds include diverticulosis, tumors, ischemic colitis, and arteriovenous malformations.

Signs of significant gastrointestinal blood loss include the presence of "coffee ground" emesis, black tarlike stools (melena), obvious blood in the emesis or stool, orthostatic hypotension, pulse greater than 100 (unless on beta-blockers), and confusion. GI bleeding in the elderly is a true emergency and requires prompt transport to an appropriate medical facility.

Bowel obstruction. Bowel obstructions in the elderly typically involve the small bowel and may be caused by tumors, prior abdominal surgery, use of certain medications, and occasionally the presence of vertebral compression fractures. The patient will typically complain of diffuse abdominal pain, bloating, nausea, and vomiting. The abdomen may feel distended when palpated. Bowel sounds may be hypoactive or absent. If the obstruction has been present for a prolonged period, the patient may have fever, weakness, various electrolyte imbalances, and shock.

An even more serious condition arises with mesenteric infarct, which occurs when a portion of the bowel does not receive enough blood to survive. Certain age-related changes—atrial fibrillation or atherosclerosis—predispose the elderly to a clot lodging in one of the mesenteric arteries serving the bowel. In addition, age-related changes in the bowel itself can promote swelling that effectively cuts off blood flow. Primary signs and symptoms include pain out of proportion to the physical exam, bloody diarrhea, some tachycardia, and abdominal distention.

A mesenteric infarct, or dead bowel, attracts interstitial and intravascular fluids, thus removing them from use and increasing the likelihood of shock. Necrotic products are released to the peritoneal cavity, leading to massive infection. The prognosis is poor, due, in part, to decreased physiologic reserves on the part of older patients.

f. Skin diseases and pressure ulcers   pp. 1699–1670

Skin diseases. Age-related changes in the immune system make the elderly more prone to certain chronic skin diseases and infections. Elderly patients commonly complain about pruritus or itching. This condition can be caused by dermatitis or environmental conditions. Keep in mind that generalized itching can also be a sign of systemic diseases, particularly liver or renal disorders.

Slower healing and compromised tissue perfusion in the elderly make them more susceptible to bacterial infection of wounds, appearing as cellutitis, impetigo, and, in the case of immunocompromised adults, staphylococcal scalded skin. The elderly also experience a higher incidence of fungal infections and suffer higher rates of herpes zoster (shingles), which peaks between ages 50 and 70.

In treating skin disorders, remember that many conditions may be drug induced. For example, antihistamines and corticosteroids are two to three times more likely to provoke adverse reactions in the elderly than in younger adults. In most cases, encourage the patient to seek a medical evaluation to rule out drug complications or an underlying disease.

Pressure ulcers. Most pressure ulcers (bedsores) occur in people over age 70. Pressure ulcers typically develop from the waist down, usually over bony prominences, in bedridden patients. They most commonly result from tissue hypoxia and affect the skin, subcutaneous tissues, and muscle. Factors that can increase the risk of this condition include external compression of tissues, altered sensory perception, maceration (caused by excessive moisture), decreased activity or mobility, poor nutrition, and friction or shear.

To reduce the development of pressure ulcers or to alleviate their condition, assist the patient in changing position frequently, especially during extended transport. Use a pull sheet to move the patient, reducing the likelihood of tearing. Reduce the possibility of shearing by padding areas of skin prone to movement. Unless a life-threatening condition exists, take time to clean and dry areas of excessive moisture. Clean ulcers with normal saline solution and cover with hydrocolloid or hydrogel dressings, if available. With severe ulcers, pack with loosely woven gauze moistened with normal saline.

g. Osteoarthritis and osteoporosis pp. 1700–1701

Osteoarthritis. Osteoarthritis is the leading cause of disability among people age 65 and older. Contributing factors to this disease include age-related wear and tear, loss of muscle mass, obesity, primary disorders of the joint (such as inflammatory arthritis), trauma, and congenital abnormalities (such as hip dysplasia).

Osteoarthritis initially presents as joint pain. As the disease progresses, pain may be accompanied by diminished mobility, joint deformity, and crepitus (grating sensations), and ultimately tenderness during passive motion or upon palpation. Prevention strategies include stretching exercises and activities that strengthen stress-absorbing tendons. Immobilization, even for short periods, can accelerate the condition. Surgery—that is, total joint replacement—is the last resort.

Osteoporosis. Osteoporosis affects an estimated 20 million Americans and is largely responsible for fractures of the hip, wrist, and vertebral bones following a fall or other injury. Risk factors include:

- *Age.* Bone mass usually starts to decline after the third decade of life, and decreased bone density generally becomes a treatment consideration at about age 50.
- *Gender.* Women are more than twice as likely as men to develop the disease, especially if they experience early menopause (before age 45) and do not take estrogen replacement therapy.
- *Race.* Whites and Asians are more likely to develop osteoporosis than African Americans and Latinos, who have higher bone mass at skeletal peak.
- *Body weight.* Increased skeletal weight is thought to promote bone density, putting thin people at greater risk of developing the disease than obese people. However, weight-bearing exercise can have the same effect.
- *Family history.* Genetic factors—that is, peak mass attainment—may affect the occurrence of the disease.
- *Miscellaneous.* Late menarche, nulliparity, and use of caffeine, alcohol, and cigarettes are all thought to be important determinants of bone mass.

Unless a bone density test has been conducted, people are usually asymptotic until a fracture occurs. Management includes prevention of fractures through exercise and drug therapy, such as administration of calcium, vitamin D, estrogen, and other medications or minerals.

h. Hypothermia and hyperthermia pp. 1702–1703

Hypothermia. Thermoregulatory emergencies represent some of the most common EMS calls involving the elderly. As a group, the elderly are vulnerable to low temperatures, suffering about 750,000 winter deaths annually, primarily from hypothermia and "winter risks" such as pneumonia and influenza. Factors that predispose the elderly to hypothermia include accidental exposure to cold, CNS disorders, head trauma, stroke, endocrine disorders (particularly hypoglycemia and diabetes), drugs that interfere with heat production, malnutrition or starvation, chronic illness, forced inactivity as a result of a medical condition, low or fixed income (which discourages use of home heating), inflammatory dermatitis, and A-V shunts.

Hypothermic patients may exhibit slow speech, cold skin, confusion, and sleepiness. In early stages, vital signs may reveal hypertension and an increased heart rate. As hypothermia progresses, however, blood pressure drops and the heart rate slows, sometimes to a barely detectable level. Keep in mind that the elderly patient with hypothermia often does not shiver. Check the abdomen and back to see if the skin is cool to the touch or, if your unit has a low-temperature thermometer, check the patient's core temperature.

Treatment is focused on rewarming the patient and rapid transport. Once the elderly develop hypothermia, they become progressively impaired, with their condition worsening other chronic medical problems. Remain alert for complications, most commonly cardiac arrest or ventricular fibrillation.

Hyperthermia. Age-related changes in the sweat glands and increased incidence of heart disease place the elderly at risk of heat stress. They may develop heat cramps, heat exhaustion, or heat stroke. Risk factors for severe hyperthermia include altered sensory output, inadequate liquid intake, decreased functioning of the thermoregulatory center, commonly prescribed medications that inhibit sweating (such as antihistamines and tricyclic antidepressants), low or fixed incomes (which may result in a lack of fans or air-conditioning), alcoholism, concomitant medical disorders, and use of diuretics (which increase fluid loss).

Early heatstroke may present with nonspecific signs and symptoms such as nausea, lightheadedness, dizziness, headache, and high fever. Prevention strategies include adequate fluid intake, reduced activity, shelter in an air-conditioned environment, and use of light clothing. If hyperthermia develops, however, rapid treatment and transport are necessary.

i. Toxicological problems, including drug toxicity, substance abuse, alcohol abuse, and drug abuse   pp. 1703–1706

Toxicological problems. Aging alters pharmacokinetics and pharmacodynamics in the elderly. Functional changes in the kidneys, liver, and GI system slow the absorption and elimination of many medications. In addition, the various compensatory mechanisms that help buffer against medication side effects are less effective in the elderly than in younger patients.

Approximately 30 percent of all hospital admissions are related to drug-induced illnesses. About 50 percent of all drug-related deaths occur in people over age 60. Accidental overdoses may occur more frequently in the aged due to confusion, vision impairment, self-selection of medications, forgetfulness, and concurrent drug use. Intentional drug overdose also occurs in attempts at self-destruction. Another complicating factor is the abuse of alcohol in the elderly.

In assessing the elderly patient, always take these steps:
- Obtain a full list of medications currently taken by the patient.
- Elicit any medications that are newly prescribed.
- Obtain a good past medical history, including prior renal or hepatic depression.
- Know your medications, their routes of elimination, and their potential side effects.
- If possible, always take all medications to the hospital along with the patient.

Some of the drugs or substances that have been identified as commonly causing toxicity in the elderly include:
- *Lidocaine.* Lidocaine is recommended for the treatment of ventricular dysrhythmias in the acute setting, especially in acute myocardial infarction and in dysrhythmias that arise from cardiac surgery or catheterization. Patients with liver or kidney problems will have problems metabolizing this drug. Lidocaine toxicity is characterized by vision disturbances, GI effects, tinnitus, trembling, breathing difficulties, dizziness or syncope, seizures, and bradycardiac dysrhythmias. Since the cardiac antidysrhythmics in general can cause a decrease in cardiac function and output, observe for shortness of breath, lightheadedness, loss of consciousness, fatigue, chest discomfort, and palpitations.
- *Beta-blockers.* Beta-blockers are widely used to treat hypertension, angina pectoris, and cardiac dysrhythmias. Elderly patients, however, are susceptible to CNS side effects such as depression, lethargy, and sleep disorders. Because geriatric patients often have preexisting cardiovascular problems that can cause decreased cardiac function and output, beta-blockers will limit the heart's ability to respond to postural changes, causing orthostatic hypotension. Beta-blockers also limit the heart's ability to increase contractile force and cardiac output whenever a sympathetic response is necessary in situations such as exercise or hypovolemia. This can be detrimental to the trauma patient who is hemorrhaging and cannot mount the sympathetic response necessary to maintain perfusion of vital organs.

  Treatment of beta-blocker overdoses includes general supportive measures, the removal of gastric contents, support of the ABCs, fluids, and administration of nonadrenergic inotropic agents such as glucagons for hypotension. Excessive bradycardia can be countered with atropine.
- *Antihypertensives/diuretics.* These medications act on the kidneys to increase urine flow and the excretion of water and sodium. They are used primarily in the treatment of hypertension and congestive heart failure. Of these drugs, furosemide is the most widely used diuretic in the elderly. The elimination half-life of furosemide is markedly prolonged in the patient with acute pulmonary edema and renal and hepatic failure. As a result, the geriatric patient is at

risk for a drug buildup. Excessive urination caused by the drug may put the elderly at risk for postural hypotension, circulatory collapse, potassium depletion, and renal function impairment. To reduce this risk, a smaller dose is often prescribed and the patient usually takes a daily potassium supplement.

- *Angiotensin-converting enzyme (ACE) inhibitors.* ACE inhibitors are used for the management of hypertension and congestive heart failure. Geriatric patients generally respond well to treatment with ACE inhibitors. However, these drugs can cause chronic hypotension in patients with severe heart failure who are also taking high-dose loop diuretics. ACE inhibitors can also cause plasma volume reduction and hypotension with prolonged vomiting and diarrhea in the elderly patient. Some hemodialysis patients can experience anaphylactic reactions if treated with ACE inhibitors. Other side effects of ACE inhibitors include dizziness or light-headedness upon standing; presence of a rash; muscle cramps; swelling of the hands, face, or eyes; cough; headache; stomach upset; and fatigue.

- *Digitalis (digoxin, lanoxin).* Digoxin is the most widely used cardiac glycoside for the management of congestive heart failure, atrial fibrillation, atrial flutter, paroxysmal atrial tachycardia, and cardiogenic shock. The drug is unique in that it has a positive inotropic effect and a negative chronotropic effect. Because digoxin has a low margin of safety and a narrow therapeutic index, the amount of drug required to produce a desired effect is very close to the toxic range. Digoxin toxicity in the elderly can result from accidental or intentional ingestion. In the renally impaired elderly patient, any change in kidney function usually warrants an alteration in the dosing of digoxin. Diuretics, which are often given to patients with congestive heart failure, cause the loss of large amounts of potassium in the urine. If potassium is not adequately replenished in the patient taking digoxin, toxicity will develop.

    Signs and symptoms of digoxin toxicity include visual disturbances, fatigue, weakness, nausea, loss of appetite, abdominal discomfort, dizziness, abnormal dreams, headache, and vomiting. Low potassium (hypokalemia) is also common with chronic digoxin toxicity due to concurrent diuretic therapy. Dysrhythmias commonly associated with digoxin toxicity include sinoatrial (SA) exit block, SA arrest, second- or third-degree A-V block, atrial fibrillation with a slow ventricular response, accelerated A-V junctional rhythms, patterns of premature ventricular contractions, ventricular tachycardia, and atrial tachycardia with A-V block.

    The management of digoxin toxicity includes gastric lavage with activated charcoal, correction of confirmed hypokalemia with K+ supplements, treatment of bradycardias with atropine or pacing, and the treatment of rapid ventricular rhythms with lidocaine. Digoxin-specific FAB fragment antibodies (Digibind), an antidote for digoxin toxicity, is used in the treatment of potentially life-threatening situations.

- *Antipsychotics/antidepressants.* Psychotropic medications comprise a variety of agents that affect mood, behavior, and other aspects of mental function. The elderly often experience a high incidence of psychiatric disorders and may take any number of medications, including antidepressants, antianxiety agents, sedative-hypnotic agents, and antipsychotics.

    Antidepressant use in the elderly may result in side effects such as sedation, lethargy, and muscle weakness. Some antidepressants tend to produce anticholinergic effects, including dry mouth, constipation, urinary retention, and confusion. Newly prescribed tricyclic antidepressants can also cause orthostatic hypotension, which can be compounded if the geriatric patient is taking diuretics or other antihypertensive medications. Side effects such as sedation and confusion may also impair the patient's cognitive abilities and possibly endanger the elderly patient who lives alone.

    Antipsychotic medications produce a number of minor side effects such as sedation and anticholinergic effects. Extrapyramidal side effects can also occur, including restlessness and involuntary muscle movements, particularly in the face, jaw, and extremities.

    Field treatment for overdose of antipsychotics and antidepressants is aimed primarily at the ABCs, with special emphasis on airway management.

- *Medications for Parkinson's disease.* Drug treatment for Parkinson's disease is aimed at restoring the balance of neurotransmitters in the basal ganglia. Toxicity of Parkinson's drugs commonly presents as dyskinesia (the inability to execute voluntary movements) and psychological disturbances such as visual hallucinations and nightmares. When these medications are first taken, orthostatic hypotension may also occur. The goal of field management is aimed at decreasing the patient's anxiety and providing a supportive environment. Remember that patients with gross involuntary motor movements are at risk for aspiration and choking.

- *Antiseizure medications.* Seizure disorders are not uncommon in the elderly, and the selection of antiseizure medication depends upon the type of seizure present in the patient. The most common side effect of antiseizure medications is sedation. Other side effects include GI distress, headache, dizziness, lack of coordination, and dermatological reactions (rashes). Recommended treatment involves airway management and supportive therapy.
- *Analgesics and antiinflammatory agents.* Treatment of pain and inflammation for chronic conditions such as rheumatoid arthritis and osteoarthritis includes narcotics and non-narcotic analgesics and corticosteroids. Adverse side effects of these drugs include sedation, mood changes, nausea, vomiting, and constipation. Orthostatic hypotension and respiratory depression may also occur. Over long periods of time, patients may develop drug tolerance and physical dependence on narcotic agents. In the case of corticosteroids, side effects may include hypertension, peptic ulcer, aggravation of diabetes mellitus, glaucoma, increased risk of infection, and suppression of normally produced corticosteroids.

Substance abuse, drug abuse, alcohol abuse. In general, the factors that contribute to substance abuse among the elderly are different than those of younger people. They include age-related changes, loss of employment, loss of spouse or partner, malnutrition, loneliness, moving from a long-loved home, and multiple prescriptions.

The elderly who become physically and/or psychologically dependent upon drugs or alcohol are more likely to hide their dependence and less likely to seek help than other age groups. Common signs and symptoms of drug abuse include memory changes, drowsiness, decreased vision/hearing, orthostatic hypotension, poor dexterity, mood changes, falling, restlessness, and weight loss. Pertinent findings for alcohol abuse include mood swings, denial and hostility (when questioned about alcohol), confusion, history of falls, anorexia, insomnia, visible anxiety, and nausea.

Treatment follows many of the same steps as for any other patient with a pattern of substance abuse. DO NOT judge the patient. Manage the ABCs and evaluate the need for fluid therapy or medications to accommodate withdrawal. Transport the patient to the hospital for further evaluation and referral.

j. Psychological disorders, including depression and suicide pp. 1707–1708

Psychological disorders. When behavioral or psychological problems develop later in life, they are often dismissed as normal age-related changes. This attitude denies an elderly person the opportunity to correct a treatable condition and may overlook an underlying physical disorder. It is important to keep in mind the emotionally stressful situations facing many elderly people—isolation, loneliness, loss of self-dependence, loss of strength, and fear of the future. The elderly also face a higher incidence of secondary depression as a result of neuroleptic medications such as Haldol and Thorazine. Some of the common classifications of psychological disorders related to age include organic brain syndrome, affective disorders, neurotic disorders, and paranoid disorders.

Depression and suicide. Up to 15 percent of the noninstitutionalized elderly experience depression. Within institutions, that figures rises to about 30 percent. In general, depressed patients should receive supportive care, with caregivers delicately raising questions about suicidal thoughts. Keep in mind that the elderly account for 20 percent of all suicides even though they only represent 12 percent of the total population. In fact, suicide is the third leading cause of non-disease related death among the elderly, following falls and car accidents.

In cases of seriously depressed patients, elicit behavior patterns from family, friends, or caregivers. Warning signs may include curtailing activities and self-care, breaking from medical or exercise regimens, grieving a personal loss, expressing feelings of uselessness, putting affairs in order, and stock-piling medications. Be particularly alert to suicide among the acutely ill, especially those in a home-care setting.

Your first priorities in the management of a suicidal elderly patient are to protect yourself and then to protect the patient from self-harm. Conduct a brief interview with the patient, if possible, to determine the need for further action. DO NOT leave the suicidal patient alone. Administer medications with caution, keeping in mind polypharmacy and drug interactions in the elderly. (Consult with medical direction.) All suicidal elderly patients should be transported to the hospital.

18. **Describe the incidence, morbidity/mortality, risk factors, prevention strategies, pathophysiology, assessment, need for intervention and transport, and management of the elderly trauma patient with:**

   a. **Orthopedic injuries** p. 1712

   The elderly suffer the greatest mortality and greatest incidence of disability from falls. Approximately 33 percent of the falls in the elderly result in at least one fractured bone. The most common fall-related fracture is a fracture of the hip or pelvis. Falls also result in a variety of stress fractures in the elderly, including fractures of the proximal humerus, distal radius, proximal tibia, and thoracic and lumbar bodies. In treating orthopedic injuries, remember to ask questions aimed at detecting an underlying medical condition.

   b. **Burns** pp. 1712–1713

   People age 60 and older are more likely to suffer death from burns than any other age group except neonates and infants. Factors that help explain the high mortality rate among the elderly include age-related changes that slow reaction time, preexisting diseases that increase the risk of medical complications, age-related skin changes (thinning) that increase the severity of burns, immunological and metabolic changes that increase the risk of infection, and reductions in physiologic function and the reduced reserves of several organ systems that make the elderly more vulnerable to systemic stress.

   Management of the elderly burn patient follows the same general procedures as other patients. However, remember that the elderly are at increased risk of shock. Administration of fluids is important to prevent renal tubular damage. Assess hydration in the initial hours after the burn injury by blood pressure, pulse, and urine output. Keep in mind that complications in the elderly may manifest themselves in the days and weeks following the incident. For serious burns to heal, the body may use up to 20,000 calories a day. Elderly patients, with altered metabolisms and complications such as diabetes, may not be able to meet this demand, increasing the chances for infection and systemic failure. Part of your job may be to prepare the family for such a delayed response.

   c. **Head injuries** p. 1713

   As people age, the brain decreases in size and weight. The skull, however, remains constant in size, allowing the brain more room to move, thus increasing the likelihood of brain injury. Because of this, the signs and symptoms of brain injury may develop more slowly in the elderly patient, sometimes over days or weeks. In fact, the patient may often have forgotten the offending incident.

   The cervical spine is also more susceptible to injury due to osteoporosis and spondylosis—a degeneration of the vertebral body. In addition, arthritic changes can gradually compress the nerve rootlets or spinal cord. Thus, injury to the spine in the elderly makes them much more susceptible to spinal-cord injury. Therefore, it is important to provide older patients with suspected spinal-cord injury, especially those involved in motor vehicle collisions, with immediate manual cervical stabilization at the time of initial assessment.

19. **Given several preprogrammed simulated geriatric patients with various complaints, provide the appropriate assessment, management, and transport.** pp. 1669–1713

   During your classroom, clinical, and field training, you will assess real and simulated geriatric patients and develop a management plan for them. Use the information presented in this text chapter, the information on assessment of geriatric patients in the field presented by your instructors, and the guidance given by your clinical and field preceptors to develop good patient assessment and care skills. Continue to refine these skills once your training ends and you begin your career as a paramedic.

©2007 Pearson Education, Inc.
Essentials of Paramedic Care, 2nd ed.

CHAPTER 43 *Geriatric Emergencies* 605

Content Self-Evaluation

MULTIPLE CHOICE

_____ 1. All of the following are responsible for the growing number of elderly people in the United States—and the projected increase in the number of elderly patients treated by EMS services—EXCEPT a(n):
   A. increase in the mean survival rate of older persons.
   B. increase in the birth rate.
   C. absence of major wars.
   D. improved health care.
   E. higher standard of living.

_____ 2. The scientific study of the effects of aging and of age-related diseases on humans is known as:
   A. geriatrics.
   B. ageism.
   C. gerontology.
   D. eldercare.
   E. gerontotherapeutics.

_____ 3. The existence of multiple diseases in the elderly is known as:
   A. functional impairment.
   B. dysphagia.
   C. comorbidity.
   D. polypharmacy.
   E. senility.

_____ 4. Common complaints in the elderly include:
   A. falls, weakness, and syncope.
   B. fractures, drowning, and diabetes.
   C. GSW, croup, and nausea.
   D. MVC, meningitis, and poisoning.
   E. fever, epiglottitis, and febrile seizures.

_____ 5. When compared to younger patients, the elderly experience fewer adverse drug reactions.
   A. True
   B. False

_____ 6. Drugs concentrate more readily in the plasma and tissues of elderly patients because of:
   A. diminished neurologic function.
   B. increased body fluid.
   C. atrophy of organs.
   D. more efficient compensatory mechanisms.
   E. increased renal function.

_____ 7. Factors that can decrease medication compliance in the elderly include all of the following EXCEPT:
   A. limited mobility.
   B. fear of toxicity.
   C. childproof containers.
   D. multiple-compartment pill boxes.
   E. sensory impairment.

_____ 8. Factors that can increase medication compliance in the elderly include:
   A. compliance counseling.
   B. a belief that an illness is serious.
   C. clear, simple directions.
   D. blister-pack packaging.
   E. all of the above

_____ 9. A lack of mobility can have detrimental physical and emotional effects on the elderly.
   A. True
   B. False

_____ 10. Which of the following is the leading cause of accidental deaths among the elderly?
   A. drownings
   B. fall-related injuries
   C. motor vehicle collisions
   D. gunshot wounds
   E. poisonings

_____ 11. Intrinsic factors that can cause an elderly person to fall include all of the following EXCEPT:
   A. dizziness.
   B. slippery floors.
   C. decreased mental status.
   D. impaired vision.
   E. CNS problems.

_____ 12. Extrinsic factors that can cause an elderly person to fall include:
   A. an altered gait.
   B. a sense of weakness.
   C. a lack of hand rails.
   D. use of certain medications.
   E. a history of repeated falls.

_____ 13. The inability to retain urine or feces because of loss of sphincter control or because of cerebral or spinal lesions is called:
   A. diarrhea.
   B. involuntary elimination.
   C. diuresis.
   D. incontinence.
   E. uremia.

_____ 14. In elderly people with cerebrovascular disease or impaired baroreceptor reflexes, efforts to force a bowel movement can lead to a transient ischemic attack.
   A. True
   B. False

_____ 15. Possible causes of elimination problems in the elderly include:
   A. diverticular disease.
   B. constipation.
   C. colorectal cancer.
   D. use of opioids.
   E. all of the above

_____ 16. One of the most common reasons that elderly patients underestimate the severity of a primary medical problem is that they have a(n):
   A. shrinkage of structures in the ear.
   B. clouding and thickening of lenses in the eyes.
   C. lowered sensitivity to pain.
   D. deterioration of the teeth and gums.
   E. altered sense of taste.

_____ 17. All of the following factors play a part in forming a general assessment of the elderly patient EXCEPT:
   A. average cost of rent.
   B. medication history.
   C. living situations.
   D. sleep patterns.
   E. level of activity.

_____ 18. Conditions that may discourage eating among the elderly include:
   A. breathing or respiratory problems.
   B. nausea or vomiting.
   C. poor dental care.
   D. alcohol or drug abuse.
   E. all of the above

_____ 19. Which of the following is a byproduct of malnutrition?
   A. electrolyte abnormalities
   B. dehydration
   C. vitamin deficiencies
   D. hypoglycemia
   E. all of the above

_____ 20. The elderly are more prone to environmental thermal problems due to changes in the sweat glands.
   A. True
   B. False

_____ 21. A medical condition in which eye pressure increases and ultimately diminishes sight is known as:
   A. Meniere's disease.
   B. tinnitus.
   C. cataracts.
   D. glaucoma.
   E. retinitis.

_____ 22. A disease of the inner ear characterized by vertigo, nerve deafness, and a roar or buzzing in the ear is called:
   A. Meniere's disease.
   B. tinnitus.
   C. cataracts.
   D. glaucoma.
   E. cerumen.

_____ 23. To improve communication with an elderly patient, you should try to:
   A. display verbal and nonverbal signs of concern.
   B. dim the room lights.
   C. avoid looking directly into the patient's eyes.
   D. first talk to family members, then the patient.
   E. remain as quiet as possible.

_____ 24. Both senility and organic brain syndrome may manifest themselves as:
   A. distractibility.
   B. excitability.
   C. hostility.
   D. restlessness.
   E. all of the above

_____ 25. When assessing an elderly person, if they are confused or disoriented, you can conclude that the patient is senile.
   A. True
   B. False

_____ 26. Changes in mental status in the elderly patient may be due to which of the following?
   A. traumatic head injury
   B. dementia
   C. decreased sugar level
   D. infection
   E. all of the above

_____ 27. To help reduce an elderly patient's fears, you should:
   A. downplay the patient's fears.
   B. ignore nonverbal messages.
   C. discourage the expression of feelings.
   D. confirm what the patient has said.
   E. instruct the patient to calm down.

_____ 28. Compared to younger people, the skin of elderly people:
   A. is thicker and oilier.
   B. heals more quickly.
   C. tears less easily.
   D. is less subject to fungal infections.
   E. perspires less.

_____ 29. The elderly have a greater risk of trauma-related complications due to a decrease in blood volume.
   A. True
   B. False

_____ 30. Age-related changes to the respiratory system include all of the following EXCEPT:
   A. increased chest wall compliance.
   B. diminished breathing capacity.
   C. reduced strength and endurance.
   D. increased air trapping.
   E. reduced gag reflex.

_____ 31. The decrease of an effective cough reflex and the activity of the _____ make the elderly more prone to respiratory infection.
   A. gag reflex
   B. alveoli
   C. cilia
   D. bronchioles
   E. vagal response

_____ 32. In treating respiratory disorders in the elderly patient, do not fluid overload.
   A. True
   B. False

_____ 33. An exaggeration of the normal posterior curvature of the spine is called:
   A. scoliosis.
   B. kyphosis.
   C. fibrosis.
   D. hypertrophy.
   E. spondylosis.

_____ 34. An increase in the size and bulk of the left ventricle wall in some elderly patients is an example of:
   A. kyphosis.
   B. anoxia hypoxemia.
   C. hypertrophy.
   D. fibrosis.
   E. Marfan's syndrome.

_____ 35. In managing elderly patients with complaints related to the cardiovascular system, take all of the following steps EXCEPT:
   A. monitor the ECG.
   B. provide high-concentration supplemental oxygen.
   C. walk the patient slowly to the rig.
   D. remain empathetic to the patient's fears.
   E. start an IV for medication administration.

_____ 36. All of the following are age-related changes to the nervous system EXCEPT:
   A. decreased reaction time.
   B. increased brain weight.
   C. impaired balance.
   D. shrinkage of brain tissue.
   E. recent memory loss.

_____ 37. The elderly are less susceptible to subdural hematomas than younger people.
   A. True
   B. False

_____ 38. Age-related changes in the gastrointestinal system include all of the following EXCEPT:
   A. impaired swallowing.
   B. diminished digestive functions.
   C. decreased liver efficiency.
   D. a predisposition to choking.
   E. increased gastric secretions.

_____ 39. A protrusion of the stomach upward into the mediastinal cavity through the diaphragm is known as:
   A. a hiatal hernia.
   B. Marfan's syndrome.
   C. a diaphragmatic hernia.
   D. an inguinal hernia.
   E. an epigastric hernia.

_____ 40. Reasons that the elderly develop pneumonia more frequently than younger people include all of the following EXCEPT a(n):
   A. decreased immune response.
   B. increased pulmonary function.
   C. abnormal or ineffective cough reflex.
   D. decreased activity of mucociliary cells.
   E. decreased colonization of the pharynx by gram-negative bacteria.

_____ 41. An elderly patient in an institutional setting is up to 50 times more likely to contract pneumonia than an elderly patient receiving home care.
   A. True
   B. False

_____ 42. The usual signs and symptoms of COPD include:
   A. cough and wheezing.
   B. dyspnea and tachypnea.
   C. exercise intolerance.
   D. pleuritic chest pain.
   E. all of the above

_____ 43. The most effective prevention of COPD involves:
   A. elimination of smoking.
   B. lowering blood sugar.
   C. reducing physical activity.
   D. lowering blood pressure.
   E. use of supplemental oxygen.

_____ 44. Your elderly patient is complaining of acute onset of sharp chest pain and shortness of breath. The patient was recently released from the hospital for a leg fracture. What is the most likely suspected disorder?
   A. pneumonia
   B. pulmonary embolism
   C. heart attack
   D. COPD
   E. pulmonary edema

_____ 45. Although all of the following can contribute to a pulmonary embolism, the condition is most frequently caused by:
   A. fat.
   B. bone marrow.
   C. blood clots.
   D. tumor cells.
   E. air.

_____ 46. The leading cause of death in the elderly is:
   A. pneumonia.
   B. stroke.
   C. cardiovascular disease.
   D. Alzheimer's disease.
   E. COPD.

_____ 47. The heart sounds in an elderly patient are generally louder than those in a young patient.
   A. True
   B. False

_____ 48. All of the following are atypical presentations of a myocardial infarction in the elderly EXCEPT:
   A. syncope.
   B. tearing chest pain.
   C. dyspnea.
   D. neck or dental pain.
   E. exercise intolerance.

_____ 49. Assessment findings specific to the elderly such as anorexia, nocturia, dependent edema, and hepatomegaly may be found in a patient with:
   A. a pulmonary embolism.
   B. heart failure.
   C. hypertension.
   D. an aneurysm.
   E. syncope.

_____ 50. An abnormal dilation of a blood vessel, usually an artery, due to a congenital defect or weakness in the wall of the vessel is called:
   A. an aneurysm.
   B. an infarct.
   C. thrombosis.
   D. an embolism.
   E. a hernia.

_____ 51. A series of symptoms resulting from decreased blood flow to the brain that are caused by a sudden decrease in cardiac output from a heart block are known as:
   A. autonomic dysfunction.
   B. Stokes-Adams syndrome.
   C. sick sinus syndrome.
   D. dying heart muscle.
   E. Marfan's syndrome.

_____ 52. Injury to or death of brain tissue resulting from interruption of cerebral blood flow and oxygenation is called a(n):
   A. subarachnoid hemorrhage.
   B. autonomic dysfunction.
   C. TIA.
   D. stroke.
   E. intracerebral hemorrhage.

_____ 53. Common causes of seizures in the elderly include all of the following EXCEPT:
   A. head trauma.
   B. alcohol withdrawal.
   C. spinal injury.
   D. stroke.
   E. hypoglycemia.

_____ 54. A progressive, degenerative disease that attacks the brain and results in impaired memory, thinking, and behavior is called:
   A. dementia.
   B. Parkinson's disease.
   C. delirium.
   D. Alzheimer's disease.
   E. aphasia.

_____ 55. A chronic, degenerative nervous disease characterized by tremors, muscular weakness and rigidity, and loss of postural reflexes is called:
   A. Parkinson's disease.
   B. Shy-Drager syndrome.
   C. Alzheimer's disease.
   D. sick sinus syndrome.
   E. grand mal seizure.

_____ 56. All of the following are forms of upper GI bleed EXCEPT:
   A. peptic ulcer disease.
   B. ischemic colitis.
   C. esophageal varices.
   D. gastritis.
   E. diverticulitis.

_____ 57. An example of a lower GI bleed is:
   A. a Mallory-Weiss tear.
   B. diverticulosis.
   C. peptic ulcer disease.
   D. a bowel obstruction.
   E. a mesenteric infarct.

_____ 58. An inflammation of the colon due to impaired or decreased blood supply is called:
   A. diverticulosis.
   B. ischemic colitis.
   C. arterio-venous malformation.
   D. colostomy.
   E. gastritis.

_____ 59. An abnormal dilation of veins in the lower esophagus common in patients with cirrhosis of the liver is called esophageal varices.
   A. True
   B. False

_____ 60. The acute skin eruption caused by a reactivation of latent varicella virus that peaks between ages 50 and 70 is known as:
   A. shingles.
   B. pruritus.
   C. maceration.
   D. herpes zoster.
   E. both A and D

_____ 61. When transporting an elderly patient with pressure ulcers, you should encourage the patient to remain still.
   A. True
   B. False

_____ 62. Risk factors for osteoporosis include all of the following EXCEPT:
   A. African or Latino ancestry.
   B. low body weight.
   C. early menopause.
   D. family history of fractures.
   E. use of caffeine, alcohol, and cigarettes.

_____ 63. In general, the kidney loses approximately one third of its weight between the ages of 30 and 80.
   A. True
   B. False

_____ 64. All of the following are signs and symptoms of hypothermia in an elderly patient EXCEPT:
   A. confusion.
   B. slow speech.
   C. shivering.
   D. skin cool to the touch.
   E. sleepiness.

_____ 65. Elderly patients with hepatic impairment and decreased renal function should receive the normal dose of lidocaine.
   A. True
   B. False

MATCHING

Write the letter of the term in the space provided next to the appropriate description.

A. epistaxis
B. varicosities
C. sick sinus syndrome
D. autonomic dysfunction
E. transient ischemic attack
F. brain ischemia
G. urosepsis
H. nocturia
I. polycythemia
J. delirium
K. senile dementia
L. vertigo
M. mesenteric infarct
N. spondylosis
O. dysphoria

_____ 66. acute alteration in mental functioning that is often reversible

_____ 67. septicemia originating from the urinary tract

_____ 68. medical term for a nose bleed

_____ 69. excessive urination, usually at night

_____ 70. death of tissue in the peritoneal fold that encircles the small intestine

_____ 71. exaggerated feeling of depression or unrest

_____ 72. excess of red blood cells

_____ 73. abnormal dilation of a vein

_____ 74. group of disorders characterized by dysfunction of the SA node

_____ 75. sensation of faintness or dizziness causing loss of balance

_____ 76. general term used to describe an abnormal decline in mental function in the elderly

_____ 77. degeneration of the vertebral body

_____ 78. abnormality of the involuntary aspect of the nervous system

_____ 79. injury to the brain tissues caused by an inadequate supply of oxygen and nutrients

_____ 80. medical condition like a stroke but reversible and commonly involving syncope

Abuse and Assault

Review of Chapter Objectives

After reading this chapter, you should be able to:

1. **Discuss the incidence of abuse and assault.**   p. 1716

   Because of underreporting, it is difficult to provide accurate statistics on the incidence of abuse and assault in the United States today. That makes the available figures even more overwhelming in their seriousness. To grasp the magnitude of the problem, consider these facts:

   - Nearly three million children suffer abuse each year and more than 1,000 die annually.
   - Between two and four million women each year are battered by their partners or spouses.
   - Elder abuse occurs at an incidence of between 700,000 and 1.1 million annually.

2. **Describe the categories of abuse.**   pp. 1716–1725

   Partner abuse
   Partner abuse results when a man or woman subjects a domestic partner to some form of physical or psychological violence. The victim may be a husband or wife, someone who shares a residence, or simply a boyfriend or girlfriend.

   Elder abuse
   There are basically two types of elder abuse—domestic and institutional. Domestic elder abuse takes place when an elder is being cared for in a home-based setting, usually by relatives. Institutional elder abuse occurs when an elder is being cared for by a person with a legal or contractual responsibility to provide care, such as paid caregivers, nursing home staff, or other professionals. Both types of abuse can be either acts of commission (acts of physical, sexual, or emotional violence) or acts of omission (neglect).

   Child abuse
   Child abuse may range from physical or emotional impairment to neglect of a child's most basic needs. It can occur from infancy to age 18 and can be inflicted by any number of caregivers—parents, foster parents, stepparents, babysitters, siblings, step-siblings, or other relatives or friends charged with a child's care.

   Sexual abuse/assault
   Sexual abuse, which is a form of physical abuse, can occur in almost any setting with a male or female of any age. It involves forced sexual contact and includes date rape and such contact within marriage. Although the legal definitions of sexual assault vary from state to state, courts generally

interpret it as unwanted sexual contact, whether it be genital, oral, rectal, or manual. Rape is usually defined as penile penetration of the genitalia or rectum (however slight) without the consent of the victim. Both forms of sexual violence are prosecuted as crimes, with rape constituting a felony offense.

3. **Discuss examples of spouse, elder, child, and sexual abuse.** pp. 1716–1725

   Examples of spouse/partner abuse

   Partner abuse can fall into several categories. The most obvious form is physical abuse, which involves the application of force in ways too many to list. In addition to direct injury, physical abuse may exacerbate existing medical conditions, such as hypertension, diabetes, or asthma. Verbal abuse, which consists of words chosen to control or harm a person, may leave no physical mark. However, it damages a person's self-esteem and can lead to depression, substance abuse, or other self-destructive behavior. As noted in objective 2, partner abuse can also take the form of sexual abuse—unwanted, forced sexual contact between two people.

   Examples of elder abuse

   Elder abuse can also be physical, verbal, or sexual. In some cases, signs of elder abuse are subtle, such as theft of the victim's belongings or loss of freedom. Other signs, such as wounds, untreated decubitus ulcers, or poor hygiene, are more obvious. (For other examples of elder abuse, see Chapter 43.)

   Examples of child abuse

   As pointed out in Chapters 41 and 42, abused children suffer every imaginable mistreatment. They can be shaken, thrown, burned or scalded, and battered with almost any kind of object. They can be denied food, clean clothing, medical care, or even access to a toilet. The damage done to a child can last a lifetime and perpetuate a cycle of violence for generations to come.

   Examples of sexual abuse/assault

   Sexual abuse/assault typically involves a male assailant and a female victim, but not always. Forced sexual contact can range from exposure to fondling to rape to sexual torture. It may involve one assailant or multiple assailants. It can be an isolated act or an ongoing occurrence. Sexual abuse/assault can result in injuries, infections, sexually transmitted diseases, and unwanted pregnancies. The psychological damage is deep and long-lasting. Shame, anger, and a lack of trust may persist for years—or even a lifetime.

4. **Describe the characteristics associated with the profile of a typical spouse, elder, or child abuser and the typical assailant of sexual abuse.** pp. 1717, 1719–1720, 1720–1721, 1725

   Profile of spouse/partner abusers

   Partner abuse occurs in all demographic groups. However, abuse is more common in lower socioeconomic levels in which wage earners have trouble paying bills, holding down jobs, or keeping pace with technological changes. Typically the abuser does not like being out of control but at the same time feels powerless to change. A spouse or partner abuser usually exhibits an overly aggressive personality—an outgrowth of low self-esteem. They often feel insecure and jealous, flying into sudden and unpredictable rages. Use of alcohol or drugs increases the likelihood that the abuser will lose control and may not even remember his or her actions.

   In the aftermath of an abusive incident, the abuser often feels a sense of remorse and shame. The person may seek to relieve his or her guilt by promising to change or even seeking help. For a time, the abuser may appear charming or loving, convincing an abused spouse or partner to think the pattern has finally been broken. All too often, however, the cycle of violence repeats itself in just a few days, weeks, or months.

   Profile of elder abusers

   Like partner abuse, elder abuse cuts across all demographic groups. As a result, it is difficult to profile the people who are most likely to abuse elders. However, there are several characteristics found in abusers of the elderly. Often, the perpetrators exhibit alcoholic behavior, drug addiction, or some mental impairment. The abuser may also be dependent upon the income or assistance of the elder—a situation that can cause resentment, anger, and, in some cases, violence. According to one study, in cases of domestic elder abuse, the most typical abusers are adult children who are overstressed by care of the elder and/or who were abused themselves.

Profile of child abusers

As with other types of abusers, you cannot relate child abuse to social class, income, or education. However, most abusers share one common trait: They were physically or emotionally abused as children. They often would prefer to use other forms of discipline, but under stress they regress to the earliest and most familiar patterns. Once they have resorted to physical discipline, the punishments become more severe and more frequent.

In cases of reported physical abuse, perpetrators tend to be men. However, the statistics for men and women even out when neglect is taken into account. Although potential child abusers can include a wide variety of caregivers, one or both parents are the most likely abusers. Frequent behavioral traits include use or abuse of alcohol and/or drugs, immaturity, self-absorption, and an inability to emotionally identify with the child.

Typical assailants of sexual abuse

Once again, sexual assailants can come from almost any background. However, the violent victimizers of children are substantially more likely than the victimizers of adults to have been physically or sexually abused as children. Many assailants, particularly adolescents and abusive adults, think domination is part of any relationship. Such thinking can lead to date rape or marital rape. In a significant number of all cases, the assailants are under the influence of alcohol or drugs.

5. **Identify the profile of the "at-risk" spouse, elder, and child.** pp. 1717–1718, 1719, 1721, 1724–1725

At-risk spouses/partners

The primary risk factor for abuse is a family history of violence toward a spouse or partner. According to studies, pregnancy also appears to play a role, with 45 percent of abused women suffering some form of abuse during pregnancy. Substance abuse and emotional disorders play a role as well.

In identifying an abusive family situation, keep in mind the generic risk factors identified in "Domestic Violence: Cracking the Code of Silence," a source cited in the DOT's National Standard Curriculum. These factors, based on research of battered women, include:
- Male is unemployed.
- Male uses illegal drugs at least once a year.
- Partners have different religious backgrounds.
- Family income is below the poverty level.
- Partners are unmarried.
- Either partner is violent toward children at home.
- Male did not graduate from high school.
- Male is unemployed or he has a blue-collar job.
- Male is between 18 and 30 years old.
- Male saw his father hit his mother.

At-risk elders

A number of factors place the elderly at risk of abuse. Some of these include increased dependency on others (as a result of longer life spans), decreased productivity in later years, physical and mental impairments (especially among the "old-old"), limited resources for long-term care of the elderly, strained family resources, and stress on middle-aged caregivers responsible for two generations—children and parents.

In general, elder abuse occurs most frequently among people who are dependent upon others for their care, especially among those elders who are mentally or physically challenged. Elders in poor health are more likely to be abused than elders in good health. This situation results, in part, from their inability to report the abuse. Yet another risk factor is family history, or a cycle of violence among family members. Finally, the potential for elder abuse increases proportionately with the personal problems of the caregivers. Abusers of the elderly tend to have more difficulties, either financial or emotional, than nonabusers.

At-risk children

As indicated in Chapter 42, abused children share several characteristics. Often, the child is seen as "special" and different from others. Premature infants and twins stand a higher risk of abuse than other children. Many abused children are less than 5 years of age. Physically and mentally challenged children as well as those with special needs are at greater risk. So are uncommunicative (e.g., autistic) children. Boys are more often abused than girls. A child who is not what the parents wanted (e.g., the "wrong" gender) is at increased risk of abuse, too.

6. Discuss the assessment and management of the abused patient. pp. 1717, 1718, 1719, 1721–1723, 1726

Your primary responsibility on a call involving an abusive situation is safety—both your own and that of the patient. You should never enter a scene if your safety is compromised, and you should leave the scene as soon as you feel unsafe.

You can expect the victims of abuse to feel threatened as a result of the violence they have suffered. One of your main duties is to provide a safe environment for an already traumatized patient. Sometimes you can provide safety merely by your official presence. Other times, you may have to move the patient to the ambulance so you can relocate to a different environment. In still other situations, you may have to summon additional personnel, such as law enforcement.

Specific assessment and management considerations will depend upon the type of abuse encountered. In cases of partner abuse, use direct questions, if possible, to convey an awareness that the person's partner may have contributed to the injury. In cases of suspected child abuse, examine the patient for identifiable patterns of physical mistreatment or neglect and record your objective observations. In cases of sexual abuse, use open-ended questions to reestablish the patient's sense of control. If possible, allow a same-sex crew member to maintain contact with the victim.

Regardless of the situation, keep in mind that the patient has been harmed by another human being, in many cases a person that he or she knows intimately. Try to transport the patient to the hospital. If you cannot do so, either because of patient refusal or intervention by the suspected abuser, be sure to report your suspicions to the appropriate authorities or agencies.

7. Discuss the legal aspects associated with abuse situations. pp. 1718, 1723, 1726–1727

Abuse and assault constitute crimes. Although their nature and the extent of the crime often depends upon local laws, you have a responsibility to report suspected cases. Because the assailants may be detained only a short time, you also have an obligation to find out about the victim and witness protection programs available in your area.

Study the local laws and protocols regarding cases of abuse and assault. All 50 states require health care workers to report suspected cases of child abuse. Some states require EMS personnel to report even a suspicion of abuse or assault. Some states allow minors to seek medical care for sexual assault without parental consent. The Joint Commission of Accreditation of Healthcare Organizations (JCAHO) mandates that hospital personnel screen incoming patients for abuse. Regardless of where you live, take time to learn the rules and regulations that affect your practice, both for your sake and for the sake of your patient.

8. Identify community resources that are able to assist victims of abuse and assault. pp. 1718, 1723, 1726–1727

Specialized resources include both private and state or federally funded programs. Make a point of learning about hospital units for the victims of sexual assault, public and private shelters for battered persons, and state agencies responsible for youth and their families. Also acquaint yourself with nurses trained as Sexual Assault Nurse Examiners (SANE). They have completed programs allowing them to perform the physical exam for sexual assaults.

9. Discuss the documentation necessary when caring for abused and assaulted patients. pp. 1723, 1726–1727

It is important that you carefully and objectively document all your findings. Your actions can affect the outcome of a case or prosecution of a crime. If the patient tells you something about the abuser or assailant, mark it with quotation marks on the patient care report. In the case of rape, patients should not urinate, defecate, douche, bathe, eat, drink, or smoke. Some jurisdictions have specific rules for evidence protection, such as using paper bags to collect evidence or placing bags over the patient's hands to preserve trace evidence. Remember that any evidence you collect must remain in your custody until you can give it directly to a law enforcement official to preserve the chain of evidence. Regardless of the emotions evoked by the call, when documenting the incident, you must be completely factual and nonjudgmental.

Content Self-Evaluation

MULTIPLE CHOICE

_____ 1. Partner abuse is defined as physical or emotional violence from a man or woman toward a co-worker.
   A. True
   B. False

_____ 2. The most widespread and best-known form of abuse involves the abuse of:
   A. women by men.
   B. children by their mothers.
   C. children by their fathers.
   D. elders by their children.
   E. same-sex partners.

_____ 3. Many victims of abuse hesitate or fail to report the problem because of a:
   A. fear of reprisal.
   B. lack of knowledge.
   C. fear of humiliation.
   D. lack of financial resources.
   E. all of the above

_____ 4. By far the most common characteristic of abusers—whether they be partner abusers, child abusers, or elder abusers—is a:
   A. history of substance abuse.
   B. lack of employment.
   C. family history of violence.
   D. lack of education.
   E. mental impairment.

_____ 5. Forty-five percent of pregnant women suffer some form of battery during pregnancy.
   A. True
   B. False

_____ 6. In assessing the battered patient, all of the following are appropriate actions EXCEPT:
   A. direct questioning.
   B. asking the victim why she or he doesn't leave.
   C. rehearsing the quickest way to leave the home.
   D. nonjudgmental questioning.
   E. reminding the patient that assault is a crime.

_____ 7. All of the following are causes of elder abuse EXCEPT:
   A. stress on middle-aged caregivers.
   B. decreased life expectancies.
   C. physical and mental impairments.
   D. limited resources for long-term care.
   E. decreased productivity in later years.

_____ 8. Which of the following are two main types of elder abuse?
   A. neglect and domestic
   B. emotional and financial
   C. domestic and institutional
   D. mental and institutional
   E. financial and domestic

_____ 9. The perpetrators of domestic elder abuse tend to be:
   A. paid caregivers.
   B. siblings.
   C. adult children.
   D. spouses.
   E. friends or neighbors.

_____ 10. In cases of child abuse, the most likely abusers are:
   A. babysitters.
   B. siblings.
   C. strangers.
   D. one or both parents.
   E. friends charged with the child's care.

_____ 11. All of the following are characteristics of abused children EXCEPT:
   A. sudden behavioral changes.
   B. neediness.
   C. absence of nearly all emotions.
   D. unusual wariness.
   E. concern over a parent's absence.

_____ 12. One of the signs of intentional scalding of a child is:
   A. staphylococcal scalded skin.
   B. hematological disorders.
   C. multiple splatter marks.
   D. multiple bruises.
   E. absence of splash burns.

_____ 13. Children rarely exhibit accidental fractures to the:
   A. head.
   B. ribs.
   C. legs.
   D. arms.
   E. hands or feet.

_____ 14. Which type of injury claims the largest number of lives among abused children?
   A. malnutrition
   B. head injuries
   C. burns
   D. chest injury
   E. abdominal injuries

_____ 15. The group most likely to be victims of sexual assault or rape are adolescent females under age 18.
   A. True
   B. False

_____ 16. The victims of rape most commonly describe their assailant as a stranger.
   A. True
   B. False

_____ 17. When talking to a rape victim, you can help the patient regain a sense of self-control by asking _____ questions.
   A. open-ended
   B. closed-ended
   C. indirect
   D. nonpersonal
   E. leading

_____ 18. Sexual Assault Nurse Examiners are specially trained health care workers who can:
   A. help with the prehospital care report.
   B. protect the patient against the assailant.
   C. provide information on the protection of evidence.
   D. protect EMS crews against legal suits.
   E. none of the above

_____ 19. In managing a rape case, honor the patient's request to bathe or shower.
   A. True
   B. False

_____ 20. All 50 states require health care workers to report suspected cases of:
   A. child abuse.
   B. rape.
   C. elder abuse.
   D. spousal abuse.
   E. partner abuse.

Chapter 45

The Challenged Patient

Review of Chapter Objectives

After reading this chapter, you should be able to:

1. **Describe the various etiologies and types of hearing impairments.** p. 1731

   There are basically two types of deafness—conductive deafness and sensorineural deafness. Conductive deafness results from any condition that prevents sound waves from being transmitted from the external ear to the middle or inner ear. The condition may be temporary or permanent. If caught early, many forms of conductive deafness may be treated and cured. Sensorineural deafness, on the other hand, is often incurable. The condition arises from the inability of nerve impulses to reach the auditory center of the brain because of nerve damage either to the inner ear or to the brain. In the case of infants and children, sensorineural deafness often results from congenital defects or birth injuries.

2. **Recognize the patient with a hearing impairment.** p. 1732

   It is very important to detect deafness early in your assessment. A partially deaf person may ask questions repeatedly, misunderstand answers to questions, or respond inappropriately. Such reactions can easily be mistaken for head injury, leading to misdirected treatment.

   The most obvious sign of deafness is a hearing aid. Unfortunately, hearing aids do not work for all types of deafness. Also, many people do not wear hearing aids, even when they have been prescribed. In addition, deaf people may have poor diction, due to hearing loss. They might use their hands to gesture or use sign language. Deaf people may ask you to speak louder or they may speak excessively loud themselves. Finally, deaf people will commonly face you so that they can read your lips.

3. **Anticipate accommodations that may be needed in order to properly manage the patient with a hearing impairment.** p. 1732

   When managing a patient with a hearing impairment, you can do several things to ease communications.

   - Begin by identifying yourself and making sure the patient knows that you are speaking to him or her.
   - Address deaf patients face to face, giving them the opportunity to read your lips and interpret your expression.
   - Speak slowly in a normal voice. Never yell or use exaggerated gestures, which often distort your facial and body language.

- Keep in mind that nearly 80 percent of hearing loss is related to high-pitched sounds. As a result, you might use a low-pitched voice to speak directly into the patient's ear.
- Make sure background noise is reduced as much as possible.
- If necessary, find or adjust a hearing aid.
- Be innovative. Put the stethoscope on the patient and try speaking into it. Don't forget the most simple and effective means of communication—a pen and paper.
- If necessary and if time allows, draw pictures to illustrate procedures.
- If the patient knows sign language, usually American Sign Language (ASL), utilize an interpreter, documenting the name of the person who did the interpreting and the information received.

4. **Describe the various etiologies and types, recognize patients with, and anticipate accommodations that may be needed in order to properly manage each of the following conditions:**

   a. **visual impairments** pp. 1732–1733

   When caring for the patient with a visual impairment, it is important to note if the impairment is a permanent disability or if it is a new symptom caused by the illness or injury for which you were called. Visual impairments have a number of etiologies—injury, disease, congenital conditions, infection (such as cytomegalovirus [CMV]), and degeneration of the retina, optic nerve, or nerve pathways.

   Depending on the degree of impairment and a person's adjustment to the loss of vision, you may or may not recognize the condition right away. In cases of obvious blindness, identify yourself as you approach the patient so that the person knows you are there. Also describe everything you are doing. Take into account any special tools that assist a visually impaired person with daily living, most notably guide dogs and/or canes. Depending upon local protocols, arrange to transport the guide dog to the hospital with the patient. If the patient is ambulatory, have the person take your arm for guidance rather than taking the patient's arm.

   b. **speech impairments** pp. 1733–1734

   When performing an assessment, you may come across a patient who is awake, alert, and oriented but cannot communicate with you due to a speech impairment. Possible miscommunication can hinder both the treatment administered and the information provided to the receiving facility. You may encounter four types of speech impairments. They include:
   - **Language disorders.** A language disorder is an impaired ability to understand the spoken or written word. In children, language disorders result from a number of causes such as congenital learning disorders, cerebral palsy, hearing impairments, or inadequate language stimulation during the first year of life (delayed speaking ability). In adults, language disorders may result from a variety of illnesses or injuries—stroke, aneurysm, head injury, brain tumor, hearing loss, or some kind of emotional trauma. The loss of ability to communicate in speech, writing, or signs is known as aphasia. Aphasia can manifest itself in the following ways.

     Sensory aphasia—a person can no longer understand the spoken word. Patients with sensory aphasia will not respond to your questions because they cannot understand what you are saying.

     Motor aphasia—a person can no longer use the symbols of speech. Patients with motor aphasia, also known as expressive aphasia, will understand what you say but cannot clearly articulate a response.

     Global aphasia—occurs when a person has both sensory and motor aphasia. These patients can neither understand nor respond to your questions. A brain tumor in the Broca's region can cause this condition.
   - **Articulation disorders.** Articulation disorders, also known as dysarthria, affect the way a person's speech is heard by others. These disorders occur when sounds are produced or put together incorrectly or in a way that makes it difficult to understand the spoken word. Articulation disorders may start at an early age, when the child learns to say words incorrectly or when a hearing impairment is involved. This type of disturbance can occur in both children and adults when neural damage causes a disturbance in the nerve pathways leading from the brain to the larynx, mouth, or lips.

- **Voice production disorders.** When a patient has a voice production disorder, the quality of the person's voice is affected. This can be caused by trauma due to overuse of the vocal cords or infection. Cancer of the larynx can also cause a speech failure by impeding air from passing through the vocal cords. A patient with a production disorder will exhibit hoarseness, harshness, an inappropriate pitch, or abnormal nasal resonance.
- **Fluency disorders.** Fluency disorders present as stuttering. Although the cause of stuttering is not fully understood, the condition is found more often in men than in women. When speaking with patients who stutter, do not interrupt or finish their answers out of frustration and do not correct the way they speak.

When speaking to a patient with a speech impairment, never assume that the person lacks intelligence. Do not rush the patient or predict an answer. Try to form questions that require short, direct answers. When asking questions, look directly at the patient. If you cannot understand what the person has said, politely ask him or her to repeat it. Never pretend to understand when you don't. You might miss valuable information related to the call. If all else fails, give the patient the opportunity to write responses to your questions.

c. obesity   pp. 1734–1736

Over 40 percent of the U.S. population are considered obese, while many more are heavier than their ideal body weight. Obesity occurs for a number of reasons. In many cases, diet, exercise, and lifestyles result in a caloric intake that exceeds daily energy needs. Genetic factors also predispose a person toward obesity. In rare cases, an obese patient may have a low basal metabolic rate, which causes the body to burn calories at a slower rate. In such cases, the condition may have been produced by an illness, such as hyperthyroidism.

Managing an obese patient presents a number of challenges. Beside the obvious difficulty of lifting and moving these patients, excess weight can exacerbate the complaint for which you were called. Obesity can also lead to a number of serious medical conditions, including hypertension, heart disease, stroke, diabetes, and joint and muscle problems. In conducting a history, you will need to question patients carefully to make sure they are not mistakenly attributing signs and symptoms to their weight.

When doing your patient assessment, you may need to accommodate for the patient's weight. It may be necessary to auscultate lung sounds anteriorly on a patient who is too obese to lean forward. If the patient's adipose tissue presents an obstruction, you may need to place ECG monitoring electrodes on the arms and thighs instead of on the chest. Also be sure to have plenty of assistance for lifting and keep in mind that many of the litters and stretchers are not rated for extremely large patients. Finally, alert the emergency department of the need for extra lifting assistance and special stretchers upon arrival.

d. paraplegia/quadriplegia   p. 1736

During your career, you may respond to a call and find that your patient is paralyzed from a previous traumatic or medical event. You will have to treat the chief complaint while taking into account the accommodations that must be made when treating a patient who cannot move some or all of his or her extremities.

A paralyzed patient may be paraplegic or quadriplegic. A paraplegic patient has been paralyzed from the waist down, while a quadriplegic patient has paralysis of all four extremities. In addition, spinal cord injuries in the area of C-3 to C-5 and above may also paralyze the patient's respiratory muscles and compromise the ability to breathe.

In managing a paraplegic or quadriplegic patient, be prepared for a number of common devices. These include a home ventilator, tracheostomy, halo traction, or colostomy. Be sure to make accommodations for these—and any other assisting devices—when you transport the patient. (For more on acute interventions for physically disabled and other chronic care patients, see Chapter 46.)

e. mental illness and mental/emotional impairments   p. 1736

Mental and emotional illnesses or impairments present a special challenge to the EMS provider. The disorders may range from the psychoses caused by complex biochemical brain diseases, such as bipolar disorder (manic depression), to the personality disorders related to personality development, to a traumatic experience. Emotional impairments can include such conditions as hysteria, compulsive behavior, or anxiety. (For a detailed discussion on the etiologies, assessment, management, and treatment of these patients, see Chapter 38 in Division 4.)

f. developmentally disabled   pp. 1736–1737

People with developmental disabilities are those individuals with impaired or insufficient development of the brain who are unable to learn at the usual rate. Developmental disabilities can occur for a variety of reasons. They can be genetic, such as Down syndrome, or they can be the product of a brain injury caused by some hypoxic or traumatic event. Such injuries can take place before birth, during birth, or anytime thereafter.

Except for patients with Down syndrome, it may be difficult to recognize someone with a developmental disability unless the person lives in a group home or other special residential setting. Remember that a person with a developmental disability can recognize body language, tone, and disrespect just like anyone else. Treat him or her as you would any other patient, listening to his/her answers, particularly if you suspect physical or emotional abuse.

If a patient has a severe cognitive disability, you may need to rely on others to obtain the chief complaint and history. Also, many children or young people with learning disabilities have been taught to be wary of strangers who may seek to touch them. You have to establish a basis of trust with the patient, perhaps by making it clear that you are a member of the medical community or by asking for the support of a person the patient does trust. Also, some people with developmental disabilities have been judged "stupid" or "bad" for behavior that results in an accident and they may try to cover up the events that led up to a call.

At all times, keep in mind that a person with a developmental disability may not understand what is happening. The ambulance, special equipment, and even your uniform may confuse or scare them. In cases of severe disabilities, it will be important to keep the primary caregivers with you at all times, even in the back of the ambulance.

g. Down syndrome   pp. 1737–1738

Down syndrome results from an extra chromosome, usually on chromosome 21 or 22. Although the cause is unknown, the chromosomal abnormality increases with the age of the mother, especially after age 40. It also occurs at a higher rate in parents with a chromosomal abnormality, such as the translocation of chromosome 21 to chromosome 14.

Typically Down syndrome presents with easily recognized physical features. They include eyes sloped up at the outer corners, folds of skin on either side of the nose that cover the inner corner of the eye, small face and features, large and protruding tongue, flattening on the back of the head, and short and broad hands.

In addition to mild to moderate developmental disability, Down syndrome patients may have other physical ailments, such as heart defects, intestinal defects, and chronic lung problems. Down syndrome people are also at high risk of developing cataracts, blindness, and Alzheimer's disease at an early age.

When assessing the Down syndrome patient, consider the level of his or her developmental delay and follow the general guidelines mentioned in objective 4f. Transport to the hospital should be uneventful, especially if the caregiver comes along.

h. emotional impairment and i. emotional/mental impairment   p. 1736

See objective 4e.

5. **Describe, identify possible presenting signs of, and anticipate accommodations for the following diseases/illnesses:**

a. arthritis   pp. 1738–1739

The three most common types of arthritis include:

- **Juvenile rheumatoid arthritis (JRA)**—a connective tissue disorder that strikes before age 16
- **Rheumatoid arthritis**—an autoimmune disorder
- **Osteoarthritis**—a degenerative joint disease, the most common arthritis seen in elderly people

All forms cause painful swelling and irritation of the joints, making everyday tasks sometimes impossible. Treatment of arthritis includes aspirin, nonsteroidal antiinflammatory drugs (NSAIDS), and/or corticosteroids. It is important for you to recognize the side effects of these medications in case you have been called upon to treat a medication side effect rather than the disease. NSAIDS can cause stomach upset and vomiting, with or without bloody emesis. Corticosteroids, such as prednisone, can cause hyperglycemia, bloody emesis, and decreased immunity. You should also take note of all the patient's medications so that you do not administer a medication that can interact with the ones already taken by the patient.

When transporting arthritis patients, keep in mind their high level of discomfort. Use pillows to elevate affected extremities. The most comfortable position might not be the best position to start an IV, but try to make the patient as comfortable as possible.

b. cancer
pp. 1739–1740

Cancer is caused by the abnormal growth of cells in normal tissue. The primary site of origin of the cancer determines the type of cancer the patient has. It may be difficult for you to recognize a cancer patient because the disease often has few obvious signs and symptoms. Rather, the treatments for the disease take on telltale signs, such as anorexia leading to weight loss or alopecia (hair loss). Tattoos may be left on the skin by radiation oncologists to mark positioning of radiation therapy equipment. In addition, physical changes, such as loss of a breast (mastectomy), may be obvious.

Management of the cancer patient can present a special challenge. Many patients undergoing chemotherapy treatments become neutropenic—a condition in which chemotherapy creates a dangerously low neutrophil (white blood cell) count. If patients have recently received chemotherapy, assume that they are neutropenic and take every precaution to protect them from infection. Keep a mask on the patient both during transport and during transfer at the emergency department.

In treating cancer patients, also keep in mind that their veins may have become scarred and difficult to access due to frequent IV starts, blood draws, and caustic chemotherapy transfusions. Cancer patients may also have an implanted infusion port, found just below the skin, with the catheter inserted into the subclavian vein or brachial artery. You need special training to access these ports and should not attempt to access them unless you have such training and the approval of medical direction.

Cancer patients may also have a peripheral access device such as a Groshong catheter or Hickman catheter. In this situation, it may simply be a matter of flushing the line and then hooking up your IV fluids to this external catheter. Whatever you decide to do, involve the patient, who has already lost a lot of control over his or her treatment, in the decision-making process.

c. cerebral palsy
p. 1740

Cerebral palsy (CP) is a group of disorders caused by damage to the cerebrum in utero or by trauma during birth. Prenatal exposure of the mother to German measles can cause cerebral palsy, as well as any condition leading to fetal hypoxia. Premature birth or brain damage from a difficult delivery can also lead to cerebral palsy. Other causes include encephalitis, meningitis, or head injury during a fall or abuse of an infant.

There are three main types of cerebral palsy—spastic paralysis, athetosis, and ataxia. In treating patients with cerebral palsy, keep this fact in mind: Many people with atheotoid and diplegic CP are highly intelligent. Do not assume that a person with cerebral palsy cannot communicate with you.

When transporting cerebral palsy patients, make accommodations to prevent further injury. If they experience severe contractions, the patients may not rest comfortably on a stretcher. Use pillows and extra blankets to pad extremities that are not in proper alignment. Have suction available if a patient drools. If a patient has difficulty communicating, make sure that the caregiver helps in your assessment. Be alert for cerebral palsy patients who sign. If you do not know how to sign, find somebody who does and alert the emergency department.

d. cystic fibrosis
p. 1741

Cystic fibrosis (CF) is an inherited disorder involving the exocrine glands primarily in the lungs and digestive system. Thick mucus forms in the lungs, causing bronchial obstruction and atelectasis in the small ducts of the alveoli. In addition, the thick mucus causes blockages in the small ducts of the pancreas, leading to decrease in the pancreatic enzymes needed to absorb nutrients.

Obtaining a complete medical history is important to the recognition of a CF patient. A unique characteristic of CF is the high concentration of chloride in the sweat, leading to the use of a diagnostic test known as the "sweat test." A CF patient may also complain of frequent lung infections, clay-colored stools, or clubbing of the fingers or toes.

Because of the high probability of respiratory distress in a CF patient, some form of oxygen therapy may be necessary. You may need to have a family member or caregiver hold blow-by oxygen (rather than use a mask) if this is all the patient will tolerate. Suctioning may be necessary to help the patient clear the thick secretions. If the patient is taking antibiotics to prevent infection and using inhalers or Mucomyst to thin secretions, bring these medications to the hospital. Above all else, keep in mind that these patients have been chronically ill for their entire lives. The last thing they or their loved ones want is another trip to the hospital.

Because of a poor prognosis, most of the CF patients that you see will be children or adolescents. A child with cystic fibrosis is still a child. So remember everything that you have learned about the treatment of pediatric patients and apply it to the developmental stage of the CF patient that you are treating.

e. multiple sclerosis   p. 1741

Multiple sclerosis (MS) is a disorder of the central nervous system that usually strikes between the ages of 20 and 40, affecting women more than men. The exact cause of MS is unknown, but it is considered to be an autoimmune disorder. Characteristically, repeated inflammation of the myelin sheath surrounding the nerves leads to scar tissue, which in turn blocks nerve impulses to the affected area.

The onset of MS is slow. It starts as a change in the strength of a muscle and a numbness or tingling in the affected muscle. Patients may develop problems with gait, slurred speech, and clumsiness. They may experience double vision due to weakness of the eye muscles or eye pain due to neuritis of the optic nerve. As symptoms progress, they become more permanent, leading the MS patient to become increasingly weak and more vulnerable to lung or urinary infections.

Transporting of the MS patient to the hospital may require supportive care, such as oxygen therapy. Make sure the patient is comfortable and help position the patient as needed. Bring any assistive devices, such as a wheelchair or cane, so that the patient can maintain as much independence as possible.

f. muscular dystrophy   pp. 1741–1742

Muscular dystrophy (MD) is a group of hereditary disorders characterized by progressive weakness and wasting of muscle mass. It is a genetic disorder, leading to gradual degeneration of muscle fibers. The most common form of MD is Duchenne muscular dystrophy, which typically affects boys between the ages of 3 and 6. It leads to progressive muscle weakness in the legs and pelvis and to paralysis by age 12. Ultimately, the disease affects the respiratory muscles and heart, causing death. The other various MD disorders are classified by the age of the patient at onset of symptoms and by the muscles affected.

Since MD is a hereditary disease, you should obtain a complete family history. You should also note the particular muscle groups that the patient cannot move. Again, since MD patients are primarily children, choose age-appropriate language. Respiratory support may be needed, especially in later stages of the disease.

g. myasthenia gravis   p. 1743

Myasthenia gravis is an autoimmune disease characterized by chronic weakness of voluntary muscles and progressive fatigue. The condition results from a problem with the neurotransmitters, which causes a blocking of nerve signals to the muscles. It occurs most frequently in women between ages 20 and 50.

A patient with myasthenia gravis may complain of a complete lack of energy, especially in the evening. The disease commonly involves muscles in the face. You may note eyelid drooping or difficulty chewing or swallowing. The patient may also complain of double vision.

In severe cases of myasthenia gravis, a patient may experience paralysis of the respiratory muscles, leading to respiratory arrest. These patients may need assisted ventilations en route to the emergency facility.

h. poliomyelitis   p. 1742

Poliomyelitis is a communicable disease affecting the gray matter in the brain and spinal cord. Although it is highly contagious, immunization has made outbreaks of polio extremely rare in developed nations. However, it is important to be aware of the disease, since many people born before development of the polio vaccine in the 1950s were affected by the disease.

Although most patients recover from polio, they are left with permanent paralysis of the affected muscles. You may recognize a polio victim by the use of assistive devices for ambulation or by the reduced size of the affected limb due to muscle atrophy. Some patients may have experienced paralysis of the respiratory muscles, requiring assisted ventilations. Patients on long-term ventilators will typically have tracheotomies.

Along with polio, you should know about a related disorder called post-polio syndrome. Post-polio syndrome affects those patients who suffered severely from polio more than 30 years ago. Patients with this condition quickly tire, especially after exercise, and develop an intolerance for cold in their extremities.

Many patients with polio or post-polio syndrome may insist on walking to the ambulance but should not be encouraged to do so. Because they may not have required hospitalization for polio since childhood, you will have to alleviate their anxiety, keeping in mind their fears of a renewed loss of independence.

i. spina bifida   pp. 1742–1743

Spina bifida is a congenital abnormality that falls under the category of a neural tube defect. It presents when there is a defect in the closure of the backbone and the spinal canal. In spina bifida occulta, the patient exhibits few outward signs of the deformity. In spina bifida cystica, the failure of the closure allows the spinal cord and covering membranes to protrude from the back, causing an obvious deformity.

Symptoms depend upon which part of the spinal cord is protruding through the back. The patient may have paralysis of both lower extremities and lack of bowel or bladder control. A large percentage of the children with this disease also have hydrocephalus, requiring a surgical shunt to help drain excess fluid from the brain.

When treating spina bifida patients, keep several things in mind. Recent research has shown that between 18 and 73 percent of children and adolescents with spina bifida have latex allergies. For safety, assume that all patients with spina bifida have this problem. In transporting spina bifida patients, be sure to bring along any devices that aid them. If you are called to treat an infant, safe transport to the hospital should be done in a car seat, unless contraindicated.

j. patients with a previous head injury   p. 1742

Patients with a previous head injury may not be easily recognized until they begin to speak. They may display similar symptoms to those of stroke, but without the hemiparesis (paralysis on one side of the body). Such patients may have aphasia, slurred speech, or loss of vision or hearing, or may develop a learning disability. They may also exhibit short-term memory loss and may not have any recollection of their original injury.

Obtaining a medical history will be extremely important, especially if you are responding to a traumatic event. Note any new symptoms the patient may be having or the recurrence of old ones. If the patient cannot speak, look for obvious physical signs of trauma or for facial expressions of pain. Treatment and transport considerations will depend upon the condition for which you were called.

6. **Define, recognize, and anticipate accommodations needed to properly manage patients who:**

a. are culturally diverse   pp. 1743–1744

Culturally diverse patients may speak a different language or have different traditions or religious beliefs from yours. What may make it difficult for you to treat culturally different patients may not be the differences per se, but your inability to understand them. Do not consider this a reason for refusing treatment. Rather, consider it a learning experience that will prepare you for a similar situation on another run.

As a paramedic, you are ethically required to take care of all patients in the same manner, regardless of their race, religion, gender, ethnic background, or living situation. Remember, the patient who has decision-making abilities has a right to self-determination and can refuse treatment. You should, however, obtain a signed document indicating informed refusal of consent. If your patient does not speak English, communication may be a problem. You may need to rely on a family member to act as an interpreter or on a translator device, such as a telephone language line for non-English speaking-people. In such cases, be sure to notify the receiving facility of the need for an interpreter.

b. **are terminally ill**   p. 1744

Caring for a terminally ill patient can be an emotional challenge. Many times, the patient will choose to die at home, but at the last minute the family compromises those wishes by calling EMS. In other cases, the patient may call for an ambulance so that a newly developed condition can be treated or a medication adjusted. (For more on caring for the terminally ill, see Chapter 46.)

c. **have a communicable disease**   p. 1744

When treating people with communicable diseases, you should withhold all personal judgment. Although you will need to take BSI precautions just as you would with any patient, keep in mind the heightened sensitivity of a person with a communicable disease. Although most of these patients are familiar with the health care setting, you should still explain that you take these measures with all patients who have a similar disease. Also, you do not need to take additional precautions beyond those required by departmental policy. The patient will generally spot these extra measures and react with feelings of shame, guilt, or anger. (For more on the etiologies and treatment of communicable diseases, see Chapter 37 in Division 4.)

d. **have a financial impairment**   p. 1744

Patients who have financial impairments, such as the homeless, sometimes refuse care because they think they cannot afford to pay the medical bills. It is your job to help these patients understand that they can receive health care regardless of their financial situation. Become familiar with public hospitals and clinics that provide services for the needy. In providing care, keep this guideline in mind: Treat the patient, not the financial condition the patient is in!

7. **Given several challenged patients, provide the appropriate assessment, management, and transportation.**   pp. 1730–1744

During your classroom, clinical, and field training, you will be presented with real and simulated challenged patients and develop management plans for them. Use the information presented in this text chapter, the information on assessing challenged patients provided by your instructors, and the guidance given by your clinical and field preceptors to develop good skills in caring for the special needs of these patients. Continue to refine newly learned skills once your training ends and you begin your career as a paramedic.

Content Self-Evaluation

Multiple Choice

1. The two main types of deafness are:
   - A. tinnitus and Meniere's disease.
   - B. conductive and sensorineural.
   - C. partial and sudden.
   - D. clinical and nonclinical.
   - E. temporary and complete.

2. A middle ear infection, frequently associated with upper respiratory infection, is:
   - A. labyrinthitis.
   - B. otitis media.
   - C. presbycusis.
   - D. otomycosis.
   - E. cerumen.

3. During the patient interview and physical exam, hearing deficits may be mistaken for:
   - A. head injury.
   - B. intoxication.
   - C. transducer infection.
   - D. effusion syndrome.
   - E. drug overdose.

_____ 4. When communicating with a deaf patient, consider all of the following strategies EXCEPT:
   A. speaking slowly in a normal voice.
   B. using a high-pitched voice to speak directly into the patient's ear.
   C. reducing background noise.
   D. using a pen and paper.
   E. putting a stethoscope on the patient and speaking into it.

_____ 5. The term for removal of the eyeball after trauma, such as a penetrating injury, or certain kinds of illnesses is:
   A. retinal detachment.
   B. enucleation.
   C. optic chiasm.
   D. orbitotomy.
   E. corneal abrasion.

_____ 6. Diabetes can slowly lead to a loss of a vision as a result of:
   A. degeneration of the optic nerve.
   B. disorders in the blood vessels leading to the retina.
   C. degeneration of the eyeball.
   D. cytomegalovirus (CMV).
   E. retinitis.

_____ 7. When approaching a patient with a seeing eye dog in a harness, pet the dog to show that you mean no harm to its owner.
   A. True
   B. False

_____ 8. All of the following are types of speech impairments, except:
   A. congenital disorders.
   B. language disorders.
   C. fluency disorders.
   D. articulation disorders.
   E. voice production disorders.

_____ 9. A language disorder that can be caused by a stroke or brain injury is known as:
   A. amnesia.
   B. ataxia.
   C. aphagia.
   D. aphasia.
   E. aphonia.

_____ 10. Stuttering is an example of a(n):
   A. dyslexic disorder.
   B. fluency disorder.
   C. auditory disorder.
   D. vocal cord disorder.
   E. voice production disorder.

_____ 11. If the adipose tissue on an obese patient presents an obstruction, you may need to place ECG monitoring electrodes on the:
   A. chest and back.
   B. hands and feet.
   C. arms and back.
   D. neck and chest.
   E. arms and thighs.

_____ 12. A quadriplegic patient has been paralyzed from the waist down.
   A. True
   B. False

_____ 13. Depression and psychoses are examples of:
   A. emotional and mental impairments.
   B. developmental disabilities.
   C. visual impairments.
   D. articulation disorders.
   E. pathological challenges.

_____ 14. People with Down syndrome are at risk of developing:
   A. cataracts.
   B. blindness.
   C. early Alzheimer's disease.
   D. heart defects.
   E. all of the above

_____ 15. Fetal alcohol syndrome (FAS) is sometimes confused with Down syndrome because they both:
   A. produce similar facial characteristics.
   B. are caused by alcohol consumption during pregnancy.
   C. are preventable birth defects.
   D. cause death at an early age.
   E. produce hyperactivity.

_____ 16. It is not uncommon for children with juvenile rheumatoid arthritis (JRA) to suffer complications involving the spleen or liver.
   A. True
   B. False

_____ 17. Cancer patients receiving chemotherapy are at high risk for:
   A. syncope.   D. weight gain.
   B. infection.   E. diminished sense of pain.
   C. altered mental status.

_____ 18. If a cancer patient has an implanted infusion port, you can generally hook up your IV fluids to this port.
   A. True
   B. False

_____ 19. When caring for cerebral palsy patients, you may need to:
   A. treat them as if they have a spinal injury.
   B. change the order of the initial assessment.
   C. use pillows and blankets to pad unaligned extremities.
   D. anticipate brief periods of apnea.
   E. both A and D

_____ 20. A group of hereditary disorders characterized by progressive weakness and wasting of muscle tissue is known as:
   A. poliomyelitis.   D. cystic fibrosis.
   B. spina bifida.   E. muscular dystrophy.
   C. multiple sclerosis.

_____ 21. Most of the cystic fibrosis patients that you see will be:
   A. adults in their 30s and 40s.
   B. elderly patients over age 60.
   C. infants 1 year old and younger.
   D. children and adolescents.
   E. women between the ages of 20 and 40.

_____ 22. A congenital abnormality in which a large percentage of children are born with hydrocephalus is:
   A. Down syndrome.   D. fetal alcohol syndrome.
   B. cerebral palsy.   E. cystic fibrosis.
   C. spina bifida.

_____ 23. A preventable disorder caused by alcohol consumption during pregnancy is:
   A. JRA.   D. TIA.
   B. FAS.   E. PE.
   C. ACE.

_____ 24. Research has shown that between 18 and 73 percent of children and adolescents with _____ have a latex allergy.
   A. cerebral palsy   D. spina bifida
   B. myasthenia gravis   E. Down syndrome
   C. poliomyelitis

_____ 25. A patient with spina bifida may have any of the following conditions EXCEPT:
  A. accumulation of fluid on the brain.
  B. loss of bladder control.
  C. paralysis of the lower extremities.
  D. loss of bowel control.
  E. paralysis on one side of the body.

_____ 26. Common complaints from a patient with myasthenia gravis include:
  A. chronic fatigue or lack of energy.
  B. nausea and headache.
  C. shortness of breath and heart palpitations.
  D. dizziness and loss of appetite.
  E. unsteady gait and double vision.

_____ 27. Accommodation of a culturally diverse population requires:
  A. patience.
  B. ingenuity.
  C. respect.
  D. use of translators.
  E. all of the above

_____ 28. When a patient refuses treatment because of religious reasons, you should:
  A. call the police to intervene.
  B. administer treatment and document your reasons.
  C. ask the person to reconsider his or her religious views.
  D. obtain a signed refusal of treatment and transportation form.
  E. leave the scene.

_____ 29. When treating people with communicable diseases, you should take additional precautions beyond those required by departmental policy.
  A. True
  B. False

_____ 30. If a homeless person is unable to afford medical bills, it is your job to help the patient get health care regardless of his or her financial situation.
  A. True
  B. False

MATCHING

Write the letter of the term in the space provided next to the appropriate description.

A. labyrinthitis
B. conductive deafness
C. motor aphasia
D. deafness
E. diabetic retinopathy
F. sensorineural deafness
G. sensory aphasia
H. otitis media
I. neutropenic
J. enucleation
K. cerumen
L. colostomy
M. mucoviscidosis
N. presbycusis
O. glaucoma

_____ 31. an inability to hear

_____ 32. progressive hearing loss that occurs with aging

_____ 33. middle ear infection

_____ 34. group of eye disorders that result in increased intraocular pressure on the optic nerve

_____ 35. ear wax

_____ 36. occurs when the patient cannot speak but can understand what is said

_____ 37. a surgical diversion of the large intestine through an opening in the skin where the fecal matter is collected in a pouch

_____ 38. a condition that results in an abnormally low white blood cell count

_____ 39. caused when there is a blocking of the transmission of the sound waves through the external ear canal to the middle or inner ear

_____ 40. slow loss of vision as a result of damage done by diabetes

_____ 41. occurs when a patient cannot understand the spoken word

_____ 42. inner ear infection that causes vertigo, nausea, and an unsteady gait

_____ 43. removal of the eyeball after trauma or illness

_____ 44. caused by the inability of nerve impulses to reach the auditory center of the brain because of nerve damage either to the inner ear or to the brain

_____ 45. cystic fibrosis of the pancreas resulting in abnormally viscous mucoid secretion from the pancreas

Chapter 46: Acute Interventions for the Chronic-Care Patient

Review of Chapter Objectives

After reading this chapter, you should be able to:

1. **Compare and contrast the primary objectives of the paramedic and the home care provider.** pp. 1748, 1752

   The paramedic's primary role is to identify and treat any life-threatening problems and transport as necessary. Home care providers, on the other hand, assume responsibility, in varying degrees, for managing a chronic condition in the home setting and for helping the patient to live as normally as possible. A paramedic provides acute interventions; a home care provider provides ongoing care per medical directives, usually from a physician.

2. **Identify the importance of home health care medicine as it relates to emergency medical services.** pp. 1747–1748

   The shift to home health care has important implications for emergency medical services. As patients assume greater responsibility for their own treatment and recovery, the likelihood of advanced life support (ALS) intervention at home for the chronic-care patient increases. Calls may come from the patient, the patient's family, or a home health care provider.

   In home care settings, you can expect to encounter a sometimes dizzying array of devices, machines, and equipment designed to provide anything from supportive to life-sustaining care. The failure or malfunction of this type of equipment has the potential to become a life-threatening or life-altering event.

   In a call involving a home care patient, you are responding to a patient who is already sick or injured in some way. A previously manageable condition may have suddenly become unmanageable or more complicated. Unlike in a hospital, the patient or home care provider cannot push a button and summon immediate help. Instead, they often summon you, the ALS provider.

3. **Differentiate between the role of the paramedic and the role of the home care provider.** pp. 1748, 1752

   As noted in objective 1, the paramedic provides acute interventions for the chronically ill patient who relies in some way on a home care provider who helps to manage his or her condition. Remember that the home care provider—whether it be a nurse, nurse's aide, family member, or friend—usually knows the patient better than anyone else. The provider will often spot subtle changes in the patient's condition that may seem insignificant to the outsider. In assessing the patient, it is crucial that you listen carefully to what this person says.

©2007 Pearson Education, Inc.
Essentials of Paramedic Care, 2nd ed.

4. **Compare and contrast the primary objectives of acute care, home care, and hospice care.** pp. 1747–1748, 1752, 1774–1775

- **Acute care**—focuses on short-term intervention aimed at identifying and managing any immediate life-threatening emergencies, using transport as needed.
- **Home care**—involves the ongoing care and supportive assistance required to help a patient manage an injury or a chronic condition, usually according to a physician's instructions or written orders; home care may be either short-term or long-term.
- **Hospice care**—provides a program of palliative care and support services that address the physical, social, economic, and spiritual needs of terminally ill patients and their families.

5. **Discuss aspects of home care that enhance the quality of patient care and aspects that have the potential to become detrimental.** pp. 1747–1748

Supporters of home health care offer several arguments in its favor. First, they point out that patients often recover faster in the familiar environments of their homes than in the hospital. They also emphasize the differences in the cost of home care versus hospital care. However, the technological devices required by many home care patients can—and do—fail. Family members may either willingly accept the responsibilities of home care or succumb to the pressure. Finally, as noted in objective 6, home care patients are susceptible to a wide variety of complications related to their particular treatments and/or conditions.

6. **List pathologies and complications in home care patients that commonly result in ALS intervention.** pp. 1748–1753, 1775–1776

A number of situations can involve you in the treatment of a home care patient—equipment failure, unexpected complications, absence of a caregiver, need for transport, the inability to operate a device, and more. Many of the medical problems that you will encounter in a home care setting are the same ones that you would encounter elsewhere in the field. Some of the typical responses involve airway complications, respiratory failure, cardiac decompensation, alterations in peripheral circulation, altered mental status, GI/GU crises, infections, and/or septic complications. (For specific information or examples of home care problems requiring acute interventions, see text pages 1748–1753.)

In providing ALS intervention, you must always keep in mind that the home care patient is in a more fragile state to begin with. A member of the medical community has already decided that the person needs extra help. A home care patient is more likely to decompensate and go into crisis more quickly than a member of the general population. As a result you need to monitor the home care patient carefully and be ready to intervene at all times.

7. **Compare the cost, mortality, and quality of care for a given patient in the hospital versus the home care setting.** pp. 1747–1748

The steady rise in hospital charges and the cost of skilled nursing facilities prompted the growth of home health care, along with other factors such as the enactment of Medicare, advent of HMOs, increased medical acceptance, and improved medical technology. With total health expenditures expected to rise by an estimated 7.5 percent in the first decade of the 2000s, the savings promised by home health care continues to speed the dismissal of patients from hospitals and nursing homes. As indicated in objective 5, there are trade-offs to be made in treating a patient in the hospital versus a home care setting.

8. **Discuss the significance of palliative care programs as related to a patient in a home health care or hospice setting.** pp. 1752, 1774–1775

A patient in the home care setting is usually receiving curative care aimed at healing the patient's illness or injury. If a patient's condition is terminal, treatment switches to palliative or comfort care. The goal is to relieve symptoms, manage pain, and give patients control over the end of their lives. Palliative care may be provided by hospice workers in the patient's home or in homes or apartments managed by hospices.

9. Define hospice care, comfort care, and DNR/DNAR as they relate to local practice, law, and policy.   pp. 1758–1759, 1774–1776

Hospice care provides a program of palliative or comfort care as well as support services that address the physical, social, economic, and spiritual needs of terminally ill patients and their families. The goal of hospice care is very different than the goal of most other branches of the health care professions, including EMS. For an ALS team, care is usually geared toward aggressive and life-saving treatment. A hospice team, on the other hand, seeks to make the patient as comfortable as possible.

For the most part, patients in hospice situations have already exhausted or declined curative resources. As a rule, family members, caregivers, and health care workers have been instructed to call a hospice rather than EMS. However, you may be summoned for intervention, particularly in situations involving transport. In such cases, you should keep in mind that the hospice patient is in an end-stage disease and has already expressed wishes to withhold resuscitation. In all likelihood the patient will probably have a Do Not Resuscitate (DNR) or Do Not Attempt Resuscitation (DNAR) order in place. However, such orders should not prevent you from performing palliative or comfort care.

Local protocols may vary in respect to DNRs, DNARs, living wills, and durable power of attorney documents. Be sure that you are familiar with these legal statements and their implications for care of the terminally ill. (For more on this topic, see Chapter 2 in Division 1.)

10. List and describe the characteristics of typical home care devices related to airway maintenance, artificial and alveolar ventilation, vascular access, drug administration, and the GI/GU tract.   pp. 1748–1749, 1750, 1752, 1757, 1761–1772

You can expect to encounter a vast number of machines and devices in the home care situation—anything from a home dialysis unit to personal care items such as a long-handled shoehorn to wheelchairs, canes, and walkers. Examples of typical equipment aimed at airway maintenance and/or ventilation include portable suctioning devices, nebulized and aerosolized medication administrators, incentive spirometers, home ventilators, apnea monitors, tracheostomy tubes or collars, and oxygen delivery systems (oxygen concentrators, oxygen masks, liquid oxygen reservoirs, regulator-flow meters, nasal cannulas, tubing, and sterile water).

Patients may also have any variety of vascular access devices (VADs). Patients may have a peripherally inserted central catheter (PICC line) or a surgically implanted medication delivery system such as a Port-A-Cath or Medi-Port. Some VADs have been permanently implanted, such as a dialysis shunt or a Hickman, Broviac, or Groshong catheter.

Yet other patients may have various long-term devices to support gastrointestinal or genitourinary functions. These include urinary catheters (Texas/condom catheters or internal/Foley catheters), urostomies, nasogastric feeding tubes, or gastrostomy tubes (with a colostomy).

As these examples show, home care devices range from the simplicity of a nasal cannula to the complexity of a home ventilator. If you encounter an unfamiliar device—which may happen at some time in your career—don't panic. Find out what it's used for, and you will then have an idea how to proceed. Don't be afraid to look foolish by asking questions. You won't. You will be foolish, and endanger the patient, if you pretend to understand a device but don't.

11. Discuss the complications of assessing each of the devices described in objective 10.   pp. 1761–1772

Discussion of the complications for the various devices can be found on the pages indicated with this objective. However, in general, keep in mind these points.

Oxygen delivery systems
Very few problems arise from oxygen delivery systems themselves. When they do occur, patients or home care providers can usually correct the situation on their own. Some technical problems include impeded oxygen flow (faulty tubing/dirty or plugged humidifier), activation of the warning buzzer on the oxygen concentrator (unplugged unit or power failure), and hissing or rapidly depleted oxygen tank (leak).

In terms of the oxygen therapy itself, follow these guidelines:
- Ensure the ability of the patient/home care provider to administer oxygen.
- Make sure the patient knows what to do in case of a power failure.
- Evaluate sterile conditions, especially disinfections of reusable equipment.
- Remain alert to signs and symptoms of hypoxemia.

Artificial airways/tracheostomies

The most common problems faced by tracheostomy patients include blockage of the airway by mucus and a dislodged cannula. Children can also have their stoma blocked by foreign objects that enter by accident or are put there by a sibling or playmate. Other complications include infection of the stoma, drying of the mucus leading to crusting or bleeding, and tracheal erosion from an overinflated cuff (causing necrosis).

If EMS is called, it means that neither the patient nor the caregiver has been able to solve the problem. If the tracheostomy patient is on a ventilator, you must rapidly determine if the problem is with the ventilator or with the airway itself. If the problem is simply a loose-fitting or disconnected tube, fix it. If the problem is not immediately apparent, do not waste time trying to troubleshoot the machine—unless you are qualified to do so. Your bag-valve device will connect directly to where the ventilator tubing connects. Remove the tubing, connect the bag-valve device to the trach connector, and ventilate.

If the problem is with the patient's airway, you will need to clear it. If the patient is hypoxic, always hyperventilate before suctioning. Remember to ensure that ventilations are directed downward toward the lungs. If you are unable to ventilate, clearing the airway is your first priority. If it appears that the inner cannula is blocked or dislodged, you may remove it. If necessary, you may intubate the stoma. Once the airway is secure, you may proceed with the rest of your assessment. It is inappropriate to proceed until you have protected the airway.

Ventilators

Ventilatory problems are traditionally easy to remedy, such as in the case of unplugged power cords or a temporary loss of electricity. If you are familiar with the ventilator, you can remedy other problems by adjusting the settings to restore or improve ventilations. However, if you are unfamiliar with the ventilator, play it safe and support ventilations with your own equipment. Remember—if a home ventilator fails, begin manual positive-pressure ventilation immediately. Whatever interventions you choose, you will have to make arrangements for home devices to be transported with you to the hospital.

Vascular access devices

In the case of patients with VADs, the most common complications result from various types of obstructions. A thrombus may form at the catheter site, or an embolus may lodge elsewhere in the body. Other obstructive problems include catheter kinking or catheter tip embolus. With central venous access devices, always be aware of the potential for an air embolus. Of course, any device implanted in the body has a risk for infection. Because these catheters provide a channel into the central circulation, patients may quickly become septic, especially if they are weakened or immunosuppressed.

Urinary devices

Most complications related to urinary tract support devices result from infection or device malfunctions. Infection is a very common problem with urinary tract devices because the area is rich with pathogens and because the catheter provides a pathway directly into the body. Remain alert to foul-smelling urine or altered urine color, such as tea-colored, cloudy, or blood-tinged urine. Also look for signs and symptoms of systemic infection, or urosepsis, as urinary infections can quickly spread in the immunocompromised patient.

Device malfunctions typically include accidental displacement of the device, obstruction, balloon ruptures in devices that use a balloon as an anchor, or leaking collection devices. Changes in the patient's anatomy, such as a shortened urinary tract or tissue necrosis, can also cause malfunctions. Ensure that the collection device is empty and record the amount of urine output. Look for kinks or other obstructions in the device and make sure the collection bag is placed below the patient.

Gastrointestinal tract devices

Complications from GI tract devices include tube misplacement, obstruction, or infection. Because misplaced tubes can obstruct the airway or GI system, you should always ensure device patency if you have any doubts about placement of the tube. First, have the patient speak to you. If he or she cannot speak, the tube may be in the airway and need to be removed. Second, to ensure patency of an NG tube, use a 60 mL syringe to insert air into the stomach. Use your stethoscope to listen over the epigastrium for air movement within the stomach. A low-pitched rumbling should be heard. You may also note stomach contents spontaneously moving up the tube or they may be aspirated with a 60 cc syringe. In such cases, patients may be repositioned to return patency, or the device reinserted.

Tubes are also prone to obstruction. Colostomies may become clogged or otherwise obstructed. Feeding tubes can become clogged due to the thick consistency of supplemental feedings or pill fragments. As a result, the tubes may require irrigation with water. In addition, the thick consistency of food may cause bowel obstructions or constipation.

As might be expected, ostomies can become infected or lose skin integrity from pressure. Look for signs and symptoms of skin or systemic infection. In addition, remember that digestive enzymes may leak from various ostomies and begin to digest the skin and abdominal contents.

12. Describe indications, contraindications, and techniques for urinary catheter insertion in the male and female patient in an out-of-hospital setting. pp. 1769–1770

There are various medical devices designed to support patients with urinary tract dysfunction. External devices, such as Texas catheters or condom catheters, attach to the male external genitalia to collect urine. Because these devices are not inserted into the urethra, they reduce the risk of infection. However, they do not collect urine in a sterile manner, nor are they adequate for long-term use.

Internal catheters, such as Foley or indwelling catheters, are the most commonly used devices for urinary tract dysfunction. They are long catheters with a balloon tip that is inserted through the urethra into the urinary bladder. The balloon is then inflated with saline to keep the device in place. Internal catheters are well tolerated for long-term use and are frequently found in hospitals, skilled nursing facilities, or home care situations.

Suprapubic catheters are similar in purpose to internal catheters. However, they are inserted directly through the abdominal wall into the urinary bladder. Suprapubic catheters may be used instead of indwelling catheters in the event of surgery or other problems with the genitalia or bladder.

In nearly all cases, insertion of urinary catheters is performed in a medical setting.

13. Identify failure of GI/GU, ventilatory, vascular access, and drain devices found in the home care setting. pp. 1761–1772

See appropriate portions of points listed in objective 11.

14. Discuss the relationship between local home care treatment protocols/SOPs and local EMS protocols/SOPs. p. 1752

In responding to a call involving a home care patient, remember that you may not be the first person to provide intervention. If home care patients have a good relationship with their home health care practitioner or physician, they may contact this person first. In fact, they may be required to do so in order to receive reimbursement for medical services. As a result, be sure to ask whether a patient has called another health care professional. If so, find out what instructions or medications have been issued. Also inquire about written orders from the physician or the physician-approved health care plan. Health care agencies resubmit these plans to physicians at least every 62 days. So check the date to see when the plan was last revised.

If the call involved a hospice patient, the situation will almost always require intervention by specially trained health care professionals. Find out the names of these people as quickly as possible and determine the advisability of consultations versus rapid transport.

15. Discuss differences in the ability of individuals to accept and cope with their own impending death. p. 1776

Each patient deals with his or her impending death in a different manner. Some can come to grips with it, while others refuse to believe they are going to die. Remember that while hospice prepares patients for their death, patients without hospice may be ill-prepared for the end stages of life. Don't assume that all terminally ill patients are under hospice care. A simple question to determine the presence of hospice may alter your course of treatment and approach to the patient.

16. List the stages of the grief process and relate them to an individual in hospice care. p. 1776

Regardless of whether a patient is in hospice or not, keep in mind the stages of the grief process—denial, anger, depression, bargaining, and acceptance. Remember that both the patient and the family will go through these stages, and, in the case of the terminally ill, the patient may have reached acceptance well ahead of those who will remain behind.

17. Discuss the rights of the terminally ill patient. pp. 1774–1776

In treating a terminally ill patient, you need to establish communication with the home care worker as quickly as possible. Your inclination may be to intubate, start a line, or administer medications. However, palliative care supersedes curative care. A hospice worker, when faced with the end stage of a disease, may do nothing in accordance with the patient's wishes, whether those wishes are expressed through a family member or a written document. If you are called to the house, it is your responsibility to respect the wishes of the patient and the ideas of hospice care.

18. Summarize the types of home health care available in your area and the services provided. pp. 1747–1753

There is a wide variety of home health care services provided in every community, ranging from professional home care agencies to unpaid volunteers. Find out what services operate in your area, using sources such as local hospitals (which arrange referrals) or county health departments (which certify and/or regulate many agencies).

19. Given a series of home care scenarios, determine which patients should receive follow-up home care and which should be transported to an emergency care facility. pp. 1753–1757

During your classroom, clinical, and field training, you will assess real and simulated patients and decide which patients should be transported to the hospital and which should receive additional care in the out-of-hospital setting. Use the information in this text chapter, the information on chronic home care patients presented by your instructors, and the guidance given by your clinical and field preceptors to develop good assessment and decision-making skills in regard to patient transport. Continue to refine these skills once your training ends and you begin your career as a paramedic.

20. Given a series of scenarios, demonstrate interaction and support with the family members/support persons for a patient who has died. pp. 1774–1776

Approaching the family members/support persons left behind after a patient has died is never easy, even if they have had the help of hospice. As noted in the text, many times the terminally ill patients are more prepared for their impending death than their family or caregivers. However, they, too, must go through the stages of grieving—denial, anger, depression, bargaining, and acceptance. Use practice scenarios to draw upon the information in this text chapter and suggestions presented by your instructors and clinical and field preceptors to develop the communication skills needed to manage this difficult situation. Continue to refine these skills once your training ends and you begin your career as a paramedic. Also find out about stress management programs provided by your agency so that you can get support after such a call has ended.

Content Self-Evaluation

MULTIPLE CHOICE

_____ 1. All of the following factors have promoted the growth of home care in recent years EXCEPT:
   A. enactment of Medicare.
   B. the advent of HMOs.
   C. an increase in malpractice lawsuits.
   D. changes in the attitudes of doctors and patients toward hospital care.
   E. improved medical technology.

_____ 2. As patients assume greater responsibility for their own treatment and recovery, the likelihood of ALS intervention for the chronic-care patient increases.
   A. True
   B. False

_____ 3. Common reasons for ALS intervention in the treatment of a home care patient include all of the following EXCEPT:
   A. inability to operate a device.
   B. absence of a caregiver.
   C. equipment failure.
   D. need for transport.
   E. pain management.

_____ 4. Home care providers can be of great assistance to EMS crews because they:
   A. have more experience in the field of prehospital medicine.
   B. will often spot subtle changes in the patient's condition.
   C. will easily grasp technical medical language.
   D. have legal authority to speak for the patient.
   E. both C and D

_____ 5. A home care patient is less likely to decompensate and will go into crisis less quickly than the general population.
   A. True
   B. False

_____ 6. Common causes of cardiac decompensation—a true medical emergency leading to shock—include all of the following EXCEPT:
   A. acute myocardial infarction.
   B. stroke.
   C. cardiac hypertrophy.
   D. sepsis.
   E. heart transplant.

_____ 7. One reason that diabetics get gangrene is due to slowed circulation to the extremities.
   A. True
   B. False

_____ 8. Signs and symptoms of sepsis in a patient with an indwelling device can include:
   A. cyanosis at the infection site.
   B. fever.
   C. increased urination.
   D. cool skin at the insertion site.
   E. all of the above

_____ 9. Home interventions such as peritoneal dialysis can alter electrolytes.
   A. True
   B. False

_____ 10. The ability of the skin to return to normal appearance after being subjected to pressure is called:
   A. capillary refill.
   B. tenting.
   C. turgor.
   D. diaphoresis.
   E. hypertrophy.

©2007 Pearson Education, Inc.
Essentials of Paramedic Care, 2nd ed.

_____ 11. Conditions that may be treated in a home care setting include:
   A. brain or spinal trauma.
   B. arthritis.
   C. AIDS.
   D. both B and C
   E. all of the above

_____ 12. Examples of commonly used medical devices in the home care setting includes all of the following EXCEPT:
   A. glucometers.
   B. tracheostomies.
   C. apnea monitors.
   D. home ventilators.
   E. dialysis units.

_____ 13. The matrix for injury prevention developed by William Haddon includes all of the following steps EXCEPT:
   A. prevent the creation of the hazard in the first place.
   B. counter the damage done by the hazard.
   C. increase the release of an already existing hazard.
   D. modify the basic qualities of the hazard.
   E. separate the hazard and that which is to be protected by a barrier.

_____ 14. It is a serious mistake to arrive on the scene with a "take-over" mentality that all but eliminates the home care provider.
   A. True
   B. False

_____ 15. In responding to any home care situation, you should remember that:
   A. any bed-bound patient may have pressure sores.
   B. hospital beds, wheelchairs, or walkers may be contaminated by body fluid.
   C. medical wastes may not be properly contained.
   D. sharps may be present.
   E. all of the above

_____ 16. In assessing home care patients, the focus of your physical exam should be on the patient's chronic condition.
   A. True
   B. False

_____ 17. Of the following acute home care situations, the one LEAST commonly encountered by paramedics is:
   A. respiratory disorders.
   B. end stages of a hospice patient.
   C. cardiac problems.
   D. GI/GU disorders.
   E. use of vascular access devices.

_____ 18. When providing intervention to home care patients with chronic respiratory diseases, remember that they usually have a low dosing regimen, which may make them more responsive to their medications.
   A. True
   B. False

_____ 19. In treating home care patients with cystic fibrosis (CF), the patient will probably be:
   A. over age 65.
   B. between 40 and 60 years old.
   C. of almost any age.
   D. under age 40.
   E. an infant.

_____ 20. Which of the following is an advantage of oxygen therapy for the home care patient?
   A. It is relatively easy to manage.
   B. Most patients tolerate it easily.
   C. Oxygen therapy adds to the quality of life.
   D. Oxygen prevents hypoxic states.
   E. all of the above

_____ 21. If a buzzer goes off on an oxygen concentrator, you would mostly likely suspect:
   A. faulty tubing.
   B. a leak in the tank.
   C. a dirty or plugged humidifier.
   D. power failure.
   E. either A or C

_____ 22. Routine care of a tracheostomy includes all of the following EXCEPT:
   A. keeping the stoma clean and dry.
   B. removing the device daily.
   C. frequent suctioning.
   D. changing the ventilator hose routinely.
   E. periodically changing/cleaning of the inner cannula.

_____ 23. Which of the following ventilatory options are you LEAST likely to find in a home care setting?
   A. PEEP
   B. CPAP
   C. BIPAP
   D. poncho-wrap
   E. both A and C

_____ 24. Patients with VADs will be much more prone to bleeding disorders than the general population.
   A. True
   B. False

_____ 25. The most common complication found in patients with VADs results from:
   A. an embolus.
   B. dehydration.
   C. a thrombus.
   D. hypertension.
   E. both A and C

_____ 26. The most commonly used device for urinary tract dysfunction is a(n):
   A. Texas catheter.
   B. urostomy.
   C. Foley catheter.
   D. suprapubic catheter.
   E. condom catheter.

_____ 27. The most common complications related to urinary tract support devices result from:
   A. obstructions.
   B. device malfunctions.
   C. infections.
   D. misplacement of devices.
   E. both B and C

_____ 28. If you have any doubts about the placement of a nasogastric feeding tube, your first step should be to:
   A. listen for air movement within the stomach.
   B. use a 60 mL syringe to insert air into the stomach.
   C. have the patient speak to you.
   D. irrigate the tube with water.
   E. immediately remove the tube.

_____ 29. In terms of providing care, the goal of hospices closely resembles the goal of EMS services.
   A. True
   B. False

_____ 30. The stages in the grief process for both the patient and those left behind are:
   A. depression, bargaining, guilt, anger, acceptance.
   B. anger, denial, bargaining, guilt, acceptance.
   C. denial, bargaining, anger, acceptance, guilt.
   D. bargaining, denial, anger, guilt, acceptance.
   E. denial, anger, depression, bargaining, acceptance.

MATCHING

Write the letter of the term in the space provided next to the appropriate description.

A. hypertrophy
B. hemoptysis
C. exocrine
D. demylenation
E. emesis
F. cellulitis
G. gangrene
H. turgor
I. cor pulmonale
J. sensorium

_____ 31. destruction or removal of the myelin sheath of nerve tissue; found in Guillain-Barré syndrome

_____ 32. death of tissue or bone, usually from an insufficient blood supply

_____ 33. disorder involving external secretions

_____ 34. an increase in the size of an organ or structure caused by growth rather than by tumor

_____ 35. ability of the skin to return to normal appearance after being subjected to pressure

_____ 36. sensory apparatus of the body as a whole; also that portion of the brain that functions as a center of sensations

_____ 37. inflammation of cellular or connective tissue

_____ 38. expectoration of blood arising from the oral cavity, larynx, trachea, bronchi, or lungs

_____ 39. vomitus

_____ 40. congestive heart failure secondary to pulmonary hypertension

SHORT ANSWER

Write out the terms that each of the following abbreviations/acronyms stands for in the space provided.

41. PEEP _____

42. CPAP _____

43. BIPAP _____

44. COPD _____

45. ARDS _____

46. PPV _____

47. VAD _____

_____

48. PICC _____

_____

49. DNAR _____

_____

50. CHF _____

_____

Chapter 47: Assessment-Based Management

Review of Chapter Objectives

After reading this chapter, you should be able to:

1. Explain how effective assessment is critical to clinical decision making. pp. 1779–1781

Assessment forms the foundation for patient care. You can't treat or report a problem that is not found or identified. To find a problem, you must gather, evaluate, and synthesize information. Based on this process, you can then make a decision and take the appropriate actions to formulate a management plan and determine the priorities for patient care.

A paramedic is entrusted with a great deal of independent judgment and responsibility for performing correct actions for each individual patient, including such advanced skills as ECG interpretation, rapid sequence intubation, and medication administration. Additionally, the medical director and hospital staff must rely on your experience and expertise as you describe the patient's condition and your conclusions about it. Consequently, the ability to reason and to reach a field diagnosis is critical to paramedic practice.

2. Explain how the paramedic's attitude and uncooperative patients affect assessment and decision making. pp. 1781–1782

Attitude
Your attitude is one of the most critical factors in performing an effective assessment. You must be as nonjudgmental as possible to avoid "short-circuiting" accurate data collection and pattern recognition by leaping to conclusions before completing a thorough assessment. Remember the popular computer mnemonic GIGO—garbage in/garbage out. You can't reach valid conclusions about your patient based on hasty or incomplete assessment. Seek to identify any preconceived notions that you may have about a group and then work to eliminate them.

Uncooperative patients
Admittedly, uncooperative patients make it difficult to perform good assessments. However, you must remember that there are many possible causes for patient belligerence. Whenever you assess an uncooperative or a restless patient, consider medical causes for the behavior—hypoxia, hypovolemia, hypoglycemia, or a head injury. Be careful not to jump to the conclusion that the patient is "just another drunk" or a "frequent flyer." The frequent flyer that you have transported for alcoholic behavior in the past may, this time, be suffering from trauma or a medical emergency.

In addition, cultural and ethnic barriers—as well as prior negative experiences—may cause a patient to lack confidence in the rescuers. Such situations make it difficult for you to be effective at the scene, and the patient in fact may refuse to provide express consent for treatment or transport. However, it is your job to increase patient confidence. Become familiar with the cultural customs of any large ethnic populations in your area. Find out about available translation services. Above all, don't permit yourself to make snap judgments about the patient.

3. **Explain strategies to prevent labeling, tunnel vision, and decrease environmental distractions.** pp. 1780–1784

    A number of factors—both internal (for example, your personal attitudes) and external (for example, the patient's attitude, distracting injuries, or environmental factors at the scene)—can affect your assessment of the patient and ultimately your decisions on how to manage treatment.

    Labeling and tunnel vision
    The dangers of labeling have been discussed in objective 2. However, another internal factor that can negatively affect your assessment is tunnel vision. Do not focus on distracting injuries, such as a scalp laceration, that look worse than they really are. Instead, resist the temptation to form a field diagnosis too early. Always take a systematic approach to patient assessment to avoid distractions and to find and prioritize care for all of the patient's injuries and conditions. In general, follow an inverted pyramid format that progresses from a differential diagnosis to a narrowing process to your field diagnosis. (For more information on the inverted pyramid format, see the diagram on page 1779 of your textbook.)

    Environmental distractions
    You've probably already experienced some of the environmental factors that can affect patient assessment and care—scene chaos, violent or dangerous situations, high noise levels, crowds of bystanders, or even crowds of responders. Limit these distractions through the careful staging of personnel (see objectives 4 and 5). In the case of a large number of rescuers, you might assign crowd control tasks to some of them or stage them nearby. They can then be brought to the scene when and if necessary. Finally, you might change environments completely. Sometimes the best way to deal with excessive environmental noise and distractions is to rapidly load the patient into the ambulance and leave the scene. You can always pull over for further assessment in a quieter environment.

4. **Describe how personnel considerations and staffing configurations affect assessment and decision making.** pp. 1782–1784

    As a rule, assessment is best achieved by one rescuer. A single paramedic can gather information and provide treatment sequentially. In the case of two paramedics, one paramedic can assess the patient, while the other provides simultaneous treatment. With multiple responders, however, assessment and history may take place entirely by "committee," which often leads to disorganized management. It can also be difficult to manage a patient if the responders are all at the same professional level and have no clear direction. Therefore, it is important to plan for these events so that personnel can have predesignated roles. These roles may be rotated among team members so no one is left out, but there must be a plan to avoid "freelancing." If there is only one paramedic, then that person must assume all ALS roles.

5. **Synthesize and apply concepts of scene management and choreography to simulated emergency calls.** pp. 1783–1784

    Points in the textbook and direction by your instructors and clinical or field preceptors will help you to manage and choreograph simulated emergency calls. When approaching these practice sessions, remember the importance of an effective preplan. In the case of a two-person team, the roles of team care leader and patient care provider can be assigned on an alternating basis. Paramedics who work together regularly may develop their own plan, but a universally understood plan allows for other rescuers to participate in a rescue without interrupting the flow. While the dynamics of field situations may necessitate changes in plans, a general "game plan" can go a long way toward preventing chaos. If field dynamics dictate a change in the preplanned roles, you are still working from a solid base.

6. Explain the roles of the team leader and the patient care person. pp. 1783–1784

In setting up a two-person team, keep in mind the general tasks performed by the team leader and patient care provider as outlined below.

Roles of Team Leader	*Roles of Patient Care Provider*
Establishes patient contact	Provides "scene cover"
Obtains history	Gathers scene information
Performs physical exam	Talks to relatives/bystanders
Presents patient	Obtains vital signs
Handles documentation	Performs interventions
Acts as EMS commander	Acts as triage group leader

7. List and explain the rationale for bringing the essential care items to the patient. pp. 1784–1785

Having the right equipment at the patient's side is essential. As a paramedic, you must be prepared to manage many conditions and injuries or changes in the patient's condition. Assessment and management must usually be done simultaneously. If you do not have the right equipment readily available, then you have compromised patient care and, in fact, the patient may die.

8. When given a simulated call, list the appropriate equipment to be taken to the patient. pp. 1784–1785

Think of your equipment as items in a backpack. Just like backpacking, you must downsize your equipment to minimum weight and bulk to facilitate rapid movement. At the same time, you need certain essential items to ensure survival—in this case, patient survival. The following is a list of the essential equipment for paramedic management of life-threatening conditions. You must bring these items to the side of every patient, regardless of what you initially think you may need.

- Infection Control
    —Infection control supplies—e.g., gloves, eye shields
- Airway Control
    —Oral airways
    —Nasal airways
    —Suction (electric or manual)
    —Rigid tonsil-tip and flexible suction catheters
    —Laryngoscope and blades
    —Endotracheal tubes, stylettes, syringes, tape
- Breathing
    —Pocket mask
    —Manual ventilation bag-valve mask
    —Spare masks in various sizes
    —Oxygen masks, cannulas, and extension tubing
    —Occlusive dressings
    —Large-bore IV catheter for thoracic decompression
- Circulation
    —Dressings
    —Bandages and tape
    —Sphygmomanometer, stethoscope
    —Note pad and pen or pencil
- Disability
    —Rigid collars
    —Flashlights
- Dysrhythmia
    —Cardiac monitor/defibrillator
- Exposure and Protection
    —Scissors
    —Space blankets or something to cover the patient

You may also pack some optional "take-in" equipment, such as drug therapy and venous access supplies. The method by which these supplies are carried may depend upon how your system is designed—e.g., paramedic ambulances versus paramedics in nontransporting vehicles. It may also depend upon local protocols, flexibility of standing orders, the number of paramedic responders in your area, and the difficulty of accessing patients because of terrain or some other problem.

9. **Explain the general approach to the emergency patient.** pp. 1785–1788

In addition to having the right equipment, you need to have the essential demeanor to calm or reassure the patient. You must look and act the professional, while exhibiting the compassion and understanding associated with an effective "bedside manner." While patients may not have the ability to rate your medical performance, they can certainly rate your people skills and service. Be aware of your body language and the messages it sends, either intentionally or unintentionally. Think carefully about what you say and how you say it—this includes your conversations with other members of the ALS team and anyone else on the scene.

Once again, it helps to preplan your general approach to the patient. This will prevent confusion and improve the accuracy of your assessment. One team member should engage in an active, concerned dialogue with the patient. This same person should also demonstrate the listening skills needed to collect information and to convey a caring attitude. Taking notes may prevent asking the same question repeatedly as well as ensuring that you acquire and pass on accurate data.

10. **Explain the general approach, patient assessment differentials, and management priorities for patients with various types of emergencies that may be experienced in prehospital care.** pp. 1779–1788

Scene Size-Up
Before approaching the patient (see objective 9), you must carefully size up the scene. The scene size-up has the following components: body substance isolation, ensuring scene safety, locating all patients, and identifying the mechanism of injury or the nature of the illness.

Initial Assessment
After you size up the scene, you quickly begin the initial assessment for the purpose of detecting and treating immediate life threats. The components of the initial assessment are:

- Forming a general impression
- Determining mental status (AVPU)
- Assessing airway, breathing, and circulation
- Determining the patient's priority for further on-scene care or immediate transport

Depending upon your findings during initial assessment, you might take either the contemplative or the resuscitative approach to patient care. You might also decide to immediately transport the patient.

Contemplative approach. In general, use the contemplative approach when immediate intervention is not necessary. In such situations, the focused history and physical exam, followed by any required interventions can be performed at the scene, before transport to the hospital.
Resuscitative approach. Use the resuscitative approach whenever you suspect a life-threatening problem, including:

- Cardiac or respiratory arrest
- Respiratory distress or failure
- Unstable dysrhythmias
- Status epilepticus
- Coma or altered mental status
- Shock or hypotension
- Major trauma
- Possible C-spine injury

In these cases, you must take immediate resuscitative action (such as CPR, defibrillation, or ventilation) or other critical action (such as supplemental oxygen, control of major bleeding, or C-spine immobilization). Additional assessment and care can be performed after resuscitation and the rapid trauma assessment and/or en route to the hospital.

Immediate evacuation. In some cases, you will need to immediately evacuate the patient to the ambulance. For example, a patient with severe internal bleeding requires life-saving interventions beyond a paramedic's skills. You might also resort to immediate evacuation if the scene is too chaotic for rational assessment or if it is too unsafe or unstable.

Focused History and Physical Exam

Following the initial assessment, you will perform the focused history and physical exam. Based on the patient's chief complaint and the information gathered during the initial assessment, you should consider your patient to belong to one of the following four categories:

- Trauma patient with a significant mechanism of injury or altered mental status
- Trauma patient with an isolated injury
- Medical patient who is unresponsive
- Medical patient who is responsive

For a trauma patient with a significant MOI or altered mental status or for an unresponsive medical patient, perform a complete head-to-toe physical examination (rapid trauma assessment for the trauma patient, rapid medical assessment for the medical patient). For a trauma patient with an isolated injury or for a responsive medical patient, perform a physical exam focused on body systems related to the chief complaint.

Ongoing Assessment and Detailed Physical Exam

The ongoing assessment must be performed on all patients to monitor and to observe trends in the person's condition—every 5 minutes if the patient is unstable, every 15 minutes if the patient is stable. Ongoing assessments must be performed until the patient is transferred to the care of hospital personnel. The ongoing assessment includes evaluation of the following:

- Mental status
- Airway, breathing, and circulation
- Transport priorities
- Vital signs
- Focused assessment of any problem areas or conditions
- Effectiveness of interventions
- Management plans

The detailed physical exam is similar to but more thorough than the rapid trauma assessment. It is generally performed only on trauma patients and only if time and the patient's condition permit.

Identification of Life-Threatening Problems

At all stages of the assessment, from initial assessment through ongoing assessments, from the scene—to the ambulance—to arrival at the hospital, you must actively and continuously look for and manage any life-threatening problems. Basically your role as a paramedic is to rapidly and accurately assess the patient and then to treat for the worst-case scenario. This is the underlying principle of assessment-based management—your guide to providing effective medical care.

11. Describe how to effectively communicate patient information face to face, over the telephone, by radio, and in writing. pp. 1788–1790

The ability to communicate effectively is the key to transferring patient information, whether in an out-of-hospital setting or within the hospital itself. Although neither basic nor advanced life-support interventions may be required for every patient, a skill that will be used on every single patient is that of presentation, whether it is over the radio or telephone, in writing, or in face-to-face transfers at the receiving facility.

Effective presentation and communication skills help establish a paramedic's credibility. They also inspire trust and confidence in patients. If you present your assessment, your findings, and your treatment in a clear, concise manner, you give the impression of a job well done. A poor presentation, on the other hand, implies poor assessment and poor patient care.

The most effective oral presentations usually meet these guidelines:

- Last less than one minute
- Are very concise and clear
- Avoid excessive use of medical jargon
- Follow a basic format, usually the SOAP format or some variation
- Include both pertinent findings and pertinent negatives
- Conclude with specific actions, requests, or questions related to the plan

An ideal presentation should include the following:

- Patient identification, age, sex, and degree of distress
- Chief complaint
- Present illness/injury
  —Pertinent details about the present problem
  —Pertinent negatives
- Past medical history
  —Allergies
  —Medications
  —Pertinent medical history
- Physical signs
  —Vital signs
  —Pertinent positive findings
  —Pertinent negative findings
- Assessment
  —Paramedic impression
- Plan
  —What has been done
  —Orders requested

12. Given various preprogrammed and moulaged patients, provide the appropriate scene size-up, initial assessment, focused assessment, and detailed assessment, then provide the appropriate care, ongoing assessments, and patient transport. pp. 1779–1791

In order to develop as an entry-level practitioner at the paramedic level, it is important to participate in scenario-based reviews of commonly encountered complaints. Laboratory-based simulations require you to assess a preprogrammed patient or mannequin. Use the information presented in the textbook, the information on assessment-based management provided by your instructors, and the guidance given by your clinical and field preceptors to develop good assessment-based management skills. Remember—the chance to practice does not stop at the classroom. While a paramedic student or the new member of a team, take advantage of every opportunity to practice your new skills.

Content Self-Evaluation

MULTIPLE CHOICE

____ 1. Which of the following gives the correct order of steps in the clinical decision making of the inverted pyramid?
   A. field diagnosis, differential diagnosis, narrowing process
   B. differential diagnosis, narrowing process, field diagnosis
   C. narrowing process, field diagnosis, differential diagnosis
   D. differential diagnosis, field diagnosis, narrowing process
   E. field diagnosis, narrowing process, differential diagnosis

____ 2. The foundation of patient care is:
   A. the detailed physical exam.
   B. BLS protocols.
   C. assessment.
   D. medication administration.
   E. ALS protocols.

____ 3. In a medical patient, the physical exam takes precedence over the history.
   A. True
   B. False

____ 4. All of the following are examples of external factors that can affect assessment EXCEPT:
   A. the attitude of family members.
   B. an uncooperative patient.
   C. distracting injuries.
   D. scene chaos.
   E. personal attitudes.

____ 5. Protocols and standing orders do not replace:
   A. good history taking.
   B. a good attitude.
   C. good judgment.
   D. the team approach.
   E. both A and C.

____ 6. A paramedic can do something to correct or lessen obstacles to performing a good assessment such as reducing:
   A. tunnel vision.
   B. labeling.
   C. cultural and ethnic barriers.
   D. preconceived notions.
   E. all of the above

____ 7. You should treat a "frequent flyer" just like you would any other patient.
   A. True
   B. False

____ 8. A team leader's roles include all of the following EXCEPT:
   A. obtains a history.
   B. performs the physical exam.
   C. handles documentation.
   D. triages patients.
   E. performs a detailed exam.

____ 9. Roles of a patient care provider include:
   A. talking to bystanders.
   B. obtaining vital signs.
   C. gathering scene information.
   D. providing scene cover.
   E. all of the above

____ 10. Patient assessment is best performed by two paramedics rather than just one.
   A. True
   B. False

_____ 11. Which of the following is probably optional "take-in" equipment carried by paramedics?
   A. rigid collars
   B. infection control supplies
   C. drug therapy
   D. space blankets
   E. sphygmomanometer

_____ 12. Components of the initial assessment include all of the following EXCEPT:
   A. forming a general impression.
   B. assessing ABCs.
   C. assessing the scene.
   D. determining the patient's priority.
   E. assessing mental status.

_____ 13. A patient with severe internal bleeding is a candidate for:
   A. the resuscitative approach.
   B. the contemplative approach.
   C. immediate evacuation.
   D. detailed physical exam.
   E. both B and D

_____ 14. In critical patients, a detailed physical exam is more important than continuing ongoing assessments.
   A. True
   B. False

_____ 15. The most effective patient presentations will:
   A. use medical jargon.
   B. follow the SOAP format.
   C. be done in writing.
   D. last 5 to 10 minutes.
   E. exclude subjective findings.

Chapter 48 Operations

Part 1: Ambulance Operations

Review of Chapter Objectives

Because Chapter 48 is lengthy, it has been divided into five parts to aid your study. Read the assigned text pages, then progress through the objectives and self-evaluation materials as you would with other chapters. When you feel secure in your grasp of the content, proceed to the next part.

After reading Part 1 of this chapter, you should be able to:

1. Identify current local and state standards that influence ambulance design, equipment requirements, and staffing of ambulances. pp. 1798–1800

Various standards, as well as administrative rules and regulations, influence the design of ambulances and the medical equipment carried on each unit. Similar guidelines determine staffing levels and deployment of EMS agencies.

Because the oversight for EMS usually falls to state governments, many of the requirements for ambulance services are written in state statutes or regulations. However, national standards and trends do have an influence on the development of these laws. Typically, state laws are broad, while corresponding regulations provide more specific guidelines or rules. For example, a public health law may authorize the state department of health to issue regulations through its EMS bureau. These regulations, known as the "state EMS code," might then handle such matters as the essential equipment to be carried on every ambulance.

In most cases, government standards tend to be generic enough so that they are "palatable," affordable, and politically feasible to all EMS agencies in the state. State standards usually set minimum standards, rather than the "gold standard," for operation. In other words, they establish the lowest level at which units will be allowed to operate. When local and/or regional EMS systems get involved in regulation, their lists tend to be much more detailed and often approach a gold standard, which is the goal when ample resources are provided.

2. Discuss the importance of completing an ambulance equipment/supply checklist. pp. 1800–1801

Routine, detailed shift checks of the ambulance can minimize the issues associated with risk management. Many services, for example, hold a "stretcher day" once a week. By performing and documenting preventative maintenance on stretchers, it is less likely that a faulty stretcher will cause a patient to be dropped or EMS personnel to injure their backs. Medications carried on the paramedic unit expire. Therefore, expiration dates should be checked each shift, and the older unexpired drugs marked appropriately so that they will be used first. In services that utilize scheduled medications such as narcotics, the paramedics should sign for these medications at the beginning and at the end of each shift. In addition, the vehicle itself should be regularly checked so that it is always in safe working order.

3. **Discuss factors used to determine ambulance stationing and staffing within a community.** pp. 1801–1802

   Deployment

   The strategy used by an EMS agency to maneuver its ambulances and crews in order to reduce response times is referred to as deployment. Deployment is based upon a number of factors—location of the facilities to house ambulances, location of hospitals, anticipated volume of calls, and the specific geographic and traffic congestion in your area.

   The ideal deployment decisions must take into account two sets of data—past community responses and projected demographic changes. The highest volume of calls, or peak load, should be described both in terms of the day of the week and the time of day.

   In communities that do not have multiple strategically located stations, services often deploy ambulances to wait for calls at specific high-volume locations. Such stationing locations are known as primary areas of responsibility (PAR).

   Some technologically sophisticated systems use computers to assist the dispatch center in relocating ambulances. Vehicle tracking systems tell the computer exactly where each ambulance is located at a given time.

   Operational staffing

   In general, ambulance staffing should take into account the peak load of the system. Some services vary shift times to ensure ample coverage for the busiest days of the week and the busiest times of day. Services should also take into account the need for reserve capacity—the ability to muster additional crews when all ambulances are on call or when a system's resources are taxed by a multiple casualty incident. Some services fulfill this need by asking off-duty personnel to carry pagers or to volunteer for backup.

   Whatever plan is adopted, each system must consider how they will deal with assigning paramedics. Clearly, an ambulance with two paramedics onboard is limited in the amount of care these two highly trained personnel can provide if they are the only available responders to cardiac arrests (meaning no backup for simultaneous additional emergencies). As a result, some communities prefer to combine an EMT-Intermediate with a paramedic to make an ALS unit. Other communities, such as New York City, specify that an ALS unit must have two paramedics so that they can back each other up in making scene decisions.

   Finally, each service needs to determine standards for ambulance operators and for driving the vehicle itself. As a rule, these standards are usually spelled out at the local service level.

4. **Describe the advantages and disadvantages of air medical transport, and identify conditions/situations in which air medical transport should be considered.** pp. 1806–1809

   Advantages of air medical transport

   - Rapid transport in situations where the time required for ground transport poses a threat to the patient's survival or recovery
   - Access to rural or remote areas
   - Access to specialty units—e.g., neonatal intensive care units, replantation units, transplant centers, burn centers, and so on
   - Access to personnel with specialized skills—e.g., surgical airway, thoracotomy, rapid sequence intubation, critical care, and more
   - Access to special supplies—e.g., aortic balloon pumps

   Disadvantages of air medical transport

   - Weather and environmental restrictions to flying
   - Altitude limitations
   - Air speed limitations

- Cabin sizes that sometimes restrict the number of crew members, the amount of onboard equipment, stretcher configuration, and the procedures that can be performed
- Lack of normal temperature control, especially in helicopters with their thin-walled fuselages
- Limited lighting (to prevent glare from entering the pilot's compartment)
- High cost of equipment, maintenance, and downtime, which puts air medical transport (especially helicopters) beyond the reach of some communities

Indications for air medical transport

- Clinical criteria
  - Trauma score < 12
  - Glasgow Coma Scale < 10
  - Penetrating trauma to abdomen, pelvis, chest, neck, or head
  - Spinal cord or spinal column injury or an injury producing paralysis or lateralizing signs
  - Partial or total amputation of an extremity (excluding digits)
  - Two or more long-bone fractures or pelvis fracture
  - Crush injury to abdomen, chest, or head
  - Major burns or burns to face, hands, feet, or perineum; burns with respiratory involvement; electrical or chemical burns
  - Patients in a serious traumatic event who are < 12 or > 55 years of age
  - Patients with near-drowning injuries
  - Adult patients with:
    - Systolic BP < 90 mmHg
    - Respiratory rate < 10 or > 35 per minute
    - Heart rate < 60 or > 120 beats per minute
    - Unresponsive to verbal stimuli
- Mechanism of injury
  - Vehicle rollover with unbelted passengers
  - Vehicle striking pedestrian > 20 mph
  - Falls > 10 feet
  - Motorcycle victim ejected at > 20 mph
  - Multiple victims
- Difficult access situations
  - Wilderness rescue
  - Ambulance egress or access impeded by road conditions, weather, or traffic
- Time/distance factors
  - Transport to trauma center > 15 minutes by ground ambulance
  - Transport time to local hospital by ground ambulance greater than transport time to trauma center by helicopter
  - Patient extrication time > 20 minutes
  - Utilization of local ground ambulance results in absence of ground ambulance coverage for local community

Content Self-Evaluation

MULTIPLE CHOICE

1. What type of ambulance standards are usually set by states?
   A. minimum standards
   B. maximum standards
   C. gold standards
   D. essential-equipment standards
   E. DOT KKK standards

_____ 2. A conventional truck cab-chassis with a modular ambulance body is a _____ ambulance design.
   A. Type I
   B. Type II
   C. Type III
   D. medium-duty
   E. heavy-duty

_____ 3. A specialty van with a forward control integral cab-body is a _____ ambulance design.
   A. Type I
   B. Type II
   C. Type III
   D. medium-duty
   E. heavy-duty

_____ 4. Which of the following agencies or organizations influence ambulance standards?
   A. Department of Transportation (DOT)
   B. National Flight Nurses Association (NFNA)
   C. National Flight Paramedics Association (NFPA)
   D. Federal Communications Commission (FCC)
   E. all of the above

_____ 5. The agency that has helped ensure equipment lists calling for disinfecting agents, sharps containers, and other protective items onboard ambulances is:
   A. NIOSH.
   B. NFPA.
   C. OSHA.
   D. CDC.
   E. NFPA.

_____ 6. The agency that provides a "gold standard" for the EMS community to follow, including a list of "essential equipment" to be carried on ambulances, is:
   A. ACS.
   B. CAAS.
   C. NFPA.
   D. NIOSH.
   E. OSHA.

_____ 7. The expiration dates on medications carried on the paramedic unit should be checked:
   A. once a day.
   B. once a week.
   C. at the start of every shift.
   D. at the start of every month.
   E. every other day.

_____ 8. An EMS agency uses deployment based on all of the following factors EXCEPT:
   A. anticipated call volume.
   B. local geographic and traffic conditions.
   C. location of hospitals.
   D. projected ethnic makeup of the population.
   E. location of facilities to house ambulances.

_____ 9. A deployment strategy that uses a computerized personnel and ambulance deployment system is known as:
   A. a peak load system.
   B. a primary area of responsibility.
   C. system status management.
   D. primary deploy management.
   E. none of the above

_____ 10. A system that allows multiple vehicles to arrive at an EMS call at different times is called a _____ system.
   A. multiple response
   B. tiered response
   C. primary response
   D. reserve capacity
   E. peak load

_____ 11. Almost all communities in the United States require two paramedics aboard an ALS unit.
   A. True
   B. False

_____ 12. According to one study, the majority of ambulance collisions occur:
   A. in patients' driveways.
   B. at intersections.
   C. backing into ambulance bays.
   D. at night.
   E. during inclement weather.

_____ 13. A legal term found in the motor vehicle laws of most states that sets up a higher standard for the operators of emergency vehicles is called:
   A. *res ispa loquitur*.
   B. exempt rights.
   C. emergency power.
   D. due regard.
   E. special status.

_____ 14. State laws typically exempt ambulance drivers who are operating in an emergency from all of the following traffic situations EXCEPT:
   A. posted speed limits.
   B. crossing railroad tracks with the gates down.
   C. posted directions of travel.
   D. parking regulations.
   E. requirements to wait for red lights.

_____ 15. Nowhere in the motor vehicle laws are drivers other than emergency vehicle operators held accountable for the safety of all other motorists.
   A. True
   B. False

_____ 16. Which of the following is NOT true about the use of lights and sirens?
   A. Motorists are less inclined to yield to an ambulance when the siren is continually sounded.
   B. Many motorists feel that the right-of-way privileges given to ambulances are abused when sirens are sounded.
   C. Inexperienced motorists tend to decrease their driving speed by 10 to 15 miles per hour when a siren is sounded.
   D. The continuous sound of a siren can possibly worsen the condition of patients by increasing their anxiety.
   E. Ambulance drivers may develop anxiety from using sirens on long runs.

_____ 17. Why do most EMS agencies no longer suggest the use of a police escort for ambulances?
   A. Ambulances and police cars have different braking distances.
   B. Motorists are often confused by escorts going through intersections.
   C. Motorists often will not see the second vehicle and pull out in front of it.
   D. Ambulance drivers may have trouble keeping up with police cars.
   E. all of the above

_____ 18. When your ambulance is the first to arrive at the scene of a motor vehicle collision, you should park:
   A. behind the wreckage.
   B. in front of the wreckage.
   C. in a staging area.
   D. next to the wreckage on the side.
   E. across the road from the wreckage.

_____ 19. Always go around cars stopped at an intersection on their right (passenger's) side.
   A. True
   B. False

_____ 20. The type of air transport that you will most likely encounter as a paramedic is fixed-wing aircraft.
   A. True
   B. False

_____ 21. The use of helicopters for medical rescue grew out of their proven benefit during:
   A. the Vietnam War.
   B. Operation Desert Storm.
   C. the Korean War.
   D. World War II.
   E. both A and C

_____ 22. All of the following are advantages of air transport EXCEPT:
   A. cost efficiency.
   B. access to remote areas.
   C. access to specialty units.
   D. rapid transport when distance is a consideration.
   E. access to specialty supplies.

_____ 23. A number of local programs require physiological abnormalities in addition to MOI findings to activate air medical transport.
   A. True
   B. False

_____ 24. A piece of equipment that can be affected by pressure changes during a flight is a(n):
   A. IV bag.
   B. capnograph.
   C. PASG.
   D. mobile radio.
   E. both A and C

_____ 25. As a rule, a helicopter requires a landing zone of approximately:
   A. 100 by 100 feet.
   B. 100 by 100 yards.
   C. 75 by 75 yards.
   D. 75 by 75 feet.
   E. 15 large steps on each side.

MATCHING

Write the letter of the term in the space provided next to the appropriate description.

A. peak load
B. primary area of responsibility
C. tiered response system
D. deployment
E. demographic
F. gold standard
G. spotter
H. reportable collisions
I. minimum standard
J. reserve capacity

_____ 26. strategy used by an EMS agency to maneuver its ambulances and crews in an effort to reduce response times

_____ 27. ultimate standard of excellence

_____ 28. lowest or least allowable standards

_____ 29. the highest volume of calls at a given time

_____ 30. pertaining to population makeup or changes

_____ 31. stationing of ambulances at specific high-volume locations

_____ 32. allows multiple vehicles to arrive at an EMS call at different times, often providing different levels of care or transport

_____ 33. the ability of an EMS agency to respond to calls beyond those handled by the on-duty crews

_____ 34. collisions that involve over $1,000 in damage or a personal injury

_____ 35. the person behind the left rear side of the ambulance who assists the operator in backing up the vehicle

Part 2: Medical Incident Management

Review of Chapter Objectives

After reading Part 2 of this chapter, you should be able to:

1. Explain the need for the Incident Management System (IMS)/Incident Command System (ICS) in managing emergency medical services incidents. pp. 1809–1810

Traditional paramedic education focuses on the relationship between one or two patient care providers and a single patient. In this setting, a paramedic has the ability to concentrate on the assessment and treatment of the patient. Occasionally, however, paramedics are called upon to treat more than one patient at a time. The multipatient incident may result from a motor vehicle collision (MVC), an apartment fire, a gang fight, or any number of other scenarios.

Based on the need for overall scene and resource management recognized at a number of major fires and other large-scale incidents in the 1970s, the fire service took the lead in organizing responses to large-scale emergencies. The result was the beginning of the modern-day Incident Command System (ICS)—a management program designed for controlling, directing, and coordinating emergency response resources. In the time since the events of September 11, 2001, and the increased potential for large-scale terrorist incidents, the ICS continues to evolve into a comprehensive, standardized National Incident Management System (NIMS). NIMS is a national system used for the management of multiple-casualty incidents, involving assumption of responsibility for command and designation and coordination of such elements as triage, treatment, transport, and staging.

2. Describe the functional components (command, finance, logistics, operations, and planning) of the incident management system. pp. 1813–1814

To familiarize yourself with the components of the incident management system, use the mnemonic C-FLOP, which stands for the first letter in each of the following functions or roles:

- **Command**—individual or group responsible for coordinating all activities and who makes final decisions on the emergency scene; often referred to as the Incident Commander (IC).
- **Finance/administration**—section responsible for maintaining records for personnel, time, and costs of resources/procurement; reports directly to the IC; rarely operates on small-scale incidents.
- **Logistics**—section that supports incident operations, coordinating procurement and distribution of all medical and other resources.
- **Operations**—section that fulfills directions from command and does the action work at an incident.
- **Planning**—section that provides past, present, and future information about an incident; operates on the principle of "anything that can go wrong, will go wrong," thus ensuring the necessary strategic support.

3. Differentiate between singular and unified command and identify when each is most applicable. pp. 1813–1814

There are at least two different types of command: singular and unified command. To distinguish between these two types of command, keep these definitions in mind:

- **Singular command**—process where a single individual is responsible for coordinating an incident.
- **Unified command**—process in which managers from different jurisdictions—law enforcement agencies, fire, EMS—coordinate their activities and share responsibility for command.

At small incidents with limited jurisdictions, singular command usually works best. Such incidents have a smaller scope and usually do not involve outside agencies. In many incidents, however, a singular command will not be feasible because of overlapping responsibilities or jurisdictions. Instead, a unified command will be established. Examples of such incidents include terrorist attacks, explosions, sniper or hostage situations, and large-scale disasters. In each of these examples, the managers from several jurisdictions, law enforcement, fire, and EMS will coordinate their activities.

4. **Describe the role of command, the need for command transfer, and procedures for transferring it.**   pp. 1811–1816

    The most important functional area in the Incident Management System is command. The Incident Commander is the individual who essentially oversees and controls the incident. The ultimate authority for decision making rests with the Incident Commander. Most agencies have a chain of authority that defines the highest-ranking official at a scene. However, establishing command at a multiagency, multijurisdictional incident can be complicated. State or local agencies often decide the issue in such situations. Otherwise, the decision should be reached by a preexisting disaster plan.

    The criteria for determining when to establish command and when to declare an MCI varies from agency to agency. As a rule, the first arriving public safety unit usually establishes command. Sometimes this unit is an ambulance and then you and your partner will most likely fill the roles of Incident Commander and Triage Officer—until other units arrive. If, or when, higher-ranking officers do arrive, command will be transferred. However, a higher-ranking officer does not become IC simply by his or her arrival. Command is only transferred face-to-face, with the current Incident Commander conducting a short but complete briefing on the incident status.

5. **List and describe the functions of the following groups and leaders in the ICS as they pertain to EMS incidents:**

    The functions differ depending on which vest is being worn at an MCI. The following are examples of the sectors for which you, the paramedic, may be responsible for at the next MCI:

    a. **Safety**   pp. 1812, 1816–1817

    The Safety Officer may hold the most important role at an MCI. This person—or, in some cases, team of people—monitors all on-scene actions and ensures that they do not create any potentially harmful conditions.

    b. **Logistics**   p. 1818

    The logistics section supports incident operations. One of its most critical functions is overseeing the Medical Supply Unit. In general, logistics coordinates the procurement and distribution of equipment and supplies at an MCI or disaster.

    c. **Rehabilitation (rehab)**   p. 1826

    Medical personnel operating in the rehabilitation section assume responsibility for monitoring the well-being of rescuers. They assure food and water are available, rescuers take rest breaks, take vital signs, and watch for signs of fatigue or incident stress. A predetermined threshold should be established so that rescuers with abnormal vitals or signs of fatigue or stress are removed from operation. This is especially important during extremely hot or cold conditions.

    d. **Staging**   p. 1825

    The Staging Officer supervises the staging area—the location where ambulances, personnel, and equipment are kept in reserve—and guards against premature commitment of resources. The Staging Officer makes every effort to prevent "freelancing" by EMS personnel.

    e. **Treatment**   pp. 1824–1825

    When the number of patients exceeds the number of ambulances available for support, you will need to collect patients in a treatment sector comprised of a red treatment unit, a yellow treatment unit, and a green treatment unit. Each of these units is supervised by a Treatment Unit Leader, who reports to the Treatment Group Supervisor—the person who controls all actions in the Treatment Group Sector.

The unit leader's job requires extreme flexibility to ensure that patients receive adequate care. Patient conditions can change and responders, equipment, or supplies may not be available in the subarea. As a result, communications must be carefully coordinated. The Treatment Group Supervisor must be apprised of activities in each subarea. He or she must also help coordinate operations with other functional areas, particularly command, triage, and transport.

f. Triage pp. 1820–1824

Because triage will drive subsequent incident operations, it is one of the first functions performed at an MCI. As a result, all personnel should be trained in triage techniques and all response units should carry triage equipment. At small incidents, you or your partner may assume the role of triage. Larger incidents may require a Triage Group Supervisor, who may either act independently or supervise the Triage Group or Sector.

g. Transportation pp. 1825–1826

The Transportation Unit Supervisor coordinates operations with the Staging Officer and the Treatment Supervisor. His or her job is to get patients into the ambulances and routed to hospitals. If you are assigned to this role, you will need to be flexible in determining the order in which patients are packaged and loaded. You may, for example, elect to place two critical patients in one ambulance for transport to a trauma center. If you decide that the ambulance provider cannot adequately care for two critical patients, you may instead decide to transport one critical and one noncritical patient.

The routing of patients to hospitals is as important as getting them into the ambulance. Communication with local hospitals is essential to avoid overloading the resources of any one unit.

h. Extrication/rescue p. 1826

In general, the Extrication/Rescue group removes patients from entanglements at the incident and arranges for them to be carried to treatment areas. The operation has many facets and may require specialized personnel and equipment.

i. Disposition of deceased (morgue) p. 1824

The Morgue Officer supervises the morgue—the area where the expectant victims of an incident are collected. This person may report to the Triage Officer or to the Treatment Officer. In many cases, these supervisors will in fact assist in selection and securing of an area for the morgue.

j. Communications pp. 1814, 1826–1827

At large-scale incidents, the Incident Management System provides for an EMS Communications Officer, also known as the EMS COM or the MED COM. This person works closely with the Transportation Unit Supervisor to notify hospitals of incoming patients. A dedicated radio channel works best for this purpose. The EMS COM will not deliver complete patient reports, which would increase communications traffic. Instead, he or she will transmit the basic information collected by the Transportation Supervisor, such as the number of Priority one patients en route to the hospital, the expected arrival time, and so on.

6. Describe the methods and rationale for identifying specific functions and leaders for the functions in the ICS. pp. 1810–1811, 1814

The rationale for dividing tasks at an MCI has already been discussed in previous objectives. However, it is equally important that everybody knows who is in charge of the various functions. For an Incident Commander to manage an MCI, all personnel must be able to recognize the IC. At smaller, single-agency events, everyone may know the IC simply by his or her voice over the radio. However, at medium- or large-scale incidents, such recognition is often impossible. As a result, the Incident Management System calls for the IC and other officers to wear special reflective vests. The vests can be color-coded to functional areas and may have the officer's title on the front and back. Such vests should be worn whenever IMS is utilized, even at smaller incidents. By making a basic set of vests, especially command and triage, available on every response unit, personnel will get in the habit of wearing and/or recognizing the vests prior to a major incident.

7. **Describe essential elements of the scene size-up when arriving at a potential MCI.** pp. 1812–1813

The first few minutes at an MCI can set the course of the next 60 minutes. The scene size-up is very important and should include three main priorities: life safety, incident stabilization, and property conservation.

Life Safety
Life safety is always the top priority. If you arrive first on the scene of a high-impact incident, you must observe and protect all rescuers, including yourself, from hazards. Then, and only then, will you attend to patients who are in immediately life-threatening situations. Keep in mind, however, that the needs of the many usually outweigh the needs of the few. If you commit to caring for the first patient that you encounter, you may neglect the other critical patients lying nearby.

Incident Stabilization
To achieve incident stabilization, quickly identify whether the situation is an open incident or a closed incident. Because an open incident can generate more patients at any time, it's better to call too many resources than to call too few.

In the case of a closed incident, the injuries have usually already occurred by the time you arrive on-scene. Yet even a so-called closed incident carries the potential for additional hazards—an undetected gas leak, a distraught family member who rushes into traffic, or further injury to patients wandering about the scene. As a result, it only makes sense for an Incident Commander to expend effort stabilizing the incident. Preventing further injuries—either of patients or rescue personnel—helps to ensure a smoother and more successful management of an MCI.

Property Conservation
At no time during an operation should rescue personnel damage property unless it is absolutely necessary for achieving the first two priorities—life safety and incident stabilization. Property conservation includes protection of the environment where operations are staged.

8. **Define the terms *multiple-casualty incident (MCI), disaster management, open or uncontained incident,* and *closed or contained incident*.** pp. 1809, 1812, 1813, 1827

- Multiple casualty incident (MCI)—incident that generates large numbers of patients and that often makes traditional EMS response ineffective because of special circumstances surrounding the event; also known as a mass casualty incident.
- Disaster management—management of incidents that generate large numbers of patients, often overwhelming resources and damaging parts of the infrastructure.
- Open (uncontained) incident—an incident that has the potential to generate additional patients; also known as an unstable incident.
- Closed (contained) incident—an incident that is not likely to generate any further patients; also known as a stable incident.

9. **Describe the role of the paramedics and EMS system in planning for MCIs and disasters.** pp. 1819, 1827–1828, 1829

The first step you can take in planning for MCIs and disasters is to familiarize yourself with the various laws, regulations, protocols, and standards that apply to EMS operations at an MCI. In the aftermath of September 11, 2001, the federal government is moving to assure that incident management is uniform throughout the country. Research the current NICS standards and assure your EMS policies and protocols conform.

With this information in mind, you can more effectively take part in developing a plan before an MCI or disaster actually occurs. Conduct a hazard analysis and then rate these hazards according to their likelihood. Anticipate any problems that could occur and work toward removing them. Anything that can be planned in advance should be planned in advance.

Once you have assessed potential hazards and any complicating problems, your agency should develop a plan that outlines the SOPs and protocols for the incidents that you have identified. Develop contingency plans for worst-case scenarios. Then, after you have completed your preplan, test it. Make sure that all personnel who could show up at any MCI or disaster are familiar with the preplan and, if possible, take part in practice drills. Start out small. Use local drills within your department to help familiarize personnel with the system. Then, aim for large-scale drills that involve outside agencies.

10. **Explain the local/regional threshold for establishing command and implementation of the Incident Management System including MCI declaration.** pp. 1809, 1811–1812

    The threshold for establishing command and implementation of the IMS may differ from agency to agency, depending on the resources available at any given time. An example would be as follows:
    Level 1: 3 to 10 patients
    Level 2: 11 to 25 patients
    Level 3: over 25 patients

11. **Describe the role of both command posts and emergency operations centers in MCI and disaster management.** pp. 1811–1816

    A command post (CP) provides a place where representatives and officers from various agencies can meet with each other and make relevant decisions. Because a command post may operate for weeks, the site should be selected carefully. Access to telephones, restrooms, and shelters should be taken into account. Also, the command post should be close enough to the scene so that officers can monitor operations, but far enough away so that they are outside the direct operational area. Persons operating on the scene, members of the media, and bystanders should not have routine access to the CP.

    The emergency operations center (EOC) is where governmental officials (municipal, county, state, and/or federal) exercise oversight of a large emergency or disaster. It is often a predesignated secure site with communications capability and informational resources to permit remote tracking, resource management, and control of the incident and the response.

12. **Describe the role of the on-scene physician at multiple-casualty incidents.** p. 1825

    At some high-impact or long-term incidents, physicians may be used outside the hospital to support EMS. Physicians may use their advanced medical knowledge and skills in several ways at an MCI. For example, they may be better able to make difficult triage decisions, perform advanced triage and treatment in the treatment area, or perform emergency surgery to extricate a patient as a last resort. Physicians also provide direct supervision and medical direction over paramedics in the treatment area, removing the need to operate under standing orders or radio contact. A contingency plan should be established outlining when and how physicians respond to and operate at an MCI.

13. **Define triage and describe the principles of triage.** pp. 1820–1824

    Triage is the act of sorting patients based upon the severity of their injuries. The objective of emergency medical services at an MCI is to do the most good for the most people. For this reason, you need to determine which patients need immediate care to live, which patients will live despite delays in care, and which patients will die despite receiving medical attention. Because triage will drive the EMS response, it is one of the first functions provided at the MCI.

14. **Describe the START (Simple Triage and Rapid Transport) method of initial triage.** pp. 1821–1822

    The most widely used triage system is START, an acronym standing for simple triage and rapid transport. START's easy-to-use procedures allow for rapid sorting of patients into the categories in objective 15. START does not require a specific diagnosis on the part of the responder. Instead it focuses on four criteria:

Ability to walk
    Able to walk—minimal (green)
Respiratory effort (if not able to walk)
    Not breathing with airway positioning—expectant—(black)
    Breathe once airway is positioned—immediate—(red)
    Spontaneous respirations > 30/minute—immediate—(red)
Pulses/perfusion (if breathing is spontaneous and < 30/minute)
    Absent radial pulse—immediate—(red)
Neurological status (if radial pulse is present)
    On command, grips both your hands—delayed—(yellow)
    On command does not grip both your hands—immediate—(red)

15. Given color-coded tags and numerical priorities, assign the following terms to each: pp. 1821–1822

    a. Immediate—patients in need of immediate treatment receive a red tag, indicating Priority–1 (P–1).

    b. Delayed—patients whose treatment can be delayed (i.e., they do not have an immediately life-threatening injury or condition) receive a yellow tag, indicating Priority–2 (P–2).

    c. Minimal—patients who do not exhibit the signs and symptoms of START can have treatment withheld, even if they are injured, until a later time. They receive a green tag, indicating Priority–3 (P–3).

    d. Expectant—patients who have mortal injuries or have died receive a black tag, indicating Priority–0 (P–0).

16. Define primary, secondary, and ongoing triage and their implementation techniques.   p. 1821

- **Primary triage**—the initial and immediate evaluation of a patient (using the START system) at an MCI.
- **Secondary triage**—a more in-depth and ongoing triage of the patient during the MCI. Also called ongoing triage.

17. Describe techniques used to allocate patients to hospitals and track them.   pp. 1825–1826

The Transportation Unit Supervisor is responsible for assessing the ability of local health care facilities (hospitals and other facilities) to care for the injured. He or she then identifies patient injury severity and special needs (such as burn care) and then distributes patients to assure an appropriate distribution of patients to the health care facilities available.

18. Describe the techniques used in tracking patients during multiple-casualty incidents and the need for such techniques.   pp. 1822–1826

Triage helps the Transportation Unit Supervisor to assign priorities for transport and to determine the types of treatment facilities to which patients should be sent. As you might suspect, the Transportation Supervisor needs to implement some type of tracking system or designation log. Ideally, the tracking sheet or log should include the following data:

- Triage tag number
- Triage priority
- Patient's age, gender, and major injuries
- Transporting unit
- Hospital destination
- Departure time
- Patient's name, if possible

The tracking sheet not only helps to organize activities at an MCI but it also proves invaluable in reconstructing the incident at a later time. In addition, this record will help document on-scene patient care.

19. Describe modifications of telecommunications procedures during multiple-casualty incidents. pp. 1814, 1826–1827

Modified Telecommunications

Communication forms the cornerstone of the Incident Management System. Once command is established, the Incident Commander has a responsibility to relay this information to dispatch. After an MCI has been declared, further communication should be moved to a secondary, or tactical, channel. The Incident Commander must be able to supply the information necessary to coordinate resources. That is the whole purpose of the Incident Management System. Use of a secondary channel will also prevent an Incident Commander from interfacing with the communications by other jurisdictions or from overwhelming the primary EMS channel.

When acting as an Incident Commander, remember that communication will involve units from different jurisdictions and perhaps different districts. One of the foundations of incident management is the use of a common terminology. When communicating, you should eliminate all radio codes and use only plain English. A radio code may have different meanings in different places. As an Incident Commander, you must eliminate any unnecessary confusion in an already complicated situation. In fact, it may be preferable to avoid radio codes even in routine operations. Then there will be no need to even think about switching to plain English when you assume command of an MCI.

Alternative Means of Communication

Also keep in mind the possibility of communications failure. Things can—and do—go wrong. Your primary radio system might not always work at an MCI. Disasters can knock out radio towers and power. Frequencies can be overwhelmed. Telephone lines can be down. Radio batteries can fail. As a result, alternative means of communication should be included in every MCI preplan and should be practiced regularly. You might use cellular phones, mobile data terminals, alphanumeric pages, fax machines, or other technology to overcome the failure of your primary radio system. When all else fails, runners can be used to hand deliver messages around the incident scene. Although there are obvious limitations, it may be your last resort. So know how to use it.

20. List and describe the essential equipment to provide logistical support to MCI operations to include: pp. 1818, 1824–1825

The treatment sector(s) of an MCI often requires large quantities of basic EMS equipment. Such equipment may be stored in a trailer for quick movement to the scene and includes materials for:

   a. **Airway, respiratory, and hemorrhage control**
      Oxygen masks and additional oxygen cylinders and regulator/flow-meters, oral and nasal airways, bag-valve-masks, and dressing and bandage materials.
   b. **Burn management**
      Clean burn sheets and dressings and intravenous fluids.
   c. **Patient packaging/immobilization**
      Short and long spineboards, cervical collars, cravats, padded board and air splints, and straps.

21. Describe the role of mental health support in MCIs. pp. 1817–1818, 1826, 1829–1830

Research has begun to demonstrate that critical incident stress debriefing has not had the intended effect on rescuers that was once thought. In fact, it may actually be detrimental. However, there is an important role for mental health personnel to provide psychological first aid to those affected by an event.

22. Describe the role of the following exercises in preparation for MCIs: p. 1829

   a. **Tabletop exercises**
      For any MCI preplan to be effective, it must be tested and practiced. Tabletop drills are a good place to begin. Once you have worked out the wrinkles, distribute the plan to everyone in your

department, the surrounding departments, local police, fire departments, hospitals—in short, to anyone who could be involved in the IMS in your area.

b. Small and large MCI drills

The next step is to make sure that all the personnel who could show up at an MCI have received training in the use of the IMS. Run or take part in drills so that you gain practice in MCI operations and large-scale use of the IMS. As mentioned in objective 4, start out small. Use local drills within your department and then plan large-scale, multiagency drills. Never say "It will never happen here." Experience has proven time and again that multicasualty incidents and disasters can occur almost anywhere and at any time.

23. Given several incident scenarios with preprogrammed patients, provide the appropriate triage, treatment, and transport options for MCI operations based on local resources and protocols. pp. 1809–1830

During your classroom, clinical, and field training, you will have the opportunity to practice the skills required for the various roles and sectors at an MCI. Use the information presented in this text chapter, the information on MCIs presented by your instructors, and the guidance given by your clinical and field preceptors to develop skills needed to implement the Incident Management System in the unit where you serve. Continue to refine these skills once your training ends and you begin your career as a paramedic.

Content Self-Evaluation

MULTIPLE CHOICE

_____ 1. An emergency event that involves more patients than paramedics to provide care or ambulances to transport may be called a(n):
   A. disaster.
   B. critical incident.
   C. multiple-casualty incident.
   D. mutual aid situation.
   E. command situation.

_____ 2. Standards being merged into a uniform command system for use at MCIs is being developed by:
   A. the Department of Homeland Security.
   B. the Environmental Protection Agency.
   C. OSHA.
   D. the National Fire Protection Association.
   E. Firescope.

_____ 3. The most important functional area in the Incident Management System is:
   A. logistics.
   B. planning.
   C. command.
   D. triage.
   E. operations.

_____ 4. On average the span of control at an MCI is around:
   A. 5.
   B. 10.
   C. 15.
   D. 20.
   E. 25.

_____ 5. Singular command, in many incidents, is not feasible because of overlapping responsibilities or jurisdictions.
   A. True
   B. False

_____ 6. A place where officers from various agencies can meet with each other and select a management staff is called a(n):
   A. command post.
   B. coordination post.
   C. incident post.
   D. Incident Management System.
   E. direct operational area.

_____ 7. At an MCI, the needs of the many usually outweigh the needs of the few.
   A. True
   B. False

_____ 8. An incident that has the potential to generate additional patients is known as a(n):
   A. open incident.
   B. MCI.
   C. closed incident.
   D. ICS.
   E. contained incident.

_____ 9. The cornerstone of the Incident Command System (ICS) is:
   A. leadership.
   B. utilizing singular command.
   C. having enough resources.
   D. practice and drilling.
   E. communication.

_____ 10. The primary role of the Incident Commander is:
   A. recognizing unified command.
   B. identifying a staging area.
   C. using common terminology.
   D. the strategic deployment of all resources.
   E. directing the efficient movement of patients to the ED.

_____ 11. To ensure flexibility, an Incident Commander should radio a brief progress report every 10 minutes until the event has been stabilized.
   A. True
   B. False

_____ 12. Before command can be transferred to another leader, it is necessary to report:
   A. face-to-face.
   B. via radio.
   C. in writing at the command post.
   D. via an indirect contact.
   E. none of the above—a higher-ranking officer automatically takes command upon arrival.

_____ 13. The management, or command, staff handles all of the following EXCEPT:
   A. public information.
   B. safety.
   C. triage.
   D. outside liaisons.
   E. mental health support services.

_____ 14. Under the Incident Management System, the Safety Officer has the authority to stop any action that is deemed as life threatening.
   A. True
   B. False

_____ 15. The person or group responsible for fulfilling the Medical Supply Unit is the:
   A. Facilities Unit.
   B. Liaison Officer.
   C. Finance/Administration Sector.
   D. Logistics Sector.
   E. Planning Officer.

_____ 16. Which of the following is the most task-specific section at an MCI?
   A. branch
   B. group
   C. division
   D. unit
   E. sector

_____ 17. The term *sector* is interchangeable for a functional or geographical area.
   A. True
   B. False

_____ 18. Triage that takes place after patients are moved to a treatment area to determine any changes in their status is referred to as:
   A. secondary triage.
   B. supplemental triage.
   C. sector triage.
   D. delayed triage.
   E. primary triage.

_____ 19. Under the START system, a Triage Officer would focus on all of the following signs and symptoms EXCEPT:
   A. ability to walk.
   B. respiration.
   C. pulses/perfusion.
   D. ability to talk.
   E. neurological status.

_____ 20. Patients with absent radial pulses should be tagged:
   A. red.
   B. yellow.
   C. green.
   D. white.
   E. black.

_____ 21. Color-coded tags that are placed on patients that have been sorted serve to:
   A. track the patient.
   B. prevent retriage of the patient.
   C. alert care providers to patient priorities.
   D. record treatment information.
   E. all of the above

_____ 22. One efficient way to speed up the triage process is to:
   A. add extra personnel to triage.
   B. not use triage tags.
   C. skip the primary triage.
   D. not triage the walking wounded.
   E. ask the IC to assist in triage.

_____ 23. An ambulance crew who is dedicated to stand by in case a rescuer becomes ill or injured is called a _____ Team.
   A. Rescue Response
   B. Rehabilitation
   C. Extrication
   D. Rapid Intervention
   E. TIP

_____ 24. As a general rule, disaster management occurs in which four stages?
   A. mitigation, planning, response, recovery
   B. request, response, react, recover
   C. mitigation, react, recovery, recall
   D. activation, planning, mitigation, recall
   E. planning, response, react, reassess

_____ 25. Mental health personnel should circulate around the scene of a high-impact incident to help meet the emotional needs of those affected by the incident.
   A. True
   B. False

MATCHING

Write the letter of the term in the space provided next to the appropriate description.

A. Public Information Officer
B. closed incident
C. planning
G. demobilized
H. span of control
D. C-FLOP
E. command post
F. scene-authority law
I. Liaison Officer
J. Staff Functions

_____ 26. mnemonic for the main functional areas within the NIMS

_____ 27. supervisory roles in the NIMS

_____ 28. coordinates all incident operations that involve outside agencies

_____ 29. the number of people a single individual can monitor

_____ 30. collects data about the incident and releases it to the media

_____ 31. an incident that is not likely to generate additional patients

_____ 32. release of resources no longer needed at an incident

_____ 33. provides past, present, and future information about the incident

_____ 34. state or local statute specifying who has authority at an MCI

_____ 35. place where command officers from various agencies can meet

SHORT ANSWER

Write out the terms that each of the following acronyms stands for in the spaces provided.

36. MCI _____

37. C-FLOP _____

38. EOC _____

39. IMS _____

40. START _____

Part 3: Rescue Awareness and Operations

Review of Chapter Objectives

After reading Part 3 of this chapter, you should be able to:

1. Define the term *rescue,* and explain the medical and mechanical aspects of rescue operations.   pp. 1830–1831

   According to the dictionary, rescue is "the act of delivering from danger or imprisonment." In the case of EMS, rescue means extricating and/or disentangling the victims who will become your patients.
   Rescue involves a combination of medical and mechanical skills with the correct amount of each applied at the appropriate time. The medical aspects of rescue involve assessment and treatment of the patient. Mechanical aspects involve the tools and skills to disentangle the victim.

2. Describe the phases of a rescue operation, and the role of the paramedic at each phase. pp. 1835–1838

There are basically seven phases in a rescue operation. They include:

Arrival and size-up. Key to the success of any rescue operation is the prompt recognition of a rescue situation and the quick identification of the specific type of rescue required. You can then quickly notify dispatch of the magnitude of the event and summon the necessary resources. Now is the time to implement the IMS, any mutual-aid agreements, and the procedures for contacting off-duty personnel or backup ALS units. In calling for support, follow this precaution: "Don't undersell overkill."

Hazard control. On-scene hazards must be identified with speed and clarity. You must often deal with these hazards before even attempting to reach the patient. To do otherwise would place you and other personnel at risk. Control as many of the hazards as possible, but don't attempt to manage any conditions beyond your training or skills. Individual acts of courage may be called for, but safety comes first. If in doubt, err on the side of safety.

Patient access. After controlling hazards, you will then attempt to gain access to the patient or patients. Begin by formulating a plan. Determine the best method to gain access and deploy the necessary personnel. Make sure that you take steps to stabilize the physical location of the patient.

As you know, access triggers the technical beginning of the rescue. While gaining access, you must use appropriate safety equipment and procedures. This is the point when you and/or the Command and Safety Officer must honestly evaluate the training and skills needed to access the patient. During this phase, key medical, technical, and command personnel must confer with the Safety Officer on the strategy they will use to accomplish the rescue.

Medical treatment. After devising a rescue plan, medical personnel can begin to make patient contact. No personnel should enter an area to provide patient care unless they are physically fit, protected from hazards, and have the technical skills to reach, manage, and remove patients safely. In general, a paramedic has three responsibilities during this phase of operation. They are:
- Initiation of patient assessment and care as soon as possible
- Maintenance of patient care procedures during disentanglement
- Accompaniment of the patient during removal and transport

Disentanglement. Disentanglement involves the actual release from the cause of entrapment. This phase may be the most technical and time-consuming portion of the rescue. If assigned to patient care during this phase of the rescue, you have three responsibilities. They are:
- Personal and professional confidence in the technical expertise and gear needed to function effectively in the active rescue zone
- Readiness to provide prolonged patient care
- Ability to call for and/or use special rescue resources

If you or another member of the rescue team cannot fulfill these requirements, reassess available rescue personnel and call for backup.

Patient packaging. After disentanglement, a patient must be appropriately packaged to ensure that all medical needs are addressed. Some forms of packaging can be more complex than others, depending upon the specialized rescue techniques required to extricate the patient—e.g., being lifted out of a hole in a Stokes by a ladder truck. In situations where the patient may be vertical or suspended in a Stokes basket, it is paramount that the rescuer know how to properly package the patient to prevent additional injury.

Removal/transport. Removal of the patient may be one of the most difficult tasks to accomplish or it may be as easy as placing the person on a stretcher and wheeling it to a nearby ambulance. Activities involved in the removal of a patient will require the coordinated effort of all personnel. Transportation to a medical facility should be planned well in advance, especially if you anticipate any delays. Decisions regarding patient transport—whether it be by ground vehicle, by aircraft, or by physical carry-out—should be coordinated based on advice from medical direction. En route to the hospital, perform the ongoing assessment and treatment per the patient's condition.

3. **List and describe the personal protective equipment needed to safely operate in the rescue environment to include:** pp. 1831–1833

   a. **Head, eye, and hand protection**

   Head. To protect the head, every unit should carry helmets, preferably ones with a four-point, nonelastic suspension system. A compact firefighting helmet that meets NFPA standards is adequate for most vehicle and structural applications. However, climbing helmets may work better for confined space and technical rescues, while padded rafting or kayaking helmets are more appropriate for water rescues.

   Eye. Two essential pieces of eye gear include goggles, vented to prevent fogging, and industrial safety glasses. These should be ANSI approved. Do not rely on the face shields found in fire helmets. They usually provide inadequate eye protection.

   Hand. Leather gloves usually protect against cuts and punctures. They allow free movement of the fingers and ample dexterity. As a rule, heavy gauntlet-style gloves are too awkward for most rescue work.

   b. **Personal flotation devices**

   All PFDs should meet the U.S. Coast Guard standards for flotation and should be worn whenever operating on or around water. The Type III PFD is preferred for rescue work. You should also attach a knife, strobe light, and whistle to the PFD so that they can be easily accessed.

   c. **Thermal protection/layering systems**

   Appropriate clothing and gear should be worn for both flame/flash protection and insulation against extreme cold. Turnout gear, coveralls, or jumpsuits all offer some arm and leg protection. However, for limited flame protection, select gear made from Nomex, PBI, or flame-retardant cotton. For protection in cold or wet situations, such as remote wilderness areas, layer your clothing. Avoid cotton and choose synthetic materials that wick away moisture. Outer layers should be made from water- and wind-resistant fabrics such as Gore-Tex or nylon. Although insulated gear or jumpsuits are helpful in cold environments, they can also increase heat stress during heavy work or in high ambient temperatures.

   d. **High visibility clothing**

   For high visibility, pick bright colors such as orange or lime and reflective trim or symbols. Some services, for example, have an SOP calling for highly visible gear and/or orange safety vests at all highway operations—both day and night.

4. **Explain the risks and complications associated with rescues involving moving water, low head dams, flat water, trenches, motor vehicles, and confined spaces.** pp. 1838–1845, 1846–1851

   Moving water. The force of moving water can be very deceptive. The hydraulics of moving water change with a number of variables, including water depth, velocity, obstructions to flow, changing tides, and more. Four swift-water rescue scenarios present a special challenge and danger to rescuers. They include:

   - **Recirculating currents**—movement of currents over a uniform obstruction; also known as a "drowning machine"
   - **Strainers**—a partial obstruction that filters, or strains, the water, such as downed trees or wire mesh; causes an unequal force on two sides
   - **Low head dams/hydroelectric intakes**—structures that create the risk of recirculating currents (dams) and strainers (hydroelectric intakes)
   - **Pins**—entrapped foot or extremity that exposes a person to the force and weight of moving water

   Flat water. The greatest problem with flat water is that it looks so calm. Yet a large proportion of drowning or near-drowning incidents take place in flat or slow-moving water. Entry into the water exposes the rescuer to some of the same risks as the patient, such as hypothermia, exhaustion, and so on. Remember: REACH-THROW-ROW-GO, with "go" being absolutely the last resort.

   Trenches. If a collapse has caused burial, a secondary collapse is likely. Therefore, your initial actions should be geared toward safety. While waiting for a rescue team to arrive, do not allow entry in the area surrounding the trench or cave-in. Safe access can take place only when proper shoring is in place.

Motor vehicles. Traffic flow is the largest single hazard associated with EMS highway operations. Studies have shown that drivers who are tired, drunk, or drugged actually drive right into the emergency lights. Spectators can worsen the situation by getting out of their cars to watch or even "help." Other hazards besides traffic flow include:
- fire and fuel
- alternative fuel systems
- sharp objects
- electric power (downed lines or underground feeds)
- energy-absorbing bumpers
- supplemental restraint systems
- hazardous cargoes
- rolling vehicles
- unstable vehicles

Confined spaces. Confined spaces present a wide range of risks. Some of the most common ones include:
- oxygen-deficient atmospheres
- toxic or explosive chemicals
- engulfment
- machinery entrapment
- electricity
- structural complications

5. **Explain the effects of immersion hypothermia on the ability to survive sudden immersion and self-rescue.** pp. 1839–1840

Immersion can rapidly lead to hypothermia. As a rule, people cannot maintain body heat in water that is less than 92°F. The colder the water, the faster the loss of heat. In fact, water causes heat loss 25 times faster than the air. Immersion in 35°F water for 15 to 20 minutes is likely to kill a person. Factors contributing to the demise of a hypothermic patient include:

- Incapacitation and an inability to self-rescue
- Inability to follow simple directions
- Inability to grasp a line or flotation device
- Laryngospasm (caused by sudden immersion) and greater likelihood of drowning

6. **Explain the benefits and disadvantages of water-entry or "go techniques" versus the reach-throw-row-go approach to water rescue.** pp. 1840–1841

The water rescue model is REACH-THROW-ROW-GO. All paramedics should be trained in reach-and-throw techniques. You should become proficient with a water-throw bag for shore-based operations. Remember: Boat-based techniques require specialized rescue training. Water entry ("go") is only the last resort—and is an action best left to specialized water rescuers. In all instances, a PFD should be worn in case you or another rescuer are pulled into the water, accidentally slip, and so on.

7. **Explain the self-rescue position if unexpectedly immersed in moving water.** pp. 1840, 1843

If people suddenly become submerged, they can assume the Heat Escape Lessening Position (HELP). This position involves floating with the head out of the water and the body in a fetal tuck. Researchers estimate that someone who has practiced with HELP can reduce heat loss by almost 60 percent, as compared to the heat expended when treading water.

8. **Describe the use of apparatus placement, headlights and emergency vehicle lighting, cone and flare placement, and reflective and high visibility clothing to reduce scene risk at highway incidents.** pp. 1846–1847

Apparatus placement. When apparatus arrives, ensure that it causes the minimum reduction of traffic flow. As much as possible, apparatus should be positioned to protect the scene. The ambulance loading area should NOT be directly exposed to traffic.

Headlights and emergency vehicle lighting. DO NOT rely solely on ambulance lights to warn traffic away. These lights are often obstructed when medics open the doors for loading. When deciding upon emergency lighting, use only a minimum amount of warning lights to alert traffic of a hazard and to define the actual size of your vehicle. Too many lights can confuse or blind drivers, causing yet other accidents. Experts strongly advise that you turn off all headlights when parked at the scene and rely instead on amber scene lighting.

Cones and flare placement. Be sure traffic cones and flares are placed early in the incident. If the police are not already on scene, this is your responsibility. As a first responder, you must redirect traffic away from the collision and away from all emergency workers. In other words, you need to create a safety zone. Make sure that you do not place lighted flares too near any sources of fuel or brush; otherwise you risk an explosion or fire. Once you light the flares, allow them to burn out. DO NOT try to extinguish them. Attempting to pick up a flare can cause a very serious thermal burn.

Reflective and high visibility clothing. As noted in objective 3, all rescuers should be dressed in highly visible clothing. Since many EMS, police, and fire agencies wear dark-colored uniforms, you should don a brightly colored turnout coat or vest with reflective tape. You can directly apply the tape at the scene.

9. **List and describe the design element hazards and associated protective actions associated with autos and trucks, including energy-absorbing bumpers, air bag/supplemental restraint systems, catalytic converters, and conventional and nonconventional fuel systems.** pp. 1848–1849

    Energy-absorbing bumpers. The bumpers on many vehicles come with pistons and are designed to withstand a slow-speed collision. Sometimes these bumpers become "loaded" in the crushed position and do not immediately bounce back out. When exposed to fire or even just tapped by rescue workers, the pistons can suddenly unload their stored energy. If you discover a loaded bumper, stay away from it unless you are specially trained to deal with this hazard.

    Air bag/supplemental restraint systems. Air bags also have the potential to release stored energy. If they have not been deployed during the collision, they may do so during the middle of an extrication. As a result, these devices must be deactivated prior to disentanglement. Auto manufacturers can provide information about power removal or power dissipation for their particular brand of SRS. Also, keep in mind that many new model vehicles come equipped with side impact bags.

    Catalytic converters. Remember that all automobiles manufactured since the 1970s have catalytic converters. They run at a temperature of around 1,200°F—hot enough to heat fuel to the point of ignition. Be especially careful when a vehicle has gone off the road into dry grass or brush. The debris can be just as dangerous as spilled fuel, especially when brought into contact with a blazing hot catalytic converter.

    Conventional fuel systems. Fuel spilled at the scene increases the changes of fire. Be very careful whenever you smell or see pools of liquid at a collision. Keep in mind that bystanders who are smoking can cause a bigger problem than the original accident if they flick lighted ashes into a fuel leak. DO NOT drive your emergency vehicle over a fuel spill—or worse yet, park on one!

    Nonconventional fuel systems. Be cautious of vehicles powered by alternative fuel systems. High-pressure tanks, especially if filled with natural gas, are extremely volatile. Even vehicles powered by electricity can be dangerous. The storage cells possess the energy to spark, flash, and more.

10. **Given a diagram of a passenger auto, identify the A, B, C, and D posts, firewall, and unibody versus frame construction.** pp. 1849–1850

    Basic Vehicle Constructions
    Vehicles can have either a unibody or a frame construction. Most automobiles today have a unibody design, while older vehicles and lightweight trucks have a frame construction. For unibody vehicles to maintain their integrity, all the following features must remain intact: roof posts, floor, firewall, truck support, and windshield.

©2007 Pearson Education, Inc.
Essentials of Paramedic Care, 2nd ed.

CHAPTER 48 *Operations* 671

Both types of construction have roofs and roof supports. The support posts are lettered from front to back. The first post, which supports the roof at the windshield, is called the "A" post. The next post is the "B" post. The third post, found in sedans and station wagons, is the "C" post. Station wagons have an additional rear post, known as the "D" post.

Firewalls

The firewall separates the engine compartment from the occupant compartment. Frequently, the firewall can collapse on a patient's legs during a high-speed head-on collision. Sometimes, a patient's feet may go through the firewall.

11. **Explain the difference between tempered and safety glass, identify its locations on a vehicle, and describe how to break it.** p. 1850

Safety Glass

Safety glass is made from three layers of fused materials: glass—plastic laminate—glass. It is found in windshields and designed to stay intact when shattered or broken. However, safety glass can still produce glass dust or fracture into long shards. These materials can easily get into a patient's eyes, nose, or mouth and/or create cuts. As a result, be sure to cover a patient whenever you remove this type of glass. Safety glass is usually cut out with a GlasMaster saw or a flat-head axe.

Tempered Glass

Tempered glass has high tensile strength. However, it does not stay intact when shattered or broken. It fractures into many small beads of glass, all of which can cause injuries or cuts. Tempered glass is usually broken using a spring-loaded center punch.

12. **Explain typical door anatomy and methods to access through stuck doors.** p. 1850

The doors of most new vehicles contain a reinforcing bar to protect the occupant in side-impact collisions. They also have a case-hardened steel "Nader" pin. Named after consumer advocate Ralph Nader, these pins help keep the doors from blowing open and ejecting the occupants. If the Nader pin has been engaged, it will be difficult to pry open the door. You must first disentangle the latch or use hydraulic jaws.

Before attempting to assist a patient through a door, you should be trained in proper extrication techniques. In general, follow these steps:

- Try all four doors first—a door is the easiest means of access.
- Otherwise, gain access through the window farthest away from the patient(s).
- Alternatively, use simple hand tools to peel back the outer sheet of metal on the door, exposing the lock mechanism. Unlock the lock and pry the cams from the Nader pin. Then pry open the door.

13. **Describe methods for emergency stabilization using rope, cribbing, jacks, spare tires, and come-a-longs for vehicles found in various positions.** pp. 1849, 1850–1851

Motor vehicles can land in all kinds of unstable positions. They can roll over onto their side or roof. They can stop on an incline or unstable terrain. They can be suspended over a cliff or a river. They can come to rest on a patch of ice or on an on-site spill or leak.

As a result, vehicles must be stabilized before accessing the patient. Sometimes vehicle stabilization can be as simple as making sure the vehicle is in "Park" and chocking the wheels so it will not roll. Other times, such as in the case of an overturned vehicle, you might need to use ropes, cribbing, jacks, or even a spare tire to help prevent it from rolling over. If a vehicle is hanging over an embankment, you might use a combination of cribbing and a come-along tied onto the guard rail (if one is present). However, only attempt these techniques if you have the skills to do so. Otherwise, you need to request the necessary stabilization crews and/or equipment.

14. **Describe electrical and other hazards commonly found at highway incidents (above and below the ground).** pp. 1848–1849

    Contact with downed power lines or underground electrical feeds can be lethal. If a vehicle is in contact with electrical lines, consider it to be "charged" and call the power company immediately. In most newer communities, electric lines run underground. However, a vehicle can still run into a transformer or an electric feed box. As a result, make sure you look under the car and all around it during your scene size-up. DO NOT touch a vehicle until you have ruled out all electrical hazards. (Other hazards commonly found at highway incidents are listed/discussed in objectives 4 and 9.)

15. **Define low-angle rescue, high-angle rescue, belay, rappel, scrambling, and hasty rope slide.** pp. 1851–1852

    - **Low-angle rescue**—rescues up to 40° over faces that are not excessively smooth; requires rope, harnesses, hardware, and the necessary safety systems
    - **High-angle rescue**—rescues involving ropes, harnesses, and specialized equipment to ascend and descend a steep and/or smooth face; also known as "vertical" rescue
    - **Belay**—procedure for safeguarding a climber's progress by controlling a rope attached to an anchor; person controlling the rope is sometimes also called the belay
    - **Rappel**—to descend by sliding down a fixed double rope, using the correct anchor, harness, and gear
    - **Scrambling**—climbing over rocks and/or downed trees on a steep trail without the aid of ropes
    - **Hasty rope slide**—using a rope to assist in balance and footing on rough terrain; rescuers do not actually "clip into" the rope as they do in low-angle and high-angle rescues

16. **Describe the procedure for Stokes litter packaging for low-angle evacuations.** pp. 1852–1854

    A Stokes litter is the standard stretcher for rough terrain evacuation. It provides a rigid frame for patient protection and is easy to carry with an adequate number of personnel. When using a Stokes litter (also called a Stokes basket stretcher) for high-angle or low-angle evacuation, take the following steps:

    - Apply a harness to the patient.
    - Apply leg stirrups to the patient.
    - Secure the patient to a litter to prevent movement.
    - Tie the tail of one litter line to the patient's harness.
    - Use a helmet or litter shield to protect the patient.
    - Administer fluids (IV or orally).
    - Allow accessibility for taking BP, performing suction, and assessing distal perfusion.
    - Apply extra strapping or lacing as necessary (for rough terrain evacuation and/or extrication).

17. **Explain anchoring, litter/rope attachment, and lowering and raising procedures as they apply to low-angle litter evacuation.** pp. 1852, 1854

    Before beginning patient removal, rescuers must ensure that all anchors are secure. They must check their own safety equipment and recheck patient packaging. They must also have the necessary lowering and hauling systems in place, again doing the recommended safety checks.

    Materials, especially ropes, should never be used if there is any question of their safety. If you see a frayed rope or any stressed or damaged equipment, do not hesitate to point it out to the rescuers in a polite, but professional, manner. Also, because hauling sometimes requires many "helpers," you may be asked to assist. Make sure you understand all directions given by the rescuers. Evacuation is a team effort.

18. **Explain techniques used in nontechnical litter carries over rough terrain.** p. 1854

    When removing a patient in a nontechnical litter over flat, rough terrain, make sure you have enough litter carriers to "leapfrog" ahead of each other to save time and to rotate rescuers. An adequate number of litter bearers would be two or, better yet, three teams of six. Litter bearers on each carry should be approximately the same height.

Several devices exist to ease the difficulty of a litter carry. For example, litter bearers can run webbing straps over the litter rails, across their shoulders, and into their free hands. This will help distribute the weight across the bearers' backs. Another helpful device is the litter wheel. It attaches to the bottom of a Stokes basket frame and takes most of the weight of the litter. Bearers must keep the litter balanced and control its motion. As you might suspect, the litter wheel works best across flatter terrain.

19. Explain nontechnical high-angle rescue procedures using aerial apparatus.   **p. 1854**

When using aerial apparatus, it is necessary to provide a litter belay during movement to a bucket. Litters, of course, must then be correctly attached to the bucket. Use of aerial ladders can be difficult because upper sections are usually not wide enough to slot the litter. The litter must always be properly belayed if being slid down the ladder. Finally, ladders or other aerial apparatus should NOT be used as a crane to move a litter. They are neither designed nor rated for this work. Serious stress can cause accidents resulting in patient death.

20. Explain assessment and care modifications (including painmedication, temperature control, and hydration) necessary for attending entrapped patients.   **pp. 1855–1856**

Protocols for extended care, which is often the case with entrapped patients, can vary substantially from standard EMS procedures. If SOPs for such situations do not already exist, procedures adopted from wilderness medical research will prove useful. Position papers written by the Wilderness Medical Society or the National Association for Search and Rescue can serve as guidelines for protocols.

In most situations, you should prepare for long-term hydration management. You should also look for signs and symptoms of hypothermia, which is not uncommon for these patients. You may have to apply nonpharmacological pain management (distracting questions, proper splinting, use of sensory stimuli) when doing painful procedures. Alternatively, you may need to turn to pharmacological pain management—morphine or nitrous oxide—depending upon the patient's condition, the length of entrapment, and/or advice from medical direction.

21. List the equipment necessary for an "off-road" medical pack.   **pp. 1833, 1856**

An off-road medical pack should contain at least the following items:

- **Airway**—oral and nasal airways, manual suction, intubation equipment
- **Breathing**—thoracic decompression equipment, small oxygen tank/regulator, masks/cannulas, pocket mask/BVM
- **Circulation**—bandages/dressings, triangular bandages, occlusive dressings, IV administration equipment, BP cuff, and stethoscope
- **Disability**—extrication collars
- **Expose**—scissors
- **Miscellaneous**—headlamp/flashlight, space blanket, added aluminum splint (SAM splint), PPE (leather gloves, latex gloves, eye shields), provisions for drinking water, clothing for inclement weather, snacks for a few hours, temporary shelter, butane lighter, and some redundancy in lighting in case of light source failure

22. Explain the different types of "Stokes" or basket stretchers and the advantages and disadvantages associated with each.   **pp. 1852, 1854**

Stokes baskets come in wire and tubular as well as plastic styles. The older "military style" wire mesh Stokes basket will not accept a backboard. Newer models, however, offer several advantages. They include:

- Generally greater strength
- Less expense per unit

- Better air/water flow through the basket
- Better flotation, an important concern in water rescues

Plastic basket stretchers are usually weaker than their wire mesh counterparts. They are often rated for only 300 to 600 pounds. However, they tend to offer better patient protection. In general, Stokes baskets with plastic bottoms and steel frames are best. These versatile units can also be slid in snow, when necessary.

23. Given a list of rescue scenarios, provide the victim survivability profile and identify which are rescue versus body recovery situations.   pp. 1830–1856

During your classroom, clinical, and field training, you will be presented with a number of rescue scenarios in which you will be called upon to provide a victim survivability profile and to distinguish between rescue and body recovery situations. Use information presented in this text, the information on rescue operations presented by your instructors, and the guidance given by your clinical and field preceptors to develop a high level of rescue awareness and the skills needed to implement the various phases of a rescue operation. Continue to refine these skills once your training ends and you begin your career as a paramedic.

24. Given a series of pictures, identify those considered "confined spaces" and potentially oxygen deficient.   pp. 1845–1846

Confined-space rescues present any number of potentially fatal threats, but one of the most serious is an oxygen-deficient environment. At first glance, most confined spaces might appear relatively safe. As a result, you might mistakenly think rescue procedures will be easier and/or less time-consuming and dangerous than they really are. Here's where rescue awareness comes in. According to NIOSH, nearly 60 percent of all fatalities associated with confined spaces are people attempting to rescue a victim.

While "confined space" can have a variety of interpretations, OSHA regulation CFR 1910 interprets the term to mean any space with limited access/egress that is not designed for human occupancy or habitation. In other words, confined spaces are not safe for people to enter for any sustained period of time. Examples of confined spaces include transport or storage tanks, grain bins and silos, wells and cisterns, manholes and pumping stations, drainage culverts, pits, hoppers, underground vaults, and the shafts of mines or caves.

Before going into a confined space, special entry teams monitor the atmosphere to determine oxygen concentration, levels of hydrogen sulfide, explosive limits, flammable atmosphere, or toxic contaminants. They are also aware that increases in oxygen content for any reason—e.g., a gust of wind—can give atmospheric monitoring meters a false reading. The bottom line is this: Confined spaces often mean hazardous atmospheres.

Content Self-Evaluation

MULTIPLE CHOICE

_____ 1. As applied to rescue operations, awareness training involves a(n):
    A. command of the technical skills to execute a rescue.
    B. ability to recognize hazards.
    C. realization of the need for additional resources.
    D. detailed knowledge of rescue specialties.
    E. both B and C

_____ 2. Most PPE used in rescue situations has been designed for the field of EMS.
    A. True
    B. False

_____ 3. The person who makes a "go/no go" decision in a rescue operation is the:
   A. medical dispatcher.
   B. Incident Commander.
   C. specialized rescue crew.
   D. Safety Officer.
   E. first responders.

_____ 4. In what phase of a rescue operation does patient access take place?
   A. first
   B. second
   C. third
   D. fourth
   E. fifth

_____ 5. The technical phase of a rescue begins with:
   A. scene size-up.
   B. medical treatment.
   C. access.
   D. hazard control.
   E. packaging.

_____ 6. During an extended rescue, take all the following steps to calm patient fears EXCEPT:
   A. explain all delays.
   B. tell the patient you will not abandon him or her.
   C. minimize the dangers of the situation.
   D. explain unfamiliar technical aspects of the operation.
   E. be sure the patient knows your name.

_____ 7. Water causes heat loss 25 times faster than the air.
   A. True
   B. False

_____ 8. Actions to delay the onset of hypothermia in water rescues include all of the following EXCEPT:
   A. use of PFDs.
   B. use of HELP.
   C. huddling together.
   D. treading water.
   E. both C and D

_____ 9. The first action you should take in a water rescue is to:
   A. reach for the patient with a pole.
   B. swim to the patient.
   C. row to the patient.
   D. throw a flotation device to the patient.
   E. talk the patient into a self-rescue.

_____ 10. At a low head dam, one of the biggest dangers to rescue is a(n):
   A. strainer.
   B. foot pin.
   C. recirculating current.
   D. eddy.
   E. large rocks.

_____ 11. Factors that affect the survival of a patient in a near-drowning accident include:
   A. age.
   B. lung volume.
   C. water temperature.
   D. posture.
   E. all of the above

_____ 12. You should attempt resuscitation on any hypothermic and/or pulseless, nonbreathing patient who has been submerged in cold water.
   A. True
   B. False

_____ 13. The primary reason confined spaces present a potentially fatal threat is because:
   A. a patient cannot get out and panics.
   B. a lack of OSHA regulations.
   C. the space is oxygen deficient.
   D. faulty retrieval devices.
   E. none of the above

_____ 14. Although all of the following present risks, the largest single hazard associated with EMS highway operations is:
   A. sharp objects.
   B. traffic flow.
   C. rollover situations.
   D. hazardous cargoes.
   E. alternative fuel systems.

_____ 15. The post that supports the roof at the windshield is the:
   A. "A" post.
   B. "B" post.
   C. "C" post.
   D. "D" post.
   E. "E" post.

_____ 16. The easiest means of accessing a motor vehicle patient is through the:
   A. windshield.
   B. door.
   C. window closest to the patient.
   D. hatch.
   E. rear window.

_____ 17. Removal of the patient from the vehicle almost always precedes patient care.
   A. True
   B. False

_____ 18. Each member of a high-angle rescue team must have complete competency in the ability to rig a hauling system.
   A. True
   B. False

_____ 19. Most Stokes stretchers are not equipped with adequate restraints.
   A. True
   B. False

_____ 20. Which of the following probably would NOT be found in a downsized backcountry pack?
   A. SAM splints
   B. small oxygen tank/regulator
   C. ECG monitor
   D. intubation equipment
   E. extrication collars

MATCHING

Write the letter of the term in the space provided next to the appropriate description.

A. recirculating currents
B. mammalian diving reflex
C. extrication
D. strainer
E. eddies
F. HELP
G. safety glass
H. active rescue zone
I. short haul
J. tempered glass

_____ 21. area where special rescue teams operate

_____ 22. use of force to free a patient from entrapment

_____ 23. an in-water, head-up tuck or fetal position designed to reduce heat loss

_____ 24. movement of currents over a uniform obstruction

_____ 25. type of glass with a high tensile strength that fractures into small beads when shattered

_____ 26. helicopter extrication technique where a person is attached to a rope that is, in turn, attached to a helicopter

_____ 27. partial obstruction that filters moving water

_____ 28. water that flows around especially large objects and, for a time, flows upstream on the downside of the object

_____ 29. a type of glass made from three layers of fused materials that is designed to stay intact when shattered

_____ 30. the body's natural response to submersion in cold water, the end process of which increases blood flow to the heart and brain

Part 4: Hazardous Materials Incidents

Review of Chapter Objectives

After reading Part 4 of this chapter, you should be able to:

1. Explain the role of the paramedic/EMS responder at the hazardous material incident in terms of the following: pp. 1857–1858

   a. **Incident size-up**
   One of the most critical aspects of any hazmat response is the simple awareness that a dangerous substance may be present. Virtually every emergency site—residential, business, or highway—possesses the potential for hazardous materials. Always keep the possibility of dangerous substances in mind whenever you approach the scene of an emergency. In addition, learn the various placard systems and the resources for identifying them (see objective 1b).

   Priorities at a hazmat incident are the same as for any other major incident: life, safety, and property conservation. However, you should be prepared for the special circumstances surrounding most hazmat emergencies. In performing early hazmat interventions, you face the challenge of avoiding exposure to the hazardous material yourself. As a result, never compromise scene safety during the early phase of a hazmat operation.

   In addition, expect a number of agencies to be involved in a hazmat incident. As a result, you should be skilled in the use of the Incident Management System (IMS) discussed in Part 2 of this chapter. As you learned in that part, you will need to quickly determine whether the hazmat emergency is an open or a closed incident. In reaching your decision, remember that some chemicals have delayed effects. Triage must be ongoing, as patient conditions can change rapidly.

   Finally, you must take into account certain conditions when choreographing the scene. The most preferable site for deploying resources will be uphill and upwind. This will help prevent contamination from ground-based liquids, high vapor density gases, run-off water, and vapor clouds. A backup plan for areas of operation must be determined early in the event. For example, what would you do if the wind direction suddenly shifted and a cloud of chlorine gas headed toward your staging area?

   b. **Assessment of toxicologic risk**
   To aid in the visual recognition of hazardous materials, two simple systems have been developed. The Department of Transportation (DOT) has implemented placards to identify dangerous substances in transit, while the National Fire Protection Association (NFPA) has devised a system for fixed facilities. When DOT placards are used on vehicles, you can spot them easily by their diamond shape. Some placards also carry a UN number—a four digit number specific to the actual chemical. For quick reference, keep in mind these general classifications.

   Hazard Classes and Placard Colors

Hazard Class	Hazard Type	Color Code
1	explosives	orange
2	gases	red or green
3	liquids	red
4	solids	red and white
5	oxidizers and organic peroxides	yellow
6	poisonous and etiologic agents	white
7	radioactive materials	yellow and white
8	corrosives	black and white
9	miscellaneous	black and white

In addition to numbers and colors, placards also use symbols to indicate hazard types. For example, a flame symbol indicates a flammable substance, and a skull-and-crossbones symbol indicates a poisonous substance.

The NFPA 704 System identifies hazardous materials at fixed facilities. Like the DOT placards, the system uses diamond-shaped figures, which are divided into four sections and colors. The top section is red and indicates the flammability of the substance. The left section is blue and indicates the health hazards. The right segment is yellow and indicates the reactivity. The bottom segment is white and indicates special information such as water reactivity, oxidizer, or radioactivity.

Flammability, health hazard, and reactivity are measured on a scale of 0 to 4. A designation of 0 indicates no hazard, while a designation of 4 indicates extreme hazard.

See objective 2 for resources used to identify toxic substances and objective 3 for levels of toxicity.

c. Appropriate decontamination methods

There are four methods of decontamination—dilution, absorption, neutralization, and isolation. The method used depends upon the type of hazardous substance and the route of exposure. In many instances, rescuers will use two or more of these methods during the decontamination process.

d. Treatment of semi-decontaminated patients

Remember that no patient who undergoes field decontamination is truly decontaminated. Field decontaminated patients, sometimes called semi-decontaminated patients, may still need to undergo a more invasive decon procedure at a medical facility.

When treating critically ill hazmat patients, it is important to perform a rapid risk-to-benefit assessment. Ask yourself these questions: How much risk of exposure will I incur by intubating a patient during decon? Does the patient really need an intravenous line established right now? Few ALS procedures will truly make a difference if performed rapidly, but one mistake can make any rescuer into a patient. Take a few moments and think before you act.

At incidents where patients are noncritical, rescuers can take a more contemplative approach, especially if they can identify the substance. Decontamination and treatment can proceed simultaneously, depending upon the substance. You might also have time to give special attention to other matters, such as containing run-off water, reclothing patients, isolating or containing patients, and so on.

e. Transportation of semi-decontaminated patients

When transporting field-contaminated patients, always recall that they still have some contamination in or on them. For example, a patient may have ingested a chemical, which can be expelled if the patient coughs or vomits. As a result, use as much disposable equipment as possible. Keep in mind that any airborne hazard will not only incapacitate the crew in the back of the ambulance, but will affect the driver as well. Although it is not practical to line the ambulance in plastic, you can isolate the patient using a stretcher decon pool. The pool can help contain any potentially contaminated body fluids. Plastic can also be used to cover the pool—yet another protective barrier.

2. Identify resources for substance identification, decontamination, and treatment information.   pp. 1862–1863

There are many sources for information that can be used to identify hazmat substances, methods of contamination, and treatment information. Some of the most common include:

- Emergency Response Guidebook (ERG)
- Shipping papers
- Material safety data sheets
- Monitors/chemical tests
- Databases (CAMEO)
- Hazmat telephone hotlines (CHEMTREC, CHEMTEL, Inc.)
- Poison control centers
- Toxicologists
- Reference books

3. **Identify primary and secondary decontamination risk.** p. 1865

Whenever people or equipment come in contact with a potentially toxic substance, they are considered to be contaminated. The contamination may be either primary or secondary.

Primary contamination occurs when someone or something is directly exposed to a hazardous substance. At this point, the contamination is limited—that is the exposure has not yet harmed others.

Secondary contamination takes place when a contaminated person or object comes in contact with an uncontaminated person or object—that is the contamination is transferred. Touching a contaminated patient, for example, can result in a contaminated care provider. Although gas exposure rarely results in secondary contamination, liquids and particulate matter are much more likely to be transferred.

4. **Describe topical, respiratory, gastrointestinal, and parenteral routes of exposure.** pp. 1865–1866

There are four ways in which a patient can be exposed to a hazardous substance. The most common method is respiratory inhalation. Gases, liquids, and particulate solids can all be inhaled through the nose or mouth. Once substances enter the bronchial tree, they can be quickly absorbed, especially in oxygen-deficient atmospheres. The substance then enters the central circulation system and is distributed throughout the body. As a result, inhaled substances often trigger a rapid onset of symptoms.

Toxic substances may also be introduced into the body through the skin, either by topical absorption or parenteral injection. Any toxic substance placed topically on intact skin and transferred into the person's circulation is considered a medical threat. In the case of injections, poisons directly enter the body via a laceration, a burn, or a puncture.

In hazmat situations, the least common route of exposure is through gastrointestinal ingestion. In occupations involving hazardous materials, people can be exposed to poisons by eating, drinking, or smoking around deadly substances. Foodstuffs can be exposed to a chemical and then eaten. People can forget to wash their hands and introduce the substance into their mouths.

5. **Explain acute and delayed toxicity, local versus systemic effects, dose response, and synergistic effects.** p. 1866

Basically, a poison's actions may be acute or delayed. Acute effects include those signs and symptoms that manifest themselves immediately or shortly after exposure. Delayed effects may not become apparent for hours, days, weeks, months, or even years.

Effects from a chemical may be local or systemic. Local effects involve areas around the immediate site and should be evaluated based upon the burn model. You can usually expect some skin irritation (topical) or perhaps acute bronchospasm (respiratory).

Systemic effects occur throughout the body. They can affect the cardiovascular, neurologic, hepatic, and/or renal systems.

Once a substance is introduced into the body, it is distributed to target organs. The organs most commonly associated with toxic substances are the liver and kidneys. The liver metabolizes most substances by chemically altering them through a process known as biotransformation. The kidneys can usually excrete the substances through the urine. However, both the liver and kidneys can be adversely affected by chemicals as are other organ systems. In such situations, the body may not be able to eliminate substances, creating a life-threatening situation.

When treating patients exposed to toxic substances, keep in mind that two substances or drugs may work together to produce an effect that neither of them can produce on its own. This effect, known as synergism, is part of the standard pharmacological approach to medicine. Before administering any medication, be sure to consult with medical direction or the poison control center on possible synergistic effects or treatments.

6. **Explain how the substance and route of contamination alters triage and decontamination methods.** pp. 1868–1869

See objective 1c.

680 ESSENTIALS OF PARAMEDIC CARE

7. Explain the employment and limitations of field decontamination procedures. pp. 1870–1871

The decontamination method and type of PPE depend upon the substance involved. If in doubt, assume the worst-case scenario. When dealing with unknowns, do not attempt to neutralize. Brush dry particles off the patient before the application of water to prevent possible chemical reactions. Next, wash with great quantities of water—the universal decon agent—using tincture of green soap, if possible. Isopropyl alcohol is an effective agent for some isocyanates, while vegetable oil can be used to decon taminate water-reactive substances.

As noted in objective 1d, field decontamination is never true contamination. Depending on the type of exposure, wounds may need debridement, hair or nails may need to be trimmed or removed, and so on. However, it is always better to deliver a grossly decontaminated living patient to the hospital than a perfectly decontaminated corpse. Just make sure that field-contaminated patients are transported to facilities capable of performing more thorough decon procedures.

8. Explain the use and limitations of personal protective equipment (PPE) in hazardous material situations. p. 1871

EMS personnel should not become involved in any hazmat situation without the proper PPE. All ambulances carry some level of PPE—even if not ideal. Hard hats, for example, protect rescuers against impacts to the head.

If the situation is emergent or the chemical unknown, use as much barrier protection as possible. Full turnout gear or a Tyvek suit is better than no gear at all. HEPA filter masks and double or triple gloves offer good protection against some hazards. Keep in mind that latex gloves are not chemically resistant. Instead, use nitrile gloves, which have a high resistance to most chemicals. Also remember that leather boots will absorb chemicals permanently, so be sure to don rubber boots.

In general, there are basically four levels of hazmat protective equipment, ranging from Level A (the highest level) to Level D (the minimum level).

- **Level A**—provides the highest level of respiratory and splash protection. This hazmat suit offers a high degree of chemical breakthrough time and fully encapsulates the rescuer, even covering the SCBA. The sealed, impermeable suits are typically used by hazmat teams entering the hot zones with an unknown substance and a significant potential for both respiratory and dermal hazards.
- **Level B**—offers full respiratory protection when there is a lower probability of dermal hazard. The Level B suit is nonencapsulating but chemically resistant. Seams for zippers, gloves, boots, and mask interface are usually sealed with duct tape. The SCBA is worn outside the suit, allowing increased maneuverability and greater ease in changing SCBA bottles. The decon team typically wears Level B protective equipment.
- **Level C**—includes a nonpermeable suit, boots, and gear for protecting eyes and hands. Instead of SCBA, Level C protective equipment uses an air-purifying respirator (APR). The APR relies on filters to protect against a known contaminant in a normal environment. As a result, the canisters in the APR must be specifically selected and are not usually implemented in a hazmat emergency response. Level C clothing is usually worn during transport of patients with the potential for secondary contamination.
- **Level D**—consists of structural firefighter, or turnout, gear. Level D gear is usually not suitable for hazmat incidents.

9. List and explain the common signs, symptoms, and treatment of exposures to: pp. 1866–1868

a. Corrosives (acids/alkalis)

Corrosives—acids and alkalis (bases)—can be inhaled, ingested, absorbed, or injected. Primary effects include severe skin burns and respiratory burns and/or edema. Some corrosives may also have systemic effects.

When decontaminating a patient exposed to solid corrosives, brush off dry particles. In the case of liquid corrosives, flush the exposed area with large quantities of water. Tincture of green soap may help in decontamination. Irrigate eye injuries with water, possibly using a topic ophthalmic anesthetic such as tetracaine to reduce eye discomfort. In patients with pulmonary edema, consider the administration of furosemide (Lasix) or albuterol. If the patient has ingested a corrosive, DO NOT induce vomiting. If the patient can swallow and is not drooling, you may direct the person to drink 5cc/kg water up to 200 cc. As with other injuries, maintain and support the ABCs.

b. Pulmonary irritants (ammonia/chlorine)

Many different substances can be pulmonary irritants, including the fumes from chlorine and ammonia. Primary respiratory exposure cannot be decontaminated. However, you should remove the patient's clothing to prevent any trapped gas from being contained near the body. You should also flush any exposed skin with large quantities of water. Irrigate eye injuries with water, possibly using tetracaine to reduce eye discomfort. Treat pulmonary edema with furosemide, if indicated. Again, treatment includes maintaining and supporting the ABCs.

c. Pesticides [(carbamates/organophosphates)]

Toxic pesticides or insecticides primarily include carbamates and organophosphates. These substances can act to block acetylcholinesterase (AChE)—an enzyme that stops the action of acetylcholine, a neurotransmitter. The result is overstimulation of the muscarinic receptors and the SLUDGE syndrome: salivation, lacrimation, urination, diarrhea, gastrointestinal distress, and emesis. Stimulation of the nicotinic receptor may also trigger involuntary contraction of the muscles and pinpoint pupils.

These chemicals will continue to be absorbed as long as they remain on the skin. As a result, decontamination with large amounts of water and tincture of green soap is essential. Remove all clothing and jewelry to prevent the chemical from being trapped against the skin. Maintain and support airway, breathing, and circulation. Secretions in the airway may need to be suctioned.

The primary treatment for significant exposure to pesticides is atropinization. The dose should be increased until the SLUDGE symptoms start to resolve. For carbamates, Pralidoxime is NOT recommended. If an adult patient presents with seizures, administer 5 to 10 mg of diazepam. DO NOT induce vomiting if the patient has ingested the chemical. However, if the patient can swallow and has an intact gag reflex, you can administer 5 cc/kg up to 200 cc of water.

d. Chemical asphyxiants [(cyanides/carbon monoxide)]

The most common chemical asphyxiants include carbon monoxide (CO) and cyanides such as bitter almond oil, hydrocyanic acid, potassium cyanide, wild cherry syrup, prussic acid, and nitroprusside. Keep in mind that both CO and cyanides are byproducts of combustion, so patients who present with smoke inhalation may need to be assessed for these substances as well.

These two chemicals have different actions once inhaled. Carbon monoxide has a high affinity for hemoglobin. As a result, it displaces oxygen in the red blood cells. Cyanides, on the other hand, inhibit the action of cytochrome oxidase. This enzyme complex enables oxygen to create the adenosine triphosphate (ATP) required for all muscle energy. Primary effects of CO exposure include changes in mental status and other signs of hypoxia such as chest pain, loss of consciousness, and seizures. Primary effects of cyanides include rapid onset of unconsciousness, seizures, and cardiopulmonary arrest.

Decontamination of patients exposed to CO and cyanide asphyxiants is usually unnecessary. However, they must be removed from the toxic environment without exposing rescuers to inhalation. Take off the patient's clothing to prevent entrapment of any toxic gases while maintaining airway, breathing, and circulatory support. Definitive treatment for CO inhalation is oxygenation. In some cases, it may be provided through hyperbaric therapy.

Definitive treatment for cyanide exposure can be provided by several interventions carried in a cyanide kit. Basically follow these steps:

- Administer an ampule of amyl nitrite for 15 seconds.
- Repeat at one-minute intervals until the sodium nitrite is ready.

- Administer an infusion of sodium nitrite, 300 mg IV push over 5 minutes.
- Follow with an infusion of sodium thiosulfate, 12.5 g IV push over 5 minutes.
- Repeat at half the original doses, if necessary.

e. Hydrocarbon solvents [(xylene, methylene chloride)]

Many different chemicals can act as solvents, including xylene and methylene chloride. Usually found in liquid form, they give off easily inhaled vapors. Primary effects include dysrhythmias, pulmonary edema, and respiratory failure. Delayed effects include damage to the central nervous system and the renal system. If the patient ingests the chemical and vomits, aspiration may lead to pulmonary edema.

Treatment varies with the route of exposure. In cases of topical contact, decontaminate the exposed area with large quantities of warm water and tincture of green soap. If the patient has ingested the solvent, DO NOT induce vomiting. If the adult patient presents with seizures, administer 5–10 mg diazepam. In the case of inhalation, maintain and support the ABCs.

10. Describe the characteristics of hazardous materials and explain their importance to the risk assessment process. pp. 1857, 1858–1863, 1869–1870

Keep in mind the definition of hazardous materials offered by the DOT. A hazardous material can be regarded as "any substance which may pose an unreasonable risk to health and safety of operating or emergency personnel, the public, and/or the environment if not properly controlled during handling, storage, manufacture, processing, packaging, use, disposal, and transportation."

Some of the characteristics that will be important to consider when doing a risk assessment of chemicals include a material's boiling point, flammable/explosive limits, flash point, ignition temperature, specific gravity, vapor density, vapor pressure, and water solubility.

These characteristics, as well as other on-scene factors and substance-specific qualities, will help you decide the best and safest mode of operation. In general, you will engage in either "fast-break" or long-term decision making. Fast-break decision making occurs at incidents that call for immediate action to prevent rescuer contamination and/or to handle obvious life threats. Long-term decision making takes place at extended events in which hazmat teams retrieve patients, identify the substance(s), and determine methods of decontamination and treatment.

11. Describe the hazards and protection strategies for alpha, beta, and gamma radiation. pp. 1864–1865

The levels of radiation and strategies for protection from their particles include:

- **Alpha radiation**—neutrons and protons released by the nucleus of a radioactive substance. These are very weak particles and will only travel a few inches in the air. Alpha particles are stopped by paper, clothing, or intact skin. They are hazardous if inhaled or ingested.
- **Beta radiation**—electrons released with great energy by a radioactive substance. Beta particles have more energy than alpha particles and will travel 6 to 10 feet in the air. Beta particles will penetrate a few millimeters of skin.
- **Gamma radiation**—high-energy photons, such as X-rays. Gamma rays have the ability to penetrate most substances and to damage any cells within the body. Heavy shielding is needed for protection against gamma rays. Because gamma rays are electromagnetic (instead of particles), no decontamination is required.

(For more information on the hazards of and protection strategies for these types of radiation, see Chapter 49.)

12. Define the toxicologic terms and their use in the risk assessment process. p. 1865

Here are the most important toxicological terms used in the field during the risk assessment process:

- **Threshold limit value/time weighted average (TLV/TWA)**—maximum concentration of a substance in the air that a person can be exposed to for 8 hours each day, 40 hours per week, without suffering any adverse health effects. The lower the TLV/TWA, the more toxic the substance. The Permissible Exposure Limit (PEL) is a similar measure of toxicity.

- **Threshold limit value/short-term exposure limit (TLV/STEL)**—maximum concentration of a substance that a person can be exposed to for 15 minutes (time weighted), not to be exceeded or repeated more than four times daily with 60-minute rests between each of the four exposures.
- **Threshold limit value/ceiling level (TLV-CL)**—maximum concentration of a substance that should never be exceeded, even for a moment.
- **Lethal concentration/lethal doses (LCt/LD)**—concentration (in air) or dose (if ingested, injected, or absorbed) that results in the death of 50 percent of the test subjects. Also referred to as the LCt50 or LD50.
- **Parts per million/parts per billion (ppm/ppb)**—representation of the concentration of a substance in the air or a solution, with parts of the substance expressed per million or billion parts of the air or solution.
- **Immediately dangerous to life and health (IDLH)**—level of concentration of a substance that causes an immediate threat to life. It may also cause delayed or irreversible effects or interfere with a person's ability to remove himself or herself from the contaminated area.

13. Given a specific hazardous material, research the appropriate information about its physical and chemical properties and hazards, suggest the appropriate medical response, and determine the risk of secondary contamination.   pp. 1862–1863

Once you have identified the hazardous material, it is necessary to research the appropriate information about the physical and chemical properties and hazards and then determine the appropriate medical response and any risk of secondary decontamination. It is strongly suggested that a number of resources be consulted in developing the plan of action. The resources include, but are not limited to, those listed in objective 2.

14. Identify the factors that determine where and when to treat a hazardous material incident patient.   pp. 1863, 1869–1870

As noted in objective 10, EMS personnel generally engage in one of two modes of operation at hazmat incidents that generate patients: "fast-break" or long-term decision making.

Fast-break decision making
At hazmat incidents where patients are conscious, contaminated victims will often self-rescue. They will walk themselves from the primary incident site to the EMS unit. In such cases, you must make fast-break decisions to prevent rescuer contamination. Keep in mind that it may take time for a hazmat team to arrive and set up operations. In the interim, the conscious, contaminated patients may try to leave the scene entirely. As a result, all EMS units must be prepared for gross decontamination. Basic personal protection equipment should be on board and all personnel should be familiar with the two-step decontamination procedures (see objective 16).

Implement this mode of decision making at all incidents with critical patients and unknown life-threatening materials. Fire apparatus often respond very quickly and carry large quantities of water that can be used for decon. Remove patient clothing, treat life-threatening problems, and wash with water. While it is preferable to use warm water to prevent hypothermia, this option is not always available. Please remember that the first rule of EMS is NOT TO BECOME A PATIENT! At no time should you and other crew members expose yourselves to contaminants—even to rescue a critically injured patient. Instead, contain and isolate the patient as best as possible until the proper support arrives.

Long-term decision making
At more extended events, you will engage in long-term decision making. Traditionally, EMS personnel have not been trained or equipped to enter a contaminated area to retrieve patients. Instead, a hazmat team is summoned promptly, and the EMS crew awaits the team's arrival. The team will

not make their entry until you or members of your crew perform the necessary medical monitoring and establish a decontamination corridor (see below). It often takes 60 minutes or more for actual team deployment.

Typically, three zones will be established at a hazmat incident:

- **Hot (red) zone:** This zone, also known as the exclusionary zone, is the site of contamination. Prevent anyone from entering this area unless they have the appropriate high-level PPE. Hold any patients that escape from this zone in the next zone, where contamination and/or treatment will be performed.
- **Warm (yellow) zone:** This zone, also called the contamination reduction zone, lies immediately adjacent to the hot zone. It forms a "buffer zone" in which a decontamination corridor is established for patients and decontamination personnel leaving the hot zone. The corridor has both a "hot" and a "cold" end.
- **Cold (green) zone:** The cold zone, or "safe zone," is the area where the incident operation takes place. It includes the command post, medical monitoring and rehabilitation, treatment areas, and apparatus staging. The cold zone must be free of any contamination. No people or equipment from the hot zone should enter until undergoing the necessary decontamination. You and your crew should remain inside this zone unless you have the necessary training, equipment, and support to enter other areas.

15. **Determine the appropriate level of PPE for various hazardous material incidents including:**   p. 1871

   a. **Types, application, use, and limitations**
   See objective 8.

   b. **Use of a chemical compatibility chart**
   When chemicals can be identified, consult a permeability chart to determine the breakthrough time on a hazmat site. No single material is suitable to all hazmat situations. Some materials are resistant to certain chemicals and nonresistant to others.

16. **Explain decontamination procedures including:**   p. 1870

   a. **Critical patient rapid two-step decontamination process**
   Use the two-step decon process for gross decontamination of patients who cannot wait for a more comprehensive decon process, usually patients at a fast-break incident. Remove all clothing, including shoes, socks, and jewelry. (Remember to have some method of accounting for personal effects BEFORE hazmat incidents occur.) Wash and rinse the patients with soap and water, making sure that they do not stay in the run-off. Repeat the process, paying particular attention to the body areas noted in objective 18.

   b. **Noncritical patient eight-step decontamination process**
   The eight-step process takes place in a complete decontamination corridor and is much more thorough. To leave the hot zone, the hazmat rescuers follow these steps:

   - **Step 1:** Rescuers enter the decon area at the hot end of corridor and mechanically remove contamination from the victims.
   - **Step 2:** Rescuers drop equipment in a tool-drop area and remove outer gloves.
   - **Step 3:** Decon personnel shower and scrub all victims and rescuers, using gross decontamination techniques. As surface contamination is removed, the run-off is conducted into a contained area. Victims may be moved ahead to Step 6 or Step 7.
   - **Step 4:** Rescuers remove and isolate their SCBA. If reentry is necessary, the team dons new SCBA from a noncontaminated side.
   - **Step 5:** Rescuers remove all protective clothing. Articles are isolated, labeled for disposal, and placed on the contaminated side.
   - **Step 6:** Rescuers remove all personal clothing. Victims who have not had their clothing removed have it taken off here. All items are isolated in plastic bags and labeled for later disposal or storage.
   - **Step 7:** Rescuers and patients receive a full-body washing, using soft scrub brushes or sponges, water, and mild soap or detergent. Cleaning tools are bagged for later disposal.

- **Step 8:** Patients receive rapid assessment and stabilization before being transported to hospitals for further care. EMS crews medically monitor rescuers, complete exposure records, and transport rescuers to hospitals as needed.

These procedures are not set in stone. Small variations may exist from system to system. You should become familiar with the specific procedures in the jurisdiction where you work.

17. Identify the four most common solutions used for decontamination. p. 1870

The most common solutions used for decontamination are water, tincture of green soap, isopropyl alcohol, and vegetable oil.

18. Identify the body areas that are difficult to decontaminate. p. 1870

Body areas that are difficult to decontaminate include:

- Scalp and hair
- Ears
- Nostrils
- Axilla
- Fingernails
- Navel
- Genitals
- Groin
- Buttocks
- Behind the knees
- Between the toes
- Toenails

19. Explain the medical monitoring procedures for hazardous material team members. p. 1872

Entry readiness
Prior to entry, you or other EMS crew members will assess rescuers and document the following information on an incident flow sheet: blood pressure, pulse, respiratory rate, temperature, body weight, ECG, and mental/neurologic status. If you observe anything abnormal, do not allow the hazmat team member to attempt a rescue.

After-exit "rehab"
After the hazmat team exits the hot zone and completes decontamination, they should report back to EMS for post-entry monitoring. Measure and document the same parameters on the flow sheet. Rehydrate the team with more water or diluted sports drink. You can use weight changes to estimate fluid losses. Check with medical direction or protocols to determine fluid replacement by means of PO or IV. Entry teams should not be allowed to reenter the hot zone until they are alert, nontachycardic, normotensive, and within a reasonable percentage of their normal body weight.

20. Explain the factors that influence the heat stress of hazardous material team personnel. p. 1872

To evaluate heat stress, you will need to take into account many factors. Primary considerations include ambient temperature and humidity. Prehydration, duration and degree of activity, and the team member's overall physical fitness will also have a bearing on your evaluation. Keep in mind that Level A suits protect a rescuer, but prevent cooling. A rescuer essentially works inside an encapsulated sauna. The same suit that seals out hazards also prevents heat loss by evaporation, conduction, convection, and radiation. Therefore, place heat stress at the top of your list of tasks for post-exit medical monitoring.

21. **Explain the documentation necessary for hazmat medical monitoring and rehabilitation operations.** p. 1872

   The documentation for hazmat medical monitoring and rehabilitation operations should include the following: blood pressure, pulse, respiratory rate, temperature, body weight, ECG, and mental status. (See objective 19.)

22. **Given a simulated hazardous substance, use reference material to determine the appropriate actions.** pp. 1862–1863

   Begin by collecting any information provided on the placards—numbers, symbols, colors, and so on. Then use several of the references identified in objective 2 to augment this information. Become familiar with the latest edition of the Emergency Response Guidebook, which should be aboard the EMS unit at all times.

23. **Integrate the principles and practices of hazardous materials response in an effective manner to prevent and limit contamination, morbidity, and mortality.** pp. 1857–1872

   As a paramedic, you will play an important role at any hazmat incident. You may establish command, make the first incident decisions, and help protect all on-scene personnel, including the hazmat team. As a result, you should practice skills that you can expect to use in most hazmat incidents.

   Here are some things that you should routinely do. Put on and take off Level B hazmat protective equipment. Set up a rapid two-step decontamination process and an eight-step decontamination process, preferably with the help of the local hazmat team. With a crew member, identify a simulated chemical, determine the correct PPE, and establish the proper decontamination methods. Practice preentry and post-exit medical monitoring and documentation. Prepare a patient and ambulance for transport. As these skills may be rarely used except in the busiest EMS systems, you should work closely with your local hazmat team to practice these skills on a regular basis.

24. **Size up a hazardous material (hazmat) incident and determine:** pp. 1858–1863, 1865–1871

   a. **Potential hazards to the rescuers, public, and environment**

   Sizing up a hazmat incident is a very difficult task. You often receive inaccurate or incomplete information. Plus events tend to develop very quickly during each phase of the incident. Also, you can expect other agencies to be involved in the event.

   As indicated in objective 1a, you must remember that almost every emergency response has the potential for hazardous materials. For example, most households keep ammonia and liquid bleach in the kitchen or laundry room. When combined, these substances can produce a toxic gas. Homes with kerosene heaters or blocked flues can be filled with carbon monoxide. Don't take any chances. Always keep the possibility of dangerous substances in mind whenever you approach the scene of an emergency.

   Transportation incidents. Be especially wary of any transportation accident—automobile, truck, or railroad. Maintain a high degree of hazmat awareness whenever you are summoned to MVCs involving commercial vehicles, pest control vehicles, tanker trucks, tractor-trailers, or cars powered by alternative fuels. Do not rule out the presence of hazardous materials just because you do not see a warning placard. Hospitals and laboratories, for example, routinely and legally transport medical radioactive isotopes in unmarked passenger cars.

   Railroad accidents merit special attention for two reasons. First, railroad cars can carry large quantities of hazardous materials. Second, there may be several tank cars hitched together on a freight train. Obviously there is a greater chance for a major incident if one or more of these tanks rupture during an accident.

   Incidents at fixed facilities. Hazmat incidents can take place in a variety of fixed facilities where hazardous substances are stored. Chemical plants and all manufacturing operations have tanks, storage vessels, and pipelines used to transport products and/or wastes. Additional fixed sites with possible hazardous materials include warehouses, hardware or agricultural stores, water treatment centers, and loading docks. If you work in a rural area, keep in mind the number of places where you can find hazardous materials on a farm or ranch—silos, barns, greenhouses, and more.

Terrorist incidents. As a last note, remember that a new type of hazmat incident has emerged in recent years in the form of terrorism. The terrorists may use any variety of chemical, biological, or nuclear devices to strike at government or high-profile targets.

b. Potential risk of primary contamination to patients

In sizing up a hazmat incident (real or simulated), remember that whenever people or equipment come in contact with potentially toxic substances they should be considered contaminated. Direct contact, as indicated in objective 3, means primary contamination.

c. Potential risk of secondary contamination to rescuers

See objectives 3 and 14. Keep in mind the high risk of secondary contaminations to rescuers in "fast-break" situations.

25. Given a contaminated patient, determine the level of decontamination necessary and: pp. 1866–1871

a. Level of rescuer PPE

See objective 8 for the information that you will be applying.

b. Decontamination methods

See objectives 1c, 7, 9, 16, 17, and 18 for the information that you will be applying.

c. Treatment

See objectives 1d, 5, 9, and 14 for the information that you will be applying.

d. Transportation and patient isolation techniques

See objective 1e for the information that you will be applying.

26. Determine the hazards present to the patient and paramedic given an incident involving a hazardous material. pp. 1857–1872

During your classroom, clinical, and field training, you will given a chance to participate in, or observe, all of the phases of a hazmat incident. Use the information presented in this text chapter, the information on hazardous materials presented by your instructors, and guidance given by your clinical and field preceptors to develop good safety skills at a hazmat incident. Continue to refine these skills once your training ends and you begin your career as a paramedic.

Content Self-Evaluation

MULTIPLE CHOICE

_____ 1. Upon arriving at the scene of a potential hazmat incident, the first step you should take is to:
  A. size up the scene.
  B. don PPE.
  C. activate the IMS.
  D. refer to OSHA CFR 1910.120.
  E. establish command.

_____ 2. Which first responders need to be trained to the hazmat Awareness Level?
  A. all EMS personnel
  B. police officers
  C. firefighters
  D. A and C
  E. A, B, and C

_____ 3. The most preferable site for deploying resources at a hazmat scene is:
  A. uphill and downwind.
  B. uphill and upwind.
  C. across the street from the incident.
  D. one mile away.
  E. 100 yards away.

_____ 4. The basic IMS at a hazmat incident will require all of the following EXCEPT a:
   A. staging area.
   B. decontamination corridor.
   C. transport zone.
   D. command post.
   E. treatment area.

_____ 5. One of the most critical aspects of any hazmat response is:
   A. working with unified command.
   B. establishing the time the incident began.
   C. transporting all patients who have been exposed.
   D. the awareness that a dangerous substance is present.
   E. treating critically injured patients.

_____ 6. A diamond-shaped graphic placed on vehicles to indicate hazard classification is a(n):
   A. placard.
   B. MSDS.
   C. UN number sign.
   D. NFPA label.
   E. ERG.

_____ 7. One of the most difficult aspects of dealing with a hazmat incident is:
   A. reading hazmat references.
   B. identifying the particular substance.
   C. working with uncooperative patients.
   D. establishing EMS command.
   E. communicating with the media.

_____ 8. Data sheets containing detailed information about all potentially hazardous substances found at a work site are called:
   A. placards.
   B. MSDS.
   C. UN number signs.
   D. NFPA labels.
   E. reactivity data sheets.

_____ 9. Shipping papers that contain accurate information about a transported substance are known as:
   A. transport vouchers.
   B. MSDS.
   C. bills of lading.
   D. cargo filing.
   E. special protection information.

_____ 10. Hazmat monitoring devices should be routinely used by EMS personnel for quick identification of a substance.
   A. True
   B. False

_____ 11. Which safety zone is also called the contamination reduction or buffer zone?
   A. hot zone
   B. warm zone
   C. cold zone
   D. treatment zone
   E. extrication zone

_____ 12. Which of the following is least likely to result in secondary contamination?
   A. acids and alkalis
   B. carbon monoxide
   C. organophosphates
   D. liquid corrosives
   E. carbamates

_____ 13. In hazmat situations, the least common route(s) of exposure is (are) through:
   A. respiratory inhalation.
   B. parenteral injection.
   C. topical absorption.
   D. gastrointestinal ingestion.
   E. both A and C

_____ 14. In a hazmat situation, the most common route(s) of exposure is (are) through:
   A. respiratory inhalation.
   B. parenteral injection.
   C. topical absorption.
   D. gastrointestinal ingestion.
   E. both B and D

_____ 15. If a patient was exposed to a hazardous gas and developed acute bronchospasm, this could be called a _____ effect.
   A. local
   B. systemic
   C. biotransformation
   D. synergistic
   E. secondary

_____ 16. The most common route of exposure of cyanides is through inhalation, although cyanides can also be ingested, absorbed, or injected.
   A. True
   B. False

_____ 17. Definitive treatment for CO inhalation is:
   A. oxygenation.
   B. hyperbaric therapy.
   C. use of a cyanide kit.
   D. infusion of sodium thiosulfate.
   E. none of the above

_____ 18. All of the following are methods of decontamination EXCEPT:
   A. stabilization.
   B. dilution.
   C. absorption.
   D. isolation.
   E. neutralization.

_____ 19. Which priority should guide your decision making while performing decontamination?
   A. life safety
   B. incident stabilization
   C. property conservation
   D. triage
   E. neutralization

_____ 20. All the following are common decontamination solvents EXCEPT:
   A. water.
   B. tincture of green soap.
   C. isopropyl alcohol.
   D. baking soda.
   E. vegetable oil.

_____ 21. Two methods for decontamination in the field are the:
   A. two-step and twelve-step processes.
   B. complete and incomplete methods.
   C. gross decon and neutralizing methods.
   D. two-step and eight-step processes.
   E. fast-break and long-term methods.

_____ 22. The lowest level of hazmat protective equipment is:
   A. Level A.
   B. Level B.
   C. Level C.
   D. Level D.
   E. Level E.

_____ 23. The highest level of hazmat protective equipment uses a(n):
   A. HEPA filter mask.
   B. air-purifying respirator.
   C. SCBA.
   D. SCUBA.
   E. PBI flash protector.

_____ 24. Which of the following should be consulted to determine the breakthrough time of a specific chemical on a hazmat suit?
   A. CAMEO website
   B. Emergency Response Guidebook
   C. permeability chart
   D. OSHA publication CFR 1910.120
   E. NFPA table

_____ 25. One of the primary roles of EMS personnel at a hazmat incident is medical monitoring of entry personnel.
   A. True
   B. False

MATCHING

Write the letter of the term in the space provided next to the appropriate description.

A. boiling point   F. ignition temperature
B. warm zone   G. cold zone
C. CHEMTREC   H. warning placard
D. hazardous material   I. MSDS
E. flash point   J. hot zone

_____ 26. any substance that causes adverse health effects upon human exposure
_____ 27. diamond-shaped graphic placed on vehicles to indicate hazmat classification
_____ 28. easily accessible sheets of detailed information about chemicals found at fixed facilities
_____ 29. Chemical Transportation Emergency Center, which maintains a 24-hour toll-free hazmat information hotline
_____ 30. the location where the hazardous material and the highest levels of contamination exist
_____ 31. the location where the decontamination corridor should be set up
_____ 32. the area at a hazardous material incident where the command post and sectors are set up
_____ 33. the lowest temperature at which a liquid will give off enough vapors to ignite
_____ 34. the temperature at which a liquid becomes a gas
_____ 35. the lowest temperature at which a liquid will give off enough vapors to support combustion

Part 5: Crime Scene Awareness

Review of Chapter Objectives

After reading Part 5 of this chapter, you should be able to:

1. **Explain how EMS providers are often mistaken for the police.**   pp. 1873–1878

   Depending upon your uniform colors and the use of badges, people might mistake you for the police—especially if you exit from a vehicle with flashing lights and a siren. They might expect you to intervene in a violent situation, or they might direct aggression toward you as an authority figure.

   When entering gang territory, you are especially at risk if your uniform resembles that of the police. Gangs with a history of arrest may in fact make every effort to prevent you from transporting one of their members to a hospital or any other place beyond their reach. Do not force the situation if your safety is at stake.

2. **Explain specific techniques for risk reduction when approaching the following types of routine EMS scenes:** pp. 1873–1879

   a. **Highway encounters**
   To make a safe approach to a vehicle at a roadside emergency, follow these steps:
   - Park the ambulance in a position that provides safety from traffic.
   - Notify dispatch of the situation, location, the vehicle make and model, and the state and number of the license plate.
   - Use a one-person approach. The driver should remain in the ambulance, which is elevated and provides greater visibility.
   - The driver should remain prepared to radio for immediate help and to back or drive away rapidly once the other medic returns.
   - At nighttime, use the ambulance lights to illuminate the vehicle. However, do not walk between the ambulance and the other vehicle. You will be backlit, forming an easy target.
   - Since police approach vehicles from the driver's side, you should approach from the passenger's side, which is an unexpected route.
   - Use the A, B, and C door posts for cover.
   - Observe the rear seat. Do not move forward of the C post unless you are sure there are no threats in the rear seat or foot wells.
   - Retreat to the ambulance (or another strategic position of cover) at the first sign of danger.
   - Make sure you have mapped out your intended retreat and escape with the ambulance driver.

   b. **Violent street incidents**
   You can encounter many different types of violence while working on the streets. Incidents can range from random acts of violence against individual citizens to organized efforts at domestic or international terrorism. In responding to the scene of any violent crime, keep these precautions in mind:
   - Dangerous weapons may have been used in the crime.
   - Perpetrators may still be on scene or could return on scene.
   - Patients may sometimes exhibit violence toward EMS personnel, particularly if they risk criminal penalties as a result of the original incident.

   When on the streets, you must remain constantly aware of crowd dynamics. Crowds can quickly become larger and volatile, especially in the case of a hate crime. Violence can be directed against anyone or anything in the path of an angry crowd. Your status as an EMS provider does not give you immunity against an out-of-control mob. Whenever a crowd is present, look for these warning signs of impending danger:
   - Shouts or increasingly loud voices
   - Pushing or shoving
   - Hostilities toward anyone on scene, including the perpetrator of a crime, the victim, police, and so on
   - Rapid increase in crowd size
   - Inability of law enforcement officials to control bystanders

   To protect yourself, constantly monitor the crowd and retreat if necessary. If possible, take the patient with you so that you do not have to return later. Rapid transport may require limited or tactical assessment at the scene, with more in-depth assessment done inside the safety of the ambulance. Be sure to document reasons for the quick assessment and transport.

   c. **Residences and "dark houses"**
   Domestic violence needs to be a consideration whenever you approach a residence and detect yelling, screaming, or any other signs of fighting. Sometimes you might spot clues such as broken glass or blood on the sidewalk. If you approach a "dark house," especially one where the front door is ajar, be very cautious—it could be a set-up. In such cases, ask the dispatcher to call the residence and request that occupants turn on lights and meet you at the front door, if possible. When entering a residence, look around for any potential weapons that may be used against you. If you are unsure of the safety of the scene, call for police backup. If there is a fight going on as you approach the residence, retreat and request police to secure the scene.

3. **Describe the warning signs of potentially violent situations.** pp. 1873–1877

You should remain alert throughout a call, especially in areas with a history of violence. You may enter the scene and spot weapons or drugs. Additional combative people may arrive on the scene. The patient or bystanders may become agitated or threatening. Even if treatment has begun, you must place your own safety first. You may have just two tactical options: quickly package the patient and leave the scene with the patient or retreat without the patient.

4. **Explain emergency evasive techniques for potentially violent situations, including:** pp. 1873–1883

    a. **Threats of physical violence**
    See objectives 2, 5, and 6.

    b. **Firearms encounters**
    See objectives 5b and 6c.

    c. **Edged weapons encounters**
    Your best tactical response to an edged weapon is observation. If you suspect violence with any kind of weapon, stay out of danger in the first place—that is retreat. Ideally you will retreat to the ambulance so that you can summon help. If the attacker pursues you, follow the evasive strategies listed in objective 6c.

5. **Explain EMS considerations for the following types of violent or potentially violent situations:** pp. 1873–1879

    a. **Gangs and gang violence**
    Street gangs can be found in big cities, suburban towns, and, lately, in rural communities. No EMS unit is totally immune from gang activity. In fact, some gangs have purposely branched out into smaller towns in an effort to escape surveillance and expand their illicit businesses. Commonly observed gang characteristics include:
    - **Appearance:** Gang members frequently wear unique clothing specific to the group. Because the clothing is often a particular color or hue, it is referred to as the gang's "colors." Wearing a color, even a bandana, can signify gang membership. Within the gang itself, members sometimes wear different articles to signify rank.
    - **Graffiti:** Gangs have definite territories or "turfs." Members often mark their turf with graffiti broadcasting the gang's logo, warning away intruders, bragging about crimes, insulting rival gangs, or taunting police.
    - **Tattoos:** Many gang members wear tattoos or other body markings to identify their gang affiliation. Some gangs even require these tattoos. The tattoos will be in the gang's colors and often contain the gang's motto or logo.
    - **Hand signals/language:** Gangs commonly create their own methods of communication. They give gang-related meanings to everyday words or create codes. Hand signals provide quick identification among gang members, warn of approaching law enforcement, or show disrespect to other gangs. Gang members often perform signals so quickly that an uninformed outsider may not spot them, much less understand them.

    Always remember that gang members are usually armed and expect your respect. Do not cut their "colors" or clothing without permission, or you will be displaying a public show of disrespect. Finally, keep in mind the attitudes toward authority mentioned in objective 1.

    b. **Hostages/sniper situations**
    The provision of care in hostage/sniper situations often necessitates risks far beyond those found on most EMS calls. Medical personnel assigned to such incidents require special training and authorization. Like hazmat teams, they must don special equipment, function with compact gear, and, in most cases, work as medical adjuncts to the police or military.

    If you find yourself in one of these situations, be sure to stage your ambulance outside the "kill zone," or the range of a typical rifle. If you are unsure of the distance, ask the police. Do not approach the scene, as you may end up being taken as a hostage also.

A good precaution for any dangerous situation is the use of prearranged verbal and nonverbal clues. Be sure to alert dispatch to the meaning of spoken clues. Choose signals that indicate a variety of circumstances while sounding harmless to an attacker. This can be a life-saving technique in situations where you find yourself, the crew, and/or the patient held hostage. Your so-called "routine" radio reports can spell out the nature of the trouble and summon help from a Special Weapons and Tactics (SWAT) team.

c. Clandestine drug labs

Drug raids on clandestine ("clan") labs have a way of turning into hazmat operations. All too often, the labs contain toxic fumes and volatile chemicals. The people on scene complicate matters by fighting or shooting at the rescuers who come to extricate them from the toxic environment. As they retreat, drug dealers may also trigger booby traps or wait for police or EMS personnel to trigger them. If you ever come upon a clan lab, take these actions:

- Leave the area immediately.
- Do not touch anything.
- Never stop any chemical reactions already in progress.
- Do not smoke or bring any source of flame near the lab.
- Notify the police.
- Initiate ICS and hazmat procedures.
- Consider evacuation of the area.

Remember that laboratories can be found anywhere—on farms, in trailers, in city apartments, and more. They may be mobile, roaming from place to place in a camper or a truck. Or they may be disassembled and stored in almost any variety of locations. The job of raiding clan labs belongs to specialized personnel—not EMS.

d. Domestic violence

Domestic violence involves people who live together in an intimate relationship. The violence may be physical, emotional, sexual, verbal, or economic. It may be directed against a spouse or partner, or it may involve children and/or older relatives who live at the residence.

When called to the scene of domestic violence, the abuser may turn on you or other members of the crew. You have two main concerns: your own personal safety and protection of the patient from further harm. For more on the indications of domestic violence and the appropriate actions of EMS crews, see Chapter 44, "Abuse and Assault."

e. Emotionally disturbed people

The prudent strategy is to retreat whenever you spot indicators of violence or physical confrontations with an emotionally disturbed person. Conduct the retreat in a calm but decisive manner. Be aware that the danger is now at your back and integrate cover into your retreat. For information on emotionally disturbed patients, see Chapter 38.

6. Explain the following techniques: pp. 1879–1883

a. Field "contact and cover" procedures during assessment and care

The concept of "contact and cover" comes from a police procedure developed in San Diego, California. When adapted to EMS practice, the procedure assigns the roles shown in the following table.

Contact Provider	*Cover Provider*
Initiates and provides direct patient care.	Observes the scene for danger while the "contact" cares for the patient.
Performs patient assessment.	Generally avoids patient care duties that would prevent observation of the scene.
Handles most interpersonal scene contact.	In small crews, may perform limited functions such as handling equipment.

As with any tactic adopted from another discipline, contact and cover has obvious correlations and drawbacks. The tactic is ideal for street encounters with intoxicated persons or subjects acting in a suspicious manner. An obvious drawback is that two medics working on a cardiac arrest will not be able to designate one person to act solely as a "cover" medic.

Perhaps the best application of this police procedure to EMS is its emphasis on the importance of observation and teamwork. A crew that works well together will assign roles—formally or informally—to guarantee safety and patient care. In its most basic form, contact and cover means that you will watch your partner's back while he or she watches yours.

b. Evasive tactics

Some specific techniques to avoid violence include:
- Throwing equipment to trip, slow, or distract an aggressor
- Wedging a stretcher in a doorway to block an attacker
- Using an unconventional path while retreating
- Anticipating the moves of the aggressor and taking counter moves
- Overturning objects in the path of the attacker
- Using preplanned tactics with your partner to confuse or "throw off" an aggressor

Key to the success of these safety tactics is your own physical well-being. Regular exercise and good health ensure that you will have the strength to outrun or, if necessary, defend yourself against an attacker. Some units provide basic training in self-defense or have protocols on its use. Make sure you take advantage of this training and/or know the protocols related to the application of force.

c. Concealment techniques

When faced with danger, two of your most immediate and practical strategies are cover and concealment. Concealment hides your body, as when you crouch behind bushes, wallboards, or vehicle doors. However, most common objects do not stop bullets. During armed encounters, seek cover by hiding your body behind solid and impenetrable objects such as brick walls, rocks, large trees, telephone poles, and the engine block of vehicles.

For cover and concealment to work, they must be used properly. In applying these safety tactics, keep in mind the following general rules.

- As you approach any scene, remain aware of the surroundings and any potential sources of protection in case you must retreat or are "pinned down."
- Choose your cover carefully. You may have only one chance to pick your protection. Select the item that hides your body adequately while shielding you against bullets.
- Once you have made your choice of cover, conceal as much of your body as possible. Be conscious of any reflective clothing that you may be wearing. Armed assailants can use it as a target, especially at night.
- Constantly look to improve your protection and location.

7. Describe police evidence considerations and techniques to assist in evidence preservation. pp. 1883–1885

When on the scene of a call where a crime has been committed, the paramedic should never jeopardize patient care for the sake of evidence. However, do not perform patient care with disregard of the criminal investigation that will follow. Remember that EMS and the police are on the same side—so work together. If you are the first person on the scene of a crime, be aware that anything you touch, walk on, pick up, cut, wipe off, or move could be evidence. Developing an awareness of evidence will even affect the way you treat patients. You will need to observe the patient carefully and to disturb as little direct evidence as possible. Also, when examining a patient, remember that you may be at risk. The patient may have a concealed weapon, such as a knife or gun.

Types of Evidence

Gathering evidence is a specialized and time-consuming job. While it is unrealistic to train EMS personnel in the details of police work, it is not unrealistic to ask them to develop an awareness of the general types of evidence that they may expect to encounter at a crime scene. Some of the main categories of evidence include prints, blood and body fluids, and particulate evidence.

On-Scene Observations

Everything that you and other members of the EMS crew see and hear can serve as evidence. Your observations on the scene will become part of the police record—and ultimately part of the court record. Be sure to look for and record the following information:

- Conditions at the scene—absence or presence of lights, locked or unlocked doors, open or closed curtains, and so on
- Position of the patient/victim

- Injuries suffered by the patient/victim
- Statements of persons on the scene
- Statements by the patient/victim
- Dying declarations
- Suspicious persons at, or fleeing from, the scene
- Presence and/or location of any weapons

Documenting Evidence

Record only the facts at the scene of a crime and record them accurately. Otherwise, they might be thrown out of court as evidence. Use quotation marks to indicate the words of bystanders and any remarks made by the patient. Avoid opinions not relevant to patient care. If the patient has died, do not offer any judgments that might contradict later findings by the medical examiner.

Finally, follow local policies and regulations regarding confidentiality surrounding any crime case. Any offhand remarks that you make might later become testimony in a courtroom, along with other documents that you prepare at the scene.

8. **Given several crime scene scenarios, identify potential hazards and determine if the scene is safe to enter, then provide care preserving the crime scene as appropriate.** pp. 1872–1885

During your classroom, clinical, and field training, you will have a chance to practice your approach to violent or potentially violent crime scenes. Use the information presented in this text chapter, the information on crime scene awareness presented by your instructors, and the guidance given by your clinical and field preceptors to develop the skills to protect yourself and your partner, as well as to preserve on-scene evidence. Continue to refine these skills once your training ends and you begin your career as a paramedic.

Content Self-Evaluation

MULTIPLE CHOICE

_____ 1. According to the Division of Violence Prevention at the National Center for Injury Prevention, arrest rates for homicide, rape, robbery, and aggravated assault are consistently higher for people ages:
   A. 10 to 14.
   B. 15 to 34.
   C. 35 to 50.
   D. 51 to 65.
   E. over age 65.

_____ 2. A computer-aided dispatch (CAD) program can assist in preventing an attack on EMS personnel by:
   A. predicting when crimes are most likely to occur.
   B. noting addresses with a history of violence.
   C. maintaining a list of known criminals.
   D. linking an EMS unit to a special forces team.
   E. all of the above

_____ 3. The EMS unit should follow the police units to the scene.
   A. True
   B. False

_____ 4. One of the main purposes of the scene survey at a crime scene is to search for:
   A. possible evidence.
   B. alleged assailants.
   C. hazards.
   D. law enforcement officials.
   E. a way to rescue the victim.

_____ 5. Even if a scene has been declared secure by the police, violence may still occur.
   A. True
   B. False

_____ 6. When approaching a residence that may be hazardous, you should:
   A. be careful not to backlight yourself.
   B. hold your flashlight to the side.
   C. take an unconventional approach to the door.
   D. keep your partner in sight.
   E. all of the above

_____ 7. Before knocking on the door, you should do all of the following EXCEPT:
   A. stand on the hinge side of the door.
   B. listen for loud noises.
   C. listen for items breaking.
   D. listen for the lack of any sounds at all.
   E. look in the windows for the presence of weapons.

_____ 8. If you must defend yourself, use the maximum amount of force possible.
   A. True
   B. False

_____ 9. To make a safe approach to a suspicious roadside emergency, you should take all of the following safety steps EXCEPT:
   A. use a one-person approach.
   B. use the ambulance lights to illuminate the vehicle.
   C. approach the vehicle from the driver's side.
   D. use the A, B, and C posts for cover.
   E. observe the rear seat.

_____ 10. According to the U.S. Department of Justice, the most common location for violent crimes is on the streets.
   A. True
   B. False

_____ 11. Crimes committed against a person solely on the basis of the individual's actual or perceived race, color, national origin, ethnicity, gender, disability, or sexual orientation are known as:
   A. bias crimes.   D. selective crimes.
   B. hate crimes.   E. none of the above
   C. nondiscriminatory crimes.

_____ 12. When responding to the scene of any violent crime, you should remember that:
   A. dangerous weapons may have been used in the crime.
   B. perpetrators may still be on scene.
   C. patients may sometimes exhibit violence toward EMS personnel.
   D. perpetrators may return to the scene.
   E. all of the above

_____ 13. Warning signs of impending danger from a crowd include all of the following EXCEPT:
   A. a rapid increase in the crowd size.   D. inability of police to control bystanders.
   B. hostility toward anyone on the scene. E. a decreasing level of noise.
   C. pushing or shoving.

_____ 14. A gang's "colors" refers to their:
   A. clothing.   D. graffiti.
   B. flag.   E. logo.
   C. language.

_____ 15. Gang activities are confined to urban areas and are of minimal concern to EMS units outside cities.
   A. True
   B. False

_____ 16. One of the most common substances manufactured in clandestine drug labs is:
   A. cocaine.
   B. methamphetamine.
   C. heroin.
   D. methadone.
   E. morphine.

_____ 17. If you ever come upon a clan lab, all of the following are appropriate actions EXCEPT to:
   A. leave the area immediately.
   B. stop any chemical reactions in progress.
   C. notify the police.
   D. initiate ICS and hazmat procedures.
   E. evacuate the area.

_____ 18. Clan labs generally have the following requirements:
   A. privacy.
   B. utilities.
   C. glassware.
   D. heating mantles or burners.
   E. all of the above

_____ 19. All of the following strategies can be employed as safety tactics in a potentially violent situation EXCEPT:
   A. retreat.
   B. cover and concealment.
   C. confrontation and interrogation.
   D. distraction and evasion.
   E. contact and cover.

_____ 20. Concealment is hiding your body behind solid and impenetrable objects such as brick walls.
   A. True
   B. False

_____ 21. Most body armor is able to stop all bullets and all but a few knives.
   A. True
   B. False

_____ 22. Which of the following describes how tactical EMS differs from normal or nontactical EMS?
   A. A major priority is patient extraction.
   B. Trauma is more frequent than medical emergencies.
   C. Treatment interventions must be coordinated with the IC.
   D. Complete assessment occurs after patient movement.
   E. all of the above

_____ 23. Which of the following is NOT appropriate when providing care at the possible crime scene?
   A. Cut through bullet or knife holes in clothing.
   B. Place clothing in paper bags.
   C. Place patient care before crime scene preservation.
   D. Wear gloves and otherwise limit any fingerprints you might leave behind.
   E. All of the above are appropriate actions at a crime scene.

_____ 24. Gloves worn by EMS providers generally limit the fingerprints left behind at the scene but will not prevent other prints from being smudged.
   A. True
   B. False

_____ 25. Which of the following is proper for documenting a crime scene response?
   A. Record only the facts at the crime scene.
   B. Use quotation marks to indicate exact words from bystanders or the patient.
   C. Do not offer opinions as to the victim's cause of death.
   D. Describe the nature and shape of a wound, not the suspected cause.
   E. all of the above

MATCHING

Write the letter of the term in the space provided next to the appropriate description.

A. TEMS
B. particulate evidence
C. concealment
D. SWAT
E. body armor
F. EMT-Ts
G. blood splatter evidence
H. cover
I. CONTOMS
J. graffiti

_____ 26. painting on walls to mark a gang's territory, membership, or threats

_____ 27. trained police unit equipped to handle hostage takers and other difficult law enforcement situations

_____ 28. hiding the body behind objects that shield a person from view but offer little or no protection against bullets or other ballistics

_____ 29. vest made of tightly woven, strong fibers that offers protection against handgun bullets, most knives, and blunt trauma

_____ 30. counter-narcotics tactical operations program that manages training and certification of EMT-Ts and SWAT-medics

_____ 31. hairs or fibers that cannot be readily seen with the human eye

_____ 32. a specially trained unit that provides on-site medical support to law enforcement

_____ 33. hiding the body behind solid and impenetrable objects that protect a person from bullets

_____ 34. pattern that blood forms when it is dropped at the scene of a crime

_____ 35. EMS personnel trained to serve with a law enforcement agency

Chapter 49

Responding to Terrorist Acts

Review of Chapter Objectives

After reading this chapter, you should be able to:

1. **Identify the typical weapons of mass destruction likely to be used by terrorists.** pp. 1891–1902

   The most likely weapon of mass destruction used by the terrorist, either foreign or domestic, is the conventional explosive. As terrorists gain greater funding and sophistication, however, the risk of terrorists using nuclear, biological, and chemical weapons is increasing. Terrorists may also use agents and mechanisms not yet mentioned as they search for new ways to terrify the public and bring attention to their causes. An example of this was crashing commercial airliners, laden with fuel, into large buildings.

2. **Explain the mechanisms of injury associated with conventional and nuclear weapons of mass destruction.** pp. 1892–1895

   Chemical reactions in the conventional explosion release tremendous amounts of heat energy in milliseconds. This energy instantaneously creates super-heated gases and results in extreme pressure at the detonation site. This pressure moves outward rapidly, first creating a pressure wave traveling at sonic speeds and then becoming a forceful blast wind. The pressure wave (called overpressure) rapidly compresses and then decompresses all with which it comes in contact. Serious injury may result to any hollow and air-filled spaces, such as those in the middle ear, the bowel, and the lungs. The blast wind can propel the explosive container parts or other debris, such as glass or wood splinters, causing injury to those it strikes. The blast wind may also throw victims, resulting in blunt trauma as they strike objects or the ground. The pressure wave and blast wind may also cause structural collapse, resulting in crushing injury and/or entrapment. Finally, the blast heat may cause serious burn injury directly or burns from combustion of material it ignites.

   The nuclear weapon releases energy as atoms are broken apart and reassembled. The energy released from a relatively small bomb is thousands of times greater than a conventional explosive of equal size. The nuclear detonation injures through the same mechanisms as the conventional explosion. The resulting injuries, however, are more extensive and serious. Additionally, the nuclear detonation releases exceptional amounts of heat energy that kills most individuals in the detonation area and causes serious burns at some distance from the blast epicenter. Lastly, the detonation emits great amounts of nuclear radiation causing direct radiation exposure and energizes dust and debris causing radioactive fallout. The fallout may travel with upper air currents and fall to earth many miles from the detonation site.

©2007 Pearson Education, Inc.
Essentials of Paramedic Care, 2nd ed.

3. **Identify and describe the major subclassifications of chemical and biological weapons of mass destruction.** pp. 1895–1902

   Chemical Weapons
   — **Nerve agents.** Nerve agents attack the central nervous system by causing an impulse transmission overload. This results in muscle spasms, convulsions, unconsciousness, and respiratory failure.
   — **Vesicants.** Vesicants are chemical agents that damage exposed skin and cause blistering. They may also damage the eyes, respiratory tract, and lung tissue and may induce general illness as well.
   — **Pulmonary agents.** Pulmonary agents attack the airway and lungs, producing inflammation and pulmonary edema. Their use frequently results in nasal and throat irritation, wheezing, cough, dyspnea, and hypoxia.
   — **Biotoxins.** Biotoxins are chemicals produced by living organisms and behave more like chemical agents. Botulinum is the most toxic, 15,000 times more potent than the worst of the nerve agents (VX).

   Biological Weapons
   — **Pulmonary or pneumonia-like agents.** Pulmonary agents are the most likely biological agents to be used by terrorists. These agents are transmitted via the respiratory system and induce cough, dyspnea, fever, and malaise.
   — **Encephalitis-like agents.** Encephalitis-like agents affect the central nervous system and present with flulike signs and symptoms. However, these biological agents usually carry a much higher mortality rate than the flu or similar diseases.

   Other Biological Agents
   Cholera and *viral hemorrhagic fever* are other biological agents terrorists may use. Cholera causes profuse diarrhea, and viral hemorrhagic fever attacks the blood's ability to coagulate.

4. **List the scene evidence that might alert the EMS provider to a terrorist attack that involves a weapon of mass destruction.** pp. 1902–1903

   Terrorists are likely to target public places where the effects of their actions are the greatest on structures that symbolize an institution they oppose. The results of a conventional or nuclear explosion make them easy to recognize but chemical and biological releases may be insidious. Whenever a large number of people appear to be complaining of similar signs and symptoms, suspect the deployment of chemical or biological weapons. In a chemical release, the effects are likely to occur immediately or shortly after exposure. Confined spaces, such as within a building or in a subway terminal, are likely targets although terrorists may release an agent upwind of a large public gathering. A biological release is even more difficult to detect. You, or more likely, Emergency Department personnel, may recognize many patients with similar generalized signs and symptoms. Only after extensive diagnostic tests and investigation may someone confirm that a weapon of mass destruction was deployed.

5. **Describe the special safety precautions and safety equipment appropriate for an incident involving nuclear, biological, or chemical weapons.** pp. 1902–1903

   The first step in responding to a possible weapon of mass destruction incident is to maintain the proper index of suspicion and to assure that you, fellow rescuers, and the public are not exposed to danger. Approach the scene from upwind and when in doubt about scene safety, request that a properly trained response team assess and enter the scene before you. Only after the response team determines the scene is safe should you enter (if at all).

   Affected patients must be properly decontaminated before you can offer care, both for your protection and theirs. This occurs whether they are brought to you or you enter the scene to treat them.

When responding to a nuclear incident, act at the direction of persons trained in radiation detection. Wear a dosimeter when appropriate and have your exposure level checked periodically. When off duty, properly decontaminate and move a good distance from the scene to limit cumulative exposure.

For biological agents, employ appropriate body substance isolation precautions. In this case, BSI usually means a properly fitted HEPA-filter mask and gloves. While it is unlikely that you will recognize the release of an agent, you may be called on to treat victims days after the initial exposure.

Chemical agent releases may present with a recognizable and immediate danger. Remain at a distance and upwind from the scene and call for the victims to self-evacuate. Only properly trained personnel wearing the appropriate protective gear (a properly trained and equipped HAZMAT team) should enter the scene. Patients must be properly decontaminated before it is safe for you to care for them.

6. **Identify the assessment and management concerns for victims of conventional, nuclear, biological, and chemical weapons.** pp. 1892–1902

Conventional. Victims of a conventional weapon detonation suffer compression injuries from the blast wave. The most serious injury is to the lungs. Any sign of compression injury such as middle ear or bowel injury signs or any dyspnea should suggest lung injury. Blast victims may also suffer penetrating and blunt injuries due to debris propelled by the blast wind or from being thrown by the wind. Finally, the victim may be injured during structural collapse.

Focus management of the blast victim on care for the respiratory injury. Administer high-flow, high-concentration oxygen. Provide intermittent positive-pressure ventilation as needed, but conservatively, as the blast may have injured the alveolar walls. Care for other blunt and penetrating injuries as indicated.

Nuclear. Victims of a nuclear blast are most likely to receive burns as their most serious injuries. Radiation exposure may come from the initial blast or from radioactive fallout at or downwind from the explosion. There will be limited signs and symptoms unless the radiation exposure was very high. With high radiation exposure, the patient will display nausea, vomiting, and malaise. The greater the radiation exposure, the faster these signs will appear following exposure.

Patient care includes decontamination and then care for thermal burns. Protection from fallout is an additional concern and best addressed by moving the victims away from the expected fallout path. Care for the patient exposed to radioactivity is mostly supportive.

If there is a recognized release of radiation through a conventional explosion or other mechanism, direct your first efforts to reduce further exposure. Then assure that the patients are properly decontaminated. Only then, concentrate your efforts on specific injury care.

Biological. It is unlikely that anyone will immediately detect the release of a biological agent. It is more likely that you or other health care workers will notice a group of people complaining of similar symptoms. These symptoms will most likely be fever, nausea, body aches, and malaise (symptoms similar to the flu).

Care for the victims of a biological agent release is first directed at reducing transmission. At the first sign of a possible biological agent (or any potentially contagious disease), don a mask and gloves and isolate the patient (or patients). Provide supportive care as for any other serious contagious disease.

Chemical. A chemical release is likely to affect its victims very quickly. They will complain of respiratory symptoms such as chest tightness or burning or possibly skin irritation. If you receive reports of several or many individuals complaining of similar symptoms, suspect a chemical release and approach the scene with great caution. Alert the fire department or the designated hazardous materials team and position your vehicle upwind from the scene. Assure the evacuation of persons downwind and decontamination of those victims brought to you for care.

Care for the victims of a chemical release includes high-flow, high-concentration oxygen, respiratory support as needed (including bag-valve masking and intubation), and antidote administration as indicated.

7. **Given a narrative description of a conventional, nuclear, biological, or chemical terrorist attack, identify the elements of scene size-up that suggest terrorism, and identify the likely injuries and any special patient management considerations necessary.** pp. 1891–1903

During your classroom training and practical skills session you will learn and practice the skills associated with recognizing, taking the proper protective precautions for you and the public, and caring for patients subject to illness or injury from weapons of mass destruction. Use this training and practice to perfect your skills of WMD care.

Content Self-Evaluation

MULTIPLE CHOICE

_____ 1. Which of the following is the most likely weapon of choice for terrorist groups?
   A. conventional explosives
   B. nuclear weapons
   C. biological agents
   D. chemical agents
   E. incendiary devices

_____ 2. Terrorists are likely to target which of the following?
   A. an embassy
   B. a symbol of government
   C. their employer
   D. corporations
   E. all of the above

_____ 3. The blast pressure wave is likely to injure all of the following EXCEPT:
   A. the lungs.
   B. the ears.
   C. the bowel.
   D. the heart.
   E. the sinuses.

_____ 4. Incendiary agents differ from conventional explosives in that they:
   A. have greater explosive energy.
   B. cause more burn injuries.
   C. consume more oxygen.
   D. are dropped from a high altitude.
   E. combine both explosive and nuclear damage.

_____ 5. Which of the following is the mechanism of injury associated with most deaths from a nuclear blast?
   A. radiation burns
   B. radiation illness
   C. cancer
   D. thermal burns
   E. pressure injuries

_____ 6. The best way to detect radiation in the absence of a Geiger counter is:
   A. by a strange taste in your mouth.
   B. a warm sensation in your muscles.
   C. immediate nausea.
   D. a tingling sensation from the exposed surface.
   E. none of the above

_____ 7. Fallout associated with nuclear detonation is not likely to be a factor until how long after the detonation?
   A. 10 minutes
   B. 30 minutes
   C. 1 hour
   D. 4 hours
   E. 2 days

_____ 8. Once a victim is exposed to nuclear radiation and debris has been properly decontaminated, he poses no danger to himself or others.
   A. True
   B. False

_____ 9. Which of the following is a symptom associated with radiation exposure?
   A. nausea
   B. fatigue
   C. malaise
   D. hypertension
   E. all of the above except D

_____ 10. Which of the following influence the delivery of a chemical weapon?
   A. wind strength
   B. the agent's specific gravity
   C. the agent's volatility
   D. precipitation
   E. all of the above

_____ 11. Which of the following is NOT a common sign or symptom of a nerve agent?
   A. dry mouth
   B. tearing eyes
   C. urination
   D. defecation
   E. vomiting

_____ 12. Blistering agents are also known as:
   A. organophosphates.
   B. vesicants.
   C. carbamates.
   D. chambering agents.
   E. none of the above

_____ 13. Which of the following is NOT a blistering agent?
   A. lewisite
   B. phosgene oxime
   C. botulinum
   D. sulfur mustard
   E. nitrogen mustard

_____ 14. One of the most toxic agents known to man is:
   A. sulfur mustard.
   B. ricin.
   C. VX gas.
   D. botulinum.
   E. none of the above

_____ 15. Which of the following suggests a chemical agent release?
   A. a strange smell
   B. numerous patients complaining of the same symptoms
   C. a cloud of dust or gas
   D. incapacitated or dead birds and insects
   E. all of the above

_____ 16. Which of the following is NOT a biological agent capable of spreading from person to person?
   A. Ebola
   B. smallpox
   C. plague
   D. anthrax
   E. cholera

_____ 17. A biological release can be recognized by which of the following?
   A. a distinctive cloud
   B. a distinctive color
   C. immediate signs and symptoms
   D. very distinct signs and symptoms
   E. all of the above

_____ 18. The most likely biological agents to be used by terrorists are:
   A. pneumonia-like agents.
   B. flulike agents.
   C. encephalitis-like agents.
   D. Ebola.
   E. all of the above

_____ 19. Almost all biological weapons are transmitted via the respiratory route; therefore, the HEPA respirator is very effective at reducing transmission.
   A. True
   B. False

_____ 20. Dangers of a conventional explosion used by terrorists include all of the following EXCEPT:
   A. the danger of a secondary explosion.
   B. inability to recognize the incident.
   C. radioactive contamination.
   D. structural collapse.
   E. all of the above

WORKBOOK ANSWER KEY

Note: Throughout Answer Key, textbook page references are shown in italic.

Division 1: Introduction to Advanced Prehospital Care

Chapter 1: Introduction to Advanced Prehospital Care

MULTIPLE CHOICE

1. C *p. 6*
2. A *p. 6*
3. E *p. 6*
4. E *p. 7*
5. D *p. 7*
6. C *p. 7*
7. B *p. 7*
8. A *p. 7*
9. E *p. 8*
10. D *p. 8*

MULTIPLE CHOICE

1. A *p. 8*
2. A *p. 9*
3. E *p. 9*
4. B *p. 10*
5. A *p. 13*
6. D *p. 13*
7. A *p. 13*
8. E *p. 14*
9. C *p. 14*
10. E *p. 14*
11. B *p. 15*
12. C *p. 16*
13. A *p. 16*
14. D *p. 16*
15. B *p. 16*
16. A *p. 16*
17. D *p. 16*
18. D *p. 17*
19. A *p. 17*
20. E *p. 17*
21. B *p. 17*
22. A *p. 18*
23. D *p. 18*
24. C *p. 18*
25. B *p. 18*
26. C *p. 19*
27. E *p. 20*
28. B *p. 20*
29. C *p. 20*
30. E *p. 20*
31. B *p. 21*
32. B *p. 21*
33. A *p. 21*
34. C *p. 23*
35. A *p. 23*

LISTING

36. U.S. DOT (National Traffic and Highway Safety Administration) *p. 18*
37. U.S. General Services Administration *p. 18*
38. American College of Surgeons Committee on Trauma *p. 18*
39. American College of Emergency Physicians *p. 18*
40. Joint Review Committee on Educational Programs for the EMT-Paramedic *p. 18*

MULTIPLE CHOICE

1. A *p. 23*
2. E *p. 23*
3. E *p. 23*
4. A *p. 24*
5. B *p. 25*
6. C *p. 26*
7. C *p. 26*
8. E *p. 26*
9. B *p. 26*
10. B *p. 27*
11. B *p. 28*
12. A *p. 29*
13. D *p. 29*
14. B *p. 29*
15. C *p. 30*

MATCHING

16. G *p. 26*
17. C *p. 25*
18. D *p. 25*
19. C *p. 25*
20. F *p. 26*
21. A *p. 23*
22. C *p. 25*
23. C *p. 25*
24. E *p. 25*
25. B *p. 24*
26. D *p. 25*
27. A *p. 23*
28. G *p. 26*
29. C *p. 25*
30. C *p. 25*

MULTIPLE CHOICE

1. C *p. 31*
2. A *p. 31*
3. A *p. 31*
4. B *p. 32*
5. C *p. 31*
6. E *p. 32*
7. A *p. 32*
8. C *p. 33*
9. E *p. 33*
10. C *p. 33*
11. A *p. 35*
12. A *p. 35*
13. D *p. 36*
14. E *p. 36*
15. B *p. 36*
16. E *p. 36*
17. E *p. 36*
18. A *p. 37*
19. E *p. 37*
20. C *p. 38*
21. C *p. 39*
22. B *p. 39*
23. B *p. 40*
24. A *p. 39*
25. A *p. 41*
26. D *p. 41*
27. D *p. 44*
28. B *p. 42*
29. B *p. 42*
30. A *p. 43*
31. E *p. 43*
32. B *p. 44*
33. E *p. 44*
34. A *p. 45*
35. C *p. 46*
36. A *p. 46*
37. A *p. 45*
38. E *p. 46*
39. B *p. 47*
40. B *p. 47*

MATCHING

pp. 35–36

41. A, B
42. A, B, D
43. A, B
44. A, C
45. A, B, D

MULTIPLE CHOICE

1. C *p. 47*
2. A *p. 47*
3. A *p. 47*
4. B *p. 48*
5. A *p. 48*
6. B *p. 50*
7. A *p. 50*
8. B *p. 50*
9. C *p. 50*
10. A *p. 51*
11. C *p. 51*
12. A *p. 51*
13. E *p. 51*
14. B *p. 52*
15. E *p. 53*

MULTIPLE CHOICE

1. A *p. 53*
2. B *p. 54*
3. D *p. 54*
4. A *p. 54*
5. D *p. 54*
6. B *p. 56*
7. A *p. 57*
8. B *p. 58*
9. A *p. 60*
10. E *p. 61*

Chapter 2: Medical/Legal Aspects of Advanced Prehospital Care

MULTIPLE CHOICE

1. B *p. 66*
2. C *p. 66*
3. C *p. 66*
4. A *p. 66*
5. E *p. 68*
6. D *p. 69*
7. B *p. 69*
8. A *p. 69*
9. D *p. 70*
10. E *p. 70*
11. C *p. 70*
12. C *p. 71*
13. E *p. 72*
14. A *p. 72*
15. B *p. 73*
16. D *p. 73*
17. E *p. 74*
18. B *p. 75*
19. C *p. 75*
20. E *p. 75*
21. B *p. 76*
22. B *p. 76*
23. E *p. 76*
24. B *p. 76*
25. B *p. 77*
26. A *p. 78*
27. D *p. 78*
28. C *p. 78*
29. D *p. 78*
30. A *p. 79*
31. E *p. 79*
32. A *p. 80*
33. A *p. 80*
34. C *p. 81*
35. C *p. 81*

Chapter 3: Anatomy and Physiology

MULTIPLE CHOICE

1. A *p. 88*
2. A *p. 88*
3. C *p. 88*
4. E *p. 89*
5. C *p. 89*
6. D *p. 89*
7. A *p. 90*
8. E *p. 91*
9. D *p. 91*
10. A *p. 92*
11. E *p. 91*
12. E *p. 92*
13. A *p. 92*
14. B *p. 92*
15. A *p. 92*
16. B *p. 93*
17. B *p. 93*
18. C *p. 94*
19. B *p. 95*
20. D *p. 95*
21. E *p. 96*
22. B *p. 96*
23. A *p. 97*
24. B *p. 97*
25. E *p. 98*
26. D *p. 98*
27. A *p. 99*
28. B *p. 99*
29. A *p. 99*
30. B *p. 101*
31. A *p. 100*
32. D *p. 101*
33. E *p. 101*
34. A *p. 101*
35. B *p. 102*
36. C *p. 102*
37. B *p. 102*
38. B *p. 102*
39. D *p. 102*
40. A *p. 103*

©2007 Pearson Education, Inc.
Essentials of Paramedic Care, 2nd ed.

MULTIPLE CHOICE

1. A	p. 105	53. C	p. 146	105. D	p. 196
2. A	p. 106	54. B	p. 151	106. D	p. 197
3. E	p. 106	55. C	p. 151	107. B	p. 198
4. A	p. 106	56. B	p. 154	108. C	p. 200
5. D	p. 106	57. A	p. 153	109. C	p. 201
6. C	p. 107	58. C	p. 154	110. E	p. 201
7. B	p. 108	59. A	p. 154	111. D	p. 204
8. C	p. 108	60. E	p. 154	112. D	p. 204
9. A	p. 109	61. B	p. 155	113. A	p. 205
10. D	p. 109	62. E	p. 155	114. B	p. 205
11. A	p. 110	63. B	p. 155	115. A	p. 207
12. E	p. 112	64. E	p. 156	116. C	p. 206
13. B	p. 113	65. C	p. 156	117. C	p. 208
14. E	p. 113	66. A	p. 157	118. D	p. 208
15. B	p. 113	67. D	p. 156	119. A	p. 208
16. E	p. 114	68. B	p. 157	120. E	p. 210
17. D	p. 114	69. E	p. 158	121. D	p. 210
18. B	p. 117	70. B	p. 158	122. A	p. 211
19. C	p. 117	71. A	p. 158	123. B	p. 212
20. B	p. 117	72. C	p. 158	124. C	p. 213
21. A	p. 117	73. D	p. 160	125. A	p. 214
22. C	p. 118	74. C	p. 160	126. E	p. 214
23. D	p. 118	75. C	p. 162	127. C	p. 215
24. A	p. 119	76. C	p. 164	128. C	p. 215
25. B	p. 119	77. A	p. 164	129. B	p. 215
26. A	p. 119	78. E	p. 164	130. A	p. 216
27. C	p. 120	79. D	p. 165	131. E	p. 216
28. A	p. 120	80. D	p. 165	132. C	p. 217
29. C	p. 134	81. A	p. 171	133. C	p. 217
30. E	p. 134	82. D	p. 174	134. A	p. 218
31. D	p. 134	83. C	p. 176	135. C	p. 218
32. A	p. 138	84. B	p. 179	136. E	p. 218
33. E	p. 139	85. A	p. 183	137. E	p. 220
34. B	p. 140	86. B	p. 184	138. B	p. 222
35. C	p. 140	87. B	p. 185	139. A	p. 222
36. E	p. 140	88. D	p. 185	140. E	p. 222
37. D	p. 140	89. B	p. 185	141. A	p. 223
38. B	p. 141	90. B	p. 186	142. B	p. 225
39. B	p. 141	91. E	p. 186	143. A	p. 227
40. A	p. 142	92. C	p. 186	144. D	p. 227
41. C	p. 142	93. B	p. 186	145. B	p. 228
42. A	p. 142	94. C	p. 186	146. B	p. 228
43. A	p. 143	95. A	p. 186	147. C	p. 230
44. E	p. 143	96. A	p. 186	148. E	p. 231
45. C	p. 143	97. A	p. 186	149. A	p. 232
46. E	p. 145	98. C	p. 188	150. B	p. 232
47. B	p. 145	99. B	p. 190	151. A	p. 232
48. C	p. 143	100. E	p. 191	152. C	p. 232
49. C	p. 145	101. A	p. 192	153. D	p. 232
50. D	p. 146	102. A	p. 193	154. C	p. 233
51. A	p. 146	103. D	p. 194	155. C	p. 234
52. A	p. 146	104. A	p. 195		

Chapter 4: General Principles of Pathophysiology

MULTIPLE CHOICE

1. B	p. 242	9. A	p. 247	17. A	p. 251
2. E	p. 242	10. E	p. 247	18. D	p. 251
3. D	p. 243	11. B	p. 248	19. E	p. 252
4. E	p. 243	12. B	p. 248	20. B	p. 253
5. E	p. 244	13. C	p. 248	21. C	p. 253
6. D	p. 245	14. A	p. 249	22. A	p. 254
7. A	p. 246	15. D	p. 249	23. D	p. 255
8. C	p. 246	16. C	p. 250	24. E	p. 255

25. C	p. 254	32. C	p. 259	39. B	p. 262
26. A	p. 256	33. C	p. 260	40. E	p. 264
27. C	p. 256	34. D	p. 260	43. D	p. 265
28. E	p. 257	35. A	p. 260	42. C	p. 263
29. C	p. 258	36. C	p. 260	43. A	p. 265
30. C	p. 258	37. D	p. 260	44. B	p. 267
31. A	p. 258	38. D	p. 260	45. E	p. 267

MATCHING

46. A	p. 261	50. E	p. 264	54. C	p. 263
47. C	p. 263	51. D	p. 265	55. B	p. 262
48. E	p. 264	52. B	p. 262		
49. D	p. 265	53. E	p. 264		

MULTIPLE CHOICE

1. B	p. 268	13. B	p. 273	25. D	p. 283
2. C	p. 269	14. E	p. 274	26. B	p. 283
3. B	p. 270	15. D	p. 275	27. A	p. 283
4. C	p. 270	16. B	p. 277	28. B	p. 283
5. B	p. 271	17. E	p. 277	29. A	p. 284
6. A	p. 271	18. A	p. 278	30. B	p. 283
7. A	p. 273	19. C	p. 278	31. E	p. 284
8. B	p. 272	20. C	p. 279	32. B	p. 284
9. E	p. 272	21. D	p. 279	33. C	p. 285
10. E	p. 273	22. D	p. 279	34. D	p. 285
11. C	p. 273	23. E	p. 281	35. B	p. 287
12. E	p. 273	24. C	p. 282		

Chapter 5: Life-Span Development

MULTIPLE CHOICE

1. D	p. 292	10. C	p. 296	19. E	p. 301
2. B	p. 296	11. A	p. 297	20. A	p. 301
3. E	p. 292	12. D	p. 297	21. E	p. 302
4. A	p. 292	13. B	p. 297	22. B	p. 302
5. B	p. 292	14. C	p. 299	23. E	p. 302
6. B	p. 292	15. C	p. 299	24. A	p. 303
7. E	p. 293	16. A	p. 299	25. A	p. 304
8. A	p. 294	17. D	p. 301		
9. C	p. 294	18. A	p. 301		

MATCHING

26. F	p. 301	30. D	p. 299	34. C	p. 297
27. G	p. 301	31. H	p. 303	35. A	p. 294
28. A	p. 295	32. D	p. 299		
29. E	p. 300	33. B	p. 297		

Chapter 6: General Principles of Pharmacology

MULTIPLE CHOICE

1. D	p. 309	15. D	p. 315	29. E	p. 321
2. A	p. 310	16. E	p. 315	30. C	p. 322
3. B	p. 310	17. D	p. 316	31. C	p. 322
4. A	p. 310	18. A	p. 316	32. B	p. 322
5. B	p. 310	19. C	p. 317	33. D	p. 323
6. B	p. 310	20. B	p. 317	34. B	p. 323
7. C	p. 311	21. D	p. 317	35. C	p. 323
8. C	p. 311	22. A	p. 318	36. A	p. 323
9. E	p. 312	23. D	p. 320	37. A	p. 324
10. B	p. 313	24. B	p. 320	38. D	p. 324
11. E	p. 313	25. D	p. 321	39. E	p. 325
12. E	p. 314	26. A	p. 321	40. C	p. 325
13. A	p. 314	27. C	p. 321		
14. B	p. 315	28. C	p. 321		

MULTIPLE CHOICE

1. E	p. 327	28. B	p. 337	55. B	p. 351
2. B	p. 327	29. A	p. 337	56. D	p. 352
3. E	p. 327	30. A	p. 337	57. C	p. 352
4. A	p. 327	31. D	p. 337	58. E	p. 353
5. D	p. 328	32. D	p. 337	59. C	p. 353
6. C	p. 328	33. C	p. 337	60. A	p. 353
7. B	p. 328	34. B	p. 337	61. C	p. 355
8. C	p. 329	35. D	p. 338	62. B	p. 355
9. C	p. 329	36. B	p. 339	63. A	p. 356
10. A	p. 329	37. D	p. 339	64. C	p. 356
11. D	p. 329	38. A	p. 341	65. E	p. 357
12. A	p. 330	39. E	p. 340	66. E	p. 358
13. B	p. 330	40. B	p. 341	67. A	p. 360
14. B	p. 331	41. D	p. 342	68. E	p. 360
15. A	p. 332	42. D	p. 341	69. A	p. 360
16. B	p. 333	43. A	p. 341	70. C	p. 360
17. A	p. 333	44. A	p. 344	71. C	p. 361
18. C	p. 333	45. B	p. 344	72. B	p. 361
19. D	p. 333	46. C	p. 345	73. B	p. 362
20. D	p. 334	47. D	p. 346	74. A	p. 362
21. D	p. 334	48. C	p. 347	75. D	p. 362
22. B	p. 334	49. C	p. 348	76. A	p. 364
23. B	p. 335	50. C	p. 349	77. B	p. 366
24. B	p. 335	51. A	p. 350	78. E	p. 366
25. A	p. 335	52. D	p. 351	79. B	p. 368
26. B	p. 335	53. B	p. 351	80. A	p. 369
27. B	p. 336	54. B	p. 351		

Chapter 7: Intravenous Access and Medication Administration

MULTIPLE CHOICE

1. A	p. 375	16. D	p. 379	31. B	p. 391
2. B	p. 375	17. B	p. 380	32. B	p. 392
3. D	p. 376	18. B	p. 382	33. A	p. 392
4. E	p. 376	19. B	p. 382	34. A	p. 392
5. A	p. 376	20. C	p. 384	35. E	p. 392
6. A	p. 376	21. A	p. 384	36. A	p. 398
7. C	p. 377	22. E	p. 384	37. C	p. 400
8. D	p. 377	23. A	p. 384	38. D	p. 402
9. A	p. 377	24. B	p. 385	39. B	p. 399
10. C	p. 378	25. A	p. 385	40. A	p. 402
11. E	p. 378	26. B	p. 386	41. D	p. 405
12. D	p. 378	27. C	p. 386	42. C	p. 402
13. C	p. 379	28. B	p. 389	43. D	p. 402
14. C	p. 379	29. D	p. 389	44. D	p. 405
15. E	p. 379	30. B	p. 390	45. B	p. 405

MULTIPLE CHOICE

1. E	p. 405	18. E	p. 412	35. A	p. 423
2. B	p. 406	19. B	p. 413	36. B	p. 430
3. E	p. 406	20. B	p. 413	37. A	p. 431
4. D	p. 407	21. D	p. 414	38. B	p. 432
5. A	p. 407	22. B	p. 414	39. B	p. 432
6. C	p. 408	23. B	p. 414	40. A	p. 431
7. E	p. 408	24. B	p. 416	41. C	p. 432
8. D	p. 408	25. A	p. 416	42. B	p. 433
9. E	p. 408	26. C	p. 416	43. C	p. 433
10. E	p. 409	27. C	p. 418	44. C	p. 434
11. B	p. 410	28. E	p. 418	45. A	p. 434
12. A	p. 409	29. E	p. 420	46. A	p. 435
13. D	p. 410	30. D	p. 421	47. C	p. 435
14. C	p. 411	31. D	p. 421	48. A	p. 435
15. A	p. 412	32. B	p. 422	49. C	p. 441
16. A	p. 412	33. D	p. 422	50. D	p. 441
17. A	p. 408	34. C	p. 422		

Chapter 8: Airway Management and Ventilation

MULTIPLE CHOICE

1. A	p. 457	23. B	p. 475	45. A	p. 494
2. C	p. 458	24. C	p. 476	46. B	p. 495
3. B	p. 459	25. C	p. 476	47. B	p. 497
4. B	p. 459	26. B	p. 478	48. B	p. 498
5. B	p. 460	27. A	p. 478	49. B	p. 502
6. E	p. 460	28. E	p. 480	50. C	p. 502
7. D	p. 461	29. B	p. 481	51. A	p. 504
8. A	p. 462	30. B	p. 481	52. A	p. 506
9. C	p. 462	31. B	p. 482	53. E	p. 507
10. C	p. 462	32. D	p. 482	54. A	p. 512
11. C	p. 464	33. E	p. 482	55. B	p. 512
12. D	p. 464	34. A	p. 482	56. A	p. 516
13. A	p. 465	35. C	p. 478	57. E	p. 521
14. B	p. 464	36. C	p. 485	58. B	p. 522
15. E	p. 466	37. E	p. 486	59. C	p. 522
16. B	p. 469	38. A	p. 487	60. C	p. 524
17. C	p. 470	39. B	p. 488	61. D	p. 524
18. D	p. 471	40. C	p. 489	62. C	p. 526
19. B	p. 472	41. E	p. 494	63. D	p. 527
20. A	p. 473	42. B	p. 494	64. A	p. 528
21. A	p. 473	43. C	p. 495	65. D	p. 528
22. C	p. 474	44. A	p. 494		

Chapter 9: Therapeutic Communications

MULTIPLE CHOICE

1. B	p. 533	6. C	p. 535	11. B	p. 539
2. A	p. 533	7. A	p. 536	12. B	p. 540
3. C	p. 533	8. B	p. 536	13. E	p. 540
4. B	p. 534	9. B	p. 538	14. A	p. 540
5. C	p. 534	10. E	p. 539	15. C	p. 542

Division 2: Patient Assessment

Chapter 10: History Taking

MULTIPLE CHOICE

1. D	p. 547	6. B	p. 551	11. C	p. 554
2. A	p. 547	7. A	p. 551	12. D	p. 554
3. A	p. 548	8. B	p. 551	13. B	p. 556
4. B	p. 548	9. C	p. 553	14. A	p. 558
5. C	p. 548	10. E	p. 554	15. A	p. 560

MATCHING

16. S	p. 552	20. P	p. 552	24. Q	p. 552
17. P	p. 551	21. O	p. 551	25. O	p. 551
18. R	p. 552	22. R	p. 552		
19. Q	p. 552	23. T	p. 552		

Chapter 11: Physical Exam Techniques

MULTIPLE CHOICE

1. A	p. 566	9. C	p. 569	17. A	p. 571
2. B	p. 569	10. B	p. 570	18. E	p. 571
3. A	p. 567	11. C	p. 570	19. B	p. 572
4. C	p. 566	12. A	p. 570	20. C	p. 572
5. B	p. 567	13. E	p. 571	21. E	p. 572
6. C	p. 567	14. A	p. 571	22. C	p. 573
7. A	p. 567	15. D	p. 571	23. D	p. 573
8. A	p. 568	16. C	p. 571	24. D	p. 573

©2007 Pearson Education, Inc.
Essentials of Paramedic Care, 2nd ed.

25. B	p. 573	32. A	p. 579	39. B	p. 585
26. B	p. 574	33. E	p. 579	40. D	p. 588
27. D	p. 578	34. D	p. 579	41. E	p. 590
28. B	p. 578	35. B	p. 582	42. A	p. 594
29. A	p. 578	36. D	p. 584	43. B	p. 594
30. E	p. 578	37. E	p. 585	44. E	p. 596
31. C	p. 578	38. A	p. 585	45. A	p. 600

MULTIPLE CHOICE

1. D	p. 605	6. C	p. 606	11. D	p. 613
2. B	p. 605	7. C	p. 608	12. B	p. 617
3. E	p. 606	8. B	p. 608	13. B	p. 617
4. B	p. 606	9. E	p. 609	14. B	p. 625
5. A	p. 606	10. D	p. 613	15. D	p. 625

MULTIPLE CHOICE

1. C	p. 627	13. A	p. 633	25. A	p. 642
2. A	p. 627	14. C	p. 633	26. C	p. 644
3. D	p. 629	15. D	p. 635	27. E	p. 644
4. E	p. 629	16. D	p. 635	28. B	p. 644
5. E	p. 629	17. E	p. 635	29. A	p. 645
6. A	p. 630	18. A	p. 635	30. B	p. 645
7. E	p. 630	19. B	p. 636	31. B	p. 645
8. B	p. 630	20. D	p. 638	32. A	p. 645
9. C	p. 630	21. C	p. 636	33. D	p. 646
10. D	p. 631	22. E	p. 638	34. E	p. 647
11. D	p. 631	23. C	p. 642	35. A	p. 647
12. B	p. 633	24. E	p. 642		

Chapter 12: Patient Assessment in the Field

MULTIPLE CHOICE

1. A	p. 653	11. A	p. 658	21. A	p. 664
2. E	p. 653	12. D	p. 661	22. E	p. 664
3. E	p. 654	13. B	p. 661	23. C	p. 664
4. B	p. 654	14. A	p. 661	24. A	p. 665
5. A	p. 655	15. B	p. 661	25. C	p. 666
6. C	p. 655	16. D	p. 661	26. A	p. 665
7. A	p. 655	17. E	p. 662	27. B	p. 666
8. E	p. 656	18. C	p. 663	28. D	p. 666
9. E	p. 656	19. E	p. 663	29. A	p. 668
10. C	p. 657	20. C	p. 663	30. C	p. 668

LISTING

p. 653
31. Scene size-up
32. Initial assessment
33. Focused history and physical exam
34. Detailed physical exam
35. Ongoing assessment

MULTIPLE CHOICE

1. C	p. 673	11. B	p. 678	21. D	p. 686
2. D	p. 673	12. D	p. 680	22. B	p. 686
3. B	p. 674	13. B	p. 680	23. E	p. 686
4. A	p. 675	14. D	p. 682	24. B	p. 687
5. E	p. 675	15. C	p. 682	25. E	p. 688
6. A	p. 676	16. E	p. 683	26. A	p. 689
7. D	p. 676	17. D	p. 684	27. E	p. 692
8. A	p. 676	18. B	p. 684	28. A	p. 692
9. B	p. 676	19. C	p. 685	29. A	p. 698
10. C	p. 676	20. A	p. 686	30. E	p. 698

Chapter 13: Clinical Decision Making

MULTIPLE CHOICE

1. A	p. 705	6. C	p. 707	11. D	p. 710
2. D	p. 706	7. A	p. 707	12. B	p. 710
3. A	p. 705	8. B	p. 707	13. A	p. 711
4. C	p. 706	9. B	p. 707	14. D	p. 712
5. D	p. 706	10. A	p. 708	15. B	p. 713

MATCHING

16. B	p. 712	20. C	p. 712	23. C	p. 712
17. D	p. 713	21. B	p. 712	24. A	p. 712
18. A	p. 712	22. A	p. 712	25. D	p. 713
19. A	p. 712				

Chapter 14: Communications

MULTIPLE CHOICE

1. E	p. 717	10. C	p. 723	19. A	p. 730
2. B	p. 718	11. E	p. 723	20. D	p. 730
3. C	p. 718	12. A	p. 724	21. E	p. 731
4. E	p. 719	13. E	p. 724	22. A	p. 731
5. D	p. 720	14. E	p. 725	23. D	p. 731
6. B	p. 721	15. A	p. 727	24. A	p. 732
7. A	p. 722	16. B	p. 727	25. C	p. 733
8. D	p. 722	17. D	p. 728		
9. E	p. 722	18. C	p. 729		

Chapter 15: Documentation

MULTIPLE CHOICE

1. E	p. 736	11. B	p. 745	21. E	p. 749
2. B	p. 736	12. A	p. 745	22. D	p. 750
3. A	p. 737	13. E	p. 747	23. E	p. 750
4. B	p. 738	14. A	p. 747	24. A	p. 748
5. B	p. 738	15. C	p. 747	25. E	p. 751
6. C	p. 743	16. B	p. 748	26. B	p. 751
7. A	p. 744	17. D	p. 748	27. A	p. 752
8. D	p. 744	18. E	p. 748	28. D	p. 752
9. C	p. 744	19. B	p. 748	29. E	p. 753
10. B	p. 745	20. A	p. 749	30. C	p. 755

MATCHING

See pp. 740–743

31. P	36. E	41. M	46. V	51. W
32. Y	37. B	42. J	47. I	52. K
33. L	38. O	43. Q	48. N	53. S
34. T	39. U	44. G	49. F	54. D
35. A	40. X	45. R	50. C	55. H

Division 3: Trauma Emergencies

Chapter 16: Trauma and Trauma Systems

MULTIPLE CHOICE

1. C	p. 761	6. D	p. 762	11. A	p. 766
2. A	p. 761	7. B	p. 762	12. A	p. 766
3. A	p. 762	8. D	p. 763	13. E	p. 766
4. A	p. 762	9. E	p. 764	14. C	p. 767
5. C	p. 762	10. B	p. 765	15. A	p. 767

Chapter 17: Blunt Trauma

MULTIPLE CHOICE

1. A	p. 771	15. C	p. 779	29. A	p. 790
2. B	p. 771	16. B	p. 779	30. E	p. 791
3. B	p. 771	17. C	p. 781	31. D	p. 791
4. D	p. 771	18. A	p. 782	32. B	p. 792
5. C	p. 772	19. E	p. 782	33. C	p. 792
6. E	p. 772	20. A	p. 782	34. A	p. 792
7. B	p. 772	21. E	p. 782	35. C	p. 793
8. E	p. 774	22. E	p. 785	36. A	p. 793
9. E	p. 774	23. B	p. 785	37. D	p. 794
10. D	p. 774	24. D	p. 786	38. B	p. 795
11. A	p. 777	25. A	p. 786	39. A	p. 796
12. B	p. 777	26. C	p. 787	40. E	p. 797
13. C	p. 778	27. E	p. 788		
14. B	p. 778	28. A	p. 788		

Chapter 18: Penetrating Trauma

MULTIPLE CHOICE

1. B	p. 803	10. A	p. 808	19. A	p. 814
2. C	p. 803	11. A	p. 810	20. D	p. 814
3. A	p. 804	12. C	p. 810	21. C	p. 815
4. C	p. 804	13. E	p. 811	22. B	p. 815
5. B	p. 804	14. A	p. 810	23. E	p. 816
6. E	p. 805	15. C	p. 811	24. D	p. 816
7. A	p. 805	16. B	p. 812	25. C	p. 818
8. A	p. 807	17. A	p. 813		
9. E	p. 807	18. A	p. 814		

Chapter 19: Hemorrhage and Shock

MULTIPLE CHOICE

1. D	p. 823	15. D	p. 830	29. C	p. 840
2. B	p. 822	16. A	p. 830	30. B	p. 841
3. A	p. 824	17. A	p. 831	31. E	p. 841
4. D	p. 824	18. A	p. 832	32. D	p. 841
5. D	p. 824	19. C	p. 833	33. A	p. 841
6. B	p. 824	20. B	p. 834	34. B	p. 843
7. E	p. 825	21. E	p. 834	35. E	p. 844
8. A	p. 825	22. E	p. 834	36. C	p. 844
9. B	p. 826	23. E	p. 835	37. E	p. 844
10. D	p. 830	24. D	p. 836	38. B	p. 845
11. A	p. 829	25. B	p. 836	39. E	p. 845
12. B	p. 830	26. B	p. 839	40. A	p. 847
13. C	p. 830	27. B	p. 839		
14. E	p. 830	28. A	p. 840		

Chapter 20: Soft-Tissue Trauma

MULTIPLE CHOICE

1. B	p. 854	13. C	p. 863	25. A	p. 868
2. E	p. 858	14. B	p. 863	26. C	p. 868
3. B	p. 855	15. A	p. 863	27. E	p. 868
4. C	p. 855	16. E	p. 864	28. D	p. 870
5. D	p. 858	17. C	p. 864	29. A	p. 871
6. E	p. 856	18. E	p. 864	30. A	p. 871
7. B	p. 857	19. A	p. 865	31. E	p. 873
8. A	p. 859	20. E	p. 866	32. B	p. 875
9. D	p. 860	21. E	p. 866	33. A	p. 877
10. B	p. 860	22. A	p. 867	34. E	p. 877
11. B	p. 862	23. A	p. 867	35. C	p. 879
12. B	p. 862	24. B	p. 867	36. B	p. 879
37. C	p. 880	42. E	p. 884	47. A	p. 886
38. D	p. 879	43. E	p. 884	48. E	p. 886
39. A	p. 881	44. D	p. 886	49. C	p. 886
40. C	p. 882	45. E	p. 886	50. E	p. 888
41. B	p. 882	46. B	p. 886		

Chapter 21: Burns

MULTIPLE CHOICE

1. A	p. 892	21. B	p. 902	41. B	p. 913
2. D	p. 892	22. C	p. 902	42. B	p. 913
3. A	p. 892	23. B	p. 904	43. B	p. 913
4. D	p. 893	24. C	p. 904	44. D	p. 913
5. B	p. 893	25. D	p. 904	45. B	p. 914
6. A	p. 893	26. E	p. 904	46. B	p. 914
7. C	p. 895	27. E	p. 904	47. B	p. 915
8. E	p. 895	28. E	p. 905	48. A	p. 915
9. A	p. 895	29. B	p. 907	49. E	p. 916
10. B	p. 896	30. A	p. 909	50. D	p. 916
11. B	p. 896	31. A	p. 909	51. B	p. 917
12. B	p. 897	32. B	p. 914	52. D	p. 918
13. C	p. 897	33. B	p. 902	53. E	p. 917
14. A	p. 898	34. E	p. 904	54. C	p. 918
15. E	p. 900	35. A	p. 911	55. B	p. 919
16. D	p. 899	36. D	p. 911	56. D	p. 919
17. B	p. 899	37. D	p. 911	57. A	p. 919
18. E	p. 900	38. D	p. 911	58. A	p. 919
19. C	p. 902	39. A	p. 912	59. E	p. 919
20. D	p. 902	40. A	p. 913	60. B	p. 920

Chapter 22: Musculoskeletal Trauma

MULTIPLE CHOICE

1. E	p. 925	18. E	p. 934	35. D	p. 944
2. A	p. 926	19. E	p. 935	36. E	p. 945
3. C	p. 927	20. C	p. 936	37. D	p. 947
4. B	p. 927	21. C	p. 937	38. E	p. 947
5. B	p. 928	22. B	p. 937	39. B	p. 948
6. A	p. 927	23. A	p. 938	40. A	p. 948
7. E	p. 930	24. A	p. 939	41. B	p. 949
8. B	p. 929	25. A	p. 939	42. C	p. 949
9. A	p. 930	26. E	p. 939	43. C	p. 950
10. A	p. 931	27. A	p. 942	44. A	p. 950
11. E	p. 931	28. D	p. 942	45. A	p. 951
12. B	p. 931	29. C	p. 941	46. B	p. 951
13. A	p. 931	30. D	p. 943	47. E	p. 952
14. C	p. 932	31. B	p. 943	48. E	p. 953
15. A	p. 933	32. B	p. 944	49. A	p. 953
16. D	p. 932	33. E	p. 944	50. B	p. 955
17. A	p. 934	34. E	p. 944		

Chapter 23: Head, Facial, and Neck Trauma

MULTIPLE CHOICE

1. A	p. 959	11. A	p. 965	21. C	p. 970
2. D	p. 959	12. D	p. 966	22. A	p. 970
3. A	p. 962	13. E	p. 966	23. E	p. 971
4. B	p. 961	14. B	p. 967	24. A	p. 971
5. E	p. 962	15. C	p. 967	25. C	p. 972
6. C	p. 962	16. E	p. 968	26. A	p. 972
7. D	p. 965	17. C	p. 968	27. A	p. 973
8. B	p. 964	18. A	p. 968	28. A	p. 973
9. B	p. 964	19. B	p. 969	29. B	p. 973
10. B	p. 964	20. C	p. 969	30. E	p. 974

©2007 Pearson Education, Inc.
Essentials of Paramedic Care, 2nd ed.

Workbook Answer Key

31. E	p. 975	41. B	p. 983	51. C	p. 990
32. A	p. 975	42. D	p. 983	52. B	p. 992
33. C	p. 980	43. E	p. 984	53. C	p. 992
34. C	p. 977	44. A	p. 986	54. B	p. 992
35. B	p. 979	45. C	p. 986	55. D	p. 993
36. E	p. 980	46. A	p. 986	56. B	p. 993
37. B	p. 980	47. A	p. 987	57. B	p. 994
38. C	p. 981	48. E	p. 989	58. E	p. 994
39. B	p. 982	49. B	p. 989	59. C	p. 995
40. E	p. 982	50. A	p. 989	60. B	p. 997

Chapter 24: Spinal Trauma

MULTIPLE CHOICE

1. E	p. 1002	11. A	p. 1009	21. B	p. 1018
2. A	p. 1004	12. C	p. 1009	22. E	p. 1019
3. A	p. 1004	13. C	p. 1010	23. A	p. 1021
4. B	p. 1005	14. A	p. 1012	24. A	p. 1022
5. C	p. 1005	15. E	p. 1012	25. A	p. 1023
6. A	p. 1006	16. A	p. 1015	26. B	p. 1023
7. E	p. 1006	17. A	p. 1015	27. A	p. 1025
8. A	p. 1006	18. E	p. 1015	28. E	p. 1026
9. D	p. 1007	19. B	p. 1016	29. D	p. 1027
10. B	p. 1008	20. B	p. 1017	30. B	p. 1027

Chapter 25: Thoracic Trauma

MULTIPLE CHOICE

1. A	p. 1031	18. E	p. 1041	35. B	p. 1048
2. C	p. 1033	19. C	p. 1042	36. E	p. 1048
3. D	p. 1035	20. A	p. 1043	37. E	p. 1049
4. B	p. 1035	21. A	p. 1043	38. A	p. 1049
5. A	p. 1035	22. A	p. 1043	39. D	p. 1051
6. A	p. 1035	23. D	p. 1045	40. E	p. 1051
7. E	p. 1036	24. A	p. 1044	41. B	p. 1051
8. B	p. 1036	25. E	p. 1045	42. B	p. 1052
9. D	p. 1037	26. B	p. 1045	43. A	p. 1055
10. B	p. 1037	27. D	p. 1045	44. C	p. 1054
11. B	p. 1038	28. A	p. 1046	45. A	p. 1054
12. E	p. 1037	29. C	p. 1046	46. B	p. 1055
13. D	p. 1040	30. B	p. 1046	47. C	p. 1055
14. B	p. 1039	31. E	p. 1047	48. A	p. 1056
15. D	p. 1040	32. C	p. 1046	49. A	p. 1056
16. D	p. 1041	33. B	p. 1047	50. E	p. 1058
17. D	p. 1041	34. A	p. 1047		

Chapter 26: Abdominal Trauma

MULTIPLE CHOICE

1. A	p. 1062	13. D	p. 1066	25. A	p. 1070
2. B	p. 1063	14. E	p. 1066	26. A	p. 1073
3. B	p. 1063	15. E	p. 1067	27. D	p. 1072
4. D	p. 1063	16. D	p. 1067	28. E	p. 1072
5. C	p. 1063	17. C	p. 1068	29. C	p. 1075
6. B	p. 1063	18. A	p. 1068	30. C	p. 1075
7. E	p. 1064	19. A	p. 1068	31. E	p. 1075
8. C	p. 1064	20. E	p. 1068	32. B	p. 1075
9. A	p. 1065	21. D	p. 1069	33. D	p. 1075
10. C	p. 1065	22. D	p. 1069	34. A	p. 1077
11. B	p. 1066	23. C	p. 1069	35. A	p. 1077
12. A	p. 1066	24. A	p. 1069		

Division 4: Medical Emergencies

Chapter 27: Pulmonology

MULTIPLE CHOICE

1. C	p. 1081	20. E	p. 1090	39. D	p. 1108
2. A	p. 1081	21. D	p. 1090	40. B	p. 1108
3. A	p. 1082	22. D	p. 1090	41. B	p. 1110
4. D	p. 1082	23. D	p. 1090	42. A	p. 1109
5. E	p. 1082	24. B	p. 1091	43. B	p. 1113
6. C	p. 1084	25. E	p. 1092	44. A	p. 1114
7. D	p. 1085	26. B	p. 1092	45. B	p. 1114
8. B	p. 1086	27. E	p. 1093	46. A	p. 1115
9. B	p. 1086	28. D	p. 1093	47. A	p. 1115
10. B	p. 1087	29. C	p. 1093	48. D	p. 1115
11. B	p. 1086	30. C	p. 1094	49. C	p. 1116
12. A	p. 1111	31. E	p. 1105	50. A	p. 1117
13. C	p. 1088	32. C	p. 1100	51. A	p. 1117
14. B	p. 1088	33. A	p. 1101	52. A	p. 1118
15. A	p. 1089	34. A	p. 1103	53. C	p. 1115
16. B	p. 1089	35. B	p. 1104	54. A	p. 1114
17. A	p. 1090	36. B	p. 1105	55. D	p. 1110
18. C	p. 1090	37. B	p. 1106		
19. A	p. 1090	38. D	p. 1107		

MATCHING

56. C	p. 1101	60. G	p. 1113
57. F	p. 1105	61. B	p. 1114
58. A	p. 1107	62. D	p. 1115
59. E	p. 1109		

Chapter 28: Cardiology

MULTIPLE CHOICE

1. C	p. 1126	16. B	p. 1133	31. A	p. 1164
2. E	p. 1126	17. A	p. 1134	32. C	p. 1165
3. C	p. 1127	18. C	p. 1135	33. D	p. 1166
4. B	p. 1128	19. B	p. 1140	34. E	p. 1168
5. B	p. 1127	20. D	p. 1141	35. B	p. 1171
6. E	p. 1128	21. C	p. 1142	36. E	p. 1169
7. A	p. 1128	22. E	p. 1143	37. B	p. 1171
8. C	p. 1233	23. C	p. 1146	38. C	p. 1173
9. D	p. 1129	24. C	p. 1147	39. E	p. 1176
10. D	p. 1129	25. D	p. 1150	40. D	p. 1177
11. E	p. 1130	26. A	p. 1155	41. B	p. 1177
12. E	p. 1130	27. B	p. 1158	42. D	p. 1181
13. B	p. 1131	28. B	p. 1161	43. A	p. 1178
14. A	p. 1131	29. A	p. 1163	44. E	p. 1182
15. E	p. 1133	30. E	p. 1164	45. E	p. 1185

MATCHING

46. B	p. 1128	50. H	p. 1128	54. B	p. 1130
47. G	p. 1128	51. C	p. 1128	55. C	p. 1130
48. D	p. 1128	52. F	p. 1129	56. A	p. 1130
49. A	p. 1128	53. E	p. 1128		

SPECIAL PROJECT: Dysrhythmia Recognition

Rhythm 1 *Regularity:* regular (slightly irregular)
Rate: 48 beats per minute
P Waves: uniform and upright; regular P–P interval
PRI: .18 seconds and constant
QRS: .12 seconds
Interp: Sinus Bradycardia (with wide QRS)

Rhythm 2 *Regularity:* irregular
Rate: approximately 80 beats per minute
P Waves: not discernible
PRI: none
QRS: .10 seconds
Interp: controlled Atrial Fibrillation

Rhythm 3 *Regularity:* regular
Rate: 50 beats per minute
P Waves: uniform and upright; regular P–P interval
PRI: .12 seconds and constant
QRS: .08 seconds
Interp: Sinus Bradycardia

Rhythm 4 *Regularity:* regular
Rate: 150 beats per minute
P Waves: P waves are not visible
PRI: none
QRS: .10 seconds
Interp: Supraventricular Tachyc

Rhythm 5 *Regularity:* regular P–P; irregular R–R
Rate: atrial rate 107 beats per minute; ventricular rate 90 beats per minute
P Waves: upright and uniform
PRI: progressively lengthens until one P wave is not conducted
QRS: .08 seconds
Interp: Wenckebach—Type I Second Degree Heart Block

Rhythm 6 *Regularity:* irregular
Rate: approximately 80 beats per minute
P Waves: uniform and upright; regular P–P interval
PRI: .14 seconds and constant
QRS: .06 seconds
Interp: Sinus Arrhythmia

Rhythm 7 *Regularity:* regular underlying rhythm interrupted by an ectopic
Rate: 58 beats per minute
P Waves: uniform; regular P–P interval
PRI: .20 seconds
QRS: .10 seconds in underlying rhythm; .18 seconds in ectopic; ectopic has bizarre configuration
Interp: Sinus Bradycardia with one PVC

Rhythm 8 *Regularity:* regular underlying rhythm interrupted by ectopics
Rate: 75 beats per minute
P Waves: uniform; regular P–P interval
PRI: .18 seconds
QRS: .12 seconds in underlying complex; .12 seconds in ectopics; ectopics have bizarre configuration
Interp: Sinus Rhythm (with wide QRS) with two PVCs

Rhythm 9 *Regularity:* regular
Rate: 136 beats per minute
P Waves: uniform and upright; regular P–P interval
PRI: .16 seconds and constant
QRS: .06 seconds
Interp: Sinus Tachycardia

Rhythm 10 *Regularity:* regular
Rate: atrial rate 100 beats per minute; ventricular rate 35 beats per minute
P Waves: uniform; regular P–P interval; more P waves than QRS complexes
PRI: the P waves are not associated with the QRS complexes
QRS: .12 seconds
Interp: Third Degree Heart Block (CHB) with ventricular escape focus

Rhythm 11 *Regularity:* regular
Rate: 107 beats per minute
P Waves: upright and uniform
PRI: .12 seconds
QRS: .08 seconds
Interp: Sinus Tachycardia

Rhythm 12 Regularity: unable to determine
Rate: 10 beats per minute or less
P Waves: none
PRI: none
QRS: .24 seconds
Interp: Idioventricular Rhythm

Rhythm 13 *Regularity:* regular
Rate: 83 beats per minute
P Waves: no visible P waves
PRI: none
QRS: .08 seconds
P Waves: no visible P waves
Interp: Accelerated Junctional Rhythm

Rhythm 14 *Regularity:* regular
Rate: 51 beats per minute
P Waves: uniform and upright; regular P–P interval
PRI: .24 seconds and constant
QRS: .10 seconds
Interp: Sinus Bradycardia with First Degree Heart Block

Rhythm 15 *Regularity:* regular
Rate: atrial rate 74 beats per minute; ventricular rate 37 beats per minute
P Waves: uniform; regular P–P interval; consistently two P waves for every QRS complex
PRI: .26 seconds and constant on conducted beats
QRS: .12 seconds
Interp: Type II Second Degree Heart Block with 2:1 conduction

Rhythm 16 *Regularity:* regular
Rate: atrial rate is 328 beats per minute; ventricular rate is 82 beats per minute
P Waves: uniform; sawtooth appearance
PRI: none
QRS: .08 seconds
Interp: Atrial Flutter with 4:1 response

Rhythm 17 *Regularity:* P–P very slightly irregular; R–R irregular
Rate: atrial rate 79 beats per minute; ventricular rate 70 beats per minute
P Waves: upright and uniform
PRI: progressively lengthens until one P wave is not conducted

©2007 Pearson Education, Inc.
Essentials of Paramedic Care, 2nd ed.

QRS: .12 seconds
Interp: Wenckebach—Type I Second Degree Heart Block (with wide QRS)

Rhythm 18 Regularity: totally chaotic baseline
Rate: cannot be determined
P Waves: none
PRI: none
QRS: none
Interp: Ventricular Fibrillation

Rhythm 19 Regularity: regular
Rate: atrial rate 115 beats per minute; ventricular rate 73 beats per minute
P Waves: non-conducted P waves are more apparent after mapping the P–P interval, since some P waves are hidden within the QRS complexes and T waves
PRI: P waves are not associated with QRS complexes
QRS: .08 seconds
Interp: Third Degree Heart Block (CHB) with junctional escape focus

Rhythm 20 Regularity: regular
Rate: 43 beats per minute
P Waves: no visible P waves
PRI: none
QRS: .08 seconds
Interp: Junctional Escape Rhythm

Rhythm 21 Regularity: regular
Rate: 40 beats per minute
P Waves: none
PRI: none
QRS: .20 seconds; bizarre configuration
Interp: Idioventricular Rhythm

Rhythm 22 Regularity: slightly irregular
Rate: approximately 30 beats per minute
P Waves: uniform and upright; irregular P–P interval
PRI: .18 seconds and constant
QRS: .08 seconds
Interp: Sinus Bradyarrhythmia

Rhythm 23 Regularity: regular
Rate: 214 beats per minute
P Waves: unable
PRI: unable
QRS: .08 seconds
Interp: Supraventricular Tachycardia

Rhythm 24 Regularity: slightly irregular
Rate: 150 beats per minute
P Waves: none visible
PRI: none
QRS: .20 seconds
Interp: Ventricular Tachycardia

Rhythm 25 Regularity: regular P–P; irregular R–R
Rate: atrial rate 65 beats per minute; ventricular rate 40 beats per minute
P Waves: upright and uniform
PRI: .20 seconds and constant on conducted beats
QRS: .08 seconds
Interp: Type II Second Degree Heart Block with variable conduction

Rhythm 26 Regularity: irregular in a pattern of grouped beating
Rate: 80 beats per minute (including ectopics)
P Waves: upright and uniform
PRI: .12 seconds
QRS: .08 seconds (both underlying rhythm and ectopics)
Interp: Sinus Rhythm with bigeminy of PACs

Rhythm 27 Regularity: regular
Rate: 35 beats per minute
P Waves: none
PRI: none
QRS: .16 seconds
Interp: Idioventricular Rhythm

MULTIPLE CHOICE

1. A p. 1187
2. B p. 1187
3. D p. 1187
4. B p. 1190
5. C p. 1193
6. E p. 1198
7. D p. 1200
8. E p. 1200
9. B p. 1200
10. C p. 1200
11. B p. 1200
12. B p. 1180
13. A p. 1201
14. B p. 1204
15. A p. 1206
16. C p. 1204
17. B p. 1211
18. A p. 1212
19. D p. 1214
20. B p. 1214
21. E p. 1224
22. B p. 1226
23. A p. 1230
24. D p. 1232
25. C p. 1234

MATCHING

26. B p. 1188
27. F p. 1155
28. E p. 1222
29. G p. 1222
30. C p. 1222
31. D p. 1233
32. A p. 1234
33. E p. 1199
34. D p. 1206
35. A p. 1198
36. B p. 1204
37. C p. 1206
38. A p. 1216
39. C p. 1213
40. B p. 1213
41. B p. 1216
42. C p. 1219
43. D p. 1220
44. B p. 1221
45. F p. 1229
46. E p. 1221
47. A p. 1222
48. G p. 1224
49. H p. 1225

Chapter 29: Neurology

MULTIPLE CHOICE

1. C p. 1245
2. B p. 1246
3. C p. 1249
4. E p. 1253
5. C p. 1257
6. B p. 1257
7. D p. 1259
8. C p. 1266
9. B p. 1266
10. B p. 1264
11. C p. 1265
12. A p. 1268
13. C p. 1268
14. C p. 1273
15. E p. 1272

MATCHING

16. B, G p. 1250
17. E, H p. 1250
18. A, D p. 1250
19. C, I p. 1250
20. F, J p. 1250
21. A, D p. 1259
22. C, E p. 1259
23. C, F p. 1258
24. B, C p. 1259

Chapter 30: Endocrinology

MULTIPLE CHOICE

1. C p. 1281
2. C p. 1282
3. C p. 1282
4. E p. 1282
5. B p. 1284
6. D p. 1285
7. E p. 1285
8. A p. 1285
9. A p. 1285
10. A p. 1285
11. C p. 1288
12. E p. 1287
13. A p. 1288
14. B p. 1289
15. A p. 1290
16. E p. 1291
17. B p. 1291
18. A p. 1292
19. B p. 1293
20. A p. 1293

Chapter 31: Allergies and Anaphylaxis

MULTIPLE CHOICE

1. B   p. 1296
2. D   p. 1296
3. B   p. 1297
4. C   p. 1297
5. D   p. 1297
6. A   p. 1296
7. C   p. 1298
8. C   p. 1299
9. C   p. 1298
10. B   p. 1299
11. A   p. 1299
12. B   p. 1300
13. C   p. 1301
14. D   p. 1301
15. D   p. 1300

Chapter 32: Gastroenterology

MULTIPLE CHOICE

1. D   p. 1307
2. A   p. 1307
3. B   p. 1310
4. E   p. 1311
5. A   p. 1311
6. C   p. 1311
7. D   p. 1313
8. B   p. 1312
9. A   p. 1314
10. E   p. 1315
11. B   p. 1315
12. A   p. 1317
13. C   p. 1317
14. D   p. 1320
15. B   p. 1324

MATCHING

p. 1308
16. C
17. E
18. A
19. B
20. A
21. E
22. A
23. D

Chapter 33: Urology and Nephrology

MULTIPLE CHOICE

1. B   p. 1329
2. C   p. 1330
3. D   p. 1331
4. B   p. 1331
5. E   p. 1332
6. B   p. 1334
7. A   p. 1334
8. A   p. 1335
9. A   p. 1335
10. A   p. 1337
11. C   p. 1339
12. D   p. 1340
13. A   p. 1340
14. C   p. 1342
15. E   p. 1344
16. C   p. 1344
17. B   p. 1345
18. C   p. 1345
19. A   p. 1346
20. A   p. 1346

Chapter 34: Toxicology and Substance Abuse

MULTIPLE CHOICE

1. C   p. 1351
2. A   p. 1352
3. D   p. 1352
4. B   p. 1353
5. A   p. 1354
6. B   p. 1356
7. E   p. 1354
8. B   p. 1354
9. B   p. 1355
10. B   p. 1355
11. C   p. 1356
12. A   p. 1356
13. D   p. 1357
14. B   p. 1358
15. A   p. 1358
16. E   p. 1362
17. A   p. 1361
18. B   p. 1363
19. A   p. 1364
20. A   p. 1351
21. E   p. 1363
22. C   p. 1367
23. E   p. 1368
24. A   p. 1366
25. B   p. 1367
26. D   p. 1370
27. E   p. 1366
28. A   p. 1371
29. A   p. 1373
30. C   p. 1381
31. A   p. 1381
32. A   p. 1383
33. A   p. 1383
34. B   p. 1386

MATCHING

35. B   p. 1353
36. H   p. 1380
37. N   p. 1350
38. M   p. 1352
39. A   p. 1350
40. O   p. 1380
41. G   p. 1365
42. P   p. 1352
43. F   p. 1386
44. L   p. 1370
45. I   p. 1354
46. J   p. 1352
47. K   p. 1380
48. D   p. 1359
49. C   p. 1380
50. E   p. 1380

Chapter 35: Hematology

MULTIPLE CHOICE

1. B   p. 1390
2. B   p. 1390
3. D   p. 1390
4. C   p. 1392
5. D   p. 1394
6. E   p. 1394
7. A   p. 1395
8. C   p. 1396
9. D   p. 1396
10. C   p. 1397
11. C   p. 1399
12. E   p. 1401
13. D   p. 1401
14. B   p. 1401
15. B   p. 1402

Chapter 36: Environmental Emergencies

MULTIPLE CHOICE

1. C   p. 1407
2. A   p. 1407
3. E   p. 1408
4. B   p. 1411
5. B   p. 1415
6. A   p. 1415
7. B   p. 1415
8. D   p. 1416
9. A   p. 1419
10. C   p. 1419
11. E   p. 1422
12. B   p. 1424
13. D   p. 1426
14. C   p. 1427
15. C   p. 1426
16. B   p. 1426
17. E   p. 1428
18. D   p. 1432
19. C   p. 1435
20. D   p. 1435

MATCHING

21. I   p. 1413
22. D   p. 1422
23. E   p. 1435
24. J   p. 1418
25. G   p. 1435
26. F   p. 1431
27. H   p. 1432
28. A   p. 1418
29. C   p. 1429
30. B   p. 1435

Chapter 37: Infectious Disease

MULTIPLE CHOICE

1. B   p. 1443
2. E   p. 1445
3. B   p. 1443
4. C   p. 1444
5. D   p. 1447
6. A   p. 1448
7. E   p. 1449
8. C   p. 1448
9. B   p. 1448
10. B   p. 1453
11. C   p. 1451
12. E   p. 1454
13. D   p. 1459
14. A   p. 1457
15. A   p. 1459
16. B   p. 1461
17. D   p. 1464
18. C   p. 1465
19. D   p. 1467
20. E   p. 1482
21. A   p. 1468
22. E   p. 1468
23. B   p. 1474
24. A   p. 1475
25. C   p. 1478

Chapter 38: Psychiatric and Behavioral Disorders

MULTIPLE CHOICE

1. B   p. 1488
2. B   p. 1488
3. C   p. 1490
4. C   p. 1490
5. B   p. 1491
6. D   p. 1490
7. E   p. 1494
8. C   p. 1495
9. C   p. 1495
10. A   p. 1492
11. C   p. 1493
12. A   p. 1493
13. A   p. 1497
14. B   p. 1504
15. B   p. 1501

MATCHING

16. J   p. 1498
17. A   p. 1493
18. D   p. 1493
19. I   p. 1499
20. E   p. 1493
21. H   p. 1496
22. F   p. 1494
23. C   p. 1493
24. G   p. 1494
25. B   p. 1493

Chapter 39: Gynecology

MULTIPLE CHOICE

1. D   p. 1510
2. B   p. 1510
3. C   p. 1511
4. C   p. 1510
5. C   p. 1511
6. A   p. 1512
7. E   p. 1513
8. B   p. 1513
9. B   p. 1514
10. D   p. 1513
11. C   p. 1513
12. B   p. 1514
13. A   p. 1515
14. A   p. 1515
15. D   p. 1515

Chapter 40: Obstetrics

MULTIPLE CHOICE

1. A p. 1519	10. A p. 1527	19. C p. 1547
2. D p. 1519	11. A p. 1528	20. A p. 1537
3. E p. 1522	12. C p. 1530	21. A p. 1543
4. D p. 1522	13. B p. 1533	22. B p. 1543
5. A p. 1524	14. E p. 1534	23. B p. 1544
6. C p. 1524	15. C p. 1539	24. C p. 1548
7. E p. 1525	16. B p. 1538	25. D p. 1550
8. C p. 1522	17. B p. 1549	
9. B p. 1528	18. C p. 1549	

MATCHING

26. D p. 1521	30. B p. 1520	34. I p. 1537
27. E p. 1519	31. G p. 1536	35. F p. 1537
28. A p. 1522	32. J p. 1536	
29. C p. 1519	33. H p. 1524	

Division 5: Special Considerations/Operations

Chapter 41: Neonatology

MULTIPLE CHOICE

1. B p. 1556	13. B p. 1560	25. A p. 1569
2. A p. 1556	14. E p. 1560	26. E p. 1570
3. C p. 1557	15. B p. 1561	27. D p. 1570
4. E p. 1557	16. E p. 1563	28. A p. 1573
5. B p. 1557	17. A p. 1563	29. A p. 1574
6. A p. 1557	18. B p. 1563	30. B p. 1575
7. A p. 1557	19. B p. 1563	31. D p. 1576
8. B p. 1559	20. D p. 1564	32. E p. 1577
9. E p. 1559	21. B p. 1566	33. A p. 1578
10. D p. 1559	22. A p. 1564	34. A p. 1579
11. B p. 1559	23. A p. 1564	35. B p. 1580
12. C p. 1559	24. C p. 1567	

Chapter 42: Pediatrics

MULTIPLE CHOICE

1. C p. 1587	16. E p. 1600	31. C p. 1628
2. D p. 1587	17. E p. 1601	32. E p. 1628
3. A p. 1588	18. A p. 1604	33. C p. 1629
4. B p. 1589	19. D p. 1605	34. A p. 1630
5. E p. 1589	20. A p. 1605	35. D p. 1633
6. C p. 1590	21. C p. 1605	36. B p. 1636
7. C p. 1590	22. D p. 1608	37. A p. 1637
8. B p. 1591	23. E p. 1609	38. B p. 1643
9. C p. 1594	24. C p. 1612	39. C p. 1645
10. E p. 1601	25. E p. 1613	40. C p. 1649
11. A p. 1595	26. C p. 1613	41. C p. 1652
12. B p. 1596	27. D p. 1617	42. C p. 1656
13. B p. 1596	28. A p. 1619	43. E p. 1658
14. B p. 1596	29. C p. 1619	44. D p. 1660
15. B p. 1598	30. B p. 1621	45. C p. 1663

Chapter 43: Geriatric Emergencies

MULTIPLE CHOICE

1. B p. 1669	23. A p. 1677	45. C p. 1688
2. C p. 1670	24. E p. 1678	46. C p. 1689
3. C p. 1672	25. B p. 1678	47. B p. 1689
4. A p. 1672	26. E p. 1679	48. B p. 1690
5. B p. 1672	27. D p. 1680	49. B p. 1690
6. C p. 1672	28. E p. 1684	50. A p. 1691
7. D p. 1672	29. A p. 1682	51. B p. 1692
8. E p. 1673	30. B p. 1680	52. D p. 1693
9. A p. 1673	31. C p. 1680	53. C p. 1694
10. B p. 1673	32. A p. 1681	54. D p. 1695
11. B p. 1673	33. B p. 1684	55. A p. 1696
12. C p. 1673	34. C p. 1682	56. B p. 1698
13. D p. 1674	35. C p. 1682	57. B p. 1698
14. A p. 1675	36. B p. 1682	58. B p. 1698
15. E p. 1675	37. B p. 1682	59. A p. 1698
16. C p. 1673	38. E p. 1683	60. E p. 1699
17. A p. 1675	39. A p. 1683	61. B p. 1700
18. E p. 1675	40. B p. 1686	62. A p. 1700
19. E p. 1676	41. A p. 1686	63. A p. 1701
20. A p. 1676	42. E p. 1687	64. C p. 1703
21. D p. 1676	43. A p. 1687	65. B p. 1704
22. A p. 1676	44. B p. 1688	

MATCHING

66. J p. 1694	71. O p. 1707	76. K p. 1695
67. G p. 1703	72. I p. 1693	77. N p. 1713
68. A p. 1692	73. B p. 1692	78. D p. 1692
69. H p. 1691	74. C p. 1692	79. F p. 1693
70. M p. 1698	75. L p. 1694	80. E p. 1675

Chapter 44: Abuse and Assault

MULTIPLE CHOICE

1. B p. 1716	8. C p. 1719	15. A p. 1724
2. A p. 1716	9. C p. 1719	16. B p. 1724
3. E p. 1716	10. D p. 1720	17. A p. 1726
4. C p. 1717	11. E p. 1721	18. C p. 1726
5. A p. 1718	12. E p. 1722	19. B p. 1726
6. B p. 1718	13. B p. 1722	20. A p. 1726
7. B p. 1718	14. B p. 1722	

Chapter 45: The Challenged Patient

MULTIPLE CHOICE

1. B p. 1731	11. E p. 1735	21. D p. 1741
2. B p. 1731	12. B p. 1736	22. C p. 1742
3. A p. 1732	13. A p. 1736	23. B p. 1738
4. B p. 1732	14. C p. 1737	24. D p. 1743
5. B p. 1732	15. A p. 1738	25. E p. 1743
6. B p. 1733	16. A p. 1738	26. A p. 1743
7. B p. 1733	17. B p. 1739	27. E p. 1743
8. A p. 1733	18. B p. 1740	28. D p. 1744
9. D p. 1734	19. C p. 1740	29. B p. 1744
10. B p. 1734	20. E p. 1741	30. A p. 1744

MATCHING

31. D p. 1730	36. C p. 1734	41. G p. 1734
32. N p. 1731	37. L p. 1736	42. A p. 1731
33. H p. 1731	38. I p. 1739	43. J p. 1732
34. O p. 1733	39. B p. 1731	44. F p. 1731
35. K p. 1731	40. E p. 1733	45. M p. 1741

Chapter 46: Acute Interventions for the Chronic-Care Patient

MULTIPLE CHOICE

1. C p. 1747
2. A p. 1747
3. E p. 1747
4. B p. 1748
5. A p. 1749
6. B p. 1749
7. A p. 1749
8. B p. 1750
9. A p. 1750
10. C p. 1750
11. E p. 1751
12. E p. 1752
13. C p. 1752
14. A p. 1754
15. E p. 1753
16. B p. 1755
17. B p. 1757
18. B p. 1759
19. D p. 1759
20. E p. 1761
21. D p. 1762
22. B p. 1763
23. D p. 1765
24. A p. 1768
25. E p. 1768
26. C p. 1769
27. E p. 1770
28. C p. 1771
29. B p. 1774
30. E p. 1776

MATCHING

31. D p. 1760
32. G p. 1749
33. C p. 1759
34. A p. 1749
35. H p. 1750
36. J p. 1750
37. F p. 1750
38. B p. 1759
39. E p. 1754
40. I p. 1759

SHORT ANSWER

41. Positive end-expiratory pressure p. 1765
42. Continuous positive airway pressure p. 1765
43. Bilevel positive airway pressure p. 1765
44. Chronic obstructive pulmonary disease p. 1758
45. Acute respiratory distress syndrome p. 1765
46. Positive-pressure ventilation 1765
47. Vascular access device p. 1767
48. Peripherally inserted central catheter p. 1767
49. Do not attempt resuscitation orders p. 1775
50. Congestive heart failure p. 1759

Chapter 47: Assessment-Based Management

MULTIPLE CHOICE

1. B p. 1779
2. C p. 1779
3. B p. 1780
4. E p. 1781
5. C p. 1781
6. E p. 1781
7. A p. 1781
8. D p. 1783
9. E p. 1784
10. B p. 1783
11. C p. 1785
12. C p. 1786
13. C p. 1786
14. B p. 1787
15. B p. 1789

Chapter 48: Operations

MULTIPLE CHOICE

1. A p. 1799
2. A p. 1799
3. C p. 1799
4. E p. 1800
5. E p. 1800
6. B p. 1800
7. C p. 1800
8. D p. 1801
9. C p. 1801
10. B p. 1802
11. B p. 1802
12. B p. 1803
13. D p. 1804
14. B p. 1804
15. A p. 1804
16. C p. 1804
17. E p. 1805
18. B p. 1805
19. B p. 1806
20. B p. 1806
21. E p. 1806
22. A p. 1807
23. A p. 1807
24. E p. 1807
25. A p. 1809

MATCHING

26. D p. 1801
27. F p. 1799
28. I p. 1799
29. A p. 1799
30. E p. 1801
31. B p. 1801
32. C p. 1802
33. J p. 1802
34. H p. 1802
35. G p. 1803

MULTIPLE CHOICE

1. C p. 1809
2. A p. 1810
3. C p. 1811
4. A p. 1811
5. A p. 1813
6. A p. 1814
7. A p. 1812
8. A p. 1812
9. E p. 1814
10. D p. 1815
11. A p. 1815
12. A p. 1815
13. E p. 1816
14. A p. 1816
15. D p. 1818
16. D p. 1819
17. B p. 1819
18. A p. 1821
19. D p. 1821
20. A p. 1821
21. E p. 1822
22. A p. 1824
23. B p. 1826
24. A p. 1827
25. A p. 1829

MATCHING

26. D p. 1811
27. J p. 1816
28. I p. 1817
29. H p. 1811
30. A p. 1817
31. B p. 1813
32. G p. 1816
33. C p. 1819
34. F p. 1810
35. E p. 1814

SHORT ANSWER

36. Multiple casualty incident p. 1809
37. Command, Finance, Logistics, Operations, Planning p. 1811
38. Emergency Operation Center p. 1811
39. Incident Management System p. 1810
40. Simple Triage and Rapid Transport p. 1821

MULTIPLE CHOICE

1. E p. 1830
2. B p. 1831
3. D p. 1833
4. C p. 1835
5. C p. 1835
6. C p. 1837
7. A p. 1839
8. D p. 1840
9. E p. 1840
10. C p. 1841
11. E p. 1843
12. A p. 1844
13. C p. 1845
14. B p. 1847
15. A p. 1849
16. B p. 1850
17. B p. 1851
18. A p. 1852
19. A p. 1854
20. C p. 1856

MATCHING

21. H p. 1837
22. C p. 1826
23. F p. 1840
24. A p. 1841
25. J p. 1850
26. I p. 1855
27. D p. 1841
28. E p. 1843
29. G p. 1850
30. B p. 1843

MULTIPLE CHOICE

1. A p. 1857
2. E p. 1858
3. B p. 1858
4. C p. 1858
5. D p. 1858
6. A p. 1859
7. B p. 1862
8. B p. 1862
9. C p. 1862
10. B p. 1862
11. B p. 1863
12. B p. 1865
13. D p. 1866
14. A p. 1865
15. A p. 1866
16. A p. 1867
17. A p. 1868
18. A p. 1868
19. A p. 1869
20. D p. 1870
21. D p. 1870
22. D p. 1871
23. C p. 1871
24. C p. 1871
25. A p. 1872

MATCHING

26. D p. 1857
27. H p. 1859
28. I p. 1862
29. C p. 1863
30. J p. 1863
31. B p. 1863
32. G p. 1863
33. E p. 1864
34. A p. 1863
35. F p. 1864

MULTIPLE CHOICE

1. B p. 1872
2. B p. 1873
3. B p. 1873
4. C p. 1874
5. A p. 1874
6. E p. 1874
7. A p. 1875
8. B p. 1875
9. C p. 1876
10. A p. 1877
11. B p. 1877
12. E p. 1877
13. E p. 1877
14. A p. 1878
15. B p. 1878
16. B p. 1879
17. B p. 1879
18. E p. 1879
19. C p. 1880
20. B p. 1880
21. B p. 1882
22. E p. 1883
23. A p. 1884
24. A p. 1884
25. E p. 1885

MATCHING

26.	J	p. 1878	30. I p. 1883	34.	G	p. 1884
27.	D	p. 1882	31. B p. 1885	35.	F	p. 1883
28.	C	p. 1880	32. A p. 1873			
29.	E	p. 1882	33. H p. 1881			

Chapter 49: Responding to Terrorist Acts

MULTIPLE CHOICE

1. A p. 1891
2. E p. 1891
3. C p. 1892
4. B p. 1892
5. D p. 1894
6. E p. 1894
7. C p. 1894
8. A p. 1894
9. E p. 1894
10. E p. 1895
11. A p. 1896
12. B p. 1896
13. C p. 1896
14. D p. 1897
15. E p. 1898
16. D p. 1900
17. E p. 1900
18. A p. 1901
19. A p. 1901
20. B p. 1902

718 ESSENTIALS OF PARAMEDIC CARE

©2007 Pearson Education, Inc.
Essentials of Paramedic Care, 2nd ed.

National Registry of Emergency Medical Technicians

Practical Evaluation Forms

The forms on the next pages are provided to help you identify common criteria by which you will be evaluated. It may be valuable to review your practical skills by using these sheets during your class practice sessions and as you review those skills before class, state, and any national testing. Evaluation forms will vary; however, many of the important elements of paramedic practice are common to all forms.

EMT-Paramedic Forms

The following skill instruments for the EMT-Paramedic level were developed by the National Registry of EMTs and have been approved for use in advanced level National Registry examinations.

- Bleeding Control/Shock Management
- Dual Lumen Airway Device
- Dynamic Cardiology
- Intravenous Therapy
- Oral Station
- Patient Assessment—Medical
- Patient Assessment—Trauma
- Pediatric Intraosseous Infusion
- Pediatric (less than 2 years) Ventilatory Management
- Spinal Immobilization (Seated Patient)
- Spinal Immobilization (Supine Patient)
- Static Cardiology
- Ventilatory Management—Adult

EMT-Paramedic Form

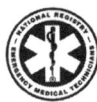

National Registry of Emergency Medical Technicians
Advanced Level Practical Examination

BLEEDING CONTROL/SHOCK MANAGEMENT

Candidate: _____ Examiner: _____

Date: _____ Signature: _____

Time Start:_____	Possible Points	Points Awarded
Takes or verbalizes body substance isolation precautions	1	
Applies direct pressure to the wound	1	
Elevates the extremity	1	
NOTE: The examiner must now inform the candidate that the wound continues to bleed.		
Applies an additional dressing to the wound	1	
NOTE: The examiner must now inform the candidate that the wound still continues to bleed. The second dressing does not control the bleeding.		
Locates and applies pressure to appropriate arterial pressure point	1	
NOTE: The examiner must now inform the candidate that the bleeding is controlled.		
Bandages the wound	1	
NOTE: The examiner must now inform the candidate that the patient is exhibiting signs and symptoms of hypoperfusion.		
Properly positions the patient	1	
Administers high concentration oxygen	1	
Initiates steps to prevent heat loss from the patient	1	
Indicates the need for immediate transportation	1	
Time End: _____ **TOTAL**	10	

CRITICAL CRITERIA

_____ Did not take or verbalize body substance isolation precautions
_____ Did not apply high concentration of oxygen
_____ Applied a tourniquet before attempting other methods of bleeding control
_____ Did not control hemorrhage in a timely manner
_____ Did not indicate the need for immediate transportation

You must factually document your rationale for checking any of the above critical items on the reverse side of this form.

© 2000 National Registry of Emergency Medical Technicians, Inc., Columbus, OH
All materials subject to this copyright may be photocopied for the non-commercial purpose of educational or scientific advancement.

p313/8-003k

EMT-Paramedic Form

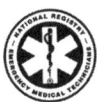

National Registry of Emergency Medical Technicians
Advanced Level Practical Examination

DUAL LUMEN AIRWAY DEVICE (COMBITUBE® OR PTL®)

Candidate: _____ Examiner: _____

Date: _____ Signature: _____

NOTE: If candidate elects to initially ventilate with BVM attached to reservoir and oxygen, full credit must be awarded for steps denoted by "**" so long as first ventilation is delivered within 30 seconds.

	Possible Points	Points Awarded
Takes or verbalizes body substance isolation precautions	1	
Opens the airway manually	1	
Elevates tongue, inserts simple adjunct [oropharyngeal or nasopharyngeal airway]	1	
NOTE: Examiner now informs candidate no gag reflex is present and patient accepts adjunct		
**Ventilates patient immediately with bag-valve-mask device unattached to oxygen	1	
**Hyperventilates patient with room air	1	
NOTE: Examiner now informs candidate that ventilation is being performed without difficulty		
Attaches oxygen reservoir to bag-valve-mask device and connects to high flow oxygen regulator [12-15 L/minute]	1	
Ventilates patient at a rate of 10-20/minute with appropriate volumes	1	
NOTE: After 30 seconds, examiner auscultates and reports breath sounds are present and equal bilaterally and medical control has ordered insertion of a dual lumen airway. The examiner must now take over ventilation.		
Directs assistant to pre-oxygenate patient	1	
Checks/prepares airway device	1	
Lubricates distal tip of the device [may be verbalized]	1	
NOTE: Examiner to remove OPA and move out of the way when candidate is prepared to insert device		
Positions head properly	1	
Performs a tongue-jaw lift	1	
☐ USES COMBITUBE® / **☐ USES PTL®**		
Inserts device in mid-line and to depth so printed ring is at level of teeth / Inserts device in mid-line until bite block flange is at level of teeth	1	
Inflates pharyngeal cuff with proper volume and removes syringe / Secures strap	1	
Inflates distal cuff with proper volume and removes syringe / Blows into tube #1 to adequately inflate both cuffs	1	
Attaches/directs attachment of BVM to the first [esophageal placement] lumen and ventilates	1	
Confirms placement and ventilation through correct lumen by observing chest rise, auscultation over the epigastrium, and bilaterally over each lung	1	
NOTE: The examiner states, "You do not see rise and fall of the chest and you only hear sounds over the epigastrium."		
Attaches/directs attachment of BVM to the second [endotracheal placement] lumen and ventilates	1	
Confirms placement and ventilation through correct lumen by observing chest rise, auscultation over the epigastrium, and bilaterally over each lung	1	
NOTE: The examiner confirms adequate chest rise, absent sounds over the epigastrium, and equal bilateral breath sounds.		
Secures device or confirms that the device remains properly secured	1	
TOTAL	**20**	

CRITICAL CRITERIA

_____ Failure to initiate ventilations within 30 seconds after taking body substance isolation precautions or interrupts ventilations for greater than 30 seconds at any time
_____ Failure to take or verbalize body substance isolation precautions
_____ Failure to voice and ultimately provide high oxygen concentrations [at least 85%]
_____ Failure to ventilate patient at a rate of at least 10/minute
_____ Failure to provide adequate volumes per breath [maximum 2 errors/minute permissible]
_____ Failure to pre-oxygenate patient prior to insertion of the dual lumen airway device
_____ Failure to insert the dual lumen airway device at a proper depth or at either proper place within 3 attempts
_____ Failure to inflate both cuffs properly
_____ **Combitube** - failure to remove the syringe immediately after inflation of each cuff
       PTL - failure to secure the strap prior to cuff inflation
_____ Failure to confirm that the proper lumen of the device is being ventilated by observing chest rise, auscultation over the epigastrium, and bilaterally over each lung
_____ Inserts any adjunct in a manner dangerous to patient

You must factually document your rationale for checking any of the above critical items on the reverse side of this form.

© 2000 National Registry of Emergency Medical Technicians, Inc., Columbus, OH
All materials subject to this copyright may be photocopied for the non-commercial purpose of educational or scientific advancement.

p304/8-003k

EMT-Paramedic Form

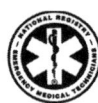

National Registry of Emergency Medical Technicians
Advanced Level Practical Examination

DYNAMIC CARDIOLOGY

Candidate: _____ Examiner: _____

Date: _____ Signature: _____

SET # _____

Level of Testing: ☐ NREMT-Intermediate/99   ☐ NREMT-Paramedic

Time Start: _____

	Possible Points	Points Awarded
Takes or verbalizes infection control precautions	1	
Checks level of responsiveness	1	
Checks ABCs	1	
Initiates CPR if appropriate [verbally]	1	
Attaches ECG monitor in a timely fashion or applies paddles for "Quick Look"	1	
Correctly interprets initial rhythm	1	
Appropriately manages initial rhythm	2	
Notes change in rhythm	1	
Checks patient condition to include pulse and, if appropriate, BP	1	
Correctly interprets second rhythm	1	
Appropriately manages second rhythm	2	
Notes change in rhythm	1	
Checks patient condition to include pulse and, if appropriate, BP	1	
Correctly interprets third rhythm	1	
Appropriately manages third rhythm	2	
Notes change in rhythm	1	
Checks patient condition to include pulse and, if appropriate, BP	1	
Correctly interprets fourth rhythm	1	
Appropriately manages fourth rhythm	2	
Orders high percentages of supplemental oxygen at proper times	1	
Time End: _____ **TOTAL**	24	

CRITICAL CRITERIA

_____ Failure to deliver first shock in a timely manner due to operator delay in machine use or providing treatments other than CPR with simple adjuncts
_____ Failure to deliver second or third shocks without delay other than the time required to reassess rhythm and recharge paddles
_____ Failure to verify rhythm before delivering each shock
_____ Failure to ensure the safety of self and others [verbalizes "All clear" and observes]
_____ Inability to deliver DC shock [does not use machine properly]
_____ Failure to demonstrate acceptable shock sequence
_____ Failure to order initiation or resumption of CPR when appropriate
_____ Failure to order correct management of airway [ET when appropriate]
_____ Failure to order administration of appropriate oxygen at proper time
_____ Failure to diagnose or treat 2 or more rhythms correctly
_____ Orders administration of an inappropriate drug or lethal dosage
_____ Failure to correctly diagnose or adequately treat v-fib, v-tach, or asystole

You must factually document your rationale for checking any of the above critical items on the reverse side of this form.

© 2000 National Registry of Emergency Medical Technicians, Inc., Columbus, OH
All materials subject to this copyright may be photocopied for the non-commercial purpose of educational or scientific advancement.

p306/8-003k

EMT-Paramedic Form

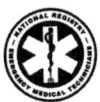

National Registry of Emergency Medical Technicians
Advanced Level Practical Examination

INTRAVENOUS THERAPY

Candidate: _____ Examiner: _____

Date: _____ Signature: _____

Level of Testing: ❏ NREMT-Intermediate/85   ❏ NREMT-Intermediate/99   ❏ NREMT-Paramedic

Time Start: _____

	Possible Points	Points Awarded

Checks selected IV fluid for:
    -Proper fluid (1 point)
    -Clarity (1 point)
	2	

Selects appropriate catheter	1	
Selects proper administration set	1	
Connects IV tubing to the IV bag	1	
Prepares administration set [fills drip chamber and flushes tubing]	1	
Cuts or tears tape [at any time before venipuncture]	1	
Takes/verbalizes body substance isolation precautions [prior to venipuncture]	1	
Applies tourniquet	1	
Palpates suitable vein	1	
Cleanses site appropriately	1	

Performs venipuncture
    -Inserts stylette (1 point)
    -Notes or verbalizes flashback (1 point)
    -Occludes vein proximal to catheter (1 point)
    -Removes stylette (1 point)
    -Connects IV tubing to catheter (1 point)
	5	

Disposes/verbalizes disposal of needle in proper container	1	
Releases tourniquet	1	
Runs IV for a brief period to assure patent line	1	
Secures catheter [tapes securely or verbalizes]	1	
Adjusts flow rate as appropriate	1	
Time End: _____ **TOTAL**	21	

CRITICAL CRITERIA
____ Failure to establish a patent and properly adjusted IV within 6 minute time limit
____ Failure to take or verbalize body substance isolation precautions prior to performing venipuncture
____ Contaminates equipment or site without appropriately correcting situation
____ Performs any improper technique resulting in the potential for uncontrolled hemorrhage, catheter shear, or air embolism
____ Failure to successfully establish IV within 3 attempts during 6 minute time limit
____ Failure to dispose/verbalize disposal of needle in proper container

NOTE: Check here (_____) if candidate did not establish a patent IV and do not evaluate IV Bolus Medications.

INTRAVENOUS BOLUS MEDICATIONS

Time Start: _____

	Possible Points	Points Awarded
Asks patient for known allergies	1	
Selects correct medication	1	
Assures correct concentration of drug	1	
Assembles prefilled syringe correctly and dispels air	1	
Continues body substance isolation precautions	1	
Cleanses injection site [Y-port or hub]	1	
Reaffirms medication	1	
Stops IV flow [pinches tubing or shuts off]	1	
Administers correct dose at proper push rate	1	
Disposes/verbalizes proper disposal of syringe and needle in proper container	1	
Flushes tubing [runs wide open for a brief period]	1	
Adjusts drip rate to TKO/KVO	1	
Verbalizes need to observe patient for desired effect/adverse side effects	1	
Time End: _____ **TOTAL**	13	

CRITICAL CRITERIA
____ Failure to begin administration of medication within 3 minute time limit
____ Contaminates equipment or site without appropriately correcting situation
____ Failure to adequately dispel air resulting in potential for air embolism
____ Injects improper drug or dosage [wrong drug, incorrect amount, or pushes at inappropriate rate]
____ Failure to flush IV tubing after injecting medication
____ Recaps needle or failure to dispose/verbalize disposal of syringe and needle in proper container

You must factually document your rationale for checking any of the above critical items on the reverse side of this form.

© 2000 National Registry of Emergency Medical Technicians, Inc., Columbus, OH
All materials subject to this copyright may be photocopied for the non-commercial purpose of educational or scientific advancement.

p309/8-003k

©2007 Pearson Education, Inc.
Essentials of Paramedic Care, 2nd ed.

EMT-Paramedic Form

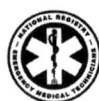

National Registry of Emergency Medical Technicians
Advanced Level Practical Examination
ORAL STATION

Candidate: _____ Examiner: _____

Date: _____ Signature: _____

Scenario: _____

Time Start: _____

	Possible Points	Points Awarded
Scene Management		
Thoroughly assessed and took deliberate actions to control the scene	3	
Assessed the scene, identified potential hazards, did not put anyone in danger	2	
Incompletely assessed or managed the scene	1	
Did not assess or manage the scene	0	
Patient Assessment		
Completed an organized assessment and integrated findings to expand further assessment	3	
Completed initial, focused, and ongoing assessments	2	
Performed an incomplete or disorganized assessment	1	
Did not complete an initial assessment	0	
Patient Management		
Managed all aspects of the patient's condition and anticipated further needs	3	
Appropriately managed the patient's presenting condition	2	
Performed an incomplete or disorganized management	1	
Did not manage life-threatening conditions	0	
Interpersonal relations		
Established rapport and interacted in an organized, therapeutic manner	3	
Interacted and responded appropriately with patient, crew, and bystanders	2	
Used inappropriate communication techniques	1	
Demonstrated intolerance for patient, bystanders, and crew	0	
Integration (verbal report, field impression, and transport decision)		
Stated correct field impression and pathophysiological basis, provided succinct and accurate verbal report including social/psychological concerns, and considered alternate transport destinations	3	
Stated correct field impression, provided succinct and accurate verbal report, and appropriately stated transport decision	2	
Stated correct field impression, provided inappropriate verbal report or transport decision	1	
Stated incorrect field impression or did not provide verbal report	0	

Time End: _____   **TOTAL**   15

Critical Criteria

_____ Failure to appropriately address any of the scenario's "Mandatory Actions"
_____ Performs or orders any harmful or dangerous action or intervention

You must factually document your rationale for checking any of the above critical items on the reverse side of this form.

© 2000 National Registry of Emergency Medical Technicians, Inc., Columbus, OH
All materials subject to this copyright may be photocopied for the non-commercial purpose of educational or scientific advancement.

p308/8-003k

EMT-Paramedic Form

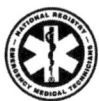

National Registry of Emergency Medical Technicians
Advanced Level Practical Examination

PATIENT ASSESSMENT - MEDICAL

Candidate: _____ Examiner: _____
Date: _____ Signature: _____
Scenario: _____
Time Start: _____

	Possible Points	Points Awarded
Takes or verbalizes body substance isolation precautions	1	
SCENE SIZE-UP		
Determines the scene/situation is safe	1	
Determines the mechanism of injury/nature of illness	1	
Determines the number of patients	1	
Requests additional help if necessary	1	
Considers stabilization of spine	1	
INITIAL ASSESSMENT		
Verbalizes general impression of the patient	1	
Determines responsiveness/level of consciousness	1	
Determines chief complaint/apparent life-threats	1	
Assesses airway and breathing 　　-Assessment (1 point) 　　-Assures adequate ventilation (1 point) 　　-Initiates appropriate oxygen therapy (1 point)	3	
Assesses circulation 　　-Assesses/controls major bleeding (1 point)　　-Assesses skin [either skin color, temperature, or condition] (1 point) 　　-Assesses pulse (1 point)	3	
Identifies priority patients/makes transport decision	1	
FOCUSED HISTORY AND PHYSICAL EXAMINATION/RAPID ASSESSMENT		
History of present illness 　　-Onset (1 point)　　　　-Severity (1 point) 　　-Provocation (1 point)　-Time (1 point) 　　-Quality (1 point)　　　-Clarifying questions of associated signs and symptoms as related to OPQRST (2 points) 　　-Radiation (1 point)	8	
Past medical history 　　-Allergies (1 point)　　-Past pertinent history (1 point)　　-Events leading to present illness (1 point) 　　-Medications (1 point)　-Last oral intake (1 point)	5	
Performs focused physical examination [assess affected body part/system or, if indicated, completes rapid assessment] 　　-Cardiovascular　　-Neurological　　-Integumentary　　-Reproductive 　　-Pulmonary　　　　-Musculoskeletal　-GI/GU　　　　　-Psychological/Social	5	
Vital signs 　　-Pulse (1 point)　　　　　-Respiratory rate and quality (1 point each) 　　-Blood pressure (1 point)　-AVPU (1 point)	5	
Diagnostics [must include application of ECG monitor for dyspnea and chest pain]	2	
States field impression of patient	1	
Verbalizes treatment plan for patient and calls for appropriate intervention(s)	1	
Transport decision re-evaluated	1	
ON-GOING ASSESSMENT		
Repeats initial assessment	1	
Repeats vital signs	1	
Evaluates response to treatments	1	
Repeats focused assessment regarding patient complaint or injuries	1	

Time End: _____
CRITICAL CRITERIA **TOTAL** 48

_____ Failure to initiate or call for transport of the patient within 15 minute time limit
_____ Failure to take or verbalize body substance isolation precautions
_____ Failure to determine scene safety before approaching patient
_____ Failure to voice and ultimately provide appropriate oxygen therapy
_____ Failure to assess/provide adequate ventilation
_____ Failure to find or appropriately manage problems associated with airway, breathing, hemorrhage or shock [hypoperfusion]
_____ Failure to differentiate patient's need for immediate transportation versus continued assessment and treatment at the scene
_____ Does other detailed or focused history or physical examination before assessing and treating threats to airway, breathing, and circulation
_____ Failure to determine the patient's primary problem
_____ Orders a dangerous or inappropriate intervention
_____ Failure to provide for spinal protection when indicated

You must factually document your rationale for checking any of the above critical items on the reverse side of this form.

© 2000 National Registry of Emergency Medical Technicians, Inc., Columbus, OH
All materials subject to this copyright may be photocopied for the non-commercial purpose of educational or scientific advancement.　　　　p302/8-003k

EMT-Paramedic Form

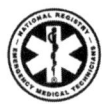

National Registry of Emergency Medical Technicians
Advanced Level Practical Examination

PATIENT ASSESSMENT - TRAUMA

Candidate: _____ Examiner: _____

Date: _____ Signature: _____

Scenario # _____

Time Start: _____   NOTE: Areas denoted by "**" may be integrated within sequence of Initial Assessment

	Possible Points	Points Awarded
Takes or verbalizes body substance isolation precautions	1	
SCENE SIZE-UP		
Determines the scene/situation is safe	1	
Determines the mechanism of injury/nature of illness	1	
Determines the number of patients	1	
Requests additional help if necessary	1	
Considers stabilization of spine	1	
INITIAL ASSESSMENT/RESUSCITATION		
Verbalizes general impression of the patient	1	
Determines responsiveness/level of consciousness	1	
Determines chief complaint/apparent life-threats	1	
Airway -Opens and assesses airway (1 point) -Inserts adjunct as indicated (1 point)	2	

Breathing
    -Assess breathing (1 point)
    -Assures adequate ventilation (1 point)
    -Initiates appropriate oxygen therapy (1 point)
    -Manages any injury which may compromise breathing/ventilation (1 point)
	4	

Circulation
    -Checks pulse (1point)
    -Assess skin [either skin color, temperature, or condition] (1 point)
    -Assesses for and controls major bleeding if present (1 point)
    -Initiates shock management (1 point)
	4	

Identifies priority patients/makes transport decision	1	
FOCUSED HISTORY AND PHYSICAL EXAMINATION/RAPID TRAUMA ASSESSMENT		
Selects appropriate assessment	1	
Obtains, or directs assistant to obtain, baseline vital signs	1	
Obtains SAMPLE history	1	
DETAILED PHYSICAL EXAMINATION		

Head
    -Inspects mouth**, nose**, and assesses facial area (1 point)
    -Inspects and palpates scalp and ears (1 point)
    -Assesses eyes for PERRL** (1 point)
	3	

Neck**
    -Checks position of trachea (1 point)
    -Checks jugular veins (1 point)
    -Palpates cervical spine (1 point)
	3	

Chest**
    -Inspects chest (1 point)
    -Palpates chest (1 point)
    -Auscultates chest (1 point)
	3	

Abdomen/pelvis**
    -Inspects and palpates abdomen (1 point)
    -Assesses pelvis (1 point)
    -Verbalizes assessment of genitalia/perineum as needed (1 point)
	3	

Lower extremities** -Inspects, palpates, and assesses motor, sensory, and distal circulatory functions (1 point/leg)	2	
Upper extremities -Inspects, palpates, and assesses motor, sensory, and distal circulatory functions (1 point/arm)	2	

Posterior thorax, lumbar, and buttocks**
    -Inspects and palpates posterior thorax (1 point)
    -Inspects and palpates lumbar and buttocks area (1 point)
	2	

Manages secondary injuries and wounds appropriately	1	
Performs ongoing assessment	1	

Time End: _____   **TOTAL**   43

CRITICAL CRITERIA

_____ Failure to initiate or call for transport of the patient within 10 minute time limit
_____ Failure to take or verbalize body substance isolation precautions
_____ Failure to determine scene safety
_____ Failure to assess for and provide spinal protection when indicated
_____ Failure to voice and ultimately provide high concentration of oxygen
_____ Failure to assess/provide adequate ventilation
_____ Failure to find or appropriately manage problems associated with airway, breathing, hemorrhage or shock [hypoperfusion]
_____ Failure to differentiate patient's need for immediate transportation versus continued assessment/treatment at the scene
_____ Does other detailed/focused history or physical exam before assessing/treating threats to airway, breathing, and circulation
_____ Orders a dangerous or inappropriate intervention

You must factually document your rationale for checking any of the above critical items on the reverse side of this form.

© 2000 National Registry of Emergency Medical Technicians, Inc., Columbus, OH
All materials subject to this copyright may be photocopied for the non-commercial purpose of educational or scientific advancement.

p301/8-003k

EMT-Paramedic Form

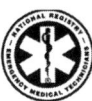

National Registry of Emergency Medical Technicians
Advanced Level Practical Examination

PEDIATRIC INTRAOSSEOUS INFUSION

Candidate: _____ Examiner: _____

Date: _____ Signature: _____

Time Start: _____

	Possible Points	Points Awarded
Checks selected IV fluid for: -Proper fluid (1 point) -Clarity (1 point)	2	
Selects appropriate equipment to include: -IO needle (1 point) -Syringe (1 point) -Saline (1 point) -Extension set (1 point)	4	
Selects proper administration set	1	
Connects administration set to bag	1	
Prepares administration set [fills drip chamber and flushes tubing]	1	
Prepares syringe and extension tubing	1	
Cuts or tears tape [at any time before IO puncture]	1	
Takes or verbalizes body substance isolation precautions [prior to IO puncture]	1	
Identifies proper anatomical site for IO puncture	1	
Cleanses site appropriately	1	
Performs IO puncture: -Stabilizes tibia (1 point) -Inserts needle at proper angle (1 point) -Advances needle with twisting motion until "pop" is felt (1 point) -Unscrews cap and removes stylette from needle (1 point)	4	
Disposes of needle in proper container	1	
Attaches syringe and extension set to IO needle and aspirates	1	
Slowly injects saline to assure proper placement of needle	1	
Connects administration set and adjusts flow rate as appropriate	1	
Secures needle with tape and supports with bulky dressing	1	

Time End: _____ **TOTAL** 23

CRITICAL CRITERIA

_____ Failure to establish a patent and properly adjusted IO line within the 6 minute time limit
_____ Failure to take or verbalize body substance isolation precautions prior to performing IO puncture
_____ Contaminates equipment or site without appropriately correcting situation
_____ Performs any improper technique resulting in the potential for air embolism
_____ Failure to assure correct needle placement before attaching administration set
_____ Failure to successfully establish IO infusion within 2 attempts during 6 minute time limit
_____ Performing IO puncture in an unacceptable manner [improper site, incorrect needle angle, etc.]
_____ Failure to dispose of needle in proper container
_____ Orders or performs any dangerous or potentially harmful procedure

You must factually document your rationale for checking any of the above critical items on the reverse side of this form.

© 2000 National Registry of Emergency Medical Technicians, Inc., Columbus, OH
All materials subject to this copyright may be photocopied for the non-commercial purpose of educational or scientific advancement.

p310/8-003k

©2007 Pearson Education, Inc.
Essentials of Paramedic Care, 2nd ed.

EMT-Paramedic Form

National Registry of Emergency Medical Technicians
Advanced Level Practical Examination

PEDIATRIC (<2 yrs.) VENTILATORY MANAGEMENT

Candidate: _____ Examiner _____

Date: _____ Signature: _____

NOTE: If candidate elects to ventilate initially with BVM attached to reservoir and oxygen, full credit must be awarded for steps denoted by "**" so long as first ventilation is delivered within 30 seconds.

	Possible Points	Points Awarded
Takes or verbalizes body substance isolation precautions	1	
Opens the airway manually	1	
Elevates tongue, inserts simple adjunct [oropharyngeal or nasopharyngeal airway]	1	
NOTE: Examiner now informs candidate no gag reflex is present and patient accepts adjunct		
**Ventilates patient immediately with bag-valve-mask device unattached to oxygen	1	
**Hyperventilates patient with room air	1	
NOTE: Examiner now informs candidate that ventilation is being performed without difficulty and that pulse oximetry indicates the patient's blood oxygen saturation is 85%		
Attaches oxygen reservoir to bag-valve-mask device and connects to high flow oxygen regulator [12-15 L/minute]	1	
Ventilates patient at a rate of 20-30/minute and assures adequate chest expansion	1	
NOTE: After 30 seconds, examiner auscultates and reports breath sounds are present, equal bilaterally and medical direction has ordered intubation. The examiner must now take over ventilation.		
Directs assistant to pre-oxygenate patient	1	
Identifies/selects proper equipment for intubation	1	
Checks laryngoscope to assure operational with bulb tight	1	
NOTE: Examiner to remove OPA and move out of the way when candidate is prepared to intubate		
Places patient in neutral or sniffing position	1	
Inserts blade while displacing tongue	1	
Elevates mandible with laryngoscope	1	
Introduces ET tube and advances to proper depth	1	
Directs ventilation of patient	1	
Confirms proper placement by auscultation bilaterally over each lung and over epigastrium	1	
NOTE: Examiner to ask, "If you had proper placement, what should you expect to hear?"		
Secures ET tube [may be verbalized]	1	
TOTAL	**17**	

CRITICAL CRITERIA

_____ Failure to initiate ventilations within 30 seconds after applying gloves or interrupts ventilations for greater than 30 seconds at any time
_____ Failure to take or verbalize body substance isolation precautions
_____ Failure to pad under the torso to allow neutral head position or sniffing position
_____ Failure to voice and ultimately provide high oxygen concentrations [at least 85%]
_____ Failure to ventilate patient at a rate of at least 20/minute
_____ Failure to provide adequate volumes per breath [maximum 2 errors/minute permissible]
_____ Failure to pre-oxygenate patient prior to intubation
_____ Failure to successfully intubate within 3 attempts
_____ Uses gums as a fulcrum
_____ Failure to assure proper tube placement by auscultation bilaterally **and** over the epigastrium
_____ Inserts any adjunct in a manner dangerous to the patient
_____ Attempts to use any equipment not appropriate for the pediatric patient

You must factually document your rationale for checking any of the above critical items on the reverse side of this form.

© 2000 National Registry of Emergency Medical Technicians, Inc., Columbus, OH
All materials subject to this copyright may be photocopied for the non-commercial purpose of educational or scientific advancement.

p305/8-003k

EMT-Paramedic Form

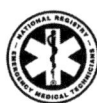

National Registry of Emergency Medical Technicians
Advanced Level Practical Examination

SPINAL IMMOBILIZATION (SEATED PATIENT)

Candidate: _____ Examiner: _____

Date: _____ Signature: _____

Time Start: _____	Possible Points	Points Awarded
Takes or verbalizes body substance isolation precautions	1	
Directs assistant to place/maintain head in the neutral, in-line position	1	
Directs assistant to maintain manual immobilization of the head	1	
Reassesses motor, sensory, and circulatory function in each extremity	1	
Applies appropriately sized extrication collar	1	
Positions the immobilization device behind the patient	1	
Secures the device to the patient's torso	1	
Evaluates torso fixation and adjusts as necessary	1	
Evaluates and pads behind the patient's head as necessary	1	
Secures the patient's head to the device	1	
Verbalizes moving the patient to a long backboard	1	
Reassesses motor, sensory, and circulatory function in each extremity	1	
Time End: _____ **TOTAL**	12	

CRITICAL CRITERIA

_____ Did not immediately direct or take manual immobilization of the head
_____ Did not properly apply appropriately sized cervical collar before ordering release of manual immobilization
_____ Released or ordered release of manual immobilization before it was maintained mechanically
_____ Manipulated or moved patient excessively causing potential spinal compromise
_____ Head immobilized to the device **before** device sufficiently secured to torso
_____ Device moves excessively up, down, left, or right on the patient's torso
_____ Head immobilization allows for excessive movement
_____ Torso fixation inhibits chest rise, resulting in respiratory compromise
_____ Upon completion of immobilization, head is not in a neutral, in-line position
_____ Did not reassess motor, sensory, and circulatory functions in each extremity after voicing immobilization to the long backboard

You must factually document your rationale for checking any of the above critical items on the reverse side of this form.

© 2000 National Registry of Emergency Medical Technicians, Inc., Columbus, OH
All materials subject to this copyright may be photocopied for the non-commercial purpose of educational or scientific advancement.

p311/8-003k

©2007 Pearson Education, Inc.
Essentials of Paramedic Care, 2nd ed.

EMT-Paramedic Form

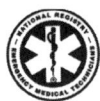

National Registry of Emergency Medical Technicians
Advanced Level Practical Examination

SPINAL IMMOBILIZATION (SUPINE PATIENT)

Candidate: _____ Examiner: _____

Date: _____ Signature: _____

Time Start: _____

	Possible Points	Points Awarded
Takes or verbalizes body substance isolation precautions	1	
Directs assistant to place/maintain head in the neutral, in-line position	1	
Directs assistant to maintain manual immobilization of the head	1	
Reassesses motor, sensory, and circulatory function in each extremity	1	
Applies appropriately sized extrication collar	1	
Positions the immobilization device appropriately	1	
Directs movement of the patient onto the device without compromising the integrity of the spine	1	
Applies padding to voids between the torso and the device as necessary	1	
Immobilizes the patient's torso to the device	1	
Evaluates and pads behind the patient's head as necessary	1	
Immobilizes the patient's head to the device	1	
Secures the patient's legs to the device	1	
Secures the patient's arms to the device	1	
Reassesses motor, sensory, and circulatory function in each extremity	1	
TOTAL	**14**	

Time End: _____

CRITICAL CRITERIA

_____ Did not immediately direct or take manual immobilization of the head
_____ Did not properly apply appropriately sized cervical collar before ordering release of manual immobilization
_____ Released or ordered release of manual immobilization before it was maintained mechanically
_____ Manipulated or moved patient excessively causing potential spinal compromise
_____ Head immobilized to the device **before** device sufficiently secured to torso
_____ Patient moves excessively up, down, left, or right on the device
_____ Head immobilization allows for excessive movement
_____ Upon completion of immobilization, head is not in a neutral, in-line position
_____ Did not reassess motor, sensory, and circulatory functions in each extremity after voicing immobilization to the device

You must factually document your rationale for checking any of the above critical items on the reverse side of this form.

© 2000 National Registry of Emergency Medical Technicians, Inc., Columbus, OH
All materials subject to this copyright may be photocopied for the non-commercial purpose of educational or scientific advancement.

p312/8-003k

EMT-Paramedic Form

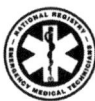

National Registry of Emergency Medical Technicians
Advanced Level Practical Examination

STATIC CARDIOLOGY

Candidate: _____ **Examiner:** _____

Date: _____ **Signature:** _____

SET #_____

Level of Testing: ☐ NREMT-Intermediate/99   ☐ NREMT-Paramedic

Note: No points for treatment may be awarded if the diagnosis is incorrect.
Only document incorrect responses in spaces provided.

Time Start: _____

	Possible Points	Points Awarded
STRIP #1 Diagnosis:	1	
Treatment:	2	
STRIP #2 Diagnosis:	1	
Treatment:	2	
STRIP #3 Diagnosis:	1	
Treatment:	2	
STRIP #4 Diagnosis:	1	
Treatment:	2	
TOTAL	12	

Time End: _____

© 2000 National Registry of Emergency Medical Technicians, Inc., Columbus, OH
All materials subject to this copyright may be photocopied for the non-commercial purpose of educational or scientific advancement.

p307/8-003k

EMT-Paramedic Form

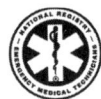

National Registry of Emergency Medical Technicians
Advanced Level Practical Examination

VENTILATORY MANAGEMENT - ADULT

Candidate: _____ Examiner: _____

Date: _____ Signature: _____

NOTE: If candidate elects to ventilate initially with BVM attached to reservoir and oxygen, full credit must be awarded for steps denoted by "**" so long as first ventilation is delivered within 30 seconds.

	Possible Points	Points Awarded
Takes or verbalizes body substance isolation precautions	1	
Opens the airway manually	1	
Elevates tongue, inserts simple adjunct [oropharyngeal or nasopharyngeal airway]	1	
NOTE: Examiner now informs candidate no gag reflex is present and patient accepts adjunct		
**Ventilates patient immediately with bag-valve-mask device unattached to oxygen	1	
**Hyperventilates patient with room air	1	
NOTE: Examiner now informs candidate that ventilation is being performed without difficulty and that pulse oximetry indicates the patient's blood oxygen saturation is 85%		
Attaches oxygen reservoir to bag-valve-mask device and connects to high flow oxygen regulator [12-15 L/minute]	1	
Ventilates patient at a rate of 10-20/minute with appropriate volumes	1	
NOTE: After 30 seconds, examiner auscultates and reports breath sounds are present, equal bilaterally and medical direction has ordered intubation. The examiner must now take over ventilation.		
Directs assistant to pre-oxygenate patient	1	
Identifies/selects proper equipment for intubation	1	
Checks equipment for: -Cuff leaks (1 point) -Laryngoscope operational with bulb tight (1 point)	2	
NOTE: Examiner to remove OPA and move out of the way when candidate is prepared to intubate		
Positions head properly	1	
Inserts blade while displacing tongue	1	
Elevates mandible with laryngoscope	1	
Introduces ET tube and advances to proper depth	1	
Inflates cuff to proper pressure and disconnects syringe	1	
Directs ventilation of patient	1	
Confirms proper placement by auscultation bilaterally over each lung and over epigastrium	1	
NOTE: Examiner to ask, "If you had proper placement, what should you expect to hear?"		
Secures ET tube [may be verbalized]	1	
NOTE: Examiner now asks candidate, "Please demonstrate one additional method of verifying proper tube placement in this patient."		
Identifies/selects proper equipment	1	
Verbalizes findings and interpretations [compares indicator color to the colorimetric scale and states reading to examiner]	1	
NOTE: Examiner now states, "You see secretions in the tube and hear gurgling sounds with the patient's exhalation."		
Identifies/selects a flexible suction catheter	1	
Pre-oxygenates patient	1	
Marks maximum insertion length with thumb and forefinger	1	
Inserts catheter into the ET tube leaving catheter port open	1	
At proper insertion depth, covers catheter port and applies suction while withdrawing catheter	1	
Ventilates/directs ventilation of patient as catheter is flushed with sterile water	1	
TOTAL	**27**	

CRITICAL CRITERIA

_____ Failure to initiate ventilations within 30 seconds after applying gloves or interrupts ventilations for greater than 30 seconds at any time
_____ Failure to take or verbalize body substance isolation precautions
_____ Failure to voice and ultimately provide high oxygen concentrations [at least 85%]
_____ Failure to ventilate patient at a rate of at least 10/minute
_____ Failure to provide adequate volumes per breath [maximum 2 errors/minute permissible]
_____ Failure to pre-oxygenate patient prior to intubation and suctioning
_____ Failure to successfully intubate within 3 attempts
_____ Failure to disconnect syringe **immediately** after inflating cuff of ET tube
_____ Uses teeth as a fulcrum
_____ Failure to assure proper tube placement by auscultation bilaterally **and** over the epigastrium
_____ If used, stylette extends beyond end of ET tube
_____ Inserts any adjunct in a manner dangerous to the patient
_____ Suctions the patient for more than 15 seconds
_____ Does not suction the patient

You must factually document your rationale for checking any of the above critical items on the reverse side of this form.

© 2000 National Registry of Emergency Medical Technicians, Inc., Columbus, OH
All materials subject to this copyright may be photocopied for the non-commercial purpose of educational or scientific advancement.   p303/8-003k

Emergency Drug Cards

The following pages contain prepared three-by-five-inch index cards. Each card represents one of the drugs commonly used by the paramedic. They identify the name and class of the drug, a brief description, its indications, contraindications, precautions, common dosages, and routes of administration.

Detach and cut out the cards and review each one in detail. Be sure that your instructor identifies which drugs are used in your system and which need to be modified to indicate your system's specific indications, contraindications, precautions, doses, and methods of administration. You may also wish to prepare cards for the drugs used in your system that are not included in this card set.

Once your cards are prepared, begin to familiarize yourself with all the information contained on the card when presented with the drug name. You will notice that the drug name appears on the back of each card. Working on just a few cards each week and then reviewing them as your course progresses will help you commit to memory the essential information you must know about each drug.

Name/Class: ACETAMINOPHEN (Tylenol, Anacin-3)/Analgesic, Antipyretic

Description: Acetaminophen is a clinically proven analgesic/antipyretic with little effect on platelet function.
Indications: For mild to moderate pain and fever when aspirin is otherwise not tolerated.
Contraindications: Hypersensitivity, children under 3 years.
Precautions: Patients with hepatic disease; children under 12 years with arthritic conditions; alcoholism; malnutrition; and thrombocytopenia.
Dosage/Route: 325 to 650 mg. PO/4 to 6 hours. 650 mg PR/4 to 6 hours.

©2007 Pearson Education, Inc.

Name/Class: ACTIVATED CHARCOAL (Actidose)/Adsorbent

Description: Activated charcoal is a specially prepared charcoal that will adsorb and bind toxins from the gastrointestinal tract.
Indications: Acute ingested poisoning.
Contraindications: An airway that cannot be controlled; ingestion of cyanide, mineral acids, caustic alkalis, organic solvents, iron, ethanol, methanol.
Precautions: Administer only after emesis or in those cases where emesis is contraindicated.
Dosage/Route: 1 g/kg mixed with at least 6 to 8 oz of water, then PO or via an NG tube.

©2007 Pearson Education, Inc.

Name/Class: ADENOSINE (Adenocard)/Antidysrhythmic

Description: Adenosine is a naturally occurring agent that can "chemically cardiovert" PSVT to a normal sinus rhythm. It has a half-life of 10 seconds and does not cause hypotension.
Indications: Narrow, complex paroxysmal supraventricular tachycardia refractory to vagal maneuvers.
Contraindications: Hypersensitivity, 2nd- and 3rd-degree heart block, sinus node disease, or asthma.
Precautions: It may cause transient dysrhythmias. COPD.
Dosage/Route: 6 mg rapidly (over 1 to 2 sec) IV, then flush the line rapidly with saline. If ineffective, 12 mg in 1 to 2 min, may be repeated. Ped: 0.1 mg/kg (over 1 to 2 sec) IV followed by rapid saline flush, then 0.2 mg/kg in 1 to 2 min to max 12 mg.

©2007 Pearson Education, Inc.

ACETAMINOPHEN

ACTIVATED CHARCOAL

ADENOSINE

Name/Class: ALBUTEROL (Proventil, Ventolin)/Sympathomimetic Bronchodilator

Description: Albuterol is a synthetic sympathomimetic that causes bronchodilatation with less cardiac effect than epinephrine and reduces mucus secretion, pulmonary capillary leaking, and edema in the lungs during allergic reactions.

Indications: Bronchospasm and asthma in COPD.

Contraindications: Hypersensitivity to the drug.

Precautions: The patient may experience tachycardia, anxiety, nausea, cough, wheezing, and/or dizziness. Vital signs and breath sounds must be monitored; use caution with elderly, cardiac, or hypertensive patients.

Dosage/Route: Two inhalations (90 mcg) via metered-dose inhaler (2 sprays) or 2.5 mg in 2.5 to 3 mL NS via nebulizer, repeat as needed. The duration of effect is 3 to 6 hours. Ped: 0.15 mg/kg in 2.5 to 3 mL NS via nebulizer, repeat as needed.

©2007 Pearson Education, Inc.

Name/Class: ALTEPLASE RECOMBINANT (tPA) (Activase)/Thrombolytic

Description: Recombinant DNA–derived form of human tPA promotes thrombolysis by forming plasmin. Plasmin, in turn, degrades fibrin and fibrinogen and, ultimately, the clot.

Indications: To thrombolyse in acute myocardial infarction, acute ischemic stroke, and pulmonary embolism.

Contraindications: Active internal bleeding, suspected aortic dissection, traumatic CPR, recent hemmorhagic stroke (6 mo), intracranial or intraspinal surgery or trauma (2 mo), pregnancy, uncontrolled hypertension, or hypersensitivity to thrombolytics.

Precautions: Recent major surgery, cerebral vascular disease, recent GI or GU bleeding, recent trauma, hypertension, patient > 75 years, current oral anticoagulants, or hemorrhagic ophthalmic conditions.

Dosage/Route: *MI and stroke:* 15 mg IV, then 0.75 mg/kg (up to 50 mg) over 30 min, then 0.5 mg/kg (up to 35 mg) over 60 min.
Pulmonary embolism: 100 mg IV infusion over 2 hours.

©2007 Pearson Education, Inc.

Name/Class: AMINOPHYLLINE (Aminophylline, Somophyllin)/Methylxanthine Bronchodilator

Description: Aminophylline is a methylxanthine that prolongs bronchodilation and decreased mucus production and has mild cardiac and CNS stimulating effects.

Indications: Bronchospasm in asthma and COPD refractory to sympathomimetics and other bronchodilators and in CHF.

Contraindications: Hypersensitivity to methylxanthines or uncontrolled cardiac dysrhythmias.

Precautions: Cardiovascular disease, hypertension, or taking theophylline, hepatic impairment, diabetes, hyperthyroidism, young children, glaucoma, peptic ulcers, acute influenza or influenza immunization, and the elderly. Watch for PVCs or tachycardia. May cause hypotension.

Dosage/Route: 250 to 500 mg IV over 20 to 30 min. Ped: 6 mg/kg over 20 to 30 min. Max 12 mg/kg/day.

©2007 Pearson Education, Inc.

ALBUTEROL

ALTEPLASE RECOMBINANT

AMINOPHYLLINE

Name/Class: AMIODARONE (Cordarone, Pacerone)/Antidysrhythmic

Description: Amiodarone is an antidysrhythmic that prolongs the duration of the action potential and refractory period and relaxes smooth muscles, reducing peripheral vascular resistance and increasing coronary blood flow.

Indications: Life-threatening ventricular and supraventricular dysrythmias, frequently atrial fibrillation.

Contraindications: Hypersensitivity, cardiogenic shock, severe sinus bradycardia, or advanced heart block.

Precautions: Hepatic impairment, pregnancy, nursing mothers, children.

Dosage/Route: 150 to 300 mg IV over 10 min, then 1 mg/min over next 6 hours. Ped: 5 mg/kg IV/IO, then 15 mg/kg/day.

©2007 Pearson Education, Inc.

Name/Class: AMRINONE (Inocor)/Cardiac Inotrope

Description: Amrinone enhances myocardial contractility, increasing output, and reduces systemic vascular resistance.

Indications: To increase cardiac output in CHF or children in septic shock or myocardial dysfunction.

Contraindications: Hypersensitivity to amrinone or bisulfites.

Precautions: CHF immediately after MI (may cause ischemia).

Dosage/Route: *CHF:* 0.75 mg/kg IV over 2 to 3 min, then drip at 5 to 15 mcg/kg/min titrated to hemodynamic response (may repeat bolus at 30 min).

Septic shock or myocardial dysfunction in peds: 0.75 to 1 mg/kg IV over 5 min, repeated up to 2 times to 3 mg/kg, then drip of 5 to 10 mcg/min IV.

©2007 Pearson Education, Inc.

Name/Class: AMYL NITRITE (Amyl Nitrite)/Vasodilator

Description: Amyl nitrite is a short-acting vasodilator similar to nitroglycerin. Binds with hemoglobin to help biodegrade cyanide.

Indications: Acute cyanide poisoning.

Contraindications: None for acute cyanide poisoning.

Precautions: None.

Dosage/Route: 0.3 mL ampule/min (crushed) until sodium nitrate infusion is ready. Ped: same as adult.

©2007 Pearson Education, Inc.

AMIODARONE

AMRINONE

AMYL NITRITE

Name/Class: ANISTREPLASE (APSAC) (Eminase)/Thrombolytic

Description: Anistreplase causes thrombolysis by converting plasminogen into plasmin, which then dissolves the fibrin and fibrinogen of the clot.

Indications: To reduce infarct size in acute MI.

Contraindications: Active internal bleeding, suspected aortic dissection, traumatic CPR, recent hemorrhagic stroke, intracranial or intraspinal surgery or trauma, tumors, pregnancy, hypertension, hypersensitivity to anistreplase or streptokinase.

Precautions: Recent major surgery, cerebral vascular disease, recent GI or GU bleeding, recent trauma, hypertension, patients over 75 years, current oral anticoagulants, or hemorrhagic ophthalmic conditions.

Dosage/Route: 30 units IV over 2 to 5 min.

Name/Class: ASPIRIN (Acetylsalicylic Acid) (Alka-Seltzer, Bayer, Empirin, St. Joseph Children's)/Analgesic, Antipyretic, Platelet Inhibitor, Antiinflammatory

Description: Aspirin inhibits agents that cause the production of inflammation, pain, and fever. It relieves mild to moderate pain by acting on the peripheral nervous system, lowers body temperature in fever, and powerfully inhibits platelet aggregation.

Indications: Chest pain suggestive of an MI.

Contraindications: Hypersensitivity to salicylates, active ulcer disease, asthma.

Precautions: Allergies to other NSAIDs, bleeding disorders, children or teenagers with varicella or influenza-like symptoms.

Dosage/Route: 160 to 325 mg PO (chewable).

Name/Class: ATENOLOL (Tenormin)/Antidysrhythmic, Antihypertensive

Description: Atenolol is a selective beta-blocker that reduces the rate and force of cardiac contraction and lowers cardiac output and blood pressure.

Indications: Non–Q-wave MI and unstable angina.

Contraindications: Sinus bradycardia, 2nd- or 3rd-degree heart block, CHF, cardiogenic failure or shock.

Precautions: Asthma, COPD, or CHF controlled by digitalis and diuretics.

Dosage/Route: 5 mg slow IV (over 5 min), if tolerated, then after 10 min repeat.
   Ped: 0.8 to 1.5 mg/kg/day PO (max 2 mg/kg/day).

ANISTREPLASE (APSAC)

ASPIRIN

ATENOLOL

Name/Class: ATRACURIUM (Tracrium)/Nondepolarizing Neuromuscular Blocker

Description: Atracurium is a synthetic skeletal muscle relaxant that produces a short-duration neuromuscular blockade.

Indications: To produce skeletal muscle relaxation to facilitate endotracheal intubation and IPPV.

Contraindications: Myasthenia gravis.

Precautions: Asthma, anaphylaxis, cardiovascular or neuromuscular disease, electrolyte or acid–base imbalance, dehydration, or pulmonary impairment.

Dosage/Route: 0.4 to 0.5 mg/kg IV. Ped: < 2 years 0.3 to 0.4 mg/kg, otherwise same as adult.

Name/Class: ATROPINE/Parasympatholytic

Description: Atropine blocks the parasympathetic nervous system, specifically the vagal effects on heart rate. It does not increase contractility but may increase myocardial oxygen demand. Decreases airway secretions.

Indications: Hemodynamically significant bradycardia, bradyasystolic arrest, and organophosphate poisoning.

Contraindications: None in the emergency setting.

Precautions: AMI, glaucoma.

Dosage/Route: *Symptomatic bradycardia:* 0.5 to 1 mg IV/2 mg ET. Repeat 3 to 5 min to 0.04 mg/kg. Ped: 0.02 mg/kg IV, 0.04 mg/kg ET, may repeat in 5 min up to 1 mg. Asystole: 1 mg IV or 2 mg ET, may repeat 3 to 5 min up to 0.04 mg/kg.
 Organophosphate poisoning: 2 to 5 mg IV/IM/IO/10 to 15 min. Ped: 0.05 mg/kg IV/IM/IO/ 10 to 15 min.

Name/Class: BRETYLIUM (Bretylol)/Antidysrhythmic

Description: Bretylium causes a release of norepinephrine, depresses ventricular fibrillation, and reduces ectopy. Bretylium also suppresses ventricular tachydysrhythmias with reentry mechanisms.

Indications: Ventricular fibrillation and ventricular tachycardia refractory to lidocaine.

Contraindications: None in the presence of life-threatening dysrhythmias.

Precautions: Digitalized patients, digitalis-induced dysrhythmias, fixed cardiac output, angina, or renal impairment. May induce postural hypotension.

Dosage/Route: 5 mg/kg IV, then 10 mg/kg/15 to 30 min, to a max 30 mg/kg. Following conversion: 1 to 2 mg/min drip. Ped: 5 mg/kg IV, repeat 10 mg/kg in 15 to 30 min.

ATRACURIUM

ATROPINE

BRETYLIUM

Name/Class: BUMETANIDE (Bumex)/Loop Diuretic

Description: Bumetanide is related to furosemide, though it has a faster rate of onset, a greater diuretic potency (40 times), shorter duration, and produces only mild hypotension.
Indications: To promote diuresis in CHF and pulmonary edema.
Contraindications: Hypersensitivity to bumetanide and other sulfonamides.
Precautions: Pregnancy (use only for life-threatening conditions).
Dosage/Route: 0.5 to 1 mg IM/IV over 1 to 2 min, repeat in 2 to 3 hours as needed.

©2007 Pearson Education, Inc.

Name/Class: BUTORPHANOL (Stadol)/Synthetic Narcotic Analgesic

Description: Butorphanol is a centrally acting synthetic narcotic analgesic about 5 times more potent than morphine. A schedule IV narcotic.
Indications: Moderate to severe pain.
Contraindications: Hypersensitivity, head injury, or undiagnosed abdominal pain.
Precautions: May cause withdrawal in narcotic-dependent patients.
Dosage/Route: 1 mg IV or 3 to 4 mg IM/3 to 4 hours.

©2007 Pearson Education, Inc.

Name/Class: CALCIUM CHLORIDE (Calcium Chloride)/Electrolyte

Description: Calcium chloride increases myocardial contractile force and increases ventricular automaticity.
Indications: Hyperkalemia, hypocalcemia, hypermagnesemia, and calcium channel blocker toxicity.
Contraindications: Ventricular fibrillation, hypercalcemia, and possible digitalis toxicity.
Precautions: It may precipitate toxicity in patients taking digoxin. Ensure the IV line is in a large vein and flushed before using and after calcium.
Dosage/Route: 2 to 4 mg/kg IV (10% solution)/10 min, as needed. Ped: 20 mg/kg IV (10% solution) repeat at 10 min, as needed.

©2007 Pearson Education, Inc.

BUMETANIDE

BUTORPHANOL

CALCIUM CHLORIDE

Name/Class: CALCIUM GLUCONATE (Kalcinate)/Electrolyte

Description: Calcium gluconate increases myocardial contractile force and increases ventricular automaticity. It is more potent than calcium chloride.
Indications: Hyperkalemia, hypermagnesemia, and calcium channel blocker toxicity.
Contraindications: Ventricular fibrillation.
Precautions: It may precipitate toxicity in patients taking digitalis, with renal or cardiac insufficiency, and immobilized patients.
Dosage/Route: 5 to 8 mL of 10% solution, repeated as necessary at 10-min intervals.

©2007 Pearson Education, Inc.

Name/Class: CHLORDIAZEPOXIDE (Librium)/Sedative, Hypnotic

Description: Chlordiazepoxide is a benzodiazepine derivative that produces mild sedation and anticonvulsant, skeletal muscle relaxant, and prolonged hypnotic effects.
Indications: Severe anxiety and tension, acute alcohol withdrawal symptoms (DTs).
Contraindications: Hypersensitivity to benzodiazepines, pregnant and nursing mothers, children under 6.
Precautions: Primary depressive disorders or psychoses, acute alcohol intoxication.
Dosage/Route: 50 to 100 mg IV/IM.

©2007 Pearson Education, Inc.

Name/Class: CHLORPROMAZINE (Thorazine)/Tranquilizer, Antipsychotic

Description: Chlorpromazine is a phenothiazine derivative used to manage psychotic episodes by providing strong sedation and moderate extrapyramidal symptoms. Produces reduced initiative, interest, and affect.
Indications: Acute psychotic episode, intractable hiccups, nausea/vomiting.
Contraindications: Hypersensitivity to phenothiazines, coma, sedative overdose, acute alcohol withdrawal, and children < 6 months.
Precautions: Agitated states with depression, seizure disorders, respiratory infection or COPD, glaucoma, diabetes, hypertension, peptic ulcer, prostatic hypertrophy, breast cancer, thyroid, cardiovascular, and hepatic impairment, and patients exposed to extreme heat or organophosphates.
Dosage/Route: 25 to 50 mg IM. Ped: 0.5 mg/kg IM or 1 mg/kg PR.

©2007 Pearson Education, Inc.

CALCIUM GLUCONATE

CHLORDIAZEPOXIDE

CHLORPROMAZINE

Name/Class: DEXAMETHASONE (Decadron)/Steroid

Description: Dexamethasone is a long-acting synthetic adrenocorticoid with intense antiinflammatory activity. It prevents the accumulation of inflammation generating cells at the sites of infection or injury.
Indications: Anaphylaxis, asthma, COPD, spinal cord edema.
Contraindications: No absolute contraindications in the emergency setting. Relative contraindications: systemic fungal infections, acute infections, tuberculosis, varicella, or vaccinia or live virus vaccinations.
Precautions: Herpes simplex, keratitis, myasthenia gravis, hepatic or renal impairment, diabetes, CHF, seizures, psychic disorders, hypothyroidism, and GI ulceration.
Dosage/Route: 4 to 24 mg IV/IM Ped: 0.5 to 1 mg/kg.

©2007 Pearson Education, Inc.

Name/Class: DEXTROSE 50% IN WATER ($D_{50}W$)/Carbohydrate

Description: Dextrose is a simple sugar that the body can rapidly metabolize to create energy.
Indications: Hypoglycemia.
Contraindications: None in hypoglycemia.
Precautions: Increased ICP. Determine blood glucose level before administration. Ensure good venous access.
Dosage/Route: 25g $D_{50}W$ (50 mL) IV. Ped: 2 mL/kg of a 25% solution IV.

©2007 Pearson Education, Inc.

Name/Class: DIAZEPAM (Valium)/Antianxiety, Hypnotic, Anticonvulsant, Sedative

Description: Diazepam is a benzodiazepine sedative and skeletal muscle relaxant that reduces tremors, induces amnesia, and reduces the incidence and recurrence of seizures. It relaxes muscle spasms in orthopedic injuries and produces amnesia for painful procedures (cardioversion).
Indications: Major motor seizures, status epilepticus, premedication before cardioversion, muscle tremors due to injury, and acute anxiety.
Contraindications: Hypersensitivity to the drug, shock, coma, acute alcoholism, depressed vital signs, obstetric patients, neonates.
Precautions: Psychoses, depression, myasthenia gravis, hepatic or renal impairment, addiction, elderly or very ill patients, or COPD. Due to a short half-life of the drug, seizure activity may recur.
Dosage/Route: *Seizures:* 5 to 10 mg IV/IM. Ped: 0.5 to 2 mg IV/IM.
 Acute anxiety: 2 to 5 mg IV/IM. Ped: 0.5 to 2 mg IM.
 Premedication: 5 to 15 mg IV. Ped: 0.2 to 0.5 mg/kg IV.

©2007 Pearson Education, Inc.

DEXAMETHASONE

DEXTROSE 50% IN WATER ($D_{50}W$)

DIAZEPAM

Name/Class: DIAZOXIDE (Hyperstat)/Antihypertensive

Description: Diazoxide is a rapid-acting thiazide nondiuretic hypotensive and hyperglycemia agent that reduces BP and peripheral vascular resistance.

Indications: Rapidly decreases BP in hypertensive crisis

Contraindications: Hypersensitivity to thiazides, cerebral bleeding, eclampsia, significant coronary artery disease.

Precautions: Diabetes, impaired cerebral or cardiac circulation, renal impairment, corticosteroid or progesterone therapy, gout, or uremia.

Dosage/Route: 1 to 3 mg/kg IV up to 150 mg, repeated/5 to 15 min, as needed. Ped: same as adult.

©2007 Pearson Education, Inc.

Name/Class: DIGOXIN (Digoxin, Lanoxin)/Cardiac Glycoside

Description: Digoxin is a rapid-acting cardiac glycoside used in the treatment of CHF and rapid atrial dysrhythmias. It increases the force and velocity of myocardial contraction and cardiac output. It also decreases conduction through the AV node, thus decreasing heart rate.

Indications: Increase cardiac output in CHF and to stabilize supraventricular tachydysrhythmias.

Contraindications: Hypersensitivity, ventricular fibrillation, or ventricular tachycardia except due to CHF.

Precautions: Reduce dosage if digitoxin taken within 2 weeks. Toxicity potentiated by an MI and with hypokalemia, hypocalcemia, advanced heart disease, incomplete heart block, cor pulmonale, hyperthyroidism, respiratory impairment, children, elderly or debilitated patients, and hypomagnesemia.

Dosage/Route: 0.25 to 0.5 mg slowly IV. Ped: 10 to 50 mcg/kg IV.

©2007 Pearson Education, Inc.

Name/Class: DIGOXIN IMMUNE FAB (Digibind)/Antidote

Description: Digoxin immune FAB is comprised of fragments of antibodies specific for digoxin (and effective for digitoxin) and prevents the drug from binding to receptor sites.

Indications: Life-threatening digoxin or digitoxin toxicity.

Contraindications: Hypersensitivity to sheep products and renal or cardiac failure.

Precautions: Patients with prior sheep or bovine antibody fragments, renal impairment, and allergies.

Dosage/Route: Dose dependent upon patient digoxin or digitoxin levels.

©2007 Pearson Education, Inc.

DIAZOXIDE

DIGOXIN

DIGOXIN IMMUNE FAB

Name/Class: DILTIAZEM (Cardizem)/Calcium Channel Blocker

Description: Diltiazem is a slow calcium channel blocker similar to verapamil. It dilates coronary and peripheral arteries and arterioles, thus increasing circulation to the heart and reducing peripheral vascular resistance.

Indications: Supraventricular tachydysrhythmias (atrial fibrillation, atrial flutter, and PSVT refractory to adenosine) and to increase coronary artery perfusion in angina.

Contraindications: Hypersensitivity, sick sinus syndrome, 2nd- or 3rd-degree heart block, systolic BP < 90, diastolic BP < 60, wide-complex tachycardia and WPW.

Precautions: CHF (especially with beta blockers), conduction abnormalities, renal or hepatic impairment, the elderly, and nursing mothers.

Dosage/Route: 0.25 mg/kg IV over 2 min, may repeat as needed with 0.35 mg/kg followed by a drip of 5 to 10 mg/hr not to exceed 15 mg/hr over 24 hours.

©2007 Pearson Education, Inc.

Name/Class: DIMENHYDRINATE (Dramamine)/Antihistamine

Description: Dimenhydrinate is related to diphenhydramine though it is most frequently used for the prevention and treatment of motion sickness and vertigo rather than any antihistamine properties.

Indications: To relieve nausea/vomiting associated with motion sickness and narcotic use.

Contraindications: None in the emergency setting.

Precautions: Seizure disorders and asthma.

Dosage/Route: 12.5 to 25 mg IV; 50 mg IM/4 hours as needed. Ped: 1.25 mg/kg/4 hours up to 300 mg/day.

©2007 Pearson Education, Inc.

Name/Class: DIMERCAPROL (BAL in Oil)/Antidote

Description: Dimercaprol is a dithiol compound that combines with the ions of various heavy metals to form nontoxic compounds that can be excreted.

Indications: Antidote for acute arsenic, mercury, lead, and gold poisoning.

Contraindications: Hepatic and severe renal impairment and poisonings due to cadmium, iron, selenium, and uranium.

Precautions: Hypertensive patients.

Dosage/Route: *Gold and arsenic*: 2.5 to 3 mg/kg IM. Ped: same as adult.
  Mercury: 5 mg/kg IM. Ped: same as adult.
  Lead: 4 mg/kg IM. Ped: same as adult.

©2007 Pearson Education, Inc.

DILTIAZEM

DIMENHYDRINATE

DIMERCAPROL

Name/Class: DIPHENHYDRAMINE (Benadryl)/Antihistamine

Description: Diphenhydramine blocks histamine release, thereby reducing bronchoconstriction, vasodilation, and edema.
Indications: Anaphylaxis, allergic reactions, and dystonic reactions.
Contraindications: Asthma and other lower respiratory diseases.
Precautions: May induce hypotension, headache, palpitations, tachycardia, sedation, drowsiness, and/or disturbed coordination.
Dosage/Route: 25 to 50 mg IV/IM.

©2007 Pearson Education, Inc.

Name/Class: DOBUTAMINE (Dobutrex)/Sympathomimetic

Description: Dobutamine is a synthetic catecholamine and beta agent that increases the strength of cardiac contraction without appreciably increasing rate.
Indications: To increase cardiac output in congestive heart failure/cardiogenic shock.
Contraindications: Hypersensitivity to sympathomimetic amines, ventricular tachycardia, and hypovolemia without fluid resuscitation.
Precautions: Atrial fibrillation or preexisting hypertension.
Dosage/Route: 2 to 20 mcg/kg/min IV. Ped: same as adult.

©2007 Pearson Education, Inc.

Name/Class: DOPAMINE (Intropin)/Sympathomimetic

Description: Dopamine is a naturally occurring catecholamine that increases cardiac output without appreciably increasing myocardial oxygen consumption. It maintains renal and mesenteric blood flow while inducing vasoconstriction and increasing systolic blood pressure.
Indications: Nonhypovolemic hypotension (70 to 100 mmHg) and cardiogenic shock.
Contraindications: Hypovolemic hypotension without aggressive fluid resuscitation, tachydysrhythmias, ventricular fibrillation, and pheochromocytoma.
Precautions: Occlusive vascular disease, cold injury, arterial embolism. Ensure adequate fluid resuscitation of the hypovolemic patient.
Dosage/Route: 2 to 5 mcg/kg/min up to 20 mcg/kg/min, titrated to effect. Ped: same as adult.

©2007 Pearson Education, Inc.

DIPHENHYDRAMINE

DOBUTAMINE

DOPAMINE

Name/Class: DROPERIDOL (Inapsine)/Antiemetic

Description: Droperidol is related to haloperidol and antagonizes the emetic properties of morphine-like analgesics. It may also produce hypotension and mild sedation.

Indications: Nausea and vomiting (second line), to produce a tranquilizing effect, and in some cases as an antipsychotic.

Contraindications: Intolerance.

Precautions: Elderly, debilitated, hypotension, and hepatic, renal, or cardiac impairment and Parkinson's disease.

Dosage/Route: 2.5 to 10 mg IV. Ped: 0.088 to 0.165 mg/kg IV.

©2007 Pearson Education, Inc.

Name/Class: ENOXAPARIN (Lovenox)/Anticoagulant

Description: Enoxaparin is a heparin derivative that prevents the conversion of fibrinogen to fibrin.

Indications: To inhibit clot formation in unstable angina and non–Q-wave myocardial infarction.

Contraindications: Hypersensitivity to the drug, pork products or heparin, major active bleeding, or thrombocytopenia.

Precautions:

Dosage/Route: *Unstable angina and non–Q wave MI:* 1 mg/kg subcutaneously.
Pulmonary embolism: 0.5 mg/kg IV.

©2007 Pearson Education, Inc.

Name/Class: EPINEPHRINE (Adrenalin)/Sympathomimetic

Description: Epinephrine is a naturally occurring catecholamine that increases heart rate, cardiac contractile force myocardial electrical activity, systemic vascular resistance, and systolic blood pressure and decreases overall airway resistance and automaticity. It also, through bronchial artery constriction, may reduce pulmonary congestion and increase tidal volume and vital capacity.

Indications: To restore rhythm in cardiac arrest and severe allergic reactions.

Contraindications: Hypersensitivity to sympathomimetic amines, narrow angle glaucoma; hemorrhagic, traumatic, or cardiac shock; coronary insufficiency; dysrhythmias; organic brain or heart disease; or during labor.

Precautions: Elderly, debilitated patients, hypertension, diabetes, hyperthyroidism, Parkinson's disease, tuberculosis, asthma, emphysema, and in children < 6 years.

Dosage/Route: *Arrest:* 1 mg of 1:10,000 IV/3 to 5 min (ET: 2 to 2.5 mg 1:1,000).
Ped: 0.01 mg/kg 1:10,000 IV/IO (ET: 0.1 mg/kg 1:1,000). All subsequent doses 0.1 mg/kg IV/IO.
Allergic reactions: 0.3 to 0.5 mg of 1:1,000 subcutaneously/5 to 15 min as needed or 0.5 to 1 mg of 1:10,000 IV if subcutaneous dose ineffective or severe reaction. Ped: 0.01 mg/kg of 1:1,000 subcutaneously/10 to 15 min or 0.01 mg/kg of 1:10,000 IV if subcutaneous dose ineffective or severe.

©2007 Pearson Education, Inc.

DROPERIDOL

ENOXAPARIN

EPINEPHRINE

Name/Class: ESMOLOL (Brevibloc)/Beta-Blocker

Description: Esmolol is an ultra–short-acting cardioselective beta-blocker that inhibits the actions of the catecholamines.
Indications: Supraventricular tachycardias with rapid ventricular responses.
Contraindications: Cardiac failure, 2nd- and 3rd-degree block, sinus bradycardia, and cardiogenic shock.
Precautions: Allergies or bronchial asthma, emphysema, CHF, diabetes, and renal impairment.
Dosage/Route: 500 mcg/kg/min IV for 1 min, loading dose, then 50 mcg/kg/min for 4 min. If unsuccessful, repeat loading dose every 4 min and increase maintenance dose by 50 mcg/kg to 200 mcg/kg/min.

©2007 Pearson Education, Inc.

Name/Class: ETOMIDATE (Amidate)/Hypnotic

Description: Etomidate is an ultra–short-acting nonbarbiturate hypnotic with no analgesic effects and limited cardiovascular and respiratory effects.
Indications: Induce sedation for rapid sequence intubation.
Contraindications: Hypersensitivity.
Precautions: Marked hypotension, severe asthma, or severe cardiovascular disease.
Dosage/Route: 0.1 to 0.3 mg/kg IV over 15 to 30 sec. Ped: children > 10 years, same as for adults.

©2007 Pearson Education, Inc.

Name/Class: FENTANYL (Sublimaze)/Narcotic Analgesic

Description: Fentanyl is a potent synthetic narcotic analgesic similar to morphine and meperidine but with a more rapid and less-prolonged action.
Indications: Induce sedation for endotracheal intubation.
Contraindications: MAO inhibitors within 14 days, myasthenia gravis.
Precautions: Increased intracranial pressure, elderly, debilitated, COPD, respiratory problems, hepatic and renal insufficiency.
Dosage/Route: 25 to 100 mcg slowly IV (2 to 3 min). Ped: 2 mcg/kg slow IV/IM.

©2007 Pearson Education, Inc.

ESMOLOL

ETOMIDATE

FENTANYL

Name/Class: FLECAINIDE (Tambocor)/Antidysrhythmic

Description: Flecainide is a local anesthetic and antidysrhythmic that slows myocardial conduction and effectively suppresses PVCs and a variety of atrial and ventricular dysrhythmias.

Indications: Atrial flutter, atrial fibrillation, AV reentrant tachycardia, or SVT associated with WPW syndrome.

Contraindications: Hypersensitivity, 2nd- or 3rd-degree heart block, right bundle branch block with left hemiblock, cardiogenic shock, or significant hepatic impairment.

Precautions: CHF, sick sinus syndrome, or renal impairment.

Dosage/Route: 100 mg PO/12 hour or 2 mg/kg IV at 10 mg/min. Ped: 1 to 3 mg/kg/day PO in three equal doses (max 8 mg/kg/day).

©2007 Pearson Education, Inc.

Name/Class: FLUMAZENIL (Romazicon)/Benzodiazepine Antagonist

Description: Flumazenil is a benzodiazepine antagonist used to reverse the sedative, recall, and psychomotor effects of diazepam, midazolam, and the other benzodiazepines.

Indications: Respiratory depression secondary to the benzodiazepines.

Contraindications: Hypersensitivity to flumazenil or benzodiazepines; those patients who take flumazenil for status epilepticus or seizures; seizure-prone patients during labor and delivery; tricyclic antidepressant overdose.

Precautions: Hepatic impairment, elderly, pregnancy, nursing mothers, head injury, alcohol and drug dependency and physical dependence on benzodiazepines.

Dosage/Route: 0.2 mg IV over 30 sec/min, up to 1 mg.

©2007 Pearson Education, Inc.

Name/Class: FOSPHENYTOIN (Cerebyx)/Anticonvulsant

Description: Fosphenytoin is a drug that, once administered, is converted to phenytoin and causes the anticonvulsant properties associated with that drug.

Indications: Seizure control and status epilepticus.

Contraindications: Hypersensitivity, seizures due to hypoglycemia, sinus bradycardia, heart block, Stokes-Adams syndrome, late pregnancy, and lactating mothers.

Precautions: Hepatic or renal impairment, alcoholism, hypotension, bradycardia, heart block, severe CAD, diabetes, hyperglycemia, or respiratory depression.

Dosage/Route: 15 to 20 mg PE/kg IV given at 100 to 150 mg PE/min (PE = phenytoin equivalent).

©2007 Pearson Education, Inc.

FLECAINIDE

FLUMAZENIL

FOSPHENYTOIN

Name/Class: FUROSEMIDE (Lasix)/Diuretic

Description: Furosemide is a rapid-acting, potent diuretic and antihypertensive that inhibits sodium reabsorption by the kidney. Its vasodilating effects reduce venous return and cardiac workload.

Indications: Congestive heart failure and pulmonary edema.

Contraindications: Hypersensitivity to furosemide or the sulfonamides, fluid and electrolyte depletion states, heptic coma, pregnancy (except in life-threatening circumstances).

Precautions: Infants, elderly, hepatic impairment, nephrotic syndrome, cardiogenic shock associated with acute MI, gout, or patients receiving digitalis or potassium-depleting steroids.

Dosage/Route: 40 to 120 mg slow IV. Ped: 1 mg/kg slow IV.

©2007 Pearson Education, Inc.

Name/Class: GLUCAGON (GlucaGen)/Hormone, Antihypoglycemic

Description: Glucagon is a protein secreted by pancreatic cells that causes a breakdown of stored glycogen into glucose and inhibits the synthesis of glycogen from glucose.

Indications: Hypoglycemia without IV access and to reverse beta-blocker overdose.

Contraindications: Hypersensitivity to glucagon or protein compounds.

Precautions: Cardiovascular or renal impairment. Effective only if there are sufficient stores of glycogen in the liver.

Dosage/Route: *Hypoglycemia:* 1 mg IM/SC repeat/5 to 20 min. Ped: 0.1 mg/kg 1 m/SC/IV for child < 10 kg; 1 mg/kg 1 m/SC/IV for child > 10 kg.
Beta-blocker overdose: 50 to 150 mg/kg IV over 1 min. Ped: 50 to 150 mg/kg IV over 1 min.

©2007 Pearson Education, Inc.

Name/Class: HALOPERIDOL (Haldol)/Antipsychotic

Description: Haloperidol is believed to block dopamine receptors in the brain associated with mood and behavior, is a potent antiemetic, and impairs temperature regulation.

Indications: Acute psychotic episodes.

Contraindications: Parkinson's disease, seizure disorders, coma, alcohol depression, CNS depression, and thyrotoxicosis, and with other sedatives.

Precautions: Elderly, debilitated patients, urinary retention, glaucoma, severe cardiovascular disease, or anticonvulsant, anticoagulant, or lithium therapy.

Dosage/Route: 2 to 5 mg IM. Ped: Children > 3 years, 0.015 to 0.15 mg/kg/day PO in 2 or 3 divided doses.

©2007 Pearson Education, Inc.

FUROSEMIDE

GLUCAGON

HALOPERIDOL

Name/Class: HEPARIN (Heparin)/Anticoagulant

Description: Heparin is a rapid-onset anticoagulant, enhancing the effects of antithrombin III and blocking the conversion of prothrombin to thrombin and fibrinogen to fibrin.

Indications: To prevent thrombus formation in acute MI.

Contraindications: Hypersensitivity; active bleeding or bleeding tendencies; recent eye, brain, or spinal surgery; shock.

Precautions: Alcoholism, elderly, allergies, indwelling catheters, elderly, menstruation, pregnancy, or cerebral embolism.

Dosage/Route: 5,000 units IV, then 20,000 to 40,000 units over 24 hours.

Name/Class: HYDRALAZINE (Apresoline)/Antihypertensive

Description: Hydralazine reduces blood pressure by arterial vasodilation, increasing cardiac output and renal and cerebral blood flow.

Indications: Hypertensive crisis and preeclampsia.

Contraindications: Hypersensitivity, coronary artery or mitral valve disease, AMI, tachydysrhythmias.

Precautions: CVA, renal impairment, and MAO inhibitor use.

Dosage/Route: 20 to 40 mg IV/IM repeated in 4 to 6 hours. Ped: 0.1 to 0.5 mg/kg/day IV/IM.

Name/Class: HYDROCORTISONE (Solu-Cortef)/Steroid

Description: Hydrocortisone is a short-acting synthetic steroid that inhibits histamine formation, storage, and release from mast cells, reducing allergic response.

Indications: Inflammation during allergic reactions, severe anaphylaxis, asthma, and COPD.

Contraindications: Hypersensitivity to glucocorticoids.

Precautions: Limited precautions in acute care.

Dosage/Route: 40 to 250 mg IV/IM. Ped: 4 to 8 mg/kg/day IV/IM.

HEPARIN

HYDRALAZINE

HYDROCORTISONE

Name/Class: HYDROXYZINE (Vistaril)/Antihistamine

Description: Hydroxyzine is an antihistamine with depressive, sedative, antiemetic, and bronchodilator properties.
Indications: Acute anxiety, nausea/vomiting.
Contraindications: Hypersensitivity.
Precautions: Elderly.
Dosage/Route: *Anxiety:* 50 to 100 mg deep IM. Ped: 1 mg/kg deep IM.
 Nausea/vomiting: 25 to 50 mg deep IM. Ped: 1 mg/kg deep IM.

©2007 Pearson Education, Inc.

Name/Class: IBUPROFEN (Advil, Motrin, Nuprin, Excedrin IB)/Nonsteroidal Antiinflammatory Drug (NSAID)

Description: Ibuprofen is the prototype NSAID with significant analgesic and antipyretic properties. It also inhibits platelet aggregation and increases bleeding time.
Indications: Reduce fever and relieve minor to moderate pain.
Contraindications: Sensitivity to aspirin or other NSAIDs, active peptic ulcer, and bleeding abnormalities.
Precautions: Hypertension, GI ulceration, hepatic or renal impairment, cardiac decompensation.
Dosage/Route: 200 to 400 mg PO/4 to 6 hours up to 1,200 mg/day. Ped: 5 to 10 mg/kg PO/4 to 6 hours up to 40 mg/kg/day.

©2007 Pearson Education, Inc.

Name/Class: IBUTILIDE (Corvert)/Antidysrhythmic

Description: Ibutilide is a short-acting antidysrhythmic that may convert atrial flutter and fibrillation or may assist with electrical cardioversion.
Indications: Recent onset atrial flutter and fibrillation.
Contraindications: Hypersensitivity, hypokalemia, or hypomagnesemia.
Precautions: CHF, low ejection fraction, recent MI, prolonged QT intervals, hepatic impairment, cardiovascular disorder other than atrial dysrhythmias, or drugs that prolong the QT interval, lactation.
Dosage/Route: 1 mg over 10 min IV. Patients < 60 kg, 0.01 mg/kg IV, may repeat in 10 min as needed.

©2007 Pearson Education, Inc.

HYDROXYZINE

IBUPROFEN

IBUTILIDE

Name/Class: INSULIN (Regular Insulin, Humulin)/Hormone

Description: Insulin is a naturally occurring protein that promotes the uptake of glucose by the cells.
Indications: Hyperglycemia and diabetic coma.
Contraindications: Hypersensitivity and hypoglycemia.
Precautions:
Dosage/Route: 5 to 10 units IV/IM/SC. Ped: 2 to 4 units IV/IM/SC.

©2007 Pearson Education, Inc.

Name/Class: IPECAC SYRUP/Emetic

Description: Ipecac syrup is a gastric irritant and acts on the emetic centers of the medulla to induce vomiting. Emesis usually occurs within 5 to 10 minutes.
Indications: Poisoning and overdose.
Contraindications: Reduced level of consciousness, corrosive ingestion, petroleum distillate ingestion, alkali ingestion, or antiemetic ingestion (especially phenothiazine).
Precautions: Monitor the airway and have suction ready. Administer activated charcoal only after emesis. Caution with heart disease patients.
Dosage/Route: 30 mL PO, followed by 1 to 2 glasses of water, repeat in 20 min as needed.
Ped: 15 mL PO followed by 1 to 2 glasses of water, repeat in 20 min as needed.

©2007 Pearson Education, Inc.

Name/Class: IPRATROPIUM (Atrovent)/Anticholinergic

Description: Ipratropium is a bronchodilator used in the treatment of respiratory emergencies that causes bronchial dilation and dries respiratory tract secretions by blocking acetylcholine receptors.
Indications: Bronchospasm associated with asthma, COPD, and inhaled irritants.
Contraindications: Hypersensitivity to atropine or its derivatives, or as a primary treatment for acute bronchospasm.
Precautions: Elderly, cardiovascular disease, or hypertension.
Dosage/Route: 500 mcg in 2.5 to 3 mL NS via nebulizer or 2 sprays from a metered dose inhaler.
Ped: 125 to 250 mcg in 2.5 to 3 mL NS via nebulizer, or 1 or 2 sprays of a metered dose inhaler.

©2007 Pearson Education, Inc.

INSULIN

IPECAC SYRUP

IPRATROPIUM

Name/Class: ISOETHARINE (Bronkosol)/Sympathomimetic Bronchodilator

Description: Isoetharine is a synthetic sympathomimetic with rapid onset and prolonged duration that relaxes the bronchial smooth muscles, decreasing airway resistance and helping clear secretions.

Indications: Bronchospasm in asthma and COPD.

Contraindications: Hypersensitivity to or use of sympathomimetic amines, preexisting tachydysrhythmias, allergy to sodium bisulfite agents.

Precautions: Elderly, hypertension, acute coronary artery disease, CHF, hyperthyroidism, diabetes, tuberculosis, or seizures.

Dosage/Route: 1 or 2 sprays via metered dose inhaler, 0.5 mL in 2 to 3 mL saline via nebulizer.
Ped: 0.01 mL/kg of 1% solution (max 0.5 mL) diluted in 2 to 3 mL saline by nebulizer.

©2007 Pearson Education, Inc.

Name/Class: ISOPROTERENOL (Isuprel)/Sympathomimetic

Description: Isoproterenol is a synthetic sympathomimetic that results in increased cardiac output by increasing the strength of cardiac contraction and somewhat increasing rate. It also reduces peripheral vascular resistance and venous return.

Indications: Bradycardia refractory to atropine when pacing is not available and for severe status asthmaticus.

Contraindications: Cardiogenic shock.

Precautions: Tachydysrhythmias and those associated with digitalis and acute myocardial infarction.

Dosage/Route: *Bradycardia:* 2 to 10 mcg/min titrated to cardiac rate. Ped: 0.1 mcg/kg/min titrated to cardiac rate.
Status asthmaticus: 1 or 2 sprays, metered dose inhaler. Ped: same as adult.

©2007 Pearson Education, Inc.

Name/Class: KETOROLAC (Toradol)/Nonsteroidal Antiinflammatory Drug (NSAID)

Description: Ketorolac is an injectable NSAID that exhibits analgesic, antiinflammatory, and antipyretic properties without sedative effects.

Indications: Mild or moderate pain.

Contraindications: Hypersensitivity to ketorolac, aspirin, or other NSAIDs, and asthma.

Precautions: Peptic ulcers, renal or hepatic impairment, or elderly.

Dosage/Route: 30 mg IV/IM (15 mg > 65 years or weighs < 50 kg)

©2007 Pearson Education, Inc.

ISOETHARINE

ISOPROTERENOL

KETOROLAC

Name/Class: LABETALOL (Trandate, Normodyne)/Beta-Blocker

Description: Labetalol is a beta-blocker with some alpha-blocker characteristics. It induces vasodilation, reduces peripheral vascular resistance, and lowers blood pressure.

Indications: Acute hypertensive crisis.

Contraindications: Asthma, CHF, 2nd- and 3rd-degree heart block, severe bradycardia, or cardiogenic shock.

Precautions: COPD, heart failure, hepatic impairment, diabetes, peripheral vascular disease.

Dosage/Route: 20 mg slow IV, then 40 to 80 mg/10 min as needed, up to 300 mg OR a continuous drip 2 mg/min up to 300 mg.

©2007 Pearson Education, Inc.

Name/Class: LIDOCAINE (Xylocaine)/Antidysrhythmic

Description: Lidocaine is an antidysrhythmic that suppresses automaticity and raises stimulation threshold of the ventricles. It also causes sedation, anticonvulsant, and analgesic effects.

Indications: Pulseless ventricular tachycardia, ventricular fibrillation, ventricular tachycardia (w/ pulse).

Contraindications: Hypersensitivity to amide-type local anesthetics, supraventricular dysrhythmias, Stokes-Adams syndrome, 2nd- and 3rd-degree heart blocks, and bradycardias.

Precautions: Hepatic or renal impairment, CHF, hypoxia, respiratory depression, hypovolemia, myasthenia gravis, shock, debilitated patients, elderly, family history of malignant hypothermia.

Dosage/Route: *Cardiac arrest:* 1 to 1.5 mg/kg IV repeated every 3 to 5 min up to 3 mg/kg, follow conversion with a drip of 2 to 4 mg/min. Ped: 1 mg/kg IV, repeat/3 to 5 min up to 3 mg/kg, follow conversion with a drip of 20 to 50 mcg/kg/min.

Ventricular tachycardia (w/ pulse): 1 to 1.5 mg/kg slow IV. May repeat at one-half dose every 5 to 10 min until conversion up to 3 mg/kg. Follow conversion with an infusion of 2 to 4 mg/min. Ped: 1 mg/kg, followed by a drip at 20 to 50 mg/kg/min.

©2007 Pearson Education, Inc.

Name/Class: LORAZEPAM (Ativan)/Sedative

Description: Lorazepam is the most potent benzodiazepine available. It has strong antianxiety, sedative, hypnotic, and skeletal muscle relaxant properties, and a relatively short half-life.

Indications: Sedation for cardioversion and status epilepticus.

Contraindications: Sensitivity to benzodiazepines.

Precautions: Narrow-angle glaucoma, depression or psychosis, coma, shock, acute alcohol intoxication, renal or hepatic impairment, organic brain syndrome, myasthenia gravis, GI disorders, elderly, debilitated, limited pulmonary reserve.

Dosage/Route: *Sedation:* 2 to 4 mg IM, 0.5 to 2 mg IV. Ped: 0.03 to 0.5 mg/kg IV/IM/PR up to 4 mg.
Status epilepticus: 2 mg slow IV/PR (2 mg/min). Ped: 0.1 mg/kg slow IV/PR (2 to 5 min).

©2007 Pearson Education, Inc.

LABETALOL

LIDOCAINE

LORAZEPAM

Name/Class: MAGNESIUM SULFATE (Magnesium)/Electrolyte

Description: Magenesium sulfate is an electrolyte that acts as a calcium channel blocker, acting as a CNS depressant and anticonvulsant. It also depresses the function of smooth, skeletal, and cardiac muscles.

Indications: Refractory ventricular fibrillation and pulseless ventricular tachycardia (especially torsade de pointes), AMI, eclamptic seizures.

Contraindications: Heart block, myocardial damage, shock, persistent hypertension, and hypocalcemia.

Precautions: Renal impairment, digitalized patients, other CNS depressants, or neuromuscular blocking agents.

Dosage/Route: *Ventricular fibrillation or tachycardia:* 1 to 2 g IV over 2 min.
Torsade de pointes: 1 to 2 g IV followed by infusion of 0.5 to 1 g/hr IV.
AMI: 1 to 2 g IV over 5 to 30 min.
Eclampsia: 2 to 4 g IV/IM.

©2007 Pearson Education, Inc.

Name/Class: MANNITOL (Osmitrol)/Osmotic Diuretic

Description: Mannitol is an osmotic diuretic that draws water into the intravascular space through its hypertonic effects, then causes diuresis.

Indications: Cerebral edema.

Contraindications: Hypersensitivity, pulmonary edema, CHF, organic CNS disease, intracranial bleeding, shock, or severe dehydration.

Precautions:

Dosage/Route: 1.5 to 2 g/kg slow IV. Ped: 0.25 to 0.5 g/kg over 60 min.

©2007 Pearson Education, Inc.

Name/Class: MEPERIDINE (Demerol)/Narcotic Analgesic

Description: Meperidine is a synthetic narcotic with sedative and analgesic properties comparable to morphine but without hemodynamic side effects.

Indications: Moderate to severe pain.

Contraindications: Hypersensitivity, seizure disorders, or acute abdomen prior to diagnosis.

Precautions: Increased intracranial pressure, asthma or other respiratory conditions, supraventricular tachycardias, prostatic hypertrophy, urethral stricture, glaucoma, elderly or debilitated patients, renal or hepatic impairment, hypothyroidism, or Addison's disease.

Dosage/Route: 25 to 50 mg IV, 50 to 100 mg IM. Ped: 1 mg/kg IV/IM.

©2007 Pearson Education, Inc.

MAGNESIUM SULFATE

MANNITOL

MEPERIDINE

Name/Class: METAPROTERENOL (Alupent)/Sympathomimetic Bronchodilator

Description: Metaproterenol is a synthetic sympathomimetic amine, similar to isoproterenol that causes smooth muscle relaxation of the bronchial tree, decreasing airway resistance, facilitating mucus drainage, and increasing vital capacity.

Indications: Bronchospasm, as in asthma and COPD.

Contraindications: Hypersensitivity to sympathomimetic agents, tachydysrhythmias, and hyperthyroidism.

Precautions: Elderly, hypertension, coronary artery disease, and diabetes.

Dosage/Route: 0.65 mg via metered dose inhaler (2 sprays); 0.2 to 0.3 mL in 2.5 to 3 mL NS via nebulizer. Ped: 0.1 to 0.2 mL/kg (5% solution) in 2.5 to 3 mL NS via nebulizer.

©2007 Pearson Education, Inc.

Name/Class: METARAMINOL (Aramine)/Sympathomimetic

Description: Metaraminol is a sympathomimetic similar to norepinephrine but less potent, with gradual onset and longer duration. It causes systemic vasoconstriction and increased cardiac contraction strength, increasing blood pressure and reducing flow to the kidneys.

Indications: Hypotension in a normovolemic patient.

Contraindications: Hypovolemia; MAO inhibitor therapy; peripheral or mesenteric thrombosis; pulmonary edema; cardiac arrest; untreated hypoxia, hypercapnia, and acidosis.

Precautions: Digitalized patients, hypertension, thyroid disease, diabetes, hepatic impairment, malaria.

Dosage/Route: 100 mg/500 mL D$_5$W or NS, titrated to blood pressure: 5 to 10 mg IM.

©2007 Pearson Education, Inc.

Name/Class: METHYLPREDNISOLONE (Solu-Medrol)/Corticosteroid, Antiinflammatoty

Description: Methylprednisolone is a synthetic adrenal corticosteroid, effective as an antiinflammatory and used in the management of allergic reactions and in some cases of shock. It is sometimes used in the treatment of spinal cord injury.

Indications: Spinal cord injury, asthma, severe anaphylaxis, COPD.

Contraindications: No major contraindications in the emergency setting.

Precautions: Only a single dose should be given in the prehospital setting.

Dosage/Route: *Asthma/COPD/anaphylaxis:* 125 to 250 mg IV/IM. Ped: 1 to 2 mg/kg/dose IV/IM.
Spinal cord injury: 30 mg/kg IV over 15 min, after 45 min an infusion of 5.4 mg/kg/hr.

©2007 Pearson Education, Inc.

METAPROTERENOL

METARAMINOL

METHYLPREDNISOLONE

Name/Class: METOCLOPRAMIDE (Reglan)/Antiemetic

Description: Metoclopramide is a dopamine antagonist similar to procainamide but with few antidysrhythmic or anesthetic properties. Its antiemetic properties stem from rapid gastric emptying and desensitization of the vomiting reflex.
Indications: Nausea and vomiting.
Contraindications: Hypersensitivity, allergy to sulfite agents, seizure disorders, pheochromocytoma, mechanical GI obstruction or perforation, and breast cancer.
Precautions: CHF, hypokalemia, renal impairment, GI hemorrhage, intermittent porphyria.
Dosage/Route: 10 to 20 mg IM; 10 mg slow IV (over 1 to 2 min). Ped: 1 to 2 mg/kg/dose.

©2007 Pearson Education, Inc.

Name/Class: METOPROLOL (Lopressor)/Beta-Blocker

Description: Metroprolol is a beta-adrenergic blocking agent that reduces heart rate, cardiac output, and blood pressure.
Indications: AMI.
Contraindications: Cardiogenic shock, sinus bradycardia < 45, 2nd- or 3rd-degree heart block, PR interval > 0.24, cor pulmonale, asthma, or COPD.
Precautions: Hypersensitivity, hepatic or renal impairment, cardiomegaly, CHF controlled by digitalis and diuretics, AV conduction defects, thyrotoxicosis, diabetes, or peripheral vascular disease.
Dosage/Route: 5 mg slow IV/5 min up to 3 times.

©2007 Pearson Education, Inc.

Name/Class: MIDAZOLAM (Versed)/Sedative

Description: Midazolam is a short-acting benzodiazepine with CNS depressant, muscle relaxant, anticonvulsant, and anterograde amnestic effects.
Indications: To induce sedation before cardioversion or intubation.
Contraindications: Hypersensitivity to benzodiazepines, narrow-angle glaucoma, shock, coma, or acute alcohol intoxication.
Precautions: COPD, renal impairment, CHF, elderly.
Dosage/Route: 1 to 2.5 mg slow IV; 0.07 to 0.08 mg/kg IM (usually 5 mg). Ped: 0.05 to 0.2 mg/kg IV: 0.1 to 0.15 mg/kg IM; 3 mg intranasal.

©2007 Pearson Education, Inc.

METOCLOPRAMIDE

METOPROLOL

MIDAZOLAM

Name/Class: MILRINONE (Primacor)/Cardiac Inotrope, Vasodilator

Description: Milrinone is related to amrinone and increases the strength of cardiac contraction without increasing rate, increasing cardiac output without increasing oxygen demand.

Indications: CHF or pediatric septic shock.

Contraindications: Hypersensitivity.

Precautions: Elderly, pregnancy, and nursing mothers.

Dosage/Route: *CHF:* 50 mcg/kg IV over 10 min, then a drip of 0.375 to 0.75 mcg/kg/min IV. Ped: (septic shock) 50 to 75 mcg/kg IV, then a drip of 0.5 to 0.75 mcg/kg/min.

©2007 Pearson Education, Inc.

Name/Class: MORPHINE SULFATE (Morphine)/Narcotic Analgesic

Description: Morphine sulfate is a potent analgesic and sedative that causes some vasodilation, reducing venous return, and reduced myocardial oxygen demand.

Indications: Moderate to severe pain and in MI and to reduce venous return in pulmonary edema.

Contraindications: Hypersensitivity to opiates, undiagnosed head or abdominal injury, hypotension, or volume depletion, acute bronchial asthma, COPD, severe respiratory depression, or pulmonary edema due to chemical inhalation.

Precautions: Elderly, children, or debilitated patients. Naloxone should be readily available to counteract the effects of morphine.

Dosage/Route: *Pain:* 2.5 to 15 mg IV; 5 to 20 mg IM/subcutaneous. Ped: 0.05 to 0.1 mg/kg IV; 0.1 to 0.2 mg/kg IM/subcutaneous.
AMI or PE: 1 to 2 mg/6 to 10 min to response.

©2007 Pearson Education, Inc.

Name/Class: NALBUPHINE (Nubain)/Narcotic Analgesic

Description: Nalbuphine is a synthetic narcotic analgesic equivalent to morphine, though its respiratory depression does not increase with higher doses.

Indications: Moderate to severe pain.

Contraindications: Hypersensitivity, undiagnosed head or abdominal injury.

Precautions: Impaired respirations, narcotic dependency.

Dosage/Route: 5 mg IV/IM/subcutaneous, repeat as 2 mg doses as needed up to 20 mg. Ped: 0.1 to 0.15 mg/kg IV/IM/subcutaneous (rarely used).

©2007 Pearson Education, Inc.

MILRINONE

MORPHINE SULFATE

NALBUPHINE

Name/Class: NALOXONE (Narcan)/Narcotic Antagonist

Description: Naloxone is a pure narcotic antagonist that blocks the effects of both natural and synthetic narcotics and may reverse respiratory depression.

Indications: Narcotic and synthetic narcotic overdose, coma of unknown origin.

Contraindications: Hypersensitivity to the drug, non–narcotic-induced respiratory depression.

Precautions: Possible dependency (including newborns). It also has a half-life that is shorter than that of most narcotics; hence the patient may return to the overdose state.

Dosage/Route: 0.4 to 2 mg IV/IM (2 to 2.5 times the dose ET), repeated/2 to 3 min as needed up to 10 mg. Ped: 0.01 mg IV/IM (2 to 2.5 times the dose ET) repeated/2 to 3 min as needed up to 10 mg.

©2007 Pearson Education, Inc.

Name/Class: NIFEDIPINE (Procardia, Adalat)/Calcium Channel Blocker

Description: Nifedipine is a calcium channel blocker that reduces coronary artery spasm in angina. It also decreases peripheral vascular resistance, blood pressure, and cardiac workload.

Indications: Severe hypertension and angina.

Contraindications: Hypersensitivity or hypotension.

Precautions: Monitor blood pressure carefully, since it can drop significantly with nifedipine use.

Dosage/Route: One 10 to 20 mg capsule SL/PO.

©2007 Pearson Education, Inc.

Name/Class: NITROGLYCERIN (Nitrostat)/Nitrate

Description: Nitroglycerin is a rapid smooth muscle relaxant that reduces peripheral vascular resistance, blood pressure, venous return, and cardiac workload.

Indications: Chest pain associated with angina and acute myocardial infarction, and acute pulmonary edema.

Contraindications: Hypersensitivity, tolerance to nitrates, severe anemia, head trauma, hypotension, increased ICP, patients taking sildenafil, glaucoma, and shock.

Precautions: May induce headache that is sometimes severe. Nitroglycerin is light sensitive and will lose potency when exposed to the air.

Dosage/Route: 1 tablet (0.4 mg) SL. May be repeated/3 to 5 min up to 3 tablets, or ½ inch of topical ointment, or 0.4 mg (one spray)SL up to 3 sprays/25 min.

©2007 Pearson Education, Inc.

NALOXONE

NIFEDIPINE

NITROGLYCERIN

Name/Class: NITROUS OXIDE (Nitronox)/Analgesic (gas)

Description: Nitrous oxide is a self-administered analgesic gas composed of 50% oxygen and 50% nitrous oxide. Its effects last only 2 to 5 minutes after administration ceases.

Indications: Musculoskeletal, burn, and ischemic chest pain and severe anxiety (including hyperventilation).

Contraindications: Possible bowel obstruction, pneumothorax or tension pneumothorax, COPD, head injury, impaired mental status, or drug intoxication.

Precautions: Use in well-ventilated area. It may cause nausea and vomiting.

Dosage/Route: It is self-administered inhalation until the pain is relieved or the patient drops the mask.

©2007 Pearson Education, Inc.

Name/Class: NOREPINEPHRINE (Levophed)/Sympathomimetic Agent

Description: Norepinephrine is a naturally occurring catecholamine and causes vasoconstriction, cardiac stimulation, and increased blood pressure, myocardial oxygen demand, and coronary blood flow.

Indications: Refractory hypotension and neurogenic shock.

Contraindications: Hypotension due to hypovolemia.

Precautions: Hypertension, hyperthyroidism, severe heart disease, elderly, MAO inhibitor therapy, patients receiving tricyclic antidepressants. Monitor blood pressure frequently and infuse the drug through the largest vein available as it may cause tissue necrosis.

Dosage/Route: 0.5 to 30 mcg/min IV, titrated to BP. Ped: 0.01 mcg/kg/min (rarely used).

©2007 Pearson Education, Inc.

Name/Class: OXYGEN/Oxidizing Agent (Gas)

Description: Oxygen is an odorless, colorless, tasteless gas, essential for life. It is one of the most important emergency drugs.

Indications: Hypoxia or anticipated hypoxia, or in any medical or trauma patient to improve respiratory efficiency.

Contraindications: There are no contraindications to oxygen therapy.

Precautions: Chronic obstructive pulmonary disease and very prolonged administration of high concentrations in the newborn.

Dosage/Route: Hypoxia: 100% by inhalation or IPPV.

©2007 Pearson Education, Inc.

NITROUS OXIDE

NOREPINEPHRINE

OXYGEN

Name/Class: OXYTOCIN (Pitocin)/Hormone

Description: Oxytocin is a naturally occurring hormone that causes the uterus to contract, thereby inducing labor, encouraging delivery of the placenta, and controlling postpartum hemorrhage.

Indications: Severe postpartum hemorrhage.

Contraindications: Hypersensitivity, prehospital administration before delivery of the infant or infants.

Precautions: Before delivery may induce uterine rupture and fetal dysrhythmias, hypertension, intracranial bleeding, or asphyxia. Uterine tone, ECG, and vital signs should be monitored during administration.

Dosage/Route: 3 to 10 units IM after delivery of the placenta. 10 to 20 units in 1,000 mL of D_5W or NS IV titrated to effect.

©2007 Pearson Education, Inc.

Name/Class: PANCURONIUM (Pavulon)/Nondepolarizing Neuromuscular Blocker

Description: Pancuronium is a nondepolarizing neuromuscular blocker that causes paralysis without bronchospasm or hypotension, it does not cause the fasciculations associated with polarizing agents.

Indications: To facilitate endotracheal intubation.

Contraindications: Hypersensitivity to pancuronium or bromides, or tachycardia.

Precautions: Debilitated patients, myasthenia gravis, pulmonary, hepatic, or renal disease, or fluid or electrolyte imbalance.

Dosage/Route: 0.04 to 0.1 mg/kg IV. Ped: same as adult.

©2007 Pearson Education, Inc.

Name/Class: PHENOBARBITAL (Luminal)/Anticonvulsant

Description: Phenobarbital is a long-acting barbiturate anticonvulsant with sedative and hypnotic effects that limits the spread of seizure activity.

Indications: Seizures, status epilepticus, and acute anxiety.

Contraindications: Hypersensitivity to barbiturates.

Precautions: Hepatic, renal, cardiac, or respiratory impairment, allergies, elderly, debilitated patients, fever, hyperthyroidism, diabetes, severe anemia, hypoadrenal function, and during labor, delivery, and lactation.

Dosage/Route: 100 to 300 mg slow IV/IM. Ped: 6 to 10 mg/kg slow IV/IM.

©2007 Pearson Education, Inc.

OXYTOCIN

PANCURONIUM

PHENOBARBITAL

Name/Class: PHENYTOIN (Dilantin)/Anticonvulsant

Description: Phenytoin is a derivative related to phenobarbital that reduces the spread of electrical discharges in the motor cortex and inhibits seizures. It also has antidysrhythmic properties that counteract the effects of digitalis.

Indications: Seizures, status epilepticus, or cardiac dysrhythmias secondary to digitalis toxicity.

Contraindications: Hypersensitivity to hydantoin products, seizures due to hypoglycemia, sinus bradycardia, heart block, and Adams-Stokes syndrome.

Precautions: Hepatic or renal impairment, alcoholism, cardiogenic shock, elderly, debilitated patients, diabetes, hyperglycemia, bradycardia, heart block, or respiratory depression.

Dosage/Route: *Seizures, status epilepticus:* 10 to 15 mg/kg slow IV. Ped: 8 to 10 mg/kg slow IV.
Dysrhythmias: 100 mg slow IV (over 5 min) to a maximum 1,000 mg. Ped: 3 to 5 mg/kg slow IV.

©2007 Pearson Education, Inc.

Name/Class: PHYSOSTIGMINE (Antilirium)/Parasympathomimetic

Description: Physostigmine inhibits the breakdown of acetylcholine, resulting in prolonged parasympathetic effects. It is sometimes used as an antidote for anticholinergic (e.g., atropine) and tricyclic antidepressant overdoses.

Indications: Tricyclic antidepressant (CNS and cardiac effects) and anticholinergic overdose.

Contraindications: Asthma, diabetes, gangrene, cardiovascular disease, or narrow-angle glaucoma.

Precautions: Reduce dose (or administer atropine) if increased salivation, emesis, or bradycardia develop.

Dosage/Route: 0.5 to 3 mg IV (not faster than 1 mg min), repeat as needed. Ped: 0.01 to 0.03 mg/kg/15 to 20 min to max 2 mg.

©2007 Pearson Education, Inc.

Name/Class: PRALIDOXIME (2-PAM)/Cholinesterase Reactivator

Description: Pralidoxime reactivates cholinesterase and reinstitutes the degrading of acetylcholine and restores normal neuromuscular transmission. It is used to reverse severe organophosphate poisoning.

Indications: Organophosphate poisoning.

Contraindications: Carbamate insecticides (Sevin), inorganic phosphates, and organophosphates having no anticholinesterase activity, asthma, peptic ulcer disease, severe cardiac disease, or patients receiving aminophylline, theophylline, morphine, succinylcholine, reserpine, or phenothiazines.

Precautions: Rapid administration may result in tachycardia, laryngospasm, and muscle rigidity. Excited or manic behavior may be noted after regaining consciousness.

Dosage/Route: 1 to 2 g in 250 to 500 mL NS infused over 15 to 30 min; or 1 to 2 g IM/subcutaneous if IV not feasible. Ped: 20 to 40 mg/kg IV/IM subcutaneous.

©2007 Pearson Education, Inc.

PHENYTOIN

PHYSOSTIGMINE

PRALIDOXIME

Name/Class: PROCAINAMIDE (Pronestyl)/Antiarrhythmic

Description: Procainamide prolongs ventricular repolarization, slows conduction, and decreases myocardial excitability.

Indications: Ventricular fibrillation and pulseless ventricular tachycardia refractory to lidocaine.

Contraindications: Hypersensitivity to procainamide or procaine, myasthenia gravis, and 2nd- or 3rd-degree heart block.

Precautions: Hypotension, cardiac enlargement, CHF, AMI, ventricular dysrhythmias from digitalis, hepatic or renal impairment, electrolyte imbalance, or bronchial asthma.

Dosage/Route: 20 to 30 mg/min IV drip up to 17 mg/kg to effect, then 1 to 4 mg/min. Ped: 15 mg/kg/IV/IO over 30 to 60 min.

©2007 Pearson Education, Inc.

Name/Class: PROCHLORPERAZINE (Compazine)/Antiemetic

Description: Prochlorperazine is a phenothiazine derivative similar to chlorpromazine with potent antiemetic properties and fewer sedative, hypotensive, and anticholinergic effects.

Indications: Severe nausea and vomiting or acute psychosis.

Contraindications: Hypersensitivity to phenothiazines coma or depression.

Precautions: Breast cancer, children with acute illness or dehydration.

Dosage/Route: 5 to 10 mg IV/IM. Ped: 0.13 mg/kg IV/IM/PR if > 10 kg or > 2 years.

©2007 Pearson Education, Inc.

Name/Class: PROMETHAZINE (Phenergan)/Antiemetic

Description: Promethazine is an anticholinergic agent that enhances the effects of analgesics and is a potent antiemetic.

Indications: Nausea and vomiting, motion sickness, to enhance the effects of analgesics, and to induce sedation.

Contraindications: Hypersensitivity to phenothiazines.

Precautions: Hepatic, respiratory, or cardiac impairment, asthma, hypertension, elderly, or debilitated patients.

Dosage/Route: 12.5 to 25 mg IV/IM/PR. Ped: 0.5 mg/kg IV/IM/PR.

©2007 Pearson Education, Inc.

PROCAINAMIDE

PROCHLORPERAZINE

PROMETHAZINE

Name/Class: PROPAFANONE (Rythmol)/Antidysrhythmic

Description: Propafanone is an antidysrhythmic that stabilizes the myocardial membranes, reduces automaticity and the rate of single and multiple PVCs, and suppresses ventricular tachycardia.

Indications: Ventricular and supraventricular dysrhythmias.

Contraindications: Hypersensitivity, uncontrolled CHF, cardiogenic shock, sick sinus syndrome, AV block, bradycardia, hypotension, bronchospastic disorders, electrolyte imbalances, non–life-threatening dysrhythmias, COPD, or nursing mothers.

Precautions: CHF, AV block, hepatic or renal impairment, elderly, or pregnancy.

Dosage/Route: 150 to 300 mg PO/8 hours or 1 to 2 mg/kg IV at 10 mg/min.

Name/Class: PROPRANOLOL (Inderal)/Beta-Blocker

Description: Propranolol is a nonselective beta-blocker affecting both bronchial and cardiac sites. It reduces heart rate, myocardial irritability, contraction force, cardiac output, and blood pressure.

Indications: Ventricular fibrillation and pulseless ventricular tachycardia refractory to lidocaine and bretylium and selected SVTs.

Contraindications: 2nd- and 3rd-degree heart blocks, CHF, cor pulmonale, sinus bradycardia, cardiac impairment, cardiogenic shock, bronchospasm, or bronchial asthma, COPD, adrenergic-augmenting psychotropic or MAO inhibitors.

Precautions: Peripheral vascular disease, bee sting allergy, mild COPD, renal or hepatic impairment, diabetes, hypoglycemia, myasthenia gravis, WPW syndrome, or major surgery.

Dosage/Route: 1 to 3 mg slow IV (over 2 to 5 min), not to exceed 1 mg/min, may repeat/2 min to 0.1 mg/kg. Ped: 0.01 mg/kg slow IV.

Name/Class: PROSTAGLANDIN E_1 (Prostin VR Pediatric)/Vasodilator

Description: Prostaglandin E_1 is derived from fatty acids and causes vasodilation, inhibits platelet aggregation, and stimulates intestinal and uterine smooth muscles. It also helps maintain ductus arteriosus patency in newborn infants.

Indications: Infant cyanotic heart disease.

Contraindications:

Precautions: Constant respiratory monitoring is required.

Dosage/Route: Infant: 0.05 to 0.1 mcg/kg/min IV/IO.

PROPAFANONE

PROPRANOLOL

PROSTAGLANDIN E$_1$

Name/Class: RACEMIC EPINEPHRINE (microNefrin, Vaponefrin)/Sympathomimetic Agonist

Description: Racemic epinephrine is a variation of epinephrine used only for inhalation to induce bronchodilation and to reduce laryngeal edema and mucus secretion.

Indications: Croup (laryngotracheobronchitis).

Contraindications: Hypersensitivity, hypertension, or epiglottitis.

Precautions: May result in tachycardia and other dysrhythmias. Patient vital signs and ECG should be monitored.

Dosage/Route: 0.25 to 0.75 mL of a 2.25% solution in 2 mL NS once by nebulizer. Ped: same as adult.

©2007 Pearson Education, Inc.

Name/Class: SODIUM BICARBONATE ($NaHCO_3$)/Alkalizing Agent

Description: Sodium bicarbonate provides vascular bicarbonate to assist the buffer system in reducing the effects of metabolic acidosis and in the treatment of some overdoses.

Indications: Tricyclic antidepressant and barbiturate overdose, refractory acidosis, or hyperkalemia.

Contraindications: None when used in severe hypoxia or late cardiac arrest.

Precautions: May cause alkalosis if given in too large a quantity. It may also deactivate vasopressors and may precipitate with calcium chloride.

Dosage/Route: 1 mEq/kg IV, then 0.5 mEq/kg/10 min. Ped: same as adult (may be given IO).

©2007 Pearson Education, Inc.

Name/Class: SODIUM NITROPRUSSIDE (Nipride)/Nitrate

Description: Sodium nitroprusside is a rapid-acting hypotensive agent producing peripheral vasodilation and a mild increase in heart rate, a decrease in cardiac output, and a slight decrease in peripheral vascular resistance.

Indications: Hypertensive crisis.

Contraindications: Compensatory hypertension or impaired cerebral circulation (head injury, stroke).

Precautions: Hepatic or renal impairment, hyponatremia, or hypothyroidism.

Dosage/Route: 0.5 to 0.1 mcg/kg/min IV drip. Ped: same as adult.

©2007 Pearson Education, Inc.

RACEMIC EPINEPHRINE

SODIUM BICARBONATE

SODIUM NITROPRUSSIDE

Name/Class: SOTALOL (Betapace)/Beta-Blocker, Antidysrhythmic

Description: Sotalol is a nonselective beta-blocker that slows heart rate and decreases AV conduction and irritability.

Indications: Ventricular and supraventricular dysrhythmias.

Contraindications: Hypersensitivity, bronchial asthma, sinus bradycardia, 2nd- and 3rd-degree heart block, long QT syndromes, cardiogenic shock, uncontrolled CHF, or COPD.

Precautions: CHF, electrolyte disturbances, recent MI, diabetes, sick sinus rhythms, or renal impairment.

Dosage/Route: 1 to 1.5 mg/kg IV at 10 mg/min or 80 mg PO bid or 160 mg PO QD.

Name/Class: STREPTOKINASE (Streptase)/Fibrinolytic

Description: Streptokinase is a fibrinolytic that acts by activating the process that converts plasminogen to plasmin and results in the degradation of fibrin and fibrinogen and decreases erythrocyte aggregation.

Indications: AMI, deep vein thrombosis (DVT), or pulmonary embolism.

Contraindications: Active internal bleeding, aortic dissection, traumatic CPR, recent stroke, intracranial or intraspinal surgery or trauma (within 2 months), intracranial tumors, uncontrolled hypertension, pregnancy, hypersensitivity to anistreplase or streptokinase.

Precautions: Recent major surgery (10 days), patients > 75 years, cerebral vascular disease, GI or GU bleeding, recent trauma, hypertension, hemorrhagic conditions, ophthalmic conditions, or oral anticoagulant use.

Dosage/Route: *AMI:* 1.5 million units IV over 1 hour.
 DVT and pulmonary emboli: 250,000 units IV over 30 min, then 100,000 units/hr.

Name/Class: SUCCINYLCHOLINE (Anectine)/Depolarizing Neuromuscular Blocker

Description: Succinylcholine is an ultra–short-acting depolarizing neuromuscular blocker.

Indications: Facilitated endotracheal intubation.

Contraindications: Hypersensitivity, family history of malignant hyperthermia, penetrating eye injury, narrow-angle glaucoma.

Precautions: Severe burn or crush injury; electrolyte imbalances; hepatic, renal, cardiac, or pulmonary impairment; fractures; spinal cord injury; dehydration; severe anemia; porphyria.

Dosage/Route: 1 to 1.5 mg/kg IV/IM. Ped: 1 to 2 mg/kg IV/IM.

SOTALOL

STREPTOKINASE

SUCCINYLCHOLINE

Name/Class: TERBUTALINE (Brethine, Bricanyl)/Sympathetic Agonist

Description: Terbutaline is a synthetic sympathomimetic that causes bronchodilatation with less cardiac effect than epinephrine.

Indications: Bronchial asthma and bronchospasm in COPD.

Contraindications: Hypersensitivity to the drug.

Precautions: The patient may experience palpitations, anxiety, nausea, and/or dizziness. Vital signs and breath sounds must be monitored; use caution with cardiac or hypertensive patients.

Dosage/Route: Two inhalations with a metered dose inhaler, repeated once in 1 min or 0.25 mg SQ repeated in 15 to 30 mins.

©2007 Pearson Education, Inc.

Name/Class: THIAMINE/Vitamin

Description: Thiamine is vitamin B_1, which is required to convert glucose into energy. It is not manufactured by the body and must be constantly provided from ingested foods.

Indications: Coma of unknown origin, chronic alcoholism with associated coma, and delirium tremens.

Contraindications: None.

Precautions: Known hypersensitivity to the drug.

Dosage/Route: 50 to 100 mg IV/IM. Ped: 10 to 25 mg IV/IM.

©2007 Pearson Education, Inc.

Name/Class: VASOPRESSIN (Pitressin)/Hormone, Vasopressor

Description: Vasopressin is a hormone with strong vasopressive and antidiuretic properties but that may precipitate angina and/or AMI.

Indications: To increase peripheral vascular resistance in arrest (CPR) or to control bleeding from esophageal varices.

Contraindications: Chronic nephritis with nitrogen retention, ischemic heart disease, PVCs, advanced arteriosclerosis, or 1st stage of labor.

Precautions: Epilepsy, migraine, heart failure, angina, vascular disease, hepatic impairment, elderly, and children.

Dosage/Route: *Arrest:* 40 units IV.
Esophageal varices: 0.2 to 0.4 units/min IV drip.

©2007 Pearson Education, Inc.

TERBUTALINE

THIAMINE

VASOPRESSIN

Name/Class: VECURONIUM (Norcuron)/Nondepolarizing Skeletal Muscle Relaxant

Description: Vecuronium is a nondepolarizing skeletal muscle relaxant similar to pancuronium with minimal cardiovascular effects.

Indications: Facilitated endotracheal intubation.

Contraindications: Hypersensitivity.

Precautions: Hepatic or renal impairment, impaired fluid and electrolyte or acid–base balance, severe obesity, myasthenia gravis, elderly, debilitated patients, or malignant hyperthermia.

Dosage/Route: 0.08 to 0.1 mg/kg IV. Ped: same as adult.

©2007 Pearson Education, Inc.

Name/Class: VERAPAMIL (Isoptin, Calan)/Calcium Channel Blocker

Description: Verapamil is a calcium channel blocker that slows AV conduction, suppresses reentry dysrhythmias such as PSVT, and slows ventricular responses to atrial tachydysrhythmias. Verapamil also dilates coronary arteries and reduces myocardial oxygen demand.

Indications: PSVT refractory to adenosine, atrial flutter, and atrial fibrillation with rapid ventricular response.

Contraindications: Severe hypotension, cardiogenic shock, 2nd- or 3rd-degree heart block, CHF, sinus node disease, and accessory AV pathways, WPW syndrome. It should not be administered to persons taking beta-blockers.

Precautions: Hepatic and renal impairment, MI with coronary artery occlusion, or myocardial stenosis.

Dosage/Route: 2.5 to 5 mg IV bolus over 2 to 3 min, then 5 to 10 mg after 15 to 30 min to a max of 30 mg in 30 min. Ped: newborn—0.1 to 0.2 mg/kg (not to exceed 2 mg), age 1 to 15—0.1 to 0.3 mg/kg (not to exceed 5 mg).

©2007 Pearson Education, Inc.

©2007 Pearson Education, Inc.

VECURONIUM

VERAPAMIL